Occupational Therapy Essentials for Clinical Competence
Second Edition

Occupational Therapy Essentials for Clinical Competence
Second Edition

Edited by

Karen Jacobs, EdD, OTR/L, CPE, FAOTA
Boston University
College of Health & Rehabilitation Sciences: Sargent College
Boston, MA

Nancy MacRae, MS, OTR/L, FAOTA
Westbrook College of Health Professions
University of New England
Portland, ME

Karen Sladyk, PhD, OTR/L, FAOTA
Bay Path College
Longmeadow, MA

Instructor materials created by Gail M. Bloom, OTD, MA, OTR/L

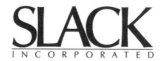

SLACK
INCORPORATED

www.Healio.com/books

ISBN: 978-1-61711-638-4

Occupational Therapy Essentials for Clinical Competence, Second Edition includes ancillary materials specifically available for faculty use. Included are Test Bank Questions and PowerPoint slides. Please visit http://www.efacultylounge.com to obtain access.

Published by: SLACK Incorporated
                  6900 Grove Road
                  Thorofare, NJ 08086 USA
                  Telephone: 856-848-1000
                  Fax: 856-848-6091
                  www.Healio.com/books

Contact SLACK Incorporated for more information about other books in this field or about the availability of our books from distributors outside the United States.

Library of Congress Cataloging-in-Publication Data

Occupational therapy essentials for clinical competence / [edited by] Karen Jacobs, Nancy MacRae, Karen Sladyk. -- Second edition.
    p. ; cm.
  Includes bibliographical references and index.
  ISBN 978-1-61711-638-4 (hardback : alk. paper)
  I. Jacobs, Karen, 1951- editor of compilation. II. MacRae, Nancy, 1944- editor of compilation. III. Sladyk, Karen, 1958- editor of compilation.
  [DNLM: 1. Occupational Therapy. 2. Accreditation--standards. 3. Clinical Competence--standards. WB 555]
  RM735
  615.8'515--dc23
                        2013045368

Printed in the United States of America.

Last digit is print number: 10 9 8 7 6 5 4 3 2 1

Dedication

To our children; grandchildren; parents; our students past, current, and future; and our professional colleagues, who continually support, inspire, and teach us.

622880

Contents

Occupational Therapy Essentials for Clinical Competence, Second Edition includes ancillary materials specifically available for faculty use. Included are Test Bank Questions and PowerPoint slides. Please visit http://www.efacultylounge.com to obtain access.

Acknowledgments

A text of this magnitude could not have been accomplished without the support of a collaborative team. Our gratitude is extended to each of the contributors to this second edition. In particular, we appreciate the new energy and insight brought by Dr. Gail Bloom, who created the PowerPoint presentations, multiple choice questions and authored the chapter on ethics.

We acknowledge the continued support of SLACK Incorporated, especially Veronica, Brien, and John.

About the Editors

Karen Jacobs, EdD, OTR/L, CPE, FAOTA is a past president and vice president of the American Occupational Therapy Association (AOTA). She is a 2005 recipient of a Fulbright Scholarship to the University of Akureyri in Akureyri, Iceland; the 2009 recipient of the Award of Merit from the Canadian Association of Occupational Therapists (CAOT); the 2003 recipient of the Award of Merit from the AOTA; and recipient of the 2011 Eleanor Clarke Slagle Lectureship Award. The title of her Slagle lecture was *PromOTing Occupational Therapy: Words, Images and Action.*

Dr. Jacobs is a clinical professor of occupational therapy and the program director of the distance education post-professional occupational therapy programs at Boston University. She has worked at Boston University for 30 years and has expertise in the development and instruction of online graduate courses.

Dr. Jacobs earned a doctoral degree at the University of Massachusetts, a Master of Science at Boston University, and a Bachelor of Arts at Washington University in St. Louis, Missouri.

Dr. Jacobs' research examines the interface between the environment and human capabilities. In particular, she examines the individual factors and environmental demands associated with increased risk of functional limitations among populations of university- and middle school–aged students, particularly in notebook computing, use of tablets such as iPads (Apple), backpack use, and the use of games such as Wii Fit (Nintendo).

In addition to being an occupational therapist, Dr. Jacobs is also a certified professional ergonomist (CPE), the founding editor in chief of the international, interprofessional journal *WORK: A Journal of Prevention, Assessment & Rehabilitation* (IOS Press, The Netherlands), and a consultant in ergonomics, marketing, and entrepreneurship.

She is the proud mother of three children (Laela, Josh, and Ariel) and Amma (grandmother in Icelandic) to Sophie, Zachary, Liberty, and Zane. Her occupational balance is through travel, photography, walking, and co-writing children's books.

Nancy MacRae, MS, OTR/L, FAOTA is an associate professor at the University of New England (UNE), in Portland, Maine, where she has taught for 23 years. She is a past president of the Maine Occupational Therapy Association and a past director of the UNE occupational therapy program.

Nancy's work experience has been within the field of developmental disabilities, primarily mental retardation, across the lifespan. Her graduate degree is in adult education, with a minor in educational gerontology. Involvement in interprofessional activities at UNE allows her to mentor and learn from future health care practitioners and to model the collaboration our health care system needs. Scholarship has centered around aging and sexuality, documentation, professional writing, and interprofessional ventures. She has been a member of the editorial board of *WORK: A Journal of Prevention, Assessment & Rehabilitation* since its inception.

Nancy is the proud mother of two sons and a 14-year-old granddaughter. Occupational balance is maintained through participation in yoga, reading, walking, baking, and basket making.

Karen Sladyk, PhD, OTR/L, FAOTA has been an occupational therapy educator in New England for over 18 years—first at Quinnipiac University and currently at Bay Path College. She "accidentally" fell into writing when she was a substitute at a focus group at an American Occupational Therapy Association (AOTA) annual meeting and conference, offering suggestions of what she thought students wanted to know. Since that time, she has edited or authored 9 textbooks targeted specifically at occupational therapy/occupational therapy assistant students' specific needs. Known as a "hard and demanding" teacher, she cares very deeply about students getting an intense and meaningful education.

Like every occupational therapist/occupational therapy assistant, she has a difficult time balancing her life, but she enjoys travel, quilting, crafts, and writing. She visited all 50 states before turning 50 herself. Karen spends time with her sisters and nephews in Connecticut and Utah and continues to collect vintage jewelry at flea markets. Lately, she has been hunting for Disney Lanyard pins.

Contributing Authors

Ali Kae Arsenault, OTR *(Chapters 8 and 9)*
Key Rehab at the Windsor Place
Coffeyville, Kansas

Bethany Augustoni, MS, OTR/L *(Chapters 8 and 9)*
Tufts Medical Center
Boston, Massachusetts

Diane P. Bergey, MOT, OTR/L *(Chapter 35)*
Belfast, Maine

Caryn Birstler Husman, MS, OTR/L *(Chapter 4)*
Coordinator and Assistant Professor of Health,
    Wellness, and Occupational Studies
University of New England
Biddeford, Maine

Roxie M. Black, PhD, OTR/L, FAOTA *(Chapter 2)*
Program Director
MOT Program
University of Souther Maine
Lewiston, Maine

Gail M. Bloom, OTD, MA, OTR/L *(Chapter 48)*
Consultant
Andover, Massachusetts

Jessica J. Bolduc, DrOT, MS, OTR/L *(Chapter 16)*
Staff Occupational Therapist
Mercy Hospital
Portland, Maine

Alfred G. Bracciano, EdD, OTR/L, FAOTA, FAIS
    (Chapter 33)
Associate Professor and Program Director
Entry-Level Distance Program
Creighton University at University of Alaska-Anchorage
Anchorage, Alaska
Department of Occupational Therapy
Creighton University Medical Center
Omaha, Nebraska

Susan C. Burwash, PhD, MSc(OT), OTR/L, OT(C)
    (Chapter 54)
Assistant Professor
Department of Occupational Therapy
Eastern Washington University
Spokane, Washington

Lisa L. Clark, MS, OTR/L, CLT *(Chapters 39 and 44)*
Clinical Faculty
Master of Occupational Therapy Program
University of Southern Maine, Lewiston-Auburn
Lewiston, Maine
Mid Coast Hospital
Brunswick, Maine

Marilyn B. Cole, MS, OTR/L, FAOTA *(Chapter 14)*
Professor Emerita
Occupational Therapy
Quinnipiac University
Hamden, Connecticut

Jeffrey L. Crabtree, OTD, MS, FAOTA *(Chapter 37)*
Associate Professor
Department of Occupational Therapy
School of Health and Rehabilitation Science
Indiana University
Indianapolis, Indiana

William R. Croninger, MA, OTR/L
    (Chapters 22, 30, and 31)
Staff Therapist
Maria Parham Medical Center
Henderson, North Carolina

Danielle J. Cropley, MSOT Student *(Chapter 21)*
University of New England
Portland, Maine

Betsy DeBrakeleer, COTA/L, ROH *(Chapters 30 and 31)*
Alpha One Enterprises
South Portland, Maine

Mary V. Donohue, PhD, OTL, FAOTA (Chapter 21)
Co-Editor, *Occupational Therapy in Mental Health*
Stony Brook University
New York University Retiree
Stony Brook, New York

Nancy Doyle, OTD, OTR/L (Chapters 10 and 38)
Online Instructor, Occupational Therapy Department
College of Health & Rehabilitation Sciences: Sargent
  College
Boston University
Boston, Massachusetts
Pediatric Occupational Therapist
Washington, DC

Julie Eldredge, MS, OTR/L (Chapters 8 and 9)
Cartenders Home Health
Andover, Massachusetts

Verna G. Eschenfelder, PhD, OTR/L (Chapter 5)
Assistant Professor of Occupational Therapy
The University of Scranton
Scranton, Pennsylvania

Thomas Fisher, PhD, OTR, CCM, FAOTA (Chapter 53)
Professor and Chairman
Department of Occupational Therapy
Indiana University School of Health & Rehabilitation
  Sciences
Indianapolis, Indiana

Erica A. Flagg, OT (Chapter 35)
Union, Maine

Kathleen Flecky, OTD, OTR/L (Chapter 7)
Associate Professor
Department of Occupational Therapy
School of Pharmacy and Health Professions
Creighton University
Omaha, Nebraska

Jan Froehlich, MS, OTR/L (Chapters 8, 9, and 21)
Associate Professor
Department of Occupational Therapy
University of New England
Portland, Maine

Heather Goertz, OTD, OTR/L (Chapter 7)
Director of Ministry
St. John's Lutheran Church
Bennington, Nebraska

Michelle Goulet, MS, OTR/L (Chapters 20 and 28)
St. Joseph's Rehabilitation and Nursing Care Center
New England Rehabilitation Hospital
Boston, Massachusetts

Kristin B. Haas, OTD, OTR/L (Chapter 13)
Associate Professor, Occupational Therapy
College of Saint Mary
Omaha, Nebraska

Dory E. Holmes, MPH, OTR/L (Chapter 39)
Director, Rehabilitation Services
MidCoast Hospital
Brunswick, Maine

Bevin J. Journey, MS, OTR/L (Chapter 27)

Tara Kaminski, MSOT Student (Chapter 24)
University of New England
Portland, Maine

Rosalie M. King, DHS, OTR/L (Chapter 1)
Associate Professor of Occupational Therapy
The University of Findlay
Findlay, Ohio

Lisa J. Knecht-Sabres, DHS, OTR/L (Chapter 17)
Associate Professor
Occupational Therapy Program
Midwestern University
Downers Grove, Illinois

*Amy Jo Lamb, OTD, OTR/L, FAOTA (Chapters 42
  and 55)*
Program Director & Assistant Professor of Occupational
  Therapy
Eastern Michigan University
Ypsilanti, Michigan
Vice President 2013-2015, American Occupational
  Therapy Association

John E. Lane, Jr., OTR/L (Chapter 30)
Owner, WorkFit Rehabilitation Services
Lancaster, New Hampshire

Barbara Larson, MA, OTR/L, FAOTA (Chapter 18)
Independent Consultant, Work and Industry
Adjunct Faculty
The College of St. Scholastica
Duluth, Minnesota

Kathryn M. Loukas, OTD, MS, OTR/L, FAOTA
  (Chapters 12, 27, 32, and 34)
Clinical Professor of Occupational Therapy
University of New England
Portland, Maine

James Marc-Aurele, MBA, OTR/L (Chapter 44)
Mid Coast Hospital
Brunswick, Maine

Scott McNeil, OTD, MS, OTR/L (Chapter 32)
Assistant Clinical Professor & Academic Fieldwork
  Coordinator
Occupational Therapy Program
University of New England
Portland, Maine

Penelope A. Moyers, EdD, OT/L, BCMH, FAOTA
  (Chapter 52)
Dean of the Henrietta Schmoll School of Health and
  Graduate College
St. Catherine University
St. Paul, Minnesota

Julie Ann Nastasi, OTD, OTR/L, SCLV, FAOTA
  (Chapters 6 and 43)
Faculty Specialist
Department of Occupational Therapy
University of Scranton
Scranton, Pennsylvania

Linda H. Niemeyer, OT, PhD (Chapter 45)
Lecturer in Occupational Therapy
Sargent College of Health and Rehabilitation Sciences
Department of Occupational Therapy
Boston University
Boston, Massachusetts

Claudia E. Oakes, OTR/L, PhD (Chapter 11)
Department of Health Sciences and Nursing
University of Hartford
West Hartford, Connecticut

Jane O'Brien, PhD, OTR/L (Chapters 23 and 29)
Associate Professor and Program Director
Occupational Therapy Department
University of New England
Portland, Maine

Carol Reinson, PhD, OTR/L (Chapter 51)
University of Scranton
Scranton, Pennsylvania

Michael E. Roberts, MS, OTR/L (Chapter 25)
Academic Fieldwork Coordinator and Lecturer
Tufts University
Medford, Massachusetts

Regula H. Robnett, PhD, OTR/L (Chapter 24)
Professor, Department of Occupational Therapy
University of New England
Portland, Maine

Jan Rowe, DrOT, OTR/L, FAOTA (Chapter 50)
Coordinator
Tourett Syndrome and Tic Disorder Program
Children's of Alabama
Birmingham, Alabama

Marie C. Roy, LCSW, OTR/L (Chapters 8 and 9)
Hospice of Southern Maine
Scarborough, Maine

Diane Sauter-Davis, MA, OTR/L (Chapter 49)
Kennebec Valley Community College
Fairfield, Maine

Julie Savoyski, MS, OTR/L, MPA (Chapter 36)
United Cerebral Palsy
Jamaica Plain, Massachusetts

Courtney S. Shufelt, MS, OTR/L (Chapters 20 and 28)
Northside Medical Center
Columbus Regional Health
Columbus, Georgia

*Wendy B. Stav, PhD, OTR/L, SCDCM, FAOTA
(Chapter 46)*
Chair and Professor
Nova Southeastern University
Fort Lauderdale, Florida

*Barbara J. Steva, MS, OTR/L (Chapter 26 and
Appendix E)*
University of New England
Portland, Maine
Community Therapy Center
Biddeford, Maine

Christine Sullivan, OTD, MS, OTR/L (Chapter 47)
Associate Professor and Program Director
Occupational Therapy Assistant Program
Mercy College
Dobbs Ferry, New York

Roseanna Tufano, LMFT, OTR/L (Chapter 15)
Clinical Associate Professor and Academic Coordinator
Occupational Therapy
Quinnipiac University
Hamden, Connecticut

Nicolaas van den Heever, BOT, OTD, OTR/L (Foreword)
Founding Dean/Program Director
Master of Science Occupational Therapy
West Coast University
Los Angeles, California

Lori Vaughn, OTD, OTR/L (Chapter 19)
Program Director and Associate Professor of
    Occupational Therapy
Bay Path College
Longmeadow, Massachusetts

John W. Vellacott, EdD, MEd, BA (Chapter 54)
Director-Intergovernmental Relations Unit
Alberta Human Services
Edmonton, Alberta, Canada

Kristin Winston, PhD, OTR/L (Chapter 34)
Assistant Professor, Director PhD Program
Nova Southeastern University
Fort Lauderdale, Florida

Patricia A. Wisniewski, MS, OTR/L, CPRP (Chapter 5)
Lecturer
Department of Occupational Therapy
University of Scranton
Scranton, Pennsylvania

Briana Youland, MS, OTR/L (Chapters 20 and 28)
Southern Oaks Nursing and Rehabilitation Facility
Pensacola, Florida

Foreword

As with the first edition, the words that capture the prospective reader's attention in the title of the second edition of the *Occupational Therapy Essentials for Clinical Competence* textbook are certainly "clinical competence." Miriam-Webster (2011) defines competence as having the "necessary ability or skills to do something well," or "well enough to meet a standard."

The process of obtaining the necessary knowledge and skills for any occupational therapy clinician certainly starts when the individual enters occupational therapy education. The Accreditation Council for Occupational Therapy Education (ACOTE) has established the academic standards necessary for accreditation of occupation therapy education programs. ACOTE also reviews programs for granting initial and continuing accreditation status. Graduation from an accredited occupational therapy education program is required to engage in occupational therapy practice.

"Doing something well enough to meet a standard" (Miriam-Webster, 2011) is therefore operationalized for occupational therapy professionals collectively through the application of knowledge and skill as designated by the 2011 ACOTE Standards.

Furthermore, the importance of possessing competence through the application of knowledge and skill is emphasized and confirmed in the Preamble of the current (AOTA, 2013) version of the ACOTE Standards and Interpretive Guide. That is, "The rapidly changing and dynamic nature of contemporary health and human services delivery systems provides challenging opportunities for the occupational therapist to use knowledge and skills in a practice area as a direct care provider, consultant, educator, manager, leader, researcher, and advocate for the profession and the consumer" (AOTA, 2013).

Establishing competence through an academic process has evolved over the years. White (1959) described competence as observable behaviors or practice gained through knowledge acquisition, which then provides the basis for performing the skills. As andragogy in higher education moved toward constructivism, changing the role of the student from passive recipient of knowledge to active participant in generating knowledge, so also did the definition and assessment of "competence" become more dynamic. Older research studies focused on Miller's Pyramid of Competence (1990)—a model that conceptualizes the essential elements of clinical competence—have placed competence at the "knows how to" level, or merely learning a related skill. Lately, competence is associated with the top level of the pyramid—"Does" or doing. The clinician is expected to perform and be assessed in the actual work place on overall performance, that is, combining the cognitive components of obtaining knowledge with the behavioral components of skill and attitude. In occupational therapy education, assessing overall performance or competence in order to prepare a student to be an entry-level generalist, is exactly attained at the "Does" level of Miller's Pyramid—applying knowledge, skill, and behavior in the actual workplace through level II fieldwork. Details of the competency elements an entry-level practitioner should possess are outlined in the Preamble of the 2011 ACOTE Standards.

This textbook, compiled by leading educators in the occupational therapy field, provides the roadmap and tools of competencies to prepare the next generation of "generalist with a broad exposure to the delivery models and systems used in setting where occupational therapy is currently practiced and where it is emerging as a service" (AOTA, 2013).

The premise of the ACOTE Content ("B") Standards is that, when included and fully operationalized in a curriculum, the student would have acquired the necessary foundational content and breadth and depth of knowledge to articulate and apply the theory of occupational therapy. Not only does this textbook provide every topic needed for generalist competency, but also links the topics with the ACOTE Content Standards. The structure and content of this book can thus serve as the foundation of a curriculum design for new programs or for curriculum restructuring of existing programs.

In order to educate occupational therapy students to render client-centered, occupation-based interventions, and to view their clients as a whole versus as parts, not only does the book provide the essential information and content, but the layout is such that it will facilitate integrative versus fragmented thinking. It will assist the student in viewing the client as a multifaceted human being, incorporating all aspects of occupational therapy's domain that will "transact to support engagement, participation and [ultimately] health" (AOTA, 2008, p. 628). Thus, incorporating the content and layout of this text in the curriculum is the pedagogical solution to the issue of creating silos of knowledge and fragmented thinking, which is counterintuitive to the process and value of occupational therapy. Furthermore, evidence-based practice is a thread throughout the content of this book, assisting the reader to explore the content in depth. The book also provides the users—instructor and student—with tools for active learning and participation, such as objectives for each chapter, critical thinking questions, self-assessments, and quizzes.

During a time in higher education where the formulation of outcomes and the subsequent data collection to provide evidence for the established outcomes are paramount, the objectives provided to the reader at the beginning of each chapter, and the accompanying ACOTE Content Standards, can be utilized as course or student learning outcomes. Learning outcomes can be met through assignments or objective testing, which can deliver data to provided evidence of students' performance and competence level. The data can further be applied to drive teaching efficacy of faculty and curriculum content, especially if paired with NBCOT pass rate data.

As competency focuses on the individual's ability to do something successfully or efficiently, the editors and contributors of this book have given the occupational therapy education community an invaluable tool that will enable them to create future occupational therapists that will be successful and efficient providers of health care. In doing so, occupational therapy practitioners will be able to meet society's occupational needs, able to act as advocates for the profession, and develop the desire to be lifelong learners (AOTA, 2013). The ability to perform at the expected level requires a process of lifelong learning. Occupational therapy practitioners must continually reassess their competencies and identify needs for additional knowledge, skills, personal growth, and integrative learning experiences. This textbook will be instrumental in facilitating and maintaining that process.

References

American Occupational Therapy Association. (2013). *2011 Accreditation council for occupational therapy education standards and interpretive guide.* Retrieved from http://www.aota.org/-/media/Corporate/Files/EducationCareers/Accredit/Draft-Standards/2011 Standards-and-Interpretive-Guide-August-2013.ashx

American Occupational Therapy Association. (2008). *Occupational therapy practice framework: domain and process.* White Plains, MD: Automated Graphic Systems.

Merriam-Webster. (2011). *Competence.* Retrieved December 8, 2013 from http://http://www.merriam-webster.com/dictionary/competence

Miller, G. E. (1990). The assessment of clinical skills/competence/performance. *Academic Medicine, 65*(9 Suppl), S63-S67.

White, R. (1959). Motivation reconsidered: The concept of competence. *Psychological Review, 66,* 297-333.

Nicolaas van den Heever, BOT, OTD, OTR/L
West Coast University
Los Angeles, California

Introduction

Occupation, theory-driven, evidence-based, and client-centered practice continues to be the core of our profession and is the central focus of the second edition of *Occupational Therapy Essentials for Clinical Competency*. Promoting the health and wellness of our clients is a crucial value for our interventions. Assisting students to learn more about the simple yet complex nature of occupation and how meaningful occupations are to our clients are primary goals of this text. We hope readers will view this book as a bridge to effective, occupation-based occupational therapy interventions.

The second edition is organized to address the *2011 Accreditation Council for Occupational Therapy Education (ACOTE) Standards* (effective July 31, 2013) master's degree–level educational program. The text intentionally follows the sequence outlined in these standards.

Every topic necessary for competence as an entry-level occupational therapy practitioner is introduced. Varied perspectives are provided in each chapter, with consistent references made to the relevance of certified occupational therapy assistant roles and responsibilities.

In this second edition, all chapters have been updated and enriched from new perspectives and evidence-based research. A number of new chapters have also been added: Interprofessional Education and Practice, Occupational Therapy Practice Framework, Meaning and Dynamic of Occupation and Activity, Evaluation and Interventions to Enhance Rest and Sleep, Emerging Areas of Practice, Telehealth, Grants, and Professional Presentations.

Based on adult learning theory, it is easier to understand concepts if they are "chunked" together or if they utilize "scaffolding" techniques to reinforce learning. This is the case for many chapters where the content and application for a topic, such as theory, is covered in multiple places throughout the book.

The second edition includes many returning authors and some new ones. We value the commitment, contributions, and voices that over 60 authors have made to this second edition. Depending on the topic, the length of a chapter will vary—some chapters are longer and more thorough than others, such as Ethics, Physical Agent Modalities, and Research.

The second edition also includes supplemental materials such as PowerPoint presentations and multiple choice questions for each chapter. We are grateful to the dedication of Dr. Gail Bloom, who created these resources for both students and faculty.

We wish you our best in learning more about occupational therapy through this textbook.

Karen, Nancy, and Karen

Introduction

I

SETTING THE STAGE

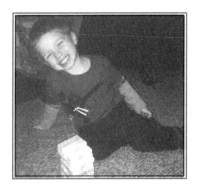

1

THE EXPERIENCE OF FLOW AND MEANINGFUL OCCUPATION

Rosalie M. King, DHS, OTR/L

ACOTE STANDARDS EXPLORED IN THIS CHAPTER

B.3.6

KEY VOCABULARY

- **Experience sampling method:** A research methodology designed to capture people's behaviors, thoughts, or feelings as they occur in real time.
- **Flow experience:** The mental state in which a person performing an activity is fully immersed in a feeling of energized focus, full involvement, and enjoyment in the process of the activity.
- **Meaningful occupation:** The ordinary, familiar things an individual does every day that are valued and have significance for that person.

- **Occupational therapy:** A health and wellness profession using occupation as both a means and an end in promoting participation, meaning, and satisfaction in all aspects of life.
- **Optimal experience:** Alternate term for "flow experience."
- **Well-being:** Judging life as positive and satisfying.

Introduction

A review of the literature indicates a relationship between the characteristics of meaningful occupation and the experience of flow. Current literature within the occupational therapy profession frequently emphasizes the importance of using occupation, and, in doing so, practicing in a client-centered, holistic manner. Although there is a strongly held belief in the profession about the value of occupation, the need to provide supporting evidence still exists. In addition, there is a paucity of evidence available to assist occupational therapy practitioners in determining what is meaningful and enjoyable to the client, and the assignment of value and meaning to occupations is subjective (Csikszentmihalyi, 1997; Persson, Erlandsson, Eklund, &

Jacobs, K., MacRae, N., & Sladyk, K. (Eds.).
Occupational Therapy Essentials for
Clinical Competence, Second Edition (pp. 3-10).
© 2014 SLACK Incorporated.

Iwarsson, 2001). People are not always able to articulate what is of particular value to them when asked directly. This review of the literature is an attempt to examine the characteristics of the concept of flow experiences and of occupations that contribute to the well-being of those we serve. In addition, because the flow construct is well established in the field of psychology, finding parallels would support the validity of the use of occupation and afford occupational therapists a larger body of knowledge upon which to build.

Flow, or *optimal experience*, is a construct studied in the discipline of social psychology and developed by Mihaly Csikszentmihalyi (1990). Flow describes a subjective state of consciousness in which one becomes totally immersed in the occupation or task at hand and from which the individual derives satisfaction and a sense of well-being. The theory has been well researched and clearly delineates the conditions that must be present in order for the flow experience to occur. A more thorough explanation of the construct will be developed to increase understanding of the prerequisite conditions for flow and the benefits to the person experiencing this state.

Occupational therapy has identified the importance of using meaningful occupation in interventions with client populations in order to increase motivation and success in achieving client goals. Christiansen, Backman, Little, and Nguyen (1999) spoke of the predominant perception that engagement in daily occupations serves to meet intrinsic and extrinsic needs and contributes to satisfaction and quality of life within the field. Founders of the profession of occupational therapy equated health and life satisfaction with balance in daily activities, a tenet we still espouse today. Yet it is true that a healthy balance varies from person to person, as does the idea of which activities and occupations are considered meaningful. Hammell (2004) also points out that occupational therapy theory tends to group occupations into the categories of self-care, leisure, and productivity, which can be limiting. Some occupations that might be meaningful do not appear to fall into these categories. This is further complicated by occupational therapy theories that do not clearly distinguish the difference between the terms "meaningful" and "purposeful." If occupations are considered meaningful only if they are goal oriented and purposeful, occupations chosen by a practitioner during intervention might have meaning (not necessarily positive) but not be meaningful (Hammell, 2004).

Because there are activities and occupations an individual may consider important that do not result in optimal experience, the idea of examining and determining occupations that do result in flow for a given person does not provide a complete recipe for successful intervention. However, exploration of the concept of flow in relation to meaningful occupation bears consideration in terms of

its potential to support the philosophical belief of occupational therapy and to learn more about how we might enable our clients to achieve a greater sense of well-being and life satisfaction.

Methodology for Searching the Literature

A search of databases including the Cumulative Index to Nursing and Allied Health Literature (CINAHL), PsycINFO, OT Search, and the journal holdings of the American Occupational Therapy Association (AOTA) was conducted using the following key terms: *meaningful occupation*, *occupational therapy*, *well-being*, and *flow experience*. The term *optimal experience* was added to increase responses. In addition, a Google search was conducted using the same key words. Retrieved abstracts and articles, as well as references cited in some of the literature, led to an additional search using the term *experience sampling method*. The search yielded 44 articles, which were narrowed down to 33 for this review. Information that did not come from a peer-reviewed source was discarded.

Review of the Literature

To address this topic, a review of the occupational therapy literature was conducted regarding the use of occupation and its role in contributing to life experience and satisfaction. Although the idea of participation in life through the activities and engagement in the occupations in which people take part every day is not new, its importance has been emphasized in the last decade as the occupational therapy profession attempts to reconnect with its roots. The psychology literature was consulted to examine optimal experience, or flow. The search yielded examples of studies conducted using the flow construct, which have been undertaken by researchers in various fields to include psychology, leisure, education, occupational therapy, technology, and business. Although flow is not a novel concept, especially in the discipline of psychology, little emphasis has been placed on it in the occupational therapy literature since the 1990s. Therefore, an exploration of both constructs seems to have merit, followed by an examination of the literature to look at a possible correlation between the two.

The Importance of Meaningful Occupation

There has been a shift in the global view of health from that of absence of disease or impairment to one that supports the idea that true health has more to do with satisfaction, quality of life, and the pursuit of health (Zemke, 2004). Numerous accounts exist of individuals who have found new meaning in life after the onset of a traumatic illness or life-altering event, which has contributed to a greater sense of purpose and well-being. Dossey (1991, as cited in Bridle, 1999) talked about individuals not only seeking meaning in their lives and in their doing, but in their debility. Celebrities such as Michael J. Fox, Christopher Reeve, and countless others have talked openly about finding a new sense of purpose and meaning as a result of injury and illness.

Finding meaning in everyday occupations is important for all human beings. As occupational therapy practitioners, we are faced with the challenge of not only discerning which occupations a client values, but also aiding the individual in discovering new sources of meaning when previously valued occupations are no longer possible.

Christiansen (1999) highlighted the importance of occupations in contributing to one's sense of identity. He discussed the need human beings have to express themselves in a unique way that gives meaning to life, viewing engagement in occupations as a vehicle to fulfill that need. He also talked about the relationship between self and others in influencing this sense of identity, stating that we both affect others and are affected by them. Our identities are closely related to the things we do, as well as how we interpret what we do in the social context. In our analysis of events, human beings look for personal meaning, and if these events are deemed significant, we respond in an emotional way and are shaped by them. Our perceptions of life are subsequently formed as well. Therefore, Christiansen stated that identity plays an important role in promoting well-being and satisfaction in life. Having a sense of control and purpose gives meaning to individuals. Bridle (1999) also discussed identity in terms of the relationship between "being" and "doing" as a dimension of holism.

In a qualitative study that examined the relationship between occupation and its contribution to competence and identity, persons with serious mental illness engaged in woodworking occupations in two community settings (Mee, Sumsion, & Craik, 2004). All participants identified engagement in occupation as the mechanism to acquire skills, a sense of competence and purpose, and a personal sense of self-worth and identity. Hvalsøe and Josephsson (2003) found that their subjects with mental illness believed it was essential that occupations met their need to be engaged in various roles and that these occupations matched their personal preferences and interests in order for them to be of value. Use of occupations that are meaningful to people and that contribute to their sense of identity only underscore the importance of employing this in our intervention strategies with clients; in doing so, practitioners will be facilitating the fulfillment of a common basic need experienced by all human beings.

Yerxa (1998) examined the relationship between health and engagement in occupation, bringing in the idea of the importance of the human spirit. She identified some of the early theorists of the occupational therapy profession, such as Reilly and Meyer, who clearly saw the connection between involvement in everyday occupations and health. Yerxa cited research studies regarding some of the creative thinkers of the world, which revealed how little attention has been paid to the idea of work being a contributor to happiness, even if a given individual lacks close personal relationships. The point is made that the drive for autonomy is just as important as the impetus to get closer to other people. What is of greater significance is that the interests pursued are those that contribute to well-being and life satisfaction.

For many individuals, the occupation of work is a source of great meaning and satisfaction, regardless of health status (Kennedy-Jones, Cooper, & Fossey, 2005). In addition to the obvious practical benefits of working for a wage to sustain one's livelihood and one's family, the occupation of work is seen as an avenue to establish one's place in society, help form self-identity, and utilize and increase skills. Work was more frequently cited than leisure in numerous studies conducted to determine which everyday occupations resulted in optimal experiences, positive feelings, and satisfaction (Csikszentmihalyi, 1997; Csikszentmihalyi & LeFevre, 1989; Gerhardsson & Jonsson, 1996; Rebeiro & Polgar, 1998). Because many clients referred for occupational therapy services experience limitations in their ability to work, it is important to recognize the importance of any life changes that negatively affect this meaningful role. Occupational therapy intervention may involve helping clients to make adaptations so that they can resume the worker role or discover meaning through different occupations.

Effective occupational therapy intervention may require drawing on past occupations that once provided meaning for an individual. When asked why certain occupations were preferred, subjects in a study that elicited the perspectives of persons with mental illness identified occupations that had evoked positive feelings in the past (Hvalsøe & Josephsson, 2003). Knowledge of occupations that have been valued by the client may serve as an impetus to continue involvement or to reintroduce that occupation into one's life. Recently during a level II fieldwork placement in the community mental health system, my student discovered that one of her clients once derived satisfaction from needlework, but had stopped engaging in this leisure occupation. Inspired by that knowledge, the student provided materials for the client to participate in a similar occupation, which proved to be meaningful and, therefore, motivating.

The founders of occupational therapy strongly believed that health and well-being could be influenced by engagement in occupation (Schwartz, 2005). Schwartz gave the following examples of the meaning occupation held for these historical figures in occupational therapy. William Rush Dunton, Jr. found that crafts had a therapeutic effect on him personally and went on to further the Arts and Crafts movement as part of the intervention in children and adults with mental illness. Meyer and Slagle espoused the importance of habits and involvement in occupations as a way to deal with problems in living. Hall focused on the importance of work, rather than rest, as an avenue toward improved health. The profession, in some respects, has come full circle in recognizing the power of occupation. Therefore, it is imperative that we continue to learn how to unleash that power.

The Concept of Flow

The theory of optimal experience based on the concept of flow was developed in the 1970s by Mihaly Csikszentmihalyi who said: "Flow [autotelic experience] is the way people describe their state of mind when consciousness is harmoniously ordered, and they want to pursue whatever they are doing for its own sake" (1990, p. 6). The experience is so enjoyable and absorbing that it becomes autotelic, meaning it is worth doing even if there is no tangible outcome (Csikszentmihalyi, 1999). Csikszentmihalyi wanted to understand the internal feeling state of individuals when they were doing what they enjoyed the most and to determine why they felt that way. He viewed this construct as a possible avenue to help improve quality of life. In addition, Csikszentmihalyi believed that the ability to experience flow, as well as hope and optimism, could be learned, which would in turn affect one's level of happiness (Csikszentmihalyi & Hunter, 2003). While research has gathered information about the kinds of experiences (e.g., leisure, work, athletics, music, religious rituals, and creative activities) that may result in flow, Csikszentmihalyi discussed the possibility of ordering one's consciousness so that any activity could result in flow and, thereby, enhance well-being (Csikszentmihalyi, 1990).

Regardless of the activity that generates the flow experience, people describe flow similarly across all cultures (Carlson & Clark, 1991; Moneta, 2004). When experiencing optimal flow, individuals become so immersed that they lose sense of time and feel joyful, motivated, creative, and intensely focused. There is a lack of self-consciousness, an escape from problems, and a clear sense of one's goal (Carlson & Clark, 1991; Csikszentmihalyi, 1990, 1999; Csikszentmihalyi & LeFevre, 1989; Gerhardsson & Jonsson, 1996; Jacobs, 1994; Rebeiro & Polgar, 1998). Process becomes more important than any outcome of this expenditure of psychic energy (Rebeiro & Polgar, 1998). It is also true that stress is an aspect of flow, the degree depending on the level of the challenge involved. Certain conditions must exist in order for flow to occur (Csikszentmihalyi, 1990; Gerhardsson & Jonsson, 1996; Jacobs, 1994; Persson, 1996; Rebeiro & Polgar, 1998).

There must be a match between one's skills and the challenge of the activity:

- There must be clear short-term goals.
- The individual needs to feel he or she has control.
- The activity must provide immediate feedback.

Csikszentmihalyi identified the following contexts of challenge and skills: anxiety, flow, boredom, and apathy (Jacobs, 1994; McCormick, Funderburk, Lee, & Hale-Fought, 2005). In the anxiety context, the individual perceives the challenge of the activity as beyond one's capacity as compared with the skills the person possesses. Flow occurs when challenges and skills are equal, with the caveat that the activity or experience requires that the individual stretch beyond usual performance. Boredom occurs when the challenges are less than the skill level as perceived by the individual. Apathy occurs when both skills and challenges are perceived as below that of the individual's perception of his or her average capability and challenge (Jacobs, 1994).

The experience sampling method (ESM) was developed as an alternative to qualitative interviews to gather data about the flow experience of individuals as they occurred in natural contexts over time (Carlson & Clark, 1991; Csikszentmihalyi, 2003; Csikszentmihalyi & LeFevre, 1989; Farnworth, Mostert, Harrison, & Worrell, 1996; Jacobs, 1994). The instrument asks about challenges the subject is experiencing in the here and now in order to identify flow and gathers information about the subjective experience of the individual regarding the quality of experience and kind of activity in which he or she is engaged. Subjects wear an electronic device that beeps randomly throughout the day, and they are asked to complete an experience sampling form (ESF) that addresses pertinent questions regarding what activities they were engaged in at the time as well as the perceived challenges and skills related to the task. This methodology for studying the experience of flow was seen as an improvement on other means of gathering these data (Farnworth et al., 1996). Time diaries have been used to collect similar data, but they do not necessarily provide direct access to the individual's internal experience, nor to the intensity of it. In addition, interviews have their limitations owing to selective remembering as well as the possibility that the subjects may skew their reports based on a desire to please the researcher in some way (Farnworth et al., 1996). Carlson and Clark (1991) highlighted the merits of this methodology as a valid way to record data to increase knowledge of how human beings are affected by ordinary activities.

To exemplify the use of the flow construct and the ESM of gathering data, some examples are given. Studies outside of the discipline of occupational therapy and within the profession are described.

In a study designed to predict boredom and anxiety in the lives of community mental health clients, McCormick et al. (2005) discovered that states of boredom and anxiety interfered with social and cognitive functioning. Through the use of the ESM, he learned that individuals with severe mental illness tend to have fewer challenges in their lives and spend most of their time engaged in activities below their skill level; this would be thought to result in boredom. However, that was not the subjective experience of the participants. Although his research indicated that there is little in the way of stimulating activity in the lives of persons with severe mental illness, it may well be that these individuals avoid anxiety by not seeking out more challenging situations. He concluded that for this population, understimulation and overstimulation could be problematic. Either way, his findings speak to the importance of balance between skills and challenge in order to promote well-being and quality of life.

To examine behaviors and habits that could be associated with happiness, Csikszentmihalyi and Hunter (2003) conducted a study of American youth using the ESM. As a premise, it was understood that events occurring outside of oneself have an effect on personal happiness, but one's values and interpretation of events also have an effect. Given the age of the subjects, weekdays were consumed with school or work activities. With regard to the time of day, the teens indicated a higher level of happiness at lunch and after school when their time was more free. The activities with which the subjects were involved at a given time, as well as their companions, also had an effect on perceived happiness. The final results indicated that younger teens of lower socioeconomic groups were happier—they tended to spend less time alone and more time in high-challenge/high-skill activities, which resulted in flow. The ESM allowed researchers to capture information about what was meaningful and fulfilling to this population.

Jacobs (1994) used the ESM to examine optimal flow experiences and job satisfaction in occupational therapy practitioners. Most of her subjects worked in physical rehabilitation settings and reported experiencing flow a relatively small percentage of time (average of 5.24 times per week). As expected, flow experiences occurred most often during the intervention process. Her intent was to gain information to enable practitioners to develop and apply strategies to enhance flow experiences for occupational therapists while at work, as well as to enable them to facilitate this experience for their clients. In her article, she reiterates the suggestions made by Csikszentmihalyi (1990) regarding how this might be accomplished.

Persson (1996) used the concepts of play and flow theories to examine the occupational process with a creative activity group for clients with chronic pain. The aim of this study was to look at theory that would emphasize a "doing" perspective and to see if the chosen theories could be used to study this process. Many of the components of both theories are congruent. The results indicated that the concepts of play and flow are useful in this context. Subjects experienced the creative activities as both serious and playful, as well as enjoyable, although frustrating at times (Persson, 1996). Some typical characteristics of flow experiences were reported by the subjects while they were engaged in the activity, including statements that pain was sometimes forgotten. Persson gave an example describing "how a meaningful activity and its possibilities and demands can arouse the energy and intention for the actor when he/she at first enters into it with skepticism" (p. 40).

Subjects with schizophrenia were engaged in a study by Gerhardsson and Jonsson (1996) designed to explore intrinsic motivation and flow experience. The participants were observed during selected activities of personal interest at three different times, followed by a semistructured interview immediately after each session. The content of the interview was designed to learn about the subject's experience of the activity and to compare his or her report with the observation report, which was based on elements of the flow experience. If the participant had experienced the activity previously, the chances of flow increased. Overall, the results suggested that the elements of the flow theory are useful in describing which aspects of a particular occupation have a therapeutic effect on an individual (Gerhardsson & Jonsson, 1996).

Csikszentmihalyi and LeFevre (1989) used the ESM in a study with adult workers to discern any differences in the quality of experience for these individuals while they were engaged in work versus leisure. Quality was measured in terms of the match of challenges and skills, as well as level of happiness, satisfaction, creativity, and motivation. Although it might seem unlikely, more subjects appeared to experience flow-like conditions while at work as opposed to when engaged in leisure pursuits. The researchers hypothesized that it may be that during free time people just need to relax and recuperate from an intense workday, or that they are unable to direct their psychic energy when time is not organized and structured. It was suggested that if people realized that they actually derived more benefits from work than they had previously thought, it might result in a reevaluation of any negative perceptions they held about their jobs. In addition, it might be that a more conscious use of leisure activities could result in experiences more conducive to flow during free time.

The explosion of technology to include social media has resulted in increasing numbers of individuals using the Internet. Online learning, researching, shopping, and gaming have become meaningful occupations for many individuals, and occupational therapists need to be mindful of this development. In exploring the literature, a significant number of researchers have conducted studies that examine the flow experience in relation to internet use and Web design. Skadberg and Kimmel (2004) found that two primary factors contributed to optimal experience or flow: attractiveness and the interactivity of the Web site. One of their most important discoveries was that telepresence (loss of awareness, intense focus) was the greatest measure of flow. Furthermore, optimal experience was associated with the context of the situational interaction in addition to gathering information on a particular topic. Pace (2004) found that informants in his study experienced time distortion, escape from concerns, and decreased awareness of the physical and social environment while they were engaged online.

Playing online games has become a valued leisure activity for many people. Flow is encouraged through online gaming in that the player receives immediate feedback, experiences enjoyment, and the activity requires concentration (Chiang, Lin, Cheng, & Liu, 2011). Teng and Huang (2012) found that skill and challenge predicted flow when subjects were engaged in gaming. Online games produce a cognitive state that facilitates flow, and players can begin at a simpler level and advance to more challenging levels, thereby increasing mastery (Cowley, Charles, Black, & Hickey, 2008). Researchers investigating what motivated customers to continue online gaming or remain loyal to a particular game found that having an optimal experience/flow experience was the greatest factor (Choi & Kim, 2004; Lee & Tsai, 2010). Flow theory plays a significant role in research related to information technology (Teng & Huang, 2012).

Discussion

Early theorists as well as current scholars in the field of occupational therapy discuss skill acquisition and providing the "just right challenge" when planning and implementing interventions for those we serve (Carlson & Clark, 1991; Mee et al., 2004; Yerxa, 1998). One of the most important criteria in producing flow is that skills must match the challenge of the activity and that there should be a certain degree of tension. An individual should have to stretch his or her capacity to expand, grow, and actualize potential. The work of Csikszentmihalyi (1989) in breaking down the ratio of skills to challenge into the contexts of anxiety, boredom, flow, and apathy provides a lens through which the occupational therapist might analyze occupational choices and occupational behavior when designing effective interventions for clients (Carlson & Clark, 1991). Another important requirement for facilitating flow is that the goals of the activity or occupation must be clear and distinct. Christiansen (1999) equated occupation with "goal-directed activity in the context of living" (p. 553), and elaborated by saying that because an individual imagines the outcome if a goal is met, that goal becomes a source of motivation. Setting

achievable goals based on client input to increase motivation is inherent in occupational therapy practice.

The concept of balance in life as a determinant of health has been germane to the field of occupational therapy since its inception. Yerxa (1998) cited leaders in the profession, to include Meyer and Reilly, as espousing the merits of a healthy balance. Csikszentmihalyi, too, saw the value of balance when he discussed the need for a match between perceived skills and the challenge of activities in the environment (Yerxa, 1998). Law (2007) saw the relevance of Csikszentmihalyi's work to occupational therapy just as her colleagues had (Carlson & Clark, 1991; Yerxa, 1998).

Christiansen (1999), in discussing the power of occupation, proposed that we create meaning in our lives through the things we do. Csikszentmihalyi (1990) devoted a chapter to the subject of meaning, stating that "creating meaning involves bringing order to the contents of the mind by integrating actions into a unified flow experience" (p. 216). Meaningful lives require challenging goals of significance that must be pursued with resolve in order to produce harmony (Csikszentmihalyi, 1990). Englehart (1986) echoed the perspective of founders of the profession by describing occupational therapists as custodians of meaning. Studies designed to validate the importance of meaningful occupation, including some cited in this chapter, have provided evidence that what we do in everyday life has a profound effect on life satisfaction and well-being. However, what is meaningful to one individual may not be to another (Persson et al., 2001). In order for occupational therapy interventions to be successful, we must learn which occupations are of value to clients because the concepts of purpose and meaning are central to therapeutic outcomes (Farnworth et al., 1996). To underscore the powerful effect the discovery of a meaningful occupation can have on an individual, Csikszentmihalyi (1997) described a woman with chronic schizophrenia who had been hospitalized for more than 10 years. In a period of study using the ESM, she reported having positive moods several times that occurred when she was caring for her fingernails. Based on those findings, the staff in the facility enlisted the aid of a professional manicurist to teach the client skills that resulted in the woman giving manicures to other clients. Not only did her mood improve, but she was able to be discharged to the community where she eventually took up the trade and became self-sufficient within a year.

Despite the similarities between the concept of flow and the philosophy of occupational therapy with respect to the value of meaningful occupation, Csikszentmihalyi's work has not been used to provide evidence in support of our work. The flow construct has been researched and utilized in the fields of psychology, leisure, education, and business. However, there was little to be found in the occupational therapy literature that referenced flow, and much of the evidence was produced more than a

EVIDENCE-BASED RESEARCH CHART

Topic	Evidence
Occupational therapy and meaningful occupation	Bridle, 1999; Christiansen, 1999; Christiansen, Backman, Little, & Nguyen, 1999; Englehardt, 1986; Hammell, 2004; Hvalsøe & Josephsson, 2003; Kennedy-Jones, Cooper, & Fossey, 2005; Law, 2007; Mee, Sumsion, & Craik, 2004; Persson, Erlandsson, Eklund, & Iwarsson, 2001; Schwartz, 2005; Yerxa, 1998; Zemke, 2004
Theory of flow	Csikszentmihalyi, 1990, 1997, 1999, 2003; Csikszentmihalyi & Hunter, 2003; Csikszentmihalyi & LeFevre, 1989
Studies about flow	Chiang, Lin, Cheng, & Liu, 2011; Choi & Kim, 2004; Cowley, Charles, Black, & Hickey, 2008; Lee & Tsai, 2010; McCormick, Funderburk, Lee, & Hale-Fought, 2005; Moneta, 2004; Pace, 2004; Skadberg & Kimmel, 2004; Teng & Huang, 2012
Flow and occupational therapy	Carlson & Clark, 1991; Farnworth, Mostert, Harrison, & Worrell, 1996; Gerhardsson & Jonsson, 1996; Jacobs, 1994; Persson, 1996; Rebeiro & Polgar, 1999

decade ago, primarily outside of the United States. It would appear that we have not taken advantage of a well-researched body of work that has considerable merit, but we have the opportunity to do so. On a macro level, the flow construct could serve to validate the importance of the role of occupational therapy in facilitating health, well-being, and quality of life. On a micro level, Csikszentmihalyi's theory could enable us to determine what is, in fact, meaningful occupation as we intervene with clients on a day-to-day basis.

Summary

The literature clearly indicates a relationship between meaningful occupation and the concept of flow. The studies described exemplify how one might use Csikszentmihalyi's work and methodology to provide further evidence on the value of occupation. Flow "is highly relevant to occupational science because it documents an everyday phenomenon that importantly relates to, among other things, happiness, self-esteem, work productivity, the enjoyment of leisure, and life satisfaction" (Carlson & Clark, 1991, p. 239).

Embracing Csikszentmihalyi's theory and capitalizing on the extensive body of evidence that has been produced primarily outside of the occupational therapy profession would lend credence to our own body of knowledge. The degree to which the relationship between these two constructs needs to be investigated is beyond the scope of this chapter. Occupational therapists need to engage in the meaningful occupation of producing evidence to validate

what we do and to increase our understanding of how we can best intervene to facilitate successful outcomes for our clients who are depending on us to assist them with improving quality of life.

Student Self-Assessment

1. List some of your favorite occupations. What are some of your usual feelings when engaged in these pursuits?

2. Do you think you experience flow when participating in any of these occupations? Which ones?

3. Evaluate your favorite occupations in terms of Csikszentmihalyi's conditions of flow listed on page 6. Do any of these pursuits meet his criteria for flow? If so, which ones? If not, which ones? Why or why not?

4. Review the challenge and skills contexts discussed on pages 6 and 7. Identify an activity or occupation in which you experience (a) anxiety, (b) boredom, and (c) apathy. How do these subjective feelings affect your motivation and sense of well-being?

5. Discuss any parallels you see between the experience of flow and occupations that are meaningful to individuals. How could you apply this to occupational therapy practice?

6. Do you think it is possible to experience flow while engaged in an activity or occupation even if all of Csikszentmihalyi's conditions are not met?

References

Bridle, M. J. (1999). Are doing and being dimensions of holism? *American Journal of Occupational Therapy, 53*(6), 636-639.

Carlson, M. E., & Clark, F. A. (1991). The search for useful methodologies in occupational science. *American Journal of Occupational Therapy, 45*(3), 235-241.

Chiang, Y., Lin, S., Cheng, C., & Liu, E. (2011). Exploring online game players' flow experiences and positive affect. *The Turkish Online Journal of Educational Technology, 10*(1), 106-114.

Choi, D., & Kim, J. (2004). Why people continue to play online games: In search of critical design factors to increase customer loyalty to online contents. *CyberPsychology & Behavior, 7*(3), 11-23.

Christiansen, C. H. (1999). The 1999 Eleanor Clarke Slagle lecture: Defining lives: Occupation as identity: An essay on competence, coherence, and the creation of meaning. *American Journal of Occupational Therapy, 53*(6), 547-558.

Christiansen, C. H., Backman, C., Little, B. R., & Nguyen, A. (1999). Occupations and well-being: A study of personal projects. *American Journal of Occupational Therapy, 53*(1), 91-100.

Cowley, B., Charles, D., Black, M., & Hickey, R. (2008). Toward an understanding of flow in video games. *ACM Computers in Entertainment, 6*(2), 20.1-20.27.

Csikszentmihalyi, M. (1990). *Flow: The psychology of optimal experience.* New York, NY: HarperCollins.

Csikszentmihalyi, M. (1997). *Finding flow: The psychology of engagement with everyday life.* New York, NY: Basic Books.

Csikszentmihalyi, M. (1999). If we are so rich, why aren't we happy? *American Psychologist, 54*(10), 821-827.

Csikszentmihalyi, M. (2003). Happiness in everyday life: The uses of experience sampling. *Journal of Happiness Studies, 4*(2), 185-199.

Csikszentmihalyi, M., & Hunter, J. (2003). Happiness in everyday life: The uses of experience sampling. *Journal of Happiness Studies, 4,* 185-199.

Csikszentmihalyi, M., & LeFevre, J. (1989). Optimal experience in work and leisure. *Journal of Personality and Social Psychology, 56*(5), 815-822.

Englehardt, T. (1986). Occupational therapists as technologists and custodians of meaning. In G. Kielhofner (Ed.), *Health through occupation* (pp. 139-144). Philadelphia, PA: F. A. Davis Company.

Farnworth, L., Mostert, E., Harrison, S., & Worrell, D. (1996). The experience sampling method: Its potential use in occupational therapy research. *Occupational Therapy International, 3*(1), 1-17.

Gerhardsson, C., & Jonsson, H. (1996). Experience of therapeutic occupations in schizophrenic subjects: Clinical observations organized in terms of the flow theory. *Scandinavian Journal of Occupational Therapy, 3*(4), 149-155.

Hammell, K. (2004). Dimensions of meaning in the occupations of daily life. *Canadian Journal of Occupational Therapy, 5*(71), 296-305.

Hvalsøe, B., & Josephsson, S. (2003). Characteristics of meaningful occupations from the perspective of mentally ill people. *Scandinavian Journal of Occupational Therapy, 10*(2), 61-71.

Jacobs, K. (1994). Flow and the occupational therapy practitioner. *American Journal of Occupational Therapy, 48*(11), 989-996.

Kennedy-Jones, M., Cooper, J., & Fossey, E. (2005). Developing a worker role: Stories of four people with mental illness. *Australian Occupational Therapy Journal, 52*(2), 116-126.

Law, M. (2007). Occupational therapy: A journey driven by curiosity. *American Journal of Occupational Therapy, 61,* 599-602.

Lee, M., & Tsai, T. (2010). What drives people to continue to play online games? An extension of technology model and theory of planned behavior. *International Journal of Human-Computer Interaction, 26*(6), 601-620.

McCormick, B. P., Funderburk, J. A., Lee, Y. K., & Hale-Fought, M. (2005). Activity characteristics and emotional experience: Predicting boredom and anxiety in the daily life of community mental health clients. *Journal of Leisure Research, 37,* 236-253.

Mee, J., Sumsion, T., & Craik, C. (2004). Mental health clients confirm the value of occupation in building competence and self-identity. *British Journal of Occupational Therapy, 67*(5), 225-233.

Moneta, G. (2004). The flow experience across cultures. *Journal of Happiness Studies, 5*(4), 115-121.

Pace, S. (2004).The roles of challenge and skill in the flow experiences of Web users. *Issues in Informing Science & Information Technology, 1,* 341-358.

Persson, D. (1996). Play and flow in an activity group—A case study of creative occupations with chronic pain patients. *Scandinavian Journal of Occupational Therapy, 3*(1), 33-42.

Persson, D., Erlandsson, L., Eklund, M., & Iwarsson, S. (2001). Value dimensions, meaning, and complexity in human occupation—A tentative structure for analysis. *Scandinavian Journal of Occupational Therapy, 8*(1), 7-18.

Rebeiro, K. L., & Polgar, J. M. (1999). Enabling occupational performance: Optimal experiences in therapy. *Canadian Journal of Occupational Therapy, 66*(1), 14-22.

Schwartz, K. (2005). The history and philosophy of psychosocial occupational therapy. In E. Cara & A. MacRae (Eds.), *Psychosocial occupational therapy: A clinical practice* (2nd ed., pp. 61-68). Florence, KY: Delmar Cengage Learning.

Skadberg, Y., & Kimmel, J. (2004). Visitor's flow experience while browsing a web site: It's measurement, contributing factors and consequences. *Computers in Human Behavior, 20*(3), 403-422.

Teng, C., & Huang, C. (2012). More than flow: Revisiting the theory of four channels of flow. *International Journal of Computer Games Technology,* 1-9. doi:10.1155/2012/724917

Yerxa, E. J. (1998). Health and the human spirit for occupation. *American Journal of Occupational Therapy, 52*(6), 412-418.

Zemke, R. (2004). The 2004 Eleanor Clarke Slagle lecture: Time, space, and the kaleidoscopes of occupation. *American Journal of Occupational Therapy, 58*(6), 608-620.

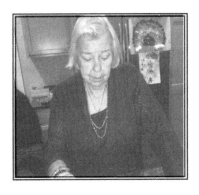

2

CULTURAL IMPACT ON OCCUPATION

Roxie M. Black, PhD, OTR/L, FAOTA

ACOTE STANDARDS EXPLORED IN THIS CHAPTER
B.1.4–B.1.6, B.2.9, B.4.0, B.4.2, B.4.4, B.4.7, B.5.0, B.5.1

KEY VOCABULARY

- **Cultural competence:** The process of actively developing and practicing cultural self-awareness, knowledge, and skill when interacting with someone culturally diverse from oneself.
- **Culturally sensitive assessment tools:** Tools and surveys that add questions that elicit information about the client's cultural beliefs and practices related to health care.
- **Culture:** The sum total of a way of living that influences the behavior(s) of a group of people.
- **Occupational justice:** The rights of people to have access to and opportunity to engage in meaningful occupations.

Introduction

The concept of culture is deeply embedded, yet readily visible, in occupational therapy. It is addressed in multiple standards from the Accreditation Council for Occupational Therapy Education (ACOTE); identified in the Occupational Therapy Practice Framework (OTPF; American Occupational Therapy Association [AOTA], 2008), as a vital context when assessing and developing interventions with occupational therapy clients; is addressed in multiple occupation-based models of practice (Christiansen & Baum, 1997; Dunn, Brown, & McGuigan, 1994; Iwama, 2006; Law, Cooper, Strong, Stewart, Rigby, & Letts, 1996; Schkade & Schultz, 2003); examined in relation to ethical practice in the OT Code of Ethics, addressed in the Centennial Vision; and found in numerous occupational therapy books and other publications. Cultural competency is a vital aspect of occupational therapy education and practice.

Jacobs, K., MacRae, N., & Sladyk, K. (Eds.).
*Occupational Therapy Essentials for
Clinical Competence, Second Edition* (pp. 11-24).
© 2014 SLACK Incorporated.

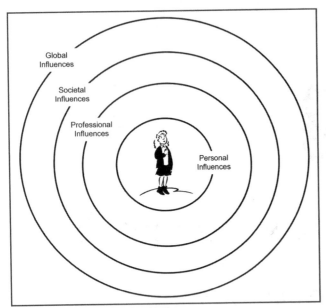

Figure 2-1. Cultural levels of influence.

The concept of culture, however ubiquitous in occupational therapy documents, is quite complex. This chapter defines culture; discusses its relevance to occupational therapy practitioners, educators, and researchers; addresses its importance in developing assessment tools and examining marginalized populations; and discusses its relevance in culturally effective care.

Culture Defined

Iwama (2004) described culture as a "slippery concept, taking on a variety of definitions and meanings, depending on how it has been socially situated and by whom" (p. 1). Some people may define "having culture" as being sophisticated and knowledgeable, whereas the term "culture" might connote racial and ethnic differences to others. A much broader definition of culture is

> the sum total of a way of living, including values, beliefs, standards, linguistic expression, patterns of thinking, behavioral norms, and styles of communication that influence the behavior(s) of a group of people that is transmitted from generation to generation. It includes demographic variables such as age, gender, and place of residence, status variables such as social, educational, and economic levels, and affiliation variables (Black & Wells, 2007, p. 5).

In addition, culture is learned. Because it is transmitted to others and following generations, aspects of one's culture—including attitudes, values, and behaviors—can be changed or adapted to meet the requirements of changing times and contexts.

As is evident in the preceding complex definition, culture is all-encompassing and influences multiple aspects

of a person's life, including occupational behaviors and occupational choices. For example, the occupation of eating breakfast varies between different cultural groups. The time we rise in the morning, the food we choose to eat (or do not eat), the utensils we use (or do not use), what time of the day we eat, how much time we take to have a meal, and whether we stand or sit, or eat alone or with others are all influenced by one's cultural group and expectations.

Not only are we influenced by the culture into which we are born (family, community, society), we are also affected by the subcultures to which we choose to belong. These may include groups from our church, synagogue, or temple; our college and occupational therapy program; our cohort of friends; our biking or hiking group; or our gym companions. Because each of these subgroups holds certain values and expectations, they also influence our behaviors and choices. Sometimes the expectations of these various cultural groups are in conflict with one another. For example, as an occupational therapy student, the faculty of your occupational therapy program may expect you to study for several hours a day or night, whereas your family or roommates may have expectations that you will be home for dinner each evening. Your occupational choice will depend on what is most important to you at that time given the context of the situation.

What is meaningful and important is culturally determined and influences occupational behaviors, choices, and performance for not only each of us, but for each client with whom we work. Recognizing the extent of cultural influence on behavior is vital for understanding the context within which our clients live and work. Therefore, "culture represents one of the most important issues facing occupational therapy today" (Iwama, 2004, p. 1).

Multiple Levels of Cultural Influence

As occupational therapy students and practitioners, culture influences us and our occupational choice on many levels, just as it does the people with whom we work. These levels begin with each of us personally, and move through several levels to the global level (Figure 2-1). We briefly examine each of these levels in this section of the chapter.

Personal Influences

Each of us develops from a particular social location. This means that our place of birth, the year of our birth, our birth order, our gender, our sexual identity, our class, family structure, ability, religion, and our ethnicity all influence who we are at birth, and, in many cases, who we will become as adults. All of these cultural characteristics influence our behavior or what we do: our occupations. For example, I was born just after the end of World War II and raised in a rural state by working-class parents. I was raised to believe in hard work, the importance of education (which my parents were unable to acquire yet knew the value of), the importance of helping others, and the love of family and nature. All of these values influence what I choose to do today, from teaching in an occupational therapy program, to spending important time with family and friends, or to one of my favorite pastimes—gardening.

Most of us are taught our cultural values by members of our families, friends, mentors, teachers, and spiritual leaders. We also learn cultural lessons from the media, such as the standard of feminine beauty, the importance of wealth, and the value of commodities. Often the messages learned from these various groups/people conflict, and we must choose what best meets our needs. For example, we may come from a large Italian family where the message of *mangia, mangia* (eat! eat!) rings in our ears; yet the print and electronic media constantly tell us that being painfully thin is the true vision of beauty in the United States. Or our peer group enjoys playing at the beach, lying in the sun and developing a deep, rich tan, whereas the message from the health community is that getting too much sun can lead to health issues. What do we do? Each of us is a unique and complex cultural being, so we will make occupational choices based on what we value, or what is important to us at that time. For these reasons, each person must be viewed as an individual.

This is also true of the people with whom we work as occupational therapy practitioners. Although there may be cultural similarities between members of a particular group, we cannot assume each member of the group holds the same beliefs, values, and occupational interests, and we cannot treat each member of a group in the same way. Certainly not all of the students in a given academic program perform the same, learn in the same manner, study the same way, or enjoy the same topics, even though the majority may be white and all female as they are in academic programs in the state of Maine. Therefore, it is imperative that the faculty understand each student as an individual, just as occupational therapy practitioners must view each client as an individual.

One reason that there is such individuality within a group or subgroup is that culture can be learned as well as unlearned. Although we are taught certain values as children, as we develop and experience more of life, we sometimes reject those earlier teachings and assume other values. For instance, we may have been taught negative things about a certain race or ethnicity, or that older people are cranky and helpless, or that women are emotional and weak, or that motorcyclists are all hoodlums. But our life experiences and/or education have refuted those lessons, and we may now perceive members of those groups in different ways. As we mature, we may choose a spiritual path or lifestyle that is different from that of our parents or cultural group, or we may move into a different

socioeconomic class—an experience that may change our perception of our world and the people in it. These changing beliefs and values will alter our occupational choices and patterns, and demonstrate the dynamic nature of our cultural influences and re-emphasize the importance of learning about people's individual and personal cultures as we work with them. Not only are we influenced by our personal beliefs and values, but what we learn as occupational therapists affects our beliefs and behaviors as well.

PROFESSIONAL INFLUENCES: CULTURE AND OCCUPATIONAL THERAPY

The concept of culture is embedded in our profession and has been since we first began recognizing clients as individuals with unique needs. The very first set of standards for occupational therapy emphasized the importance of providing treatment to each client as an individual (Standards of the National Society for the Promotion of Occupational Therapy, 1925). Although a client's "cultural influences" may not have been the language used at that time, as we sought to understand each unique person's interests, beliefs, and needs, we were actually examining aspects of his or her culture. Over the last 9 decades we have continued to view each recipient of occupational therapy services as an individual, although many concepts within the field developed and changed. Some of the more current notions and language related to occupational therapy and culture are identified in the following text.

Culture and the Occupational Therapy Practice Framework

Several educational standards refer to culture as being part of the context of a client's life. That language derives from the framework (AOTA, 2008), which describes the domain of occupational therapy practice as "supporting health and participation in life through engagement in occupation" (p. 626). Occupational therapy recognizes the importance of the context of a person's life to support engagement in occupation. The OTPF states that "[c]ontext refers to a variety of interrelated conditions within and surrounding the client...[that] exert a strong influence on performance" (AOTA, 2008, p. 642). This document identifies two environmental and four contextual conditions that an occupational therapy practitioner must consider when working with a client. One of these is culture. The OTPF defines culture as the "customs, beliefs, activity patterns, behavior standards, and expectations accepted by the society of which the individual is a member" (p. 642).

The OTPF (AOTA, 2008) not only identifies the domain of occupational therapy practice and the process by which we provide interventions, but it also guides practice. As such, this document highlights the importance of considering the culture of the people with whom we work, and mandates that we consider the clients' cultural influences on their occupational performance.

Client-Centered Care

Another important concept in occupational therapy theory and practice that supports cultural consideration of clients is client-centered care. This notion arose from Rogers' (1951) theoretical belief that a client is a partner in the client/therapist dyad, and should and must be part of the decision-making process regarding his or her own treatment. The therapist or practitioner must respect the client, recognize the client as the first authority on what he or she needs, and try to see the world through the client's eyes as well as through those of the authoritative health professional. Since the early 1990s, occupational therapists have adopted Rogers's ideas and have been redefining them to support and frame occupational therapy practice (Law, 1998; Law, Baptiste, & Mills, 1995; Pollack, 1993; Sumsion, 1993, 1999). Many of these authors suggest that for client-centered care to occur, the occupational therapy practitioner must understand the client's medical, social, and occupational history as well as his or her beliefs and values so that the client and practitioner can collaboratively determine an intervention approach that is meaningful to the client. In other words, the practitioner must understand the client's culture and the cultural influences on his or her performance. Understanding another's culture is one aspect of cultural competence and part of culturally competent care. I had previously made the argument that client-centered care must, by its definition, be culturally competent care (Black, 2005).

Cultural Competence and Culturally Competent Care

To provide culturally competent care, occupational therapists and occupational therapy assistants must be culturally competent. "For good outcomes in health care, cultural competence is needed at the individual, team, organizational, and systemic levels" (Srivastava, 2007, p. 23). Although "cultural competence" is often used when talking about race and ethnicity, the changing demographics of the United States ensures a greater increase in the multiple diversities of our clients. Diversity is apparent in race and ethnicity, in class and socioeconomic levels, in age and ability, in religion and political views, in lifestyle choices, and in gender and sexual identity. If we understand culture to incorporate all of the preceding and more, then cultural competence is appropriate when working with all people, not just those who are racially or ethnically different from ourselves (Black, 2005).

Within the occupational therapy literature, cultural competence is described "as the process of actively developing and practicing appropriate, relevant, and sensitive strategies and skills in interacting with culturally different persons" (AOTA Multicultural Task Force, 1995). An often-used definition from Cross, Bazron, Dennis, and Isaacs (1989) states that cultural competence is "a set of congruent behaviors, attitudes, and policies that come together in a system, agency, or among professionals and enable that system, agency, or those professionals to work effectively in cross-cultural situations" (p. 13). As might be extrapolated from these definitions, cultural competence is more than just understanding the culture of our clients. It incorporates three distinct characteristics: cultural self-awareness, cultural knowledge, and cross-cultural skills (Black & Wells, 2007).

Cultural self-awareness may be the most important of the three characteristics of cultural competence (Black & Wells, 2007; Harry, 1992; Lynch & Hanson, 1998). It means recognizing yourself as a cultural being who sees the world through a unique cultural lens. This awareness assists us in knowing where we fit in the sociocultural matrix of the dominant culture, especially if we are a person of color, female, poor, old, physically or mentally impaired, or have a sexual identity other than heterosexuality. Being culturally self-aware means recognizing our privileged status if we are part of the dominant culture, acknowledging our biases and prejudices, and knowing how, from where, and from whom we learned these.

It is extremely important to do the hard work of cultural self-exploration because knowing ourselves in this way will make us more sensitive when working with a client who is culturally different from ourselves. Without that awareness, unexplored biases may become a barrier when working with certain clients with a culture different from our own, and may lead to ineffective, unethical, or inappropriate interventions. In the worst case, it might lead to discriminatory behaviors that might harm the client in some way.

Cultural knowledge, the second characteristic of cultural competence, is the information we gather about a client's culture, which includes customs, traditions, body language, values, beliefs about health and wellness, and the meaning of illness. It may mean learning a little of their language if it differs from our own. Trying to speak to people in their own language connotes respect for them and—in my experience—is always appreciated. In addition, cultural knowledge includes understanding the sociocultural "status" of this person's culture, and understanding the oppression and discrimination she or he might face. Taking the time to learn about a client's culture is vital in establishing rapport and providing client-centered care.

The third characteristic of cultural competence, *cross-cultural skill,* is what differentiates cultural competence from cultural sensitivity. To develop this skill you must actively engage in communicating and interacting with others who differ from yourself. You must be willing to "put yourself out there," to be open to differing ideas and beliefs, and to make mistakes (Black, 2002). You must also learn how to recover from those mistakes.

Successful cross-cultural communication means understanding non-verbal communication as well as negotiating conflict. All three of these characteristics—cultural self-awareness, cultural knowledge, and cross-cultural skill—must be developing or in place in order to provide culturally competent care.

In order for occupational therapy practitioners to understand the client's perspective of his or her illness or condition, we need to learn to ask the right questions through a culturally sensitive assessment approach, which will be discussed later in this chapter, and to listen carefully to the answers. We cannot assume that a culturally diverse client believes and thinks the same way we do. Therefore, it is important to constantly ask for clarification of ideas and meaning. Assuming that we understand what the client means without clarification can result in miscommunication and inadequate or poor intervention.

Culture and Occupational Justice

Occupational justice is a fairly new term found in occupational therapy literature that connotes that individuals have a right to access and engage in meaningful occupations. "Occupational injustices exist when, for example, participation is barred, confined, segregated, prohibited, undeveloped, disrupted, alienated, marginalized, exploited, or otherwise devalued" (Whiteford & Townsend, 2011, p. 69). Much of the literature on occupational justice and injustice has been written outside of the United States about groups of people who are socially oppressed. However, the terminology and ideas are increasingly and appropriately used in this country as well, as many individuals and groups in the United States are also barred from engaging in activities that have meaning for them. Prisoners, street people and the homeless, people with mental illness, and others in institutions are a few examples. Many of these individuals come from a sociocultural background that differs from that of the occupational therapy practitioners who work with them—the majority of whom are white, middle-class, and highly educated women. To recognize occupational injustices and to provide the best interventions, occupational therapy practitioners will have to provide effective client-centered and culturally competent care as meaningful occupations are culturally defined.

SOCIETAL INFLUENCES

The next level of cultural influence is the societal level. Every society has its own cultural beliefs and customs. Lewis (2002) writes that "culture is constructed by humans in order to communicate and create community" (p. 13). In the United States, we are guided by the principles of the United States Constitution, which extol the value of and rights to freedom, equality, and the pursuit of happiness for all. However, the dominant culture of the United States includes English-speaking, White,

middle-class, heterosexual people who have become the "standard" by which others are measured, and most of us recognize that those constitutional promises are realized by more members of the dominant group than by the nondominant members of our society. Those of us who fall within the dominant categories have more privilege than others and easier access to goods and services. (McIntosh, 1988)

Therefore, although all citizens of the United States may be governed by the same principles and beliefs, our experiences and perceptions of our world may differ because of our cultural characteristics and the societal hierarchy within our country. Our opportunities will differ from one another, leading to varied choices and occupational behaviors. For example, the daily activities of a widowed 79-year-old white woman living in low-income housing in a small city in the northeast region of the United States may differ significantly from that of a Puerto Rican woman of the same age living with her daughter and her family in the same geographical area. The first woman may be far more isolated, especially in the winter. Her occupations may include watching favorite television shows, doing crossword puzzles, reading biographies and nonfiction literature, talking on the telephone with family and friends, and doing light housework. Because she cannot afford a car, this woman rarely leaves her housing development, having to rely on others to take her grocery shopping or to do errands. Her children and grandchildren call often and see her regularly every few weeks or so. Nevertheless, she keeps busy, and although sometimes lonely, is fairly satisfied with her life (Figure 2-2).

The second woman, who is nearly the same age as our first example, comes from Puerto Rico, and a cultural background where it is common for older individuals to live with extended family and where being an older adult has value. She continues to have an important place in this family, and her occupations reflect that. She often cooks and helps to clean up after meals, assists with laundry and babysitting for the older children, and has become a confidante to her granddaughter. She watches her favorite television shows with the family in the evenings and is included in family excursions on the weekends. She reads to the younger children and tells them stories of their parents and grandparents and of times in the "old country." Although she goes to bed fairly exhausted in the evening, and sometimes wishes for a little more time to herself, this woman is also quite satisfied with her life (Figure 2-3).

Both of these women live full, but very different, lives. If we were to receive them as clients in our practice, we could not effectively work with them in the same way, nor could we expect their occupations to be alike just because they are women in their 70s living in the same region of the United States. The life of each woman is influenced by societal expectations, yet their personal and family

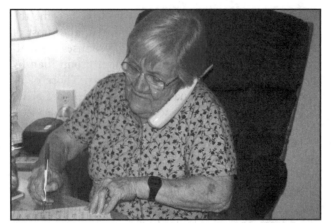

Figure 2-2. Enjoying the solitary occupation of doing a cross-word puzzle while socially interacting with a friend on the telephone.

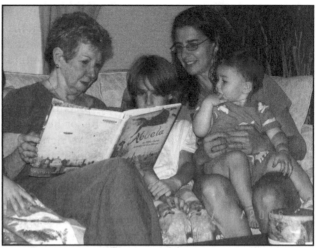

Figure 2-3. Enjoying family time by reading a favorite story to grandchildren.

cultures allow them to be individuals, and they must be respected as such.

Within the health professions, our behaviors are influenced not only by the larger societal expectations, but also by federal and state rules and regulations and our organizations' codes of ethics. Among these regulations are the National Standards for Culturally and Linguistically Appropriate Services (CLAS) in health care (United States Department of Health and Human Services, 2000). This collective set of fourteen mandates, guidelines, and recommendations was developed to inform, guide, and facilitate required and recommended practices related to culturally and linguistically appropriate health services for health care organizations and their employees. As occupational therapy practitioners, these standards will help guide our work with people and groups that are culturally diverse.

GLOBAL INFLUENCES

The broadest level of cultural influence on occupations, and perhaps the least apparent for many, comes from the larger, global world. Oftentimes, many people are ethnocentric and exclusionary, and do not seem interested in what is going on outside of his or her own country; nor do they believe they are affected by events beyond their shores. Yet, there is an impact on each of us. There is an old saying that goes something like this: the flutter of a butterfly's wings in one part of the world can spawn a hurricane in another. Our occupations may change in significant or subtle ways owing to events happening around the world.

The war in Afghanistan, for instance, has changed the occupations of not only the men and women from the United States who are fighting overseas, but also those of their families and friends who spend more time writing letters or emails, searching for and sending appropriate gifts, or—in the worst case—going to hospitals or funeral homes. Returning veterans with and without injuries struggle to pursue predeployment occupations and may have difficulty resuming roles that once were easy for them. Families work at adjusting to the return of these men and women. Others who did not have friends or family members who were deployed may have spent more time watching newscasts, reading newspapers and news magazines, or campaigning for favorite politicians as a result of the conflicts. Many of us engaged in new occupations as a direct result of the war.

When the tsunami hit Indonesia and Sri Lanka in 2005, many from the United States traveled there to help, began campaigns to send supplies or money as aid, or, again, stayed glued to their television sets to watch the latest news or increased the amount of time they spent reading newspapers and other news to follow the event.

The earthquake in Japan in March 2011, which caused damage at the Fukushima nuclear facility, brought officials from the United States to examine the structure. As the evening television news, newspapers, and blogs published information in the United States on a daily basis for months about the effects and the cleanup of the disaster, politicians and lawmakers in the United States worked diligently to develop new policies to try to avert the same kind of manmade disaster in this country (Remy, 2012). Again, many people in this country engaged in new occupations as a result of an event on the other side of the world.

Before the prevalence of new technology, people could ignore what was happening outside of their own communities or country. With television, social networking sites, and print media in most homes in the United States today and with email, smart phones, instant messaging, and other technological advances in communication, people not only know what is going on around the world, but have knowledge of events as they occur (Black & Wells, 2007). As a result, because we are more aware of world events, we become a more active part of our global culture and may choose to act on those events.

In summary, the multiple levels of cultural influences affect each of us in unique ways, shaping our own identities, the identities of the people with whom we work, and the manner in which we engage in occupational pursuits. How we understand and use this important information informs and guides our occupational therapy practice.

Culturally Effective Occupational Therapy Practice

As outlined by the OTPF, the occupational therapy "process includes evaluation, intervention, and outcome monitoring" (AOTA, 2008, p. 646). Perhaps the most important of these steps is evaluation which includes selecting and administering the most appropriate assessment tool(s) to determine the needs of the client. Although there is a multitude of evaluation tools from which occupational therapy practitioners may choose, it is important for occupational therapy students and practitioners to also consider the best culturally sensitive assessment tool as part of their assessment "tool box."

CULTURALLY SENSITIVE ASSESSMENT TOOLS

Many occupational therapy assessment tools have been developed for, and are biased toward, the sociocultural norms of a white, middle-class population, and have incorporated Western values, ethics, theories, and standards as part of their development. Although some have taken culture into consideration, notably the Loewenstein Occupational Therapy Cognitive Assessment (LOTCA) battery (Josman, Abdallah, & Engel-Yager, 2011), the Canadian Occupational Performance Measure (COPM; Fisher, 2005), and the Assessment of Motor and Process Skills (AMPS; Buchan, 2002), most have not been standardized for ethnic populations (Black & Wells, 2007). Because these assessments are not so standardized, the results of these tests may be less than optimal and could be unproductive or even harmful when administered to some individuals. For example, there are limited mental health data for the Somali population owing to the lack of appropriate assessment tools (Bhui et al., 2003). Somalis do experience mental health symptoms but traditionally believe that these symptoms are related to spirit possession (Lewis, 1998), and they endure this emotional discomfort in a somewhat fatalistic manner. Using a culturally sensitive approach to assessment might help practitioners more deeply understand the beliefs of this population of clients, resulting in more effective intervention.

The OTPF (AOTA, 2008) suggests beginning the evaluation process by using an occupational profile, which would include gathering information "that describes the client's occupational history and experiences, patterns of daily living, interests, values, and needs" (p. 649). This is a client-centered and collaborative approach that guides intervention. Adding specific questions that elicit information about the client's cultural beliefs and practices related to health care will enrich and deepen the understanding that the therapist has of the client, and will strengthen the therapist/client relationship.

There are several culturally sensitive assessment tools that the occupational therapist can choose from. These include the approach used by Black and Wells (2007), titled "Eliciting Cultural Information in Clinical Interactions" (p. 258). The authors suggest beginning with an opening paragraph that clearly explains the purpose of the questions, followed by questions regarding the client's current illness, questions regarding health beliefs and practices, and questions regarding cultural beliefs and values (Table 2-1). Using these questions to help expand the narrative and life history of the client "allows the provider to frame the problems and limitations in a cultural context" (Black & Wells, 2007, p. 257).

Other culturally sensitive tools and models include the Sunrise Model by Leininger (1988), the ETHNIC Cultural Assessment (Levin, Like, & Gottlieb, 2000), and the BELIEF Cultural Assessment (Dobbie, Medrano, Tysinger, & Olney, 2003; see Table 2-1).

Madeleine Leininger, the nurse educator who developed much of the theory related to transcultural nursing (1988), believed that the intake or interview questions that should be asked of a client be broadly conceived, and cover the following areas:

- Cultural values and lifeways
- Religious, philosophical, and spiritual beliefs
- Economic factors
- Educational factors
- Technological factors
- Kinship and social ties
- Political and legal factors

The Sunrise Model, which developed from Leininger's theory (2002; Leininger's Sunrise Model, n.d.; Figure 2-4), has been applied in nursing practice for years and provides an interesting approach that could be adopted by other health care professionals, including occupational therapy practitioners.

The ETHNIC (Levin et al., 2000) and BELIEF (Dobbie et al., 2003) assessments are similar culturally relevant interviewing instruments that address clients' beliefs and perspectives about their illness and/or health condition (see Table 2-1). Both are useful in identifying cultural beliefs and values and enhancing occupational therapy

Table 2-1.		
CULTURALLY SENSITIVE ASSESSMENT MODELS, TOOLS, AND QUESTIONNAIRES		
Authors	**Instrument**	**Reference**
Black & Wells	Cultural Information Questionnaire Opening statement Questions about current illness Health beliefs and practices Cultural beliefs and values	Black, R. M., & Wells, S. A. (2007). *Culture & occupation: A model of empowerment in occupational therapy.* Bethesda, MD: AOTA Press.
Leininger	The Sunrise Model Cultural values and lifeways Religious, philosophical, and spiritual beliefs Economic factors Educational factors Technological factors Kinship and social ties Political and legal factors	Leininger, M. (1988). Leininger's theory of nursing: Cultural care diversity and universality. *Nursing Science Quarterly, 1*(4), 152-160.
Levin, Like, & Gottlieb	The ETHNIC tool E: Explanation (How do you explain your illness?) T: Treatment (What treatment have you tried?) H: Healers (Have you sought any advice from folk healers?) N: Negotiate (mutually acceptable options) I: (Agree on) intervention C: Collaboration (with patient, family, and healers)	Levin, S. J., Like, R. C., & Gottlieb, J. E. (2000). ETHNIC: A framework for culturally competent clinical practice. *Patient Care, 9*(special issue), 188.
Dobbie, Medrano, Tysinger, & Olney	The BELIEF tool B: Health beliefs (What caused your illness/problem?) E: Explanation (Why did it happen at this time?) L: Learn (Help me understand your belief/opinion.) I: Impact (How is this illness/problem impacting your life?) E: Empathy (This must be very difficult for you.) F: Feelings (How are you feeling about it?)	Dobbie, A. E., Medrano, M., Tysinger, J., & Olney, C. (2003). The BELIEF instrument: a preclinical teaching tool to elicit patients' health beliefs. *Family Medicine, 35*(5), 316-319.

Adapted from Dobbie, A. E., Medrano, M., Tysinger, J., & Olney, C. (2003). The BELIEF instrument: A preclinical teaching tool to elicit patients' health beliefs. *Family Medicine, 35,* 316-319.

assessment that would support and influence culturally effective client-centered practice.

As well as identifying and using an effective culturally sensitive assessment tool, practitioners must be aware of some of the cultural characteristics that have the potential to become barriers to effective cross-cultural interactions.

Cultural Characteristics That Affect Effective Cross-Cultural Interactions

There are many unique characteristics and beliefs that individuals from various cultures may possess that, if not examined, may interfere with effective client-centered

and culturally effective care. As a point of illustration, this chapter briefly examines three of these characteristics: self-concept, perceptions of power and authority, and temporal issues.

SELF-CONCEPT

In North America and much of Europe, the notion of self-concept was thought to be about the individual, where identity is developed as something unique and differentiated from others, often referred to *individualism* (Brewer & Gardner, 2004). Cross-cultural research, however, identified another approach to the development of self-concept and identity—one that relied on a social identity that "reflects internalizations of the norms and characteristics of important reference groups and consists of cognitions about the self that are consistent with that group identification" (Brewer & Gardner, 2004, p. 68). This type of identity is called *collectivism*. Although few people develop a sense of self apart from others (Brewer & Gardner, 2004), and every person is unique, in many cultures, belief systems and ideals strongly emphasize one or the other of these approaches.

Individualism

Banks (1997) states, "individualism as an ideal is extreme in the United States core culture" (p. 9). In an individualistic society, the focus is on "I" rather than on the family, group, or community. People are taught to be strong and tough and take care of themselves, and seeking out help or advice from others is sometimes seen as weakness. Consider the icons in traditional American culture that represent this ideal: the strong, independent "Marlboro Man" and heroes like John Wayne. Independence and autonomy are valued, and people who are ill or disadvantaged are often told to "tough it out" or "pull themselves up by their bootstraps." The Protestant work ethic, with the belief that hard work is morally good and that sloth is sinful, has contributed to the individualistic ideal (Banks, 1997). "Doing" something is more important than talking, and practicality and efficiency are important values for people from these cultures. The individualism is often future-oriented, resulting in a sense of comfort with change (Lattanzi & Purnell, 2006).

When working with someone who holds individualistic beliefs, the occupational therapy practitioner must remember the following concepts:

- Illness is a major threat to this person's independence.
- It is important to consult the person on every decision so he or she will have some sense of control.
- This person will appreciate "working hard" toward recovery.
- It is important to respect the person's privacy.
- Seek permission before entering this person's space.
- Set individual goals to increase independence.

Because many of the values of occupational therapy were developed from a Western, individualistic ideal (Iwama, 2006), working with a client with these values should not cause much conflict with U.S. practitioners.

Collectivism

Many Eastern cultures, including the Chinese and Japanese, have more of a collectivist worldview. People from these cultures generally develop the identity of the larger society and self-concept and identity focus on the "we." One is expected to be committed first to the family and group and then to self (Banks, 1997). Interdependence is valued, and decisions are usually made by group consideration rather than individually. Health may be measured by one's ability to function within the group.

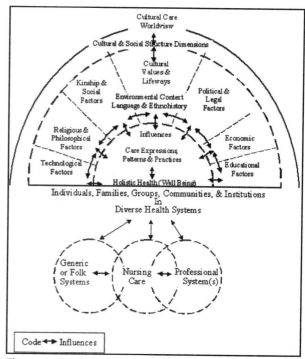

Figure 2-4. Leininger's Theory of Culture Care Worldview Image. (Reprinted from PBworks.)

Human interaction is valued over time, and cooperation is important. The past and tradition are important and authority is respected (Lattanzi & Purnell, 2006).

When working with people with a collectivist viewpoint, practitioners will want to consider the following:

- Practitioners may seek someone who knows the client to introduce them.
- Once rapport is established, the practitioner may be expected to provide all the answers as the authority figure.
- It will be important to work closely with family and group members regarding decisions about the client's interventions.
- Remember to emphasize the team approach to effective and safe care.

PERCEPTIONS OF POWER AND AUTHORITY

Another characteristic that is culturally determined is one's perception of power and authority. The way in which people view authority figures and the power inherent within those positions often influences relationships and occupational behaviors. The perception of personal power is the sense of one's ability to impact the environment, which allows one to feel good about oneself and to believe that he or she is important, and for others to recognize his or her worth (Glasser, 1984). Personal power affects our own sense of authority and our ability to control others. It is often internalized and unconscious.

The perception of power informs one's degree of the acceptance of inequality. For instance, if we accept the inequality of power, authority, and privilege as a given, then we will not see ourselves as having the need or power to change it. If we do not accept inequality as a given, and instead believe that everyone should be treated equally, we perceive a need for change in an unequal context. Geert Hostede's (1981, 2001) research with people from 40 different nations resulted in a description of *power distance*, which is "the extent to which the less powerful members of organizations and institutions (like the family) accept and expect that power is distributed unequally" (Clearly Cultural, n.d., Para. 1). Hostede identifies the difference in high power distance (HPD) and low power distance (LPD) cultures, stating that "the basic issue involved, which different societies handle differently, is human inequality" (2001, p. 79).

High Power Distance Cultures

HPD defines a culture in which inequality is accepted. Members of the culture believe that each person has a rightful place, and that superiors and subordinates treat each other differently and do not mix socially. Members of these cultures do not challenge power and authority (Hofstede, 1980, 2001). It is important to recognize these cultural characteristics in occupational therapy practice, as they will affect the relationship that practitioners have with diverse clients. When working with people from HPD cultures, one must consider the following:

- They are more conscious of the hierarchy in the health care system.
- They will want to know their place in that hierarchy and how the health care facility works.
- They may relate to people differently based on age, gender, and professional role.
- Authority is important to them, and they will tend to look to the professional for decisions and directions.
- It may be important for practitioners to share their credentials and accomplishments with the client so that authority may be established.
- It may be more difficult to provide a client-centered approach to interventions because of the expectation that the authority figure (the practitioner) will make the decisions.
- It may be more difficult to develop an empowered or participatory power relationship with the client.

Low Power Distance Cultures

In LPD cultures, the majority of the members feel that any inequality in the society should be minimized. Members believe in equal rights and that the existence of hierarchy is only for the convenience of accomplishing tasks in an organization. Many people from LPD cultures believe that education increases power and that people can move within this fluid system (Hostede, 1980). With the client from a LPD culture, consider the following:

- This person will expect to be treated on an equal basis and may want to be treated as a peer when not in a professional role.
- He or she may challenge authority and, in turn, expect to be challenged; this is seen as a sign of respect.
- It is important to keep this client apprised of the progress of therapy.
- This client is usually a good candidate for client-centered occupational therapy.

Hostede developed a power distance index (PDI), which determined the relative power distance of various nations (Clearly Cultural, n.d.). Of interest, Austria has a PDI of 11 (very low), whereas Malaysia's PDI is 104 (very high). Many Central American countries and the Philippines fall in the 90s, the PDI of Arab nations is 80, and the United States falls somewhere in the middle with a PDI of 40 (Clearly Cultural). Occupational therapy practitioners must be aware of and recognize this important cultural characteristic in their clients for effective cross-cultural interactions.

TEMPORAL ISSUES

Although the characteristics previously identified are culturally defined and important to recognize, one aspect that causes a tremendous amount of difficulty in business and health care is the difference in the concept of time between the employer and employee and therapist and client. All cultures have unique concepts of time, and much has been written about this cultural characteristic. Although several authors discuss the difference between future, present, and past temporal orientations (Bonder, Martin, & Miracle, 2002; Lattanzi & Purnell, 2006) and its impact on health care, this section of the chapter addresses the relationship of monochronic and polychronic time and how it may affect cross-cultural interactions.

Monochronic Time

There are cultures and people who perceive time as linear, and can do only one thing at a time. These monochronic people are schedule dominated, tending to live by the clock. They see the world in segmented compartments and even tend to sequence communications as well as tasks (O'Hara-Devereaux & Johansen, 1994). According to O'Hara-Devereaux and Johansen, these individuals would be disinclined to interrupt a telephone conversation to greet a third person. Efficiency and convenience are important factors for monochronic people (Table 2-2).

Table 2-2. COMMON TEMPORAL DIFFERENCES	
Monochronic Cultures	**Polychronic Cultures**
Do one thing at a time	Do many things at once
Concentrate on a task	Highly distractible; accepts interruptions
Time commitments (such as deadlines and schedules) are taken seriously	Time commitments to be achieved only if possible
Low context; needs information	High context: Has information
Committed to the task	Committed to people
Religious adherence to plans	Changes plans often and easily
Follows rules of privacy and consideration; doesn't want to disturb others	More concerned with relations (families, friends, colleagues) than with privacy
Emphasizes promptness	Base promptness on the relationship
Adapted from Hall, E. T., & Hall, M. R. (1990). *Understanding cultural differences: Germans, French, and Americans.* Boston, MA: Nicholas Brealey Publishing and from O'Hara-Devereaux, M., & Johansen, R. (1994). *Globalwork: Bridging distance, culture, and time.* San Francisco, CA: Jossey-Bass.	

Within a therapeutic relationship with a monochronic patient, consider the following:

- The client may not be interested in a holistic approach.
- The client will be interested in information about schedules, interventions, and time of discharge.
- The practitioner must follow the schedules as closely as possible; inform the client if you must be late to the appointment.
- If the client is highly stressed, give him or her permission to relax; schedule time for relaxation.

Polychronic Time

In contrast to the preceding characteristics, a polychronic person can accomplish multiple activities at the same time and will not cut a discussion short if "out of time," according to his or her schedule. "Polychronic time is open-ended; completing the task or communication is more important than adhering to a schedule" (O'Hara-Devereaux & Johansen, 1994, p. 37). These people can and often will carry on several conversations simultaneously. Polychronic people are relationship dominated; their strength is an emphasis on interactions with others and they enjoy non-linear, creative tasks.

Within a therapeutic setting, remember the following:

- Developing rapport and a comfortable relationship with the client is primary.
- Always relate to the person in some way before and during the intervention.
- Expect there to be family and friends in the treatment room.

- You may have to remind the client about the schedule and follow-up home activities.

As occupational therapy practitioners, providing effective cross-cultural care is vital when working with diverse clients. Being aware of the characteristics identified previously and addressing them with the client in an effort to minimize misunderstandings will move the practitioner toward cultural competence and the client to a place of trust, both of which will result in more effective and respectful care.

Research Evidence on Culture, Cultural Competence, and Culturally Effective Care

Over the last decade, there has been a significant increase in the occupational therapy literature on issues of culture, cultural competence, and culturally competent care (Black & Wells, 2007; Bonder & Martin, 2013; Gray & McPherson, 2005; Kirsh, Trentham, & Cole, 2006; Pooremamali, Persson, & Eklund, 2011; Stedman & Thomas, 2011). However, several of the articles written continue to be concept papers or descriptions of programs. Although this body of literature provides significant value in developing dialogue in this area, there is limited reported research on the importance of the knowledge of culture, on aspects of cultural competence, and on the effectiveness of culturally competent care in occupational therapy practice.

EVIDENCE-BASED RESEARCH CHART

Topic	Issue	Evidence
Culture	Cultural safety	Gerlach, 2012; Gray & McPherson, 2005; Jull & Giles, 2012; Whiteford, 2012
	Western viewpoints and occupational identity	Bourke-Taylor & Hudson, 2005; Rudman & Dennhardt, 2008
Culturally effective/ competent care	Responses from therapists	Stedman & Thomas, 2011
	Responses from clients	Kirsh, Trentham, & Cole, 2006
Cultural competence	Of occupational therapy practitioners	Munoz, 2007; Saurez-Balcazar et al., 2009; Wray & Mortenson, 2011
	Of occupational therapy students	McAllister, Whiteford, Hill, Thomas, & Fitzgerald, 2006; Murden et al., 2008; Rasmussen, Lloyd, & Wielandt, 2005; Taylor-Ritzler et al., 2008
	Educational pedagogy to develop cultural competence	Ekelman, Bello-Haas, Bazyk, & Bazyk, 2003; Price et al., 2005; Taylor-Ritzler et al., 2008; Velde, Wittman, & Mott, 2007
	Cultural competence assessment tools and models	Kumas-Tan et al., 2007; Balcazar, Suarez-Balcazar, & Taylor-Ritzler, 2009

Some notable exceptions include the developing research literature on cultural safety (Gerlach, 2012; Gray & McPherson, 2005; Jull & Giles, 2012; Stedman & Thomas, 2011). Cultural safety emphasizes relationships of trust in which the patient determines if the care is safe or not. For occupational therapy practitioners, this is about positive attitudinal change that enables occupational therapists to "offer a more appropriate and effective service to clients from diverse cultures" (Gray & McPherson, p. 34). Another area of research includes studies that examine the efficacy of education on the development of cultural competence (Musolino et al., 2009; Suarez-Balcazar et al., 2009; Velde, Wittman, & Mott, 2007), whereas a third research focus examines the occupational lives of immigrants and refugees (Black, 2011; Hon, Sun, Suto, & Forwell, 2011; Martins & Reid, 2007; Nayar, Hocking, & Giddings, 2012; Suto, 2009).

These developing areas of study are exciting, but there continues to be a need for further research in occupational therapy practice to provide the evidence that supports culturally competent or culturally effective care. According to the Center on an Aging Society, "cultural competence is not an isolated aspect of medical care, but an important component of overall excellence in health care delivery" (2004, p. 11). Providing "excellence in health care delivery" is an important goal of occupational therapy practice, but we must increase the amount of research that is completed and published in order to provide evidence to further support this aspect of our practice. Selected studies from occupational therapy literature are included in the evidence-based research chart.

References

American Occupational Therapy Association. (2008). Occupational therapy practice framework: Domain and process. *The American Journal of Occupational Therapy, 62*(6), 625-683.

American Occupational Therapy Association Multicultural Task Force. (1995). *Definition and terms.* Bethesda, MD: AOTA Press.

Balcazar, F. E., Suarez-Balcazar, & Taylor-Ritzler, T. (2009). Cultural competence: Development of a conceptual framework. *Disability & Rehabilitation, 31*(14), 1153-1160.

Banks, J. A. (1997). Multicultural education: Characteristics and goals. In J. A. Banks & C. A. M. Banks (Eds.). *Multicultural education: Issues and perspectives* (3rd ed., pp. 3-31). Boston: Allyn and Bacon.

Bhui, K., Abdi, A., Abdi, M., Pereira, S., Dualeh, M., Robertson, D...Ismail, H. (2003). Traumatic events, migration characteristics, and psychiatric symptoms among Somali refugees: Preliminary communication. *Social Psychiatry and Psychiatric Epidemiology, 38*, 35-43.

Black, M. (2011). From kites to kitchens: Collaborative community-based occupational therapy with refugee survivors of torture. In F. Kronenberg, N. Pollard, & D. Sakellariou *Occupational therapy without borders Vol. 2: Towards an ecology of occupation-based practice* (pp. 217-225). Edinburgh: Churchill Livingstone Elsevier.

Black, R. M. (2002). *The essence of cultural competence: Listening to the voices of occupational therapy students. Unpublished Dissertation.* Cambridge, MA: Lesley University.

Black, R. M. (2005). Intersections of care: An analysis of culturally competent care, client centered care, and the feminist ethic of care. *WORK: A Journal of Prevention, Assessment & Rehabilitation, 24*(4), 409-422.

Black, R. M., & Wells, S. A. (2007). *Culture & occupation: A model of empowerment in occupational therapy.* Bethesda, MD: AOTA Press.

Bonder, B., & Martin, L. (2013). *Culture in clinical care: Strategies for competence.* (2nd ed.). Thorofare, NJ: SLACK Incorporated.

Bonder, B., Martin, L., & Miracle, A. (2002). *Culture in clinical care.* Thorofare, NJ: SLACK Incorporated.

Bourke-Taylor, H., & Hudson, D. (2005). Cultural differences: The experience of establishing an occupational therapy service in a developing community. *Australian Journal of Occupational Therapy, 52*(3), 188-198. doi:10.1111/j.1440-1630.2005.00493.x

Brewer, M. B., & Gardner, W. (2004). Who is this 'We?' Levels of collective identity and self representations? In M. J. Hatch and M. Schultz (Eds.), *Organizational identity: A reader.* New York: Oxford University Press.

Buchan, T. (2002). The impact of language and culture when administering the Assessment of Motor and Process Skills: A case study. *British Journal of Occupational Therapy, 65*(8), 371-373.

Center on an Aging Society. (February, 2004). *Cultural competence in health care: Is it important for people with chronic conditions?* Issue Brief No. 5. Georgetown University. Retrieved May 30, 2008 from http://ihcrp.georgetown.edu/agingsociety/pubhtml/cultural/cultural.html

Christiansen, C., & Baum, C. (Eds.). (1997). *Occupational therapy: Enabling function and well-being* (2nd ed.). Thorofare, NJ: SLACK Incorporated.

Clearly Cultural (n.d.). Retrieved January 19, 2013, from http://www.clearlycultural.com/geert-hofstede-cultural-dimensions/power-distance-index/

Cross, T., Bazron, B., Dennis, K., & Isaacs, M. (1989). *Towards a culturally competent system of care,* (Vol. 1). Washington, D.C.: Georgetown Center.

Dobbie, A. E., Medrano, M., Tysinger, J., & Olney, C. (2003). The BELIEF instrument: a preclinical teaching tool to elicit patients' health beliefs. *Family Medicine, 35,* 316-319.

Dunn, W., Brown, C., & McGuigan, A. (1994). The ecology of human performance: A framework for considering the effect of context. *American Journal of Occupational Therapy, 48,* 595-607.

Ekelman, B., Bello-Haas, V. D., Bazyk, J., & Bazyk, S. (2003). Developing cultural competence in occupational therapy and physical therapy education: A field immersion approach. *Journal of Allied Health, 32*(2), 131-137.

Fisher, S. (2005). The Canadian Occupational Performance Measure: Does it address the cultural occupations of ethnic minorities? *British Journal of Occupational Therapy, 68*(5), 224-234.

Gerlach, A. J. (2012). A critical reflection on the concept of cultural safety. *Canadian Journal of Occupational Therapy, 79*(3), 151-158. doi:10.2182/cjot.2012.79.3.4

Glasser, W. (1984). *Take effective control of your life.* New York: Harper and Row.

Gray, M., & McPherson, K. (2005). Cultural safety and professional practice in occupational therapy: A New Zealand perspective. *Australian Occupational Therapy Journal 52,* 34-42. doi: 10.1111/j.1440-1630.2004.00433.x

Hall, E. T., & Hall, M. R. (1990) *Understanding cultural differences: Germans, French and Americans.* Boston: Intercultural Press.

Harry, B. (1992). Developing cultural self awareness: The first step in values clarification for early interventionists. *Topics in Early Childhood Special Education, 12,* 333-350.

Hofstede, G. (1980). *Culture's Consequences: International Differences in Work-Related Values.* Beverly Hills, CA: Sage Publications.

Hofstede, G. (2001). *Culture's Consequences: Comparing Values, Behaviors, Institutions and Organizations Across Nations, Second Edition.* Beverly Hills, CA: Sage Publications.

Hon, C., Sun, P., Suto, M., & Forwell, S. J. (2011). Moving from China to Canada: Occupational transitions of immigrant mothers of children with special needs. *Journal of Occupational Science, 18*(3), 223-236. doi:org/10.1080/14427591.2011.581627

Iwama, M. (2004). Meaning and inclusion: Revisiting culture in occupational therapy. (Guest editorial). *Australian Occupational Therapy Journal, 51*(1), 1-2.

Iwama, M. (2006). *The KAWA model: Culturally relevant occupational therapy.* Montreal: Churchill Livingston.

Josman, N., Abdallah, T. M., & Engel-Yeger, B. (2011). Using the LOTCA to measure cultural and sociodemographic effects on cognitive skills in two groups of children. *The American Journal of Occupational Therapy, 65*(3), e29-e37. doi:10.5014/ajot.2011.09037

Jull, J. E. G., & Giles, A. R. (2012). Health equity, Aboriginal peoples and occupational therapy. *Canadian Journal of Occupational Therapy, 79,* 70-76. doi:10.2182/cjot.2012.79.2.2

Kirsh, B., Trentham, B., & Cole, S. (2006). Diversity in occupational therapy: Experiences of consumer who identify themselves as minority group members. *Australian Occupational Therapy Journal, 53,* 302-313. doi:10.1111/j.1440-1630.2006.00576.x

Kumaş-Tan, Z., Beagan, B., Loppie, C., MacLeod, A., & Frank, B. (2007). Measures of cultural competence: Examining hidden assumptions. *Academic Medicine, 82*(6), 548-557. doi:10.1097/ACM.0b013e3180555a2d

Lattanzi, J. B., & Purnell, L. D. (2006). *Developing cultural competence in physical therapy practice.* Philadelphia: F.A. Davis. Company.

Law, M. (Ed.). (1998). *Client-centered occupational therapy.* Thorofare, NJ: SLACK Incorporated.

Law, M., Baptiste, S., & Mills, J. (1995). Client-centered practice: What does it mean and does it make a difference? *Canadian Journal of Occupational Therapy, 62,* 250-257.

Law, M., Cooper, B., Strong, S., Stewart, D., Rigby, P., & Letts, L. (1996). The person-environment-occupation model: A transactive approach to occupational performance. *Canadian Journal of Occupational Therapy, 63,* 9-23.

Leininger, M. (1988). Leininger's theory of nursing: Cultural care diversity and universality. *Nursing Science Quarterly, 1*(4), 152-160. doi:10.1177/089431848800100408

Leininger, M., & McFarland, M. R. (2002). *Transcultural nursing: Concepts, theories, research and practice* (3rd ed). New York, NY: McGraw-Hill.

Levin, S. J., Like, R. C., & Gottlieb, J. E. (2000). ETHNIC: A framework for culturally competent clinical practice. *Patient Care, 9* (special issue), 188.

Lewis, I. M. (1998). *Saints and Somalis: Popular Islam in a clan-based society.* Lawrenceville, NJ: Red Sea Press.

Lewis, J. (2002). *Cultural studies: The basics.* London: Sage Publications.

Lynch, E. W., & Hanson, M. J. (1998). *Developing cross-cultural competencies: A guide for working with children and their families* (2nd ed.). Paul H. Brooks Publishing Co.

Martins, V., & Reid, D. (2007). New-immigrant women in urban Canada: Insights into occupation and sociocultural context. *Occupational Therapy International, 14*(4), 203-220.

McAllister, L., Whiteford, G., Hill, B., Thomas, N., & Fitzgerald, M. (2006). Reflection in intercultural learning: Examining the international experience through a critical incident approach. *Reflective Practice: International and Multidisciplinary Perspectives, 7*(3), 367-381. doi:10.1080/14623940600837624

McIntosh, P. (1988) White privilege and male privilege: A personal account of coming to see correspondences through work in women's studies (Working Paper No. 189). Wellesley, MA: Wellesley College, Center for Research on Women.

Munoz, J. P. (2007). Culturally responsive caring in occupational therapy. *Occupational Therapy International, 14*(4), 256-280. doi:10.1002/oti.238

Murden, R., Norman, A., Ross, J., Sturdivant, E., Kedia, M., & Shah, S. (2008). Occupational therapy students' perceptions of their cultural awareness and competency. *Occupational Therapy International, 15*(3), 191-203. doi:10.1002/oti.253

Musolino, G. M., Babitz, M., Burkhalter, S. T., Thompson, C., Harris, R., Ward, R. S., & Chase-Cantarini, S. (2009). Mutual respect in healthcare: Assessing cultural competence for the University of Utah interdisciplinary health sciences. *Journal of Allied Health, 38*(2), 54E-62E(9).

Nayar, S., Hocking, C., & Giddings, L. (2012). Using occupation to navigate cultural spaces: Indian immigrant women settling in New Zealand. *Journal of Occupational Science, 19*(1), 62-75. doi:org/a0.1080/14427591.2011.60262

O'Hara-Devereaux, M., & Johansen, R. (1994). *Globalwork: Bridging distance, culture and time*. San Francisco: Jossey-Bass. Excerpt retrieved on June 7, 2008 from http://www.csub.edu/TLC/options/resources/handouts/fac_dev/culturalbarriers.html.

PBworks. http://nur2932009.pbworks.com/w/page/5730137/Leininger's%20Theory%20of%20Culture%20Care%20Diversity%20and%20Universality image by: herkules.oulu.fi/isbn9514264312/html/x215.html

Pollack, N. (1993). Client centered assessment. *American Journal of Occupational Therapy, 47*, 298-301.

Pooremamali, P., Persson, D., & Eklund, M. (2011). Occupational therapists' experience of working with immigrant clients in mental health care. *Scandinavian Journal of Occupational Therapy, 18*(2), 109-121. doi:10.3109/11038121003649789

Price, E. G., Beach, M. C., Gary, T. L., Robinson, K. A., Gozu, A., Palacio, A., . . . Cooper, L. A. (2005). A systematic review of the methodological rigor of studies evaluating cultural competence training of health professionals. *Academic Medicine, 80*(6), 578-586.

Rasmussen, T. M., Lloyd, C., & Wielandt, T. (2005). Cultural awareness among Queensland undergraduate occupational therapy students. *Australian Journal of Occupational Therapy, 52*(4), 302-310. doi:10.1111/j.1440-1630.2005.00508.x

Rogers, C. (1951). *Client-centered care*. Boston: Houghton-Mifflin.

Rudman, D. L., & Dennhardt, S. (2008). Shaping knowledge regarding occupation: Examining the cultural underpinnings of the evolving concept of occupational identity. *Australian Journal of Occupational Therapy, 55*(3), 153-162. doi:10.1111/j.1440-1630.2007.00715.x

Schkade, J. K., & Schultz, S. (2003). Occupational adaptation. In E. Crepeau, E. Cohn, & B. A. B. Schell (Eds.). *Willard and Spackman's occupational therapy* (10th ed., pp. 200-203). Philadelphia: Lippincott.

Standards of the National Society for the Promotion of Occupational Therapy. (1925). (Available from the AOTA Wilma L. West Library, Bethesda, MD).

Stedman, A., & Thomas, Y. (2011). Reflecting on our effectiveness: Occupational therapy interventions with Indigenous clients. *Australian Occupational Therapy Journal, 58*, 43-49. doi: 10.1111/j.1440-1630.2010.00916.x

Suarez-Balcazar, Y., Rodawoksi, J., Balcazar, F., Taylor-Ritzler, T., Portillo, N., Barwacz, D., & Willis, C. (2009). Perceived levels of cultural competence among occupational therapists. *The American Journal of Occupational Therapy, 63*(4), 498-595. doi: 10.5014/ajot.63.4.498

Sumsion, T. (1993). Reflections on . . . Client-centered practice: The true impact. *Canadian Journal of Occupational Therapy, 60*(1), 6-8.

Sumsion, T. (Ed.). (1999). *Client-centered practice in occupational therapy: A guide to implementation*. New York: Churchill Livingstone.

Suto, M. (2009). Compromised careers: The occupational transition of immigration and resettlement. *WORK, 32*, 417-429. doi:10.3233/-/WOR-2009-0853.

Srivastava, R. (2007). *The healthcare professional's guide to clinical cultural competence*. Toronto, ON: Elsevier Canada.

Taylor-Ritzler, T., Valcazar, F., Dimpfl, S., Suarez-Balcazar, Y., Willis, C., & Schiff, R. (2008). Cultural competence training with organizations serving people with disabilities from diverse cultural backgrounds. *Journal of Vocational Rehabilitation, 29*(2), 77-91.

United States Department of Health and Human Services Office of Minority Health (2000). *National Standards for Culturally and Linguistically Appropriate Services in Health Care*. Washington, D.C.: Author.

Velde, B. P., Wittman, P. P., & Mott, V. W. (2007). Hands-on learning in Tillery. *Journal of Transformative Education 5*(1), 79-92.

Whiteford, G., & Townsend, E. (2011). Participatory occupational justice framework (POJF 2010): Enabling occupational participation and inclusion. In F. Kronenberg, N. Pollard, & D. Sakellariou *Occupational therapies without borders: Volume 2* (pp. 65-84). Edinburgh: Churchill Livingstone Elsevier.

Whiteford, G. E. (2012). Other worlds and other lives: A study of occupational therapy student perceptions of cultural difference. *Occupational Therapy International, 2*(4), 291-313. doi: 10.1002/oti.6150020407

Wray, E. L., & Mortenson, P. A. (2011). Cultural competence in occupational therapists working in early intervention therapy programs. *Canadian Journal of Occupational Therapy, 78*(3), 180-186. doi: http://dx.doi.org/10.2182/cjot.2011.78.3.6

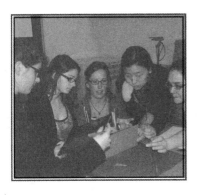

3

INTERPROFESSIONAL EDUCATION AND PRACTICE

A CURRENT NECESSITY FOR BEST PRACTICE

Nancy MacRae, MS, OTR/L, FAOTA

ACOTE STANDARDS EXPLORED IN THIS CHAPTER
Preamble, B.5.21

KEY VOCABULARY

- **Interprofessional:** A group of professionals for which communication is collaborative, goals are shared, and all are responsible for team efforts (MacRae & Dyer, 2005).

- **Interprofessional education:** "... When two or more professions learn with, from, and about each other to improve collaboration and the quality of care" (Center for the Advancement of Interprofessional Education, 2010).
- **Interprofessional practice:** Interprofessional implementation of interprofessional intervention.

Introduction

The movement toward interprofessional education (IPE) is gaining strength (Reeves, Tassone, Parker, Wagner, & Simmons, 2012). Although occupational therapists have been engaged in practice with other professions from the beginning of our profession (Jacobs, 2012), the extent to which this has occurred and how effective such collaboration efforts have been depended on a number of factors. Some of these factors included the context or type of practice, the experience and cooperative and collaborative nature of the practitioner, and administrative support.

With the increased complexity of practice and the need for accountability, safety, and improved outcomes for clients, there has been a renewed effort to educate aspiring occupational therapy practitioners about how to be an effective and efficient member of an interprofessional team (Reeves et al., 2012). This emphasis on being an effective interprofessional team member is reflected in the 2012 Accreditation Council for Occupational Therapy

25

Jacobs, K., MacRae, N., & Sladyk, K. (Eds.).
*Occupational Therapy Essentials for
Clinical Competence, Second Edition* (pp. 25-30).
© 2014 SLACK Incorporated.

(ACOTE) Standards: first in the ACOTE Preamble and then in Standard B.5.21. Although the occupational therapist has entered the IPE arena late in terms of requirements, it has been in practice for some time.

In its 2001 report, the Institute of Medicine (IOM) called for professionals to be educated about working collaboratively. Both the United States and Canada have seen this skill as a necessity, and have created collaboratives to facilitate this call for action and identify the skills necessary for interprofessional practice (IPP).

The United States version, created in 2010 by the Interprofessional Education Collaborative, devised core competency domains for collaborative practice. The domains consist of the following (Interprofessional Education Collaborative Expert Panel, 2011):

- Values/ethics for IPP
- Roles/responsibilities
- Interprofessional communication
- Teams and teamwork

This report also produced a learning continuum, which is composed of exposure (introduction) to immersion (development) to competence (entry to practice), and was founded on reflection, learning, and formative assessment (Core Competencies for Interprofessional Practice, 31.) Building teamwork competencies was stressed, as was transforming ways of knowing, from absolute to transitional, to independent, to contextual (Medical University of South Carolina, 2007).

The Canadian Interprofessional Health Collaborative (CIHC), created in 2011, also devised a national interprofessional competency framework consisting of the following six competency domains:

1. Interprofessional communication
2. Patient/client/family/community-centered care
3. Role clarification
4. Team functioning
5. Collaborative leadership
6. Interprofessional conflict resolution

Although the U.S. and Canadian versions present some differences, the primary purpose of preparing professionals to work in an interprofessional manner to facilitate clients' improvement and health is clearly paramount. The currently accepted definition of IPE is "when two or more professions learn with, from, and about each other to improve collaboration and the quality of care" (definition from Center for the Advancement of Interprofessional Communication, 2010). This definition differentiates the term *interprofessional*, where communication is collaborative, goals are shared, and all are responsible for team efforts, from that of *multiprofessional*, where team members share client information but decisions are made independently (MacRae & Dyer, 2005).

For IPE endeavors to be successful, they need to be fully supported by the administration and faculty also need to be involved and feel a sense of ownership. Effective IPE programs have occurred when they are not dictated by the administration but instead developed and embraced by faculty (Graybeal, Long, Scalise-Smith, & Zeibig, 2010). IPE courses can be elective, which initially helps maneuver around scheduling difficulties, but a combination of elective and mandatory classes elevates IPE to a higher status.

Application of Interprofessional Education and Interprofessional Practice

There are many ways that students/practitioners can learn about IPP. Efforts to inform can begin prior to, during, or after professional socialization. What is critical are creating opportunities to practice the components of IPP. To gain the skills necessary to be a fully participating and effective team member, a person must be capable of clear communication. This involves both clearly articulating and actively listening. An understanding of the parameters of your profession and those of others with whom you will likely work helps teams to gain a holistic perspective of a client and how his or her challenges can be effectively addressed by the appropriate profession. Being able to explain your professional viewpoint without using acronyms or words others will not understand becomes paramount, as does the need to question anything that is not understood. This type of clarity and questioning can break down professional barriers and strengthen the confidence of an interprofessional team. This same kind of plain language also applies to communication with clients and central team members, who need to comprehend their medical situations (Stableford, 2010).

With the health care system becoming more complex, one profession cannot adequately address most clients' concerns. Drinka and Clark (2000) contend that IP teams are needed when clients present "wicked problems." A client with a clear-cut problem, such as a hip fracture, for which there is an established clinical protocol or pathway, would not require the time and expertise of an IP team. However, an older adult with multiple diagnoses, some chronic and some acute, needs the focus of an IP team to help decipher the most appropriate care for the best client outcomes.

Safety issues and achieving positive client outcomes have been particularly important goals as accountability has become more pronounced, not only in health care, but throughout society. Having more than one profession assuming responsibility for the totality of care/intervention for a client increases the likelihood that areas will not be missed and errors will not occur. Instituting a rotating leadership of the team can ensure responsibility as a team member, dedication to problem solving, and creating the best plan of intervention for the client. It can also minimize hierarchy and power differentiation by encouraging everyone's voice to be heard.

Health Literacy

Health literacy, the client's ability to understand verbal and written materials, becomes critical especially with medication schedules, precautions, and following prescribed routines. Ensuring that clients understand—without patronization or being made to feel ashamed about their poor literacy—is important for teams to consider. Consistent use of plain language among team members facilitates the use of such language with clients (Smith & Gutman, 2011; Stableford, 2010).

Interprofessional Education Development

Students can be placed in IPE teams at the initiation of their health care career education. They can truly learn with, from, and about each other from discussing a case. As students gain more information about their profession they can begin to formulate more holistic and detailed intervention plans. Finally, they can be provided with opportunities to first watch experienced practitioners provide intervention and then to provide it themselves. This type of trajectory follows adult education principles that facilitate student learning and immediate application (Cross, 1984; Knowles, 1980). Reflection on all of these potential experiences allows students to analyze their skills and areas for change, and to begin to integrate and think about how best to apply what has been learned.

An array of applied IPE examples follow, ordered from fairly simple to the more complex programs:

- At the University of New England, students from one profession teach students from another profession; nursing students teaching occupational therapy students about taking blood pressures and pulses, and occupational therapy students teaching physician assistant students about adaptive equipment are examples of one profession teaching another.
- *Readers Theater*, where interprofessional players read a health-related script to an interprofessional audience of students, with considerable time allowed after the reading to discuss the issues that were highlighted during the production, exemplifies multiprofessions exploring one topic (MacRae & Pardue, 2007).
- University of New England's collaboration with Maine Medical Center, a tertiary care hospital, to expose students to other professional roles in the complex, acute hospital environment via specific learning activities and including videoconferencing technology (Sheldon, et al., 2012) exemplifies partnership of academia and a specific medical community.
- Collaborative program between two University of New England professions, social work and physical therapy, to develop person-centered health care communication skills using evidence-based principles and shared learning methods (Cavanaugh & Cohen-Konrad, 2012) exemplifies two professional students groups learning with and from each other.
- Community volunteer effort at the University of New England: Oxford Shelter for homeless men in Portland, Maine, where students from a number of professions staff educational sessions and simple interventions (foot care) for a group of homeless men exemplifies varied health care profession students providing service to a specific community program.
- The Community Aid, Relief, Education and Support Clinic (C.A.R.E.S) is an interprofessional learning experience for occupational therapy, physical therapy, physician assistant, pharmacy, and medicine students at the Medical University of South Carolina. Students learn from and with each other as they provide much needed health care to a specified community: an underinsured population from a tricounty area (personal communication, P. Coker-Bolt, December 28, 2012). This is an example of multiple health care professions involved in a community project.
- Strategies to Nurture Aging Persons (SNAP), an interprofessional fall prevention program between academia (University of New England) and the community, which uses a generic syllabus and student reflective narratives, is delivered by students from a number of professions to a group of independent-living older adults (Gray & MacRae, 2012), exemplifies interprofessional health care students participating in an academic/community partnership.
- The Interprofessional Geriatric Education Program, coordinated by the University of New England, is a program where physician assistant, occupational therapy, dental externs, and physical therapy students learn from each other and their older adult teachers by using interprofessional assessment and participation in rounds, the Objective Standardized Clinical Exams (OSCE) student evaluation method, and reflective journals (MacRae, 2012). This is an

example of interprofessional students collaborating with the community in providing services to older adults.

- Thomas Jefferson University's Health Mentors Program is a 2-year person-centered team-based curriculum, which involves medical nursing, occupational therapy, physical therapy, pharmacy, and couple and family therapy students. The students work and learn together as a team and complete four learning modules where they produce a comprehensive life history, wellness plan, assessment of patient safety, and a close look at self-management support and healthy behavior (personal communication, S. Kerns and A. Herge, December 7, 2012). This is an example of IPE centering around a specific client.

- Eastern Pennsylvania–Delaware Geriatric Education Center for Clinical Skills Scenario (CSS) provides medical and health profession students with an opportunity to work together as a team. Teams of students focus on an elderly woman patient and develop a plan of care for discharge, conduct a family meeting with standardized patients and caregivers, and then receive a faculty debriefing. The importance of communication, roles and responsibilities, and a team approach for discharge planning are the narrative themes (personal communication, S. Kerns and A. Herge, December 7, 2012). This is an example of interprofessional students focusing on one client and her family and the skills necessary to develop and implement a plan.

- Thomas Jefferson University holds an interprofessional symposium that focuses on communication in family-centered care. Students from occupational therapy, physical therapy, couple and family therapy, medicine, nursing, and pharmacy compose the teams. The students are challenged to deal with end-of-life decisions. Videos, team discussions, and an expert panel (including standardized patients), assist with student learning (personal communication, S. Kerns and A. Herge, December 7, 2012). This is an example of interprofessional students focusing on communication in family-centered care as they deal with a number of issues.

- Occupational Therapy and Dental Medicine Oral Hygiene Program, a program at the Medical University of South Carolina, addresses the special oral health problems of children with multiple disabilities and the training of future practitioners. A pilot interprofessional oral health program for special needs children was developed and included weekly visits to a targeted school, the development of individual oral health kits for the children, and the creation of an oral hygiene toothbrushing video

for use by teachers and teaching assistants (personal communication, P. Coker-Bolt, December 28, 2012). This is an example of two sets of professional students working on special oral health problems of children with multiple disabilities.

- A transcultural, interprofessional health mission experience in Ghana for building cultural proficiency among individual University of New England students and their teams through intense cultural immersion, including students from nursing, pharmacy, physician assistant, physical therapy, and occupational therapy departments, exemplifies a health mission to another country, with services provided by interprofessional students (Morton, 2012).

- Camp Hand to Hands is a program developed by the Medical University of South Carolina for children with hemiplegic cerebral palsy and unilateral motor weakness. Occupational and physical therapy students use constraint-induced movement therapy (CIMT) to remediate the effects of "learned nonuse." In a modified camp environment, children receive 6 hours of specific task training each day over five consecutive camp days. Students plan the theme-based camp activities, review the research evidence about pediatric CIMT, learn principles of such therapy, and practice handling and other treatment techniques. Each child works with one occupational therapy student and one physical therapy student for a 2:1 ratio (personal communication, P. Coker-Bolt, December 28, 2012). This is an example of two sets of professional students working to devise and provide an intensive CIMT camp to children with hemiplegic cerebral palsy and unilateral muscle weakness.

Summary

As these examples show, many educational and experiential efforts are underway to assist future occupational therapy practitioners in developing effective teamwork skills, all to enhance the quality of intervention and outcomes for clients. Embracing both IPE and IPP concepts adds value to team approaches and helps to ensure quality care and positive client outcomes while minimizing medical errors. The occupational therapy profession needs to continue to encourage entry level and experienced practitioners to understand the importance of collaboration and to continue to refine their team and problem solving skills in order to enhance the value and quality of the ever-increasing complexity of care they provide to their clients.

EVIDENCE-BASED RESEARCH CHART

Topic	Evidence
Interprofessional competencies	Canadian Interprofessional Health Collaborative, 2010; Interprofessional Education Collaborative Expert Panel, 2011
Interprofessional learning models	Cavanaugh & Cohen-Konrad, 2012; Gray & MacRae, 2012; MacRae, 2012; Morton, 2012; Sheldon et al., 2012
Health literacy	Smith & Gutman, 2011; Stableford, 2010

Student Self-Assessment

1. Choose one of the following topics and, in a small group, design an interprofessional education program.

   a. Fall prevention program

   b. Diabetes education program

   c. Sexuality program for developmentally disabled teenagers

   d. Energy conservation program for adults recovering from stroke

2. Discuss the challenges of working with other students and deciding which professions should do what in your chosen program.

3. How might the development of the program have gone more smoothly?

4. What did you learn about yourself and the team as a result of this exercise?

References

Canadian Interprofessional Health Collaborative (Feb. 2010). *A national interprofessional competency framework*. Vancouver, BC: Canadian Interprofessional Health Collaborative.

Cavanaugh, J. T., & Cohen-Konrad, S. (2012). Fostering development of effective person-centered healthcare communication skills: An interprofessional shared learning model. *WORK, 41*(3), 293-301.

Center for the Advancement of Interprofessional Education (2010). *Interprofessional Education: A definition*. Retrieved from: www.caipe.org.uk/us/defining-ipe.

Cross, K. P. (1984). *Adults as learners*. San Francisco: Jossey-Bass Publishers.

Drinka, J. K., & Clark, G. P. (2000). *Health care teamwork: Interdisciplinary practice and teaching*. Westport, CT: Auburn House.

Gray, B., & MacRae, N. (2012). Building a sustainable academic-community partnership: Focus on fall prevention. *WORK, 41*(3), 261-267.

Graybeal, C., Long, R., Scalise-Smith, D., & Zeibig, E. (Fall 2010). The art and science of interprofessional education. *Journal of Allied Health, 39*(3, part 2), 232-237.

Interprofessional Education Collaborative Expert Panel. (2011). *Core competencies for interprofessional collaborative practice: Report of an expert panel*. Washington, DC: Interprofessional Education Collaborative.

Institute of Medicine. (2001). *Crossing the quality chasm: A new health system for the 21st century*. Washington, DC: National Academies of Science

Jacobs, K. (2012). Promoting occupational therapy: Words, images, and actions. *American Journal of Occupational Therapy, 66*(6), 652-671.

Knowles, M. S. (1980). *The Modern Practice of Adult Education: From Pedagogy to Andragogy*. Chicago: Association Press, Follett Publishing Company.

MacRae, N. (2012), Turf, team, and town: A geriatric interprofessional education program. *WORK, 41*(3), 285-292.

MacRae, N., & Dyer, J. (2005). Collaborative teaching models for health professionals. *Occupational therapy in health care, 19*(3), 93-103.

MacRae, N, & Pardue, K. T. (2007). Use of readers theater to enhance interdisciplinary geriatric education. *Educational gerontology, 33*(6), 529-526.

Medical University of South Carolina (Feb 2007). *Creating collaborative care (C3): A quality enhancement plan (QEP)*. Charleston, SC: Author.

Morton, J. (2012). Transcultural healthcare immersion: A unique interprofessional experience poised to influence collaborative practice in cultural settings. *WORK, 41*(3), 303-312.

Reeves, S., Tassone, M., Parker, K., Wagner, S., & Simmons, B. (2012). Interprofessional education: An overview of key developments in the past three Decades. *WORK, 41*(3), 233-245.

Sheldon, M., Cavanaugh, J. T., Croninger, W., Osgood, W., Robnett, R., Seigle, J., & Simonson, L. (2012). Preparing rehabilitation healthcare providers in the 21st century: Implementation of interprofessional education through an academic-clinical site partnership. *WORK, 41*(3), 269-275.

Smith, D. L., & Gutman, S. A. (2011). Health literacy in occupational therapy practice and research, *The American Journal of Occupational Therapy, 65*(4),367-369.

Stableford, S., (2010). The last word: Health literacy and clear health communication. In R. H. Robnett & W. C. Chop (Eds.), *Gerontology for the health care professional,* 2nd edition, (pp. 373-383). Sudbury, MA: Jones and Bartlett Publishers.

II

BASIC TENETS OF OCCUPATIONAL THERAPY

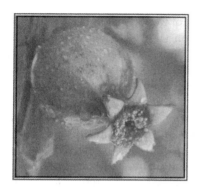

4

HISTORY AND PHILOSOPHY

Caryn Birstler Husman, MS, OTR/L

ACOTE STANDARDS EXPLORED IN THIS CHAPTER
B.2.1, B.3.4, B.3.6

KEY VOCABULARY

- **Humanism:** Philosophy that emphasizes the value of humans.
- **Moral treatment:** A humanistic treatment for people with mental illness.
- **Occupation:** Meaningful and purposeful human engagement.

- **Rehabilitation movement:** Provided opportunities for people with disability and injury to regain function and health.
- **Wellness:** Positive state of health.

Introduction

Contemporary occupational therapy is a complex and varied practice. Although the untrained eye at first may be unable to recognize the connections among occupational therapies in all forms, therapists understand that the golden thread is occupation. Occupation has been described as work, work-like activities and recreation (Meyer, 1977). Occupation has been related to concepts such as activity, task, and environment, as well as more complex notions, including social and temporal contexts (Crepeau, Cohn, & Schell, 2009). Put simply, occupation is meaningful and purposeful human engagement. Bing (1981) further called occupation the "union between the mind and the body." Faust

(1979) went so far as to say that life itself is the process of engagement in occupation.

Occupational therapy is the application of occupation as a therapeutic modality (Nelson, 1997). Therapists know that occupation has the power to facilitate change and growth in a person. Within occupational therapy, occupation is the process as well as the goal (Gray, 1998). Through the humanistic desire to attend to the well-being of others and a holistic view of each individual, occupational therapy practitioners seek to apply the core values of the profession: altruism, equality, freedom, justice, dignity, truth, and prudence (Peloquin, 2007). Let us explore how the profession has evolved, from its earliest roots to the diverse contemporary practice it has become through the influences of historical context, historical

33

Jacobs, K., MacRae, N., & Sladyk, K. (Eds.).
*Occupational Therapy Essentials for
Clinical Competence, Second Edition* (pp. 33-41).
© 2014 SLACK Incorporated.

movements, innovative health care providers, and the progression of the medical field.

Moral Treatment

The earliest use of occupation in therapy can be found in *moral treatment*, a term first used by the French physician Philippe Pinel in 1801 that described a revolutionary treatment for individuals with mental illness based upon humanism's belief that all humans have inherent value. Prior to that time, people who had mental illnesses were subjected to terrible living conditions and horrifying "treatments." The treatment reflected the idea that individuals with mental illnesses were influenced by negative supernatural forces. The philosophy of moral treatment encouraged the respect of patients and routines of typical daily activities, physical exercise, and work (Bing, 1981). Patients with mental illness were offered a variety of occupations, including exercise, work, religious services, and diversional leisure. Occupations were provided in the context of routine to provide the stability the patients needed to begin recovery (Peloquin, 1989).

William Tuke was another early adopter of moral treatment. In the late 18th century, he founded the York Retreat in England in response to the deplorable conditions at the York Hospital. He applied the concepts of the treatment philosophy by infusing a wide range of occupations into patients' daily lives. Samuel Tuke, grandson of William, recorded the successes of moral treatment in *The Retreat* in 1813. This work, along with Pinel's writings, sparked implementation of reforms in hospitals across England and America that included a strong emphasis on daily occupations (Bing, 1981).

Throughout the early 19th century, hospitals and asylums were founded that applied the philosophy of moral treatment. In these treatment centers, patients received humane treatment and engaged in a physician-prescribed routine of work and leisure (Peloquin, 1989). Moral treatment became an effective means to recovery from mental illness, and its effectiveness may be attributed to the comprehensive program of daily occupations (Bockoven, 1971). The implementation of moral treatment paved the way for the use of occupation as a healing modality and set a course for the emerging profession of occupational therapy.

Arts and Crafts Movement

The Arts and Crafts movement was an early 19th century cultural phenomenon in the United States that promoted the benefits of occupation. At this time, industrialization resulted in mass production of lower quality products and excessive materialism (Levine, 1981). In addition, industrialization altered the cultural landscape: people moved out of traditional family farming cultures and into cities in search of work (Peloquin, 1989), thereby eroding their connection with meaningful occupations. John Ruskin, the father of the Arts and Crafts movement, believed that machination and factory work resulted in deep unhappiness. He alleged that reliance on machines, poor working conditions, and displacement of human skill caused a deterioration of physical health as well as the common complaints of disease, anxiety, and fatigue. Society responded by applying a "do-it-yourself" mentality and making products by hand. Proponents of the Arts and Crafts movement advocated for a return to a meaningful lifestyle, which included farming, using natural materials, and producing and purchasing items that were simple in design. For many, the Arts and Crafts movement symbolized a return to human dignity and quality of life as well as a return to occupations of handicraft (Levine, 1981).

At the same time, the medical profession was building a scientific foundation for treatment of disease. Although this allowed for new treatment of disease, some physicians were unsatisfied with a reductionist view of health and were inspired by the Arts and Crafts movement to investigate the effects of human occupation. Three such physicians were Herbert J. Hall, Adolf Meyer, and William Rush Dunton, Jr. (Levine 1987).

Herbert Hall used work as an alternative to bed rest and created sheltered workshops where patients designed and created useful products to be sold in local shops. Hall promoted the workshops with the intent to employ people to earn a living through the production of handmade objects, provide spiritual support to professional craftsmen, and employ people with physical and mental disabilities (Levine, 1981).

Adolf Meyer was a leader in the medical profession of his day. Meyer collaborated with social worker Julia Lathrop to bring craftwork to chronically mentally ill patients (Levine, 1981). He believed that providing patients with opportunities to work, plan, create, and learn how to use materials was necessary to maintain a balance between work, play, rest, and sleep. He stated that a balance between these four factors helped promote achievement in healthy harmony with human nature. Meyer went on to present the first organized model of occupational therapy in 1921. His lecture, "The Philosophy of Occupational Therapy," was the first article in the *Archives of Occupational Therapy* (Meyer, 1977).

William Rush Dunton, Jr., was a psychiatrist who recommended exercise, work, and recreation for his patients with mental illness. He promoted goal-directed occupations and structured his patients' occupations through the use of arts and crafts. He sought training in craftsmanship so that he could provide education in the production of crafts that interested his patients (Peloquin, 1991a).

As the health benefits of craftwork became clear, the concepts of the Arts and Crafts movement were applied to meet the rehabilitation goals of patients with both physical and mental disabilities. Furthermore, arts and crafts became a central focus of early occupational therapy practice. Early therapists recognized that healthy individuals used arts and crafts occupations to maintain and improve their health (Levine, 1981). Therapists then used their humanitarian philosophy to recognize the healing that arts and crafts could bring to less fortunate individuals and those with chronic illnesses and disabilities.

National Society for the Promotion of Occupational Therapy: Early Pioneers of Occupational Therapy

In 1917, a small group gathered to officially found occupational therapy as a distinct profession in the first meeting of the National Society for the Promotion of Occupational Therapy (NSPOT). The founders were a diverse collection of doctors, nurses, and craftsmen whose ideas regarding occupational therapy and health shaped the foundation of the complex practice it has become. Although each founder brought their unique perspective, they shared a common philosophy: engagement in occupation facilitated health and healing. During the early 20th century, the founders worked to describe what distinguished occupational therapy from other types of treatment, determine the type of education that would be suitable for occupational therapists, and carve out the role of occupational therapy in the medical realm (Peloquin, 1991a). The following passages provide insight into how each of the pioneers of the profession helped to shape the profession in its early evolution.

George Edward Barton was an architect with background knowledge in nursing and medicine. Following foot surgery, he experienced paralysis and was treated at a solarium where he experienced the healing effect of occupation. He believed that occupation could provide mental as well as physical benefit. Barton asserted that individuals could become self-sufficient and productive through occupational therapy, and further that occupational therapy should provide clients with a means to work and support themselves despite illness and disability. Barton saw a strong connection between the medical field and occupation, and that occupation should be prescribed and taught by a medical professional trained in occupation (i.e., an occupational nurse). He called for a thorough evaluation before the prescription of occupational therapy and for the therapist to monitor occupation's effects. He further believed that occupation that enhanced the medical prescription through the by-product of the occupation, such as the exposure to helpful chemicals in an industrial plant, should be prescribed (Peloquin, 1991a).

William Rush Dunton, Jr., was a psychiatrist who was president of the NSPOT in 1917. He asserted that occupational therapy was the continuation of moral treatment. Dunton extolled the merits of occupation, stating it was vital to human life (Peloquin, 1991b). He believed that the power of occupation lies in its ability to give purpose to the patient, rather than to make marketable products (Peloquin, 1991a). Dunton strongly believed that occupational therapists should be medical professionals, and created a training program for nurses based on the work of Susan Tracy. Dunton described three distinct types of occupation: invalid occupation, occupational therapy, and vocational training. Invalid occupation was viewed as a diversion to provide respite from illness. Occupational therapy was intended to restore function that was lost through physical or mental illness. Vocational training was viewed as a means to provide restoration of function for people who had disabilities. Dunton also recommended occupational engagement for well people, being the first to recognize occupation's role in health maintenance (Peloquin, 1991b).

Eleanor Clarke Slagle became a strong leader in the burgeoning profession of occupational therapy. She was elected vice president at the first meeting of the NSPOT and, over time, held every office. She was instrumental in the training of nurses, attendants, and occupational therapists, created 3-week training courses for nurses, and founded the Henry B. Favill School of Occupations (Peloquin, 1991b). As she provided intervention, she noted that teaching occupation was a distinct form of therapy (Licht, 1967). Slagle believed that a physician should prescribe the outcome needed, but the occupational therapist should be independent in determining the specific occupation that would meet the patient's needs. Slagle's unique contribution to the profession included the application of habit training to chronically ill patients. She found that by using daily occupations in a routine fashion, significantly ill patients could begin to show progress (Peloquin, 1991b). As the profession progressed, Slagle held several offices of the American Occupational Therapy Association (AOTA) and assisted in the formation of the first list of qualified therapists (Punwar & Peloquin, 2000). She was such a strong leader in the field of occupational therapy and a pioneering woman that her contribution was honored by the presence of Eleanor Roosevelt and Adolf Meyer at her retirement party. Furthermore, the AOTA honored her by creating an annual Honorary Guest Lectureship in her name, henceforth known as the Eleanor Clarke Slagle Lectureship (Schwartz, 2009) and commonly known to contemporary occupational therapists as the "Slagle."

Susan C. Johnson was a high school teacher of the arts who believed in the healing power of occupation. She demonstrated that engagement in occupation could facilitate health, morality, and self-sufficiency for inmates in hospitals and almshouses. Johnson contributed greatly to occupational therapy through her focus on the education of practitioners and the process of teaching occupations to patients. She published several articles regarding training of occupational practitioners and the role of occupational therapy within the hospital setting. She asserted that occupational therapists needed education in psychology, teaching methods, and the medical field. She viewed the path of the occupational practitioner as between that of an educator and that of a nurse (Peloquin, 1991b).

Thomas B. Kidner was a Canadian architect who was committed to the health and rehabilitation of soldiers returning from war and people injured in industrial accidents. He believed in the power of occupation to cure patients and valued that power more than creating products to generate income. He argued that the value was in the process rather than the product. Kidner was a strong leader in the NSPOT as it evolved into the AOTA, and he served as president for six terms. During his tenure, standards for occupational therapy education were set. At that time, a training course of 6 hours daily for a minimum of 12 months was required. Occupational therapy education was further required to include psychology, anatomy, kinesiology, orthopedics, mental diseases, tuberculosis, and general medical concerns in addition to handicrafts (Peloquin, 1991b).

Susan Elizabeth Tracy is considered an incorporator of the profession even though she was not in attendance at the first meeting of the NSPOT. She did, however, have a strong influence on the early shaping of the profession. Tracy was a nurse who recognized the healing power of occupation in her patients and promoted a holistic definition of the word "cure" that included the patient's emotional state. Tracy was one of the first educators of occupational therapy and wrote several books that included the ideology, including the landmark *Studies of Invalid Occupations: A Manual for Nurses and Attendants* (1912). Tracy asserted that occupational therapy should be included in the realm of medication, and occupation should be prescribed by physicians. She felt that the occupational needs of very sick patients should be attended to by a nurse, but that less ill individuals could be served by non-medically trained individuals who had compassion and a desire to help others. Tracy focused on the purpose and quality of objects made by patients, rather than the ability to earn money through their production. Tracy was one of the first to educate medical professionals in teaching occupations to patients. She also promoted adaptation of occupations to meet the abilities of the client and wrote specifically about how to teach individuals who had physical disabilities or limitations in movement. Tracy even noted the healing effect of occupational therapy on the practitioner who provided the service (Peloquin, 1991a).

Herbert J. Hall is also considered an influential "near-founder" of occupational therapy (Peloquin, 1991b, p. 738). He studied the use of occupation for individuals with neurasthenia at Harvard University in 1906. He believed in the power of using one's hands in the production of products, the power of occupation to provide peace of mind, and the strong influence of work on happiness. He believed that industry should be created to hire and thus meet the occupational needs of people who had disabilities (Peloquin, 1991b). Hall believed in the medical prescription of occupation and called occupational therapy the "science of prescribed work" (as quoted in Peloquin, 1991b).

World War I

William Rush Dunton, Jr., indicated that World War I was a turning point for the early profession. He believed that the war assisted therapists in refining their ideals and purpose in the medical field (Peloquin, 1991b). Before World War I, occupational therapists worked primarily with individuals who had mental illnesses. However, the war created populations of people with physical disabilities and thus provided a new treatment milieu for occupational therapists (Punwar & Peloquin, 2000)

Occupational therapists were initially not recognized as part of the treatment team on the battlefield. Dr. Frankwood Williams, a military psychiatrist, was the first to recognize the utility of occupational therapy in the war zone (Punwar & Peloquin, 2000). Although he was unable to convince his superiors to enlist occupational therapists, he found openings for civilian workers, known as scrub-aides or reconstruction aides, and convinced a small group of occupational therapy workers to join the medical team under this guise (Peloquin, 1991b). Some reconstruction aides were artists or craftsmen who received short wartime courses to provide a modicum of medical background. Few reconstruction aides were occupational therapists. All were women, reflecting the cultural idea that women were best suited to inspire and provide refuge for the all-male military (Peloquin, 1991b).

The occupational reconstruction aides used what materials they could find first to assist men stricken with neuroses from the war horrors they had seen. Through woodwork and metalwork, the aides provided opportunities for diversion and healing. The aides were well recognized for their positive impact on the soldiers, and the power of occupation began to receive wide support (Low, 1992). As the war continued, occupational workers began to assist those who had been physically injured in rehabilitation and use of work adaptations. Furthermore, adaptive devices were created to promote independence in daily tasks such as self-care (Peloquin, 1991b).

The war years had a profound effect on the profession. Perhaps the greatest effect the war had on occupational therapy was the increase in the population served. Following the positive results that occupational therapy generated with injured soldiers in the field, occupational therapy gained new acceptance and was widely prescribed in the expanding numbers of Army and Navy hospitals (Woodside, 1971). During the war, occupational therapy began to distinguish itself from nursing, as there were too few nurses at the time and they were busy attending strictly to the medical needs of injured patients. The relationship between the occupational therapist and the patient became understood as part of the curative aspect of therapy. The war experience also helped to solidify the view that the value of occupation lies not just in the product, but also in the process of engagement. Similarly, the role of occupational therapists in returning patients to functional tasks became evident. In addition, the process of adapting and modifying tasks and equipment to facilitate function in an individual with a physical disability began to take hold (Peloquin, 1991b). At the same time, occupational therapy literature began to embrace scientific advances in knowledge, and the leaders in the field recognized that therapists required intensive education that went beyond handicrafts to include emphasis on the medical model (Levine, 1994; Peloquin, 1991b).

Post-War Boom

The 1920s increased the practice of occupational therapy, started the shift from volunteer work to medical service, and sparked the development of higher educational standards. The economic boom of the 1920s resulted in a significant increase in the number of hospitals and, in turn, a greater need for occupational therapists (Cole & Tufano, 2008). Legislation also increased the need for occupational therapy. The Smith-Bankhead Bill of 1920 established the basis for federal vocational rehabilitation by emphasizing that people with disabilities could be rehabilitated through vocational training (Woodside, 1971). The Federal Industrial Rehabilitation Act of 1923 required hospitals to employ occupational therapists to rehabilitate patients following industrial accidents and illnesses. By the end of the 1920s, occupational therapy was formally recognized as a medical ancillary service (Rerek, 1971). Occupational therapy was now required through physical prescription, and medical record keeping standards were developed (Quiroga, 1995).

With the increase in occupational therapy services provided in the hospital setting, the AOTA looked toward the American Medical Association to assist in the establishment of standards for training institutions and accreditation of educational facilities. Susan Cox Johnson and Elizabeth Upham Davis sought to standardize educational requirements, create a means of professional development for practitioners, and further research the medical conditions for which occupational therapy was prescribed. In 1923, the "Minimum Standards for Courses of Training in Occupational Therapy" was adopted by the AOTA by a unanimous vote. The standards addressed prerequisites for admission and the length and content of courses (Quiroga, 1995).

By the mid-1920s, the official scope of occupational therapy included the use of activity to facilitate recovery from illness or injury and to socialize individuals with chronic illnesses. Occupations were used to prepare for future employment and improve the mental well-being of the sick. The process of engagement in occupation was valued more than the product, and the selection of occupations was based on individual interests, abilities, and need. The ability to teach patients and provide a positive relationship and outlook were valued traits in the therapist (Levine, 1981).

The Great Depression and World War II

The expansion and gains of occupational therapy were halted with the stock market crash of 1929 and the depression that followed. Overall, health care services saw a decline (Rerek, 1971). Budget cuts as a result of the Depression and the National Economy Act of 1933 resulted in decreases in occupational therapists and closing of clinics and occupational therapy schools (Hopkins & Smith, 1993). When World War II began, the profession was not prepared to meet the needs of soldiers on the battlefield or at home. Because occupational therapists did not reach military status during World War I, funding was not available to provide service during the Second World War, which resulted in a shortage of occupational therapists. During World War II, there were 12 individuals in the United States Army working in occupational therapy, only 8 of whom were registered therapists (Hopkins & Smith, 1993). As veterans returned home, few facilities were available for rehabilitation or long-term care, and institutions for community reintegration did not exist. Veterans and their families soon sought the care they deserved and the government responded (Rerek, 1971). Among the changes was the elevation of occupational therapists to military status (Messick, 1947). Funding for occupational therapy was provided through the New Deal (Cole & Tufano, 2008), which provided social security income for people who had disabilities, and the GI Bill, which provided funding for vocational training. Furthermore, the Vocational Rehabilitation Act and amendments of 1943 allowed for the payment of medical services, including occupational therapy (Harvey-Krefting, 1985). Recognizing the health care system's inability to respond to the number of wounded veterans returning from the war, society pushed for the rehabilitation movement.

Rehabilitation Movement

The rehabilitation movement occurred from 1942 to 1960 (Punwar & Peloquin, 2000). The movement began by recognizing that, with proper care and rehabilitation, individuals with disabilities could be independent and contributing members of the community (Mosey, 1971). Rehabilitative occupational therapy consisted primarily of technical intervention, including training and fitting of prosthetics and orthotics, activities of daily living, and resistive exercises to improve strength. At this time, occupational therapy was practiced with little connection to theory or guiding models of practice. Education was increasingly medically based, and therapy became more specialized and deficit-focused (Punwar & Peloquin, 2000).

In the 1950s, the profession responded to the growing need for rehabilitation by expanding to include the first occupational therapy assistants. In 1958, the first training program for occupational therapy assistants began, consisting of 3 months of education focused on mental health intervention. Education expanded to include other areas of occupational therapy practice in the 1960s (Punwar & Peloquin, 2000). Leaders in the profession added to the knowledge base through the application of psychoanalytic and sensory motor frames of reference. Advances in neurology led to new treatment techniques, including Rood's sensorimotor reflex model and Bobath's neurodevelopmental therapy (Cole & Tufano, 2008).

The 1960s

The 1960s were an era of great social and political change in the United States. Advances in technology and changes in the family structure altered the professional and social landscape. The United States government made health care available to citizens who were economically disadvantaged or disabled through the enactment of Medicare and Medicaid legislation (Coombs, 2005). The Community Mental Health Act of 1963 expanded the breadth of mental health services to include a variety of levels and venues of service (Cole & Tufano, 2008).

During the 1960s, the field of medicine was becoming increasingly advanced and specialized. Survival rates for individuals with injuries and infants with severe medical conditions skyrocketed, resulting in significantly larger populations of people living with disabilities. Occupational therapy showed a significant movement toward specialization as well, with new focus on advanced practice areas such as hand therapy, spinal cord injury rehabilitation, and sensory integration. New practice areas such as schools, clinics, and community settings emerged. In addition, occupational therapy responded to the new social challenges of substance abuse and addiction, and the increasing prevalence of stress-related illness (Punwar & Peloquin, 2000).

The 1970s and 1980s

As the medical advances of 1970s and 1980s continued to quicken in pace, medical care itself became increasingly expensive. A trend of hospitalization for only the most significant treatment and deinstitutionalization for individuals with mental illnesses and intellectual disabilities resulted (Punwar & Peloquin, 2000). Occupational therapists quickly noted the value of working outside of the medical system, and the shift toward the community model began. The 1975 Education for All Handicapped Children Act ensured that children with disabilities received public education and marked the entrance of occupational therapy into the public school system as a related service (P.L. 94-142).

Philosophically, a holistic view of the client and an occupational focus was called forth by leaders in the field, such as Kielhofner and Burke (1980), who developed the Model of Human Occupation, one of the most widely used models of practice today. The profession also began to shift its scope of practice to include wellness and disease prevention (Punwar & Peloquin, 2000).

On an organizational level, the AOTA sought to unify the profession through the development and refinement of the Uniform Terminology of Occupational Therapy. This document delineated the roles of the occupational therapist and clarified knowledge of occupation by introducing the concepts of performance components and performance areas. The document also provided terminology for uniform documentation (Cole & Tufano, 2008).

During this era, occupational therapy education continued to become more in-depth and refined. Increasing numbers of graduate programs were founded to meet the needs of therapists entering an increasingly broad field of practice (Punwar & Peloquin, 2000). The economic challenges of providing medical care ushered in an age when justification for services and accountability for outcomes emerged (Cole & Tufano, 2008). The AOTA sought to address this need for knowledge and validation of therapeutic intervention through research (Punwar & Peloquin, 2000). Standardized assessment also emerged as a justification for service. State regulation of licensure was adopted to ensure the quality of therapists practicing across the United States (Cole & Tufano, 2008).

The 1990s

During the late 20th century, the expense of medicine and increasing numbers of chronically ill individuals continued to tax the economic system. The right of individuals to make their own decisions regarding their health care entered the social consciousness, while at the same time health management organizations (HMOs) were developed to determine what services would be rendered to people with medical insurance (Punwar & Peloquin, 2000).

The profession of occupational therapy responded with a movement into health care services rendered in the home and rehabilitation in nursing facilities. The Individuals with Disabilities Education Act of 1990 ensured public education and services, including occupational therapy, to assist students in accessing their education (United States Department of Education, n.d.; P.L. 108-446). The Americans with Disabilities Act (ADA) of 1990 also increased the need for occupational therapists (United States Equal Employment Opportunity Commission, n.d.). The ADA prohibited discrimination of people with disabilities and addressed architectural barriers and environmental modification to ensure that all buildings were accessible to people of all abilities (U.S. Equal Employment Opportunity Commission, n.d.). ADA compliance, environmental modification, advocacy for those with disabilities, and quality of life constituted new areas of practice for contemporary therapists (Punwar & Peloquin, 2000).

In the 1990s, theoretical foundations for practice and clinical reasoning were recognized as highly important facets of occupational therapy practice, most notably with the development of a framework for clinical reasoning through the work of Mattingly and Fleming (1994). In addition, occupational performance–focused models added to the practice knowledge, including, among others, the Canadian Model of Occupational Performance (1991) and Person-Environment-Occupational Performance Model (Punwar & Peloquin, 2000). Furthermore, a new field of scientific inquiry known as *occupational science* was developed to examine the nature of occupation itself (Clark et al., 1991) and to provide basic scientific knowledge regarding occupation from which the practice of occupational therapy could draw (Yerxa et al., 1990).

Education continued to move forward in the 1990s as well. Prior to this time, advanced degrees in occupational therapy were not available. Therefore, academics held degrees in related fields (Clark et al., 1991). In order to move the profession forward academically, an advanced clinical doctorate was developed to feature an emphasis on advanced occupational therapy practice (Pierce & Peyton, 1999). The first post-professional clinical doctorate was offered in 1994 at Nova Southeastern University. Creighton University went on to create the first entry-level Occupational Therapy Doctorate (OTD). Entry- and post-professional programs continue to proliferate at universities, such as Boston University and Washington University, among others (Griffiths & Padilla, 2006; Jacobs, personal communication, January 26, 2013).

Occupational Therapy in the 21st Century

With the entrance into the 21st century, society began to focus more on health and wellness promotion and the prevention of disease. The definition of health as the ability to live a full and productive life despite physical or societal limitations became recognized by such institutions as the World Health Organization (WHO) (Schwartz, 2009). In response to the changing view of health and the nearing 100-year anniversary of occupational therapy, practitioners developed the Centennial Vision for the profession. This vision connects with the founding philosophy regarding the value of occupation, and it further expands the definition of occupation by including the social context. The vision also promotes the prevention and dissolution of barriers to participation in occupation. The Centennial Vision calls for continued research and validation of the therapeutic interventions. Furthermore, the vision acknowledges that occupation is an integral vehicle for the health of all people throughout the global community (Schwartz, 2009).

In the 21st century, leaders in the profession again sought to increase the standard for professional education. In 2007, educational institutions were required to phase out remaining baccalaureate occupational therapy degrees and provide post-baccalaureate or entry-level master's degrees. This change addressed the need for advanced clinical reasoning, a high level of knowledge across a wide therapeutic milieu, a depth of knowledge in research, and autonomous practice in a variety of settings (Griffiths & Padilla, 2006).

During this second decade of the 21st century, occupational therapists are called to connect with our heritage. Practitioners, educators, and students alike strive to blend science with humanism (Schwartz, 2009) and expound the value of occupation as a health-promoting and disease-preventing force. We aim to elevate our professional status through education and research and by acting as leaders in social and medical arenas (Baum, 2006). We continue to strive for the best possible education by providing education with an occupation focus (Pierce, 2000) and expanding knowledge with PhD programs focused specifically on occupational therapy and occupational science. As our theoretical knowledge is ever expanding, we must also work to connect theories and research with practice (Pierce, 2000). We must all the while hold close our humanistic roots that remind us that all people deserve the ability to live healthy and productive lives within their scope of interest and ability. Occupational therapy facilitates this core value for the people we serve.

EVIDENCE-BASED RESEARCH CHART

Topic	Evidence
Occupation	Crepeau et al., 2009; Gray, 1998; Nelson, 1997; Peloquin, 2007; Pierce, 2000; Yerxa, 1990
Moral treatment	Bing, 1981; Bockoven, 1971; Peloquin, 1989
Reconstruction aide	Low, 1992; Peloquin, 1991b; Punwar & Peloquin, 2000

Student Self-Assessment

1. Describe moral treatment and its influence on the use of occupation in therapy. How do you think the philosophy continues to influence contemporary practitioners?

2. Explain the impact of the Arts and Crafts movement on the development of the profession.

3. Name the founders of the NSPOT and the key contributions of each.

4. Explain the effect of World War I on the profession.

5. Describe the rehabilitation movement. Did the movement limit or facilitate growth for occupational therapists?

6. Describe the shift from the medical model to the community model. In what ways did the shift change occupational therapy?

7. Explain the tenets of the Centennial Vision for occupational therapy. How will you apply these to your future practice?

References

Baum, M. C. (2006). Presidential Address, 2006: Centennial challenges, millennium opportunities. *American Journal of Occupational Therapy, 60*(6), 609-616.

Bing, R. K. (1981). Eleanor Clarke Slagle Lectureship—1981. Occupational therapy revisited; A paraphrastic journey. *American Journal of Occupational Therapy, 35*(8), 499-517.

Bockoven, J. S. (1971). Occupational therapy—a historical perspective. Legacy of moral treatment—1800s to 1910. *American Journal of Occupational Therapy, 25*(5), 223-225.

Clark, F. A., Parham, D., Carlson, M. E., Frank, G., Jackson, J., Pierce, D., Wolfe, R. J., & Zemke, R. (1991). Occupational science: Academic innovation in the service of occupational therapy's future. *American Journal of Occupational Therapy, 45*(4), 300-310.

Cole, M. B., & Tufano, R. (2008). *Applied theories in occupational therapy: A practical approach.* Thorofare, NJ: SLACK Incorporated.

Coombs, J. G. (2005). *The rise and fall of HMO's: An American health care revolution.* Madison, WI: The University of Wisconsin Press.

Crepeau, E. B., Cohn, E. S., Schell, B. A. B. (2009). *Willard and Spackman's occupational therapy* (11th ed.). Philadelphia, PA: J. B. Lippincott.

Faust, L. (1979). Therapy and function: An issue of professional direction. *American Journal of Occupational Therapy, 33*(11), 725-727.

Gray, J. M. (1998). Putting occupation into practice: Occupation as ends, occupation as means. *American Journal of Occupational Therapy, 52*(5), 354-364.

Griffiths, Y., & Padilla, R. (2006). National status of the entry-level doctorate in occupational therapy (OTD). *American Journal of Occupational Therapy, 60*(5), 540-550.

Harvey-Krefting, L. (1985). The concept of work in occupational therapy: A historical review. *American Journal of Occupational Therapy, 39*(5), 301-307.

Hopkins, H. L. & Smith, H. D. (1993). *Willard and Spackman's occupational therapy* (8th ed.). Philadelphia, PA: J. B. Lippincott.

Kielhofner, G., & Burke, J. (1980). A model of human occupation, Part 1: Conceptual framework and content. *American Journal of Occupational Therapy, 34*, 572-581.

Levine, R. (1981). The influence of the arts and crafts movement on the professional status of occupational therapy. *American Journal of Occupational Therapy, 41*(4), 248-254.

Licht, S. (1967). The founding and founders of the American Occupational Therapy Association. *American Journal of Occupational Therapy, 21*(5), 269-277.

Low, J. F. (1992). The reconstruction aides. *American Journal of Occupational Therapy, 46*(1), 38-43.

Mattingly, C., & Flemming, M. (1994). *Clinical reasoning: Forms of inquiry in a therapeutic practice.* Philadelphia, PA: F.A. Davis Company.

Messick, H. E. (1947). The new women's medical specialist corps. *American Journal of Occupational Therapy, 1*(5), 298-300.

Meyer, A. (1977). The philosophy of occupation therapy. *American Journal of Occupational Therapy, 31*(10), 639-642.

Mosey, A. C. (1971). Involvement in the rehabilitation movement 1942-1960. *American Journal of Occupational Therapy, 25*(5), 234-236.

Nelson, D. L. (1997). Why the profession of occupational therapy will flourish in the 21st century. *American Journal of Occupational Therapy, 51*(1), 11-24.

Peloquin, S. M. (1989). Moral treatment: Contexts reconsidered. *American Journal of Occupational Therapy, 43*(8), 537-544.

Peloquin, S. M. (1991a). Occupational therapy service: Individual and collective understandings of the founders, part 1. *American Journal of Occupational Therapy, 45*(4), 352-360.

Peloquin, S. M. (1991b). Occupational therapy service: Individual and collective understandings of the founders, part 2. *American Journal of Occupational Therapy, 45*(8), 733-744.

Peloquin, S. M. (2007). A reconsideration of occupational therapy's core values. *American Journal of Occupational Therapy, 61*(4), 474-478.

Pierce, D. (2000). Occupational by design: Dimensions, therapeutic power and creative process. *American Journal of Occupational Therapy, 55,* 249-259.

Pierce, D., & Peyton, C. (1999) A historical cross-disciplinary perspective on the professional doctorate in occupational therapy. *American Journal of Occupational Therapy, 53,* 64-71.

Punwar, A. J., & Peloquin, S. M. (2000). *Occupational Therapy Principles and Practice* (3rd ed.). Baltimore, MD: Lippincott Williams & Wilkins.

Quiroga, V. A. M. (1995). *Occupational therapy: The first 30 years, 1900 to 1930.* Bethesda, MD: AOTA Press.

Rerek, M. D. (1971). The depression years—1929-1941. *American Journal of Occupational Therapy, 25*(5), 231-233. Schwartz, K. B. (2009). Reclaiming our heritage: Connecting the founding vision to the centennial vision. *American Journal of Occupational Therapy, 63*(6), 681-690.

United States Department of Education. (n.d.). *Individuals with Disabilities Education Act.* Retrieved from http://idea.ed.gov

United States Equal Employment Opportunity Commission. (n.d.). *Americans with Disabilities Act (ADA): 1990-2002.* Retrieved from http://www.eeoc.gov/ada

Woodside, H. H. (1971). The development of occupational therapy 1910-1929. *American Journal of Occupational Therapy, 25*(5), 226-230.

Yerxa, E. J., Clark, F., Frank, G., Jackson, J., Parham, D., Pierce, D., Stein, C., and Zemke, R. (1990). An introduction to occupational science, a foundation for occupational therapy in the 21st century. *Occupational Therapy in Health Care, 6*(4), 1-18.

Suggested Readings

The Education of Handicapped Children Act of 1975. (P.L. 94-142).

Yerxa, E. J. (1980). Occupational therapy's role in creating a future climate of caring. *American Journal of Occupational Therapy, 34,* 533.

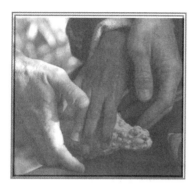

5

THE OCCUPATIONAL THERAPY PRACTICE FRAMEWORK
DOMAIN AND PROCESS, 2ND EDITION

Verna G. Eschenfelder, PhD, OTR/L and Patricia A. Wisniewski, MS, OTR/L, CPRP

ACOTE STANDARDS EXPLORED IN THIS CHAPTER
Preamble

KEY VOCABULARY

- **Activity demands:** Required features of an activity that influence a client's engagement in an occupation including objects and their properties, space and social demands, sequence and timing, performance skills, body functions, and body structures (AOTA, 2008).
- **Areas of occupation:** Common occupations people may engage in including activities of daily living, instrumental activities of daily living, rest and sleep, education, work, play, leisure, and social participation (AOTA, 2008).
- **Client factors:** The physiological and psychological aspects that reside within a client and body structures that may affect occupational performance (AOTA, 2008).

- **Context and environment:** Contextual and environmental influences both internal and external to a client that influence occupational performance including, physical and social environment and cultural, personal, temporal, and virtual context (AOTA, 2008).
- **Performance patterns:** A client's habits, routines, rituals, and roles that support engagement, participation, and health (AOTA, 2008).
- **Performance skills:** External actions or behaviors, observed when participating in meaningful occupations (AOTA, 2008).

Jacobs, K., MacRae, N., & Sladyk, K. (Eds.).
Occupational Therapy Essentials for
Clinical Competence, Second Edition (pp. 43-56).

Introduction

The Occupational Therapy Practice Framework: Domain and Process, 2nd Edition (OTPF-II), is an official document of the American Occupational Therapy Association (AOTA). It is designed to summarize constructs that define and guide occupational therapy practice and to articulate the profession's contribution to the promotion of health and participation of people, organizations, and populations through engagement in occupation (AOTA, 2008). This chapter provides a review of the OTPF-II as it relates to the scope and delivery of occupational therapy services. Included in this chapter is a description of the evolution of the OTPF-II and the ways in which it contributes to and supports the language of the profession. By the end of the chapter, the reader should understand basic factors that led to the development of the OTPF-II, recognize the interrelatedness of the domain and process of the framework, and begin to apply this knowledge to the delivery of occupational therapy practice. With guidance from an instructor, the student will apply the OTPF-II to a hypothetical case study involving a client named Marie to facilitate understanding of the complexity inherent in the framework.

Evolution of a Language for Occupational Therapy

From its beginnings, occupational therapists placed a great emphasis on the relationship between active engagement in occupation and an individual's health and well-being (Fidler & Fidler, 1978; Meyer, 1922). Toward the middle of the 20th century, the profession became increasingly aligned with the medical model of practice that involved a more reductionistic approach to treating clients. While this alignment with medicine led to a number of advancements for the profession, occupational therapists became increasingly focused on decreasing impairment and de-emphasized the importance of engagement in occupation. Over the last several decades, leaders in the profession have increased efforts to better articulate the importance of occupation as a unique contribution of the profession for the clients occupational therapists treat (Bing, 1981; Gilfoyle, 1984).

This most recent paradigm shift for the profession has resulted in a return to occupational therapy's holistic roots that place value on the relationship between occupation and health. In 1979, the Representative Assembly of the American Occupational Therapy Association (AOTA) developed the Uniform Terminology document, which sought to unify occupational therapy under one set of guidelines (Punwar, 1994). The 2nd Edition of Uniform Terminology (UT-II) was published in 1989 and set out to advance a commonly defined language for the profession.

UT-II outlined two domains of practice—the first being performance areas, which closely relate to today's areas of occupation, and the second consisting of performance components, which are currently reflected in the performance skills and client factors found in the OTPF-II. In 1994, the AOTA published Uniform Terminology, 3rd Edition (UT-III), which further expanded the document to incorporate contextual aspects of performance (AOTA, 1994). The UT-III provided definitions and a structure for the practice of occupational therapy.

In 1999, the Commission on Practice (COP) of the AOTA determined the need to develop a document that retained the initial intent of UT-III, but better reflected current occupational therapy practice. This effort resulted in the first edition of the Occupational Therapy Practice Framework: Domain and Process in 2002. The framework was designed to better articulate and differentiate that which occupational therapists do along with a process describing how practice was implemented. The authors of the framework placed great importance on occupation as the cornerstone for the profession (AOTA, 2002). Leaders in the profession recognized the need to improve on this original framework in an attempt to refine the document's domains, more clearly describe the process of evaluation and intervention, and place greater emphasis on the impact of occupational engagement on health (AOTA, 2008; Gutman, Mortera, Hinojosa, & Kramer, 2007).

The OTPF-II was published in 2008 and was designed by its authors to articulate occupational therapy's contribution to promoting the health and participation of individuals, organizations, and populations through engagement in occupation (AOTA, 2008). Pendleton and Schultz-Krohn (2013) explain the fit between the OTPF-II and the World Health Organization's (WHO), International Classification of Functioning, Disability and Health (ICF). The authors describe the change in focus from "consequences of disease" to "components of health and participation in activities of life" of the ICF as being well related to the OTPF-II focus on "supporting health and participation in life through engagement in occupation" (p. 4; AOTA, 2008, p. 660). The framework is organized into domain and process sections, with an emphasis on the interrelatedness of both components. Just as occupational therapy is an evolving profession, the OTPF-II must remain an evolving document. The AOTA COP reviews all official documents on a regular basis. In 2012, the COP initiated a process of reviewing and updating the OTPF-II. As a part of this process, the COP is working with occupational therapists as well as external groups in order to guide the revisions of the OTPF-II. The COP currently intends to maintain the integrity of the document while updating and refining it to better reflect the values of the profession.

While the OTPF-II is not designed as taxonomy, with strictly ordered categories and classification of terms

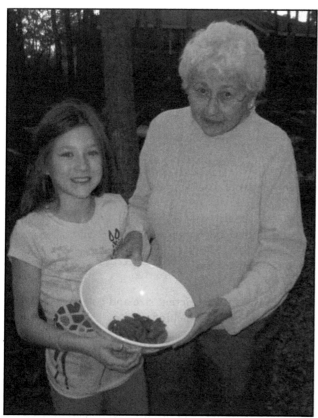

Figure 5-1. Collecting peppers from the vegetable garden.

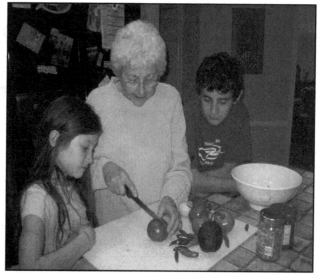

Figure 5-2. Preparing a meal for the family using vegetables from the garden.

for occupational therapy, it does "include language and concepts relevant to current and emerging occupational therapy practice" (AOTA, 2008, p. 625). The OTPF-II is intended for both internal and external audiences, and serves to increase understanding of the language used by occupational therapists. The internal language promotes professional identity, consistency, and understanding of the scope of occupational therapy practice. The external language serves to increase understanding of the occupational therapy process by clients and their families, the interprofessional community, third party payers, and administrative or regulatory agencies. The following sections describe the domain and the process of occupational therapy as described in the OTPF-II.

The Domain of Occupational Therapy

The domain of occupational therapy provides a common language used to describe the scope of occupational therapy practice. The domains are categorized into six groups that include areas of occupation, client factors, performance skills, performance patterns, contexts and environments, and activity demands. In the following paragraphs, the domains of the OTPF-II are applied to the activity of tending to a vegetable garden (Figure 5-1).

AREAS OF OCCUPATION

The OTPF-II identifies the following eight areas of occupation: activities of daily living (ADL), instrumental activities of daily living (IADL), rest and sleep, education, work, play, leisure, and social participation. Areas of occupation include categories of activities or occupations in which people, organizations, and populations engage on a regular basis (AOTA, 2008). The authors of the OTPF-II describe ADL as the activities a person completes in order to care for their self or body (AOTA, 2008, p. 631). ADL typically includes basic activities required of a person to support personal health and well-being, such as bathing and showering, bowel and bladder management, dressing, eating, feeding, functional mobility, personal device care, personal hygiene and grooming, sexual activity, and toilet hygiene.

IADL refers to activities that support occupational performance in context. These activities are typically more complex in nature and include care of others; care of pets and child rearing; shopping; preparing meals (Figure 5-2); management of home, finances, and health; along with participation in religious observances. Additional IADL, which are often necessary for successful occupational engagement, include communication management, community mobility, and maintenance of safety. Using the activity of planting a vegetable garden as an example, a gardener establishes and maintains a garden throughout the growing season, uses gardening tools safely to prevent injury, and eventually can use the produce to prepare healthy meals.

Rest and sleep is an area of occupation new to the OTPF-II. The activities included in this category include rest, sleep, sleep preparation, and sleep participation. These are "activities related to obtaining restorative sleep

Table 5-1.

AREA OF OCCUPATION ASSOCIATED WITH PLANTING A VEGETABLE GARDEN

- IADL—Home establishment and management
- Work—The job of a farmer or a volunteer at a community vegetable co-op
- Leisure—Hobby
- Social participation—Contributing to a community garden
- Informal education—Reading gardening magazines, attending gardening education seminars, sharing gardening expertise with others
- Social participation—Gardening with family members to share enjoyable experiences
- Play exploration—Including children by structuring play opportunities in the garden, such as digging for worms, picking green beans off the inside walls of the play teepee, and watering the plants

that supports healthy active engagement in other areas of occupation" (AOTA, 2008, p. 632). Restful sleep is imperative for productive engagement in occupations requiring attention, judgment, motor processing, and safety.

Education is the fourth area of occupation and includes formal and informal education as well as activities that promote exploration of personal interests. These activities are considered necessary for learning and participating in one's environment (AOTA, 2008, p. 632). A gardener, for example, might use past experiences and new knowledge obtained by reading publications or accessing informative media broadcasts in order to decide what to plant and how to obtain a bountiful harvest. Thereafter, the gardener might then choose to share their successful tips with others.

Work, as an area of occupation, can involve any activity in which one engages for the purpose of gaining some form of remuneration, including volunteer activities (AOTA, 2008, p. 632). The OTPF-II identifies employment interests and pursuits, employment seeking and acquisition, job performance, preparation and adjustment for retirement, and exploration and participation in volunteer opportunities as activities that compose the work area of occupation. Gardening can be work if the harvest is sold as a means to support one's family, or it can be considered volunteer work if the gardener offers his or her services to support the upkeep of a local community garden.

Play, which is often regarded as the work of childhood, is described as play exploration and play participation in the OTPF-II (AOTA, 2008). Play can be described as any spontaneous or organized activity, the primary goal of which is to provide enjoyment or diversion (Parham & Fazio, 1997). A garden can be a place for children to explore and play. Numerous games and unplanned activities can be engaging and entertaining such as digging for

treasure, collecting different size and colored rocks, and playing hide-and-seek behind plants.

Leisure is "a nonobligatory activity that is intrinsically motivated and engaged in during discretionary time, that is, time not committed to obligatory occupations such as work, self-care, or sleep" (Parham & Fazio, 1997, p. 250). The authors of the OTPF-II divide leisure activities into leisure exploration and leisure participation (AOTA, 2008). Feeling a breeze against your skin, smelling the scents of nature, and listening to nature's sounds are some of the appealing aspects that make gardening a relaxing leisure interest.

Mosey (1996) provides the definition of social participation used in the framework as "organized patterns of behavior that are characteristic and expected of an individual or a given position within a social system" (p. 340). The social participation area of occupation is organized by the contexts in which and with whom a person might engage and may include communities, families, peers, or friends (AOTA, 2008). Gardeners often share their hobby and leisure interests with others. Gardening can be a co-occupation among family members, friends, or a community who help with maintaining the garden or preparing the harvest for eating by washing, cooking, freezing, or canning the produce.

Table 5-1 summarizes the areas of occupation associated with planting a vegetable garden. While neither ADL or rest and sleep are included in the activity of gardening, these activities are necessary in order for a person to fully engage in the occupation. A person must not only be dressed, groomed, and otherwise prepared to go outside to the vegetable garden, but the person must also be rested and able to safely focus on related activities and tasks.

CLIENT FACTORS

Client factors are abilities, qualities, or characteristics that dwell within the person and influence performance

Table 5-2.
CLIENT FACTORS ASSOCIATED WITH PLANTING A VEGETABLE GARDEN

- Values—Nutritional content of the vegetables, pesticide-free gardening, and opportunity for fun aerobic exercise
- Beliefs—Homegrown vegetables taste better than store bought and saves money
- Spirituality—Leisure activity that offers an outlet for stressful life experiences, feeling connected with the earth, reminiscence about past gardening experiences, and a sense of enjoyment from nurturing and cultivating plants throughout the growing cycle
- Body structures
  - Structures related to movement—Muscles, hands, arms, legs
- Body functions
  - Mental functions
    - Concept formation—Divided and selective attention, working memory, perception of sensations (tactile, visual, vestibular-proprioceptive), sensory memory, spatial relationships, recognition, categorization, generalization, appropriate thought content execution of learned movements, level of consciousness
  - Sensory functions and pain
    - Visual detection/registration, visual modulation, and integrating sensations from the body and environment, vestibular functions, proprioceptive functions, touch functions, pressure if kneeling for prolonged periods
  - Neuromusculoskeletal and movement-related functions
    - Joint mobility, postural alignment and stability, muscle power, muscle tone, extremity and body strength, muscle endurance, righting reflexes, eye-hand coordination, bilateral integration, crossing the midline, fine and gross motor coordination, oculomotor control
  - Cardiovascular, hematological, immunological, and respiratory function
    - Stamina and stable blood pressure secondary to frequency of bending
    - Voice and speech functions—None
    - Digestive, metabolic, and endocrine system functions—None
    - Genitourinary and reproductive functions—None
  - Skin and related structure functions
    - Intact skin

in areas of occupation (AOTA, 2008). Client factors are categorized into values, beliefs, and spirituality; body functions; and body structures. Values are principles, standards, or qualities considered desirable by the individual client, whereas beliefs are ideas and concepts the client regards as true (AOTA, 2002, p. 623). Spirituality, which was part of the context in the first edition of the framework, is now considered a client factor in the OTPF-II and is described as "the fundamental orientation of a person's life, that which inspires and motivates that individual" (AOTA, 2002, p. 623; AOTA, 2008). Body functions include mental functions; sensory functions and pain; neuromusculoskeletal and movement-related functions; cardiovascular, hematological, immunological, and respiratory system functions; voice and speech functions; digestive, metabolic, and endocrine system functions; and genitourinary and reproductive functions. Body structures refer to the anatomical parts of the body such as the organs, limbs, and related components that support body function (AOTA, 2008). Table 5-2 identifies client factors associated with planting a vegetable garden.

PERFORMANCE SKILLS

Fisher (2006) defines performance skills as observable, concrete, goal-directed actions clients use to engage in daily life occupations (p. 375). Performance skills are described in the OTPF-II as being interrelated with each of the six domains. Performance skills include motor and praxis skills, sensory-perceptual skills, emotional regulation skills, cognitive skills, and communication and social skills (AOTA, 2008, p. 639). It is important to note that performance skills of the individual client are greatly influenced by and dependent on pre-existing or necessary client factors. Table 5-3 describes specific performance skills in relation to planting a vegetable garden.

PERFORMANCE PATTERNS

Performance patterns refer to the habits, routines, roles and rituals in which engagement in occupation is most often grounded. Performance patterns, such as fulfillment of roles and participation in rituals, are commonly associated with occupations deemed most meaningful to individual clients (Eschenfelder, 2005). Table 5-4 identifies examples of how performance patterns might relate to planting a vegetable garden as an organized activity.

Table 5-3.

PERFORMANCE SKILLS ASSOCIATED WITH PLANTING A VEGETABLE GARDEN

- Motor and praxis skills
  - Bending and kneeling to plant the flowers in the ground
  - Reaching to gather the plant and place in the hole
  - Grasping the plants and garden tools
  - Calibrating the amount of muscle power needed to carry the plants
  - Coordinating both hands working together
  - Coordinating the fingers to compact soil around the plant
  - Maintaining balance while walking in soft soil
  - Adjusting body posture in response to bending and reaching all the areas
- Sensory-perceptual skills
  - Visually detecting the plant in the hole so it is upright
  - Visually determining the depth of the hole
  - Judging the distance between each plant
  - Maintaining balance based on vestibular input from position changes
  - Modulating amount of strength needed according to the task: carry heavy items, digging a hole, and handling the seedlings
  - Discriminating between shapes and colors of each to discern between the plants
- Cognitive skills
  - Sequencing the steps of planting in the correct order
  - Selecting the correct plant
  - Determining the correct distance between each plant
  - Determining the depth of the hole
  - Create a diagram indicating where to plant according to the specific needs of each plant (light, drainage, soil type)
- Emotional regulation skills
  - Persisting in the task despite difficulties
  - Control display of frustration if the ground is compacted or if unexpected events occur
  - Communication and social skills—None, if performed as a solitary activity
- Communication skills—None if performed as a solitary activity

Table 5-4.

PERFORMANCE PATTERNS ASSOCIATED WITH PLANTING A VEGETABLE GARDEN

- Habits—Applying sunscreen and put gardening gloves on; buying seedlings or planting from seed
- Routines—Following the sequence of steps in preparing for and planting a vegetable garden
- Roles—Parent, grandparent, spouse, or friend wanting to grow their own vegetables
- Rituals—Canning vegetables using the recipes used by ancestors

CONTEXT AND ENVIRONMENT

People engage in occupations within a particular context and environment. There exists much interaction and interdependence between context and environment factors and other domains of the OTPF-II. The environment is composed of elements considered external to the client, such as the physical or nonhuman environment and the social environment. Contexts are thought of as being both within and surrounding the individual (AOTA, 2008, p. 642). Components of the context and environment domain include the physical environment, the social environment, cultural contexts, personal contexts, temporal contexts, and virtual contexts (AOTA, 2008). Table 5-5 describes contextual and environmental factors that play a role in supporting or hindering the ability to plant a vegetable garden in one's backyard.

Table 5-5.

CONTEXT AND ENVIRONMENT ASSOCIATED WITH PLANTING A VEGETABLE GARDEN

- Cultural—Cultivating one's own food, sharing or selling produce
- Personal—Age and gender of the person
- Temporal—Seasonal factors affecting gardening
- Virtual—Researching plants and creating the layout of the garden on the computer
- Physical—A sunny area in the backyard with soil space favorable for growing vegetables
- Social—Sharing vegetables with others or financial support or incentives to produce vegetable as a part of a co-op

Table 5-6.

ACTIVITY DEMANDS ASSOCIATED WITH PLANTING A VEGETABLE GARDEN

- Objects used and their properties
  - Variety of vegetable seedlings, garden tools, measuring tape, or string to measure distances between each plant and depth of each hole
- Space demands
  - Outdoor area large enough to accommodate the seedlings, soil free of grass and weeds, sufficient organic matter, good drainage, 6 to 8 hours of sun
- Social demands
  - None
- Sequencing and timing—Assuming the soil has been prepared, approximate size 15 × 15 foot garden
  - Gather plants—15 minutes
  - Design a plan designating where each vegetable or seed will be planted—30 minutes
  - Dig a hole—3 to 5 minutes per plant
  - Plant the vegetable seedling—5 minutes per plant
- Required actions and performance skills
  - Refer to Table 5-3
- Required body functions
  - Refer to Table 5-2
- Required body structures
  - Refer to Table 5-2

ACTIVITY DEMANDS

Activity demands include objects and their properties, space demands, social demands, sequence and timing, required actions and performance skills, required body functions, and required body structures. According to the authors of the OTPF-II, activity demands refer to "specific features of an activity that influence the type and amount of effort required to perform the activity" (AOTA, 2008, p. 634). In addition, "occupational therapists analyze activities to understand what is required of the client and determine the relationship of the activity's requirements to engagement in occupation" (AOTA, 2008, p. 634). Table 5-6 shows how the components of the activity demand domain are related to the activity of planting a vegetable garden.

The Process of Occupational Therapy

The process of occupational therapy outlines the way in which occupational therapists provide services to clients. It is a nonlinear, dynamic process that requires knowledge, experience, and clinical and professional reasoning on the part of the occupational therapist (AOTA, 2008, p. 647; Schell & Schell, 2007). Crucial to successful occupational therapy practice is the collaboration required between the client and the therapist. To the extent possible, given the client's current capacities and abilities and their personal meanings, the client's needs and desired outcomes must be central to the process of occupational therapy. The process of occupational therapy begins with evaluation, which is ongoing throughout

Case Study: Marie's Story

Marie is a 68-year-old woman who lives with her husband of 48 years in a small ranch-style home in Florida. Marie has two married daughters and two grandchildren, all living nearby. Marie was diagnosed with early onset dementia at the age of 55. Although Marie loved being an elementary school teacher, she retired at age 57 secondary to complications associated with diminished memory, mood fluctuations, and word finding difficulties.

Since her diagnosis, Marie has responded encouragingly to medical intervention. In addition, Marie established a daily routine to help keep her mind active and reduce anxiety by doing things she enjoyed, which is believed to have helped minimize the progression of the disease. Marie cares for her two grandchildren, ages 8 and 12, during the summer and after school during the school year. Marie has been gardening for more than 30 years and continues to tend to her vegetable garden on a daily basis, often including her granddaughters in a variety of gardening tasks. Marie is proud that she is able to donate vegetables to the local food bank and enjoys the annual ritual of making homemade spaghetti sauce to freeze, canning crushed tomatoes, and pickling a variety of fresh vegetables with her daughters. On the weekends, Marie goes to the senior center for Bingo and attends church faithfully on Sunday mornings with her husband.

Over the past year, Marie's family has been noticing a decline in her ability to independently and safely participate in her usual daily occupations. Marie is having problems with gross motor coordination, attending to conversation with others, balancing the family checkbook, and omitting ingredients from favorite recipes. Last month, while helping her mother balance her checkbook, Marie's daughter found that she has made significant monetary donations to numerous organizations despite the family's limited income. Although she has always been frugal with the family's finances, Marie is unclear about her reasons for contributing so much money to these organizations.

Recently, Marie experienced a fall which led to a right proximal humeral fracture that required an open reduction and internal fixation to stabilize the upper extremity. Marie is right-hand dominant and has experience functional limitations, which have significantly impaired her ability to complete basic ADL. Marie is experiencing severe bouts of depression, which the family believes to be related to the disruption in her daily routine and participation in meaningful activities, such as caring for her granddaughters and gardening. Marie is spending the majority of her time in bed, neglecting her ADL, and experiencing periods of emotional lability. In addition, her family expresses concerns regarding Marie's level of insight into her decline in occupational performance. Marie was referred to occupational therapy home-health services for evaluation and treatment shortly after her hospital discharge.

the process; intervention planning, implementation, and intervention review follow; and the process concludes or is renegotiated based on focus, selection, and measurement of outcomes that support health and participation in life through engagement in occupation (AOTA, 2008, p. 646).

EVALUATION

Clinical reasoning, which includes constant reflection and renegotiation of aggregate information obtained throughout the process of occupational therapy, is fundamental to successful occupational therapy practice (AOTA, 2008; Hinojosa, Kramer, & Crist, 2010). The OTPF-II describes an occupation-based evaluation as consisting of the occupational profile and analysis of occupational performance. Section IV of this text examines the evaluation process in detail. The following paragraphs describe the occupational profile and analysis of occupational performance and apply the related information to the case study of Marie (Case Study: Marie's Story).

Occupational Profile

The OTPF-II defines the occupational profile as "a summary of information that describes the client's occupational history and experiences, patterns of daily living, interests, values and needs" (AOTA, 2008, p. 649). The occupational therapist uses a client-centered approach by collaborating with the client to discover those occupations most important and meaningful to the individual client. For occupational therapists, the client-centered approach focuses on occupations and barriers to occupational engagement rather than dysfunction alone. "Once the profile data are collected and documented, the occupational therapist reviews the information; identifies the client's strengths, limitations, and needs; and develops a working hypothesis regarding possible reasons for identified problems and concerns" (AOTA, 2008, p. 650).

Table 5-7 lists questions that the occupational therapist addresses to obtain information for the occupational profile. In the case study of Marie, the occupational therapist will seek to understand her personal occupational history, which includes meaningful occupations and roles, and concerns that she has regarding her ability to engage in personally meaningful occupations such as care of others and tending to her vegetable garden. The

Table 5-7.

QUESTIONS ADDRESSED DURING THE OCCUPATIONAL PROFILE

- Who is the client and what services are being sought?
- What are the client's occupational concerns?
- Which areas of occupation are successful and which are problematic for the client?
- "Which contexts and environments facilitate or inhibit engagement in desired occupations?" (AOTA, 2008, p. 650)
- What is the client's occupational history and what are the associated meaning?
- "What are the client's priorities and desired outcomes?" (AOTA, 2008, p. 650)

Information compiled from American Occupational Therapy Association. (2008). Occupational therapy practice framework: Domain and process (2nd ed). *American Journal of Occupational Therapy, 62,* 625-683.

Table 5-8.

STEPS USED TO ANALYZE OCCUPATIONAL PERFORMANCE

- Identify areas of occupation and context that need to be addressed.
- Observe and evlauate the client's performance during occupationally relevant activities.
- Select appropriate assessments related to the OTPF-II domains.
- Interpret the assessment data to determine factors that support or inhibit occupational performance.
- Explore strengths and limitations related to occupational performance.
- Collaborate with the client to create goals that address the client's desired outcomes.
- Identify appropriate outcome measures of intervention.
- Identify potential intervention approaches based on best practice and existing evidence.

Information compiled from American Occupational Therapy Association. (2008). Occupational therapy practice framework: Domain and process (2nd ed). *American Journal of Occupational Therapy, 62,* 625-683.

therapist might include information from Marie as well as from close family members to obtain the most accurate and currently relevant information. From the information provided in the case study, the therapist might find that Marie sees herself as unable to participate in her role of grandmother and friend since she has not been able to garden and care for her grandchildren. Marie may also indicate that she is having trouble bathing and dressing, and that not completing these tasks makes it hard for her to feel "up to" going outside and being in her garden or participating in activities with family and friends.

Analysis of Occupational Performance

The analysis of occupational performance may include interviews, observations, review of records, occupation-based activity analysis, and direct assessment of specific client factors (AOTA, 2008; Table 5-8). For an occupational therapist working in collaboration with Marie, the therapist would use information collected during the occupational profile. If Marie indicates that bathing is a barrier that prohibits engagement in a desired occupation such as gardening, the occupational therapist would analyze the task of bathing further and develop interventions accordingly. The occupational therapist may also modify gardening activities in order to observe

and analyze Marie's performance during this adapted activity to compensate for limited range of motion. The occupational therapist will consider specific assessments that can be used to support the therapy plan and measure outcomes. In collaboration with Marie, the occupational therapist will create goals and intervention strategies to address Marie's specific wants and needs.

INTERVENTION

The use of occupation-based interventions is central to authentic occupational therapy practice. Included here is the idea that occupation can be used as an end or as a means for occupational therapy (Nelson, 1996; Trombly, 1995). The occupational therapist, in collaboration with the client, plans, implements, and continuously reviews the occupational therapy intervention. Occupational therapists must continuously utilize and update information gathered during the evaluation process and renegotiate the intervention plan and targeted outcomes during the process of occupational therapy. While intervention will be discussed in detail in Section V of this text, the following paragraphs will describe each phase of the intervention process in relation to the case study involving Marie.

Table 5-9.

PLANNING THE INTERVENTION

The occupational therapist must do the following:
- Develop objectives and measurable goals that include a time frame for goal achievement.
- Select occupational therapy intervention approaches that are theoretically sound and based on best available evidence.
- Identify service delivery mechanisms that best fit the client's needs and available resources.
- Develop and continuously update a plan for discharge based on the client's needs and progress.
- Select outcome measures that appropriately reflect the client's desired outcomes.
- Make recommendations for health and community based referral and follow-up as needed.

Adapted from American Occupational Therapy Association. (2008). Occupational therapy practice framework: Domain and process (2nd ed). *American Journal of Occupational Therapy, 62,* 648.

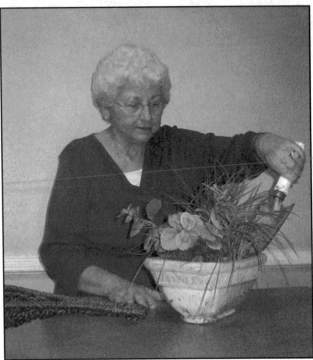

Figure 5-3. Planting a tabletop herb garden.

Intervention Plan

During intervention planning, the occupational therapist sets measurable goals and selects an intervention approach based on his or her knowledge base, theory, and evidence. Table 5-9 shows an outline of intervention planning as described in the OTPF-II. Approaches to occupation-based intervention include creating or promoting occupation; establishing or restoring a skill that has not yet developed or has been impaired; maintaining performance that has been gained or is at risk due to progression of a disease or illness; modifying context and environmental factors or activity demands; and preventing disability for clients who are at risk for occupational performance problems (AOTA, 2008, pp. 658-659). The intervention planning phase also must include initial discharge planning needs, selection of outcome measures,

and plans for making recommendations or referrals that will enhance the client's outcomes (AOTA, 2008).

When planning an intervention for Marie, goals of therapy might relate to restoration of her ability to bathe and dress safely and independently or with a defined level of assistance. Marie might also benefit from modifying the activity demands of gardening in order to allow her to participate in this self-determined and meaningful occupation (Figure 5-3). Due to Marie's decline in cognitive status, appointing an assistant to balance the family checkbook and the use of lists of favorite recipes could help Marie maintain performance abilities in her home. Discharge needs for Marie might include home safety assessment, family education, and additional assistance in the home to complete more complex or risk-laden tasks. Outcome measures should relate to Marie's expressed desires and be based on assessment and reassessment of Marie's performance skills and performance patterns as she progresses in therapy. In addition, Marie might benefit from a list of written recommendations related to her transition home and a referral to a gerontologist who specializes in dementia.

Intervention Implementation

Intervention implementation is the process of putting the intervention plan into action. The therapist employs therapeutic use of self and therapeutic use of occupations and activities during this phase of intervention (AOTA, 2008, p. 653). The occupational therapist is responsible for directing, monitoring, and supervising the implementation of intervention in a safe and efficacious manner (Schultz-Krohn & Pendleton, 2013). The type of intervention to be used and the way in which the therapist monitors the client's response according to ongoing assessment and reassessment must also be determined (AOTA, 2008, p. 648).

Occupations and activities used during Marie's occupational therapy intervention may include ADL such as bathing, grooming, and dressing; IADL related to her role as grandmother such as baking cookies (Figure 5-4); and a modified leisure activity such as tabletop gardening. Marie's therapy process will likely include all six types

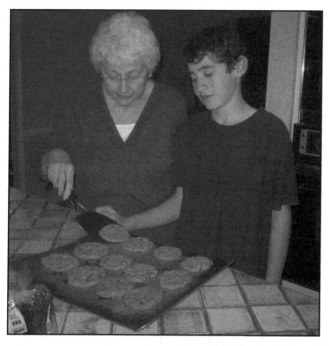

Figure 5-4. Baking cookies with grandson.

Table 5-10.

TYPES OF OCCUPATIONAL THERAPY INTERVENTION

Type and Purpose	Examples
Occupation-based intervention: "the client engages in client directed occupation that matches goals" (AOTA, 2008, p. 653).	• Completing bathing, dressing, and morning hygiene using adaptive devices • Attending a class on gardening • Bake cookies that she can share with others
Purposeful activity: "the client engages in specifically selected activities that allow the client to develop skills that enhance occupational engagement" (AOTA, 2008, p. 653).	• Practicing the use of rails, tub bench, and nonslip floor mats needed for safe bathing • Practicing how to make a grocery list that includes all ingredients needed to make cookies • Practicing the use of a memory book to help a client plan activities
Preparatory methods: "the occupational therapist selects directed methods and techniques that prepare the client for occupational performance. These methods are used in preparation for or concurrently with purposeful and occupation-based activities" (AOTA, 2008, p. 653).	• Providing splints needed to support and facilitate safe movement • Providing strengthening and range of motion exercises • Providing sensory stimulation to promote alertness and orientation
Consultation: "the occupational therapist shares their knowledge with the client to help solve problems, create solutions, or adapt occupations or environments to overcome barriers" (AOTA, 2008, p. 654).	• Providing alternative ways to garden safely at home to compensate for decreased range of motion • Suggesting ways to modify the activity of gardening to reduce the risk of falling secondary to poor balance
Education: "the occupational therapist shares information with the client and others involved that supports engagement in occupations" (AOTA, 2008, p. 654).	• Providing information on the healing process for bone fracture • Providing information on Alzheimer's and how to monitor for changes
Advocacy: "the occupational therapist promotes occupational justice and empowering the client to utilize resources that enable participating in life" (AOTA, 2008, p. 654).	• Collaborating with the client's family members to inquire about community resources for respite care • Researching community services available to older individuals that may support Marie's nurturing personality, such as participating in a day program where she can share her garden produce and skill of cooking

EVIDENCE-BASED RESEARCH CHART

OTPF-II Topic	Evidence	Area of Practice
ADL, Play, Education	Dunn, Cox, Foster, Mische-Lawson, & Tanquary, 2012	Pediatrics
ADL	Mennem, Warren, & Yuen, 2012	Low vision
ADL	Sackley et al., 2012	Rehabilitation
ADL, IADL	Walker, Gladman, Lincoln, Siemonsma, & Whiteley, 1999	Rehabilitation
IADL, Performance Skills Performance Patterns, Context and Environment, Activity Demands, & Client Factors	Gibson, D'Amico, Jaffe, & Arbesman, 2011	Mental health
IADL	Orellano, Colón, & Arbesman, 2012	Geriatrics
IADL, ADL, Leisure, Work, Social Participation	Stav, Hallenen, Lane, & Arbesman, 2012	Geriatrics, wellness
Rest/Sleep	Brown, Swedlove, Berry, & Turlapati, 2012	Pediatrics
Rest/Sleep	Gibbs & Klinger, 2011	Rehabilitation
Play	Wilkes, Cordier, Bundy, Docking, & Munro, 2011	Pediatrics
Education	Reid, Chiu, Sinclair, Wehrmann, & Naseer, 2006	Pediatrics
Work	Darragh, Harrison, & Kenny, 2008	Workplace, ergonomics
Work	Paquette, 2008	Work rehabilitation
Work, Performance Skills, Client Factors, Outcome Process of OTPF-II	Schene, Koeter, Kikkert, Swinkels, & McCrone, 2007	Mental health, workplace, treatment efficacy
Leisure	Ball, Corr, Knight, & Lowis, 2007	Geriatrics
Leisure, Play, Intervention Process	Kolehmainen et al., 2011	Pediatrics
Leisure	Wensley & Slade, 2012	Wellness
Social Participation	Donohue, Hanif, & Berns, 2011	Mental health
Social Participation	Griswold & Townsend, 2012	Pediatrics
Social Participation	Price, Stephenson, Krantz, & Ward, 2011	Rehabilitation, community-based

of interventions described in Table 5-10. Marie might require fabrication of a fracture brace or splint following her upper arm fracture. She also may be issued adaptive devices and asked to practice using these devices to help her perform ADL and other desired activities. As a part of her occupational therapy intervention, Marie might also engage in practicing how to gather ingredients for baking cookies and then actually baking cookies with supervision or assistance by the occupational therapist or family members.

Intervention Review

Intervention review is described in the OTPF-II as "the continuous process of reevaluating and reviewing the intervention plan, the effectiveness of its delivery and the progress toward outcomes" (AOTA, 2008, p. 656). During this ongoing phase, the therapist reevaluates the plan to determine its effectiveness in leading to achievement of desired outcomes. Modifications to the plan are made to improve effectiveness of intervention as

the client's occupational performance changes or as new information is uncovered. Intervention review is crucial in determining the need for continued changes to the types or approaches of intervention being used (see Table 5-10). In addition, intervention review also helps occupational therapists determine when intervention should be discontinued and what recommendations or referrals should be made.

OUTCOMES

Achievement of outcomes that support the client's health and participation in life through engagement in occupation is central to occupational therapy practice. Outcomes are the end-result of the occupational therapy process and serve to describe the value and impact of occupational therapy intervention for clients (AOTA, 2008). Outcome measures must be selected early and modified as needed during the evaluation and intervention phases of the occupational therapy process. The outcome measures that are selected should be congruent with the client's desired goals. The occupational therapist must consider the appropriateness of subjective or qualitatively assessed outcomes as well as more quantitatively measurable outcomes, based on the client's individual condition and situation. The movement toward establishing an evidentiary basis for occupational therapy has made significant gains. While occupational therapists continue to be challenged in this regard, the evidence-based research chart identifies published research related to the framework. While this chart contains only a fragment of available articles, it does serve as a starting point for those interested in investigating the aspects of the OTPF-II.

Electronic Resources

- AOTA Occupational Therapy Practice Framework: Domain and Process: http://ajot.aotapress.net/content/56/6/609.full.pdf
- AOTA Official Documents: http://www.aota.org/Practitioners/Official/Guidelines/41089.aspx?FT=.pdf
- AOTA Position Paper—Occupational Therapy's Perspective on the Use of Environments and Contexts to Support Health and Participation in Occupations: http://www.aota.org/Practitioners/Official/Position/Position.aspx?FT=.pdf
- AOTA Statement—The Philosophical Base of Occupational Therapy: http://www.aota.org/Practitioners/Official/Statements/41098.aspx?FT=.pdf
- World Health Organization—International Classification of Functioning, Disability and Health. http://www.who.int/classifications/icf/training/icfchecklist.pdf

Student Self-Assessment

1. Use the OTPF-II to identify the impact of Early Onset Dementia and the recent fall and fracture on Marie and her family.
2. Identify the Areas Of Occupations that have been affected by Marie's fall.
3. Identify the Performance Skills and Client Factors that are related Marie's ability to prepare a small, tabletop herb garden.
4. Describe how the recent fracture may impact Marie's Performance Patterns.
5. Describe how Context and Environment factors may hinder or support Marie's recovery.

6. Develop a list of questions that you would use to facilitate completion of an Occupational Profile for Marie.
7. Identify the types of occupational therapy intervention that you would consider using with Marie during early, mid, and later phases of treatment.
8. Consider how the domains of the OTPF-II relate to the evaluation, intervention, and outcome processes associated with occupational therapy services for Marie.

References

American Occupational Therapy Association. (1994). Uniform terminology for occupational therapy (3rd ed.). *American Journal of Occupational Therapy, 48,* 1047-1054.

American Occupational Therapy Association. (2002). Occupational therapy practice framework: Domain and process. *American Journal of Occupational Therapy, 56,* 609-639.

American Occupational Therapy Association. (2008). Occupational therapy practice framework: Domain and process (2nd ed). *American Journal of Occupational Therapy, 62,* 625-683.

Bing, R. K. (1981). Occupational therapy revisited: A paraphrastic journey: 1981 Eleanor Clarke Slagle Lecture. *American Journal of Occupational Therapy, 35,* 499-518.

Eschenfelder, V. G. (2005). Shaping the goal setting process in occupational therapy: The role of meaningful occupation. *Physical and Occupational Therapy in Geriatrics, 23,* 67-82.

Fidler, G. S., & Filder, J. W. (1978). Doing and becoming: Purposeful action and self-actualization. *American Journal of Occupational Therapy, 32,* 305-310.

Fisher, A. (2006). Overview of performance skills and client factors. In H. Pendelton & W. Schultz-Krohn (Eds.), *Pedretti's occupational therapy: Practice skills for physical dysfunction* (6th ed). St. Louis, MO: Mosby-Elsevier: 372-402.

Gilfoyle, E. M. (1984). Transformation of a profession: 1984 Eleanor Clarke Slagle Lecture. *American Journal of Occupational Therapy, 38,* 575-584.

Gutman, S. A., Mortera, M. H., Hinojosa, J., & Kramer, P. (2007). Revision of the Occupational Therapy Practice Framework. *American Journal of Occupational Therapy, 61,* 119-126.

Hinojosa, J., Kramer, P., & Crist, P. (2010). Evaluation: Where do we begin? In: J. Hinojosa, P. Kramer & P. Crist (Eds.), *Evaluation: Obtaining and interpreting data* (3rd ed). Bethesda, MD: AOTA Press: 1-20.

Kolehmainen, N., Francis, J. J., Ramsay, C. R., Owen, C., McKee, L., Ketelaar, M., & Rosenbaum, P. (2011). Participation in physical play and leisure: developing a theory- and evidence-based intervention for children with motor impairments. *BMC Neurology, 11,* 100.

Mattingly, C., & Fleming, M. H. (Eds.). (1994). *Clinical reasoning: Forms of inquiry in a therapeutic practice.* Philadelphia, PA: F.A. Davis Company.

Mennem, T. A., Warren, M., & Yuen, H. K. (2012). Brief report—preliminary validation of a vision-dependent activities of daily living instrument on adults with homonymous hemianopia. *American Journal of Occupational Therapy, 66,* 478-482.

Meyer, A. (1922). The philosophy of occupational therapy. *Archives of Occupational Therapy, 1*, 1-10.

Mosey, A. C. (1996). *Applied scientific inquiry in the health professions: An epistemological orientation* (2nd ed.). Bethesda, MD: AOTA Press.

Nelson, D. L. (1996). Therapeutic occupation: A definition. *American Journal of Occupational Therapy, 50*, 775-782.

Parham, L. D., & Fazio, L. S. (Eds.). (1997). *Play in occupational therapy for children.* St. Louis, MO: Mosby-Elsevier.

Pendleton, H. M., & Schultz-Krohn, W. (2013). The occupational therapy practice framework and the practice of occupational therapy for people with physical disabilities. In W. Schultz-Krohn & H. M. Pendleton (Eds.), *Pedretti's occupational therapy: Practice skills for physical dysfunction* (7th ed.). St. Louis, MO: Mosby-Elsevier: 1-17.

Punwar, A. J. (1994). *Occupational therapy: Principles and practice* (2nd ed.). Baltimore, MD: Williams & Wilkins.

Schell, B. A. B., & Schell, J. W. (Eds.). (2007). *Clinical and professional reasoning in occupational therapy.* Philadelphia, PA: Lippincott, Williams & Wilkins.

Schultz-Krohn, W., & Pendleton, H. M. (2013). Application of the Occupational Therapy Practice Framework to physical dysfunction. In W. Schultz-Krohn & H. M. Pendleton (Eds.), *Pedretti's occupational therapy: Practice skills for physical dysfunction* (7th ed.). St. Louis, MO: Elsevier-Mosby: 28-54.

Trombly, C. A. (1995). Occupation: Purposefulness and meaningfulness as therapeutic mechanisms: 1995 Eleanor Clarke Slagle Lecture. *American Journal of Occupational Therapy, 49*, 960-972.

Suggested Readings

Ball, V., Corr, S., Knight, J., & Lowis, M. J. (2007). An investigation into the leisure occupations of older adults. *British Journal of Occupational Therapy, 70*, 393-400.

Brown, C., Swedlove, F., Berry, R., & Turlapati, L. (2012). Occupational therapists' health literacy interventions for children with disordered sleep and/or pain. *New Zealand Journal of Occupational Therapy, 59*, 9-17.

Butts, D. S., & Nelson D. L. (2007). Agreement between Occupational Therapy Practice Framework classifications and occupational therapist's classifications. *American Journal of Occupational Therapy, 61*, 512-518.

Darragh, A. R., Harrison, H., & Kenny, S. (2008). Effect of an ergonomics intervention on workstations of microscope workers. *American Journal of Occupational Therapy, 62*, 61-69.

Donohue, M. V., Hanif, H., & Berns, L. W. (2011). An exploratory study of social participation in occupational therapy groups. *Mental Health Special Interest Section Quarterly, 34*, 1-3.

Dunn, W., Cox, J., Foster, L., Mische-Lawson, L., & Tanquary, J. (2012). Impact of a contextual intervention on child participation and parent competence among children with autism spectrum disorders: A pretest–posttest repeated-measures design. *American Journal of Occupational Therapy, 66*, 520-528.

Gibbs, L. B., & Klinger, L. (2011). Rest is a meaningful occupation for women with hip and knee osteoarthritis. *Occupational Therapy Journal of Research, 31*, 143-150.

Gibson, R. W., D'Amico, M., Jaffe, L., & Arbesman, M. (2011). Occupational therapy interventions for recovery in the areas of community integration and normative life roles for adults with serious mental illness: A systematic review. *American Journal of Occupational Therapy, 65*, 247-56.

Griswold, L. A., & Townsend, S. (2012). Assessing the sensitivity of the evaluation of social interaction: Comparing social skills in children with and without disabilities. *American Journal of Occupational Therapy, 66*, 709-717.

Kolehmainen, N., Francis, J. J., Ramsay, C. R., Owen, C., McKee, L., Ketelaar, M., & Rosenbaum, P. (2011). Participation in physical play and leisure: developing a theory- and evidence-based intervention for children with motor impairments. *BMC Neurology, 11*, 100.

Mattingly, C., & Fleming, M. H. (Eds.). (1994). *Clinical reasoning: Forms of inquiry in a therapeutic practice.* Philadelphia, PA: F.A. Davis Company.

Mennem, T. A., Warren, M., & Yuen, H. K. (2012). Brief report—preliminary validation of a vision-dependent activities of daily living instrument on adults with homonymous hemianopia. *American Journal of Occupational Therapy, 66*, 478-482.

Orellano, E., Colón, W. I., & Arbesman, M. (2012). Effect of occupation- and activity-based interventions on instrumental activities of daily living performance among community-dwelling older adults: A systematic review. *American Journal of Occupational Therapy, 66*, 292-300.

Paquette, S. (2008). Return to work with chronic lower back pain: Using an evidence-based approach along with the occupational therapy framework. *WORK, 31*, 63-71.

Price, P., Stephenson, S., Krantz, L., & Ward, K. (2011). Beyond my front door: The occupational and social participation of adults with spinal cord injury. *Occupational Therapy Journal of Research, 31*, 81-88.

Reid, D., Chiu, T., Sinclair, G., Wehrmann, S., & Naseer, Z. (2006). Outcomes of an occupational therapy school-based consultation service for students with fine motor difficulties. *The Canadian Journal of Occupational Therapy, 73*, 215-224.

Sackley, C. M., Burton, C. R., Herron-Marx, S., et al. (2012). A cluster randomised controlled trial of an occupational therapy intervention for residents with stroke living in UK care homes (OTCH): Study protocol. *BioMedCentral Neurology, 12*, 52.

Schene, A. H., Koeter, M. W., Kikkert, M. J., Swinkels, J. A., & McCrone, P. (2007). Adjuvant occupational therapy for work-related major depression works: Randomized trial including economic evaluation. *Psychological Medicine, 37*, 351-362.

Stav, W. B., Hallenen, T., Lane, J., & Arbesman, M. (2012). Systematic review of occupational engagement and health outcomes among community-dwelling older adults. *American Journal of Occupational Therapy, 66*, 301-310.

Walker, M. F., Gladman, J. R. F., Lincoln, N. B., Siemonsma, P., & Whiteley, T. (1999). Occupational therapy for stroke patients not admitted to hospital: A randomised controlled trial. *The Lancet, 354*, 278-280.

Wensley, R., & Slade, A. (2012). Walking as a meaningful leisure occupation: The implications for occupational therapy. *British Journal of Occupational Therapy, 75*, 85-92.

Wilkes, S., Cordier, R., Bundy, A., Docking, K., & Munro, N. (2011). A play-based intervention for children with ADHD: A pilot study. *Australian Occupational Therapy Journal, 58*, 231-240.

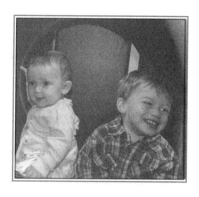

6

MEANING AND DYNAMIC OF OCCUPATION AND ACTIVITY

Julie Ann Nastasi, OTD, OTR/L, SCLV, FAOTA

ACOTE STANDARDS EXPLORED IN THIS CHAPTER
B.2.2, B.2.4, B.2.7

KEY VOCABULARY

- **Activity:** A specific task that is completed for an end result.
- **Co-occupations:** Activities that involve the social interaction of two or more persons.
- **Occupational performance:** The ability to complete an occupation or activity successfully.
- **Occupations:** Everyday activities that are purposeful and meaningful to persons, organizations, or populations.

- **Organizations:** Not limited to, but includes agencies, businesses, corporations, industries, for-profits, non-profits, or practices that receive occupational therapy services or consultations.
- **Persons:** Recipients of occupational therapy services such as clients, spouses, partners, families, siblings, caregivers, employers, teachers, and other relevant individuals.
- **Populations:** Groups within communities that have a commonality such as, but not limited to brain injury, diabetes, refugees, or prisoners of war that receive occupational therapy services.

Introduction

This chapter explores the meaning and dynamics of occupation and activity. An overview of the history of occupation is provided, as well as an in-depth analysis of occupation, which is the core of the profession of occupational therapy. By the end of the chapter, you will be able to understand how occupations encompass everyday activities in which persons, organizations, and populations participate. You will be able to distinguish the areas of occupation, performance skills,

Jacobs, K., MacRae, N., & Sladyk, K. (Eds.).
*Occupational Therapy Essentials for
Clinical Competence, Second Edition* (pp. 57-70).
© 2014 SLACK Incorporated.

performance patterns, activity demands, contexts and environments, and client factors as they relate to occupational performance.

Investigation of Occupation

The profession of occupational therapy is thought to have emerged from the moral treatment movement that occurred during the late 18th and early 19th centuries. During the movement, a humane approach was adopted for individuals with mental illness (Wilcock, 2001). This included addressing the physical, temporal, and societal aspects of the environment to facilitate the individual's participation in occupations (Kielhofner, 2009). Over time, occupational therapy has expanded and now addresses persons, populations, and organizations in a variety of contexts and environments (AOTA, 2008).

Occupational therapy was officially named as a profession in 1917 when George Barton, William Dunton, Jr., Eleanor Clark Slagle, Susan Cox Johnson, Thomas Kidner, and Isabel Newton met in Clifton Springs, New York, and produced a certificate of incorporation for the National Society for the Promotion of Occupational Therapy (NSPOT). NSPOT remained the name of the association until 1921, when the membership voted and changed the name to the American Occupational Therapy Association [AOTA] (O'Brien & Hussey, 2012). AOTA continues to be our profession's national association. AOTA plays a vital role in ensuring the growth and the future of our profession. The concept of occupation, and using occupation for health and wellness, date back before the naming of the profession of occupational therapy. Human occupations have existed since the beginning of time. For example, stories of occupation for health have been found in the Bible. Wilcock's (2001) *Occupation for Health, Volume 1* identified "the fall of humankind" in Genesis where "people were condemned to work for their survival and health" after eating the forbidden fruit (p. 30). Other Bible passages identified in the book include Deuteronomy's "accounts of people cultivating and harvesting grain, olives and grapes" (Wilcock, 2001, p. 33). Attention was given to how different occupations contributed to society. Reitz (2010) shared stories of the early philosophers, Pythagorus and Thales, who used music as a therapeutic modality. Reitz (2010) also identified how the Chinese in 2600 B.C. used activities for prevention and treatment. Occupations and activities play a vital role in the health and participation of persons, organizations, and populations (AOTA, 2008), both before the naming of the profession and since the official incorporation of the profession.

Occupation Versus Activity

"The profession of occupational therapy uses the term *occupation* to capture the breadth and meaning of everyday activity" (AOTA, 2008, p. 628). Occupations are complex and have multiple dimensions, whereas activities typically refer to a specific task. Occupations may require persons, organizations, or populations to complete many activities within an occupation. The definitions of occupation vary, but generally they encompass the concepts of an activity or activities that are purposeful and meaningful with some type of goal as the end result. The *Occupational Therapy Practice Framework: Domain and Process, 2nd Edition* (AOTA, 2008) states that "the term occupation encompasses activity" (p. 629). In practice, occupational therapy practitioners often use the terms *occupation* and *activity* interchangeably.

Meaning and Dynamics of Occupation and Activity

Occupations and activities can range from very simple to very complex in nature. It is the occupational therapist's role to promote "the health and participation of people, organizations, and populations through engagement in occupation" (AOTA, 2008, p. 625). This is done through the client-therapist collaborative process of evaluation, intervention, and outcomes. During evaluation, the occupational therapist creates an occupational profile from which the therapist gains an understanding of the client's occupational history and experiences. The client identifies the problems and concerns that are affecting his or her ability to complete occupations and activities. The occupational therapist then analyzes the client's occupational performance. Occupational performance refers to "the act of doing and accomplishing a selected activity or occupation that results from the dynamic transaction among the client, the context, and the activity" (AOTA, 2008, pp. 672-673). The occupational therapist and the occupational therapy assistant then work with the client to improve the client's engagement in occupations or activities (AOTA, 2008). Client factors include their values, beliefs, spirituality, body functions, and body structures, and they all play a role in a client's occupational performance, as well as environment or context where the activity takes place and the demands of the activity. In the next sections, the dynamics and meaning of occupation will further be explored.

Areas of Occupation

The areas of occupation refer to the broad categories of occupations or activities in which clients engage. The eight areas of occupation are: activities of daily living (ADL), instrumental activities of daily living (IADL), rest and sleep, education, work, play, leisure, and social participation (AOTA, 2008). Specific activities associated with each category are discussed in the following text

Table 6-1.
ACTIVITIES OF DAILY LIVING

Activity and Definition	Example of Activities
Bathing/ showering: obtaining and using supplies; soaping, rinsing, and drying body parts; maintaining bathing position; and transferring to and from bathing positions (AOTA, 2008, p. 631).	Jane turns on the water and enters the shower. In the shower, Jane obtains her shampoo, conditioner, and body wash. She uses the products to clean her hair and body. Jane maintains her balance throughout the activity, and then turns off the water once she has finished bathing herself. Jane dries herself and then exits the shower.
Bowel and bladder management: includes completing intentional control of bowel movements and urinary bladder and, if necessary, using equipment or agents for bladder control (AOTA, 2008, p. 631).	Sean had a spinal cord injury and needs to use adaptive equipment to control bowel movements and void his bladder. Sean uses a digital stimulator to facilitate his bowel movements on a schedule. In addition, Sean completes self-catheterization and cares for his catheter.
Dressing: selecting clothing and accessories appropriate to time of day, weather, and occasion; obtaining clothing from storage area; dressing and undressing in a sequential fashion; fastening and adjusting clothing and shoes; and applying and removing personal devices, prostheses, or orthoses (AOTA, 2008, p. 631).	Wendy selects the outfit that she is going to wear to work. She considers the weather and selects an outfit that is appropriate to wear. Wendy then obtains the clothes, put the clothes on in the correct order, and fastens items. At the end of the day, Wendy undresses from her work clothes and changes into sleep wear.
Eating: the ability to keep and manipulate food or fluid in the mouth and swallow it (AOTA, 2008, p. 631).	Rob is eating a hot dog and drinking a soda. Rob is able to keep his food in his mouth while he chews and swallows the food. Rob is also able to keep his drink in his mouth as he swallows the drink.
Feeding: the process of setting up, arranging, and bringing food (or fluid) from the plate or cup to the mouth (AOTA, 2008, p. 631).	Julie has arranged her food and drink in front of her. She has set up the food so she is able to bring the food and drink from her plate and cup to her mouth. Julie enjoys a cup of tea (Figure 6-1).
Functional mobility: moving from one position or place to another (during the performance of everyday activities), such as in-bed mobility, wheelchair mobility, and transfers (AOTA, 2008, p. 631).	Mike broke his leg and is unable to walk on it. He has learned how to move from one position to another without using his injured leg. He transfers in and out of bed with a sliding board to his wheelchair. He also uses the sliding board to transfer to the car, toilet, and shower.
Personal device care: using, cleaning, and maintaining personal care items, such as hearing aids, contact lenses, glasses, orthotics, prosthetics, adaptive equipment, and contraceptive and sexual devices (AOTA, 2008, p. 631).	Janice rinsed her contact lenses and stored them in the case her doctor provided.
Personal hygiene and grooming: obtaining and using supplies; removing body hair; applying and removing cosmetics; washing, drying, combing, styling, brushing, trimming hair; caring for nails; caring for skin, ears, eyes, nose; applying deodorant; cleaning mouth, brushing and flossing teeth; or removing, cleaning, and reinserting dental orthotics and prosthetics (AOTA, 2008, p. 631).	Wesley brushes his teeth before bed (Figure 6-2).
Sexual activity: engaging in activities that result in sexual satisfaction (AOTA, 2008, p. 631).	Dave had a total hip replacement and maintained his total hip precautions during sexual intercourse.
Toilet hygiene: obtaining and using supplies; clothing management; maintaining toileting position; transferring to and from toileting position; cleaning body; and caring for menstrual and continence needs (AOTA, 2008, p. 631).	Marlene maintained her back precautions while transferring on and off the commode and obtaining toilet paper to clean herself.

and in the *Occupational Therapy Practice Framework: Domain and Process, 2nd Edition* (AOTA, 2008).

ACTIVITIES OF DAILY LIVING

ADL are activities that are typically oriented toward caring for one's self. These activities are typically performed before leaving one's home, but are not restricted to being performed in the home. See Table 6-1 for the activities and their definitions from the *Occupational Therapy Practice Framework: Domain and Process, 2nd Edition*, and an example of each activity.

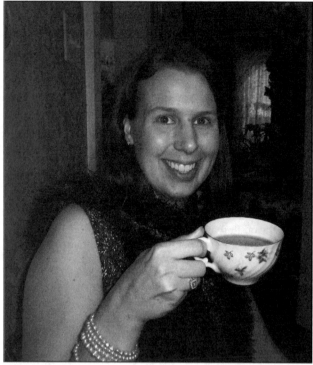

Figure 6-1. Enjoying a cup of tea.

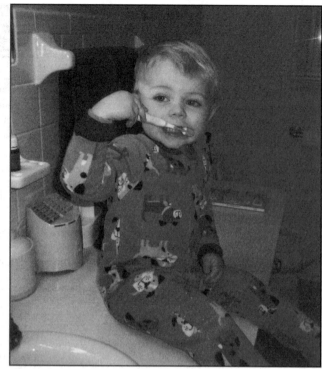

Figure 6-2. Toddler brushing his teeth before bed.

INSTRUMENTAL ACTIVITIES OF DAILY LIVING

IADL are more complex than ADL. They typically are completed at home and in the community. By nature they require more complex interactions and may involve other persons, organizations, or populations. See Table 6-2 for the activities and their definitions from the *Occupational Therapy Practice Framework: Domain and Process, 2nd Edition,* and an example of each activity.

REST AND SLEEP

Rest and sleep refer to all of the activities that are involved in preparing to fall asleep, sleeping, and gaining the energy to participate in other areas of occupation (AOTA, 2008). Rest and sleep include the following: rest, sleep, sleep preparation, and sleep participation. During rest, the client refrains from activities and relaxes in a quiet, calm environment. In order to successfully fall asleep, the client may complete the activities of sleep preparation and sleep participation. Sleep preparation includes the routines performed prior to going to bed (i.e., grooming, changing clothes). During sleep participation, the client takes care of the needs of others in order to be able to sleep through the night. This may mean giving a baby a bottle so the baby will not wake during the night. Finally, after successfully completing the other activities, the client obtains the goal of sleep, which refers to going to sleep and maintaining sufficient sleep to be able to actively participate in activities upon waking. See Table 6-3 for the activities and their

definitions from the *Occupational Therapy Practice Framework: Domain and Process, 2nd Edition,* and an example of each activity.

EDUCATION

Education refers to activities that are needed for learning and participating in the environment (AOTA, 2008). This includes formal education participation, informal personal education needs or interest exploration, and informal personal education participation. See Table 6-4 for the activities and their definitions from the *Occupational Therapy Practice Framework: Domain and Process, 2nd Edition,* and an example of each activity.

WORK

Work refers to employment and volunteer activities. This includes employment interests and pursuits, employment seeking and acquisition, job performance, retirement preparation and adjustment, volunteer exploration, and volunteer participation (AOTA, 2008). Occupational therapy practitioners work with clients on all aspects of paid and voluntary work (Figure 6-3). See Table 6-5 for the activities and their definitions from the *Occupational Therapy Practice Framework: Domain and Process, 2nd Edition,* and an example of each activity.

PLAY

Play refers to activities that are planned or unplanned that provide enjoyment or entertainment (AOTA, 2008). Play is divided into play exploration and play

Table 6-2.

INSTRUMENTAL ACTIVITIES OF DAILY LIVING

Activity and Definition	Example of Activities
Care of others: arranging, supervising, or providing care for others (AOTA, 2008, p. 631).	John cares for his wife, Beth, who has dementia. He watches over her so she is able to remain at home. When he is unable to supervise her, he arranges for a visiting nurse to come to their house.
Care of pets: arranging, supervising, or providing the care for pets and service animals (AOTA, 2008, p. 631).	Bill feeds his dog twice a day. He walks his dog before and after work, and has a doggie door so his dog can go into the fenced-in area in the backyard.
Communication management: sending, receiving, and interpreting information from a variety of systems and equipment, including writing tools, telephones, typewriters, audiovisual recorders, computers, communication boards, call lights, emergency systems, Braille writers, telecommunication devices for the deaf, augmentative communication systems, and personal digital assistants (AOTA, 2008, p. 631).	Erin checks her work email account multiple times a day and returns emails as appropriate to the senders. Erin also sends new emails when she needs to contact coworkers at different locations in different time zones.
Community mobility: moving around in the community and using public transportation, such as driving, walking, bicycling, or accessing and riding in buses, taxi cabs, or other transportation systems (AOTA, 2008, p. 631).	Jen took a taxi to the train station and then rode the train to work.
Financial management: using fiscal resources, including alternate methods of financial transaction and planning and using finances with long-term and short-term goals (AOTA, 2008, p. 631).	Aaron opted to pay for his bills online to reduce mailing expenses.
Health management and maintenance: developing, managing, and maintaining routines for health and wellness promotion, such as physical fitness, nutrition, decreasing health risk behaviors, and medication routines (AOTA, 2008, p. 631).	Michelle placed all of her medications into a pill box that organized her medications for the week. She removes her medications on a daily basis from the organizer.
Home establishment and management: obtaining and maintaining personal and household possessions and environment, including maintaining and repairing personal possessions and knowing how to seek help or whom to contact (AOTA, 2008, p. 631).	James called the roofer to repair the leak in his roof.
Meal preparation and cleanup: planning, preparing, and serving well-balanced, nutritional meals and cleaning up food and utensils after meals (AOTA, 2008, p. 631).	Kate gathered the ingredients from the refrigerator and her shelves to bake a chicken. After preparing and making the chicken, she carved the chicken and served it to her family. After the meal, she cleaned the roasting pan and supplies she used to make the chicken.
Religious observance: participating in religion (AOTA, 2008, p. 631).	Luke attends church services every Sunday.
Safety and emergency maintenance: knowing and performing preventative procedures to maintain a safe environment as well as recognizing sudden, unexpected hazardous situations and initiating emergency action to reduce the threat to health and safety (AOTA, 2008, p. 631).	Mrs. Smith heard the fire alarm go off in her classroom. She gathered her students and led them safely out of the building to the location where they were supposed to wait until the building was cleared for re-entry.
Shopping: preparing shopping lists; selecting, purchasing, and transporting items; selecting methods of payment; and completing money transactions (AOTA, 2008, p. 631).	Mary made a list of groceries that she needed from the local supermarket. At the supermarket, she gathered all of the items on her list and proceeded to the cash register where she paid for her groceries.

participation. The activity of play is typically associated with children (Figures 6-4 and 6-5). See Table 6-6 for the activities and their definitions from the *Occupational Therapy Practice Framework: Domain and Process, 2nd Edition,* and an example of each activity.

LEISURE

Leisure activity might be considered the play of adults. It is an intrinsically motivating and engaging activity that is completed in free time. Leisure is divided into leisure

Table 6-3.

REST AND SLEEP

Activity and Definition	Example of Activities
Rest: quiet and effortless actions that interrupt physical and mental activity resulting in a relaxed state (AOTA, 2008, p. 632).	Sarah sits in her recliner, closes her eyes, and listens to the sounds of waves crashing outside.
Sleep: a series of activities resulting in going to sleep, staying asleep, and ensuring health and safety through participation in sleep involving engagement with the physical and social environments (AOTA, 2008, p. 632).	Jason checks the room temperature and makes sure it is 70 degrees. He then fluffs his pillow, gets into bed under the covers, and he pulls the covers to his neck and falls asleep. Jason needs the room temperature to be at 70 degrees, and needs his fluffed pillow and blankets in order to fall asleep and stay asleep.
Sleep preparation: engaging in routines that prepare the self for a comfortable rest, such as grooming and undressing, reading or listening to music to fall asleep, saying goodnight to others, and meditation or prayers (AOTA, 2008, p. 632).	Ashley brushes her teeth and changes into her sleepwear prior to falling asleep.
Sleep participation: taking care of personal need for sleep such as cessation of activities to ensure onset of sleep, napping, dreaming, sustaining a sleep state without disruption, and nighttime care of toileting needs or hydration (AOTA, 2008, p. 632).	Sean stops drinking at 7 PM to ensure that he does not wake to go to the bathroom during the night. Right before going to bed, Sean goes to the bathroom one last time to void his bladder. This routine allows Sean to sleep through the night.

Table 6-4.

EDUCATION

Activity and Definition	Example of Activities
Formal education participation: including the categories of academic, nonacademic, extracurricular, and vocational participation (AOTA, 2008, p. 632).	Anna's formal education activities include studying for classes, playing intramural soccer for her college, and helping out in the occupational therapy clinic on her campus.
Informal personal education needs or interests exploration (beyond formal education): identifying topics and methods for obtaining topic-related information or skills (AOTA, 2008, p. 632)	Kristen is knitting a scarf for the first time; she knitted the length that she desired for the scarf. Kristen went on her computer and looked up a video online on how to end the scarf. Kristen watched the video and then completed her scarf.
Informal personal education participation: participating in classes, programs, and activities that provide instruction/training in identified areas of interest (AOTA, 2008, p. 632).	Jim attended a CPR course to learn how to complete CPR, since he wanted to know what to do if something happened to a member of his family.

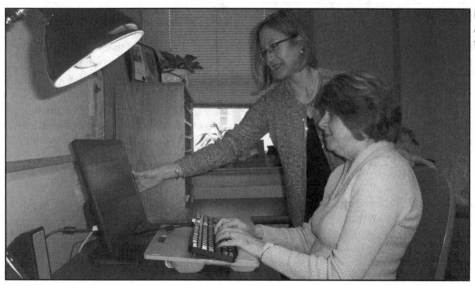

Figure 6-3. An occupational therapist evaluates a client's work setting.

Table 6-5.

WORK

Activity and Definition	Example of Activities
Employment interests and pursuits: identifying and selecting work opportunities based on assets, limitations, likes, and dislikes relative to work (AOTA, 2008, p. 632).	Jake participates in a transition program. He and other high school students attend a class where they identify the types of activities that they like to do and those that they do not. Based on their likes and dislikes, they look up jobs that match their desires.
Employment seeking and acquisition: identifying and recruiting for job opportunities; completing, submitting, and reviewing appropriate application materials; preparing for interviews; participating in interviews and following up afterward; discussing job benefits; and finalizing negotiations (AOTA, 2008, p. 632).	Colleen flips through an occupational therapy magazine and cuts out an ad for a position that she would like. Colleen reviews and completes the materials that she needs to submit for the position. Colleen attends her interview and sends a thank you note after the interview. The employer calls Colleen and offers her the position. Colleen negotiates her pay and benefits and sets up her start date.
Job performance: job performance including work skills and patterns; time management; relationships with co-workers, managers, and customers; creation, production, and distribution of products and services; initiation, sustainment, and completion of work; and compliance with work norms and procedures (AOTA, 2008, p. 632).	Part of Pattie's job is to evaluate her coworkers' workstations. Pattie's coworker was complaining about wrist strain at her computer. Pattie evaluated her coworker's workstation and provided her coworker with an adapted keyboard (see Figure 6-3).
Retirement preparation and adjustment: determining aptitudes, developing interests and skills, and selecting appropriate avocational pursuits (AOTA, 2008, p. 632).	Janet plans to retire at the end of the school year. She thinks about what activities she would like to participate in after retiring. She knows that she likes to work out, and plans to work out daily. She also likes quilting and decides that she will enroll in some quilting classes.
Volunteer exploration: determining community causes, organizations, or opportunities for unpaid 'work' in relationship to personal skills, interests, location, and time available (AOTA, 2008, p. 632).	Mary Alice retired from the local elementary school and is exploring the possibility of volunteering at her old school. She would like to assist the teachers by volunteering in their classrooms and providing extra help to children who need one-on-one attention. She contacts the principal to see if any of the teachers would like a volunteer.
Volunteer participation: performing unpaid 'work' activities for the benefit of identified selected causes, organizations, or facilities (AOTA, 2008, p. 632).	Jack volunteers at the local hospital. He visits the patients in their rooms and drops off the daily newspaper to patients who would like to read it.

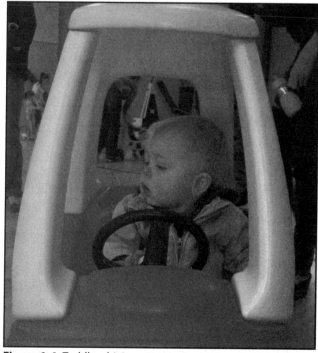

Figure 6-4. Toddler driving a toy car.

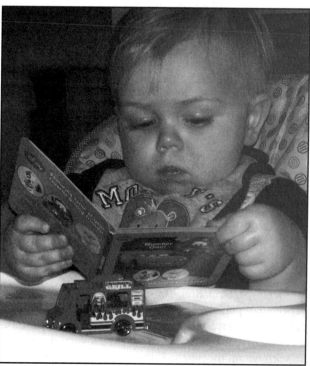

Figure 6-5. Toddler reading a book.

Table 6-6.

PLAY

Activity and Definition	Example of Activities
Play exploration: identifying appropriate play activities, which can include exploration play, practice play, pretend play, games with rules, constructive play, and symbolic play (AOTA, 2008, p. 632).	Tommy searches his playroom for toys. He thinks that he wants to play doctor so he looks for his toy stethoscope and doctor bag.
Play participation: participating in play; maintaining a balance of play with others areas of occupation; and obtaining, using, and maintaining toys, equipment, and supplies appropriately (AOTA, 2008, p. 632).	Lauren invites her friend Stephanie over to play a board game. Lauren gets the game from the closet and sets it up for them to play. After playing the game, Lauren packs up the game and returns it to the closet.

Table 6-7.

LEISURE

Activity and Definition	Example of Activities
Leisure exploration: "identifying interests, skills, opportunities, and appropriate leisure activities" (AOTA, 2008, p. 632).	Joe's coworker goes fishing on the weekends and invites him to join him. Joe thinks he would like fishing because he likes the outdoors, is pretty athletic, and likes fish. Joe goes to a local sporting goods store and looks into what equipment he will need to go fishing with his coworker.
Leisure participation: planning and participating in appropriate leisure activities; maintaining a balance of leisure activities with other areas of occupation; and obtaining, using, and maintaining equipment and supplies as appropriate (AOTA, 2008, p. 632).	Nicole likes yoga and participates in a yoga class two nights a week. When she is not in yoga class, she incorporates some of the breathing techniques into her daily activities.

Table 6-8.

SOCIAL PARTICIPATION

Activity and Definition	Example of Activities
Community: engaging in activities that result in successful interaction at the community level (AOTA, 2008, p. 633).	Lisa participates in her town's 5K run, which raises money for events in her community.
Family: engaging in activities that result in successful interaction in specific required and/or desired familial roles (AOTA, 2008, p. 633).	Grandma invites her whole family over for Sunday pasta suppers and chocolate cake.
Peer/friend: engaging in activities at different levels of intimacy, including engaging in desired sexual activity (AOTA, 2008, p. 633).	Courtney started dating Chris and they had their first kiss under the maple tree on their college campus.

exploration and leisure participation. Table 6-7 shows the activities and their definitions from the *Occupational Therapy Practice Framework: Domain and Process, 2nd Edition*, and an example of the activities.

SOCIAL PARTICIPATION

Social participation consists of behaviors that are expected of persons as members of society. Social participation takes place at the peer/friend, family, and community levels. Behaviors and expectations vary depending on with whom the person is interacting. See Table 6-8 for

the activities and their definitions from the *Occupational Therapy Practice Framework: Domain and Process, 2nd Edition*, and an example of the activities.

SUMMARY

Persons, organizations, and populations are involved in different occupations. Knowing and understanding the different areas of occupation helps occupational therapy practitioners to identify relevant areas to address with clients. Occupation can be used as an end or as a means during therapy (Trombly, 2011). Occupation-as-end refers to

Table 6-9.

PERFORMANCE SKILLS

Performance Skills and Definitions	Example of Performance Skills
Motor and praxis skills • Motor: planning and sequencing movements in order to interact with different tasks and objects in different contexts and environments. • Praxis: the ability to organize, plan, and carry out different actions.	Motor: Sue reaches up to the cabinet door and grabs the handle on the door to pull it open. Sue opens the cabinet and grabs a cup from within the cabinet. Praxis: Sue plans the steps of raising her shoulder into forward flexion while extending her elbow and wrist, and flexing her fingers around the door knob.
Sensory-perceptual skills: actions or behaviors a client uses to locate, identify, and respond to sensations and to select, interpret, associate, organize, and remember sensory events based on discriminating experiences through a variety of sensations that include visual, auditory, gustatory, and vestibular (AOTA, 2008, p. 640).	Allison has low vision and cannot see objects in her environment. Allison uses the back of her hand to feel her counter surface and guide herself to her refrigerator. Allison organizes the objects in her refrigerator so they are easy to find. Allison opens and smells her milk to ensure she does not drink spoiled milk. Allison knows the shape of the milk bottle so she can identify it from other bottles.
Emotional regulation skills: actions or behaviors a client uses to identify, manage, and express feelings while engaging in activities or interacting with others (AOTA, 2008, p. 640).	Tim gets upset when other students bump into him in line at school. His occupational therapist taught him to go to the end of the line so he can watch his classmates and to take deep breaths when students bump into him. Tim lines up at the end of the line and practices deep breaths when students bump into him.
Cognitive skills: actions or behaviors a client uses to plan and manage performance of an activity (AOTA, 2008, p. 640).	Jean realizes that she needs to balance her checkbook and pay her monthly bills. She organizes her receipts in a sequential order and then checks her checkbook entries. After checking her checkbook balance and paying her bills, she identifies she has $300 left. Jean thinks about a few different things that she needs and prioritizes which things she will buy this month, and what things can wait until next month.
Communication and social skills: actions or behaviors a person uses to communicate and interact with others in an interactive environment (AOTA, 2008, p. 641).	Amanda and Sue are sitting in a coffee shop, catching up on their lives since college. Sue smiles as Amanda shares a story about her kids. Amanda touches Sue's hand as Sue tells her about the death of a friend. The two take turns sharing stories and enjoying each other's company.

persons completing an occupation for the sake of being able to complete the occupation. Occupation-as-means refers to using different occupations to build performance skills and patterns needed in order to achieve a specific occupational performance related to the client's goals. The next sections will further explore performance skills and performance patterns.

Performance Skills

Performance skills are "the abilities that clients demonstrate in the actions they perform" (AOTA, 2008, p. 673). These include the following: motor and praxis skills, sensory perceptual skills, emotional regulation skills, cognitive skills, and communication and social skills. Acquisition and development of these skills allow persons, organizations, and populations to successfully complete different occupations. Deficits or deficiencies in performance skills can hinder and prevent successful participation in occupations. See Table 6-9 for the performance skills and their definitions from the *Occupational Therapy Practice Framework: Domain and Process, 2nd Edition,* and an example of each skill.

Performance Patterns

Performance patterns are the habits, rituals, roles, and routines that persons, organizations, and populations engage in during their occupations and activities. Habits are automatic behaviors that are engaged in, whereas rituals are symbolic actions that have meaning and awareness. Habits are found only at the person level. Rituals, roles, and routines are found at the person, organization, and population levels. Rituals are completed because of the cultural, social, or spiritual meaning of the action or behavior. Roles, like rituals, also have a social aspect. Roles are formed based on societal expectations and how the person, organization, or population defines the societal expectations, whereas routines create order and a sequence for occupations (AOTA, 2008). Routines may be created to promote healthy occupations and activities to participate in while avoiding occupations or activities

Table 6-10.	
PERFORMANCE PATTERNS	
Performance Patterns and Definitions	**Example of Performance Patterns**
Habits: automatic behavior that is integrated into more complex patterns that enable people to function on a day-to-day basis (AOTA, 2008, p. 643).	**Person:** Jill automatically locks the door to her home immediately after entering the home.
Rituals: symbolic actions with spiritual, cultural, or societal meaning, contributing to…and reinforcing values and beliefs (AOTA, 2008, p. 643).	**Person:** The Jones family has a special birthday celebration plate that is used as the birthday person's dinner plate on their birthday. The plate has been used from generation to generation. **Organization:** XYZ company holds an annual New Year's Eve party for all of its employees. **Population:** April is occupational therapy month.
Roles: a set of behaviors expected by society, shaped by culture, and may be further conceptualized and defined by the person, organization, or population (AOTA, 2008, p. 643).	**Person:** Grandmother of four grandchildren ranging from 2 to 14 years of age. **Organization:** Non-profit organization protecting the rights of individuals with low vision and blindness. **Population:** Mothers Against Drunk Driving fighting to stop drunk driving.
Routines: patterns of behavior that are observable, regular, repetitive, and that provide structure to daily life (AOTA, 2008, p. 643).	**Person:** Every day Julie goes into work, unlocks the office and file cabinets, turns on the copy machine, drops off her coat, and pulls her files for the day. **Organization:** Company ABC holds in-services for its occupational therapy department the second and fourth Tuesdays of every month. **Population:** Every fall, people are reminded that they should get their annual flu shot.

that have negative effects on persons, organizations, and populations. See Table 6-10 for the performance patterns and their definitions from the *Occupational Therapy Practice Framework: Domain and Process, 2nd Edition,* and an example of the skills.

Activity Demands

Every occupation or activity has certain requirements for the occupation or activity to be completed. Activity demands refer to the objects and their properties, space demands, social demands, sequence and timing, required actions and performance skills, required body functions, and required body structures for an activity (AOTA, 2008). The demands are specific to each activity. As occupational therapy practitioners, we pay a lot of attention to the activity demands when working with our clients. Occupational therapy practitioners are skilled at grading and adapting the activity demands to allow the client to successfully complete the activity. For example, Mary enjoys going to her grandson's football games. Mary recently had a total hip replacement and needs to maintain her total hip precautions. Mary and her occupational therapist discussed the activity demands required for Mary to go to the football games. Mary will need to use her cane and bring a cushion to sit on at the stadium (objects and properties). Mary will need to walk

200 yards from the parking lot to the open stadium on a paved path using her cane and carrying her cushion (space demands). Mary will need to be aware of the kids and families also going to the game while she walks to and from the stadium and while seated in the bleachers (social demands). Mary's occupational therapist recommends that Mary arrives early to the games and then waits until the stadium has almost cleared in order to avoid people bumping into Mary as she walks along the path (sequencing and timing). Mary will need strength and endurance to travel the 200 yard distance in both directions, as well as remain aware of her total hip precaution (required actions and performance skills, required body functions, and required body structures).

Contexts and Environments

The contexts and environments in which occupations take place may facilitate or hinder occupational performance. The environment refers to the physical and social aspects, whereas the contexts refer to the cultural, personal, temporal, and virtual aspects (AOTA, 2008). The physical environment and social environment were first addressed in the area of activity demands in this chapter. The physical environment includes the built and non-built objects with which persons, organizations, and populations interact, whereas the social environment includes the relationships of the persons, organizations, and populations. When the physical environment is built using concepts of universal design, it promotes occupational performance of all (Ringaert, 2003). Buildings without ramps or elevators hinder the participation of persons who are unable to ambulate. Social aspects may also facilitate or hinder occupational performance. Persons with family members who are able to assist them allow for a supportive environment. Persons without supports or with negative supports may have fewer opportunities to participate in activities and occupations that require more than one person.

Cultural, personal, temporal, and virtual contexts may also facilitate or hinder occupational performance. Cultural aspects are customs and beliefs held by society; for instance, in the United States, people stand for the national anthem and men remove their hats. Personal aspects refer to the specifics about the person, organization, or population. This may be the age, gender, race, origin, sexuality, religious status, economic status, political status, or educational status of the person, organization, or population. The temporal aspects refer to time (e.g., the amount of time until a certain period in life, the amount of time to complete an activity or occupation, and a specific date or time of day). Finally, virtual aspects are communications without physical presence. This is achieved through computers, tablets, radios, telephones, and cell phones, among others. Understanding the contexts helps identify how the contexts may be used to facilitate or how they may hinder occupational performance. One client may benefit from using applications on a tablet; however, this client may not have access to using or purchasing a tablet. Another client may come from a culture where family members step in and provide for the client all of the assistance needed to allow the client to complete occupations and activities.

Client Factors

"Client factors are specific abilities, characteristics, or beliefs that reside with the client and may affect performance in areas of occupation" (AOTA, 2008, p. 630). Client factors include the values, beliefs, and spirituality of the person, organization, or population. They also include the body functions and body structures that play a role in occupational performance. Occupational therapists gather information about the client's factors during the evaluation. Knowing and understanding the values, beliefs, and spirituality of the client as well as the current status of the client's body functions and body structures helps provide a holistic picture of the client as well as an appropriate treatment plan. Persons, organizations, and populations are complex and transactional relationships that occur between the areas of occupation, performance skills, performance patterns, activity demands, contexts

and environments, and client factors. Understanding all of these areas allow occupational therapy practitioners to assist clients in living a life of occupational balance.

Occupational Balance

Occupational balance has been one of the tenets of occupational therapy since its foundation (Backman, 2004). Originally, occupational balance was considered a balance among different daily occupations that promoted well-being and health (Anaby, Backman, & Jarus, 2010). However, because of its complexity, definitions of occupational balance differ (Wagman, Hakansson, & Bjorklund, 2012). Current definitions define occupational balance as "a balance of engagement in occupation that leads to well-being" (Wilcock, 2006, p. 343). As occupational therapy practitioners, we need to work with our clients for them to obtain their unique occupational balance. If a client is not getting enough sleep, it can lead to inability to complete other occupations. By obtaining an understanding of the client's occupations during the evaluation stage, interventions to allow for occupational balance during the treatment stage can take place to allow for health and wellness.

Task Analysis to Formulate an Intervention Plan

As occupational therapy practitioners who use occupation as the basis of our intervention plans, we have a lot to ponder. Although occupations and activities seem simple to the untrained eye, occupational therapists and occupational therapy assistants are constantly analyzing occupations and activities to maximize clients' occupational performance. Intervention plans must address the areas of occupation, performance skills, performance patterns, activity demands, contexts and environments, and client factors in order to maximize the success for our clients. Occupational therapy practitioners use the therapeutic use of self and therapeutic use of occupations and activities to accomplish this. Purposeful activities use activities that develop the client's skills for occupational engagement. Occupation-based interventions utilize engagement in specific occupations to match the client's goals for occupational performance in specific areas of occupation. All activities should be goal-directed and purposeful and meaningful to the client (AOTA, 2008).

When approaching the intervention, the occupational therapist will choose one or more of the following approaches: create/promote occupation, establish/restore skills, maintain occupational performance, modify activities/environment, or prevent performance problems. See Table 6-11 for the intervention approaches and their definitions from the *Occupational Therapy Practice*

Table 6-11.

INTERVENTION APPROACHES

Approaches and Definitions	Example of Approach
Create/promote: an intervention approach that does not assume a disability is present or that any factors would interfere with performance. This approach is designed to provide enriched contextual and activity experiences that will enhance performance for all persons in the natural contexts of life (AOTA, 2008, p. 657).	Create a transition class for high school seniors to promote exploration of vocations and education programs.
Establish/restore: an intervention approach designed to change client variables to establish a skill or ability that has not yet developed or to restore a skill or ability that has been impaired (AOTA, 2008, p. 657).	Develop a craft class for individuals with low vision and blindness that develops other sensory skills (hearing function, vestibular function, taste, smells, proprioceptive function, touch, and temperature/pressure) through the participation in different craft activities (see Figures 6-6 and 6-7).
Maintain: an intervention approach designed to provide supports that will allow clients to preserve the performance capabilities they have regained, that continue to meet their occupational needs, or both. The assumption is that, without continued maintenance intervention, performance would decrease, occupational needs would not be met, or both, thereby affecting health and quality of life (AOTA, 2008, p. 658).	Provide a low vision support group to individuals with low vision and blindness to maintain functional independence.
Modify: an intervention approach directed at finding ways to revise the current context or activity demands to support performance in the natural setting, [including] compensatory techniques, [such as]…enhancing some features to provide cue or reducing other features to reduce distractibility (AOTA, 2008, p. 658).	Use a box mix to reduce the number of steps to make brownies.
Prevent: an intervention approach designed to address clients with or without a disability who are at risk for occupational performance problems. This approach is designed to prevent occurrence or evolution of barriers to performance in context. Interventions may be directed at client, context, or activity variables (AOTA, 2008, p. 659).	Prevent repetitive strain injuries by teaching stretching techniques and training the person to take breaks prior to feeling pain.

Framework: Domain and Process, 2nd Edition, and an example of the intervention approach (Figure 6-6 and Figure 6-7).

Summary

Occupations and activities are complex and multidimensional. By understanding all of the dimensions of occupation and activity, we are able to maximize occupational performance for our clients. Our clients are persons, organizations, and populations. Although occupational therapy has traditionally had a large impact at the person level, it is also extremely influential in working at the organization and population levels to support "health and participation in life through engagement in occupation" (AOTA, 2008, p. 626). As our profession continues to grow, we will continue to maximize all our clients' lives, allowing them to live life to the fullest.

Electronic Resources

- American Occupational Therapy Association: www.aota.org
- Society for the Study of Occupation: USA: www.sso-usa.org

Student Self-Assessment

1. Select an ADL or IADL that you complete on a regular basis. What are the activity demands for it? How would the demands differ if you were unable to walk? What approach would you use to obtain occupational performance in this activity? Why?

2. Using the activity selected for the first question, describe two other environments or contexts in which the activity could be completed. How would the activity be the same and how would it be different in those environments or contexts?

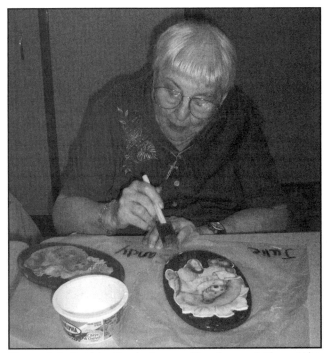

Figure 6-6. Participating in Sensory Development Class at the Lackawanna Blind Association.

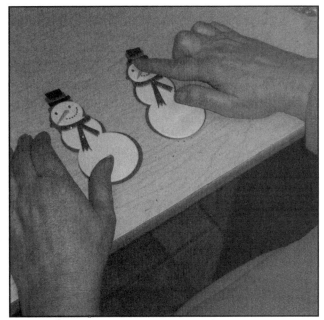

Figure 6-7. Participating in Sensory Development Class at the Lackawanna Blind Association.

EVIDENCE-BASED RESEARCH CHART

Occupational balance	Anaby, Backman, & Jarus, 2010; Backman, 2004; Wagman, Hakansson, & Bjorklund, 2012
Occupation-based practice	AOTA, 2008; Baker, Jacobs, & Tickle-Degnen, 2003; DeGrace, 2003; Fisher, 2003; Lysaght & Wright, 2005; Nelson & Mathiowetz, 2004

3. Create an example of how you might work with a client at the organization or population level.

References

American Occupational Therapy Association. (2008). Occupational therapy practice framework: Domain and process (2nd ed.). *American Journal of Occupational Therapy, 62,* 625-683.

Anaby, D., Backman, C., & Jarus, T. (2010). Measuring occupational balance: A theoretical exploration of two approaches. *Canadian Journal of Occupational Therapy, 77,* 280-288.

Backman, C. (2004). Occupational balance: Exploring relationships among daily occupations and their influence on well-being. *Canadian Journal of Occupational Therapy, 71,* 202-209.

Kielholhofner, G. (2009). *Conceptual foundations of occupational therapy practice* (4th ed.). Philadelphia, PA: F.A. Davis Company.

O'Brien, J., & Hussey, S. (2012). *Introduction to occupational therapy.* St. Louis, MO: Mosby-Elsevier.

Reitz, S. M. (2010). Historical and philosophical perspectives of occupational therapy's role in health promotion. In M. E. Scaffa, S. M. Reitz, & M. A. Pizzi (Eds.), *Occupational therapy in the promotion of health and wellness* (pp. 1-21). Philadelphia, PA: F.A. Davis Company.

Ringaert, L. (2003). Universal design of the built environment to enable occupational performance. In L. Letts, P. Pigby, & D. Stewart (Eds.), *Using environments to enable occupational performance* (pp. 97-115). Thorofare, NJ: SLACK Incorporated.

Trombly, C. (2011). Occupation: Purposeful and meaningfulness as therapeutic mechanisms. In R. Padilla, & Y. Griffiths (Eds.), *A professional legacy.* Bethesda, MD: AOTA Press.

Wagman, P., Hakansson, C., & Bjorklund, A. (2012). Occupational balance as used in occupational therapy: A concept analysis. *Scandinavian Journal of Occupational Therapy, 19,* 322-327.

Wilcock, A. (2006). *An occupational perspective of health.* Thorofare, NJ: Thorofare, NJ: SLACK Incorporated.

Wilcock, A. (2001). *Occupation for health* (Vol. I). London, United Kingdom: British Association and College of Occupational Therapists.

Suggested Readings

Baker, N., Jacobs, K., & Tickle-Degnen, L. (2003). A methodology for developing evidence about meaning in occupation: Exploring the meaning of work. *OTJR: Occupation, Participation and Health, 23,* 57-66.

DeGrace, B. (2003). Occupation-based and family-centered care: A challenge for current practice. *The American Journal of Occupational Therapy, 57,* 347-350.

Fisher, A. (2003). Why is it so hard to practice as an occupational therapist? *Australian Occupational Therapy Journal, 50,* 193-194.

Lysaght, R., & Wright, J. (2005). Professional strategies in work-related practice: An exploration of occupational and physical therapy roles and approaches. *The American Journal of Occupational Therapy, 59,* 209-217.

Nelson, D., & Mathiowetz, V. (2004). Randomized controlled trials to investigate occupational therapy research questions. *The American Journal of Occupational Therapy, 58,* 24-34.

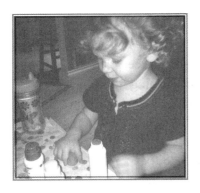

OCCUPATIONAL PERFORMANCE AND HEALTH

Kathleen Flecky, OTD, OTR/L and Heather Goertz, OTD, OTR/L

ACOTE STANDARDS EXPLORED IN THIS CHAPTER
B.2.5, B.2.6

KEY VOCABULARY

- **Activity:** "Culturally defined and general class of human actions" (Pierce, 2001, p. 137).
- **Areas of occupation:** "Various kinds of life activities in which people engage, including the following categories: ADL, IADL, rest and sleep, education, work, play, leisure, and social participation" (AOTA, 2008, p. 669).
- **Body functions and structures:** "The physiological functions of body systems, including psychological functions (WHO, 2001, p. 65) and the anatomical parts of the body such as organs, limbs, and their components" (WHO, 2001, p. 111).
- **Disability:** "Dynamic interaction between an individual (with a health condition) and that individual's contextual factors (environmental and personal factors" (WHO, 2001, p. 190).

- **Disease:** "An illness or disorder of the functioning of the body, or of certain tissues, organs or systems" (Slee, Slee, & Schmidt, 2008, p. 145).
- **Environmental factors:** "Physical, social and attitudinal environment in which people live and conduct their lives" (WHO, 2001, p. 22).
- **Function:** "Positive aspects of the interaction between an individual (with a health condition) and the individual's contextual factors (environmental and personal factors" (WHO, 2001, p. 190).
- **Health:** "Aiming for a balance of physical, mental, and social well-being attained through valued occupation" (Wilcock, 2006, p. 112); state of complete physical, mental and social well-being and not merely the absence of health (WHO, 1946).

(continued)

Jacobs, K., MacRae, N., & Sladyk, K. (Eds.).
*Occupational Therapy Essentials for
Clinical Competence, Second Edition* (pp. 71-83).

KEY VOCABULARY (CONTINUED)

- **Health promotion:** "[T]he process of enabling people to increase control over, and to improve, their health. To reach a state of complete physical, mental, and social well-being, and individual or a group must be able to identify and realize aspirations, to satisfy needs, and to change or cope with the environment" (WHO, 1986, as cited in AOTA, 2008).
- **Impairments:** "Problems in body function or structure as a significant deviation or loss" (WHO, 2001, p. 15).
- **International Classification of Diseases (ICD-10):** "International classification of diseases including a diagnosis of diseases, disorders or other health conditions" (WHO, 2001, p. 4).
- **International Classification of Functioning, Disability and Health (ICF):** "Unified and standard language and framework for the description of health and health-related states" (WHO, 2001, p. 3).

- **Occupational performance:** "The act of doing and accomplishing a selected activity or selected occupation that results from the dynamic transaction among the client, the context, and the activity" (AOTA, 2008, p. 673).
- **Participation:** "Involvement in a life situation" (WHO, 2001, p. 19).
- **Partnerships in health:** Community groups, organizations, agencies and institutions that collaborate to improve the health and well-being of individuals and populations within a community.
- **Personal factors:** "Particular background of an individual's life and living, and comprise features of the individual that are not part of the health condition or health status" (WHO, 2001, p. 23).
- **Wellness:** "An active process through which individuals become aware of and make choices toward a more successful existence" (Hettler, 1984, p. 1117, as cited in AOTA, 2008).

Introduction

What does it mean to be healthy and well? Occupational therapy professionals generally view persons as more than their disease processes. Two people can have the same disease or condition and differ widely in terms of physical, mental, social, and spiritual well-being. An individual's state of health is considered within the context of their ability to participate in needed and desired roles and to meet occupational lifestyle goals and tasks. Disease, illness, injury, and trauma can create occupational disruption that may lead to conditions of impairment, dysfunction, and disability.

Occupational therapy professionals analyze information about diseases, impairments, and other health conditions in terms of how these health states affect performance in life's roles and routines (Hansen & Atchinson, 2000). We value a perspective of health that includes the consideration of one's ability to participate in meaningful occupations. According to Wilcock (2006), an occupational perspective of health encompasses "aiming for a balance of physical, mental, and social well-being attained through valued occupation" (p. 112).

This chapter discusses health, disease, and disability within the context of occupational functioning and performance. In addition, the effects of physical and mental health, inheritable diseases, predisposing genetic conditions, disability, disease processes, and injury on the individual will be analyzed in terms of health and health promotion.

Health perspectives from a sampling of occupational therapy students have been provided to begin this chapter. In 2007, the American Occupational Therapy Association (AOTA, 2007) reported an enrollment of 10,861 students in occupational therapy programs across America. As occupational therapy students embrace concepts of health and disease, it is important to understand that health and disease are complex and that there is much more information about these concepts that exists beyond the scope of this chapter. This section introduces the discussion by exposing students to different viewpoints of health and disease.

Let us begin this discussion by reviewing occupational therapy students who individually completed a survey about their opinions of health and disease characteristics. They were not given health definitions prior to completing the survey. The students granted permission to have their comments shared with others when asked the following questions:

- Describe health.
- Describe your own personal characteristics of occupational performance when you are healthy.
- Have you ever had a major disease or illness? If yes, explain.
- Describe your own personal characteristics of occupational performance when you were affected by disease or illness.

The following sidebars highlight four students' views related to health, disease, and occupational performance. Following these views is a description of several themes identified through analysis of the students' narratives.

As the student narratives reveal, health and wellness are multidimensional concepts that include physical, emotional, social, and spiritual aspects. Definitions of health vary individually depending on one's personal values, cultural beliefs, societal values, and experiences. Other factors that influence our conceptualizations of health, as well as what it means to be ill or disabled, may include age, gender, race, ethnicity, socioeconomic status, and current and past medical status. In summary, terms such as health and well-being are difficult to define because they are personally and socially constructed. They have evolved over time as society has revised notions of health, disease, and disability. For example, the constructs of health, as described by these occupational therapy students, represented the following characteristics as shown in Table 7-1.

An awareness of your personal views of health constructs is vital to understanding how you will collaborate with your clients. Imagine standing in line at a grocery store behind a person in a wheelchair. Do you consider this person to be impaired? Why or why not? The answers to these questions are based largely on perceptions and life experiences and not necessarily on the unique lived experience of that person. An exploration of personal presuppositions and assumptions, beliefs, values, past experiences, and historical perspectives, as well as asking and clarifying client views, will enhance your professional skills at analyzing the effects of health and disease on occupational performance.

This chapter does not seek to examine every different view of health, but it introduces the concept of health by discussing historical perspectives of health, impairment, disease, and disability. For you to appreciate the complexity of health and disease, we have chosen to examine the historical views of impairments. Whether you have

Shelly's View

Health is mind, body, and spiritual wellness. I have balance in my life between work, school, friends, self-care, and leisure. When I let one take over, I usually stress about the others. If I allow time for everything, I feel I have a better handle on my life and I do a better job at each individual component. I have not experienced a major disease or illness.

Joseph's View

Health is physical, mental, and emotional balance and general wellness. I feel more productive, I can multitask, and I feel pretty confident in the work I am completing. I had chronic pain and depression. It was harder to complete schoolwork on time, and sometimes I just did the bare minimum. I slept a lot more, and sometimes my occupations didn't seem important. Reading, cooking, and exercising were discontinued in favor of sleep.

Elisa's View

Health is a state of being at an optimal weight, not having high blood pressure, exercising, eating right, and having no illness or disease. When I am healthy, I can function at a high level, perform at my best, focus, be sweet to others, and feel good about myself. I had atrioventricular nodal reentrant tachycardia. I needed help getting out of bed. I felt dependent on others and paid closer attention to how everyone treated me.

Amber's View

Health is the physical absence of disease or sickness with a mental balance and stability. I have more energy and motivation, I work toward goals, and I have a balance of occupations and leisure when I am healthy. I have Crohn's disease. The following are some characteristics of my occupational performance when I am ill: lack of energy and motivation, preoccupation with being physically ill and knowing that occupational performance is limited, difficulty focusing on working hard at school and balancing that with a social life, all while I feel that I can't physically and mentally perform up to my potential.

learned to recognize impairment as just a normal part of daily life or whether you feel sorry for the lady next door because she walks so slowly and painfully, occupational therapy professionals recognize that society has classified and categorized persons who are different from the norm. The consequences of these categorizations is that experts

	STUDENT SURVEY RESPONSES		
Student Survey Categories	**Disease Thematic Characteristics**	**Health Thematic Characteristics**	**Occupational Performance Characteristics**
Responses from 24 occupational therapy students	Difficulty completing work on time Increased sleep Occupations do not seem important Lack of energy and motivation Preoccupation with being physically ill Easily frustrated Dependent on others	Well-being of physical or bodily, mental, spiritual, and emotional health An absence of disease A harmonious state All of the above	Balanced life Alert Well rested Productive Energetic Active Motivated Goal oriented Happier Determined

Table 7-1.

have identified and defined who is impaired, diseased, or disabled rather than the people being categorized. Lack of attention to personal experiences of persons with impairments, diseases, and disabilities has led to marginalization, stigmatization, and exclusion (Depoy & Gilson, 2004; Oliver, 1996). It is necessary to recognize that contemporary perceptions of health, impairments, diseases, and disabilities exist within a historical context; where we are today is based largely on where we have been. Therefore, three predominant health models are described in the next section, and these illustrate how persons have been viewed as different, atypical, or abnormal owing to disease, impairment, and disability. Historical background is provided with these models of health in order to show how perspectives of health and disability are influenced by the cultural, social, spiritual, economic, and political contexts.

Historical Perspectives on Health and Disability

Throughout the history of the Western civilization, the predominant cultural and religious values along with social, political, and economic contexts influenced how persons with disease, impairment, and disability were viewed by society (Altman, 2001; Stiker & Sayers, 2000). A multitude of health perspectives have been advanced to define and describe health, but this section focuses on three predominant models: the religious, medical, and social perspectives, as identified in Table 7-2.

Prior to the Enlightenment Era of the 1600s, disablement or abnormality in general—whether due to illness, injury, disease, or mental or physical impairment—was based on a religious model of disability (Stiker & Sayers, 2000). Within the religious approach, personal impairments and limitations were attributed to moral or supernatural causes. Illnesses and disease were manifestations of either sinfulness or a special spiritual relationship with higher powers or with God (Braddock & Parish, 2001). With increased scientific and medical knowledge and with the influence of industrialization, atypicality was increasingly viewed as an individual affliction that limited one's ability to be a productive member of society. The impairment or disease required one to be fixed or restored through the care of others (Llewellyn & Hogan, 2000; Oliver, 1996). Charitable and medical care systems worked to either rehabilitate the disabled for the purpose of returning them to society or they confined them to custodial care within institutions (Braddock & Parish, 2001; Llewellyn & Hogan, 2000).

Initially, the occupational therapy profession was grounded in the social charitable movements of the early 20th century (Quiroga, 1995). The use of arts and crafts activities and habit training were incorporated into the everyday lives of those persons considered unproductive because of physical and mental impairments. During World War I and World War II, occupational therapy flourished within the milieu of the medical model of disablement by treating those with physical and mental disabilities (Quiroga, 1995). Our profession aligned with the medical model, which explained health, disease, and illness as bodily entities intrinsic to the person and treatable through either remediation or compensation for the effects of disease or injury (Kielhofner, 2004).

By the 20th century, medical diagnostic classification systems were created to categorize illnesses, diseases, and conditions based on health conditions, impairments, and limitations. Further advancement in medicine increased the survival rate for those with illness, injury, disease, impairment, and disability, which led to progressively more complex delineation of medical diagnoses and categories (Longmore & Umansky, 2001; Oliver, 1996). Health, ability, and disability became a function of one's

Features	Religious Model	Medical Model	Social Model
		HEALTH MODELS	
Views of health	Individual Based on spiritual or supernatural factors A reward for living a good life or a punishment for sinfulness	Individual Based on intrinsic biological factors Biological interactions and processes lead to health or ill health	Individual and environmental Based on interaction of intrinsic and extrinsic factors Social and physical environments influence health
Views of disability	Afflictions due to either sinfulness and deviancy, or impairments that indicated a special relationship with higher powers	Impairments and disability are a result of disease, illness, injury, and other abnormal health conditions; impairments are the cause of disability	Social, economic, and political factors create disability along with individual characteristics

Table 7-2.

individual health condition status rather than the capacity or opportunity to participate in desired life activities. Moreover, social, economic, and political policies based on these classifications created a climate of exclusion from participation from work and other valued life experiences for persons who had certain health conditions or impairments (Altman, 2001; Falk, 2001; Longmore & Umansky, 2001).

More recently, civil rights and social movements in Western societies advocating for self-determination and equal opportunity for all persons influenced both the development of a rights-based model of disability and the disability movement. Furthermore, legislation and disability advocacy and activism promoted a conceptual shift in disability as a medical construct to disability as a social construct (Donoghue, 2003; Oliver, 1996). In contrast to the medical model of disability, an individual with a disability was considered impaired or limited not based on individual attributes, but by an unaccommodating environment and society (Barnes, Mercer, & Shakespeare, 1999; Gill, 2001). Through the advocacy effort to enhance opportunities for participation in society, provisions for protective legislation and resources were established to prevent discrimination based on disability (Albrecht, 2001; Hahn, 1993).

World Health Organization Classifications

The need for a universal classification system for increasingly complex medical categorizations and consequences of health, disease, and disability led to the development of the family of World Health Organization (WHO) classifications. As part of this classification system, the International Classification of Impairments, Disabilities, and Handicaps (ICIDH) was developed in an effort to create a universal framework to describe the consequences of disease and disorders that included

definitions of impairment, disability, and handicap (WHO, 2001).

In the new millennium, the WHO recognizes the importance of revisions to the ICIDH constructs of impairment, disability, and handicap to include a more comprehensive view of health that reflects both medical and social models of health and disability (WHO, 2001). It encompasses components of health for all persons, not just those with disease, illness, or disability. According to the International Classification of Functioning, Disability, and Health (ICF), elements of health, functioning, disease, and disability, termed *health conditions*, are organized according to two dimensions: body structures and function as one dimension, and activities and participation as a second dimension (WHO, 2001).

Moreover, contextual factors, including personal and environmental factors, are significant components of health, functioning, and disability. Health and functioning are affected by contextual factors in an interactive and dynamic manner to impact health and functioning, and biological, personal, and sociocultural dimensions are included in a more holistic picture of health. In this way, these dimensions are linked to each other in a nonlinear manner to demonstrate the impact of change of one dimension on another (Figure 7-1; WHO, 2001).

Body functions and structures in ICF denote the anatomy, physiology, and psychology of the body systems in terms of degree of impairment or problems in body structure or function (WHO, 2001). The ICF recognizes that health and disability are not only internal to the individual, but also involve factors that define the ability to function and participate in life situations. Activities are defined as actions or tasks being executed by an individual, whereas participation describes the level of involvement of an individual in performing actions and tasks in everyday life (WHO, 2001). Examples of activities and participation are shown in Table 7-3.

Contextual factors are recognized as an important aspect of health, functioning, and disability. The ICF was

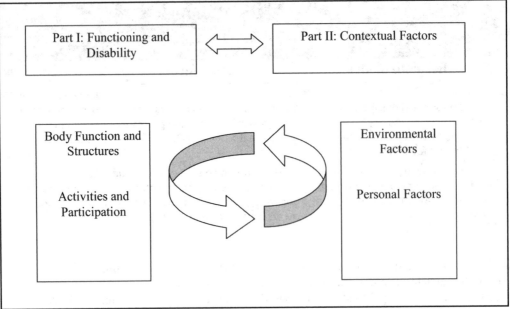

Figure 7-1. ICF: Multidimensional aspects of health and functioning. (Adapted from World Health Organization. (2001). *ICF: International Classification of Functioning, Disability, and Health.* Geneva, Switzerland: Author.)

Table 7-3.

INTERNATIONAL CLASSIFICATION OF FUNCTIONING, DISABILITY, AND HEALTH ACTIVITIES AND PARTICIPATION

- Learning and applying knowledge (e.g., school occupations)
- General tasks and knowledge (e.g., coordinating multiple tasks)
- Communication
- Mobility
- Self-care
- Domestic life (e.g., obtaining a place to live)
- Interpersonal interactions and relationships
- Major life areas (e.g., work occupations)
- Community, social, and civic life

Adapted from World Health Organization. (2001). *ICF: International Classification of Functioning, Disability and Health.* Geneva, Switzerland: Author.

developed to blend a medical model of disability with a socioecological model. Instead of classifying health, disease, and disability only as intrinsic aspects of the individual, these domains are viewed as having intrinsic and extrinsic components that have multiple interactions with the environment (WHO, 2001). Therefore, contextual factors involve both environmental and personal factors. The ICF views environmental factors as extrinsic to the individual, such as the physical and social environment, but personal factors are considered intrinsic to the individual and include features such as age, gender, genetics, personality, education, sociocultural background, and past and current life experiences (WHO, 2001). Examples

of personal and environmental factors from the ICF are shown in Table 7-4.

The interactions among body structures, body functioning, personal factors, and environmental factors are evident in the way genetics and the environment influence the nature of human disease. For example, in the United States, racial and ethnic groups display differences in incidence, progression, and severity of disease. Although there are differences in genetic frequencies that contribute to these disparities, most of the differences are due to the effects from the physical and social environment (Race, Ethnicity, and Genetics Working Group, 2005).

Disease and illness are components of health that reflect the interplay of factors intrinsic and extrinsic to

Table 7-4.

INTERNATIONAL CLASSIFICATION OF FUNCTIONING, DISABILITY, AND HEALTH PERSONAL AND ENVIRONMENTAL FACTORS

Personal Factors	Environmental Factors
Gender, age, other health conditions, coping style, social background, education, profession, past experience, character style	Products, relationships, institutions, social norms, culture, built environment, political factors, nature

Adapted from World Health Organization. (2001). *ICF: International Classification of Functioning, Disability and Health.* Geneva, Switzerland: Author.

the individual. Genetics, biology, personality, temperament, age, and gender impact the potential to experience disease and illness. Environmental factors, including physical and sociocultural aspects, can interact with intrinsic factors in both positive and negative ways to tip the balance toward health and well-being or toward ill health (AOTA, 2008; Edelman & Mandle, 2006). Alternatively, having a disease, illness, or disability does not by necessity mean that an individual is disabled or has limited opportunities to engage in meaningful occupations (Altman, 2001; Brownson & Scaffa, 2001).

International Classification of Functioning, Disability, and Health and Occupational Performance

The Framework (AOTA, 2008) has much in common with the ICF, with its emphasis on health and functioning as related to participation in life tasks and activities. Both frameworks provide a shared language regarding the domains of health, functioning, disability, participation, and activity (AOTA, 2008; WHO, 2001). In the framework, body function and body structures as described in the ICF are situated within client factors. In addition, the ICF conceptualizes activities and participation as centrally located within areas of occupation. Finally, ICF environmental factors are congruent with the framework constructs of context (AOTA, 2008; WHO, 2001). Both the framework and the ICF acknowledge the central role of participation and the environment as contributors to health and disability (AOTA, 2008; WHO, 2001). The framework further asserts that the essence of occupational engagement is a vital link to health and participation. Occupational performance becomes an interactive and dynamic engagement of an individual within environments that support and/or inhibit health and well-being (AOTA, 2008).

Importance of Occupation in Relation to Health

In order to promote health, it is necessary to discover the occupations that are meaningful to the individual in the community. Personal motivation is reflective of an established meaning in life and the roles and routines of one's lifestyle. Referring back to the occupational therapy student narratives of health, the students who indicated that they were healthy used self-descriptors such as active, motivated, energetic, and goal oriented. However, when students commented on disease characteristics, they used self-descriptors that included the terms unmotivated, exhausted, and preoccupied. It is possible for illness to be exacerbated or reduced depending on our ability to participate in meaningful occupations (Bridle, 1999). In addition, it is possible for individuals with terminal illness to maintain well-being when they are actively engaged in occupations (Lyons, Orozovic, Davis, & Newman, 2002).

Consider how you feel when you are ill. How does being ill change your daily routines and your lifestyle? Occupational therapy professionals play a key role in health promotion with individuals in the community through promoting healthy lifestyles, incorporating occupation into existing health programs, and advocating for community and individual needs. It is important to remember that health promotion is an approach that "does not assume a disability is present or that any factors would interfere with performance" (Brownson & Scaffa, 2001, p. 657). AOTA identifies various interventions that may enhance the occupational therapist and occupational therapy assistant's role in health promotion. Examples of health promotion interventions include advocating for safe playgrounds, promoting policies that support economic self-determination for all persons, and training business personnel about disability etiquette (Brownson & Scaffa, 2001).

Health promotion is relevant within the context of occupational performance because the effects of illness and disease are influenced by environmental factors, and such factors influence personal health. Individuals rely on community supports and resources for optimal performance. Partnerships in health are critical for the overall well-being of individuals in community with others. Healthy People 2010, now updated to Healthy People 2020, a joint document developed by the United States Public Health Service and the United States Department of Health and Human Services (HHS), encourages partnerships in health and delineates core health objectives to increase quality and years of healthy life and to eliminate health disparities (HHS, 2000).

Partnerships for Health: Health Promotion and Disease Prevention

Health promotion from an occupational perspective involves not only the prevention and reduction of illness, injury, trauma, and disability, but also the enhancement of health and well-being of all persons through the promotion of healthy lifestyle practices and healthy communities (Brownson & Scaffa, 2001).

Acknowledging Wilcock's (1998) occupational perspective relating to health and occupational performance is essential. She articulated that, for health and well-being to be present in individuals and communities alike, the following must occur for engagement in occupation (p. 123):

- Have meaning and be balanced between capacities.
- Provide optimal opportunity for desired growth in individuals or groups.
- Be flexible enough to develop and change according to context and choice.
- Be compatible with sustaining ecology and sociocultural values.

Occupational therapists and occupational therapy assistants should be mindful of the preceding qualities in order to improve the effects of health and disease on clients' performance. We also encourage practitioners to ask many questions until they arrive at a comfortable knowledge of the occupational profile of their clients. It is through such questioning or interviews that we develop a trusting relationship between the therapist and client. Mutual interview is preferred in order to honor collaboration with occupational therapists, occupational therapy assistants, and clients. Hence, the therapist is sharing stories and examples of his or her own experiences to guide the client toward sharing his or her experiences. Some other traits that we have found to be transforming in the therapist-client relationship are to recognize that health and/or disease is a normal part of the client's life and to look for the client's strengths and positive health indicators rather than focusing on disease specifics.

Occupational therapists and occupational therapy assistants are in a position to advocate for health promotion regardless of a person's current impairment. For instance, imagine that you are working with a client that has a wrist fracture and a long history of major depressive disorder. She is also obese and inactive. The physician referral calls for upper extremity rehabilitation, including strengthening, functional and home safety assessments, and a medication maintenance plan. However, you, the therapist, know that more services are necessary to improve this person's overall health. Therefore, you request and are granted additional referrals for nutrition and activity planning that will promote healthy living at home. Partnering with other professionals and seeking external resources would be necessary for this client's well-being.

We have worked collaboratively with multiple organizations and agencies including school systems, nonprofits, businesses, and institutions as consultants and trainers in health promotion. We have chosen three case studies to help you better understand perspectives of health and disability. In these examples, composites of persons have been used and client names and identifying information have been removed. You will meet Carrie, Salvatore, and Thomas, who exemplify the effects of health, disease, and disability on occupational performance within their own cultural context.

Summary

This chapter examined health as a dynamic process that is ever changing based on the individual, his or her occupational performance, and the environment. You should be able to discuss the importance of health, disease, and disability from multiple perspectives both intrinsic and extrinsic to the person. Persons are more than their disease processes, as explained through the occupational therapy perspective and the WHO's ICF framework. We encourage occupational therapy students to continue learning about health promotion and disability along with the effects occupational performance can have on well-being. Understanding the role of occupation in health promotion is necessary early on in your education, such that you may appreciate the complexity of health when collaborating and advocating for and with clients.

Student Self-Assessment

1. The ICF provides a framework that describes functioning as an interaction between health conditions and the environment. Compare and contrast an occupational perspective of health with perspectives within the ICF.

Carrie's Story: Case Study

Carrie is an artist who experienced a stroke several years ago. She currently is not able to work as a mortgage broker at a bank owing to frequent seizures and difficulties in speaking. Carrie uses her work as an artist as a means to support herself and as an expression of her feelings and experiences as a person with a disability. Carrie is a mentor and partner with occupational therapy students who are learning about environmental strengths and barriers to persons with disabilities who are participating in their local arts and entertainment venues. As Carrie and the students visit an art gallery to investigate physical and social barriers and make recommendations, they realize that the staff has not been trained in disability etiquette. Carrie also notes that the gallery brochure, labels for exhibits, and other signage would not be accessible to persons with visual concerns. The students and Carrie discussed with the staff that if disability etiquette staff training and minor signage changes were put in place, the gallery would be more welcoming to all persons, not just persons without disabilities. This case is an example of how the physical and social environments interact with individual capacities and abilities in a way that could disable an individual by limiting access and participation.

This case is an example of how the physical and social environments can interact with individual capacities and abilities in a way that promotes exclusion and marginalization by limiting access and participation to certain individuals. Due to her personal experiences, disability training, and previous interactions with persons with disabilities, Carrie had an increased awareness and knowledge of potential problems that persons might encounter in enjoying the gallery offerings. The occupational therapy students were skilled in analyzing client personal factors, environmental factors, and activity demands in terms of how these interact with client occupations. Together, Carrie and the students discussed how the contexts or interrelated environmental conditions, such as the physical, personal, social, cultural, and attitudinal aspects of the gallery impact a visitor's ability to both gain access and fully engage in desired activities.

Salvatore's Story: Case Study

Below is a letter that Salvatore wrote about his experience with West Nile virus. West Nile virus is spread by infected mosquitoes and can cause serious, life-altering, and even fatal disease.

Hello Family and Friends,

Get ready for this: I am now an official number at the CDC—one of over 30 cases this year. I have seen the West Nile virus and I have survived! Twenty days ago I began feeling a bit tired and my tummy was out of sorts. One morning I woke up with the worst headache I've ever had. It not only hurt inside but also outside! I had no desire to eat and the couple times I did it squirted right back out one end or the other. I was getting chills that had my teeth chattering. My mouth was desert-dry! My coffee cup felt so heavy! My weight had lessened and my thermal output was heightened to 101 degrees. On trip 2 to the doctor, I found out I had lost the ability to sign my name. Sonya, my wife, got me loaded into the car for another trip to the emergency room. They got me in quick while doctor #3 got me one of those glorious IVs heated to perfection.

He ordered up a CAT and spinal tap and then sent me home to wait for results. The weekend passed by and I began feeling a little bit better every day, but the external tenderness persisted. I came home at lunch and had to stay. My doctor finally called at 4:45 PM on Friday and said the results were positive for West Nile. She couldn't understand why I was so happy. I said, "Mystery finally solved. Now you can get me healed." I hadn't been out of the house in 2 weeks except for work, so I went and enjoyed watching high school football on a glorious late summer evening, played games on my computer, and then looked at emails around 1 AM and stumbled upon these messages that Sonya "The Wise, Well-Connected, Always-By-My-Side, Fleet-of-Foot, Medically Savvy, Persistent, Morbid, Well-Stashed, and Truthful" had been circulating. I guess Salvatore "The Night Owl" is back!

Thanks for your prayers,

Salvatore

Salvatore's story exemplifies the need for external support. In this case, his wife was his primary health advocate. There were many unknowns about his condition (i.e., diagnosis, unexplainable symptoms), along with many occupations that motivated him to heal. Health literacy—the degree to which individuals have the capacity to obtain, process, and understand the basic health information and services needed to make appropriate health decisions—was a factor in this case (HHS, 2000).

Health and wellness services can be population specific. Many communities focus on population-specific care for cohorts including adolescents, refugees, or human immunodeficiency virus/acquired immunodeficiency syndrome (HIV/AIDS) survivors. Thomas's story comes from a class of occupational therapy students that served as mentors through a community-based course.

Thomas's Story: Case Study

Occupational therapy students participated in a service-learning experience that involved developing a health promotion program with teenagers. Their semester-long efforts resulted in the "Health Through Photography" project. This project's goal was to empower teenagers to develop a new skill of photography while learning about healthy lifestyles through a camera's lens. Thomas, a quiet, polite teen, expressed some potential interest in photography. The teens took photos of numerous health objects and settings and brought this all together in an art portfolio for which they earned high school art credit. The concentrated effort toward health promotion encouraged Thomas to develop a trusting relationship with a group of college students while exploring various environments. The neighborhood, the city's downtown, and a college fitness center were some examples of the locations visited. During such visits, Thomas learned the importance of nutrition, physical fitness, hygiene, and environments on healthy lifestyles. He increased his trust in others and developed confidence in acquiring new skills (i.e., photography). His school then acknowledged this new skill by asking him to be the photographer for a special event at the end of the semester. The following photographs are samples of this project (Figures 7-2 and 7-3).

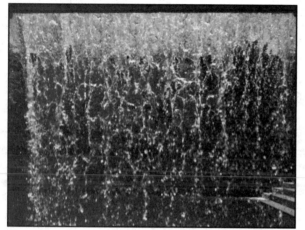

Figure 7-2. This waterfall photo was taken by a teen who was exploring environmental influences on health.

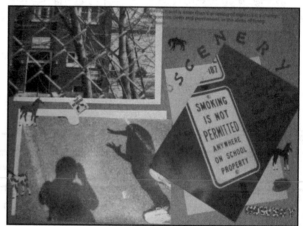

Figure 7-3. A page from the portfolio designed collaboratively by high school students and occupational therapy students.

For this project, the students chose an adolescent-specific population because there are numerous health risks facing youth (i.e., mental illness, asthma, sexually transmitted diseases, and obesity). The most common causes of disability, disease, and premature death may result from adolescents' individual choices and behaviors. Thomas is an example of the success that health promotion can have on an individual's occupational performance even in the absence of disease.

2. Going back to Carrie's case study, what are strategies that Carrie and the students could suggest to the gallery owners that have the potential to enhance participation and occupational engagement in this cultural venue? Many strategies can enhance participation for all persons, not just people with disabilities. How could the strategies you described in Question 1 be beneficial for others?

3. Going back to Salvatore's case study, how is the health status of Salvatore influenced by his occupations? If health and illness are dynamic and viewed as a continuum of interaction among many factors, which factors seem to facilitate health for Salvatore? Which are barriers to health?

4. Going back to Thomas's case study, explain the importance of population-specific interventions for the occupational therapy profession. How does health promotion benefit individuals who are not affected by a specific disease or impairment? If you were Thomas, how might your thinking about your abilities have changed through the "Health Through Photography" project?

5. As indicated in this chapter, student self-examination of their perceptions about health and disease enhances their understanding of occupational performance in relationship to health. Return to the student health survey. Compare and contrast your personal health experiences with the student responses. What interactions have you had with persons with different health conditions? How did you respond to these differences? How have the concepts discussed in this chapter enhanced your

EVIDENCE-BASED RESEARCH CHART

Issue	Evidence
Health, participation, and wellness	Baum, 2003; Goldworth, 2005; Letts, 2011; Shaw & MacKinnon, 2004; Stav, Hallenen, Lane, & Arbesman, 2012; Suarez-Balcazar, 2005; Wilcock, 1993, 2005
Health promotion and occupational therapy	AOTA, 2001, 2008; Duque, 2004; Mallinson, Fischer, Rogers, Ehrilich-Jones, & Chang, 2009; Matuska, Giles-Heinz, Flinn, Neighbor, & Bass-Haugen, 2003; Scriven & Atwal, 2004; Thibodaux, 2005
Prevention of disease, injury, and disability	AOTA, 2001; Clark et al., 1997; Hogan et al, 2013; Kroll, Jones, Kehn, & Neri, 2006; Michaud, Murray, & Bloom, 2001; Nakasato & Carnes, 2006
Disability constructs	Donoghue, 2003; Gitlow & Flecky, 2005; Llewellyn & Hogan, 2000; Lutz & Bowers, 2005; Mitra, 2006; Taylor, 2005; Temple, McLeod, Gallinger, & Wright, 2001; Vrkljan, 2005
International Classification of Functioning, Disability and Health (ICF)	Battaglia et al., 2004; Cramm, Aiken, & Stewart, 2012; Grill Stucki, Boldt, Joisten, & Swoboda, 2005; Hemmingsson & Jonsson, 2005; Kuijer, Brouwer, Preuper, Groothoff, & Dijkstra, 2006; Pettersson, Pettersson, & Frisk, 2012; Stamm, Cieza, Machold, Smolen, & Stucki, 2006
Health promotion and partnerships	Hemming & Langille, 2006; Hodge & Nandy, 2011; King, Tucker, Baldwin, & LaPorta, 2006; Suarez-Balcazar et al., 2005
Occupational performance despite impairment	Bedell, Cohn, & Dumas, 2005; Chan, 2004; Kirsh, Cockburn, & Gewutz, 2005; Reid, 2002; Rice & Thomas, 2000; Schenker, Coster, & Parush, 2005; Wilkins, Jung, Wishart, Edwards, & Norton, 2003

understanding about differences related to health, disease, and disability?

6. Encourage students to explore diversity in health, disease, and disability. Ask them to complete a health application in another language. For example, you may access a form for children's health insurance in Spanish by going to www.hhs.state.ne.us/med/spanish%20application.pdf.

7. Review concepts and definitions from the ICF framework and compare definitions of activity and participation to the AOTA practice framework's definitions of activity, occupation, and participation.

8. Give examples of personal and environmental factors that affect occupational performance, function, and participation.

Electronic Resources

- Office of Disease Prevention and Health Promotion: www.odphp.osophs.dhhs.gov
- Community Campus Partnerships for Health: www.ccph.info
- Disability History Museum: www.disabilitymuseum.org
- Health Literacy Consulting: www.healthliteracy.com

- World Health Organization and ICF link: www.who.int/en or www.who.int/classifications/icf/en

References

Albrecht, G. L., Seelman, K. D., & Bury, M. (2001). Introduction: The formation of disabilities studies. In G. L. Albrecht, K. D. Seelman, & M. Bury (Eds.), *Handbook of disabilities studies* (pp. 1-8). Thousand Oaks, CA: Sage Publications.

Altman, B. M. (2001). Disability definitions, models, classification schemes, and application. In G. L. Albrecht, K. D. Seelman, & M. Bury (Eds.), *Handbook of disability studies* (pp. 97-122). Thousand Oaks, CA: Sage Publications.

American Occupational Therapy Association. (2007). *Academic programs annual data: Academic year 2006-2007.* Retrieved December 12, 2007, from http://www.aota.org/Educate/EdRes/OTEdDAta.

American Occupational Therapy Association. (2008). Occupational therapy practice framework: Domain and process, second edition. *American Journal of Occupational Therapy, 62,* 625-683.

Barnes, C., Mercer, G., & Shakespeare, T. (1999). *Exploring disability: A sociological introduction.* Cambridge, UK: Polity Press.

Braddock, D. L., & Parish, S. L. (2001). An institutional history of disability. In G. L. Albrecht, K. D. Seelman, & M. Bury (Eds.), *Handbook of disability studies* (pp. 11-68). Thousand Oaks, CA: Sage Publications.

Bridle, M. J. (1999). Are doing and being dimensions of holism? *American Journal of Occupational Therapy, 53*(6), 636-639.

Brownson, C. A., & Scaffa, M. E. (2001). Occupational therapy in the promotion of health and the prevention of disease and disability statement. *American Journal of Occupational Therapy, 55*(6), 656-660.

Depoy, E., & Gilson, S. F. (2004). *Rethinking disability: Principles for professional and social change.* Belmont, CA: Brooks/Cole.

Donoghue, C. (2003). Challenging the authority of the medical definition of disability: Analysis of the resistance to the social constructionist paradigm. *Disability and Society, 18,* 199-208.

Edelman, C. L., & Mandle, C. L. (Eds.). (2006). *Health promotion throughout the lifespan* (6th ed.). St. Louis, MO: Mosby-Elsevier.

Falk, G. (2001). *Stigma: How we treat outsiders.* Amherst, NY: Prometheus Books.

Gill, C. J. (2001). Divided understandings: The social experience of disability. In G. L. Albrecht, K. D. Seelman, & M. Bury (Eds.), *Handbook of disability studies* (pp. 351-372). Thousand Oaks, CA: Sage Publications.

Hahn, H. (1993). The politics of physical differences: Disability and discrimination. In M. Nagler (Ed.), *Perspectives on disability* (2nd ed., pp. 37-42). Palo Alto, CA: Health Markets Research.

Hansen, R. A., & Atchinson, B. (2000). *Conditions in occupational therapy: Effect on occupational performance* (2nd ed.). Baltimore, MD: Lippincott Williams & Wilkins.

Kielhofner, G. (2004). *Conceptual foundations of occupational therapy* (3rd ed.). Philadelphia, PA: F.A. Davis Company.

Llewellyn, A., & Hogan, K. (2000). The use and abuse of models of disability. *Disability & Society, 15*(1), 157-165.

Longmore, P., & Umansky, L. (2001). *The new disability history: American perspectives (history of disability).* New York, NY: New York University Press.

Lyons, M., Orozovic, N., Davis, J., & Newman, J. (2002). Doing, being, becoming: Occupational experiences of persons with life-threatening illnesses. *American Journal of Occupational Therapy, 56*(3), 285-295.

Oliver, M. (1996). *Understanding disability: From theory to practice.* New York, NY: Palgrave Macmillan.

Pierce, D. (2001). Untangling occupation and activity. *American Journal of Occupational Therapy, 55,* 138-146.

Quiroga, V. A. M. (1995). *Occupational therapy: The first 30 years: 1900 to 1930.* Bethesda, MD: AOTA Press.

Race, Ethnicity, and Genetics Working Group, National Human Genome Research Institute. (2005). The use of racial, ethnic, and ancestral categories in human genetics research. *American Journal of Human Genetics, 77*(4), 519-532.

Slee, D. A., Slee, V. N., & Schmidt, H. J. (2008). *Health care terms* (5th ed.). Sudbury, MA: Jones and Bartlett.

Stiker, H. J., & Sayers, W. (Trans.). (2000). *A history of disabilities* (Corporealities: Discourses of Disability). Ann Arbor, MI: University of Michigan Press.

Wilcock, A. A. (1998). *An occupational perspective of health.* Thorofare, NJ: SLACK Incorporated.

Wilcock, A. A. (2006). *An occupational perspective of health* (2nd ed.). Thorofare, NJ: SLACK Incorporated.

World Health Organization. (2001). *International classification of functioning, disability, and health (ICF).* Short version. Geneva, Switzerland: Author.

Suggested Readings

Battaglia, M., Russo, E., Bolla, A., Chiusso, A., Bertelli, S., Pellegri, A., et al. (2004). International Classification of Functioning, Disability, and Health in a cohort of children with cognitive, motor, and complex disabilities. *Developmental Medicine and Child Neurology, 46*(2), 98-106.

Baum, C. M. (2003). Participation: Its relationship to occupation and health. *OTJR: Occupation, Participation and Health, 23*(2), 46-47.

Bedell, G. M., Cohn, E. S., & Dumas, H. M. (2005). Exploring parents' use of strategies to promote social participation of school-age children with acquired brain injuries. *American Journal of Occupational Therapy, 59,* 273-284.

Chan, S. C. C. (2004). Chronic obstructive pulmonary disease and engagement in occupation. *American Journal of Occupational Therapy, 58,* 408-415.

Clark, F., Azen, S. P., Zemke, R., Jackson, J., Carlson, M., Mandel, D., et al. (1997). Occupational therapy for independent-living older adults. A randomized controlled trial. *Journal of the American Medical Association, 278*(16), 1321-1326.

Cramm, H., Aiken, A. B., & Stewart, D. (2012). Perspectives on the International Classification of Functioning, Disability, and Health: Child and Youth Version (ICF-CY) and occupational therapy practice. *Physical & Occupational Therapy in Pediatrics, 32*(4), 388-403.

Duque, R. L. (2004). Health promotion and the values of occupational therapy. *World Federation of Occupational Therapy Bulletin, 49,* 5-8.

Gitlow, L., & Flecky, K. (2005). Integrating disability studies concepts into occupational therapy education using service learning. *American Journal of Occupational Therapy, 59*(5), 546-553.

Goldworth, A. (2005). Disease, illness, and ethics. *Cambridge Quarterly of Healthcare Ethics, 14*(3), 346-351.

Grill, E., Stucki, G., Boldt, C., Joisten, S., & Swoboda, W. (2005). Identification of relevant ICF categories by geriatric patients in an early post-acute rehabilitation facility. *Disability and Rehabilitation, 27*(7-8), 467-473.

Hemming, H. E., & Langille, L. (2006). Building knowledge in literacy and health. *Canadian Journal of Public Health, 97*(suppl 2), S31-S36.

Hemmingsson, H., & Jonsson, H. (2005). An occupational perspective on the concept of participation in the International Classification of Functioning, Disability and Health—Some critical remarks. *American Journal of Occupational Therapy, 59*(5), 569-576.

Hettler, W. (1984). Wellness-The lifetime goal of a university experience. In J. D. Matarazzo, S. M. Weiss, J. A. Herd, N. E. Miller, & S. M. Weiss (Eds.), *Behavioral health: A handbook of health enhancement and disease prevention.* (p. 1117) New York: Wiley,

Hodge, F. S., & Nandy, K. (2011). Predictors of wellness and American Indians. *Journal of Health Care for the Poor and Underserved, 22,* 3, 791-803. doi:10.1353/hpu.2011.0093.

Hogan, V. K., Culhane, J. F., Crews, K., J., Mwaria, C. B., Rowley, D. L., et al. (2013). The impact of social disadvantage on preconception health, illness, and well-being: An intersectional analysis. *American Journal of Health Promotion, 27*(3), eS32-eS42.

King, G. A., Tucker, M. A., Baldwin, P. J., & LaPorta, J. A. (2006). Bringing the life needs model to life: Implementing a service delivery model for pediatric rehabilitation. *Physical and Occupational Therapy in Pediatrics, 26*(1-2), 43-70.

Kirsh, B., Cockburn, L., & Gewutz, R. (2005). Best practice in occupational therapy: Program characteristics that influence vocational outcomes for people with serious mental illness. *Canadian Journal of Occupational Therapy, 72,* 265-279.

Kroll, T., Jones, G. C., Kehn, M. E., & Neri, M. T. (2006). Barriers and strategies affecting the utilization of primary preventive services for people with physical disabilities: A qualitative inquiry. *Health & Social Care in the Community, 14*(4), 284-293.

Kuijer, W., Brouwer, S., Preuper, H. R., Groothoff, J. W., Geertzen, J. H., & Dijkstra, P. U. (2006). Work status and chronic low back pain: Exploring the International Classification of Functioning, *Disability and Health. Disability and Rehabilitation, 28*(6), 379-388.

Letts, L., Edwards, M., Berenyi, J., Moros, K., O'Neill, C., O'Toole, C., et al. (2011). Using occupations to improve quality of life, health and wellness, and client and caregiver satisfaction for people with Alzheimer's disease and related dementias. *American Journal of Occupational Therapy, 65,* 497-504. doi:10.5014/ajot.2011.002584.

Lutz, B. J., & Bowers, B. J. (2005). Disability in everyday life. *Qualitative Health Research, 15*(8), 1037-1054.

Mallinson, T., Fischer, H., Rogers, J. C., Ehrlich-Jones, L., & Chang, R. (2009). The issue is human occupation for public health promotion: New directions for occupational therapy practice with persons with arthritis. *American Journal of Occupational Therapy, 63,* 220-226.

Matuska, K., Giles-Heinz, A., Flinn, N., Neighbor, M., & Bass-Haugen, J. (2003). Outcomes of a pilot occupational therapy wellness program for older adults. *American Journal of Occupational Therapy, 57*(2), 220-224.

Michaud, C. M., Murray, C. J., & Bloom, B. R. (2001). Burden of disease: Implications for future research. *Journal of the American Medical Association, 285*(5), 535-539.

Mitra, S. (2006). The capability approach and disability. *Journal of Disability Policy Studies, 16*(4), 236-247.

Nakasato, Y. R., & Carnes, B. A. (2006). Health promotion in older adults: Promoting successful aging in primary care settings. *Geriatrics, 61*(4), 27-31.

Pettersson, I., Pettersson, V., & Frisk, C. (2012). ICF from an occupational therapy perspective in adult care: An integrative literature review. *Scandinavian Journal of Occupational Therapy, 19,* 260-273.

Reid, D. T. (2002). Critical review of the research literature of seating interventions: A focus on adults with mobility impairments. *Assistive Technology, 14,* 118-129.

Rice, M. S., & Thomas, J. J. (2000). Perceived risk as a constraint on occupational performance during hot and cold water pouring. *American Journal of Occupational Therapy, 54,* 525-532.

Schenker, R., Coster, W. J., & Parush, S. (2005). Neuroimpairments, activity performance and participation in children with cerebral palsy mainstreamed in elementary schools. *Developmental Medicine and Child Neurology, 47*(12), 808-814.

Scriven, A., & Atwal, A. (2004). Occupational therapists as primary health promoters: opportunities and barriers. *British Journal of Occupational Therapy, 67*(10), 424-429.

Shaw, L., & MacKinnon, J. (2004). A multidimensional view of health. *Education for Health, 17*(2), 213-222.

Stamm, T. A., Cieza, A., Machold, K. P., Smolen, J. S., & Stucki, G. (2005). An exploration of the link of conceptual occupational therapy models and the International Classification of Functioning, *Disability and Health. Australian Occupational Therapy Journal, 53*(1), 9-17.

Stav, W. B., Hallenen, T., Lane, J., & Arbesman, M. (2012). Systematic review of occupational engagement and health outcomes among community-dwelling older adults. *American Journal of Occupational Therapy, 66,* 301-310. http://dx.doi.org/10.5014/ajot.2012.003707.

Suarez-Balcazar, Y. (2005). Empowerment and participatory evaluation of a community health intervention: Implications for occupational therapy. *OTJR: Occupation, Participation and Health, 25*(4), 133-142.

Suarez-Balcazar, Y., Hammel, J., Helfrich, C., Thomas, J., Wilson, T., & Head-Ball, D. (2005). A model of university-community partnerships for occupational therapy scholarship and practice. *Occupational Therapy in Health Care, 19,* 47-70.

Taylor, R. R. (2005). Can the social model explain all of disability experience? Perspectives of persons with chronic fatigue syndrome. *American Journal of Occupational Therapy, 59*(5), 497-506.

Temple, L. K., McLeod, R. S., Gallinger, S., & Wright, J. G. (2001). Essays on science and society. Defining disease in the genomics era. *Science, 293*(5531), 807-810.

Thibodaux, L. R. (2005). Habitus and the embodiment of disability through lifestyle. *American Journal of Occupational Therapy, 59*(5), 507-515.

United States Department of Health and Human Services, Public Health Service. (2000). *Healthy people 2010: Volume 1: Understanding and improving health. Objectives for improving health* (2nd ed.). Washington, DC: U.S. Government Printing Office.

Vrkljan, B. H. (2005). Dispelling the disability stereotype: Embracing a universalistic perspective of disablement. *Canadian Journal of Occupational Therapy, 72*(1), 57-59.

Wilcock, A. A. (1993). Biological and sociocultural aspects of occupation, health and health promotion. *British Journal of Occupational Therapy, 56*(6), 200-203.

Wilcock, A. A. (2005). Occupational science: Bridging occupation and health. *Canadian Journal of Occupational Therapy, 72*(1), 5-12.

Wilkins, S., Jung, B., Wishart, L., Edwards, M., & Norton, S. G. (2003). The effectiveness of community-based occupational therapy education and functional training programs for older adults: A critical literature review. *Canadian Journal of Occupational Therapy, 70,* 214-225

World Health Organization. (1946). Preamble to the Constitution of the World Health Organization, *Official Records of the World Health Organization, 2,* p. 100. Retrieved from http://who.int/about/definitions/en/print.html

World Health Organization. (1986). The Ottawa Charter for Health Promotion. *First International Conference on Health Promotion, Ottawa.* Retrieved from http://www. who. int/healthpromotion/conferences/previous/ottawa/en/print.html

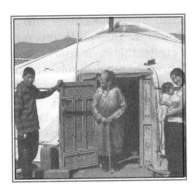

8

EFFECTIVE COMMUNICATION

Jan Froehlich, MS, OTR/L; Marie C. Roy, LCSW, OTR/L; Bethany Augustoni, MS, OTR/L; Ali Kae Arsenault, OTR; and Julie Eldredge, MS, OTR/L

ACOTE STANDARDS EXPLORED IN THIS CHAPTER
B.5.18

KEY VOCABULARY

- **Effective communication:** The artful interplay between listening and speaking with attention to both verbal and nonverbal communication coupled with an awareness and sensitivity to human diversity.
- **Nonverbal communication:** Communication through eye contact, tone of voice, facial expression, body language, and posture.

- **Organizations:** Not limited to but includes agencies, businesses, corporations, industries, for-profits, nonprofits, or practices that receive occupational therapy services or consultations.
- **Populations:** Groups within communities that have a commonality such as, but not limited to, brain injury, diabetes, refugees, or prisoners of war that receive occupational therapy services.
- **Occupational performance:** The ability to complete an occupation or activity successfully.

Introduction

The importance of communication competency in the provision of quality health care has been increasingly recognized (Alpert, 2011; Boschma et al., 2010; Fisher et al, 2007; O'Sullivan, Chao, Russell, Levine, & Fabiny, 2008; Reisdorff et al., 2006; Sargent, MacLeod, & Murray, 2011; Taylor, 2008). Furthermore, evidence shows that single communication actions can affect health outcomes (Robinson & Heritage, 2006). Effective communication is essential to the occupational therapy process, yet communicating well with a wide range of clients, family, significant others, colleagues, and other health providers and the public can be challenging.

Jacobs, K., MacRae, N., & Sladyk, K. (Eds.).
Occupational Therapy Essentials for
Clinical Competence, Second Edition (pp. 85-112).
© 2014 SLACK Incorporated.

Every occupational therapy practitioner, like every human, has undoubtedly experienced many successes and failures in communication. Nonetheless, much can be learned about how to make the communication process increasingly effective. The artful interplay between listening and speaking, coupled with awareness and sensitivity to human diversity, is at the heart of effective communication. For some occupational therapy practitioners, listening comes more easily than speaking. For others, sharing information may come easily, whereas listening is the greater challenge. For still others, the greater challenge is to communicate with confidence and ease when they are with someone from a background that is different from their own. A challenge for all health care practitioners is the thoughtful integration of technology in health care communication.

The Challenge to Truly Listen

As Alpert (2011) noted, "The commonest failure in communicating information is the result of inattentive or inaccurate listening" (p. 381). "Listening" has been ranked as the most important behavior of health professionals by clients (Harris & Templeton, 2001). Although listening appears to be a simple skill, it has many complexities that are worth exploring. Client-centered therapy requires good listening (Law, Baptiste, & Mills, 1995). Only when the therapist can listen well enough to his or her clients to understand their real concerns can client-centered therapy occur. On a basic level, listening involves learning to not interrupt the individual to whom we are listening. In everyday interactions between people, interruptions are frequent (Jackins, 1981). This occurs because, as humans, we all want and need to be listened to. Not surprisingly, it is also true that, as humans, we all need and want to listen to others. Sometimes, we find ourselves in relationships where there is a natural balance between listening and being listened to. Other times, we find ourselves in relationships were we are the listener or the talker most of the time. Unless these are client/therapist relationships in which we expect to be the primary listener, imbalanced relationships may not be as rewarding as those where there is a natural balance between listening and talking.

In many communication exchanges, if examined closely, we will find there is often frequent interrupting going on in the communication process. Interruptions often take the form of telling one's own story that is similar or giving unsought advice. These interruptions often arise as an inherent need for reciprocity. As humans, our minds are hardwired to connect with those around us, to share information that provides commonality with whoever is speaking. However, as a health practitioner, listening can be challenging when the therapist feels that the therapist/client relationship does not hold true to this principle of reciprocation. It is important that the therapist recognize that the reciprocity of effective listening comes in the ease of the therapeutic process. It is when the practitioner creates this environment for the client that the client can begin to problem solve through his or her own obstacles, thus providing the client with a sense of self-efficacy.

Given the frequent interruptions that characterize human conversations, step one in becoming an effective communicator is first noticing how much we interrupt others as we communicate, and step two is to stop interrupting. Unfortunately, this may be easier said than done. It may be particularly challenging to do this, unless we know that we too will get a turn to be listened to without interruption. Listening partnerships can assist with this challenge.

Listening Partnerships

Studies show that the communication skills of health professionals do not necessarily improve over time or with clinical experience (Fallowfield, Jenkins, Farewell, Saul, Duffy, & Eves, 2002; Fellowes, Wilkinson, & Moore, 2004). Health professional communication skills can improve with formal communication skills training. Although lectures appear to have limited use in teaching communication skills, effective methodology include small and large group discussion, role play, videotapes, feedback, skill practice, multidisciplinary panels, objective structured clinical examination (OSCE), and interactive theatre (Berkhof, van Rijssen, Schellart, Anema, & van der Beek, 2011; Boschma et al., 2010; Harmsen et al., 2005; O'Sullivan, Chao, Russell, Levine, & Fabiny, 2008; Sargeant, MacLeod, & Murray, 2011; Shield, Tong, & Beesdine, 2011).

Froehlich and her colleagues have used listening partnerships extensively in small group intercultural communication seminars for over 20 years (Froehlich & Nesbit, 2004), and occupational therapy students and faculty have generally found them to be an invaluable learning tool. Listening partnerships, which involve taking turns listening and speaking with a peer for a mutually agreed upon amount of time, are borrowed from the theory and practice of co-counseling, also known as *re-evaluation counseling* (Jackins, 1981; Kauffman & New, 2004). Taking turns listening allows listeners to develop better mental focus. Knowing one will have a turn to be listened to can enable one to listen better. New occupational therapy practitioners have noted the following about the value of listening partnerships:

- "Practicing the art of listening through listening partnerships truly taught me how to 'be in the moment.' Too often I would catch my mind wandering during daily conversations with friends and family rather than be fully devoted to the exchange at hand. These assignments not only showed me the importance of truly hearing and listening to a person, they allowed me to refine my effective communication skills for my personal life and clinical practice."

- "These partnerships have taught me multiple tools that I carry with me to this day and know that I will carry and take with me throughout my professional career. Being able to listen to my clients as well as coworkers makes for a better, safer, and more effective environment."

Because it is not possible to become a better communicator without actual practice, the reader will gain the most from this chapter if he or she sets up a listening partnership with a peer or peers who are also reading this text. Pairs are ideal, but small groups can work as well. Meeting with different partners for each meeting over the course of several weeks is recommended for optimal skill development. Then, establishing an agreement to meet with the same person on a regular basis (a regular listening partner) can further enhance the development of effective communication skills. In addition, these partnerships will only go well if the listener keeps time and notifies the speaker when time is up, and if both parties can agree to two kinds of confidentiality:

1. Nothing said in the listening partnership will be shared with anyone outside the listening partnership with the person's name attached.

2. Once a listening partnership is completed, the listener needs permission from the speaker to bring up anything said in the listening partnership.

This chapter is arranged in the following three sections: enhancing interpersonal communication skills; intercultural communication; and teamwork, technology, and other communication challenges. Focused questions are provided for listening partnerships on the following topics:

1. Enhancing interpersonal communication skills
   ◊ Not interrupting
   ◊ Nonverbal communication
   ◊ Asking questions and allowing for silences
   ◊ Listening to emotions
   ◊ Self-awareness/life story
   ◊ Restatement, reflection, summarizing, clarification/more life story
   ◊ Redirection
2. Intercultural communication
   ◊ Developing cultural competence
   ◊ Gender
   ◊ Sex and sexual orientation
   ◊ Disability
   ◊ Age
   ◊ Culture and ethnicity

◊ Religion/spiritual beliefs and heritage
◊ Socioeconomic class
◊ Race
◊ Interpreters, cultural brokers, and health literacy

3. Interprofessional teamwork, technology, and other communication challenges
   ◊ Assertiveness, interprofessional teamwork, and conflict resolution
   ◊ Other communication challenges
   ◊ Technology and communication

Time allotments are recommended for initial listening partnerships, but the learners may increase or decrease the suggested meeting times as they see appropriate. Discussion/journal questions are also provided so that at the end of each listening partnership pairs will have an opportunity to reflect both orally and in writing on what they have learned from their exchange and to provide feedback to each other on their communication skills. Although discussions are not to be timed exchanges, it will be important to ensure that each person is listened to without interruption during discussions. Journaling will offer an opportunity for students to express and clarify their thinking. Murphy (2004) found focused reflection and articulation actually promotes clinical reasoning. Furthermore, Elbow (2000) has documented that journaling can enhance writing skills—another important form of communication for occupational therapists.

Effective Communication and Cultural Competence Survey

Prior to practicing listening partnerships, the reader is encouraged to complete the communication survey (Table 8-1) and the cultural competence survey (Table 8-2). Both surveys are based on extensive literature reviews, continuing education on intercultural communication, and experience teaching culturally competent communication. They have been piloted on students who have reviewed them favorably. A number of students indicated that by simply completing the communication survey they became more aware communicators. Refinement and content validity of the communication survey was established by a panel of experts from the disciplines of psychology, counseling, nursing, social work, and medical education; intrarater reliability and content validity are currently being evaluated. The psychometric properties of the cultural competence survey have not yet been established, but students report that the survey helps them identify which cultural groups they need to learn more about. Once both surveys are completed, the learner is encouraged to proceed to practicing listening partnerships.

Table 8-1.

EFFECTIVE COMMUNICATION SURVEY

Developing effective interpersonal communication is an ongoing process for health practitioners. The purpose of this survey is to help you identify your strengths, areas for improvement, and goals related to effective interpersonal communication. Please circle the number that best reflects your agreement with the following statements so you can clarify where you need to work to be a more effective communicator.

- 1—Strongly Disagree, Much Improvement Needed
- 2—Disagree, Moderate Improvement Needed
- 3—Agree, Some Improvement Needed
- 4—Strongly Agree, Little Improvement Needed

I can listen without interrupting. 1 2 3 4	I can judge when to redirect someone in a conversation. 1 2 3 4
I can keep my mind free of distractions while listening. 1 2 3 4	I can convey hopefulness. 1 2 3 4
I can allow for silences. 1 2 3 4	I can summarize what someone has shared in a conversation. 1 2 3 4
When appropriate, I can offer steady eye contact while listening. 1 2 3 4	I can judge when someone is ready to hear information or advice. 1 2 3 4
I am aware of body language while listening. 1 2 3 4	I am concise when I speak. 1 2 3 4
My posture and facial expression show interest and caring. 1 2 3 4	I am clear when I speak. 1 2 3 4
I do not fidget while listening. 1 2 3 4	I can be appropriately assertive in interactions with others. 1 2 3 4
I can build rapport with others. 1 2 3 4	I can use humor effectively. 1 2 3 4
I appropriately maintain confidentiality. 1 2 3 4	I can judge when to use touch during conversations. 1 2 3 4
I can maintain compassion while listening. 1 2 3 4	I understand the importance of seeking an interpreter when I do not understand the language of a client. 1 2 3 4
I can determine when to ask open and closed-ended questions. 1 2 3 4	I can communicate effectively with people from different cultural groups. 1 2 3 4
I can identify and reflect emotional and verbal content. 1 2 3 4	
I can maintain mental focus when listening to someone who is upset. 1 2 3 4	
I can effectively use restatement and clarification in a conversation. 1 2 3 4	

Score: _____/100

Communication skills I want to improve (progress reported on goals in post-survey):

1.

2.

3.

© Jan Froehlich, MS OTR.L, Associate Professor, University of New England, Portland, ME 04103

Table 8-2.

CULTURAL COMPETENCE SURVEY

Developing cultural competence is an ongoing process. The purpose of this survey is to help you identify your strengths, areas for improvement, and goals related to cultural competence. Please circle the number that best reflects your agreement with the following statements so you can clarify in which areas you need to work to become more culturally competent.

- 1—Strongly Disagree, Much Improvement Needed
- 2—Disagree, Moderate Improvement Needed
- 3—Agree, Some Improvement Needed
- 4—Strongly Agree, Little Improvement Needed

I am aware that culture encompasses many human experiences related to gender, race, class, ethnicity, disability status, sexual orientation, religion, etc…
    1   2   3   4

I am aware of my own ethnic heritage (national origin of my ancestors).
    1   2   3   4

I am aware of why my ancestors came to this country, or if I am indigenous, I am aware of my tribal heritage.
    1   2   3   4

I am aware of the strengths and challenges of being of Native American heritage.
    1   2   3   4

I am aware of the strengths and challenges of being of African heritage.
    1   2   3   4

I am aware of the strengths and challenges of being of Asian heritage.
    1   2   3   4

I am aware of the strengths and challenges of being of Arab heritage.
    1   2   3   4

I am aware of the strengths and challenges of being of Latina/Latino heritage.
    1   2   3   4

I am aware of the strengths and challenges of being of Pacific Island heritage.
    1   2   3   4

I am aware of the strengths and challenges of being of White European heritage.
    1   2   3   4

I am aware of the strengths and challenges of being Jewish or of Jewish heritage.
    1   2   3   4

I am aware of the strengths and challenges of being Catholic or of Catholic heritage.
    1   2   3   4

I am aware of the strengths and challenges of being Muslim or of Muslim heritage.
    1   2   3   4

I am aware of the strengths and challenges of being Buddhist or of Buddhist heritage.
    1   2   3   4

I am aware of the strengths and challenges of being Protestant or of Protestant heritage.
    1   2   3   4

I am aware of the strengths and challenges of being Hindu or of Hindu heritage.
    1   2   3   4

I am aware of the strengths and challenges of being currently or raised poor.
    1   2   3   4

I am aware of the strengths and challenges of being currently or raised working class.
    1   2   3   4

I am aware of the strengths and challenges of being currently or raised middle class.
    1   2   3   4

I am aware of the strengths and challenges of being currently or raised upper class.
    1   2   3   4

I am aware of the strengths and challenges of being female.
    1   2   3   4

I am aware of the strengths and challenges of being male.
    1   2   3   4

I am aware of the strengths and challenges of being gay.
    1   2   3   4

I am aware of the strengths and challenges of being lesbian.
    1   2   3   4

I am aware of the strengths and challenges of being bisexual.
    1   2   3   4

I am aware of the strengths and challenges of being trans-gendered or queer.
    1   2   3   4

I am aware of the strengths and challenges of being a person with a visible disability.
    1   2   3   4

I am aware of the strengths and challenges of being a person with a hidden disability.
    1   2   3   4

I am aware of the strengths and challenges of being a large person.
    1   2   3   4

I am aware of stigma associated with mental illness.
    1   2   3   4

I am aware of the strengths and challenges of being an older adult.
    1   2   3   4

I am aware of the strengths and challenges of being an adult.
    1   2   3   4

I am aware of the strengths and challenges of being a young adult.
    1   2   3   4

I am aware of the strengths and challenges of being a teen.
    1   2   3   4

I am aware of the strengths and challenges of being a young person.
    1   2   3   4

(continued)

Table 8-2 (continued).	
CULTURAL COMPETENCE SURVEY	

I understand that culture impacts all life activities including health and wellness.
    1   2   3   4
	I refrain from acting on biases and prejudices I have toward other groups.
	    1 2 3 4

I am aware of the sociocultural determinants of health.
    1   2   3   4
	I value relationships with people from cultures different from my own.
	    1 2 3 4

I understand that cultural norms may influence all aspects of communication.
    1   1   3   4
	I am comfortable interacting with people from groups different from my own.
	    1 2 3 4

I do not impose my cultural beliefs and value systems on others.
    1   2   3   4
	I have learned from mistakes I have made in my interactions with people from different groups.
	    1 2 3 4

I am aware of biases and prejudices I have toward other groups.
    1   2   3   4
	I take action when I notice that someone is being oppressive to another human.
	    1 2 3 4

Score: /180
In terms of cultural competence, I want to improve:
1.
2.
3.

© Jan Froehlich, MS OTR.L, Associate Professor, University of New England, Portland, ME 04103

Enhancing Interpersonal Communication Skills

LISTENING PARTNERSHIP: NOT INTERRUPTING (1 MINUTE EACH WAY)

Starting with a 1-minute each way exchange of listening is often enough for an initial listening partnership. Because many of us are not used to being given another person's full attention, it may feel awkward to have someone listen to us without interrupting. On the other hand, others will feel a great sense of relief to finally have someone listen without interruption. It may also feel difficult to listen without saying anything for an entire minute. We may want to say things to reassure the other person or to give them advice or to let them know we have been through a similar experience so they know that we are indeed listening. As hard as it may be, it is important to simply listen and say nothing in this first listening partnership and to then discuss with your partner how it went afterward. Students report that in this initial listening partnership, they learn to "bite their tongue" before they speak. Increased awareness of the pattern of interrupting in conversations occurs immediately. It will be important to take turns listening not only during the formal listening partnership, but during the discussion as well.

Discussions will differ from the partnerships in that no one will be timing the shared exchanges.

Clinical Examples of Not Interrupting

- Bethany found that learning to not interrupt a client is invaluable in every practice setting. For example, clients who are experiencing agitation, frustration, or anger often redirect themselves when someone truly listens to them. The previously listed behaviors are demonstrated when a client has a lot to say and does not understand how to express these internal thoughts. Allowing a client to speak freely without interruption often allows the client to guide their mind to the real problem.

- While working on an inpatient psychiatric unit, Julie was able to learn firsthand what it was like to have a conversation without even speaking. Julie was working with Mark, who was suffering from drug addiction. Julie introduced herself and explained her role as Mark's occupational therapist and her role in his plan of care, but before Julie could explain any further, Mark began describing his dilemmas and family problems and, before the session was over, Mark had solved his problems without advice. "Well, I guess all I needed to do was just think it all through," said Mark. Even though Julie did not offer professional advice or problem solving, Mark was able to think through his thoughts and actions without being interrupted and took charge of his own problem solving strategies.

Partnership Topics

1. What were/are communication patterns like in your family?
2. Are you more comfortable listening or speaking?

Discussion/Journal Questions

1. What was it like to listen for 1 minute without interrupting?
2. Were you able to be successful at not saying anything?
3. What was it like to be listened to for 1 minute without interruption?
4. Would you have preferred more or less time?
5. Would you have preferred that your listener say something? If so, what?
6. What kind of nonverbal communication did you use that was effective at conveying to your partner that you were listening?

LISTENING PARTNERSHIP: NONVERBAL COMMUNICATION (2 TO 5 MINUTES EACH WAY)

This leads us to the next important skill necessary for effective communication. In addition to learning not to interrupt, one needs to learn effective nonverbal communication (Davis, 2011; Mueller, 2010; Taylor, 2008). Tone of voice, posture, body language, touch, eye contact, and facial expressions often speak louder than our words to the person we are assisting. The more we can show we care about the person who is speaking, the more they are likely to open up and share what is on their minds and in their hearts. Eye contact is a good place to begin. Offering our eye contact to someone who is sharing what is on his or her mind is one important way to let the person know you are there and you are listening. This can be hard for the beginning therapist to do—especially if making eye contact was not done much in one's family of origin or cultural group. As many people speak and share what is on their minds, they themselves do not maintain eye contact, but it is important for them to know that if they do look out, the listener's gaze is available. With practice in listening partnerships, this skill can be obtained quickly. With that said, it is important to note that for some occupational therapy clients too much eye contact will interfere with the therapy relationship. This may be true of people from some cultural groups and some people with disabilities. The observant therapist will pay attention to what works and does not work in offering eye contact.

Beyond eye contact, the facial expression of an effective listener will show approval, respect, and interest toward the person sharing. A relaxed, confident attitude toward the speaker will enable the person to share his or her concerns. Some of us are not aware of what our facial expressions communicate to others. We may convey an attitude of tension and criticism without being aware of this. Seeking feedback on our facial expressions from those who will give us honest feedback on how we are perceived will assist us in refining our nonverbal communication. Again, listening partnerships are a good way to seek feedback and refine our nonverbal communication skills. Lastly, it is essential to recognize that everyone has a unique nonverbal language. One person may make only brief eye contact, so when he or she chooses to hold your gaze it is worth noting. In addition, increased awareness of nonverbal language can be transferred into understanding the body language of group members.

Understanding tone is a crucial element to understanding the person in a listening partnership, as well as any client. Much of the time the word *affect* is used. However, it is essential to know that each person's tone, affect, and emotional state is ever-changing. When someone is speaking, listen to the tone embedded within their words. At times, people's words may not match their affect. Ask yourself why that may be. Specific medications often mask emotion or cause emotional liability. Being aware of potential reasons that a person's words are not matching their demeanor may help guide practitioners in a direction of more holistic and encompassing therapy.

Clinical Examples of Effective Nonverbal Communication

- Marie was working with a client with dementia who was a fluent speaker of English, but who began to speak her first language, Italian. Although Marie did not understand Italian, the more she offered her eye contact and a warm facial expression, the more animated her client became. Family reported they had not seen that level of animation in a long time. Eventually, she grabbed Marie's arm and was ready to walk again. She had not walked without her walker in many weeks. Marie attributes her client's progress to her skilled nonverbal communication.

- Tillie worked with a Sudanese woman who began to share that she had lost nine children in the war in her country. She found that simply by leaning in and showing her caring nonverbally, the woman began to speak in her mother tongue and started to sob about her loss. Tillie found that it did not matter that she did not understand the words her client spoke, she just listened. Her client was then ready to engage in therapy.

Partnership Questions

1. What have you noticed about your nonverbal communication?

2. What is it like to make eye contact as a listener or a speaker?

3. What have you noticed about the nonverbal communication of others?

4. Have there been times when you did not feel listened to because of someone's nonverbal behavior?

5. What kinds of nonverbal communication have enabled you to open up to a friend, family member, or professional?

Discussion/Journal Questions

1. Was this listening partnership any easier than the first one?

2. Were you conscious of your nonverbal behavior as you were the listener?

3. What did your partner do well in terms of nonverbal communication?

4. Were you able to continue practicing not interrupting?

LISTENING PARTNERSHIP: ASKING QUESTIONS AND ALLOWING FOR SILENCES (5 MINUTES EACH WAY)

Naturally, beyond learning not to interrupt and learning to provide effective nonverbal communication, the artful communicator learns to ask relevant questions to draw out the speaker. Robinson and Heritage (2005) found that physicians who began with open-ended general inquires—"What can I do for you today?" or "Tell me what's going on"—compared with physicians who initiated visits with closed ended requests for confirmation of symptoms or conditions were more positively evaluated by their clients in the affective-relational dimension of communication. The literature on motivational interviewing emphasizes the skillful use of open-ended questions, yet also identifies a place for closed-ended questions (Rollnick, Miller, & Butler, 2008). A good open-ended question to begin listening partnerships with is "What is new and good?" Many of us go through much of our lives with our attention on our worries and frustrations rather than on what is going well in our lives. It is useful to take a few moments to notice what is going well in our lives. There may be times when it is hard to come up with something new and good in our lives, yet the client listener will give the speaker time to think about something that is new and good. Equally important follow-up questions are, "What is upsetting or challenging in your life?" or "Where do you need a hand?" A flexible communicator may notice that some people are more responsive to being asked to share a "rose and thorn"—a rose being something going well and a thorn being something challenging—or, similarly, a "joy and a concern."

As we try out these questions, we may note that the speaker pauses or runs out of things to say. Many beginning listeners have a hard time allowing for silences and feel compelled to say something when a speaker pauses. In fact, when we allow for silences, the person talking often has more to say with no more prompting than simply having a listener at hand who can stay relaxed around silences. Much magic occurs around grief and loss related to disability when the therapist can pause for silence. The client can fill the space with what weighs heavily on them. After allowing for a few seconds of silence, if the speaker is struggling with what else to say, a simple "Tell me more," or "What else?" may be all the speaker needs to hear in order to continue talking about what is on his or her mind.

Clinical Example of Allowing for Silences

- I was working in an outpatient pediatric clinic and had been treating a young boy, Lucas, for gravitational insecurity. We had been working together for a few weeks when I had the opportunity to consult with both his mother and father after a treatment session. I simply asked, "How are things going?" At first, their responses were broad, but as I allowed for silence, Lucas's parents began to express new concerns they had not yet shared with me. I learned that Lucas had only slept in his own bed a handful of times throughout his life—which was tiresome and frustrating for both him and his parents. I collaborated with the family to incorporate this new information into a revised plan of care.

Partnership Questions

1. What is new and good in your life?

2. What is hard or challenging in your life right now? Or, where do you need a hand? Tell me more.

Discussion/Journal Questions

1. What went well in this listening partnership?

2. What could have made it even better for both individuals?

LISTENING PARTNERSHIP: LISTENING TO EMOTIONS (5 MINUTES EACH WAY)

As listening partners feel increasingly comfortable with each other, more and more emotions may be shared. Emotions are neither good nor bad; they just are. However, it has been found that expression of emotions can decrease stress and tension and foster re-evaluation of one's situation. Crying can release grief and depression; laughter can release fear, tension, and embarrassment; yawning can release physical tension and exhaustion; trembling and shaking can release fear; and raging can release anger and indignation (Jackins, 1981).

Despite the emotional healing and re-evaluations that can occur with emotional release, other than young children, most humans are somewhat inhibited from emotional expression. Many of us grew up in households where emotions were not welcome or where only certain emotions were allowed. For example, in some families, it was acceptable for women to show grief and sadness and for men to show their anger. Others of us learned to only express our emotions privately, and others grew up in families where they were encouraged to express a whole range of emotion. In order for occupational therapy practitioners to work effectively with a wide range of clients, it is important for them to be comfortable listening to a wide range of emotional expression. In addition, they may find it helpful to vent to a good listener so they can think more flexibly about each new situation they are in.

Clinical Examples of Listening to Emotions

- Marie was assisting a gentleman with dementia in transitioning to a new residence. He had incontinence and started to cry and stated, "I am so embarrassed that I wet my pants in front of you." Marie shared that it was not his fault and he cried more. She reassured him that it is okay to cry, that this is a big change for him.

- Jen was working in a skilled nursing facility with Rachel, a 78-year-old woman who was experiencing episodes of incontinence. Rachel was embarrassed by these episodes and cried each time they occurred. Jen sat by Rachel's side and said, "I am here to help. This is my job. Let's try to think of some strategies to help decrease these episodes. I know I am not a doctor but I know of a few tricks to help. I can't tell you that I understand, but let me try." From then, Rachel was open to strategies and techniques to assist with the episodes. Jen listened to Rachel's emotions, impacting and limiting her ability to participate in rehab.

- Ali was conducting an evaluation in response to a referral for a 4-year-old girl, Mila, with signs of sensory integration difficulties and resistance to transitions; consequently, Mila had some challenging behaviors. She used a variety of evaluation tools and, after an hour, was able to draw preliminary conclusions about her new client. Ali discussed the session with Mila's mother and invited her to express any questions or concerns. Mila's mother began to share her anxiety and exasperation with the situation. As she continued to speak she became more visually frustrated. Ali validated her emotions and assured her that occupational therapy could help Mila engage with her environment and transition appropriately.

Each of these vignettes illustrates how listening to emotions is a crucial role in which occupational therapy plays an important part. When therapists listen to clients' emotions, they can dig deeper into treatment plans that truly will make a difference in each client's life. Emotions allow therapists to see a person at a moment where they need assistance and we as therapists need to provide this help.

Partnership Questions

1. What was emotional expression like in your family as you were growing up?

2. Were there any gender differences in the expression of emotion?

3. What do you currently do when you feel upset? Is there anyone you can turn to if you need to cry?

4. What have you noticed when you have had a chance to laugh, cry, shake, or rage? Have you been able to listen to someone when they cried hard?

5. Which emotions are the easiest for you to listen to?

Discussion/Journal Questions

1. Would you feel comfortable venting painful emotion with your listening partner?

2. What do you anticipate it will be like to listen to future clients share painful emotion?

3. What positive feedback and suggestions for improvement can you offer your listening partner at this point?

LISTENING PARTNERSHIP: SELF-AWARENESS AND LIFE STORIES (15+ MINUTES EACH WAY)

Occupational therapy practitioners generally listen to pieces of our client's life story, yet, on some occasions, we listen to long narratives about the ups and downs of our client's life (Frank, 1995; Frantis, 2008; Kielhofner, 2008). In order to listen well to life stories, we need to first have opportunities to share and reflect upon our own life story (Davis, 2011). Because our lives are filled with both wonderful experiences and many hardships, it may only feel safe to share certain pieces of our life story with certain people. Each person gets to choose what they feel safe sharing and with whom. A good way to begin to share life stories is to reflect first on positive memories from childhood. As increased safety is created within listening partnerships, it will be useful to share some of the things that were hard when we were young. The more relaxed our listening partner is in listening to the hardships we have endured, the more we will be able to share with him or her. In addition, the more our listening partner can listen to a range of emotional experiences, the more we will feel comfortable sharing the difficulties we have faced. Lastly, it is important to be aware that everyone has more depth than meets the eye. No one ever fully knows the life or unique experiences of the person to whom they are speaking. Therapists should understand and evaluate their own personal limits so that they can be prepared to hear things that are often challenging.

Clinical Examples of Listening to Life Stories

- Claire was working in home care and asked her client to share a little of her life history. Her client, who was in her 90s, began, "When I was born in 1914, and my parents owned a farm..." Claire knew she had to think fast. She did not have time to hear her client's full life story, so she validated several of her memories and then asked her to share more about her current situation and her current goals.

- When working on an inpatient psychiatry unit, Linda, an occupational therapist, approached one of her clients who rarely spoke and appeared shaken. When asked about what was bothering her, her client proceeded to tell her fragments of her life story—details of the unspeakable horrors done to her by her ex-husband.

As illustrated in each of these clinical examples, life stories can come out in unexpected ways. When asking a question, even a simple one, occupational therapists need to be prepared for how to address unexpected challenges or emotional releases by clients. Claire quickly realized she needed to skillfully use redirection after validating her older client's memories. Redirection will be addressed further in a future listening partnership. As Linda's situation illustrates, an occupational therapist may be the first individual to whom a survivor of abuse feels comfortable disclosing this aspect of her life history. Recommendations for seeking support after listening to a client's trauma is becoming increasingly noted in the field of social work and is relevant for occupational therapists (Bell, Kulkarni, & Dalton, 2003).

Partnership Questions

1. What are some pleasant memories of your childhood?

2. What are some pleasant memories of elementary school?

3. What did you love to play?

4. Who did you like to play with?

5. What was difficult or challenging about your childhood within your family, school, or neighborhood?

Discussion Questions

1. What made this partnership go well?

2. What could have made it even better?

3. Could you have talked longer?

4. What was it like to listen for 15 minutes?

5. Were you able to stay in each role as listener and as a speaker?

6. Were you able to allow for silences?

7. Were there emotions shared? If so, were both the listener and speaker comfortable with the emotions shared?

LISTENING PARTNERSHIP: RESTATEMENT, REFLECTION, CLARIFICATION, AND SUMMARIES IN LISTENING TO LIFE STORIES (15+ MINUTES EACH WAY)

In addition to learning to ask relevant questions, the skilled communicator offers restatement, reflection, clarification, and summaries so the listener knows they are being listened to (Davis, 2011; Rollnick, Miller, & Butler, 2008). Restatement, or stating back almost exactly what the speaker has said, is used when the listener wants the speaker to know that a very important piece of information they shared has been clearly heard. It is often used as a question so the client can report whether or not the listener heard exactly what was being communicated. For example, one of many events a client shared about their adolescence may have been, "Things were so bad that I ran away from home." Using restatement, the listener might ask, "Things were that bad at home that you ran away?" This invites the speaker to confirm the information and to say more. Many of us use restatement without even thinking about it in our everyday conversations. Naturally, restatement can be overused and, if so, it can be annoying to anyone speaking. The beginning listener will want to notice when he or she uses restatement in everyday interactions as well as listening partnerships and evaluate its effectiveness.

A more complex skill is reflective listening. In reflective listening, the listener listens not only to the content being shared, but also for the emotions that underlie that content (Davis, 2011; Rollnick et al., 2008). This requires that the listener be very attentive not only to what a person is sharing verbally but also nonverbally. Nonverbal communication, including tone of voice, posture, facial expression, and eye contact, gives us great insight into what a person might be feeling. When our speaker pauses, it may be helpful to reflect back to them both the content of what they said and the emotions that we detected. For example, if in sharing her life story, our listening partner looks sad and discloses that she felt left out in high school because she did not make the cheerleading squad, you might reflect this back by saying, "It sounds like it was really hard for you when you didn't make the cheerleading squad."

Reflection such as this may invite an outpouring of even more emotion than our partner had previously shared. The beginning listener often refrains from such reflective questions exactly for this reason. They know their speaker will feel more emotion if such a statement is made. This type of statement conveys a real empathy for what our partner has experienced and may deepen the trust within the listening partnership. Furthermore, as was noted earlier, despite all the societal taboos on crying, release of old grief and resentments can clear our thinking and propel our lives forward in a positive direction (Jackins, 1981).

Natural follow-ups to the listening skill of reflection are clarification and summarization. As we listen closely to our listening partner, we may notice they have shared a great deal of information. Clarification and summarizing involve identifying the key issues the individual has expressed and having the individual focus on what is most important or most significant (Davis, 2012; Rollnick, Miller, & Butler, 2008). Often, there will be a "ring" in the voice of the speaker as they discuss their most significant experiences. The skilled listener listens for this ring and refers back to the content that generated the ring for clarification and more information.

Clinical Example of Restatement, Reflection, Clarification, and Summarizing in Listening to a Life Story

- Clarice was in the hospital for a decompressive laminectomy surgery. She was being evaluated by her occupational therapist, Ali, for functional mobility and to determine the most appropriate setting for her upon discharge from acute care. This type of evaluation was typically straight-forward and brief. As Ali and Clarice discussed her history, Clarice became weepy-eyed and emotional. Clarice began sharing with Ali an extensive life story about how she had been battling cancer for 10 years, her consequential deteriorated health, and how her medical complications weighed on her family. Ali spent over 1 hour at Clarice's bedside listening to her story. Having no medical complications, children, or comparable experience of her own, Ali could only listen and reflect what Clarice was sharing with her. Ali could see the comfort on Clarice's face from sharing her story. It was not mobility training Clarice needed at that moment, but instead a caring human presence to truly listen to her.

Partnership Questions

1. What are some pleasant memories of your adolescence?

2. What was your favorite activity?

3. Talk about your first job. What was difficult or challenging about being an adolescent within your family, school, church, community, or neighborhood?

4. What is/was great/challenging about being a young adult? What is great/challenging about being an adult?

Discussion/Journal Questions

1. Was it helpful to continue to discuss life stories?

2. Did you use restatement, reflection, or clarification as you listened to your partner?

3. If so, did it work well from your partner's point of view?

4. Are you comfortable receiving both positive and constructive feedback from your partner?

LISTENING PARTNERSHIP: REDIRECTION (5 MINUTES EACH WAY)

Practitioners must build rapport with their clients, develop individualized plans of care, and carry out treatment plans while acting in accordance with heavy caseload demands, productivity requirements, and time constraints. As was noted in the section on life stories, it is befitting for practitioners to develop tactful and tasteful methods for redirecting or concluding conversations with clients at appropriate times (Taylor, 2008).

Clinical Examples of Redirection

- Ali describes her first fieldwork rotation in an acute care setting—it was a fast-paced environment that required prioritization and time-management skills:

  I quickly learned that my friendly disposition made it difficult to end conversations once they progressed from clinical relevance to being sociable. For me, one of the most effective methods to politely end a conversation was to say, "Thank you for your time today, Mrs. Smith. I've enjoyed chatting with you, but, unfortunately, I have some other business to attend to." My clients appreciated the few minutes of extra time and understood I had other responsibilities.

- Julie was working in a skilled nursing facility when she met John, a 43-year-old male with a traumatic brain injury from a fall as well a right cerebral vascular accident resulting in left hemiparesis. John wanted to tell Julie his life story when he saw her each day. Julie quickly learned that this gentleman needed to be redirected in order to continue his skilled treatment session. Social cues were difficult for John to understand secondary to his brain injury and stroke, but Julie was able to redirect John by looking him in the eyes and explaining how important it was to focus on the task at hand. Julie stated, "Each time we complete an activity together, I want you to tell me one aspect of your life." John agreed and was able to continue on with therapy.

Partnership Questions

1. Discuss a time when you wanted to redirect someone and were or were not successful. What was this like?

2. Do you recall a time when you were redirected in a conversation? What was this like?

Discussion/Journal Questions

1. What do you anticipate it will be like to redirect clients in your future practice?

2. What clients in what types of situations will be harder to redirect?

Intercultural Communication

LISTENING PARTNERSHIP: DEVELOPING CULTURAL COMPETENCE (15+ MINUTES EACH WAY)

As humans, we are much more alike than we are different. Yet the societies that we live in tend to emphasize our differences in the areas of gender, race, class, culture, religion, physical ability/disability, country or origin, languages, body size, and sexual orientation (Rothenberg, 1998; Royeen & Crabtree, 2006). All of us have intersecting identities—we may be of African heritage, a female lawyer, and have a physical disability; or a working class Jewish male who is a truck driver. Each identity is significant, and the intersection of identities is also significant. The reader is referred to the work of Balcazar, Suarez-Balcazar, Taylor-Ritzler, and Keys (2010) for a thorough analysis of the nexus of race, culture, and disability in rehabilitation.

Although some of us may feel proud of our different identities, many of us are mistreated and made to feel badly about our differences through prejudice, discrimination, social conditioning, and oppression. Jackins (1997) defines oppression as "the systematic mistreatment of a group of people by the society and/or by another group of people who serve as agents of the society, with the mistreatment encouraged or enforced by society and its culture" (p. 151). Internalized oppression occurs when groups of oppressed people begin to believe the negative messages, lies, and misinformation that society has directed toward them. With this action, they invalidate not only themselves, but also other members of their group (Kauffman & New, 2004). This process, also called *horizontal violence*, has received significant attention in the nursing field to address the phenomenon of nurses mistreating other nurses (St. Pierre & Holmes, 2008).

As listening partners begin to feel more comfortable with each other, they will find it useful to explore diversity within themselves. In doing so, they can look at both what has been positive about being a member of a particular group and what has been challenging about being a member of a particular group. Ultimately, by engaging in this type of self-examination with a supportive listener, they can begin to heal from any mistreatment they have endured as members of different groups and take greater pride in all aspects of themselves (Brown & Mazza, 1997). In addition, as Black and Wells (2007) have pointed out, engaging in this type of self-reflection is an important step in becoming a culturally competent therapist. One cannot be responsive and sensitive to diversity in others if one has not first looked at diversity within oneself. Therefore, the next several listening partnerships will give the reader many opportunities to explore diversity within themselves and learn about diversity within their peers. In addition, since knowledge gathering is an essential component of cultural competence, many sources are cited in this chapter for additional information on human diversity.

Partnership Questions

1. Were you ever in the minority in your neighborhood, school, church, or social situation as you were growing up? If so, what was this like?

2. Were there ever times that you felt mistreated as a member of a particular group? What was this like?

3. Talk about times that you made friends with someone that crossed a line of gender, race, class, culture, sexual orientation, age, physical ability or disability, language, or country of origin, etc.

Discussion/Journal Questions

1. What was it like to dialogue about diversity?

2. How much time did your need for this partnership?

LISTENING PARTNERSHIP: GENDER— SHARING SOME OF YOUR OWN LIFE STORY AS YOU ARE LISTENING (15+ MINUTES EACH WAY)

The beauty of listening partnerships is that both individuals agree to take turns listening to one another. Knowing you will have a turn to be heard enables many beginner listeners to refrain from sharing his or her life story while listening to the life story of another. Yet the question always arises: might it not be helpful for me to share my life story with the person I am listening to while I am listening? The answer is sometimes. Sometimes when we are listening to someone share his or her life story it reminds us of similar experiences of our own. We feel eager to let the speaker know that we have been through something similar. On occasion, by sharing a little bit about our experience that is similar to the person speaking, we enable them to keep sharing about their experience. What we need to be mindful of is not turning this into our own listening turn. Again, knowing that we will get our chance when our listening partner has finished telling their story can enable us to wait for our turn.

When men and women begin to dialogue about gender in listening partnerships, they often have quite a bit to say on the subject. It can be challenging in listening partnerships to listen without sharing our own experience. An important question for the listener to always consider is, "Is what I am saying helping my partner to continue to do most of the talking?" Another important fact to keep in mind is that listening does not mean agreement. We can listen to someone for a long time and not agree with what they are saying.

The forces of gender oppression attempt to ascribe rigid roles to both men and women (Froehlich, Hamlin, Loukas, & MacRae, 1992). Both groups are mistreated by gender oppression, but in different ways. Some of the key features of women's oppression include the assumption that women are less intelligent or less capable than men, lower pay for equal work (Froehlich, 2005; MacRae, 2005), obsession with appearance, lack of pay or recognition for the significant work of mothering (Crittenden, 2001; Pierce & Frank, 1992; Primeau, 1992), violence and sexual abuse, limited access to positions of influence within businesses and governments, discrediting for being too emotional, and the assumption that mothering and care giving are our ultimate contributions.

Society has only recently begun to recognize that men are also oppressed—not by women but by the society as a whole (Jackins, 1999). Socialization to be violent and competitive begins early in the lives of boys within the family and it is reinforced in the media. At an early age, boys learn they may be called upon to kill other men for their country. In preparation for this role, boys are systematically humiliated when they show their grief or tenderness, causing them to be hardened early. Boys and men are also socialized to believe they can only have closeness with one significant partner and that sex is the ultimate closeness. Boredom and substance use are more prevalent among men (Corvinelli, 2005). Lastly, the worker role weighs heavily on men. Mossakowski (2009) found that the association between being out of the work force and depressive symptoms was stronger for men than for women.

Even though individual families work hard to break this conditioning for males and females, society continues to oppress us in these ways. As was mentioned previously, one of the worst consequences of oppression is internalized oppression. Once we internalize gender conditioning about ourselves, we oppress ourselves and members of our own group.

Listening partnerships offer an opportunity to free ourselves from internalized oppression—especially when we can first share about our experiences with someone from a similar background (i.e., women with women and men with men). By listening well to each other's experience, we can challenge and dispel the internalization of oppression. After we have shared with someone from a similar background, it is often rich and rewarding to hear the perspective from other groups.

Clinical Examples of Communicating With Awareness and Sensitivity to Gender

- Ali was working in a hospital when she had a new evaluation on the intensive care unit. She approached the darkened room, knocked on the door, and quietly entered the room. Her new client, Li, was in bed with a battered, swollen face, bruised arms, and blood still under her fingernails. According to Li's chart, her live-in boyfriend beat her up the night before after having too many drinks. Li suffered bruises, broken bones, and displaced teeth. The first session was composed mainly of an interview and test of standing tolerance. Li was honest with her therapist and disclosed intimate details about the past night's events and her relationship with her abuser. Li was born and raised in China and had come to the states for college. She was a full-time student and lived with her boyfriend, unbeknownst to her family back home. Li confessed that this was not the first time her boyfriend abused her. She refused to call her parents or friends in the area for help and planned on returning to her apartment after discharge. Ali struggled with her own convictions that Li needed additional help and should leave her abusive relationship. However, Ali was aware that Li's situation had complexities that she did not fully understand and that Li had the right to autonomy and the freedom to make her own choices. Ali could only offer herself as a resource and work with the interprofessional team in making appropriate referrals for support around domestic violence.

- Claudette, an 86-year-old French Canadian Catholic woman, was being seen in her home after a mild stroke. Her occupational therapist noted that she was extremely modest in allowing assistance with self-care. Across several occupational therapy visits, Claudette discussed the recent loss of her husband and shared that he had been physically and sexually abusive to her and that she had been sexually abused as a child. She also proudly shared that one night when her husband was very drunk, she shaved a cross on his chest. When he awoke, he thought it was a sign from God and the drinking and abuse stopped for a while.

Male individuals are not inherently dominating, but boys learn at an early age that it will be their job to dominate and control women. Although many men resist the pull to re-enact violence they endured as boys, there is a tendency to re-enact childhood violence on intimate partners as adults (Whitfield, Anda, Dube, & Felitti, 2003). The reader is referred to the work of Javaherian, Krabacher, Adnriacco, and German (2007) and the *American Occupational Therapy Association Occupational Therapy Services for Individuals Who Have Experienced Domestic Violence (Statement)* published in 2011 for more guidance on the occupational therapy role in addressing the complexities of domestic violence.

Partnership Questions

1. What is great about being male/female?
2. What is challenging about being male/female?
3. What do you not like about your own gender?
4. When have you stood up to gender oppression?
5. When have you been an effective ally to the other gender?

Discussion Questions

1. What was it like to engage in this listening partnership?
2. Were you able to listen to your partner without interrupting?
3. Did you or your partner find that it was useful to share any of your own story as your partner was speaking?
4. Can you decide to ask these questions of someone of the other gender who is not a listening partner?

LISTENING PARTNERSHIPS: SEX AND SEXUAL ORIENTATION (15+ MINUTES EACH WAY)

Regardless of one's sexual orientation, we all grow up with some confusions and embarrassments about sex and sexuality. In attempting to communicate with us about sex when we were young, family members, clergy, and teachers did their best to share helpful information, but generally also shared some embarrassment, awkwardness, and perhaps even misinformation. Because sexuality is a part of life that many occupational therapy practitioners address in their interventions with clients, it is important to work toward increasing comfort with the subject so that open communication can occur.

In addition, increased comfort with the subject of human sexuality will most likely increase one's comfort in discussing sexual orientation. A number of occupational therapy practitioners have identified that homophobia is a barrier to gay, lesbian, bisexual, transgendered, and queer (GLBTQ) individuals in receiving optimum occupational

therapy services (Jackson, 1995; Kelly, 2000; Kingsley & Molineux, 2000). Although, much progress has been made in eliminating oppression of sexual minorities; for example, the recent legalization of gay marriage in a number of states in the United States, and suicide among gay, lesbian, and bisexual adolescents continues to be a public health concern (Kitts, 2005). Because oppression continues to threaten the security of people who are GLBTQ, many choose not to be "out" about their sexual identity in their communities. Therefore, as occupational therapy practitioners, it is important for heterosexuals not to make assumptions about the sexual orientation of people with whom they are interacting.

Listening partnerships between two individuals who are GLBTQ can provide a safe place for venting about and discrimination or hurtful experiences. Internalized oppression, which places divisions between people, can be challenged. It will be useful for heterosexual people to get together with other heterosexual people to talk about all their experiences with GLBTQ individuals so they are less awkward in relating to them. As increased safety is gained, it will be richly rewarding for GLBTQ people to be able to share about their experiences with heterosexuals, and for heterosexuals to be strong allies for GLBTQ individuals in combating gay oppression.

Clinical Examples of Communicating With Awareness and Sensitivity to GLBTQ Issues

- Sarah was working on an inpatient psychiatric unit when she met Alex, a transgendered female. Alex was screaming and yelling at the nursing staff and was very difficult to redirect. Sarah was nervous to begin the initial evaluation with Alex so she approached her gently. Alex agreed to speak with Sarah in a private room. Alex began to cry when Sarah asked why she was so upset. Alex cried out that she was a "male trapped in a female's body." Alex stated that she wanted to have a baby before she became a man, but no one around her supported her decision. Sarah decided to help Alex make a pros and cons list to attempt to help with this decision. When Alex began sobbing again, Sarah touched Alex's hand, knowing that no contact was supposed to be made between practitioner and client on the psychiatric unit, but she knew that a simple touch could mean a world of difference to Alex. When Alex wiped her tears and looked at Sarah and said, "Thanks," Sarah knew she had made the right decision.

- Larry, a 36-year-old gay man, was dying of AIDS. Larry shared with Claire, his occupational therapist, that his biggest wish was for his family to accept his partner, but they never did accept him. In the end, Larry's family also did not honor Larry's wishes for his partner to inherit any of his belongings. His occupational therapist noted that now that gay marriage is legal in Maine, other GLBTQ people will have greater protections than Larry did.

Sarah's story, also shared in Chapter 9, is presented here because of the sensitivity Sarah demonstrated to GLBTQ issues in communicating with her client. Claire, obviously, also created a great deal of safety for Larry to share his struggles as a gay man.

Partnership Questions

1. While you were growing up, what attitudes were communicated to you about sex by family, clergy, teachers, and friends?

2. Were you able to talk openly about sex with anyone?

3. Share your experiences with people who are gay, lesbian, bisexual, and transgendered. If you are gay, lesbian, or bisexual and out, what has been good about your identity and what has been challenging?

4. If you are heterosexual, what has been good about this identify and what has been challenging?

Discussion/Journal Questions

1. If you have a friend who is gay, lesbian, or bisexual, what would it be like for you to ask them what it has been like to his or her identity?

2. What do you and your listening partner appreciate about each other?

LISTENING PARTNERSHIP: DISABILITY (15+ EACH WAY)

Studies have shown that occupational therapy practitioners tend to have positive attitudes toward people with disabilities, yet there is still room for improvement (Coffey, 2001; White & Olson, 1998). Occupational therapy practitioners who have had people with disabilities in their lives as friends or family members tend to have the most positive attitudes toward people with disabilities (Benham, 1988). People with positive attitudes toward people with disabilities easily notice the shared humanity between themselves as able-bodied people and their friends with disabilities.

The inclusion movement has created many more opportunities for people with disabilities and able-bodied people to form relationships. People from the United States can be particularly proud of the Americans with Disabilities Act (ADA) of 1990. Enacting a law that ensures that people with disabilities receive reasonable accommodations in employment, telecommunications, transportation, and public services has increased the inclusion of people with disabilities in the United States. Despite these advances, discrimination and oppression toward people with disabilities persist and are magnified at the intersection of race and disability (Clay, Seekins, & Castillo, 2010). The field of disabilities studies (Craddock, 1996a, 1996b; Kielhofner, 2005) promises to further break stereotypes about people with disabilities and move us all

toward even greater inclusion of people with disabilities in all facets of society.

Clinical Example of Communicating With Awareness and Sensitivity to Disability

- Jen worked on an acute rehabilitation floor for amputees and burn clients when she met Bill. Bill had just had a left, above-knee amputation secondary to poor circulation. Bill owned a local pizza shop and now had to deal with how he was going to be able to go home and work to support his family "with only one leg." Jen assumed that Bill was going to experience a tough battle with losing his identity when he lost his leg. She knew it was her role as his occupational therapist to create adaptations and modifications to his house and work place prior to his discharge home to assist Bill in keeping and even changing or adapting his identity. Jen helped Bill plan certain changes that needed to be made and Bill had a surprisingly positive response to planning by stating, "I have been a planner my whole life." Jen learned from Bill not to make assumptions about disability and identity.

In addition to communicating with awareness and sensitivity to disability, occupational therapists often need to address the complex communication needs of clients with neurological impairments. Hemesley, Balandin, and Worral (2011) found that some nurses perceive that communicating with people with complex communication needs takes too much time, whereas others find that spending more time in communication and using adaptive communication techniques are efficient practices that improve care. Speech and language pathologists and occupational therapists often have specialized training in communicating with people with complex communication needs and can play a significant role in assisting other professionals with increasing their skill and comfort in communicating with our clients with complex communication needs.

Autism is associated with communication impairment and is coined *autism spectrum disorder* because it runs on a continuum. People with autism may be mildly or severely impacted by the condition. Autism is characterized by difficulty with social interactions and impaired verbal and nonverbal communication. It is important for practitioners to be mindful that, although their clients may not be able to communicate with words, they can express their needs, wants, and ambitions in other ways. Therefore, it is crucial for practitioners to develop effective communication skills and to incorporate therapeutic use of self into his or her practice.

Clinical Example of Communicating With a Client With Complex Communication Needs

- Tyler is a 3-year-old boy who is attending a school for children with autism. He has sensory seeking behaviors and is nonverbal. He is just beginning to use a picture exchange system for communication. His one-on-one behavioral health professional (BHP) expressed concerns to the occupational therapist about figuring out what Tyler needs or wants because of his lack of communication. The occupational therapist established rapport with Tyler, observed his preferences and dislikes, and used her therapeutic use of self to effectively communicate with him. By observing his behavior she was able to determine the best methods for communication for both her and the BHP to use. The consultation allowed the BHP to feel more confident when working with Tyler.

Partnership Questions

1. Talk about a disability you currently have or an accident, injury, or disability you have had in the past, describing both the positive and challenging aspects of your situation.

2. Share all the experiences you have had, both positive and challenging, with people with disabilities. What disability would be the most challenging for you to have and why?

3. What client population will be the hardest for you to work with and why?

Discussion/Journal Questions

1. Have you noticed any students with disabilities on your campus?

2. What would it be like to reach out to this person or people?

LISTENING PARTNERSHIP: AGE DIFFERENCES (15+ MINUTES EACH WAY)

It is actually great to be any age we are. Yet the societies we live in parcel out respect differentially according to age. Young people, teenagers, young adults, and older adults experience less respect than adults in their thirties and forties. Although adults in their thirties and forties experience greater respect than people of other ages, they tend to be overburdened with work and family responsibilities. Therefore, there are certain hardships associated with being any age.

Because many occupational therapists work with individuals across the lifespan, it behooves us to reflect on our experiences with people of all ages so we can build on any positive experiences we had and leave behind any negative experiences. In particular, examining any mistreatment we have experienced as a young person can assist us in being mindful of not perpetuating disrespect toward other young people.

Although all human communication is complex, communication with young people has an added complexity because few children like to sit down and talk about their concerns. Because play is the primary occupation of children, listening through play, or "playlistening," is an effective communication process with children (Cohen, 2002; Greenspan, 1998; Wipfler, n.d.). One of the primary tenets of playlistening is to turn the table on the power dynamic where adults are always in charge and to offer time-limited opportunities for a young person to take the lead in play and have the adult follow.

Clinical Example of Communicating With Awareness and Sensitivity to Children

- Some practitioners have the misconception that just because children are young they lack the knowledge and insight to contribute to their own plans of care. In my experience, many children can acknowledge what is difficult for them and aid in their own treatment. I worked with John, a young boy with incoordination problems. He was hesitant to begin therapy. I utilized playful listening to better understand what intrigued him. I could use this information to create an environment that promoted success without making John feel like he was "working." John was able to take the lead in constructing an obstacle course. He became proud of what he was making and was willing to work hard to complete the course while simultaneously challenging his coordination. Because John felt empowered, he continued to provide input during therapy.

Partnership Questions

1. Have you ever been mistreated for being a particular age?

2. What is it like to relate to children?

3. Is it particularly challenging to relate to young people of a particular age? If so what was your life like at that age?

4. What is it like to relate to adults? What have been positive and negative experiences with adults?

5. What concerns you about growing older?

6. What have been your experiences, positive and negative, with elders?

7. How would you like to be treated as an elder?

Discussion Questions

1. Would you like to have a regular listening partner at this point?

2. What have you noticed about yourself as a listener and talker now that you have engaged in many listening partnerships?

LISTENING PARTNERSHIP: RELIGIOUS/ SPIRITUAL BELIEFS AND HERITAGE (15+ MINUTES EACH WAY)

Religion and spirituality can be a powerful source of hope, inspiration, connection, and meaning in people's lives. Yet, at the same time, humanity remains divided around religion. People are oppressed for their particular religious or spiritual beliefs, wars continue to be fought on the basis of these differences, and some religious and spiritual traditions enforce hurtful rigidities upon its participants.

Egan and Swedersky (2003) and Farrar (2001) note that, despite considerable literature describing the potential place of spirituality in occupational therapy practice, many occupational therapists continue to be uncomfortable with the concept of spirituality in practice. Listening partnerships can help occupational therapy practitioners become more comfortable discussing religion and spirituality. As we become more aware of any strengths and challenges associated with our own religious or spiritual heritage, the more we can listen to others and appreciate the strengths and challenges of their traditions.

Clinical Example of Communicating With Awareness and Sensitivity to Religion and Spiritual Beliefs

- I have found that honoring clients' religious and spiritual beliefs is crucial for the delivery of effective treatment in all settings. Incorporating spirituality and religion into treatments and interactions can either make or break a person's involvement with therapy. Involving these beliefs allows clients to feel honored and respected. If we, as therapists, try to take religion and spirituality out of a person's daily activities, we are asking them to change as a person on the inside and out. If one of our clients watches the rosary being said on television at 10 AM, we should respect that routine and schedule their therapy for before or after the rosary hour. I have noticed that for the elderly spirituality and religion can be very important to their everyday routines and their souls.

Partnership Questions

1. Describe your religious/spiritual heritage and current practices.

2. What are the strengths of your religious heritage and what are any challenges or hardships that are part of your religious background?

3. What has it been like to develop relationships from people of other religious/spiritual backgrounds?

Discussion/Journal Questions

1. What do you want to know about other religions or spiritual practices?

LISTENING PARTNERSHIP: ETHNICITY AND CULTURE (15+ MINUTES EACH WAY)

We all have a rich cultural heritage that is important to recognize. The United States has historically forced people to give up their cultural/ethnic heritage in favor of assimilating and becoming "American." People have lost connections with their language and many fine cultural traditions as a result of assimilation. As with religion and spirituality, as we each deepen our awareness and appreciation of our cultural/ethnic heritage, we can appreciate the cultural heritage of others. This will be important in occupational therapy interactions with people from diverse backgrounds (Awaad, 2003; Black, 2002; Black & Wells, 2007; Chiang & Carlson, 2003; Forwell, Whiteford, & Dyck, 2001; Iwana, 2003; Odawara, 2005; Richardson, 2004; Suarez-Balcazar et al., 2009; Velde & Wittman, 2001; Whiteford & St. Clair, 2002; Wittman & Velde, 2002). For those of us who identify as citizens of the United States, it is also important to fully claim this identity and any nuances related to being from a particular part of the country.

Clinical Examples of Communicating With Awareness and Sensitivity to Culture

- Julie notes that working in an acute rehabilitation setting in a large urban area opened up opportunities to work with people from a variety of different cultural and ethnic backgrounds. Listening to what was most important to each individual gave her insight into many cultures. Creating a cooking group with other Indian women and having Julie cook a meal from her culture enhanced her occupational performance because she felt more at home.

- Claire noted many cultural variances as she worked in home care. In working with a Cambodian child, Claire was impressed with the involvement of the extended family in caring for the child. Interdependence and collective decisions appeared highly valued. When she was referred to work with a Sudanese man, she discovered that only another male could touch a Sudanese male and work with him on personal care. When she worked with a Muslim man in prison for a wrist injury, she was impressed with his strong self-advocacy for accommodations around food restrictions and fasting during Ramadan.

Listening to determine a meaningful context for engagement in occupation can change the way an intervention session is heading. People from different cultures have different habits, routines, and rituals that we, as therapists, have to try to understand, honor, and continuously learn about every day. Listening to understand about differences is essential.

Partnership Questions

1. What is your cultural/ethnic background?

2. Why did you or your ancestors come to the United States?

3. What can you take pride in from your cultural heritage?

4. What are some challenges associated with your cultural background?

5. What makes you proud to be an American and how would you like the United States to be different?

Discussion Questions

1. If you have a regular listening partner at this point? If so, how has this changed your listening partnerships?

LISTENING PARTNERSHIP: CLASSISM (15+ MINUTES EACH WAY)

Jackins (1990) describes how classism has existed as long as humans have functioned in organized societies. The vicious classism that existed under slavery gave way to a slightly less vicious form of classism under feudalism. Despite a few attempts at alternatives, feudalism was eventually replaced by capitalism—or owning class/working class societies in most parts of the world. Under capitalism, a small percentage of the population owns and controls most of the wealth and means of production while the rest of the population works for a living. In the United States, the wealthiest 1% owns more than the bottom 95% (Galbraith, 2003).

The working class has many subdivisions that include the middle class, blue/pink collar workers (or what has been traditionally thought of as the working class), working poor people, and unemployed people. None of the divisions between classes is clear-cut. People can often identify with more than one class background, so individual stories become more meaningful than labels associated with class background.

As Hawes (1996) points out, class society permeates everything and the contradictions of capitalism are manifested in the lives of all individuals. People within the working class are often pitted against one another—the middle class is given extra privileges and more status than working class and poor people in exchange for carrying out oppressive roles. An example of this dynamic is Jewish people, who transcend all classes, yet have historically been used by owning class leaders as scapegoats. They have been made to appear as the controllers of wealth and power by the owning class so whenever working class people organize and fight their own oppression, they target Jews rather than the actual owning class (Jackins, 1990). Jewish oppression persists in the forms of stereotyping, denial of anti-Semitism, and continued scapegoating of Jewish people.

Regardless of their class background, most occupational therapists function in the middle class as professionals. Yet class is fluid under capitalism. Job cuts, disability, medical issues, divorce, single parenting, etc., can change one's socioeconomic class status virtually overnight. Increased awareness related to class will be beneficial to future occupational therapy practitioners on both a personal and professional level (Baum et al., 1996; Bottomley, 2001; Finlayson, Baker, Rodman, & Hertzberg, 2002; Froehlich, 2005; Humphrey, 1995; Neufeld & Lysack, 2004; Padilla, Gupta, & Liotta-Kleinfeld, 2004; Tryssenaar, Jones, & Lee, 1999; VanLeit, Starrett, & Crowe, 2006; Von Zuben, Crist, & Mayberry, 1991). For the occupational therapy practitioner who was raised poor or working class, dialoguing about class can promote pride in one's heritage and assist the transition to the middle class. For the occupational therapy practitioner who was raised middle class, dialoguing about class can increase awareness of the strengths and challenges present in middle class life. Sensitivity and awareness of class can promote open communication and caring relationships between professional occupational therapists and clients of all class backgrounds.

Clinical Example of Communicating With Awareness and Sensitivity to Class

- John was a homeless man who came to a long-term rehabilitation facility due to worsening Korsakoff's syndrome; he was also exhibiting Parkinsonian symptoms. John required constant support and assistance, as he was not able to return to the shelter from where he came. Julie, his occupational therapist, was working with him for about a month when she realized that he did not have any clothes; he had been in hospital gowns since admission. John did have a few visitors who would bring him snacks and candy, but never clothes. Julie was torn. Was she able to bring in old clothes from her basement for John so he was more comfortable? Was it her place? Julie battled with the idea until she decided to bring in extra clothes for John and wrote his name on the tags and assisted him with dressing. Julie knew that she would not want to see her own father, uncle, or grandfather living in hospital gowns for this long. John could not take the smile off of his face as he received his new clothes. "Thank you—thank you, I can't believe it," said John to Julie as she walked out the door.

It is often difficult for therapists to witness the poverty some of our clients endure. Julie's kind actions and respectful interactions made a difference in not only John's life, but also in her own life because she knows she did the right thing by bringing in clothing for him. No matter what someone's socioeconomic background, humans often have an object, a place in nature, a house, or something else that symbolizes "home." When working on discharge planning or conducting home safety evaluations, it is crucial to remain unbiased with respect to the person's living environment. As long as the person's environment is safe, the therapist should remember that this is "home" to the client, regardless of the way it appears to the therapist. Respectful verbal and nonverbal communication is extremely important in all therapy interactions, but particularly so when therapists interact with people from lower socioeconomic backgrounds.

Partnership Questions

1. Talk about your class background including the educational level and type of work that your grandparents and parents had and engaged in.

2. Did your family have less than enough, enough, or more than enough when you were growing up?

3. Did your family's financial resources fluctuate?

4. What are the strengths and challenges associated with your class background?

5. Have you ever encountered anti-Semitism? If so, talk about it. Did you stand up against it or did anyone else? What do you remember about learning about the Holocaust?

Discussion Questions

1. What was it like to talk about class background?

2. Were there taboos in your family regarding discussion of money and class?

LISTENING PARTNERSHIP: RACISM (15+ MINUTES EACH WAY)

There is really only one human race, yet racism would have us believe otherwise. Racism is a vicious form of classism whereby people of color (also known as the people of the global majority) are treated as less than White people or people of European heritage. In terms of global economics, people who reside in the Southern Hemisphere are mostly people of color, tend to be the poorest people in the world, and are also the global majority (Powell & Udayakumar, 2000). The United States, founded on the enslavement of people of African heritage and the genocide of Native American people, continues to struggle with enduring effects of racism and internalized racism.

Many of the effects of racism on people of color, particularly those of African heritage, are obvious in terms of media stereotyping, racial profiling, poverty, violence, lack of access to higher education (Alexander, 2012), poor access to health care and poor health (Centers for Disease Control and Prevention, 2011). Occupational therapy practitioners have begun to acknowledge and dismantle racism within occupational therapy (Beagan & Etowa, 2009; Black, 2002; Cena, McGruder, & Tomlin, 2002; David, 1995; Evans, 1992; Matlala, 1993; Nelson, 2007; Odawara, 2005; Wells & Black, 2000). The effects of racism on White people is also damaging, but in different and less obvious ways. It is damaging for White people to grow up in a society where they are bombarded with negative stereotypes about people of color and told they cannot be close to people of color. No White child was born racist, but when White children first learn about race, they are often confronted with awkwardness and guilt on the part of White adults who are challenged to communicate about race. They grow up to be young adults and adults who also feel bad about racism and awkward about discussing it (Jackins, 2002). The implicit association test shows that even people who think they are not racist tend to carry unaware racist attitudes (Greenwald, Poehlman, Uhlmann, & Banaji, 2009). Listening partnerships on racism can foster new awareness about racism, assist in healing from internalized racism, and deepen relationships between White people and people of color.

Clinical Example of Communicating With Awareness and Sensitivity to Race

*   While working in an inpatient psychiatric unit, Julie was introduced to racism in ways she had never seen before. She heard clients scream racial slurs and saw them cause a scene because their nurse or roommate was of African descent. Julie found it useful to offer apologies and a listening ear to colleagues and clients who experienced overt racism. She also experienced prejudice in other ways. A client of Hispanic descent would not work with Julie because she was White. Because racism affects people of every background, it is important to work on creating a safe environment for all clients and staff.

Partnerships Questions

1. How has racism affected you?

2. What is your earliest memory of noticing someone with a skin color other than yours?

3. Scan all your memories of Native Americans, Asians, Latinos/Latinas, Arabs, people of African heritage, people of European Heritage.

4. Have you ever witnessed racism or oppression? Did you stand up against it? If so, what was it like to take a stand against racism? If not, what held you back from taking a stand against racism?

5. Can you envision a world without racism?

Discussion/Reflection Questions

1. What conditions enable you to talk freely about racism?
2. What has it been like, overall, to engage in listening partnerships on diversity?

LISTENING PARTNERSHIP: INTERPRETERS, CULTURAL BROKERS, AND HEALTH LITERACY

Occupational therapists are increasingly working with clients from different ethnic backgrounds with different spoken languages. Although interpreter services are increasingly available in many practice settings, a newer concept in enhancing communication between people of different cultural groups is the concept of a cultural broker. Cultural brokers serve not only as interpreters when there are language barriers, but they also help health practitioners understand subtle and not so subtle cultural differences that can influence health outcomes. A complementary development in health communication is increasing recognition of the significance of health literacy. Health literacy is the concept of ensuring that verbal and written health information is presented at a level that is understandable to clients. A systematic analysis by Berkman, Sheridan, Donahue, Halpern, and Crotty (2011) shows that health literacy is highly correlated with health outcomes. All health care professionals need to refrain from the overuse of jargon and integrate health literacy and cultural competence in health interactions. Occupational therapists are no exception to this rule.

Clinical Examples of Communicating Using Interpreters and Cultural Brokers

- In working with people of Native American heritage, Deb noted that her clients were often quiet and reserved around her. She filled in the silences with questions and "chit chat." Fortunately, one Native American woman served as a cultural broker and cared enough about Deb and her work to let her know that she was alienating people on the reservation with all her questions and chatter. Deb appreciated the feedback and modified her behavior by allowing for long silences and learning to just be, rather than speak and ask questions. Occupational therapy interventions proceeded much more smoothly with Deb's modified communication style.

- Marie was working with a young Sudanese child with developmental disabilities. A Sudanese interpreter was brought in for a family meeting, but he happened to be from a Sudanese tribe that was at war with the family's tribe. He was immediately dismissed and a phone interpreter services were utilized until an acceptable match was found. The interprofessional team found that making minimal eye contact with the interpreter allowed him to optimally perform his services.

Interprofessional and Intraprofessional Teamwork, Technology, and Other Communication Challenges

LISTENING PARTNERSHIP: ASSERTIVENESS, CONFLICT RESOLUTION, AND INTERPROFESSIONAL AND INTRAPROFESSIONAL TEAMWORK

As was noted in the introduction to this chapter, studies show that effective interprofessional communication within health care teams can improve the quality of client care. Meade, Brown, and Trevan-Hawke (2005) found that teamwork, maintaining collegial relationships with coworkers, and gaining respect and recognition from others were among the top factors contributing to job satisfaction among occupational therapists. Curtis, Tzannes, and Rudge (2011) note that hierarchical relationships, increasing workload, differing perceptions, language, and prior experience may pose conflict and barriers to effective interprofessional communication and teamwork. Intraprofessional teamwork, or teamwork within a given profession, can also pose challenges in the workplace (Dillon, 2001).

Conflict occurs both between members of a particular group and between people from different groups. As was noted, internalized oppression or horizontal violence plays a role in conflict as members of oppressed groups mistreat each other (i.e., women versus women; poor people targeting other poor people; nurses versus other nurses and nursing staff, or occupational therapists versus certified occupational therapy assistants). Obviously, conflict between people across different groups (i.e., doctors and nurses, men and women, occupational and physical therapists, and different religious groups) also continues to be a challenge. Fortunately, increased awareness of the experiences of people from groups other than our own, combined with increased awareness of the mechanism of internalized oppression or horizontal violence, can begin to decrease conflict and assist in its resolution (Brown & Mazza, 1997).

Many of us have negative associations with conflict, yet, in reality, conflict can be an opportunity for increased communication, brainstorming, problem-solving, and new learning. Negative associations with conflict often stem from our early experiences with conflict in our families and can be re-evaluated in listening partnerships. When we free ourselves from some of the negative emotions associated with early conflict, we can more skillfully handle conflict in the present (Brown & Mazza, 1997).

Each conflict one encounters requires flexible, on-the-spot thinking. When appropriate, the skilled communicator knows how to use both assertiveness and listening as conflict resolution tools. It is important to remember that listening does not mean agreement. Listening means seeking to understand another point of view. If the reader has practiced the listening partnerships in this chapter, he or she may be ready to not only listen to someone with whom they are in conflict, but also to assert that they themselves deserve to be listened to as well. It may be necessary to teach the party one is in conflict with to listen without interruption.

Finding our voice in situations of conflict can be particularly challenging in hierarchical relationships or relationships between members of oppressed and oppressor or dominant groups. Davis (2011) underscores the challenges that women face in asserting themselves in the presence of men. Sometimes it works to vent aggressive feelings we have toward an individual with a supportive listening partnership and note whether this person reminds us of someone from our past so that we can clear our mind and act assertively in the present (Brown & Mazza, 1997).

Studies have shown that occupational therapists (Landa-Gonzalez, 2008; Sheirton, Mu, & Lohman, 2003) and nurses (Curtis et al., 2011)—both female-dominated professions—have difficulty asserting themselves in interprofessional, hierarchical relationships. Ethical or internal dilemmas often arise during practice. Therapists may ask questions such as "Should I tell the doctor about this change in status?" When a client's safety has potential to be compromised there is no negotiating of reporting to this to someone higher up in the specific organization. Therapists who truly advocate for their clients will own the emotion of concern for their client's well-being and will go to a source where they know the problem will be addressed.

Similarly, certified occupational therapy assistants (COTAs) may feel barriers in communicating with occupational therapists (OTs). Dillon (2001) conducted a phenomenological study on the relationships between 22 pairs of OTs and COTAs. Themes that emerged from interviews highlighted the importance of mutual respect, two-way communication, and professionalism in every aspect of the job as essential to effective OT/COTA relationships. Communication themes that emerged included becoming familiar with each other's communication styles, having in-person communication, communicating openly, and providing each other with regular feedback. These individuals indicated that building effective intraprofessional relationships required concerted effort, but

ultimately allowed them to provide a higher quality of occupational therapy services and feel a greater sense of personal satisfaction in their work.

Improved assertiveness can enhance both interprofessional and intraprofessional communication. Davis (2011) describes the work of Bower and Bower in identifying a process, abbreviated DESC, for asserting oneself that involves the following steps:

1. Describing the specific behavior that is bothersome.
2. Expressing how this behavior made you feel.
3. Specifying the desired changes in behavior
4. Consequences that will occur as a result of the behavioral change.

Curtis et al. (2011) suggest a graded approach to assertiveness for nurses that is also relevant for occupational therapists:

- Level I: Express initial concern with an "I" statement.
- Level II: Make an inquiry or offer a solution.
- Level III: Ask for an explanation.
- Level IV: A definitive challenge demanding a response.

Another form of assertive communication generated from the nursing profession is use of the ISBAR, an acronym that stands for Introduction, Situation, Background, Assessment, and Recommendation. ISBAR has been validated as an effective way to improve the clarity and content of clinically based communication (Marshall, Harrison, & Flannigan, 2009).

Clinical Examples of Assertiveness, Conflict Resolution, and Teamwork

- Conflict within a professional team can stimulate improved communication and generate novel ideas. People with different ideas can offer a variety of solutions to a problem. For example, I was working as part of an interprofessional team in an acute care setting. Our client had just experienced a severe stroke. She was nonverbal, dependent in all activities of daily living, and was beginning to form contractures of the upper and lower extremities. Each team member had specific suggestions for how to prevent these contractures. Each practitioner's viewpoint was slightly different based on their professional and clinical backgrounds, but each team member shared the same goal of providing client-centered care. As we worked out our different opinions, the team ultimately chose splints and orthotics that were best suited for the client.

Working in a skilled nursing facility has taught me how important assertiveness is to ensure that my patients are receiving the best care that can be provided from everyone involved in their plan of care. I have learned that being an advocate for my clients has allowed me to be an advocate for myself in making sure that I am doing what is right for my clients. Assertiveness is crucial in working in health care and with many other professionals who have vast knowledge. When responsibility increases, assertiveness must increase. My responsibility is to my clients. When I walk by a room and notice that a client with severe chronic obstructive pulmonary disease (COPD) is unhooked from her oxygen machine, I assume responsibility for finding out why it is unhooked and making sure the staff understands the importance of her oxygen being connected to her at all times. I find that I intuitively use ISBAR for communication, as illustrated in the following example:

- Judy, who has severe COPD, was experiencing dizziness and shortness of breath while lying in bed. I checked her oxygen and noted that she was at 79% oxygen on 3 liters of oxygen. I immediately contacted the nurse and described the situation and provided background on the client, and I stated that I recommended getting blood oxygen levels to see if there was an underlying problem. I used my professional opinion to speak with the nurse and I was open to listening to her recommendations and assisting her with finding a solution to this problem.

Each of these clinical examples highlights the importance of assertiveness, interprofessional teamwork, and conflict resolution. Now that the reader has learned to listen well to others, it might be important to assert that others learn to listen to you. For example, using the DESC formula you might say:

- Describe: I have noticed you interrupt me when I am trying to speak.
- Emotions: I am bothered when I do not get to complete a thought.
- Specify: How about if you listen to me for 5 minutes without saying anything?
- Consequence: Then I will listen to you for 5 minutes without interruption and we might find our relationship works better.

Partnership Questions

1. How was conflict handled in your family as you were growing up?

2. Talk about times when you successfully handled conflict. What is challenging for you in situations of conflict? How would you like to handle conflict differently?

3. Are you able to assert yourself, or do you tend be passive and quiet or aggressive in situations of conflict?

Discussion Questions

1. Can you make a decision to use listening skills as a conflict resolution skill?

2. Do you have a goal regarding assertive communication?

LISTENING PARTNERSHIP: OTHER CHALLENGING COMMUNICATION

Although communicating across cultural differences and hierarchical relationships can be challenging, there are many additional challenges that occupational therapists will encounter in their practice. Based on extensive interviews with occupational therapists, Taylor (2008) has identified the following categories of inevitable interpersonal events of therapy:

- Expressions of strong emotion
- Intimate self-disclosures
- Power dilemmas
- Nonverbal cues
- Crisis points
- Resistance and reluctance
- Boundary testing
- Empathic breaks
- Emotionally charged therapy tasks and situations
- Limitations of therapy
- Contextual inconsistencies

Although effective listening can play a role in handling interpersonal events, the inquisitive occupational therapy practitioner will seek multiple strategies for addressing these interpersonal events and is encouraged to read Taylor's book, *The Intentional Relationship Model: Occupational Therapy and Use of Self.* In addition to offering a listening ear in some challenging encounters, because these encounters can be distressing to the occupational therapist, seeking an opportunity to be listened to may be equally important. Whether hearing a life story of illness, trauma, and loss or feeling slighted or disrespected by a colleague, client, or interprofessional team member, it is important for occupational therapists to practice self-care. Venting to a supervisor or person who cares can make a significant difference in the therapist's ability to proceed effectively after challenging communication encounters.

Clinical Example of Handling Communication Challenges

- Hazel was a new therapist working in an inpatient psychiatric unit and approached a 16-year-old girl,

Maribeth, to see if she was interested in participating in occupational therapy. Maribeth proceeded to scream and utter profanities at Hazel and insisted that she leave her room. Hazel calmly left her room and sought support from her supervisor who encouraged Hazel not to take Maribeth's behavior personally and informed her that it was not uncommon for agitated clients to respond in this way. Hazel checked in with Maribeth the next day and Maribeth was eager to participate in occupational therapy.

Partnership Questions

1. Describe any communication challenges you have faced.

2. What did you do that was effective, and could improved listening skills have made a difference?

Discussion/Journal Questions

1. Who can you turn to for support when you encounter a communication challenge?

2. What has it been like to offer support to a peer around communication challenges?

Technology and Communication

Whether typed or handwritten, journaling is a form of communication that facilitates an individual's independent thought process; it can enhance clarity of thought and writing skills (Elbow, 2000). If the reader has engaged in journaling while reading this chapter, their writing skills may have improved—particularly if he or she had the opportunity to share journals and feedback with a partner.

Many clinicians are currently expected to write clear and concise notes utilizing technology for documentation and other forms of health communication. Although technology facilitates communication in a multitude of ways, the mindful therapist will continually evaluate whether technology is enhancing or inhibiting effective communication (Mueller, 2010). Nonverbal communication can be compromised when the therapist needs to log notes while engaged in a conversation with a client. Lost nonverbal communication can contribute to declining rapport, which may, in turn, result in poor interpersonal communication and the loss of important health information. Nonetheless, some overworked therapists are finding that communication technology reduces the stress of too much paperwork.

Although some clients may not disclose any information about themselves if the therapist is using a computer, others may feel that what they are saying is significant because the therapist is typing their words on a computer. Younger clients exposed to technology may be more responsive to a therapist who uses technology. Dialogue among interprofessional teams can aid in generating creative solutions regarding how to best integrate technology with health care communication.

Although smart phone technology, email, and social media have enabled increased communication and connection between humans, they also present barriers when the use of such forms of communication become addictive and a substitute for face-to-face human communication. Young people who have grown up with smart phones and social media appear to be particularly vulnerable to overuse of these technologies and may find listening partnerships with their cell phones turned off to be particularly useful.

CLINICAL EXAMPLES OF TECHNOLOGY AND COMMUNICATION

- Marie was working with a 90-year-old retired lobsterman who noted her computer and said, "Get that damn thing out of here. If I see that again you can take yourself and your computer out of here for good." Marie quickly put the computer away and focused her attention so she could remember what her client shared. Another 102-year-old gentleman responded to her computer similarly saying, "That's the problem with today's world. People are more interested in that than people." Marie validated his perspective and closed the computer once again. In contrast, when she worked with children with disabilities, she found they were intrigued by technology and it was a great asset to the therapy relationship.

Partnership Questions

1. How have technology and social media enhanced your interpersonal communication?

2. Discuss whether or not technology and social media have interfered with interpersonal communication.

Discussion/Journal Questions

1. What is the longest period of time you have gone without the use of technology or social media and what was this like? Is it useful to identify breaks from technology?

Summary

As Ueland (2006) stated, "When we are listened to, it creates us, makes us unfold and expand. Ideas actually begin to grow within us and come to life." Over 20 years of experience teaching occupational therapy students to use listening partnerships for the enhancement of their communication skills has enabled me to witness the unfolding and expansion of my students. Students who have had the opportunity to engage in multiple listening partnerships report in journals and papers that not only do they become much better listeners, but they also become more confident thinkers, speakers, and writers. Although they initially find it difficult to stay in the role as listener or speaker, over time this becomes natural. As the class progresses, students generally report they notice how much others do not listen and many decide to teach friends and family to listen to them.

In addition, listening partnerships focused on diversity have a positive impact on students' awareness and comfort with human diversity within themselves and their peers. Oftentimes, students from oppressed groups find enough caring, trust, and safety in their listening partnerships to vent about their experiences of mistreatment and discrimination. Students from dominant groups, such as heterosexual, gentile, and White middle-class men and women report that they have been deeply enriched by the stories of students of color, students from countries outside the United States, students with disabilities, students raised poor and working class, and students who are Jewish or Buddhist. Male and female students are riveted by what others have to say about their experiences. The occupational therapy student who applies weekly time and practice to listening partnerships will make great steps toward becoming an effective, culturally competent communicator, which is a necessity for forming effective relationships with clients, family, significant others, colleagues, and other health providers and the public.

Student Self-Assessment

The following learning activities will help the learner consolidate their skills in effective communication. These activities can be done in both listening partnerships and in a journal format.

1. Complete the communication and cultural competence surveys again and reflect on how your communication skills have changed as a result of reading this chapter and completing some of the listening exercises. Describe to a peer or in a journal any changes you have noticed in your listening skills, with attention to both verbal and nonverbal behavior. Have peers, family, or coworkers given you any feedback on your communications skills? If so, what have they said? Have you noticed any changes in your ability to express your ideas verbally and in writing? If so, describe these changes.

2. What, in particular, stands out in your mind with regard to journaling and engaging in listening partnerships on diversity? Can you identify some next steps with regard to becoming a culturally competent communicator? If so, what are they?

3. Describe your thoughts regarding the concept of internalized oppression and reflect on any of your own struggles with self-invalidation and invalidation of members of your own group.

4. Have you attempted to teach other people to refrain from interrupting you or others as they are speaking? If so, what has this been like?

5. Have you used either listening or the DESC approach in conflict resolution? If so, what were your results? If not, discuss your feelings about potentially using either of these approaches.

EVIDENCE-BASED RESEARCH CHART

Area	Component(s)	Evidence
Interprofessional and intraprofessional teamwork	Conflict resolution and assertiveness	Curtis et al., 2011; Landa-Gonzalez, 2008; Marshall et al., 2009; Meade, Brown, & Trevan-Hawke, 2005; St. Pierre & Homes, 2008; Scheirton, Mu, & Lohman, 2003
	OT/COTA relationships	Dillon, 2001
Culturally competent communication: The process	Awareness/knowledge/skills	Awaad, 2003; Black, 2002; Black & Wells, 2007; Chiang & Carlson, 2003; Iwana, 2003; Odawara, 2005; Royeen & Crabtree, 2006; Velde & Wittman, 2001; Wells & Black, 2000; Whiteford & St. Clair, 2002*; Wittman & Velde, 2002
Cultural competent communication: Self-awareness/knowledge of others	Life story/narrative	Davis, 2011; Frank, 1995; Frantis, 2005; Kielhofner, 2008; Taylor, 2008; Wells & Black, 2007
	Gender	AOTA, 2011; Crittenden, 2001; Froehlich, 2005; Froehlich, Hamlin, Loukas, & MacRae, 1992; Jackins, 1999; Javaherian et al., 2007*; MacRae, 2005; Moussakowski, 2009*; Pierce & Frank, 1992; Primeau, 1992
	Sexual orientation	Kelly, 2000; Kingsley & Molineaux, 2000; Kits, 2005; Jackson, 1995
	Disability	Balcazar et al., 2010; Benham, 1998*; Clay, Seekin, & Castillo, 2010; Coffey & Velde, 2001*; Craddock, 1996a, 1996b; Frantis, 2005; Hemesly, Balandin, & Worral, 2011*; Kielhofner, 2005; White & Olson, 1998*
	Religion/spirituality	Egan, 2003; Farrar, 2001*
	Culture and ethnicity	Awaad, 2003; Balcazar et al., 2010; Chiang & Carlson, 2003; Iwana, 2003; Odawara, 2005; Richardson, 2004; Suarez-Balcazar et al., 2009; Velde & Wittman, 2001; Wells & Black, 2007; Whiteford & St. Clair, 2002; Wittman & Velde, 2002
	Class	Bottomley, 2001; CDC, 2011*; Finlayson, Baker, Rodman, Hertzberg, 2002*; Froehlich, 2005; Galbraith, 2003; Hawes, 1996; Humphrey, 1995; Jackins, 1990; Neufeld & Lysac, 2004; Padilla, Gupta, & Liotta-Kleinfeld, 2004; Tryssenaar, Jones, & Lee, 1999; Van Leit, Starrett & Crowe, 2006*; Von Zuben, Crist, & Mayberry, 1991*
	Race	Balcazar et al., 2010; Beagan & Etowa, 2009*; Black, 2002; Cena, McGruder, & Tomlin, 2002*; Clay, Seekin, & Castillo, 2010; David, 1995*; Evans, 1992; Greenwald, Doehlman, Uhlmann, & Banaii, 2009*; Matlala, 1993; Nelson, 2007; Powell & Udayakumar, 2006
	Age	Bottomley, 2001; Cohen, 2002; Greenspan, 1998; Wipfler, 2012
Health literacy		Berkman, Sheridan, Donahue, Halpern, & Crotty, 2011*
Listening skills	Nonverbal and verbal communication	Alpen, 2011; Davis, 2011; Fisher, Emerson, Firpo, Ptak, Wonn, & Bartolacci, 2007*; Froehlich & Nesbit, 2004; Jackins, 1981; Kauffman & New, 2004; Robinson & Heritage, 2005*; Rollnick, Miller, & Butler, 2008; Taylor, 2008
Written communication	Journaling	Elbow, 2000; Murphy, 2004*

* = research papers; papers without * are conceptual papers

References

Alexander, M. (2012). *The new Jim Crow: Mass incarceration in the age of color blindness.* New York, NY: The New Press.

Alpert, J. (2011). Some simple rules for effective communication in clinical teaching and practice environments. *The American Journal of Medicine, 124*(5), 381-382.

American Occupational Therapy Association. (2011). Occupational therapy services for individuals who have experienced domestic violence. *American Journal of Occupational Therapy, 65,* S32-S45. doi:10.5014/ajot.2011.65S32.

Awaad, T. (2003). Culture, cultural competency, and occupational therapy: A review of the literature. *British Journal of Occupational Therapy, 66*(8), 356-362.

Balcazar, F., Suarez-Balcazar, Y., Taylor-Ritzler, T, & Keys, C. B. (Eds.). (2010). *Race, culture and disability: Rehabilitation science and practice.* Sudbury, MA: Jones and Bartlett Publishers.

Baum, C., McGeary, T., Pankiewicz, R., Braford, T., & Edwards, D. (1996). An activity program for cognitively impaired low-income inner city residents. *Topics in Geriatric Rehabilitation, 12*(2), 54-62.

Beagan, B. L., & Etowa, J. (2009). The impact of everyday racism on the occupations of African Canadian women. *Canadian Journal of Occupational Therapy, 76*(4), 285-293.

Bell, H., Kulkarni, S., & Dalton, L. (2003). Organizational prevention of vicarious trauma. *Families in Society, 84*(4) 463-470. doi:10.1606/1044-3894.131

Benham, P. K. (1988). Attitudes of occupational therapy personnel toward persons with disabilities. *American Journal of Occupational Therapy, 42*, 305-311.

Berkhof, M., van Rijssen, J., Schellart, A. J. M., Anema, J. R., & van der Beek, A. J. (2011). Effective training strategies for teaching communication skills to physicians: An overview of systematic reviews. *Patient Education Counseling, 84*(2) 152-162.

Berkman, N. D., Sheridan, S. L., Donahue, K. E., Halpern, D. J., & Crotty, K. (2011). Low health literacy and health outcomes: and updated systematic review. *Annals of Internal Medicine, 155*(2), 97-107. doi:10.1059/0003-4819-155-2-201107190-00005.

Black, R. M. (2002). Occupational therapy's dance with diversity. *American Journal of Occupational therapy, 56*, 140-148.

Black, R. M., & Wells, S. A. (2007). *Culture and occupation: A model of empowerment for occupational therapy.* Bethesda, MD: AOTA Press.

Boschma, G., Einboden, R., Groening, M., Jackson, C., MacPhee, M. Marshall, H., et al. (2010). Strengthening communication education in an undergraduate nursing curriculum. *International Journal of Nursing Education Scholarship, 7*(1), 1-14.

Bottomley, J. M. (2001). Health care and homeless older adults. *Topics in Geriatric Rehabilitation, 17*(1), 1-21.

Brown, C. R., & Mazza, G. J. (1997). *Healing into action: A leadership guide for creating diverse communities.* Washington, DC: National Coalition Building Institute (NCBI).

Cena, L., McGruder, J., & Tomlin, G. (2002). Representations of race, ethnicity, and social class in case examples in the American Journal of Occupational Therapy. *American Journal of Occupational Therapy, 56*, 130-139.

Centers for Disease Control and Prevention (2011). *CDC health disparities and inequality report—United States.* Retrieved from http://www.cdc.gov/mmwr/pdf/other/su6001.pdf

Chiang, M., & Carlson, G. (2003). Occupational therapy in multicultural contexts: Issues and strategies. *British Journal of Occupational Therapy, 66*(12), 559-567.

Clay, J., Seekins, T., & Castillo, J. (2010). Community infrastructure and employment opportunities for Native Americans and Alaska Natives. In F. E. Balcazar, Y. Balcazar, F. E., Suarez-Balcazar, Y. Taylor-Ritzler, T. Keys, C. B. (Eds.), *Race, culture and disability: Rehabilitation science and practice.* Sudbury, MA: Jones and Bartlett Publishers.

Cohen, L. J. (2002). *Playful parenting.* New York, NY: Ballantine Publishing Group.

Coffey, D. M., & Velde, B. P. (2001). The experience of being an occupational therapist with a disability: What about being a student? *American Journal of Occupational Therapy, 55*, 353-363.

Corvinelli, A. (2005). Alleviating boredom in adult males recovering from substance use disorder. *Occupational Therapy in Mental Health, 21*(2) 1-11.

Craddock, J. (1996a). Responses of the occupational therapy profession to the perspective of the disability movement, part 1. *British Journal of Occupational Therapy, 59*(1), 17-24.

Craddock, J. (1996b). Responses of the occupational therapy profession to the perspective of the disability movement, part 2. *British Journal of Occupational Therapy, 59*(2), 73-78.

Crittenden, A. (2001). *The price of motherhood: Why the most important job in the world is still the least valued.* New York, NY: Henry Holt and Company.

Curtis, K., Tzannes, A., & Rudge, T. (2011). How to talk to doctors—a guide for effective communication. *International Nursing Review, 58*, 13-20.

David, P. A. (1995). Service provision to black people: A study of occupational therapy staff in physical disability teams within social services. *British Journal of Occupational Therapy, 58*(3), 98-102.

Davis, C. M. (2011). *Patient practitioner interaction: An experiential manual for developing the art of health care* (5th ed.). Thorofare, NJ: SLACK Incorporated.

Dillon, T. (2001). Practitioner perspectives: effective intraprofessional relationships in occupational therapy. *Occupational Therapy in Health Care, 14*(3/4), 1-15.

Egan, M., & Swedersky, J. (2003). Spirituality as experienced by occupational therapists in practice. *American Journal of Occupational Therapy, 57*(5), 525-533.

Elbow, P. (2000). *Everyone can write: Essays toward a hopeful theory of writing and teaching writing.* New York, NY: Oxford Press.

Evans, J. (1992). What occupational therapists can do to eliminate racial barriers to health care access. *American Journal of Occupational Therapy, 46*, 676-766.

Fallowfield, L., Jenkins, V., Farewell, V., Saul, J., Duffy, A., & Eves, R. (2002) Efficacy of a cancer research UK communication skills training model for oncologists: A randomized controlled trial. *The Lancet, 359*(9307), 650-656.

Farrar, J. E. (2001). Addressing spirituality and religious life in occupational therapy. *Physical & Occupational Therapy in Geriatrics, 18*(4),65-85.

Finlayson, M., Baker, M., Rodman, L., & Hertzberg, G. (2002). The process and outcomes of a multimethod needs assessment at a homeless shelter. *American Journal of Occupational Therapy, 56*, 313-321.

Fisher, G. S., Emerson, L., Firpo, C., Ptak, J., Wonn, J, & Bartolacci, G. (2007). Chronic pain and occupation: An exploration of the lived experience. *American Journal of Occupational Therapy, 61*, 290-303.

Forwell, S. J., Whiteford, G., & Dyck, I. (2001). Cultural competence in New Zealand and Canada: Occupational therapy students' reflections on class and fieldwork curriculum. *Canadian Journal of Occupational Therapy, 68*(2), 90-103.

Frank, G. (1995). Life histories in occupational therapy clinical practice. *American Journal of Occupational Therapy, 50*, 251-263.

Frantits, L. E. (2005). Nothing about us without us: searching for the narrative of disability. *American Journal of Occupational Therapy, 59,* 577-579.

Froehlich, J. (2005). Steps toward dismantling poverty for working poor women. *WORK: A Journal of Prevention, Assessment & Rehabilitation, 24*(4), 401-408.

Froehlich, J., Hamlin, R. B., Loukas, K. M., & MacRae, N. (1992). Special issue on feminism as an inclusive perspective. *American Journal of Occupational Therapy, 46,* 967-1044.

Froehlich, J., & Nesbit, S. (2004). The aware communicator: Dialogues on diversity. *Occupational Therapy in Health Care, 18*(1/2), 171-182.

Galbraith, J. K. (2003). Why Bush likes a bad economy. *Progressive, 67,* 26-29.

Greenspan, S. (1998). *The child with special needs.* Reading, MA: Perseus Books.

Greenwald, A. G., Poehlman, T. A., Uhlmann, E., & Banaji, M. R. (2009). Understanding and using the implicit association test: III. Meta-analysis of predictive validity. *Journal of Personality and Social Psychology. 97*(1), 17-41

Harmsen, H., Bernsen, R., Meeuwesen, L., Thomas, S., Dorrenboom, G., Pinto, D., & Bruijnzeels, M. (2005). The effect of educational intervention on intercultural communication: Results of a randomized controlled trial. *British Journal of General Practice, 55,* 343-350.

Harris, S. R., & Templeton, E. (2001). Who's listening? Experiences of women with breast cancer in communicating with physicians. *The Breast Journal, 7*(6), 444-469.

Hawes, D. (1996). Against postmodernism: A Marxist perspective. *British Journal of Occupational Therapy, 59*(3), 131-132.

Hemsley, B., Balandin, S., & Worrall (2011). Nursing the patient with complex communication needs: time as a barrier and a facilitator to successful communication in hospital. *Journal of Advanced Nursing, 6891,* 116-126. doi: 10.1111/j/1365-648.2011.05722.x

Humphrey, R. (1995). Families who live in chronic poverty: Meeting the challenge of family-centered services. *American Journal of Occupational Therapy, 49,* 687-493.

Iwana, M. (2003). The issue is—Toward a culturally relevant epistemologies in occupational therapy. *American Journal of Occupational Therapy, 57,* 582-588.

Jackins, H. (1981). *The art of listening.* Seattle, WA: Rational Island Publishers.

Jackins, H. (1990). *Logical thinking about a future society.* Seattle, WA: Rational Island Publishers.

Jackins, H. (1997). *The list.* Seattle, WA: Rational Island Publishers.

Jackins, H. and others. (1999). *The human male.* Seattle, WA: Rational Island Publishers.

Jackins, T. and others. (2002). *Working together to end racism: Healing from the damage caused by racism.* Seattle, WA: Rational Island Publishers.

Jackson, J. (1995). Sexual orientation: Its relevance to occupational science and the practice of occupational therapy. *American Journal of Occupational Therapy, 49,* 669-679.

Javaherian, H., Krabacher, V., German, D. (2007). Surviving domestic violence: Rebuilding one's life. *Occupational Therapy in Health Care, 21*(3), 35-59.

Kauffman, K., & New, C. (2004). *Co-counselling: The theory and practice of re-evaluation counseling.* New York, NY: Brunner-Routledge.

Kelly, G. (2000). Rights, ethics and the spirit of occupation. *British Journal of Occupational therapy, 58*(4), 176.

Kielhofner, G. (2005). Special issue—Disability studies. *American Journal of Occupational Therapy, 61,* 481-600.

Kielhofner, G. (2008). *Model of human occupation* (3rd ed.). Philadelphia, PA: Lippincott Williams & Wilkins.

Kingsley, P., & Molineux, M. (2000). True to our philosophy? Sexual orientation and occupation. *British Journal of Occupational Therapy, 63*(5), 205-210.

Kitts, R. (2005). Gay adolescents and suicide: understanding the association. *Adolescence, 40*(159), 621-628.

Landa-Gonzalez, B. (2008). To assert or not to assert: conflict management and occupational therapy students. *Occupational Therapy in Health Care, 22*(4), 54-70.

Law, M., Baptist, S., & Mills, J. (1995). Client-centered practice: What does it mean and does it make a difference? *Canadian Journal of Occupational Therapy, 62,* 250-257.

MacRae, N, (2005). Women and work: A ten year retrospective. *WORK: A Journal of Prevention, Assessment & Rehabilitation, 24*(4), 331-340.

Marshall, S., Harrison, J., & Flannigan, B. (2009). The teaching of a structured tool improves the clarity and content of interprofessional clinical communication. *Quality & Safety in Health Care, 18,* 137-140.

Matlala, M. R. (1993). Race relations at work: A challenge to occupational therapy. *British Journal of Occupational Therapy, 56*(12), 434-436.

Meade, L., Brown, G. T., & Trevan-Hawke, J. (2005). Female and male occupational therapists: A comparison of their job satisfaction level. *Australian Occupational Therapy Journal, 52,* 136-148.

Mossakowski, K. N. (2009). The influence of past unemployment duration on symptoms of depression among young women and men in the United States. *American Journal of Public Health, 99*(10), 1826-1832.

Mueller, K. (2010). *Communication from the inside out: Strategies for the engaged professional.* Philadelphia, PA: F.A. Davis Company.

Murphy, J. (2004). Using focused reflection and articulation to promote clinical reasoning: an evidence-based teaching strategy. *Nursing Education Perspectives, 25*(2), 226-231.

Nelson, A. (2007). Seeing white: a critical exploration of occupational therapy with Indigenous Australian people. *Occupational Therapy International, 14*(4), 237-255. doi:10.1002/oti

Neufeld, S., & Lysack, C. (2004). Allocation of rehabilitation services: Who gets a home evaluation. *American Journal of Occupational Therapy, 58,* 630-638.

Odawara, E. (2005). Cultural competency in occupational therapy: Beyond a cross-cultural view of practice. *American Journal of Occupational Therapy, 59,* 325-334.

O'Sullivan, P., Chao, S., Russell, M., Levine, S., & Fabiny, A. (2008). Development and implementation of an objective structured clinical examination to provide formative feedback on communication and interpersonal skills in geriatric training. *Journal of the American Geriatric Society, 56,* 1730-1735.

Padilla, R., Gupta, J., Liotta-Kleinfeld, L. (2004). Occupational therapy and social justice: A school-based example. *Occupational Therapy Practice, 9*(Suppl. 16), CE1-CE8.

Pierce, D., & Frank, G. (1992). A mother's work: Two levels of feminist analysis of family-centered care. *American Journal of Occupational Therapy, 46,* 972-980.

Powell, J. A., & Udayakumar, S. P. (2000). Race, poverty, and globalization. Retrieved from: http://www.globalexchange.org/campaigns/econ/globalization072000.htm.pdf

Primeau, L. A. (1992). A woman's place: unpaid work in the home. *American Journal of Occupational Therapy, 46,* 981-988.

Reisdorff, E. J., Hughes, M. J., Castaneda, C., Carlson, D. J., Donohue, W. A., Fediuk, T. A., & Hughes, W. P. (2006). Developing a valid evaluation for interpersonal and communication skills. *Academy of Emergency Medicine, 13*(10), 1056-1061.

Richardson, P. (2004). How cultural ideas help shape the conceptualization of mental illness. *Mental Health Occupational Therapy, 9*(1), 5-8.

Robinson, J. D., & Heritage, J. (2006). Physicians' opening questions and patients' satisfaction. *Patient Education and Counseling, 60*(3), 279-285.

Rollnick, S., Miller, W. R., & Butler, C. (2008). *Motivational Interviewing in health care: helping patients change behavior.* Guilford Press

Rothenberg, P. S. (1998). *Race, class and gender in the United States: An integrated study* (4th ed.). New York, NY: St. Martin Press. Fellowes, D. Wilkinson, S., & Moore, P. (2004). Communication skills training for health care professionals working with cancer patients, their families and/or carers. *Cochrane Database Systematic Review,* (2), CD003751.

Royeen, M., & Crabree, J. L. (2006). *Culture in rehabilitation: From competency to proficiency.* Upper Saddle River, NJ: Pearson-Prentice Hall.

St. Pierre, I., & Holmes, D. (2008). Managing nurses through disciplinary power: A Foucauldian analysis of workplace violence. *Journal of Nursing Management, 16*(3), 352-359.

Sargent, J., MacLeod, T., & Murray, A. (2011). An interprofessional approach to teaching communication skills. *Journal of Continuing Education in the Health Professions, 31*(4) 265-267.

Shield, R. R., Tong, I., Tomas, M., & Besdine, R. W. (2011). Teaching communication and compassionate care skills: An innovative curriculum for pre-clerkship medical students. *Medical Teacher, 33,* e408-e416.

Scheirton, L., Mu, K., & Lohman, H. (2003). Occupational therapists' responses to practice errors in physical rehabilitation settings. *American Journal of Occupational Therapy, 57,* 307-314.

Suarez-Balcazar, Y., Rodakowski, J, Balcazar, F., Taylor-Ritzler, T., Portillo, N., Barwacz, D, et al. (2009). Perceived levels of cultural competence among occupational therapists. *American Journal of Occupational Therapy, 63,* 498-505.

Taylor, R. (2008). *The intentional relationship model: occupational therapy and use of self.* Philadelphia, PA: F.A. Davis Company.

Tryssenaar, J. , Jones, E. J., & Lee, D. (1999). Occupational performance needs of a shelter population. *Canadian Journal of Occupational Therapy, 66*(4), 188-196.

VanLeit, B., Starrett, R., & Crowe, T. K. (2006). Occupational concerns of women who are homeless and have children: An occupational justice critique. *Occupational Therapy in Health Care, 20*(3/4), 47-62. doi:10.1300/J003v20n03_04

Velde, B. P., & Wittman, P. P. (2001). Helping occupational therapy students and faculty develop cultural competence. *Occupational Therapy in Health Care, 13*(3/4), 23-32.

Von Zuben, M. V., Crist, P. A., & Mayberry, W. (1991). A pilot study of differences in play behavior between children of low and middle socioeconomic status. *American Journal of Occupational Therapy, 45,* 113-118.

White, M. J., & Olson, R. S. (1998). Attitudes toward people with disabilities: A comparison of rehabilitation nurses, occupational therapists, and physical therapists. *Rehabilitation Nursing, 23*(2), 126-131.

Whiteford, G., & St. Clair, V. W. (2002). Being prepared for diversity in practice: Occupational therapy students' perceptions of valuable intercultural learning experiences. *British Journal of Occupational Therapy, 65*(3), 129-137.

Whitfield, C. L., Anda, R. F., Dube, S. R., & Felitti, V. J. (2003). Violent childhood experiences and the risk of intimate partner violence in adults: Assessments in a large health maintenance organization. *Journal of Interpersonal Violence, 18*(2), 165-185.

Wittman, P., & Velde, B. P. (2002). Attaining cultural competence, critical thinking and intellectual development: A challenge of occupational therapists. *American Journal of Occupational Therapy, 56*(4), 453-456.

Ueland, B. (2006). *The art of listening.* Retrieved August 3, 2006 from: http://traubman.igc.org/listenof.htm

Wipfler, P. (n.d.). *Playlistening.* Retrieved January 15, 2013 from: http://www.handinhandparenting.org/news/56/64/Playlistening

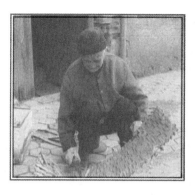

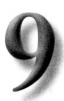

THERAPEUTIC USE OF SELF

Jan Froehlich, MS, OTR/L; Marie C. Roy, LCSW, OTR/L; Bethany Augustoni, MS, OTR/L; Julie Eldredge, MS, OTR/L; and Ali Kae Arsenault, OTR

ACOTE STANDARDS EXPLORED IN THIS CHAPTER

B.5.7

KEY VOCABULARY

- **Caring:** A set of feelings, attitudes, and actions that convey respect, hope, and care toward others.
- **Client-centered practice:** A partnership between a client and therapist that serves to empower a client toward reaching goals of his or her own choosing.
- **Counter-transference:** When one person, usually the therapist, accepts the role the client has placed on him or her.

- **Effective communication:** The artful interplay between listening and speaking coupled with awareness and sensitivity to human diversity.
- **Empathy:** A process of reaching for true understanding of the experiences and feelings of another person.
- **Transference:** When one person, usually the client, places a role on another, usually the therapist.

Introduction

Jody, the occupational therapist, has tried many strategies with Annabelle, but none have motivated her to get out of bed. Exasperated, Jody asks, "How about if I wear my wedding dress to work tomorrow, will you get out of bed for me then?" Jody wears her wedding dress to the nursing home the next day, and sure enough, Annabelle chuckles as she gets out of bed and engages in occupational therapy interventions related to her self-care.

Caring

One of the most rewarding aspects of being an occupational therapy practitioner is that we get to care about our clients. Every time we show our caring toward our clients we are using ourselves as therapeutic tools. Sometimes therapeutic use of self is the most profound aspect of the therapy process or, conversely, if we have not achieved therapeutic use of self with a given client, the most expert techniques may be ineffective. Taylor, Lee,

Jacobs, K., MacRae, N., & Sladyk, K. (Eds.).
Occupational Therapy Essentials for
Clinical Competence, Second Edition (pp. 113-125).
© 2014 SLACK Incorporated.

Kielhofner, and Ketkar (2009) found that more than 80% of survey respondents rated therapeutic use of self as the most important determinant of the outcome of therapy. Graybeal (2007) cites mounting evidence that the therapeutic alliance matters most in predicting psychotherapy outcomes.

Jody was able to inspire Annabelle to engage in occupational therapy because she cared enough about her to try something as outlandish as wearing her wedding dress to work to get Annabelle out of bed. Allowing ourselves to care for our clients comes naturally to many occupational therapy practitioners. We chose occupational therapy as our profession because we wanted to make a difference in the lives of clients in need of our services. We show our caring for our clients in a variety of ways. On a most basic level, occupational therapy practitioners are required to care for our clients by providing technically competent occupational therapy services that are based on sound judgment. Beyond providing technically competent care, some practitioners show their caring by spending time creating adaptive equipment for their clients or engaging in research on a particular occupational therapy intervention or assessment instrument. Others, like Jody, have a talent for bringing humor to the occupational therapy relationship. Still others deepen the therapeutic relationship by allowing themselves to cry right alongside their clients as tragedies and losses are expressed and faced. Many offer deep hope to clients who find little meaning and hope in their lives.

Obviously, there are a multitude of different ways that occupational therapists show their caring for their clients, and the way we show our caring is in part related to our personality. There is no one right way to care for our clients. Often, caring occurs right from the start in a therapy relationship, and many times it deepens over the course of the therapy relationship. Other times, we may find ourselves not being able to notice we like or care for a particular client, yet we offer our care just the same. Paradoxically, we can care about people even if we do not feel like we like them.

To elucidate the nature and importance of caring in occupational therapy, the 60th American Occupational Therapy Association (AOTA) conference theme was on caring. At that conference, Gilfoyle (1980) identified the importance of knowledge, skill, and attitudes in caring. She emphasized how important it is to truly know who our client is—what his or her strengths, limitations, and needs are and what will enable him or her to grow and change. In addition, she felt knowledge must include the ability to know how to respond to another person's needs and to know your own abilities and limitations as a practitioner. Flexibility was identified as a key skill in caring as we continually assess and reassess our effectiveness. Patience, honesty, trust, humility, hope, and courage were identified as the attitudes we bring to caring.

King (1980) challenged therapists to provide both effective and creative caring in occupational therapy. Like Gilfoyle, she also emphasized the importance of knowledge in caring, yet she highlighted the importance of the practitioner's engagement in independent thinking and examination of the broad issues related to therapy. Generating creative alternatives in occupational therapy was stressed as a deep form of caring.

A few years later, Devereaux (1984) described occupational therapy practitioners as specialists in making caring and connection happen. She highlighted seven elements of the caring, therapeutic relationship: competence, belief in the dignity and worth of the individual, belief in an innate potential for change and growth, effective communication, values, touch, and humor. Many other scholars have applied their own fresh thinking to therapeutic use of self and caring in occupational therapy. Peloquin (2002, 2003) and Abreu (2011) have emphasized empathy in therapeutic relationships. Many therapists have contributed to the development of client-centered practice in occupational therapy (Law, 1998). Black and Wells (2007) stand out for inspiring occupational therapy practitioners to develop cultural competence. Schwartzberg (2002) has articulated the nature of interactive reasoning in occupational therapy. Tickle-Degnen (2002) has interwoven the principles of client-centered practice and therapeutic use of self with the use of evidence-based research. Black (2005) draws an intersection of caring between client-centered practice, culturally competent care, and the feminist ethic of caring. Taylor (2008) has developed an intentional relationship model for occupational therapists.

From the authors' experience, Devereaux's seven elements of a caring, therapeutic relationship are still important today, yet they can be expanded on by the rich contributions of many other scholars from within and outside of occupational therapy. Each of these elements will now be explored and expanded on from the perspective of multiple scholars. This will be done in the context of occupational therapy clinical examples drawn from the authors' own clinical experience and occupational therapy colleagues in Northern New England, so the readers can gain an increasing appreciation and understanding of therapeutic use of self in occupational therapy.

Belief in the Dignity and Worth of the Individual: Respect

The first client I (J. F.) worked with on an inpatient psychiatric unit was Kenny, a 15-year-old boy who had stabbed his mother to death. He was psychotic at the time and believed his mother was poisoning him. As a new therapist, I found it a little challenging to notice that I did not like this client, but I could offer my care and respect. As his life story unfolded before me, I never doubted that when the entire situation was taken into account, he had done his best. I grew to like this client over time, yet right from the beginning, I cared about his well-being. Occupational therapy sessions aimed at boosting his self-confidence regarding his ability to master a variety of age-appropriate social, leisure, and pre-vocational activities were effective.

The most effective occupational therapy practitioners approach their clients with an attitude of deep respect and belief in the dignity and worth of every individual. Respect can be offered even when we do not feel like we like somebody. This respect generally acknowledges that the client we are assisting has probably been through many ups and downs in his or her life and has done their best with the cards they have been dealt. Jackins (1993) expresses this well in the following quote: "Every single human being, when the entire situation is taken into account, has always, at every moment, done the very best that he or she could do, and so deserves neither blame nor reproach from anyone, including self" (p. 3).

A caring attitude that communicates respect is one that separates people from their problems, behaviors, and distresses. In my work with Kenny, not only did I offer respect, but in my mind, I made a sharp distinction between who he is and what his problems and distresses were at that time. I held a mental picture of him as a smart, caring boy who had many hard experiences in his lifetime. Yet, at the same time, I did not forget that, in a distressed and psychotic state, he had killed his mother. I did not respect his distress.

Not confusing our clients with their distresses or problems is a crucial element in maintaining respect for a client and for enhancing the therapeutic use of self. I worked with a young woman, Martha, who after experiencing whiplash from a car accident, had bilateral wrist and foot drop that was a conversion disorder. In other words, her physical disability was in her mind. Her paralysis followed no neurological pattern. She was dependent on others for all her self-care needs, including toileting. My gut response to this situation was judgmental. However, I quickly checked that response at the door and replaced it with an attitude of respect for her as a human, not for her distresses. I assumed that when the entire situation was taken into account this woman was doing her best. Therapy proceeded well, because I could separate Martha as a human being from her problems or distresses. Using a physical rehabilitation approach and a caring attitude, Martha regained complete independence with her self-care and decided it was time to begin exploring childhood trauma in psychotherapy.

In addition to not confusing our clients with their distresses or problems, we also need to not confuse our clients with people of whom they remind us. *Transference* is the process by which one person places a role on another because they remind the individual of a significant relationship from their own past. Counter-transference is when one person accepts the role that has been placed on him or her. Both are handled by reflection on the part of the therapist combined with skillful communication and limit setting when appropriate with the client (Schwartzberg, 2002).

Ella was working on an inpatient psychiatric unit when she met Sean, a man battling alcoholism. During a group treatment session, Sean began discussing his threatening actions and feelings toward his two daughters, ages 23 and 16, as well as his wife, to whom he has been married to for 27 years. Ella began feeling anger toward this man because of the way he was describing what he has said and done to these women, but also because she had experienced an alcoholic parent. She knew that Sean had a disease and that she needed to take a deeper look into him to learn who he was as a person, separate from the alcoholism and negative behavior and separate from her own experiences with an alcoholic father, in order to create a successful treatment plan.

A supportive listener, counselor, or supervisor can aid in addressing transference and counter-transference or any other situation when a therapist finds it hard to care for or respect a given client. When a therapist finds he or she cannot work therapeutically with a particular client, it is important to address this with a supervisor and, in some cases, find a different therapist for that client.

Belief in Our Clients' Innate Potential for Change and Growth

I worked with Alice for several months on an inpatient psychiatric unit. She was lethally suicidal (attempted to hang herself) as she recalled the trauma of sexual abuse in her early life. The team and I worked with her and were able to separate Alice from her distresses and problems. She was a very intelligent, witty, attractive young woman, yet she battled with irrational thoughts in her mind that she was no good and should die. We communicated our belief in Alice that she could face the trauma of her past and move on to a brighter future. With plenty of psychotherapy, occupational therapy, expressive therapy, and assistance from a social worker, Alice was able to reconstruct a new life. After discharge from a long hospitalization, she completed a bachelor's and a master's degree and worked as a victim's advocate for years before marrying and becoming a mother of two children.

Meili was from China and lived with her husband, her husband's family, and her newborn baby. She was hospitalized on my unit for multiple serious suicide attempts and postpartum depression. She was frequently told by her husband's family that her depression was nonexistent and that her character was "weak." Meili would come to groups in my inpatient psychiatry unit but rarely speak. During individual treatments we would ask her to try and use simple mantras or phrases that began with "I am." Meili was unable to identify any of her strengths with the exception of her ability to draw. "We know that you do not believe in yourself," we told her, "so we will do that for you until you have that strength." Meili, through intensive occupational therapy and collaborative psychiatric efforts, was discharged home with a plane ticket back to China with her husband and baby. On the last day in our unit she came to us and said, "Thank you, I am strong."

Ali inherited a young client, Lily, when she began a fieldwork rotation at a pediatric outpatient clinic. Lily had been coming to the clinic because she had gravitational insecurity and general developmental delays. Ali first observed Lily using the clinic's suspended equipment and obstacle course. Lily was extremely hesitant exploring new equipment and negotiating different floor surfaces. She requested help from Ali when climbing on and off the equipment despite having the physical capabilities to do so independently. Ali began providing unconditional positive regard toward Lily's potential to conquer the clinic's equipment. Over the following weeks, Lily came in for treatment with a newfound confidence to try things she had been so afraid to do before. By the end of their time together, Lily was jumping from a loft into a ball pit with safety and without hesitation. Ali had believed in Lily's potential for growth and, in turn, Lily believed it too.

Each of these case vignettes illustrates the importance of our belief in our clients' ability to have a better life. Psychiatric rehabilitation literature (Anthony, 1993; Anthony, Cohen, Farkas, & Gagne, 2002) provides us with a compelling picture of the power of believing in the ability of our clients with psychiatric challenges to recover. The recovery perspective—which assumes psychiatric clients can find new meaning and hope in their lives—can be used in pediatrics and physical rehabilitation as well.

It appears that many occupational therapy practitioners intuitively offer hope to their clients, even those with the most disabling conditions. The simple statement that we frequently use in occupational therapy, "You can," is a strong contradiction to the despair that many people with disabilities feel about their ability to gain or regain function, occupation, meaning, and purpose in their lives. We need to follow this statement with a reminder that it may take a great deal of work to achieve particular goals a client has identified.

Many clients who are experiencing any form of depression often have lost sight of the worth they hold within their own world. Believing in them takes on a new complexity and looms as a daunting task to those who are struggling to remember who they are or what value they still hold. Providing clients with verbal confirmation that someone else believes in them allows individuals time to focus their remaining energy elsewhere. When we notice we are not feeling hopeful about a particular client with whom we are working, it is useful for us to seek supervision so we can explore any personal roadblocks to being hopeful about particular clients.

Effective Communication: Listening and Empathy

Claire worked on a general medical acute inpatient unit. She introduced herself to her client, Robert, to let him know she would work with him in the afternoon. Robert perceived Claire's kind attention and began right then to talk about his situation. He was a chiropractor who had a son who had been in a car accident and needed extensive rehabilitation. Unable to find life worth living with his disability, his son committed suicide. Robert felt betrayed by his son and shameful that this could have happened to him, a man so knowledgeable about disability. He had never told anyone his son had killed himself prior to this moment with Claire. He cried heavily with Claire and she gently touched his shoulder and let him cry for a while. She thanked him for sharing his difficult story and said she would be back later. As she was leaving, a nurse came in and Robert said, "That is the best damn occupational therapist I have ever met."

Claire was able to listen not only to Robert's story, but also to all the emotions that accompanied them. She was able to know Robert in ways he had never shared with anyone before. Caring is a feeling and an attitude, yet it is also expressed through listening. One of the most profound actions that a practitioner may offer his or her clients is the gift of listening and paying attention so we can reach for the true knowing that Gilfoyle (1980) described.

As Schwartzberg (2002) suggests, the therapist's job is to facilitate the flow of communication and to validate the person as the meaning and the content come forth. If we return to Alice, my client who was lethally suicidal, over time, more and more of her trauma experiences were shared with members of the treatment team who could listen to what she endured and all the emotions that accompanied those experiences while validating her for surviving her childhood. As Isham (2006) stated, "Listening is an attitude of the heart, a genuine desire to be with another which both attracts and heals."

Empathy is closely linked to caring and is an important part of the listening process (Davis, 2011). Abreu (2011) describes empathic interactions as one of the most important factors in occupational therapy interventions. Peloquin (2002, 2003) described empathy as a process of reaching for both the hands and the heart of our client. In doing so, we enter the experience of our clients through a communication partnership that is often deeply moving and inspiring. This partnership changes both the client and the therapist. Claire will never forget her time with Robert, nor will I forget my time with Alice. Alice expressed deep grief, fear, and anger as her life story unfolded. I was able to listen to her well by allowing myself to enter her experience and shed a few tears of my own, voice my own indignation at what had occurred, while laughing with relief that it was all in the past. This level of empathy deepened the effectiveness of the occupational therapy process. Yet, as much as I allowed myself to enter Alice's experience as I listened to her, I was also able to remind both of us the abuse was in the past and that she had survived.

The chapter on effective communication provides the reader with a process for becoming an increasingly effective listener (see Chapter 8).

Effective Communication: Client-Centered Therapy and Empowerment

Janey, a 4-year-old girl at a center for children with disabilities, had hypoglossia-hypodactylia which presented with the absence of hands and feet. She was a brilliant and determined little girl who was eager to participate in the world by using all kinds of utensils and craft tools. Bilateral activities were extra challenging for Janey, but 6 months into therapy she expressed with vehemence that she really wanted to use scissors. With some trial and error, her occupational

therapist, Marie, created a custom scissor block with mounted spring-loaded scissors angled so gravity assisted in cutting. This scissor block enabled Janey to use one residual limb to stabilize the paper and the other to actively cut. When Janey saw the scissor block and tried it for the first time, Marie said, "She lit up like a Christmas tree." Despite being a shy girl, she proclaimed to everyone in her class, "Look at me, look at what I can do!" She wanted to cut paper grass for spring baskets for all eight of her peers.

Client-centered occupational therapy has been defined as "an approach to service which embraces a philosophy of respect for, and partnership with, people receiving services" (Law, Baptiste, & Mills, 1995, p. 253). Canadian occupational therapists have developed and disseminated seminal thinking about the nature of client-centered practice in occupational therapy. The key concepts of client-centered practice include the following: respect for clients, clients have the ultimate responsibility for decisions about occupations and occupational therapy, person-centered communication with an emphasis on provision of information, physical comfort and emotional support, facilitation of client participation in all aspects of occupational therapy, flexible and individualized occupational therapy service delivery which enables clients to solve occupational performance issues, and a focus on the person-environment-occupation relationship (Law, 1998).

It would appear obvious that Marie engaged in client-centered occupational therapy that empowered Janey to achieve her goals. Tickle-Degnen (2002) describes the client-centered relationship as involving the formation of two types of relationship bonding: rapport building and a working alliance. The working alliance is formed when client and therapist collaborate with one another to develop common goals and as they develop a sense of shared responsibility for working on tasks that are involved in achieving those goals. In order for a practitioner to ascertain what a client's true concerns are and therefore be client-centered, he or she must be able to first build rapport and then listen well enough to accurately know what these concerns are. Marie quickly bonded with Janey as they instantly took a great liking to one another. They saw each other 5 days a week for 2 years. The working alliance between them was strong because Marie was deeply respectful and listened well to Janey's wishes and goals, which, besides using scissors, included working with markers, feeding herself with a spoon, and learning to hang onto a swing independently.

Randy had been given the diagnosis of a rare disease whose symptoms presented similarly to a spinal cord injury. With little known about his prognosis, occupational and physical therapy worked collaboratively by providing extensive upper and lower extremity strengthening exercises and adaptive equipment in order to work toward his goal of walking once around the rehabilitation gym. One day, while working with another client, I (B. A,) saw Randy standing with a walker. The physical therapist had a gait belt and thera-bands around him and was assisting him in taking his first steps. His upper body stood tall and his hands grasped firmly around the walker. The people present in the gym watched in awe as Randy began taking supported steps to complete his goal of walking around the rehabilitation gym. "Keep pushing me, keep pushing me," he said through his tears. "I know what it is like to work hard and this was all I wanted."

As Jackins (1993) stated, "Happiness is the overcoming of obstacles on the way to a goal of one's own choosing" (p. 34). As a therapist, learning to adapt to a client's goal while incorporating a site-specific protocol can often be a challenging task. However, a client's goal can be embedded within the foundation of the practice setting. For Randy, it would have been difficult to justify the goal of "walking"; however, by using the right upper extremity strengthening exercises and adaptations, the goals of independent dressing, feeding, and leisure could be addressed in conjunction with Randy's goal of walking around the gym. The more occupational therapy practitioners can truly listen to their clients to find out what their real goals and concerns are, the more they will be able to engage in client-centered occupational therapy that is satisfying to their clients. Not surprisingly, a number of studies have reported that client satisfaction does increase when therapists truly use a client-centered approach (Calnan et al., 1994; Henbest & Fehrsen, 1992; Wasserman, Inui, Barriatua, Carter, & Lippincott, 1984). However, as Maitra and Erway (2006) have demonstrated, there is still a gap between occupational therapists' perception of their use of client-centered therapy and clients' perceptions of how involved they were in decisions about occupational therapy. As occupational therapy practitioners continue to refine their communication skills, client-centered therapy will be more readily achieved.

Humor

Florence was attempting to get her client Carla, who had mild mental retardation and depression, to increase her engagement in self-care and social activities in her residence. Carla was so unmotivated one day that she opened the door to allow Florence into her apartment and then began walking back to her bedroom, stating that she wasn't going to cook today; she was just going to lie down. Florence ran ahead of her and got in her bed before Carla could lie down. Carla laughed and asked, "OK, what are we cooking today?"

Julie was working with Maria, an 89-year-old woman with late-stage dementia that caused her to live in the past and demonstrate inability to grasp reality. Maria was very hard to motivate and did not want to participate in therapy outside of her bedroom because of her increased confusion and, at times, nonsensical speech. Maria's family brought in the Sound of Music soundtrack to play while Maria was in bed or relaxing in her chair. Julie pressed play on the CD player and began to dance and yodel to the Goat Herd song. Before she knew it, Maria was by her side dancing, smiling, and singing along while holding Julie's hands.

Like Jody, Florence and Julie conveyed their caring by using humor to break their clients' depressed states. Physician and clown, Patch Adams, states that the greatest success in health care involves caring for others and that fun is as important as love (Adams & Mylander, 1993). He finds that humor contributes to the success of many professional and social relationships because we deepen connections when we laugh together. The therapeutic value of humor and laughter has been noted by many health professionals (Berk, 2001; Capps, 2006; Martin and Lefcourt, 2004). Laughter increases the secretion of catecholamines and endorphins, natural chemicals in the brain that make people feel good. Laughter also enhances immune function by decreasing cortisol secretion. Although when we initially laugh our heart rate and blood pressure rise, as our arteries relax, both heart rate and blood pressure decrease, resulting in a general relaxation response. After a hearty laugh, this therapeutic response can last up to 45 minutes (Adams & Mylander, 1993). Dunbar et al. (2011) found that social laughter is correlated with an elevated pain threshold.

Adams and Mylander (1993) suggest we all learn to cultivate our sense of humor by paying closer attention to what makes ourselves and those around us laugh. Workshops on humor and health care are well worth attending so we can learn to bring laughter to even the most trying and difficult situations we encounter as occupational therapists. Ultimately, we will enhance and deepen our relationships in occupational therapy by cultivating our own sense of humor.

Values

At his mother's insistence, John, a young adult man with schizoaffective disorder, was receiving home health occupational therapy to increase his participation in daily routines and to work with him in becoming more independent. An initial interview using the Canadian Occupational

Performance Measure revealed the most important goal for John was going to the gym to increase his strength and endurance. His second most important goal was learning some social skills so he could make friends. Goals important to his mother, but less important to John, were learning to cook, manage his money, and find an apartment. The second week into therapy, Florence, his occupational therapist, successfully assisted John in establishing a routine of working out at one of the local gyms 3 times a week. Other goals were eventually achieved as they became important to John.

Altruism, equality, freedom, justice, dignity, truth, and prudence are the core ethical values of occupational therapy (American Occupational Therapy Association, 2010), and they provide the foundation for a caring, therapeutic relationship. In the case of John, Florence valued his own freedom of choice regarding his engagement in occupation, and because of this, she was successful and client-centered therapy was achieved. Each core value of occupational therapy has significant implications for how we relate to our clients. The reader is referred to Chapter 48 for a review of the meaning of each of these values and is reminded of the commitment we make to upholding these values as occupational therapists.

Touch

Marie works with children with severe developmental disabilities. One of the greatest aspects of her job is that she gets to be physically close to young people all day while helping them be active participants in the world. They rely on her physical presence and caring touch for external support in order to explore textures, to activate switches connected to toys, to experience movement by bouncing on a ball or riding a horse, to be in water, or to use a paint brush or a spoon. They experience great joy and exuberance with many of these occupations. Marie finds that there is a touch that is custodial, such as wiping a mouth or nose, and then there is a whole other kind of touch that is affectionate, playful, and facilitates experiencing the world. There is also touch that is comforting and consoling and it is often more acceptable to give this kind of touch to young children.

Sarah was working on an inpatient psychiatric unit when she met Alex, a transgendered female. Alex was screaming and yelling at the nursing staff and was very difficult to redirect. Sarah was nervous to begin the initial evaluation with Alex so she approached her gently. Alex agreed to speak with Sarah in a private room. Alex began to cry when Sarah asked why she was so upset. Alex cried out that she was a "male trapped in a female's body." Alex stated that she wanted to have a baby before she became a man, but no one around her supported her decision. Sarah decided to help Alex make a pros and cons list to attempt to help with this decision. When Alex began sobbing again, Sarah touched Alex's hand, knowing that no contact was supposed to be made between practitioner and client on the psychiatric unit, but she knew that a simple touch could mean a world of difference to Alex. When Alex wiped her tears and looked at Sarah and said "Thanks," Sarah knew she had made the right decision.

As humans, we all need close physical contact. Young people instinctively seek out large amounts of physical closeness and touch. Infants often protest loudly when they are not held. It is only as we mature through childhood that we become resigned to less and less physical contact and loving touch. In adolescence, human closeness becomes less available, and in many societies, it becomes sexualized. In the United States, the sexualization of closeness has resulted in increased homophobia or fear of closeness with someone of the same gender. The net result has been less physical closeness and touch for many people (D'Arc, 2003).

Despite some of the societal taboos on closeness, health care workers often have opportunities to use touch in thoughtful and caring ways as Marie and Sarah described. Purtilo and Haddad (2002) speak of touching privileges that are granted to health care professionals. Comforting touch, such as Claire touching Robert's shoulder, has particular legitimacy and may speak more loudly than the kindest words. Yet on the other hand, some health care professionals may provide only functional touching because of concerns about a client's misinterpretation of their touch. Through extensive interviews, Chang (2001) identified that touch has physical, emotional, social, and spiritual dimensions. Hertenstein, Holmes, McCullough, and Keltner (2009) found that even blindfolded subjects could decode the emotions behind touch. The work of Kim and Buschman (1999) demonstrates that touch can lower anxiety levels and decrease episodes of dysfunctional behavior in patients with dementia. Guided by our ethics as a practitioner and paying close attention to the nonverbal and verbal communication of our clients, occupational therapists can determine what is appropriate therapeutic touch.

Carol, a 65-year-old woman who had experienced a stroke, exhibited global aphasia and a right neglect. She was aware of her deficits and would frequently get frustrated. She was given a lot of proprioceptive cues in order to bring attention to her right side. These cues were much more *effective when accompanied with understanding tones and kind touch. Carol would be unresponsive or become agitated when people talked with her in a way she found offensive.*

Touch, although often used solely as a comfort measure, is also used in transfers, neurodevelopmental treatment, and for proprioceptive purposes. When touch is used with the well-being of the client in mind, it can act as a powerful catalyst in promoting physical and emotional safety.

Competence

Dom worked in a rehabilitation hospital with an elderly gentleman, William, who was recovering from a stroke. William was despondent and shut down. Doctors and therapists could not engage him in therapy routines. Aware of how withdrawn William was, Dom went into his room and got down on his knees near his bed and said, "I can hardly imagine how hard this is for you. I know it has been hard for you to want to participate in therapy. What did you enjoy doing in the past?" The gentleman mentioned he used to enjoy reading and writing and that some of his poetry had been published. As Dom listened to William, he decided that he was going to the library to check-out his book. He brought it into work with him the next day and read to William one of his own poems about living life well. Dom read the first few sentences and William recited the rest from memory. He closed the book and with gratitude said, "Thank you for reminding me that I want to live." He got up and began to engage in occupational therapy.

Many of the chapters in this text address the development of theoretical, technical, and practical competence in the delivery of occupational therapy services. As Devereaux (1984) pointed out, this is one of the most fundamental aspects of the occupational therapy relationship. Every client deserves an occupational therapy practitioner who is technically competent. In addition, every client also deserves a therapist who is competent in developing a therapeutic relationship. Dom's work with William beautifully demonstrates such competence.

Taylor (2008) has developed an intentional relationship model to assist practitioners with refining their interpersonal competence with clients. She proposes that therapists tend to adopt a preferred mode of relating to and caring for their clients. These modes include advocating, collaborating, empathizing, encouraging, instructing, and problem solving. Although practitioners tend to have a preference for a particular mode, nonpreferred modes can be developed and enhanced. In

the preceding example, Dom exemplifies an encouraging mode with William. By reading some of William's own poetry about the value of life, Dom encouraged William to move forward in his own life and in therapy.

As Taylor notes, every therapist is presented with inevitable interpersonal events where we are challenged to relate effectively with our clients. The most effective therapists are able to handle inevitable interpersonal events by shifting modes in their practice. For example, when clients are admitted to a hospital, they are not functioning at their highest performance capacity. Not only is their inner drive and volition low, but they are also experiencing a disruption in their everyday habituation (Kielhofner, 2008). Thus, as a clinician, it is essential to remain flexible in thought and action rather than rigid in routine. Becoming stuck in the use of only one mode, for example, instructing mode, can cause interactions with clinicians to be seen as a hierarchy rather than a collaborative approach to treatment. Yet with other patients, such as a client who is experiencing mania, it may be important to utilize a mode that provides balance to a chaotic mind. Thus, the Intentional Relationship Model and its modes remain a dynamic part of the therapeutic use of self and can be used in conjunction with concrete practice models.

John was a truck driver who had recently had an above-knee amputation. He had a sense of humor that was hard to understand at times, and although his intentions were well-meant, he would often make inappropriate sexual innuendos and comments. It was not long before I (B.A.) figured out that John's "rough around the edges" personality was seeking praise, humor, and someone to match his outspoken comments. It took me a while to understand that working with John required a lot of mode shifting. It was important to be instructing when he had crossed a line. However, it was also essential that he saw that his clinicians were multifaceted people just like himself. He responded well to brief uses of empathy but would then seek a collaboration mode when trying to decide which adaptive equipment would work best upon discharge.

Cultural competence is also a critical ingredient in competent therapeutic use of self. Black (2005) has found that much of the literature on cultural competence agrees that a culturally competent individual exhibits cultural self-awareness, knowledge of diverse groups, and skill in relating to diverse groups of people. Obviously, cultural competence is an ongoing process as health care providers continually learn new information about different cultures, so an open mind and willingness to learn are also essential. The following example illustrates a therapist's willingness to re-evaluate her work with someone from a different culture.

Kazuki, a Japanese man in his late sixties, found himself at an acute rehabilitation hospital after a bilateral knee replacement. He was in incredible shape and was always willing to push himself. Kazuki spoke no English and we needed a translator to communicate. This was often hard because crucial information got lost within translation. Upon initial evaluation, I (B.A.) was going through home management tasks when he stated he did not even go into the kitchen. He was quick to participate in exercises that required extreme strength, often wanting to do exercises other clients found too difficult. I spent many sessions addressing dressing but rarely did he show interest. One day, when doing a shower activity of daily living (ADL) assessment, his wife came and took over. She began dressing him and stated that she did all the housework and usually helped him with whatever he needed. It was at this moment I realized I had to backtrack. I began to see that I had pushed my own agenda as a therapist without understanding the unique cultural differences that defined Kazuki's routines.

Oftentimes within specific practice settings it is easy to lose sight of the differences in cultural values when site protocol wants everything done in a similar way. Individual cultural practices, values, or traditions do not inhibit the therapy process. Oftentimes they open different venues for carrying out more individually relevant occupational-based interventions. Chapter 2 on culture more fully addresses cultural competence and Chapter 8 on effective communication will guide the reader through a process of becoming a culturally sensitive communicator.

Therapeutic Use of Self in Group Work

Bethany was working with Sara, a 19-year-old woman from Colombia. Sara was sensitive, reserved, and caring, and came to the unit after a suicide attempt following the loss of her mother. During a group session about simple pleasures in a life, another member brought up food. There was a pause in the group that was soon filled by Sara's crying. The entire dynamic of the group shifted in that moment. A moment that had previously only brushed the surface of human emotion quickly turned to one that encompassed depth. Sara continued crying and explained how had she followed through with her suicide attempt she never would have been able to eat another meal. She went on to explain that even the things

humans find so simple can hold so much meaning when there is a threat of it being taken away.

Bethany's story is an example of how listening and empathy are not only essential in individual interactions but also in the facilitation of group dynamics. It is important to allow individuals within a group to be a part of a healing process for another group member. In Sara's case, the members of the group listened with patience, understanding, and empathy. By doing this, Sara's peers not only gave her the gift of their listening and attention, but they also gave themselves feelings of satisfaction and worth by knowing they had helped her.

Although caring, listening, and empathy will enhance therapeutic use of self as a group leader, Bethany's success in this group situation was also based on her group leadership skills, including an understanding of group development, fostering mutual support, and handling challenging group behaviors.

Group Development

Groups often take on a life of their own and group dynamics can be complex. A number of theorists have described group development, yet perhaps the ideas of Tuckman (1965, 1977) are most well known. He identified five stages to group development: forming, storming, norming, performing, and adjourning. In the forming stage, group members are often somewhat anxious as they become acquainted with one another and become more aware of the nature and the purpose of the group. They are often very dependent on the group leader. In the storming stage, conflict occurs as group members challenge the rules, expectations, tasks, and leadership of the group. During the norming stage, these conflicts are resolved and relationships deepen as the group learns to work together. The performing stage occurs when group members work together on mutually agreed upon goals in a manner that is supportive and growth promoting. Attention to the adjourning phase, or the termination of a group, is important for consolidation of gains made in a group.

Based on her work in leading groups primarily composed of women, Schiller (2003) constructed a relational model of group development that is somewhat different. The relational model has a stronger emphasis on the development of relationships within groups, and consequently, the stage of conflict is replaced by one of challenge and change. It includes the following stages: preaffiliation, establishing a relational base, mutuality and interpersonal empathy, challenge and change, and separation. Similar to Tuckman's forming stage, in the preaffiliation stage, group members are somewhat anxious and try to determine with whom they can relate and be close. During the stage of establishing a relational base, group members seek out friendship and support and begin to share openly about themselves. During the phase of mutuality and interpersonal empathy, trust is deepened and group members take greater risks in sharing their experiences. Commonalities are noted and empathy for each other is experienced. The challenge and change stage occurs when group members feel safe enough with each other to challenge each other, yet at the same time maintain connections and relationships. The separation stage is identified as an important part of the overall group, and time is spent reviewing both positive and challenging experiences in the group and saying goodbye. Schiller finds her model of group development occurs not only in groups that are all female, but in groups that have both men and women when the leader adopts a relational perspective. The relational perspective intentionally fosters caring and connection between group members.

Fostering Mutual Support

Occupational therapy practitioners may find some of the groups that they lead follow the relational model of group development and others follow Tuckman's model. This may have to do with the practitioner's leadership style, the focus of the group, or it may have to do with the membership of a particular group. Regardless, practitioners will be effective group leaders with many different kinds of groups when they can foster mutual support within their groups as Bethany did. When it is possible, the formation of groups is made easier when the leader or orchestrator of the group uses a relational approach by getting to know members on an individual as well as a group basis. Many individuals adapt their behavior in order to take on a group role that they may not demonstrate as an individual. On an acute inpatient psychiatry unit, for example, groups will run more smoothly when individuals feel that the clinician has made an effort to understand them prior to attending a group.

As the group leader or facilitator models therapeutic use of self with each client in a group, he or she can, at the same time, support group members in relating to each other therapeutically as well. Bethany achieved this and enabled group members to play a profound role in empowering each other.

In order for clients in a group to play an empowerment role for each other, it is useful to establish group norms at the beginning of a group regarding confidentiality and respect. In addition, group members can be taught the importance of truly listening to each other without interrupting. A useful guideline for groups is that no one person is permitted to speak twice unless each person in the group has had a chance to speak once. It is then the group leader's job to ensure every voice is heard in a group. It is generally tedious for all group members when one group member tends to dominate with his or her ideas or experiences. A simple way to intervene in this situation is to simply thank the group member who is dominating for speaking and then asking what other group members think about a given subject. Giving each group member a particular amount of time to speak on a particular topic or experience can assist group members in truly getting to know each other and thereby develop empathy and support.

Supporting the leadership development of group members by giving them specific tasks and responsibilities will enhance group member empowerment as well. Group member tasks and responsibilities may include leading an opening circle or an icebreaker, sharing thoughts on a reading, or organizing clean-up or refreshments.

Handling Challenging Group and Individual Behaviors

The first group I (B.A.) ever led began with a poem. I was working on an acute inpatient psychiatry unit and had spent the previous night preparing. I figured the more prepared I was, the less that could go wrong. After reading the poem to begin the group, I asked what the members thought about it. Instantly one of my clients said, "I thought it was stupid." Initially I was taken aback, almost offended. I had tried so hard to do well and had come up short. After asking her why she felt that way, I attempted to listen carefully to her response. When I put my own ego aside I realized that she made good and insightful points. This particular member seemed shocked that I went on to validate what she said. After that moment she felt free to speak within the group. However, this time her comments were kind. Creating a safe space for clients often involves the practitioner coming out of his or her comfort zone. No preparation will ever prepare you for what others are going to say. Ultimately, there is powerlessness over others; however, the control lies in the way practitioners choose to respond to group members' reactions.

Julie handled criticism from her group member artfully. By listening to her client's concerns, she validated her perspective and the group was able to move forward. This approach does not always work. There is much to learn about how to flexibly and effectively handle challenging group behaviors such as criticism or attacks toward the group leader or facilitator, group member conflict, the silent nonparticipating group member, the hostile group member, and other forms of disruptive behavior. Use of the Intentional Relationship Model will facilitate appropriate mode shifting to handle challenging group behaviors (Taylor, 2013). Vroman (2013) also offers excellent insights into managing challenging group behavior. Based on many years of leading a variety of groups, the following are good general guidelines for leading groups so that conflict is productive and empowerment of group members occurs:

- Whenever possible, involve the group in determining group norms.
- Listen, listen, listen to find out where people are coming from.
- Be respectful of people, but not any negative patterns of behavior.
- When a group member is very challenging, you can always ask the group to take a break or discuss a particular topic in pairs while you discuss with that person what you need from them in order for them to stay in your group.
- When workable, use humor to assist in conflict resolution.
- Do not assume that someone who appears not to be participating is not gaining things from your group.
- Use work or discussion in pairs to foster new interconnections.
- Allow a range of behaviors that are not disruptive or distracting.
- Always remember that as a group leader, you have the right to ask someone to leave your group if they are making it impossible for you to lead.

Humor is a very important tool in Julie's occupational therapy tool box. When working on an inpatient psychiatric unit, Julie used humor in most, if not all, of her treatments, when deemed appropriate. When conducting a group on positive affirmations, patients voiced their strong opinion on how this was "the dumbest worksheet ever" and "really, we are not 5 years old." Julie knew that she was stuck and had to think of something quick to say: "OK, I know this is pretty silly but give me a chance. If you fill these out and discuss them with me, I will get you all ice cream." After that, the 10 members of the group sat quietly filling out the sheets and completed a very detailed discussion on positive affirmations. Julie was validating the patients' responses, and in doing so, the patients felt as though she was "on their side and understood them."

The reader is referred to the work of Yalom and Leszcz (2005) for an overview of integrating psychotherapy principles in the leadership of groups. O'Brien and Solomon's (2013) *Occupational Analysis and Group Process,* Cole's (2012) *Group Dynamics in Occupational Therapy,* and Schwartzberg, Howe, and Barnes' (2008) *Groups: Applying the Functional Group Model* are recommended for an understanding of the theoretical underpinnings of group work in occupational therapy.

Summary

Ultimately, in caring, therapeutic relationships, we bring together our minds and our hearts. Every time we think about how to offer our assistance to our clients so they can live better lives, we are caring for them as individuals. Much can be learned about how to enhance therapeutic use of self in occupational therapy by continually refining our technical, cultural, and interpersonal competence. In doing so, we need to recommit to the core values of occupational therapy and hold firm to our belief in the dignity and worth of the individual and our belief in an innate potential for change and growth. We need to continually refine our use of empathy, touch, humor, and listening as important aspects of client-centered practice. The novice and experienced occupational therapy practitioner alike can expect to experience many successes and to make mistakes as they attempt to build rapport and a working alliance with their clients. As Gilfoyle (1980) suggested, skill in caring is achieved by continually assessing and reassessing our practice. Having opportunities to reflect on these experiences with supportive peers and/or a supervisor will prove invaluable in refining therapeutic use of self in occupational therapy.

Student Self-Assessment

Use the following questions to either guide a discussion with a peer or to guide your thoughts in a journal regarding therapeutic use of self in occupational therapy.

1. Describe what caring means to you and how you will use caring in occupational therapy.

2. Can you respect someone even if you do not like him or her? What do you think of the Jackins' (1993) quote, "Every single human being, when the entire situation is taken in to account, has always, at every moment, done the very best that he or she could do, and so, deserves neither blame nor reproach from anyone, including self" (p. 3)?

3. What will it be like to offer hope to your future occupational therapy clients? Are there some people you will find it difficult to be hopeful about? Has it been helpful to you when someone offered you his or her hope? If so, discuss this time.

4. Describe a time you noticed you felt empathy for someone or that someone felt empathy for you.

5. Have you ever been assisted in pursuing a goal of your own choosing? Describe what was and was not effective in this situation.

6. Pay attention to what makes you laugh and what makes other people laugh and journal about this on a daily basis for a week. Do you have any new insights about humor from this exercise? How confident are you about using humor as an occupational therapist?

EVIDENCE-BASED RESEARCH CHART

Elements	Key Concepts	Evidence
Caring	Knowledge, skills, and attitude	Devereaux, 1984; Gilfoyle, 1980; King, 1980; Peloquin, 2002
Competence	Cultural	Black, 2005; Black & Wells, 2007
	Interpersonal	Taylor, 2008
Effective communication	Empathy	Abreu, 2011; Davis, 2011; Peloquin, 2002; Taylor, 2008
	Listening	Jackins, 1981; Rollnick, Miller, & Butler, 2008; Schwartzberg, 2002; Taylor, 2008
	Client-centered practice and empowerment	Calnan et al., 1994*; Henbest & Fehrsen, 1992*; Law, 1998; Law, Baptiste, & Mills, 1995; Maitra & Erway, 2006*; Tickle-Degnen, 2002; Wasserman, Inui, Barriatua, Carter, & Lippincott, 1984*
Group work	Group development	Cole, 2012; O'Brien & Solomon, 2013; Schiller, 2003; Schwartzberg, Howe, & Barnes, 2008; Taylor, 2013; Tuckman, 1965; Tuckman & Jensen, 1977; Vroman, 2013; Yalom & Leszcz, 2005
Humor	Therapeutic effects	Adams & Mylander, 1993; Dunbar et al., 2011*
Respect	Belief in the dignity and worth of our clients	Devereaux, 1984
Therapeutic relationships	Evidence on significance	Graybeal, 2007*; Taylor, Lee, Kielhofner, & Ketkar, 2009*
Touch	Comforting and functional	Chang, 2001*; Hertenstein, Holmes, McCullough, & Keltner, 2009*; Kim & Buschman, 1999*; Purtilo & Haddad, 2002
Values	Altruism, equality, freedom, justice, dignity, truth, and prudence	AOTA, 2010

*Evidence-based research

7. What is your own comfort level with touch? Describe how this varies in different situations.

8. In friendships, do you tend to be an encourager, empathizer, instructor, problem solver, advocate, or collaborator? Describe a situation when you functioned in one of these interpersonal modes.

9. Describe a time when you have interacted with someone from a different cultural group. Did you gain any new insights from this interaction? Once you know what your future clinical site will be, find out about the different ethnic populations served by your site and do some research to become better informed about those groups.

10. Describe how a group that you have participated in followed either Tuckman's or Schiller's model of group development.

References

Abreu, B. C. (2011). Accentuate the positive: Reflections on empathic interpersonal interactions. *American Journal of Occupational Therapy, 65,* 623-634. doi:10.5014/ajot.2011.656002

Adams, P., & Mylander, M. (1993). *Gesundheit: Bringing good health to you, the medical system, and society through physician service, complementary therapist, humor and joy.* Rochester, VT: Healing Arts Press.

American Occupational Therapy Association. (2010). *American Occupational Therapy Association: Occupational therapy code of ethics and ethics standards, 2010.* Retrieved from http://www.aota.org/Practitioners/Ethics/Docs/Standards/38527.aspx

Anthony, W. A. (1993). Recovery from mental illness: The guiding vision of the mental health service system in the 1990s. *Psychosocial Rehabilitation Journal, 16*(4), 11-23.

Anthony, W., Cohen, M., Farkas, M., & Gagne, C. (2002). *Psychiatric rehabilitation* (2nd ed.). Boston, MA: Center for Psychiatric Rehabilitation.

Berk, R. A. (2001). The active ingredients in humor: psychophysiological benefits and risks for older adults. *Educational Gerontology, 27(3-4),* 323-339.

Black, R. M. (2005). Intersections of care: An analysis of culturally competent care, client centered care, and the feminist ethic of care. *WORK: A Journal of Prevention, Assessment & Rehabilitation , 24*(4), 409-422.

Black, R. M., & Wells, S. A. (2007). *Culture and occupation: A model of empowerment for occupational therapy.* Bethesda, MD: AOTA Press.

Capps, D. (2006). The psychological benefits of humor. *Pastoral psychology, 54(5),* 393-411.

Calnan, M., Katsouyiannopoulos, V., Ovcharov, V. K., Prokhorskas, R., Ramic, H., & Williams, S. (1994). Major determinants of consumer satisfaction with primary care in different health systems. *Family Practice, 11*(4), 468-478.

Chang, S. O. (2001). The conceptual structure of physical touch in caring. *Journal of Advanced Nursing, 33*(16), 820-827.

Cole, M. B. (2012). *Group dynamics in occupational therapy: The theoretical basis and practice application of group intervention* (4th ed.). Thorofare, NJ: SLACK Incorporated.

D'Arc, J. (2003). *Allies to gay/lesbian/bisexual/transgendered workshop.* China Lake, ME.

Davis, C. M. (2011). *Patient practitioner interaction: An experiential manual for developing the art of health care* (5th ed.). Thorofare, NJ: SLACK Incorporated. Devereaux, E. B. (1984). Occupational therapy's challenge: the caring relationship. *American Journal of Occupational Therapy, 38,* 791-798.

Dunbar, R. I. M., Baron, R., Frangou, A., Pearce, E., van Leeuwin, E. J. C., Stow, J., Partridge, G., & van Vugt, M. (2011). Social laughter is correlated with an elevated pain threshold. *Proceedings of the Royal Society: Biological Sciences, 279*(1731), 1161-1167. Retrieved from http://rspb.royalsocietypublishing.org/content/279/1731/1161. DOI:10.1098/rspb.2011.1373

Gilfoyle, E. M. (1980). Caring: A philosophy for practice. *American Journal of Occupational Therapy, 34,* 517-521.

Graybeal, C. T. (2007). Evidence for the art of social work practice. *Families in Society, 88*(4), 513-523.

Henbest, R. J., & Fehrsen, G. S. (1992). Patient-centeredness: Is it applicable outside the West? Its measurement and effect on outcomes. *Family Practice, 9,* 311-317.

Hertenstein, M. J., Holmes, R. McCulough, M., & Keltner, D. (2009). Communication of emotion via touch. *Emotion, 9*(4), 566-573. doi:10.1037/a0016108

Isham, J. (2006). *Quotes of the heart.* Retrieved August 3, 2006, from http://www,heartquotes.net/Listening.html

Jackins, H. (1993). *Quotes.* Seattle, WA: Rational Island Publishers.

Kim, E. J., & Buschmann, M. T. (1999). Effect of expressive physical touch on patients with dementia. *International Journal of Nursing Studies, 36*(3), 235-243.

Kielhofner, G. (2008). *Model of human occupation: Theory and application* (4th ed.). Philadelphia, PA: Lippincott Williams & Wilkins.

King, L. J. (1980). Creative caring. *American Journal of Occupational Therapy, 34,* 522-534.

Law, M. (1998). *Client-centered occupational therapy.* Thorofare, NJ: SLACK Incorporated.

Law, M., Baptiste, S., & Mills, J. (1995). Client-centered practice: What does it mean and does it make a difference? *Canadian Journal of Occupational Therapy, 62,* 250-257.

Maitra, K. K., & Erway, F. (2006). Perception of client-centered practice in occupational therapists and their clients. *American Journal of Occupational Therapy, 60,* 298-310.

Martin, R. A., & Lefcourt, H. M. (2004). Sense of humor and physical health: Theoretical issues, recent findings, and future directions. *Humor. 17(1/2),* 1-20.

O'Brien, J. C., & Solomon, J. W. (2013). *Occupational analysis and group process.* St. Louis, MO: Mosby-Elsevier.

Peloquin, S. (2002). Reclaiming the vision of reaching for heart as well as hands. *American Journal of Occupational Therapy, 56,* 517-526.

Peloquin, S. (2003). The therapeutic relationship: manifestations and challenges in occupational therapy. In E. B. Crepeau, E. S. Cohn, & B. A. Boyt Schell (Eds.), *Willard and Spackman's occupational therapy* (10 ed., pp. 157-170). Philadelphia, PA: Lippincott Williams & Wilkins.

Purtilo, R., & Haddad, A. (2002). *Health professional and patient interaction* (6th ed.). Philadelphia, PA: W. B. Saunders & Co.

Schiller, L. Y. (2003). Women's group development from a relational model and a new look at facilitator influence on the group. In A. Mullender & M. B. Cohen (Eds.), *Gender and groupwork* (pp. 16-40). London, England: Routledge Press.

Schwartzberg, S. (2002). *Interactive reasoning in the practice of occupational therapy.* Upper Saddle River, NJ: Pearson Education, Inc.

Schwartzberg, S. L., Howe, M. C., & Barnes, M. A. (2008). *Groups: Applying the functional group model.* Philadelphia, PA: F.A. Davis Company.

Taylor, R. (2008). *The intentional relationship model: occupational therapy and use of self.* Philadelphia, PA: F.A. Davis Company.

Taylor, R. (2013). Therapeutic use of self: Applying the intentional relationship model in group therapy. In J. C. O'Brien, & J. W. Solomon (Eds.), *Occupational analysis and group process* (pp. 36-52). St. Louis, MO: Mosby-Elsevier.

Taylor, R. R., Lee, S. W., Kielhofner, G., & Ketkar, M. (2009). Therapeutic use of self: A nationwide survey of practitioners. *American Journal of Occupational Therapy, 63,* 198-207.

Tickle-Degnen, L. (2002). Evidence-based practice forum: Client-centered practice, therapeutic relationship, and the use of research evidence. *American Journal of Occupational Therapy, 56,* 470-479.

Tuckman, B. (1965). Developmental sequence in small groups. *Psychological Bulletin, 63,* 384-399.

Tuckman, B., & Jensen, M. (1977). Stages of small-group development revisited. *Group Organizational Management, 2*(4), 419-427.

Vroman, K. (2013). Managing and facilitating groups. In J. C. O'Brien, & J. W. Solomon (Eds.), *Occupational analysis and group process* (pp. 63-74). St. Louis, MO: Mosby-Elsevier.

Wasserman, R. C., Inui, T. S., Barriatua, B. S., Carter, W. B., & Lippincott, B. A. (1984). Pediatric clinician's support for parents makes a difference: An outcome-based analysis of clinician-parent interaction. *Pediatrics, 74*(6), 1047-1053.

Yalom, I., & Leszca, M. (2005). *The theory and practice of group psychotherapy* (5th ed.). New York, NY: Basic Books.

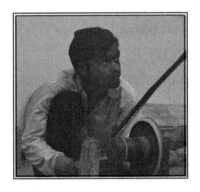

10

TEACHING, LEARNING, AND HEALTH LITERACY

Nancy Doyle, OTD, OTR/L

ACOTE STANDARDS EXPLORED IN THIS CHAPTER
B.5.4, B.5.18–B.5.21

KEY VOCABULARY

- **Health literacy:** Ability to find, understand, and use information to make health-related decisions.
- **Learner characteristics:** Features of a learner that may influence his or her learning experience and retention of information.

- **Teaching-learning process:** Interactive work of a teacher and student with the end goal of increasing the student's knowledge or skill.
- **Transfer of learning:** Ability to apply what one has learned in a different context or occupation.

Introduction

Occupational therapy's main focus is on "supporting health and participation in life through engagement in occupation" (AOTA, 2008, p. 626) at all client levels: individuals, organizations, and populations (AOTA, 2008). Our work affords many active teaching and learning opportunities regarding occupation, health, and participation (AOTA, 2007b). For example, we may teach an individual one-handed adaptations for gardening, a company about promoting occupational balance within its organization, and populations who are homeless about strategies to address and alleviate occupational deprivation. In each scenario and at each client level, we must strive to provide the most effective and efficient teaching-learning process for our clients. Just as in all areas of occupational therapy practice, our challenge is to provide not only the best clinical intervention but also the best education possible guided by theory, based in evidence, and infused with our clinical reasoning (AOTA, 2008, 2010).

When we look at education in occupational therapy, we must consider a variety of audiences and contexts. There are three main teaching audiences in occupational therapy: students, practitioners, and clients, which includes their family members, significant others, caregivers, and community. Such audiences can be at individual or group levels, and at organization or population levels. Teaching contexts are highly varied. We teach students

Jacobs, K., MacRae, N., & Sladyk, K. (Eds.).
*Occupational Therapy Essentials for
Clinical Competence, Second Edition* (pp. 127-136).
© 2014 SLACK Incorporated.

in the classroom and in fieldwork settings, practitioners in post-professional and continuing education courses, and clients and those around them in a variety of clinical and community settings. Yet despite the differences in learners and contexts, there are four commonalities that we can discuss in relation to the teaching-learning process for all: the learners' characteristics, the process of learning, teaching theories and methods, and assessment of learning. In this chapter, we highlight the teaching, learning, and health literacy of occupational therapy clients. However, similar considerations can be extended to occupational therapy students and practitioners.

Occupational Therapy Research on Teaching and Learning

Although there has been recent recognition that, like all areas of practice, the educational experiences we provide must be client-centered (Sharry, McKenna, & Tooth, 2002) and evidence-based (AOTA, 2007b; Bondoc, 2005; Stern, 2005), we are still working to build a body of evidence specific to occupational therapy education. This includes education for three main groups: students, continuing education of practitioners, and education of clients. There is a growing body of literature about how to educate occupational therapy students (Crist, Scaffa, & Hooper, 2010). Less is written about evidence-based continuing education strategies for occupational therapy practitioners. With regard to client education, the literature is often focused on specific conditions, such as for clients with stroke (Gustafsson et al., 2010) or for individuals with traumatic brain injury (Radomski et al., 2009). Until all three areas of education research are firmly established within our profession, we must employ the best available evidence and theories from not only occupational therapy, but also allied health and general education literatures. In doing so, we can provide the most evidence-based and effective teaching-learning experiences possible.

What is critical is that as we educate students, professionals, and clients, we study and document our efforts to contribute to the scholarship of teaching and learning (AOTA, 2009). These efforts will add to the occupational therapy literature on how to best provide learning opportunities for students, clients, family, significant others, colleagues, other health providers, and the general public. By doing so we will help achieve the Centennial Vision to become a powerful force supporting the health and wellness of individuals, organizations, and populations by working to meet their occupational needs (AOTA, 2007a).

Occupational Therapy Education and the Practice Framework

The elements of the teaching-learning process are easily embedded in the Occupational Therapy Practice Framework (AOTA, 2008) process, which guides all occupational therapy practice. For example, as we develop clients' occupational profiles and analyze their occupational performance, we can also gather information about their learning needs and characteristics. As we establish a therapeutic relationship with the client, we promote an open environment where genuine goals for both occupational participation and learning can be discussed and collaboratively formulated. The learning process and teaching methods we select for each client are then embedded in the occupational therapy intervention we provide. And just as the intervention strategies are guided by theory and evidence, so are the teaching-learning process and methods we select. Finally, assessing what has been learned can be included seamlessly in the review of the occupational therapy intervention and outcomes.

Learner Profile

In order for the educator or clinician to engage in the teaching-learning process with students or clients, it is helpful to first identify and understand the characteristics of the learner—something we may describe as the learner profile. Two main questions guide the development of these profiles: (1) What are the clients' learning needs? and (2) What are the learners' characteristics? First, we must determine with clients and their significant others what they need to know. Then, we work to understand characteristics of the learners that will help us in developing the most successful learning experience possible. These profiles consider the specific abilities, readiness, and motivation of the learners. They also include evaluation of the developmental and literacy levels of the learners, their contexts and cultures, and any other supports or barriers to learning. The process of understanding these learner characteristics is easily embedded in the process of developing a client's occupational profile. By working through the evaluation stage of the occupational therapy process (AOTA, 2008), we will come to understand the client's occupations, their occupational desires and barriers, and their learning needs and characteristics.

LEARNER NEEDS

In order to create successful learning experiences for our clients, we must first work with them to determine their learning needs. These are what information, processes, adaptations, habits, and routines the client needs to achieve or enhance their occupational goals. For example, if a client is recovering from a rotator-cuff tear and has a goal to return to cooking daily meals for his family, he may have a need to learn one-handed adaptations in the kitchen and recipe short-cuts. If a business is working with an occupational therapist to reduce work-related injuries, learning needs may include ergonomic information and education about the importance of new work habits, such as regular rest and stretch breaks. If an occupational therapist is contributing to public health efforts to combat childhood obesity, he or she may provide education about occupational balance as well as the importance of providing not only discussion of but also actual opportunities within a program for building new routines that incorporate physical activity, healthy cooking and eating, and rest and leisure occupations. Once learning needs such as these have been determined, other learner characteristics can be examined in order to plan the best client education possible.

LEARNER ABILITIES

As we assess a client, we are looking for their abilities, strengths, and challenges. Included in this assessment are abilities for learning. Perhaps the client has strong visual skills but difficulty with multistep directions. Or the client self-regulates attention levels well but has difficulty hearing. As you assess the client factors, performance skills, and performance patterns, many of the same abilities, strengths, and challenges you note in occupational performance will also affect the client's ability to learn.

In addition to learning abilities that would be evaluated during the occupational therapy process (AOTA, 2008), additional considerations may include cognitive and learning styles. Although both style types will benefit from continued basic and applied research to better understand the constructs and their application in educational settings (Coffield et al., 2004; Kozhevnikov, 2007; Pashler et al., 2009; Peterson et al., 2009), a basic understanding of their concepts allows occupational therapy professionals to further tailor learning experiences to the strengths and abilities of their clients.

Cognitive styles are generally defined as relatively stable ways of processing information from an individual's environment (Kozhevnikov, 2007). They include whether an individual tends to focus holistically or analytically on new information. For example, does a client prefer to discuss the whole occupational therapy process—from evaluation, to intervention, to outcomes—initially, or would the client prefer to focus on just one aspect at a time? Another cognitive style, termed *field (in)dependence*, looks at whether or not a person relies heavily on the environment to interpret information. Someone who relies heavily on environmental cues may benefit from working in a group setting where social cues may enhance the intervention process.

Learning styles and preferences are factors that affect learning behavior specifically. The experiential learning theory (Kolb & Kolb, 2005) describes learning as a process where an experience is grasped through concrete experience or abstract conceptualization and then transformed into new knowledge for an individual through reflective observation or active experimentation. In other words, a client may prefer to consider home modifications to prevent falls by actively practicing these strategies in the clinic or by more abstractly talking through them with an occupational therapist. Then they may prefer to take some time to reflect on these strategies before implementing them, or prefer to experiment with these strategies at home between occupational therapy sessions.

Clients may have preferences for the perceptual mode in which they learn. Some clients may prefer to learn visually with pictures and diagrams, aurally through audio recordings or discussions, visually through reading written text, or kinesthetically through active manipulation of learning materials (Fleming & Bonwell, 2006). Clients may, for example, prefer to complete a home program with a video, written, or audio guide depending on their learning preferences.

LEARNER READINESS

After understanding the learning needs and abilities of clients, it is important to assess their readiness. The student or client must see a need to learn what is being taught and be ready to engage in the learning process. Readiness to learn will be affected by a variety of factors both internal and external to the client. Because learning depends on readiness levels in different parts of the brain (National Research Council, 2000), internally the individual's systems, especially sensory systems, need to be functioning at an appropriate level so that information can be both received and processed (Ayres, 1973). Cognitive, emotional, and psychological readiness are also aspects of learner readiness. Clients who are, for example, currently stressed by an acute health problem may find their readiness to learn and their ability to retain information affected (Gustafsson et al., 2010). Externally, it is important to determine whether the context and conditions for working with a client are also ready for the teaching-learning process. If the environment is too noisy or the number of sessions is limited, it is important to consider what learning can be completed in these scenarios with a client who is ready to engage in the teaching-learning process.

LEARNER MOTIVATION

Motivation and readiness facilitate the teaching-learning process. When a client is both able to grasp new learning and is motivated to do so, learning will be more successful. Clients may be motivated extrinsically by rewards or consequences; motivation may be intrinsic, in that clients engage in learning for their own satisfaction or self-improvement. Generally, intrinsic motivation is most potent (Radel, Sarrazin, Legrain, & Wild, 2010). If the new learning is personally relevant, functional, utilitarian, or contributes to helping others, it is often more meaningful to the learner. In addition, materials that are neither too hard nor too easy, but instead are at the "just-right challenge" for a client, will avoid frustration or boredom and promote motivation. Motivation can also be contagious; learners often become motivated to learn if they sense genuine excitement and investment in the teaching-learning process by instructors or their peers (Radel et al., 2010). This speaks to the potential power of occupational therapy professionals and peers to motivate learners in a wide variety of contexts including group treatment, continuing education courses, and classrooms.

DEVELOPMENTAL STAGES OF LEARNING

Identifying the developmental level at which a client or student functions will help the therapist or teacher tailor the teaching-learning process appropriately. Development from infancy through old age must be considered (Bastable & Dart, 2011), including typical development, delays in development, and possible regression in the case of an injury or illness such as brain injury or dementia. Psychosocial and cognitive development are commonly considered. In order, Erikson's stages of psychosocial development focus on the development of trust, autonomy, initiative, industry, identity, intimacy, generativity, and ego integrity (Bastable & Dart, 2011). Piaget's stages of cognitive development look at learning from sensorimotor, preoperational, concrete operations, and formal operations perspectives (Piaget, 1954). When working with an infant, the focus may be on developing trust in new movement patterns through exploring toys with the therapist and caretakers; when working with an adult, more abstract discussion of roles and routines may help a client consider their contributions, successes, and areas for modification in his or her occupational plans for the future.

Another perspective on development may be in terms of the four levels of thinking: dualism, multiplicity, contextual relativism, and commitment within relativism (Perry, 1968). A dualistic thinker views knowledge as either correct or incorrect. This type of thinker is challenged by ambiguity and uncertainty and wants and needs structure and concrete examples. The new Level II fieldwork student will likely need structure to know what to do and how to do it. Beginning client expectations would be similar: the need for concrete, real examples and practice within a structured environment to support learning and transfer. A learner at the multiplicity level is learning to think with support from evidence, sees peers as legitimate sources of knowledge, and values independent thought. A student at this level desires evidence to support opinions and may balk at structure, while a client may ask for justification or proof that the approach being used is valid. Those within the contextual relativism level find all knowledge to be contextual, use metacognition, seek out many opinions, and look for connections. They insist on choice and commitment and may seek help from an authority figure. Clinically, this is the client who may combine traditional therapy with complementary approaches. The commitment within relativism stage would be represented by the expert clinician who has made professional commitments. Clinically, it would be represented by a client who has committed to providing education and support to those clients with similar diagnoses. Knowing at which Perry level students or clients are performing provides some of the information needed to design an appropriate learning environment.

LITERACY LEVEL

Assessing the learning needs of a client includes determining his or her literacy level. This includes gathering information about the primary language of communication, their general ability to comprehend spoken and written language, as well as their literacy in health information. Smith and Gutman (2011) report that the average American reads at a 6th grade level, much lower than the 10th grade level in which most information is communicated. This indicates a huge gap in what we say or write and what our clients may understand. We have a responsibility to be sure that what we communicate is at the appropriate literacy level so that our clients are able to fully grasp the information we provide to them.

When it comes to health literacy specifically, or the "ability of individuals to gather, interpret, and use information to make suitable health-related decisions" (Pizur-Barnekow & Darragh, 2011, p. 1), approximately half of all Americans have low health literacy. That is, they have "difficulty understanding and acting on health information" (Smith & Gutman, 2011, p. 367). We need to be sure that our services include advancing clients' health literacy, if necessary. For example, if a client with diabetes is unable to read and follow multistep directions to test insulin levels and take medication appropriately, we have a role in improving their ability to carry out these health-promoting activities. Just as we complete activity analyses to determine client needs in daily occupations, we can "deconstruct health activities" (Smith & Gutman, 2011, p. 368) and how they interact with clients' unique environments. We can then work to educate clients in the difficult areas of their health activities, thereby increasing intervention effectiveness (Smith & Gutman, 2011) as well as their health literacy and ability to make appropriate and optimal health choices (Pizur-Barnekow & Darragh, 2011).

It is best to assess health literacy confidentially and informally. Formal testing of literacy skills may upset or isolate clients. Instead, a question such as "How confident are you filling out medical forms by yourself?" (Cornett, 2009, p. 5) may be sufficient for determining that a client could benefit from assistance with health information. Additional behavioral cues (Cornett, 2009) may include patients' avoidance of reading pamphlets or filling out forms while in occupational therapy sessions, stating that they have forgotten their glasses, or their eyes are tired, or that they will do this at home. Clients with low literacy may not complete intake forms, or may do so incorrectly. When provided written information, their eyes may wander over but not focus on reading material. Clients with low literacy may miss appointments, and may be anxious, confused, or indifferent about written and health information. By attending to such potential indicators of low literacy, we can choose words and handouts most appropriate to the literacy needs of our clients in our teaching-learning process.

CONTEXT AND CULTURE

After looking at a client's specific learning characteristics, it is useful to look more broadly at their context and culture. This will help to situate their learning needs and appropriately design culturally sensitive teaching approaches. It is important to examine the cultural, personal, temporal, virtual, physical, and social contexts (AOTA, 2008) of the client and consider their relation to client education. Understanding whether a company works on a traditional 8-hour day or uses a different temporal rhythm for workers can affect how and when an occupational therapist provides educational sessions for administration and staff. For example, when working with refugee women from another country, it is important to understand the cultural roles, expectations, and aspirations of the clients. Whether their cultural context is based on a matriarchy or patriarchy can affect how new information is presented and whether it is presented just to the women or also to the men. When working to promote healthy occupational participation for at-risk youth, it is important to note if the physical environment includes safe playgrounds, community centers, or libraries that could promote healthy occupational choices.

In addition to considering the client's context and culture, it is important to be attuned to the context in which the teaching-learning process will occur. Learning environments need to be as authentic as possible, as posited by the situated learning theory (Lave & Wagner, 1991). Social and cultural components of a learning environment also need to be carefully considered. The amount and quality of learning can be helped or hindered by social support, dependent on the individuals' perception of the social factors. The opportunity to develop collaborative goals and the freedom to safely err may be among the norms of such an environment and therefore foster learning in a safe place.

Learning Content and Materials

Once the learner profile has been completed, the next step is to design the teaching-learning process and its content. The content is determined largely by the needs of the learner. It often includes client-centered teaching of new occupational skills (Sharry et al., 2002) and should be supported by a strong evidence base. For example, some recent literature points to the importance of providing information about a client's health conditions and how to manage them as part of client education (Radomski et al., 2009). As summarized by Radomski and colleagues (2009), clients with mild traumatic brain injury who received such education during occupational therapy sessions reported fewer symptoms and shorter symptom duration.

The occupational therapy literature in areas such as stroke rehabilitation (Gustafsson et al., 2010), adult physical disabilities (Sharry et al., 2002), and mild traumatic brain injury (Radomski et al., 2009) emphasizes the importance of providing multisensory and repetitious learning opportunities for clients. That is, clients can benefit from information being presented verbally as well as in written form (Radomski et al., 2009; Sharry et al., 2002), and from demonstration of and active practice or engagement with new learning (Gustafsson et al., 2010). Repetition of the new information may be useful for some learners. Some clients may benefit from teaching opportunities to be provided across occupational therapy sessions, particularly if their cognitive or other learning capacities increase over time or their learning needs change as they progress through various stages of therapy (Gustafsson et al., 2010).

When considering a client at the organization or population level, it seems particularly important to provide learning opportunities that target a variety of learning preferences. This will provide a more inclusive learning experience for clients with different learning and cognitive styles within the targeted organization or population.

Process

In addition to the learning content, it is important to plan how, when, and where the teaching-learning process takes place. Much of this is determined by the information gathered in the learner profile about clients' abilities, readiness, motivation, developmental stage, literacy level, context, and culture. This planning can be done concretely with the client and significant others by setting objectives for the learning in addition to those for the occupational therapy intervention. These objectives may include the amount of time and practice needed for learning, and whether and where transfer of learning should be promoted for the clients we are serving.

In addition to learning objectives, the teaching-learning process is guided by carefully selected pedagogy, educational approaches, and health behavior change theories appropriate to specific clients, their needs, and their characteristics. Just as we select theories and models to guide our occupational therapy interventions, we should choose teaching-learning theories that support our efforts to educate our clients in various areas and topics.

Learning Objectives

As objectives for occupational therapy intervention are developed with the client, specific objectives for learning new information may be included. It is important to consider not only the content of what the client desires to learn, but also the timing and sequence of the teaching-learning process. For example, the learning objectives may describe when new information will first be presented and how often it will be reinforced in the provision of therapy services (Gustafsson et al., 2010). Learning objectives should include the following: (1) where the learning will take place, (2) the duration of the teaching-learning process, (3) what the learner will demonstrate at the end of the teaching-learning process, and (4) how well the learner will perform at the end of the teaching-learning process.

Additional considerations for learning objectives might include whether the new knowledge or skill will be transferred to new situations or occupations. The amount of time and the pace of learning should be considered in relation to the complexity or volume of material and the client's learning characteristics. And finally, the amount of practice needed to master new aspects of occupational performance should also be considered when writing learning objectives and carrying out the teaching-learning process.

Pedagogy and Andragogy

The teaching-learning process may be approached differently depending on the age of the learner. Typically, a pedagogical approach is selected for children. This is where the teacher instructs by imparting knowledge to the learner. The teacher decides what is to be learned, when it is to be learned, and designs an appropriate environment in which the learning can occur.

When working with adults, a different approach may be useful. *Andragogy*, or the teaching of adults, is where the teacher assumes the role of a facilitator or a guide in the learning process. In this format, the learner assumes more responsibility for the learning, often choosing what is to be learned. The teacher and learner may be learning together, rather than the traditional transfer of knowledge from expert to novice. In this approach, the teacher may also challenge the learner to progress to higher levels of cognition (Bloom, 1956) and personal development (Cross, 1984).

An awareness of adult learning principles (Knowles, 1980) factors into using andragogy effectively. Hallmarks of adult learners are their need to know and be self-directed. They exhibit a readiness to learn, want to be involved in their learning, and are thus strongly internally motivated. They also want to immediately apply what they have learned, often to solve a problem that spawned their interest in learning. Adult learners bring a host of experiences and often a problem-centered approach to their learning. They assume responsibility for their learning; they desire choices as to how they will learn and, often, what they will learn. They want to voice what they already know, based on their life experience, and build on that knowledge. They value the experience of others, are willing to take risks, and are committed to lifelong learning (Cross, 1984; Knowles, 1980). These concepts may apply to occupational therapy students, participants in continuing education courses, and adult clients who are the experts on their lives and know what they want, but may need help strategizing how to get there.

The typical role of an occupational therapist is to facilitate learning during the therapeutic process by clarifying the goal, designing appropriate learning environments, teaching strategies for acquiring learning, providing feedback, and structuring practice opportunities to enhance transfer (Trombly, 1995). In the provision of occupational therapy services, the practitioner may need to make use of both teaching approaches and their varied concepts. Whether pedagogy or andragogy is selected may depend on the client and the progress of therapy. When working with a client or fieldwork student, the occupational therapy professional may find that it is necessary to use a pedagogical approach to structure the environment at the beginning of therapy or a fieldwork placement and, with progress, have the client or student choose which task to work on and self-structure the environment.

Educational Frames of Reference

Education has a number of teaching and learning theories and embedded frames of reference that need to be understood to design the environment that will best meet the needs of the client or student. Block and Chandler (2005) identify three frames of reference often used in schools: behaviorism, cognitivism, and constructionism. Behaviorism grew out of stimulus-response and classical and operant conditioning theories; it promotes the teacher or therapist to design the structure of the classroom or clinic and the goals for students or clients. Cognitivists encourage discovery within a less-structured environment. Constructivists believe that learners construct their own meaning and thus create their own learning.

A behaviorist approach may be used with clients who have problems controlling their behavior, such as clients with brain injury and children with emotional problems. Students may need more of this behaviorist approach as they begin to learn about the traits of an occupational therapy professional, with a lessening structure occurring as they progress in their learning. Graduate level occupational therapy education, particularly after clinical experience, would encourage a constructionist approach, providing choices for focused learning goals and the opportunity to reflect on and integrate the resulting learning. A clinical example would be encouraging clients during the last stages of community reintegration to choose a specific occupational performance issue to address and then recount his or her success or problems in performance.

Teaching-Learning Models

Once the appropriate educational approach—or progression of approaches from behaviorism through constructivism—has been selected, specific models for promoting health behavior changes are used to guide specific learning processes. These models describe how we can work with a client to think about, learn about, and implement behaviors that are health-promoting. Examples of such models include the health belief model, transtheoretical theory, social cognitive theory, diffusion of innovations, and ecological models.

Health Belief Model

The health belief model describes how the client reacts to a perceived health threat and how he or she determines the benefits and barriers to making a change in the health behavior (Champion & Skinner, 2008). This model also discusses how a client's self-efficacy, or belief in his or her ability to make changes, affects the client's ability to make the needed change. For example, when a client receives a diagnosis of diabetes, he or she is faced with choices as to how to maintain or improve health status. A belief in the ability to be successful with instituting healthy behaviors will allow for a more successful outcome.

Transtheoretical Theory

The transtheoretical theory (Prochaska et al., 1994) is a model of an individual's readiness to change a health behavior. The model describes five progressive stages of change. In the precontemplation stage, an individual may not be considering a health change even if there is a health problem. In the contemplation stage, the individual considers making a health change to address a health concern. In the preparation phase, the individual prepares and may even begin to implement some elements of a behavior change. In the action phase, the individual makes the identified behavior change and continues with the new behavior short-term, such as less than 6 months. In the maintenance phase, the individual continues with the new health-promoting behavior in the long-term or for more than 6 months. In this model, it is the educator's position to match the readiness stage of the client to what is being taught and learned. When working in an organization, providing educational sessions about implementing healthy workplace ergonomics may require a variety of sessions at the various stages of change in order to target individuals who are at different stages to consider, implement, and sustain healthy ergonomic behaviors.

Social Cognitive Theory

Social cognitive theory (Bandura, 1977) examines the interdependent relationships of the person, their environment, and the psychosocial determinants of their health behaviors. This theory takes into account the individual self-efficacy and expectations for health that an individual possesses, and how their social environment affects their health behaviors. It describes how people can learn from observing others and how environmental influences, such as policies or resources, may influence their behavior. In other words, the individual does not engage in health behaviors in isolation, but is influenced by his or her environment as well as his or her internal determinants to engage in certain health behaviors. For example, the professional behavior of occupational therapy students will be molded not just by their individual capacities and beliefs but also by learning from the behavior of occupational therapy professionals with clients and other colleagues in their fieldwork experiences.

Diffusion of Innovations

This theory looks at how new ideas, practices, or innovations are spread throughout a community or population. It models the diffusion, or spread, of the innovations in relation to their relative advantage over pre-existing innovations, their compatibility with the community, the complexity of the innovation, whether the innovation can be tried before it is adopted, and whether the results of the innovation are easily observable or measurable (Oldenburg & Glanz, 2008). This model is particularly helpful in working with communities or populations to influence behavior change.

Ecological Models

There are a variety of ecological models that look at health behavior. These models view people as embedded in multiple levels of influence on their health behaviors: environmental, policy, social, and psychological (Sallis, Owen, & Fisher, 2008). All levels can interact with one another, and interventions that target multiple levels are considered most effective for changes in health behavior. An example might be exploring the multiple levels of influence of older adults in an assisted living facility and targeting environmental, administrative policy, and group and individual attitudes and resources to enhance healthy occupational participation of all residents.

It is important to note that different health behavior change models can be used in combination (Christiansen & Baum, 2005). A combination allows for factors such as motivation, attitude, self-efficacy, and social support to be addressed simultaneously for the greatest likelihood of success.

Assessment of Learning

As in all areas of practice, assessment of teaching-learning sessions is as important as the planning and implementation of these sessions. Such assessment is best done by both sides: the therapist and the client, or the educator and the student. The following questions need to be addressed: (1) Were learning objectives met? (2) What was the quality of performance? and (3) How much more practice and variability are needed to guarantee transfer of learning? Gaining the client's perception of the session provides valuable information for future sessions and encourages self-reflection by the client. Pre-test and post-test assessments may provide valuable information about the teaching-learning process. For example, the Canadian Occupational Performance Measure (Law et al., 1998) can reflect elements of new learning as clients report on whether their satisfaction and performance of prioritized areas of occupational performance have improved. When working with families or significant others, time to absorb the material presented and time for questions become critical for carry-over at home. The same is true for students. They need to be able to consider carefully what has been discussed and pose any queries they may have. Taking such time can facilitate clients and their families and students grasping the critical concepts presented and improve the likelihood of appropriate application. The success of therapy and education hinges on a meaningful understanding of what is being taught and the ability to transfer that knowledge to situations when it is needed.

Summary

This chapter presented an overview of some of the important issues involved in teaching and learning. These include building a learner profile, understanding a client's health literacy, utilizing evidence-based teaching methods, selecting appropriate teaching-learning theories, and assessing learning. Occupational therapy

practitioners need to be aware of these issues, understand them, and incorporate them into their clinical and educational interventions for clients, families, students, colleagues, and the general public. Doing this allows for the development of optimal learning environments, ones that foster successful learning and growth, which are the cornerstones of enhanced independence and understanding.

Electronic Resources

- American Occupational Therapy Association: www.aota.org
- Occupational Therapy in Health Care: http://informahealthcare.com/loi/ohc—This journal periodically publishes research articles advancing occupational therapy education.
- NIH's Clear Communication Initiative: http://www.nih.gov/clearcommunication/healthliteracy.htm
- U.S. Department of Health and Human Services, Health Resources and Services Administration: http://www.hrsa.gov/publichealth/healthliteracy

Student Self-Assessment

1. Do you view occupational therapy practitioners as educators? Consider examples such as your professors and your fieldwork site supervisors. Why or why not? Has this chapter changed your view, and if so, with what content?

2. Consider your most recent or upcoming fieldwork experience. What elements of the learner profile do you think should be included in the occupational profile of clients in this setting?

3. Describe health literacy in your own words. Do you think it is important to promote the health literacy of your clients? How would you propose doing this with clients in your desired area of practice?

4. You are asked to put together a 5-minute presentation on creating effective client education experiences. What information can you share about appropriate verbal and written presentation of information to clients?

Acknowledgments

I would like to thank Nancy MacRae, MS, OTR/L, FAOTA for contributions to this chapter from her "Training, Education, Teaching, and Learning" chapter in the first (2010) edition of this textbook.

EVIDENCE-BASED RESEARCH CHART

Topic	Evidence
Client education	Gustafsson et al., 2010; Radomski et al., 2009; Sharry et al., 2002
Health literacy	Cornett, 2009; Pizur-Barnekow & Darragh, 2011; Smith & Gutman, 2011
Student education	AOTA, 2007a, 2009; Bondoc, 2005; Crist et al., 2010; Stern, 2005
Teaching-learning models	Bandura, 1977; Champion & Skinner, 2008; Christiansen & Baum, 2005; Oldenburg & Glanz, 2008; Prochaska et al., 1994; Sallis et al., 2008

References

American Occupational Therapy Association. (2007a). AOTA's Centennial Vision and executive summary. *American Journal of Occupational Therapy, 61,* 613-614.

American Occupational Therapy Association. (2007b). Philosophy of occupational therapy education. *American Journal of Occupational Therapy, 61,* 678.

American Occupational Therapy Association. (2008). Occupational therapy practice framework: Domain and process (2nd ed.). *American Journal of Occupational Therapy, 62,* 625-683.

American Occupational Therapy Association. (2009). Scholarship in occupational therapy. *American Journal of Occupational Therapy, 63,* 790-796.

American Occupational Therapy Association. (2010). Occupational therapy code of ethics and ethics standards. *American Journal of Occupational Therapy, 64,* S14-S24.

Ayres, A. J. (1973). *Sensory integration and learning disorders.* Los Angeles, CA: Western Psychological Services.

Bandura, A. (1977). Self-efficacy: Toward a unifying theory of behavioral change. *Psychological Review, 84,* 191-215.

Bastable, S. B., & Dart, M. A. (2011). Developmental stages of the learner. In S. B. Bastable., P. Gramet, K. Jacobs, & D. L. Sopczyk (Eds.), *Health professional as educator: Principles of teaching and learning* (pp. 151-197). Sudbury, MA: Jones & Bartlett Learning.

Block, M., & Chandler, B. E. (2005). Understanding the challenge: Occupational therapy and our schools. *OT Practice, 10*(1), CE1-CE8.

Bloom, B. S. (1956). *Taxonomy of educational objectives in the classification of educational goals: Cognitive domain* (handbook 1). New York, NY: McKay.

Bondoc, S. (2005). Occupational therapy and evidence-based education. *Education Special Interest Section Quarterly, 15,* 1-4.

Champion, V. L., & Skinner, C. S. (2008). The health belief model. In K. Glanz, B. K. Rimer, & K. Viswanath (Eds.), *Health behavior and health education: Theory, research, and practice* (pp. 45-65). San Francisco, CA: Jossey-Bass.

Christiansen, C. H., & Baum, C. M. (2005). *Occupational therapy: Performance, participation and well-being.* Thorofare, NJ: SLACK Incorporated.

Coffield, F., Moseley, D., Hall, E., & Ecclestone, K. (2004). *Learning styles and pedagogy in post-16 learning: A systematic and critical review.* London: Learning and Skills Research Centre.

Cornett, S. (2009). Assessing and addressing health literacy. *The Online Journal of Issues in Nursing, 14,* manuscript 2.

Crist, P., Scaffa, M., & Hooper, B. (2010). Occupational therapy education and the Centennial Vision. *Occupational Therapy in Health Care, 24,* 1-6.

Cross, P. K. (1984). *Adult learners: Increasing participation and facilitating learning.* San Francisco, CA: Jossey-Bass.

Fleming, N. D., & Bonwell, C. C. (2006). *VARK questionnaire, version 7.0.* Retrieved from http://www.vark-learn.com/english/page.asp?p=questionnaire

Gustafsson, L., Hodge, A., Robinson, M., McKenna, K., & Bower, K. (2010). Information provision to clients with stroke and their carers: Self-reported practices of occupational therapists. *Australian Occupational Therapy Journal, 57,* 190-196.

Knowles, M. (1980). *The modern practice of adult education.* Chicago, IL: Follett Publishing.

Kolb, A. Y., & Kolb, D. A. (2005). *The Kolb learning style inventory—Version 3.1 2005 technical specifications.* Boston, MA: Hay Resources Direct.

Kozhevnikov, M. (2007). Cognitive styles in the context of modern psychology: Toward an integrated framework of cognitive style. *Psychological Bulletin, 133,* 464-481.

Lave, J., & Wagner, E. (1991). *Situated learning: Legitimate peripheral participation.* Cambridge, MA: Cambridge University Press.

Law, M., Baptiste, S., Carswell, A., McColl, M. A., Polatajko, H., & Pollock, N. (1998). *Canadian occupational performance measure* (3rd ed.). Thorofare, NJ: SLACK Incorporated.

National Research Council. (2000). *How people learn: Brain mind, experience and school, expanded edition.* Washington, DC: National Academy Press.

Oldenburg, B., & Glanz, K. (2008). Diffusion of innovations. In K. Glanz, B. K. Rimer, & K. Viswanath (Eds.), *Health behavior and health education: Theory, research, and practice* (pp. 313-333). San Francisco, CA: Jossey-Bass.

Pashler, H., McDaniel, M., Rohrer, D., & Bjork, R. (2009). Learning styles: Concepts and evidence. *Psychological Science in the Public Interest, 9,* 105-119.

Perry, W. G. (1968). *Forms of intellectual and ethical development in the college years: A scheme.* New York, NY: Holt, Rinehart and Winston.

Peterson, E. R., Rayner, S. G., & Armstrong, S. J. (2009). Researching the psychology of cognitive style and learning style: Is there really a future? *Learning and Individual Differences, 19,* 518-523.

Piaget, J. (1954). *The construction of reality in the child.* New York, NY: Psychology Press.

Pizur-Barnekow, K., & Darragh, A. (2011). *AOTA's societal statement on health literacy.* Retrieved from: http://www.aota.org/Practitioners/Official/SocietalStmts/Health-Literacy.aspx?FT=.pdf

Prochaska, J. O., Velicer, W. F., Rossi, J. S., Goldstein, M. G., Marcus, B. H., Rakowski, W., et al. (1994). Stages of change and decisional balance for 12 problem behaviors. *Health Psychology, 13,* 39-46.

Radel, R., Sarrazin, P., Legrain, P., & Wild, T. C. (2010). Social contagion of motivation between teacher and student: Analyzing underlying processes. *Journal of Educational Psychology, 102,* 577-587.

Radomski, M. V., Davidson, L., Voydetich, D., & Erickson, M. W. (2009). Occupational therapy for service members with mild traumatic brain injury. *American Journal of Occupational Therapy, 64,* 646-655.

Sallis, J. F., Owen, N., & Fisher, E. B. (2008). Ecological models of health behavior. In K. Glanz, B. K. Rimer, & K. Viswanath (Eds.), *Health behavior and health education: Theory, research, and practice* (pp. 465-485). San Francisco, CA: Jossey-Bass.

Sharry, R., McKenna, K., & Tooth, L. (2002). Brief report—Occupational therapists' use and perceptions of written client education materials. *American Journal of Occupational Therapy, 56,* 573-576.

Smith, D. L., & Gutman, S. A. (2011). Health literacy in occupational therapy practice and research. *American Journal of Occupational Therapy, 65,* 367-369.

Stern, P. (2005). A holistic approach to teaching evidence-based practice. *American Journal of Occupational Therapy, 59,* 157-164.

Trombly, C. A. (1995). *Occupational therapy for physical dysfunction* (4th ed.). Baltimore, MD: Williams & Wilkins.

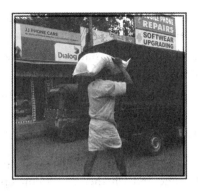

11

SAFETY AND SUPPORT

Claudia E. Oakes, OTR/L, PhD

ACOTE STANDARDS EXPLORED IN THIS CHAPTER
B.2.8, B.2.9

KEY VOCABULARY

- **Safety:** The state of being protected from injury or harm.
- **Standard precautions:** Steps to reduce the transmission of diseases.
- **Support:** To sustain or maintain so that an individual may participate in meaningful occupation.

Introduction

This chapter addresses ways in which occupational therapy practitioners and students can take steps to optimize their personal safety and the safety of their clients. It also addresses ways in which practitioners support clients' occupational performance to promote satisfaction and well-being.

Although individual health care facilities provide routine training on safety issues, this chapter provides an overview of the basic issues related to safety. It is not intended to serve as a replacement for individualized safety training specific to a particular setting. All practitioners have a responsibility to receive ongoing training and to adhere to institutional policies and procedures related to safety.

Safety and support, in the context of occupational therapy, are multifaceted concepts encompassing elements of the person, the environment, the activity, and interaction between them (Holm, Rogers, & James, 1998). The "person" in the context of safety may refer to the occupational therapy practitioner or the client. Any activity may fall on a continuum of risk from "not safe at all" to "very safe." However, it is the interaction between the person, the activity, and the environment that largely dictates whether an activity is safe. For example, consider the activity of meal preparation. There is minimal safety risk for a person without impairments who is making a simple meal in an uncluttered kitchen

Jacobs, K., MacRae, N., & Sladyk, K. (Eds.).
*Occupational Therapy Essentials for
Clinical Competence, Second Edition* (pp. 137-148).

using appliances that are in optimal working condition. However, meal preparation does present a safety risk for a person with impaired vision (interaction between the person and the activity) or for a person who is attempting to cook in a cluttered or inadequately lit work space (interaction between the person and the environment). The Occupational Therapy Practice Framework (OTPF) from the American Occupational Therapy Association (AOTA) identifies "safety and emergency maintenance" as instrumental activities of daily living (IADL) that involve "knowing and performing preventive procedures to maintain a safe environment as well as recognizing sudden, unexpected hazardous situations and initiating emergency action to reduce the threat to health and safety" (AOTA, 2008, p. 620).

This definition can be applied to practitioners for use in their daily practice, as well as to clients who are addressing issues related to functional independence. Safety concerns are present across the continuum of settings in which occupational therapy practitioners work. Although the safety issues that emerge in acute care, rehabilitation, skilled nursing facilities, schools, or home care may differ, practitioners must be vigilant in their efforts to maximize safety. Practitioners support clients' independence by providing a safe context for participants to explore and master their chosen occupations. Practitioners' efforts to support the functional independence of clients must always be balanced with efforts to maintain clients' safety.

General Safety Principles

When initiating contact with a client, practitioners and students must take steps to ensure that they are working with the correct client. For hospitalized clients, this may include checking wrist bands or confirming the identity with the client, a family member, or staff. Therapists must have accurate, up-to-date information about our clients. This may involve reading the medical chart or consulting with other staff members in preparation for the therapeutic encounter. If there is a question with respect to a client's status or his or her ability to engage in therapy (e.g., there may be conflicting information in a client's medical chart), clarification must be obtained before initiating contact with the client. Practitioners must be aware of any precautions or contraindications for intervention, such as the following:

- Orthopedic precautions (e.g., do not flex hips greater than 90 degrees)

- Cardiac precautions (e.g., stop activity if heart rate increases more than 20 beats per minute over baseline)

- Positioning precautions (e.g., do not raise head of bed greater than 30 degrees)

- Weight-bearing precautions (e.g., no more than toe-touch weight bearing on left lower extremity)

- Precautions related to feeding status (e.g., fluid restrictions, thickened liquids only)

- Supervision precautions (e.g., do not leave client unattended)

- Infection control precautions (e.g., don mask, gloves, and gown before entering the client's room)

Practitioners must be aware of any procedures that the client may have undergone and whether any follow-up precautions must be observed. For example, clients may be required to remain on bed rest for a set amount of time following an angiography (Gall, Tarique, Natarajan, & Zaman, 2006). In addition, therapists must be aware of the effects of drugs and associated common side effects that might relate to occupational therapy. Practitioners should know how to interpret common laboratory values with respect to a client's ability to engage in therapy.

Physical hazards in the environment should be reduced in order to support occupational performance. The space should be visually inspected to ensure that falling hazards have been eliminated, sharp objects from previous sessions have been stored, and potentially dangerous objects have been removed. Floors should be clear of liquid and debris.

Practitioners are required to make judgments about what is safe for each individual client. Judgments about materials such as sharp-edged scissors, needles, knives, ovens, and stoves need to be made on a case-by-case basis with each client. The dynamic nature of clients' status requires therapists to continually reassess clients' ability to safely engage in a particular occupation on a given day.

Furthermore, in order to fully support clients in performing their occupational roles and responsibilities, the practitioner must support the cultural, physical, social, personal, spiritual, temporal, and virtual contexts in which the clients are engaged. For example, some clients may need both safety education and social support to explore the Internet. The therapist must use clinical reasoning during the evaluation and intervention of both safety and support to enhance clients' quality of life.

Practitioners must consider the physical, cognitive, and emotional demands of activities to determine whether participation has the potential to compromise the client's safety. Ongoing occupation analysis helps to ensure an appropriate "fit" between the client, the occupation, and the materials that are needed. Adapting an occupation in order to provide an appropriate challenge is a fundamental step in providing support for clients and in keeping them safe while allowing them to advance their functional status.

Impaired cognition presents serious safety concerns across intervention settings. Practitioners must be aware of clients' awareness of and ability to respond to potentially dangerous situations. In order to maintain safety, clients must demonstrate adequate attention, memory, judgment, temporal awareness, problem solving, decision making, and the ability to initiate actions in a timely manner. Occupational therapists are often called upon to determine if a client can safely perform an activity independently. Part of that decision making involves determining the client's ability to respond to unsafe conditions in an effective manner and what supports might be needed to maximize safe performance. Supports may be environmental (e.g., grab bars), social (e.g., "friendly visitors"), or virtual (e.g., daily email contact).

Following interactions with clients, therapists must use our best judgment when making decisions about how and where to leave clients. For example, some clients may be left alone in their hospital room, whereas others must be supervised at all times. Some will need assistance with transport to another therapy session. It is important to know each client's status with respect to his or her ability to manage independently after a therapy session.

Suicide Risk

As health and rehabilitation workers who treat clients with a wide range of diagnoses and stressors, therapists must be alert to the risk of suicide. Practitioners must be able to accurately assess whether clients have made a suicide attempt, the risk of repetition, if suicidal ideation is present, and if the client feels hopelessness or is likely to act impulsively (Bruce & Borg, 2002). If a client makes indirect comments that suggest he or she has considered suicide, ask directly if there is a plan to commit suicide. Any statement about suicide should be taken seriously and shared with other members of the interprofessional team.

A client who appears to be suicidal should not be left unattended. The practitioner should inform the client that he or she has a responsibility to alert the physician immediately. It is critical to document any statement the client has made relative to a suicide threat, as well as any action that has been taken.

Infection Control

Infection control is a basic component of clinical practice for all practitioners and students regardless of the practice setting. Therapists must be vigilant in our efforts to curb the spread of infection and reduce our personal risk of becoming infected with contaminated materials as well as be aware of the risk of drug-resistant pathogens.

Methicillin-resistant *Staphylococcus aureus* (MRSA), vancomycin-resistant *Enterococci* (VRE), and some gram-negative bacilli (GNB) are microorganisms that are resistant to one or more classes of antibiotics. Because there are limited intervention options if an infection develops from one of these organisms, it is critical that all health care workers take steps to reduce the spread of infection. The Centers for Disease Control and Prevention (CDC) has developed a campaign that is available online to help hospital workers reduce the risk of spreading drug-resistant pathogens (www.cdc.gov/drugresistance/healthcare/default.htm). Guidelines differ for hospitalized adults, adults receiving dialysis, hospitalized children, long-term care clients, and surgical clients (CDC, 2002).

Therapists should routinely follow standard precautions which include thorough hand washing and the use of workplace procedures to reduce the risk of transmission of infectious agents. Workplace procedures, or the way tasks are performed, can minimize risk. Workplace procedures include proper waste disposal; appropriate laundry handling; and the proper use of personal protective equipment (PPE) such as gloves, eye protection, face shields, masks, and gowns.

Standard precautions are a combination of universal precautions and body substance isolation (BSI). Universal precautions were developed in the 1980s to prevent the transmission of blood-borne pathogens such as human immunodeficiency virus (HIV; Occupational Safety and Health Administration [OSHA], 2002a). BSI precautions were developed to minimize the risk of transmission of pathogens from moist body substances such as infected respiratory secretions or urine. The CDC developed standard precautions based on the assumption that all blood, body fluids, secretions, excretions (other than sweat), nonintact skin, and mucous membranes may contain infectious agents that could be transmitted to other people (Siegel, Rhinehart, Jackson, Chiarello, & Healthcare Infection Control Practices Advisory Committee, 2007). Some standard precautions are detailed in the following section.

Hand Hygiene

When properly performed, hand washing can be the single most important way to prevent the spread of disease (Potter & Perry, 2004). Hands should be washed before and after contact with every client. In addition, hand washing should be completed after coming into contact with blood, body fluids, secretions, excretions, or any client care equipment. If contact with these substances takes place, practitioners should wash their hands even if gloves were worn. The correct technique involves rubbing the hands together under running water for at least 15 seconds using a mild soap (Boyce, Pittet, Healthcare Infection Control Practices Advisory Committee, & HICPAC/SHEA/APIC/IDSA Hand Hygiene Task Force, 2002). Rub vigorously under the nails, in between the fingers, and on both surfaces of the hands. Rinse thoroughly under running water. Leave the water running while drying hands and use a clean paper towel to turn off the water. Waterless, alcohol-based, antiseptic rubs are acceptable substitutes for routine hand washing when no visible soil is present. Such rubs may be used when running water is not accessible or convenient, although hands should be washed under running water at the earliest opportunity. The CDC guidelines for hand washing are available online in an interactive video format at http://www.cdc.gov/handhygiene/Basics.html.

GLOVES

Gloves are a critical component of PPE used to reduce the risk of transmission of infectious agents. Therapists should don gloves before coming into contact with blood, body fluids, secretions, excretions, and contaminated items and before touching mucous membranes or non-intact skin. For occupational therapy practitioners, it is appropriate to don gloves during sessions involving wound care, oral hygiene, or toileting. Remove gloves immediately after use. The proper technique for removing gloves involves pulling the first glove off by grasping the outer surface of the glove to be removed (not the surface touching the skin) and slipping the glove inside out as it is pulled off the hand. To remove the second glove, slip a nongloved finger under the remaining glove and pull it off while turning it inside out. Dispose of both gloves by touching only the inner glove surface. Do not touch noncontaminated items before removing gloves. Hands should be washed immediately after removing gloves (Boyce et al., 2002).

MASKS, EYE PROTECTION, AND FACE SHIELDS

Masks, eye protection, and face shields may be needed if it is anticipated that blood, body fluids, secretions, or excretions will splash during interaction with the client. These pieces of PPE protect the practitioner's eyes, nose, and mouth from exposure to sprayed microorganisms.

GOWNS

A nonsterile gown is used for protecting skin and clothing during interactions when splashes are likely to occur. The cuffs of the gown should be tucked into the top of the gloves. After the session, the gown should be untied, held away from the body while being removed, rolled inside out, and then disposed of in an appropriate container. Hands should be washed immediately after the gown and gloves are removed.

CLIENT CARE EQUIPMENT

Care must be taken to prevent the spread of microorganisms on equipment that is used by and with clients. Equipment should be cleaned after use with an approved solution according to institutional policy. Mat tables and adaptive equipment should be cleaned according to departmental policy. Single-use items should be discarded appropriately.

LINENS

Practitioners should take steps to minimize skin and mucous membrane exposure to soiled linens. Practitioners may encounter soiled linens when performing activities of daily living (ADL) with clients. Gloves should be worn to remove soiled linens; then soiled linens should be placed in an appropriate leak-proof container for transport to laundry.

OTHER PRECAUTIONS

Additional practices, including airborne infection isolation rooms, contact precautions, and droplet precautions, are used to prevent transmission of infectious agents spread by direct or indirect contact with a client or the client's environment (CDC, 2004). These practices reflect a higher standard of infection control than standard precautions. Private rooms, negative airflow pressure, and respiratory protection devices add extra levels of infection control for clients placed under these precautions. Appropriate signage will alert practitioners of the need to follow special precautions.

RESPIRATORY HYGIENE/COUGHING ETIQUETTE

This recent addition to standard precautions (Siegel et al., 2007) broadly applies to all people who enter health care settings, including visitors. For example, a client's family member may have a cough and should therefore use coughing etiquette (e.g., covering the mouth, preferably by coughing into a bent elbow) to reduce the spread of undiagnosed infection. Respiratory hygiene requires people with coughs or respiratory discharge to cover their mouths when coughing, dispose of used tissues, and wash hands as soon as possible after doing so; wear masks if tolerated; and maintain greater than 3 feet distance from others.

VACCINATIONS

The hepatitis B virus (HBV) presents a serious risk of infection for health care workers (CDC, 2011). The HBV series reduces the risk of infection and is available, free of charge, to hospital employees who are at risk of exposure (OSHA, 2003). Health care workers may be asked to sign a declination if they choose not to receive the vaccine. The CDC (2011) recommends that health care workers receive annual influenza vaccinations. Health care workers are advised to get the immunization for measles, mumps, and rubella (MMR) in the absence of laboratory proof of immunity. Health care professionals should not get the varicella vaccination if they have proof from a health care provider that they have either had the illness or can prove through laboratory testing that they are immune (CDC, 2011). In addition, the CDC (2004) recommends periodic skin testing to detect the presence of tuberculosis for health care workers at risk of exposure.

Basic First Aid

Occupational therapy practitioners and students should demonstrate competence with basic first aid. It is important to keep current with training, as the standards periodically change.

Contact the American Red Cross (www.redcross.org) for the most up-to-date information and for information about training sessions.

BURNS

Therapists should take care to ensure that burns do not occur during the course of splinting, cooking, or bathing with clients. First-degree thermal burns, which result in reddened skin, should be treated by putting the burned area under cool, running water for 5 minutes. The burned area should be covered with a clean or sterile dressing. Creams or ointments should not be applied. Any more serious injury should be immediately reported and treated by other health care professionals (American Red Cross, 2005).

BLEEDING

In the event of bleeding, therapists should don gloves and then apply pressure with a sterile dressing. Tourniquets should not be used due to the risk of injury to nerves and/or muscles because of problems associated with ischemia. If a client has a laceration, running water should be applied for up to 5 minutes to clear the area of any foreign matter (American Red Cross, 2005). Professional judgment is necessary to determine if further medical assistance is necessary.

ALLERGIES

Latex Allergy

Latex allergies emerged as a significant public health issue in the late 1980s and into the early 1990s. During the 1990s, some estimates suggested that 1 in 10 health care workers had latex allergy, but a shift to powder-free, low-protein latex has resulted in a significant decline in the incidence of allergy (Beezhold & Sussman, 2005). However, even with this reduction, practitioners need to be aware of the symptoms of latex allergy, which include redness and itching (typically on hands); difficulty breathing; wheezing; swelling of skin, lips, and tongue; and shortness of breath. If a person exhibits these symptoms after exposure to latex products, emergency medical attention is required. Be aware that some supplies in the occupational therapy department may contain latex, such as gloves and resistance bands. Latex-free versions of many products are available for clients with latex sensitivities.

Food Allergies and Anaphylaxis

It is estimated that in the United States, three million children younger than the age of 18 have been diagnosed with food allergies (Branum & Lukacs, 2009). It is important for occupational therapy practitioners to be aware of the presence of food allergies in their clients. Allergies should be taken into account when working with feeding, meal preparation, certain craft activities, or when going on food-related outings. Be aware of the symptoms of an allergic reaction: hives, swelling of lips or tongue, vomiting, trouble breathing, or a drop in blood pressure (anaphylaxis). Should these symptoms develop, emergency medical attention is required. To prevent accidental ingestion of allergens, always read labels when completing meal preparation activities. Avoid cross-contamination when engaging in cooking activities by keeping utensils separate. For example, always use separate utensils for peanut better and jelly. Be aware of each client's emergency protocol in the event of accidental ingestion. Reactions to food allergies are commonly treated with an auto-injector of epinephrine (Epi-Pen; DEY, L. P.). It is important to know where the Epi-Pen is located and who is trained in its use.

ORTHOSTATIC HYPOTENSION

A client with orthostatic hypotension (OH) demonstrates a decrease in blood pressure of more than 20 mm Hg in systolic and of more than 10 mm Hg in diastolic, while also experiencing a 20% increase in heart rate (Goodman, Fuller, & Boissonnault, 2003). A client may experience confusion, dizziness, visual blurring, and possibly fainting when coming to stand. Practitioners must be aware of the potential causes of OH in order to prevent its onset. Some common causes include dehydration, venous pooling, side effects of certain medications, and prolonged immobility. To minimize the risk of OH in a client who is coming to stand from a supine or seated position, instruct the client to rise slowly, flex and extend the ankles, and lift the arms overhead while tightening the abdominal muscles and exhaling through pursed lips. If symptoms develop, help the client into a supine position with the legs elevated, unless contraindicated. Monitor the client's vital signs including pulse, blood pressure, and respiratory rate. This is particularly important in clients with chronic obstructive pulmonary disease who may not tolerate the "legs elevated" position.

Be aware of the risk of fainting for others in the health care environment. Visitors, including students and volunteers, may be at risk of fainting. This is due to emotional stress and the tendency of blood to pool in the lower extremities while standing with knees locked, as is often the case when observing intervention sessions. To prevent fainting, keep legs moving by marching in place or crossing legs. Warn visitors to alert a staff member if they feel lightheaded or dizzy. Provide assurance that visitors should feel free to leave the immediate area if they feel faint.

Seizures

If a client has a generalized tonic-clonic or grand mal seizure during an occupational therapy session, the practitioner is responsible for ensuring the client is not injured and that an open airway is maintained. These types of seizures generally last approximately 2 minutes and are characterized by a loss of consciousness, rigidity, jerky movements, and shallow breathing. The client should be gently lowered to the ground, mat table, or bed. Do not make any attempt to prevent the client from biting his or her tongue. Loosen clothing around the client's neck to ensure adequate airflow. Do not restrain the client. After the seizure is complete, place the client in the recovery position, lying on his or her side with his or her hand in front. Call for medical assistance (American Red Cross, 2005). A seizure that lasts for more than 15 minutes, or a series of seizures that lasts for 20 minutes without regaining consciousness in between may suggest status epilepticus. This is a medical emergency and assistance should be sought at once.

Diabetes

When working with clients who have diabetes, it is important for practitioners to differentiate between signs and symptoms of low blood sugar (hypoglycemia) and high blood sugar (hyperglycemia). Low blood sugar occurs when blood glucose falls below optimal levels and can occur if a client is engaging in physical activity, if there is too much systemic insulin, or if the client has ingested too little food. Some oral medications used to treat diabetes can also cause low blood sugar. Symptoms are variable and may include shakiness, a sense of weakness, a feeling of anxiety and confusion, dizziness, headache, blurred vision, and/or sweating. Practitioners should be aware that therapy sessions may interrupt the usual meal or snack time and therefore result in hypoglycemia. If a client displays symptoms of hypoglycemia, he or she should have a small snack that has a fast-acting source of sugar, such as juice or hard candy. After the snack, the client should check his or her blood sugar level and then contact a nurse or physician if levels are not within the client's acceptable parameters.

High blood sugar may be caused by overeating, poor coordination of eating, medication, infection, or stress. Clients with hyperglycemia may experience fatigue, low energy levels, frequent urination, and/or excessive thirst. High blood sugar may lead to diabetic ketoacidosis, which is a medical emergency. It is caused by inadequate insulin, vast deviation from diet, fever, or infection. The client may have gradual-onset weakness, stomach pain, body aches, labored breathing, fruity breath, dry mouth, nausea, and/or vomiting. Should these symptoms occur, contact medical professionals at once, immediately test blood sugar, and provide the client with plain water (Ross, Boucher, & O'Connell, 2005).

Cardiac Arrest and Choking

Occupational therapy practitioners should maintain cardiopulmonary resuscitation (CPR) certification to treat a person who is choking or who is experiencing cardiac arrest. Local chapters of the American Red Cross (n.d.) or the American Heart Association (2005; www.americanheart.org) may be contacted for information about training courses. Protocols are constantly changing as best practices are updated. A thorough description of these procedures is beyond the scope of this chapter.

Client Care Equipment

Clients may be connected to intravenous (IV) lines, arterial lines, central lines, feeding tubes, chest tubes, ventilators, catheters, and/or a variety of monitors. It is essential that the occupational therapy practitioner be aware of the purpose of various tubes and monitors. The practitioner should identify all lines and where they connect. In general, it is wise to avoid tugging, pulling, or occluding lines and to ensure adequate slack before moving the client. If any tension is felt, it is recommended that the practitioner stop and check to determine the cause.

Precautions for each tube, line, or monitor must be identified. For example, an arterial line is a catheter that is placed in the radial artery to continually measure blood pressure. Extra caution must be taken to prevent dislodging an arterial line, as dislodging one will cause profuse bleeding (Potter & Perry, 2004). The practitioner must be aware of institutional policies regarding specific equipment and of any particular precautions for an individual client. In addition, it is important that the practitioner is aware of the parameters for any monitors that are providing information about a client's physiologic state. For example, it is generally recommended that activity be stopped if oxygen saturation is below 90%, as measured by a pulse oximeter. The acceptable saturation may be lower in some clients with chronic pulmonary disease (Goodman et al., 2003).

Hazardous Materials

Therapists should always be aware of the presence of hazardous materials in the occupational therapy department. It is important to know where the Material Safety Data Sheets (MSDS) are stored. These sheets are required by OSHA (www.osha.gov). They contain useful information about proper storage of hazards, ways in which products are toxic, and information on how to clean a spill, or how to administer first aid if accidental exposure occurs.

Fire Safety

Therapists should be familiar with the fire safety procedures at our facility. This includes knowing the floor map of the facility, the areas for zone evacuation, the location of fire pulls, and the specifics of any emergency plan (OSHA, 2002b). In general, the acronym RACE is helpful to recall in the event of a fire (Potter & Perry, 2004):

- R—Remove all persons who are in immediate danger.
- A—Activate the pull station and call 911.
- C—Close doors to prevent the spread of fire. This includes fire doors, smoke doors, and doors to client rooms.
- E—Extinguish the fire as dictated by department policy.

If a practitioner is called upon to use a fire extinguisher, the acronym PASS guides technique:

- P—Pull the pin to break the glass.
- A—Aim the extinguisher at the base of the fire.
- S—Squeeze the handles together.
- S—Sweep from side to side at the base of the fire.

It is essential that the correct extinguisher is used for the specific type of fire. Labels on extinguishers identify whether they are best used for combustibles, flammable liquids, or electrical fires. More information can be obtained on the OSHA Web site at www.osha.gov/SLTC/ etools/ evacuation/portable_use.html.

Fire Safety in Clients' Homes

Practitioners working in home care settings should ensure that clients have smoke detectors in their homes. There should be at least one smoke detector on each level of the home, including the basement. Batteries should be checked twice a year, at a minimum. Smoke detectors should be replaced every 8 to 10 years. Therapists should review fire plans with members of the household, which should include:

- How to exit the house.
- Where to meet outside.
- Who is responsible for any person who may need extra help.

There should be two methods of egress in every dwelling, and this may include a window (United States Fire Administration, 2012). It is recommended that people with disabilities notify members of local fire departments in order to facilitate assistance in the event of an emergency.

Emergency Preparedness and Disaster Response

Natural and man-made disasters require therapists to respond in an efficient and effective manner in order to ensure the safety and well-being of clients, family members, and other team members. In the event of a disaster (such as a hurricane) that may limit the ability of health care employees to travel to and from the facility, practitioners may be asked to remain on-site to ensure continuity of care. This may involve sleeping at the facility overnight to ensure adequate staffing during the next scheduled shift, or remaining on-site to perform other essential functions that are within the scope of practice. This may include transporting patients or assisting with toileting or feeding patients. In the event that the facility needs to be evacuated (perhaps during a flood or power outage), therapists may be needed to assist in moving patients down flights of stairs if the elevators are out of service. It is critical to be aware of the emergency response plan at your place of employment (United States Department of Health and Human Services, 2012). For example, in some facilities, the rehabilitation department may be used as temporary place to hold patients if patient care areas have been damaged.

In addition, occupational therapy practitioners are ideally suited to assist community leaders in preparing for disasters. For example, many towns have plans in place to convert town properties into shelters during mass power outages. Because therapists are aware of the needs of people with a range of disabilities, they can provide useful suggestions about accessibility of shelters, equipment to have available, and ways to assess physical and mental capabilities of residents who occupy the temporary shelter. In the hours and days following disasters, therapists are suited to assist survivors in dealing with stress, maximize safety, and develop routines to facilitate wellness (AOTA, 2011).

When working with clients in their homes, therapists can remind them about the importance of preparing an emergency kit that contains first aid supplies, flashlights/ batteries, nonperishable food, water, medication list, and emergency documents. The Red Cross has a complete list of items online, including specific information for older adults, people with disabilities, and children. It is available at http://www.redcross.org/prepare/location/ home-family/get-kit.

Safety During Transfers and Mobility

Therapists should be familiar with the parts of hospital beds, mechanical lifts, and mobility aids before performing transfers or mobility with clients. It is critical to be aware of the procedure for locking bed and wheelchair locks to keep the objects in place. Each client should be positioned in a way that is consistent with precautions specific to his or her condition. Adjusting the height of the bed can ease transfers, requiring less effort for clients and ensuring safety for the practitioner who is assisting.

It is important to have adequate room to work, whether in clients' rooms, in the clinic, or in clients' homes. Practitioners should avoid working in small spaces as much as possible. They should also clear unneeded equipment such as bedside tables, extra wheelchairs, or other mobility aids in order to have adequate room.

Any equipment belonging to an occupational therapy department should be properly maintained. This includes cleaning, ensuring that locks work, and ensuring that all working parts are intact. Routine checks to ensure that every piece of equipment works properly and is stable are important preventive steps to ensure client safety (Kangas, 2002).

The use of proper body mechanics when transferring clients minimizes the risk of injury to practitioners or others who are assisting in the transfer. In general, this involves positioning one's self close to the person being transferred, maintaining a wide base of support, using large muscle groups to move the person, and avoiding twisting movements (Pierson, 1999). In addition, it is important to be aware of any conditions that may affect the client's performance during transfers, such as fragile skin, OH, amputations, pain, or spasms. Furthermore, it is essential that the practitioner stay current with any precautions or contraindications related to transfers, as these are subject to change. Practitioners must take the time to be aware of best practices regarding injury prevention. For example, research does not support a commonly held belief that back belts reduce injuries caused by lifting (Wassell, Gerdner, Landsittel, Johnston, & Johnston, 2001). It is recommended, however, that practitioners use a gait belt with clients when performing transfers or ambulation, unless contraindicated (e.g., after abdominal surgery; Pierson, 1999). A gait belt prevents the practitioner from having to grasp body parts or clothing when providing assistance with mobility. It can also be instrumental in controlling the speed and direction of a fall if the client cannot support his or her own body weight.

Working with clients who are extremely overweight poses potential safety concerns for health care workers and for the clients themselves. Of particular concern is the use of transfer devices and bathroom equipment. Special equipment designed for the bariatric population may be ordered to ensure safety when transferring, bathing, and toileting (Foti & Littrel, 2004). Typically, the weight capacity of durable medical equipment is listed in the ordering information. The practitioner should also consider the distribution of the client's weight, his or her preferred methods of movement, and any anxiety related to mobility.

Fall Prevention and Restraint Use

Minimizing the incidence of client falls is an important safety consideration for occupational therapy practitioners. This is especially true for older adults and persons with chronic illness who are at an elevated risk. The consequences of a serious fall may include head injury, hip fracture, psychological harm, or death. Falls may be caused by many factors including medications; age-related changes (such as an increased need to urinate at night); visual, balance, strength, or cognitive impairments; or environmental obstacles. Fall prevention efforts are context-specific, but generally include multiple interventions such as balance and gait training, medication management, environmental modifications, and attention to health concerns such as postural hypotension (American Geriatrics Society, British Geriatrics Society, & American Academy of Orthopedic Surgeons, 2001).

The Centers for Medicare and Medicaid Services (CMS) defines *restraints* as any manual method, physical or manual device, material, or equipment that immobilizes or reduces the ability of a client to move his or her arms, legs, body, or head freely; or a drug or medication when it is used as a restriction to manage the client's behavior or restrict the client's freedom of movement and is not a standard intervention or dosage for the client's condition (CMS & HHS, 2006).

Historically, restraints were thought to reduce the risk of falling, but research has shown that restraints are ineffective in reducing fall risk. In fact, they can pose serious threats to safety including incontinence, physical injury, and in some cases, death (Evans & Strumpf, 1990; Miles & Irvine, 1992). Physicians or other licensed independent practitioners are permitted to order physical restraints to treat medical symptoms. The client or surrogate decision makers must consent to their use. Physician's orders must include the circumstances and duration of restraint use, and clients must be carefully monitored while restraints are in use.

Occupational therapy practitioners can play an important part in carefully analyzing a client's fall risk to determine if there are less-restrictive options available. A variety of physical and social supports can minimize reliance on external restraints. In the event that physical restraints are in use, practitioners must ensure that the restraints are applied correctly each time they are fastened in order to prevent accidental injury. Restraints should be fastened to the frame of the bed or wheelchair rather than to a moveable part, such as a bed rail or arm rest. A strap attached to a bed rail, for example, may tighten when the rail is lifted or lowered, causing injury to the client (Potter & Perry, 2004).

Home Safety

Working in clients' homes provides an opportunity for the practitioner to make recommendations to enhance safety within the home. Every client presents with different safety needs owing to the complex interaction between individual impairments, unique elements of the physical and social environment, and the range of activities performed (Clemson, 1997). When working in clients' homes, practitioners have the ability to observe how activities are performed in their own context, how their social supports influence participation in occupations, and how routines and habits enhance or impede safety.

The following list is a useful starting point for addressing physical safety in clients' homes:

- Ensure adequate lighting throughout the home. While assessing lighting, also consider blocking light to minimize the effects of glare.

- Ensure adequate support during mobility. This may include hand rails on stairs, grab bars in bathrooms, and/or bed mobility aids.

- Minimize tripping hazards such as obstacles on floor, unsecured rugs, unfastened sills or uneven flooring, and electrical cords.

- Ensure safe and simple access to commonly used items around the home.

- Reduce the risk of scalding injuries by setting the water heater thermostat to no more than 120 degrees.

- Prevent electrical injuries by covering outlets, using surge protectors, and keeping electrical cords intact by storing them out of the way of foot traffic.

Personal Safety in Home Care Contexts

Working in clients' homes poses a unique set of safety concerns. Practitioners must take precautions to ensure personal safety when working in the home care environment. It is a safe practice to call before going to a client's home to confirm your arrival. In addition, practitioners should use an escort if there is a perceived threat to personal safety. This is a common service available through many home care agencies. A mobile phone should be readily available (on your person, if possible) in the event of an emergency.

As a means of infection control, it is recommended that practitioners refrain from placing personal items or therapy equipment bags on the ground. Rather, they should be placed over a chair back. Therapy equipment should be appropriately disinfected after each client encounter.

Areas of Competence

Therapists have a responsibility to "work within their areas of competence" (Reitz et al., 2006, p. 654) and to be aware of their personal limitations in knowledge or expertise. To maintain safe practices, assistance should be sought before performing an evaluation or intervention beyond one's skill set. Additional training, coursework, or education may be needed before working with certain groups of clients. For example, an *American Journal of Occupational Therapy* paper describes the advanced knowledge and skill required for occupational therapy practice in neonatal intensive care units (Vergara et al., 2006). The complexity of this practice setting is compounded by the unique nature of the medical diagnoses, medication regimens, technology, and the family and team dynamics that are present. It is therefore not a recommended practice context for occupational therapy assistants, entry-level therapists, or therapists without prior pediatric experience.

It is imperative for practitioners to allow only authorized personnel to provide intervention. Family members, volunteers, or other unqualified persons should not assist with or carry out interventions they are not capable of completing. When providing caregiver education and training, the practitioner should document his or her competence before allowing the caregiver to complete a task independently. In addition, occupational therapists have a duty to be clear about the roles and responsibilities of the occupational therapy assistant.

Occupational therapy practitioners should report any potentially unsafe practices to a supervisor and work within their means to ensure that the practices are not carried out in the interim. Careful documentation of adverse incidents is necessary. Proper reporting procedures dictated by your institution should be used.

Summary

Occupational therapy practitioners are instrumental in ensuring that the physical and social environments provide support for client functioning while minimizing the risk of adverse events. Careful attention to the interaction between the person, the environment, and the activity allows practitioners to create situations in which

Figure 11-1. Talking on a mobile phone while driving is hazardous to the driver, other passengers in the car, and to others on the road. The solution is to pull off to the side of the road to make or receive a phone call.

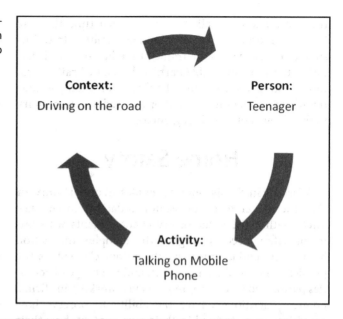

Context:	Person:
Driving on the road	Teenager
	Activity:
	Talking on Mobile Phone

EVIDENCE-BASED RESEARCH CHART

Topic	Evidence
Home modifications to support safety/function	Clemson et al., 2008; Gitlin et al., 2006
Emergency preparedness and disaster response	AOTA, 2011; WFOT, 2011
Restraint use	Evans & Strumpf, 1990; Miles & Irvine, 1992
Infection control	Boyce, Pittet, Healthcare Infection Control Practices Advisory Committee, & HICPAC/SHEA/APIC/IDSA Hand Hygiene Task Force, 2002

clients can successfully engage in meaningful occupations and enhance their quality of life.

Practitioners must engage in lifelong learning to maintain competence in safety-related issues. It is critical to keep current regarding institutional policies and procedures, clients' conditions, and the physical and social environments in order to optimize safety.

Student Self-Assessment

1. Become a keen observer of safety in a variety of contexts. Identify safety hazards in a variety of contexts:

    ◊ In your own living environment
    ◊ At the mall
    ◊ In a waiting room
    ◊ On a playground
    ◊ On a road or sidewalk in your neighborhood

    Attend to the interaction between different people in the environment (children, adults, older adults),

the activities (walking, driving, cooking), and elements of the context (mobile phones, branches in the road, shoes on the floor). Identify the threats to safety and make recommendations to improve safety. See Figure 11-1 for an example.

2. Practice washing your hands according to the CDC standards. Notice how long 15 seconds of scrubbing feels. Also practice donning and doffing PPE according to the standards.

3. Develop a fire escape plan for your current living conditions. Be sure to have two methods of egress. Be sure the dwelling has smoke detectors with intact batteries. If there is an extinguisher present, read the directions to identify the type of fire it can be used on and the procedure for use. Identify the actions suggested by the acronyms RACE and PASS.

Electronic Resources

• Centers for Disease Control and Prevention: www.cdc.gov

- Occupational Safety and Health Administration: www.osha.gov
- American Red Cross: www.redcross.org
- American Heart Association: www.americanheart.org
- Joint Commission: www.jointcommission.org
- National Safety Council: www.nsc.org

References

American Geriatrics Society, British Geriatrics Society, & American Academy of Orthopedic Surgeons Panel on Falls Prevention. (2001). Guidelines for the prevention of falls in older persons. *Journal of the American Geriatrics Society, 49*(5), 664-672.

American Heart Association. (2005). *First aid. Circulation, 112: IV-196-IV-203.* Retrieved from http://circ.ahajournals.org/content/112/24_suppl/IV-196.   doi:10.1161/CIRCULATIONAHA.105.166575

American Occupational Therapy Association. (2008). Occupational therapy framework: Domain and process, second edition. *American Journal of Occupational Therapy, 62,* 625-683.

American Red Cross. (2005). *First aid. Circulation, 112*(Suppl. I), IV-196-IV-203. Retrieved from http://circ.ahajournals.org/cgi/reprint/112/24_suppl/IV-196

American Red Cross. (n.d.) *Get a kit.* Retrieved from http://www.redcross.org/prepare/location/home-family/get-kit

Beezhold, D., & Sussman, G. (2005). *Lessons learned from latex allergy. Business briefing: Global surgery—Future directions 2005.* Retrieved from http://www.touchbriefings.com/pdf/1438/beezhold[1].pdf

Boyce, J. M., Pittet, D., Healthcare Infection Control Practices Advisory Committee, & HICPAC/SHEA/APIC/IDSA Hand Hygiene Task Force. (2002). Guideline for hand hygiene in health-care settings: Recommendations of the Healthcare Infection Control Practices Advisory Committee and the HICPAC/SHEA/APIC/IDSA Hand Hygiene Task Force. *MMWR: Recommendations and Reports, 51*(RR-16), 1-45.

Branum, A. M., & Lukacs, S. L. (2009) . Food allergy among children in the United States. *Pediatrics,* (124), 1549-1555.

Bruce, M. A. G., & Borg, B. (2002). Suicidal behavior: Critical information for clinical reasoning. In M. A. G. Bruce, & B. Borg (Eds.), *Psychosocial frames of reference: Core for occupation-based practice* (3rd ed., pp. 323-324). Thorofare, NJ: SLACK Incorporated.

Centers for Disease Control and Prevention. (2002). CDC's campaign to prevent antimicrobial resistance in health-care settings. *MMWR: Morbidity and Mortality Weekly Report, 51*(15), 343. Retrieved from http://www.cdc.gov/drugresistance/healthcare/default.htm

Centers for Disease Control and Prevention. (2004). *Surveillance for tuberculosis infection in health care workers.* Worker Health Chartbook 2004. NIOSH Publication No. 2004-146. Retrieved from http://www.cdc.gov/niosh/docs/2004-146/appendix/ap-a/ap-a-19.html

Centers for Disease Control and Prevention. (2011). Immunization of health-care personnel: Recommendations of the Advisory Committee on Immunization Practices (ACIP). *MMWR: Recommendations and Reports, 7*(60), 1-48.

Centers for Medicare & Medicaid Services, Department of Health and Human Services. (2006). *Medicare and Medicaid Programs; Hospital conditions of participation: Patients' rights: Final rule. Federal Register, 71*(236), 71377-71428.

Clemson, L. (1997). *Home fall hazards: A guide to identifying fall hazards in the homes of elderly people and an accompaniment to the assessment tool, the Westmead Home Safety Assessment.* West Brunswick, Victoria, Australia: Coordinates Publication.

Evans, L. K., & Strumpf, N. E. (1990). Myths about elder restraint. *Image: Journal of Nursing Scholarship, 22*(2), 124-128.

Foti, D., & Littrel, E. (2004). Bariatric care: Practical problem solving and interventions. *Physical Disabilities Special Interest Section Quarterly, 27,* 1-6.

Gall, S., Tarique, A., Natarajan, A., & Zaman, A. (2006). Rapid ambulation after coronary angiography via femoral artery access: A prospective study of 1000 patients. *Journal of Invasive Cardiology, 18,* 106-108.

Goodman, C. C., Fuller, K. S., & Boissonnault, W. G. (2003). *Pathology: Implications for the physical therapist* (2nd ed.). Philadelphia, PA: Saunders-Elsevier.

Holm, M. B., Rogers, J. C., & James, A. B. (1998). Treatment of occupational performance areas. In M. E. Neidstadt & E. B. Crepeau (Eds.), *Willard & Spackman's occupational therapy* (9th ed., pp. 323-390). Philadelphia, PA: Lippincott Williams and Wilkins.

Kangas, K. M. (2002). Managing transfers and lifting with the complicated patient. *Gerontology Special Interest Section Quarterly, 25,* 1-4.

Miles, S. H., & Irvine, P. (1992). Deaths caused by physical restraints. *Gerontologist, 32*(6), 762-766.

Occupational Safety and Health Administration. (2002a). *Healthcare wise hazards: Lack of universal precautions.* Retrieved from http://www.osha.gov/SLTC/etools/hospital/hazards/univprec/univ.html

Occupational Safety and Health Administration. (2002b). *Fact sheet: Fire safety in the Workplace.* Retrieved from http://www.osha.gov/OshDoc/data_General_Facts/FireSafetyN.pdf

Pierson, F. M. (1999). *Principles and techniques of patient care* (2nd ed.). Philadelphia, PA: W.B. Saunders Company.

Potter, P. A., & Perry, A. G. (2004). *Fundamentals of nursing* (6th ed.). St. Louis, MO: Mosby-Elsevier.

Reitz, S. M., Austin, D. J., Brandt, L. C., DeBrakeller, B., Franck, L. G., & Homenko, D. F., et al. (2006). Guidelines to the occupational therapy code of ethics. *American Journal of Occupational Therapy, 60*(6), 652-658.

Ross, T. A., Boucher, J. L., & O'Connell, B. S. (Eds.). (2005). *ADA guide to diabetes medical nutrition therapy and education.* Chicago, IL: American Dietetic Association.

Siegel, J. D., Rhinehart, E., Jackson, M., Chiarello, L., & Healthcare Infection Control Practices Advisory Committee. (2007). *2007 guideline for isolation precautions: Preventing transmission of infectious diseases in healthcare settings.* Atlanta, GA: Centers for Disease Control and Prevention. Retrieved from http://www.cdc.gov/ncidod/dhqp/pdf/guidelines/Isolation2007.pdf

United States Department of Health and Human Services. (2012). *Healthcare preparedness capabilities: National guidance for healthcare system preparedness.* Retrieved from http://www.phe.gov/preparedness/planning/hpp/reports/documents/capabilities.pdf

United States Fire Administration (2012). *Home fire prevention and safety tips.* Retrieved from http://www.usfa.fema.gov/citizens/home_fire_prev/

Vergara, E., Anzalone, M., Bigsby, R., Gorga, D., Holloway, E., & Hunter, J., et al. (2006). Specialized knowledge and skills for occupational therapy practice in the Neonatal Intensive care unit. *American Journal of Occupational Therapy, 60*(6), 659-668.

Wassell, J. T., Gardner, L. I., Landsittel, D. P., Johnston, J. J., & Johnston, J. M. (2001). A prospective study of back belts for prevention of back pain and injury. *Journal of the American Medical Association, 284*(21), 2727-2732. Retrieved from www.cdc.gov/niosh/jamapapr.html

Suggested Readings

American Occupational Therapy Association. (2011). The role of occupational therapy in disaster preparedness, response, and recovery. *American Journal of Occupational Therapy, 65*(suppl.), S11-S25. doi:10.5014/ajot.2011.65S11

Clemson, L., Mackenzie, L., Ballinger, C., Close, J. C., & Cumming, R. G. (2008). Environmental interventions to prevent falls in community-dwelling older people: A meta-analysis of randomized trials. *Journal of Aging and Health, 20,* 954-971.

Gitlin, L. M., Winter, L., Dennis, M. P., Corcoran, M., Schinfeld, S., & Hauck, W. W. (2006). A randomized trial of multicomponent home interventions to reduce functional difficulties in older adults. *Journal of the American Geriatrics Society, 54,* 809-816.

Occupational Safety and Health Administration. (2011). *Fact sheet: Bloodborne pathogens.* Retrieved from http://www.osha.gov/OshDoc/data_BloodborneFacts/bbfact01.pdf

Occupational Safety and Health Administration. (2012). *Hospital eTool: Bloodborne illnesses: Hepatitis B virus.* Retrieved from http://www.osha.gov/SLTC/etools/hospital/hazards/bbp/bbp.html#HepatitisBVirus

Sicherer, S. H. (2006). *Understanding and managing your child's food allergies.* Baltimore, MD: The Johns Hopkins University Press.

World Federation of Occupational Therapists. (2011). *Disaster preparedness and response.* Retrieved from http://www.wfot.org/practice/disasterpreparednessandresponsedpr.aspx

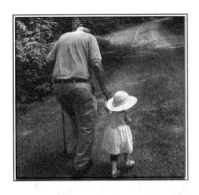

12

OCCUPATIONAL PERFORMANCE IN NATURAL ENVIRONMENTS

DYNAMIC CONTEXTS FOR PARTICIPATION

Kathryn M. Loukas, OTD, MS, OTR/L, FAOTA

ACOTE STANDARDS EXPLORED IN THIS CHAPTER

B.5.17

KEY VOCABULARY

- **Context:** The wide variety of complex and interrelated internal and external factors that affect occupational performance (AOTA, 2008).
- **Inclusion:** Full participation in life events and naturally occurring environments for and with people of all abilities.
- **Interdependence:** Functioning with the input from others in a complex and interconnected manner.

- **Least restrictive environment:** The context in which humans participate in daily occupations; the environment that best supports occupational participation.
- **Natural environments:** Contexts that occur in the daily lives of human beings in a society.
- **Nonlinear dynamics:** Complex, open systems that interact in unpredictable flow dynamics versus in a more rigid, linear, cause-effect manner (Champagne, 2008).

Occupational therapy has evolved in the use of context in intervention planning. Through the history of occupational therapy we have moved from the context of institutional settings that began with the moral treatment paradigm (Letts, Rigsby & Stewart, 2003), to a focus on occupation (Kielhofner, 1992), to practice utilizing the Person-Environment-Occupational Performance Model which emphasizes natural contexts (Christiansen & Baum, 1991). Early in our history, occupational therapy primarily occurred in the institutional setting. This institutionalization provided a closed system that discouraged individuals from participating in

Jacobs, K., MacRae, N., & Sladyk, K. (Eds.).
Occupational Therapy Essentials for
Clinical Competence, Second Edition (pp. 149-157).
© 2014 SLACK Incorporated.

real life situations in natural settings; it kept our clients and our work invisible to society and inhibited occupational justice and performance (Reed, 2006; Whalley Hammell, 2003). In her landmark Eleanor Clark Slagle lecture, Grady (1995) encouraged occupational therapy practitioners to reach out and build inclusive communities through accessibility, adaptations, hope, and social supports. Our profession continues to move forward toward this ultimate goal.

Today, engagement in purposeful, real life occupations has become the goal of occupational therapy intervention in most practice settings. *The Occupational Therapy Practice Framework* advocates occupational therapy practitioners to support participation in occupation in context (AOTA, 2002, 2008). Occupational therapy has made a paradigm shift from the medical model to the community model in order to help clients participate in the occupations of "real life" (Scaffa, 2001). Increasing the level of independence is a factor in intervention planning, but not always the ultimate goal. Occupational therapy practitioners need to also recognize and embrace the concept of interdependence. A client who wishes to live in their own natural environment may need the assistance of family or caregivers, and that is a worthy goal in achieving occupational life satisfaction. A client who is functioning in the natural rhythm of life, even with assistance, may be achieving an individual goal of occupational performance (Hinojosa & Blount, 2000).

Occupational therapy practitioners often use simulation in clinical settings to achieve occupational based goals. A rehabilitation-based occupational therapy practitioner might use the therapy room kitchen to help a client prepare to return home, an occupational therapy practitioner in work re-entry therapy might use devices that simulate work tasks such as driving or lifting, and a therapist working in early intervention may simulate a play environment in the occupational therapy room to prepare a child to use a playground in the future. Simulations prepare clients for real life, but use of the actual environment is always best for the final goals and discharge planning (Letts, Rigby, & Stewart, 2003). Natural environments are those where the client would actually engage in the occupation in context. These occupations carry with them important social meaning and occupational roles (Pierce, 2003). Typical natural environments include the home, workplace, day care settings, school, places of leisure and recreation, group homes, and the community, including private and public transportation (Hinojosa & Blount, 2000).

Natural contexts for occupational practice include the following (Perr & Bell, 2000):

- The home
- The outdoor environment
- The workplace
- Day care settings, head-start programs, developmental preschools for early intervention
- School-based inclusion in the least restrictive environment
- Community resources for play and leisure, recreation, worship, shopping, dining, and social and community events
- Private and public transportation

Chaos, Complexity, and Nonlinear Dynamics

Chaos theory and the study of nonlinear dynamics is an emerging perspective in the social sciences (Chamberlain & Butz, 1998; Kelso, 1995) and in occupational therapy (Champagne, 2008; Lazzarini, 2004; Royeen, 2003). Dynamic systems theory reflects the importance of the interaction of the complex internal and external systems that make up the whole human being (Case-Smith, 2005; Humphry & Wakeford, 2006; Thelen, 2000). Zoltan (2007) describes the dynamic interactional approach to cognition as "an ongoing production or outcome of the interaction among the individual, the task, and the environment" (p. 16). The environment plays a significant role in the occupations and occupational development of human beings, leading emerging occupational therapy approaches to emphasize contextualism (Humphry & Wakeford, 2006). This contextualism emphasizes the interconnected and inseparable nature of human beings with their environment. According to nonlinear dynamic theory, human beings and behavior are unpredictable, self-organizing systems, each with their own unique initial conditions (Chamberlain & Butz, 1998; Champagne, 2008; Kelso, 1995; Lazzarini, 2004; Royeen, 2003). The person, environment, and occupation are engaged in a transactional relationship, much as the Person-Environment-Occupational Performance Model (Christiansen & Baum, 1991) elucidates, but in a more interactive, holistic, and unpredictable manner. It is essential that occupational therapy practitioners understand the science of chaotic, complex, nonlinear dynamic systems in natural environments. Through this understanding occupational therapists can facilitate meaningful self-organization of clients in the context of dynamic everyday occupations (Champagne, 2008; Lazzarini, 2004; Royeen, 2003).

OCCUPATIONAL THERAPY APPLICATIONS

Early Intervention

Early intervention programs are designed to enhance the development of children in occupational tasks. The Individuals with Disabilities Education Act (IDEA) man-

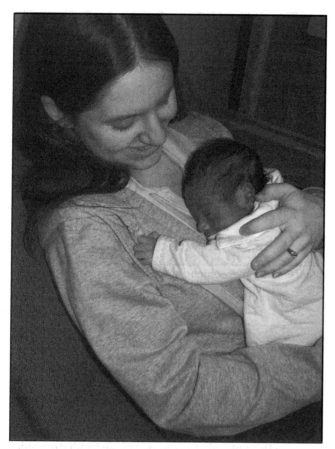

Figure 12-1. An early natural environment of Kangaroo Care is used by a new mother to bond and soothe an infant.

Case Example: Lola

Lola is the 9-month-old child of Celeste, a 19-year-old single mother living in a small house with her mother. Lola is a child who is developmentally delayed and just beginning to sit up and roll over. Lola also has some difficulty with eating and feeding and does not sleep well. Samantha, the occupational therapist, facilitated Celeste to self-organize a routine for the day, including times for feeding, developmental play, and sleep. As a therapeutic activity, Celeste and Samantha worked together to establish a realistic and meaningful routine and put this schedule on the refrigerator with magnets. Samantha's gentle influence regarding the nature of developmental activities facilitated Celeste to find a playgroup for Lola. The dynamic, social, and interactive nature of the playgroup of children and parents began to transform their isolation and improved community participation for both mother and child. The occupational therapy practitioner helped Celeste embed specially selected developmental play activities to enhance motor development into Lola's environment. This served to establish an interconnected bond between mother and child. The context of this play included setting up environments that facilitate development in the living room and outdoors. Sensory modulation input was natural and was included to facilitate Lola's nervous system prior to feeding and to inhibit her system prior to bedtime. As the natural environment of the home became child-development centered, Celeste began to grow in her role as a confident and nurturing mother and Lola began to thrive.

---

dates these services occur in "natural environments" and in a family-centered context (AOTA, 2006; Stephens & Tauber, 2005). Natural environments in early intervention include kangaroo care of the newborn resting on the parent's abdomen (Figure 12-1); transdisciplinary play environments including play groups, day care centers, preschool, and developmental groups (Loukas, Whiting, Ricci, & Cohen-Konrad, 2012); cultural and religious activities and contexts; and community settings such as shopping or service appointments. The most natural setting occupational therapy could address for a client in the 0- to 3-year-old age range is the family and home environment. Understanding the initial conditions, context, culture, and occupational patterns of the dynamic family system is important and should influence the occupational therapy intervention plan (Figure 12-2).

School-Based Practice

Current IDEA legislation requires that therapy occur in natural environments (Wrights Law, 2013) and for education to occur in the least restrictive environment (AOTA, 2006). The school has many natural environments, all of which are dynamic contexts for occupational performance. These include the classroom, the school bus, the playground, the cafeteria, the gym, the art room, the computer room, and the library. Occupational thera-

py intervention can occur in all these contexts as direct inclusive therapy or in a consultative approach. The schools have evolved from a model of specialized schools, such as the school for the deaf or the cerebral palsy center to "mainstreaming," which put children under the same roof as their typical peers to facilitation of full participation of children in the school environment and routine, which is now termed "inclusion." Occupational therapy as a profession is dedicated to inclusion and believes all members of society contribute to creating an inclusive community (AOTA, 2009; Dunn et al., 1995b). Inclusion asserts that all children engage in the same activities in the same environments, although some may need assistance or adaptations to participate.

To be effective in this complex system, the school-based occupational therapy practitioner must evaluate and affect change in complex and unpredictable ways. This requires facilitating the child, teacher, occupations, and natural environments to support learning and social development in context (Figure 12-3).

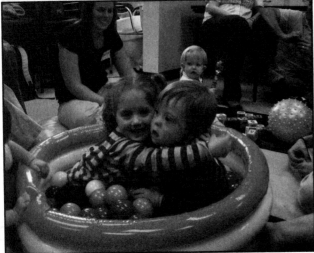

Figure 12-2. Early intervention inclusive contexts promote social participation and development.

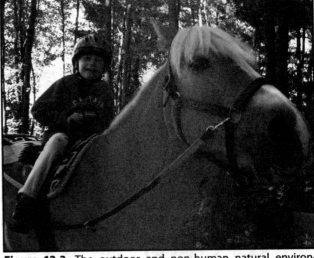

Figure 12-3. The outdoor and non-human natural environments facilitate wellness and joy.

Work-Based Programs

Return to work programs, workplace safety initiatives, ergonomics, sheltered work, employment coaching, and overall rehabilitation are part of occupational therapy practice and can occur in natural environments (AOTA, 2011). The workplace is where many of us spend most of our weekday hours engaging in productive activities. Clients who are interested in employment may find the natural environment of the workplace to be stimulating and motivating. In addition, the occupational therapy practitioner can see how the environment can be adapted, do an actual task analysis of the work to be done, and engage the client in the natural positions and conditions needed for the job. This is an effective way to address work-based goals in occupational therapy. Because of time and distance constraints, often occupational therapy practitioners cannot bring their clients to the workplace. If this is the case, the best alternative is to simulate the work situation as closely as possible in order to maximize the therapeutic impact of intervention. Occupational therapy practitioners should also consider using a volunteer position as a precursor to the work role. This may serve as a vehicle toward self-actualization and productivity for people with disabling conditions.

Aging in Place

Older adults who wish to age in natural environments, thus "aging in place," may turn to occupational therapy for assistance in that goal (AOTA, 2008; Clark et al., 1997). Occupational therapy is dedicated to developing livable communities where people of all abilities can fully participate (AOTA, 2008). Occupational therapy can occur in this natural environment while facilitating older adults to participate in community programs such as adult day programs, in-home assistance, religious or culturally based activities, and social networks. It is important for older people to stay in their natural environment in order to maintain the habits, routines, and memories associated with their own home and lifestyle. Changing locations can inhibit an older person, particularly those with cognitive impairments, to regress in their overall functioning and quality of life and may even affect mortality (Edvardsson & Nordvall, 2008). Aging in place allows older adults to maintain their habits, familiar surroundings, and social networks for occupational performance. The occupational therapy practitioner, adopting an adaptation/compensation contextual approach, can assist elders to function in their home through home adaptations, cueing systems, self-organization of the day, and memory enhancement. An emphasis on safety and supported functioning should be established. An occupational therapy practitioner can also train family members or other caretakers on how to best assist older adults with their independent or interdependent functioning (Dunn et al., 1995a; Figure 12-4).

Case Example: Curtis

Curtis is a child in the second grade. He is full of life and loves to have fun with other children. Curtis is living with cerebral palsy that affects his left side with hemiparesis, but cognitively he is at grade level. Curtis has functional mobility difficulties with negotiating the playground, sitting on the backless benches of the cafeteria, and getting on and off the school bus. He also has fine motor difficulties, which render handwriting and art projects frustrating and very difficult. The occupational therapy practitioners were committed to including Curtis in all activities and settings of the school and adopted an adaptation/compensation contextual approach in his individual education plan (IEP) to enable Curtis to participate successfully in all aspects of the school curriculum. John, the occupational therapy assistant, played with Curtis and his peers on the playground, facilitating Curtis to make good choices in equipment selection and offering ideas on how to safely get on and off the swings and slides. A chair was used at the end of the cafeteria table enabling Curtis to have supportive seating but still eat with his peers. Curtis was given physical assistance on and off the bus for safety reasons. This was facilitated by the occupational therapy practitioners in a manner that was meaningful and social to Curtis, his family, and other children involved. Curtis' classrooms were equipped with a computer with a key guard and elbow supports for school-based written work and some art projects. Dynamic occupational therapy intervention occurred in all school contexts and included the interdisciplinary team, teachers, parents, and other children in the second grade curriculum for social participation in natural activities of daily living, play, and work contexts.

Case Example: Ralph

Ralph is a 54-year-old plumber who lost his left (non-dominant) thumb and index finger at the proximal interphalangeal (PIP) joint in a work-related accident. He is now two months post amputation, participating in outpatient rehabilitation, and has quite a bit of hypersensitivity in the stump areas of his left hand. Ralph is a man who values work at home and the workplace. He is concerned he will not be able to support his family and is anxious to return to his job. Doris, his occupational therapy practitioner, noticed he is not motivated by use of simulations in the outpatient clinic. She tried to set up make-shift plumbing projects, but Ralph insists they are not close to realistic. Doris decides to set up a work-based program on the pipes in Ralph's home. Ralph becomes motivated to use his left hand as a functional assist and the hypersensitivity begins to diminish. As Ralph shows he can still do many plumbing tasks, his wife, Mary, begins to ask about different jobs needed around the house. Ralph complains to her in a good natured way, but the therapist can see he is pleased to be back in the role of "Mr. Fix It" in his home. Doris sets up further sessions in the plumbing shop and home environments to facilitate Ralph's return to former performance patterns of work and functional use of the left hand. This dynamic approach to work improves Ralph's relationships, self-image, and mood as his life roles and routines become meaningful again.

BEST PRACTICE AND SAFETY CONSIDERATIONS IN NATURAL SETTINGS

Because natural settings are not as structured or predictable as those performed in a clinic, they can pose more of a safety risk for clients both physically and psychosocially. It is important to consider a number of recommended practices to ensure positive outcomes. The following recommendations are adapted from Noonan and McCormick (2006) in their work with young children in natural environments:

1. Specialize instructional techniques to the client in the natural environment. This can be accomplished by goals that embed meaningful activities in the client's natural environment, making sure that the challenges are not dangerous or too difficult. Task analysis and careful planning are needed for successful therapy in natural environments.

2. Ensure that interventions are culturally sensitive and relevant. This may require outside investigation and questions to the client and family members.

3. Cultivate team and family involvement. Positive outcomes are more likely to occur with support by the team and the family. Build strong relationships

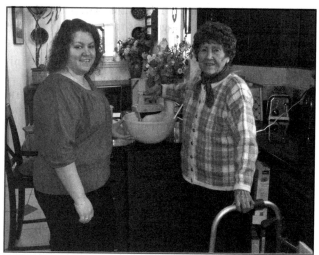

Figure 12-4. An occupational therapy practitioner assists an older adult with cooking in the natural environment of the client's home.

with the therapy team and work collaboratively to support this practice.

4. Ecological and contextual assessment. The occupational therapy practitioner should do a thorough ecological assessment for the safety of the client and the therapist. Questions to ask include the following:

   ◊ What are the intervention goals and objectives?

   ◊ Where should the intervention be provided?

   ◊ How should the intervention be provided?

   ◊ When should the intervention be provided?

   ◊ How can the intervention be evaluated? (Noonan & McCormick, 2006, p. 21)

5. Positive behavioral support. The occupational therapy practitioner should not provide therapy alone in a natural environment when the behavior of the client/family or safety considerations are questionable. Be sure support is present in any situation that warrants it. Relationship difficulties can also make for difficult or unsafe situations for the client and/ or should be closely examined prior to the planning of the context of intervention.

RECOMMENDATIONS FOR ESTABLISHING AN ETHICAL CLIMATE FOR PRIVACY AND CONFIDENTIALITY IN A COMMUNITY-BASED PRACTICE SETTING

1. Know and follow the Health Insurance Portability and Accountability Act (HIPAA) and Family Educational Rights and Privacy Act (FERPA) regulations, and encourage others to do the same, including notification of privacy procedures to clients and client families.

2. Avoid all "hall talk." Establish confidential places to discuss private client matters, and remember casual conversations can quickly turn into conversations with confidential information sharing.

3. Make sure your clients understand what is private and what is not, as research indicates many clients do not understand confidentiality (Sankar et al., 2003). For our young clients, involve them in decisions using plain language they understand.

4. Make all efforts to keep private, professional information confidential. Do not carry confidential reports or files casually, do not leave them in the bathroom or your open car. Transport confidential items only when absolutely necessary. Keep your computer encrypted or password sensitive for all client-related information.

5. Respond "naturally" to questions that occur in typical settings, but be careful not to violate privacy

---

Case Example: Marjorie

Marjorie is a 68-year-old woman in the midstages of Alzheimer's disease. Her husband, George, age 70, has been very distraught with his wife's behavior and forgetfulness. George works part time as a sales representative and would like to continue his work. The family sought occupational therapy through a center on aging. Nancy, the occupational therapy practitioner at the center, helped the family find resources in the community to assist them. They found an adult day care center for the days George works and through this became involved with a support group for caretakers of people with Alzheimer's disease. As George learned more about the importance of taking care of himself, his wife, and his home, he began to self-organize. He hired someone to clean the house, as that had really become a burden for him. In addition, they were able to hire an attendant to sleep over to deal with Marjorie's night wandering and allow George to sleep. Nancy helped George and Marjorie maintain previous routines through a picture calendar for Marjorie. This also helped George effectively engage and interact with his wife in meaningful home tasks that used to be delegated only to her, such as cooking and gardening. While engaging in these occupational tasks, Nancy is able to role-play ways of dealing with Marjorie when she becomes disoriented, belligerent, or confused. These new interactions facilitate George and their children to deal with Marjorie in social and community settings. Due to this occupational therapy intervention, George and Marjorie are able to participate in their home and community in an interdependent manner further in the future.

---

or confidentiality. Make sure paraprofessionals understand their obligations to privacy and do not give more information than is needed.

6. Communicate with your clients and their families about what you need to provide best practice as a therapist and what participation in natural environments might entail. Ask about mentioning the disability or educating others; involve them in decisions and discussion. Help clients and parents understand your need for full disclosure of medical information.

7. Implicit consent and reasonable expectations of privacy are part of practice when the client and family are involved in a community-based environment. The family and client need to be informed and "agree" to the setting and approach to intervention through an IEP, individual family service plan (IFSP), or other legal document (J. Boyden, personal communication, July 10, 2006).

EVIDENCE-BASED RESEARCH CHART

Program/Context	Intervention	Evidence
Inclusive preschool	Outdoor play guided by the interdisciplinary Ecology of Human Performance model	Anecdotal and occupational objectives achieved – parent satisfaction (Ideishi et.al., 2006)
Family involvement in intervention with clients who have physical disabilities, developmental disabilities, and mental health issues	Questionnaire to occupational therapist's regarding family involvement	Family involvement needs to be expanded. Scheduling is the biggest obstacle. More continuing education and articulation of occupational therapy work with families in mental health is needed (Humphrey et al., 1993)
The effect of context on skill acquisition	Students without disabilities were taught to use chop sticks in and out of context	Natural context elicited improvement of success significantly. Natural context found to facilitate motor learning (Ma, Trombly, & Robinson-Podolski, 1998)
Constructing daily routines of mothers with young children with disabilities	Qualitative research in naturalistic environments on daily routines in self-care or skill performance	Development of self-care is shaped by eco-cultural influences and anticipation of future possibilities (Kellegrew, 2000)
Family routines and rituals	Family daily routines, interviews of stories, daily routines and occupation focuses on morning activities	Family routines are important for organization and meaning in self-care of children (Segal, 2004)
Multicontexts used for brain injury intervention	Single case study incorporating functional tasks in natural environments and contexts of daily life	Brain injury intervention may be enhanced to include the contexts of everyday life (Landa-Gonzalez, 2001)
Occupational therapy role in keeping community-based older adults in their homes	Use of assistive devices and focus on safety in functional mobility and overall home-based tasks Group of 361 culturally diverse, independent-living elders participated in occupational therapy groups over a 9-month period; results were favorable when compared to control group	Seventeen efficacy studies focusing on decreasing falls, increasing home safety, social participation, and quality of life (Stuetjens et al., 2004) Preventive occupational therapy benefits independent-living elders across the domains of health, function, and quality of life (Clark et al., 1997)
Occupation-based intervention in homelike environments	Single case study demonstrates behavioral, neurological, and qualitative changes in a client with stroke following occupation-based intervention	Study supports use of the occupation-based practice in a homelike environment (Skubik-Peplaski, Carrico, Nicols, Chelette, & Sawaki, 2012)
Gardens found to be therapeutic	Access to nature important for healing in an institutional setting	Review of literature supporting therapeutic gardening (Mitrione, 2008)

8. Establish an ethical climate in the community through modeling, educating, and sponsoring workshops with experts. Consider establishment of an ethics program. Use an ethical decision-making model such as the six step process to assist with difficult decisions (Purtilo & Doherty, 2011; Solum & Schaffer, 2003).

Summary

Occupational therapy has historically been practiced in a number of contexts from institution, hospital, school, and home. However, emergent best practice indicates the closer we can get our intervention to the natural environment, the more meaningful and effective the occupational performance of our clients will become. This can be accomplished in many settings by finding the best "real-life" context for the occupation in which our client is engaging or wishes to engage. It is important to make sure the safety of the client and therapist are in place through environmental analysis and/or team collaboration. The chaos, complexity, and nonlinear dynamics of interactive systems are essential to consider when using the natural context in intervention planning. Finally, mandatory privacy and confidentiality issues need to be respected in the natural environment. This can be challenging and confusing in the dynamic, unpredictable natural setting, but should be highly respected for ethical best practice. Occupational participation occurs in the natural occurring contexts and environment of life, not in a contrived clinic environment. The ultimate goal of occupational therapy practice is to facilitate the client to fully participate in all life contexts of individual interest and importance.

Student Self-Assessment

1. Imagine some of your favorite pastimes and write down three of them. Include the activity and the context in which you like to do that activity.

    a. Describe how your therapist could best simulate that activity if you ever had occupational therapy.

    b. Describe how an occupational therapist could modify or assist you to perform that activity in the context you most enjoy it, if you were experiencing:

        *   Hemiparesis of your dominant side
        *   Severe visual impairment
        *   Social anxiety and panic attacks
        *   Cognitive impairments including impulsivity and short-term memory deficits

2a. Name some potential safety risks inherent in the following settings:

    ◊   The kitchen of a client's home
    ◊   Community mobility with an elder who has Parkinson's disease
    ◊   The playground
    ◊   A school field trip to another town
    ◊   The school bus
    ◊   The YMCA pool
    ◊   A summer camp
    ◊   A group home
    ◊   A shelter for battered women

2b. Now think critically and problem-solve potential precautions to put in place in each of the preceding settings to ensure safety and best practice.

3. Class discussion: Why is privacy and confidentiality more of a concern in natural, "uncontrolled" environments? Please give specific examples.

4. Name three ways that a practitioner can help to achieve an ethical climate of privacy in a natural setting during an activity that promotes real life social participation.

References

American Occupational Therapy Association. (2006). *The New IDEA: Summary of the Individuals with Disabilities Education Improvement Act of 2004* (P.L. 108-446). Retrieved from www.aota.org

American Occupational Therapy Association. (2008). *AOTA's societal statement on livable communities.* Retrieved from http://www.aota.org/practitioners-Section/Official-Docs.aspx

American Occupational Therapy Association. (2009). *Occupational therapy's commitment to non-discrimination and inclusion.* Retrieved from http://www.aota.org/practitioners-Section/Official-Docs.aspx

American Occupational Therapy Association. (2011). *Occupational therapy services in facilitating work performance.* Retrieved from http://www.aota.org/practitioners-Section/Official-Docs.aspx

Case-Smith, J. (2005). Development of childhood occupations. In J. Case-Smith (Ed.), *Occupational therapy for children* (5th ed., pp. 88-116). St. Louis, MO: Mosby-Elsevier.

Chamberlain L. L., & Butz, M. R. (1998). *Clinical chaos: A therapist's guide to nonlinear dynamics and therapeutic change.* Philadelphia, PA: Brunner/Mazel.

Champagne, T. (2008). *Sensory modulation & environment: Essential elements of occupation* (3rd ed.). Southampton, MA: Champagne Conferences & Consultation.

Christiansen, C., & Baum, C. M. (1991). *Occupational therapy: Enabling function and well-being* (2nd ed.). Thorofare, NJ: SLACK Incorporated.

Clark, F., Azen, S. P., Zemke, R., Jackson, J., Carlson, M., Mandel, D., et al. (1997). Occupational therapy for independent-living older adults. *Journal of the American Medical Association, 278*(16), 1321-1326.

Dunn, W., Foto, M., Hinojosa, J., Boyt-Schell, B., Thomson. L., & Hertfelder, S. (1995a). Independence position paper: The American Occupational Therapy Association: Broadening the construct of independence. *American Journal of Occupational Therapy, 49,* 1014.

Dunn, W., Foto, M., Hinojosa, J., Boyt-Schell, B., Thomson. L., & Hertfelder, S. (1995b). Occupational Therapy: A profession in support of full inclusion. In *Reference Manual of the Official Documents of the American Occupational Therapy Association, Inc.* Bethesda, MD: AOTA Press.

Edvardsson, D., & Nordvall, K. (2008). Lost in the present but confident of the past: Experiences of being in a psycho-geriatric unit as narrated by persons with dementia. *Journal of Clinical Nursing, 17*(4).

Grady, A. P. (1995). Building inclusive community: A challenge for occupational therapy. *American Journal of Occupational Therapy, 49,* 300-310.

Hinojosa, J., & Blount, M. L., (2000). *The texture of life purposeful activities in occupational therapy.* Bethesda, MD: AOTA Press.

Humphry, R., & Wakeford, L., (2006). An occupation-centered discussion of development and implications for practice. *American Journal of Occupational Therapy, 60,* 258-267.

Kelso, J. A. S. (1995). *Dynamic patterns: The self-organization of brain and behavior.* Cambridge, MA: The MIT Press.

Kielhofner, G. (1992). *Conceptual foundations of occupational therapy.* Philadelphia, PA: F.A. Davis Company.

Lazzarini, I. (2004). Neuro-occupation: The nonlinear dynamics of intention, meaning and perception. *British Journal of Occupational Therapy, 67*(8), 1-11.

Letts, L., Rigby, P., & Stewart, D. (2003). *Using environments to enable occupational performance.* Thorofare, NJ: SLACK Incorporated.

Loukas, K. M., Whiting, A., Ricci, E., & Cohen-Konrad, S. (2012). Transdisciplinary playgroup: Interprofessional opportunities in early intervention practice education. *OT Practice, 17*(3), 8-13.

Noonan, M. J., & McCormick, L. (2006). *Young children with disabilities in natural environments.* Baltimore, MD: Brookes Publishing Co.

Perr, A., & Bell, P. F. (2000). Moving from simulation to real life. In J. Hinojosa, & M. L. Blount (Eds.), *The texture of life purposeful activities in occupational therapy* (pp. 234-257). Bethesda, MD: AOTA Press.

Pierce, D. (2003). *Occupation by design: Building therapeutic power.* Philadelphia, PA: F.A. Davis Company.

Purtilo, R., & Doherty, R. (2011). *Ethical dimensions in the health professions* (5th ed.). St. Louis, MO: Saunders-Elsevier.

Reed, K. L. (2006). Occupational therapy values and beliefs, the formative years: 1904-1929. *OT Practice, April 17,* 21-25.

Royeen, C. B. (2003). Chaotic OT: Collective wisdom from a complex profession. *American Journal of Occupational Therapy, 57*(6), 609-624.

Sankar, P., Moran, S., Merz, J. F., & Jones, N. L. (2003). Patient perspectives on medical confidentiality. *Journal of General Internal Medicine, 18*(8), 659-669.

Scaffa, M. (2001). *Occupational therapy in community-based settings.* Philadelphia, PA: F.A. Davis Company.

Solum, L. L., & Schaffer, M. A. (2003). Ethical problems experienced by school nurses. *Journal of School Nursing, 19*(6), 330-337.

Stephens, L. C., & Tauber, S. K. (2005). Early intervention. In J. Case-Smith (Ed.), *Occupational therapy for children* (5th ed., pp. 771-793). St. Louis, MO: Mosby-Elsevier.

Thelen, E. (2000). Motor development as foundation and future of developmental psychology. *International Journal of Behavioral Development, 24*(4), 385-397.

Whalley Hammell, K. (2003). Changing institutional environments to enable occupation among people with severe physical limitations. In L. Letts, P. Rigby, & D. Stewart (Eds.), *Using environments to enable occupational performance* (pp. 35-53). Thorofare, NJ: SLACK Incorporated.

Wrights Law. (2013). *Special Education Law.* Retrieved from http://wrightslaw.com/

Zoltan, B. (2007). *Vision, perception, and cognition: A manual for the evaluation and treatment of the adult with acquired brain injury* (4th ed.). Thorofare, NJ: SLACK Incorporated.

Suggested Readings

Humphrey, R., Gonzalez, S., & Taylor, E. (1993). Family involvement in practice: Issues and attitudes. *American Journal of Occupational Therapy, 47,* 587-593.

Ideishi, S. K., Ideishi, R. I., Gandhi, T., & Yuen, L. (2006). Inclusive preschool outdoor play environments. *School system special interest section quarterly, 13*(2). Bethesda, MD: AOTA Press.

Kellegrew, D. H. (2000). Constructing daily routines: A qualitative examination of mothers with young children with disabilities. *American Journal of Occupational Therapy, 54,* 252-259.

Landa-Gonzalez, B. (2001). Multicontextual occupational therapy intervention: A case study of traumatic brain injury. *Occupational Therapy International, 8*(1), 49.

Law, M., Cooper, B., Strong, S., Stewart, P., Rigby, P., & Letts, L. (1996). The person-environment-occupation model: A transactive approach to occupational performance. *Canadian Journal of Occupational Therapy, 63,* 9-23.

Ma, H., Trombly, C. A., Robinson-Podolski, C. (1998). The effect of context on skill acquisition and transfer. *American Journal of Occupational Therapy, 53,* 138-144.

Mitrione, S. (2008). Therapeutic responses to natural environment using gardens to improve health care. *Minnesota Medicine.* Retrieved from http://www.minnesotamedicine.com/PastIssues/March2008/ClinicalMitrioneMarch2008/tabid/2488/Default.aspx

Segal, R. (2004). Family routines and rituals: A context for occupational therapy interventions. *American Journal of Occupational Therapy, 58,* 499-508.

Skubik-Peplaski, C., Carrico, C., Nichols, L., Chelette, K., & Sawaki, L. (2012). Behavioral, neurophysiological, and descriptive changes after occupation-based intervention. *American Journal of Occupational Therapy, 66,* e107-e113. Retrieved from http://dxdoi.org/10.5014/ajot.2012.003590

Stuetjens, E. M., Dekker, J., Bouter, L. M., Jellena, S., Bakker, E. B., & van den Ende, C. H. M. (2004). Occupational therapy for community dwelling elderly people. A systematic review. *Age and Aging, 33,* 453-460.

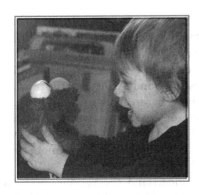

13

CLINICAL REASONING

Kristin B. Haas, OTD, OTR/L

ACOTE STANDARDS EXPLORED IN THIS CHAPTER
B.2.10, B.2.11

KEY VOCABULARY

- **Clinical reasoning:** "Thinking through the various aspects of patient care to arrive at a reasonable decision regarding the prevention, diagnosis, or treatment of a clinical problem in a specific patient" (Hawkins, Elder, & Paul, 2010, p. 3).
- **Experiential learning:** "Involves hands-on experience in a practical setting to test information learned in didactic coursework in an actual practice environment" (Coker, 2010, p. 281).

- **Narrative reasoning:** "The process through which occupational therapy practitioners make sense of people's particular circumstances; prospectively imagine the effect of illness, disability, or occupational performance problems on their daily lives; and create a collaborative story that is enacted with clients and families through intervention" (Schell & Schell, 2008, p. 446).
- **Professional reasoning:** "The process that practitioners use to plan, direct, perform, and reflect on client care" (Schell, 2009, p. 314).
- **Reflection:** Critical analysis of knowledge and feelings leading to a better understanding of the situation.

Jacobs, K., MacRae, N., & Sladyk, K. (Eds.).
Occupational Therapy Essentials for
Clinical Competence, Second Edition (pp. 159-166).
© 2014 SLACK Incorporated.

Introduction

Clinical reasoning skills can assist occupational therapy practitioners to be successful. The skill sets involved in clinical reasoning are many and varied. Being able to clinically reason is important to the success of the profession, the success of clients, and becoming a vital part of the health care team. Defining and articulating clinical reasoning can be difficult for even the most seasoned occupational therapy practitioner. Clinical reasoning is a multifaceted cognitive process that involves several different layers of thought, evidence, and experience. It is a concept that may be a challenge for students and new occupational therapy practitioners to fully grasp because even experienced occupational therapy practitioners have a difficult time describing the complete process for their own clinical reasoning and decision making. Research suggests that using a clinical reasoning frame to organize clinical observations is an effective method to help entry-level occupational therapy students learn and apply clinical reasoning concepts (Neistadt, 1998). The findings from the American Occupational Therapy Association's (AOTA) Clinical Reasoning Study (Mattingly, 1991; Mattingly & Fleming, 1994) indicated that occupational therapy practitioners use several types of reasoning during the process of clinical reasoning. The cognitive process of clinical reasoning includes narrative, procedural, interactive, and conditional reasoning. Mattingly and Fleming (1994) concluded that experienced practitioners seem to shift from one mode of thinking to another during the therapeutic intervention process. Other literature indicates the following types of reasoning that enter into the clinical reasoning process as scientific, pragmatic, ethical, and diagnostic (Schell, 2009). Moreover, reflection has been noted as being an important aspect of clinical reasoning (Plack & Santasier, 2004).

In addition to these types of reasoning, occupational therapy practitioners must use their personal experiences, evidence-based practice, and information about the specific client and his or her context in order to develop clinical reasoning skills. The use of theory can also assist occupational therapy practitioners in developing a high level of clinical reasoning. Hawkins, Elder, and Paul (2010) define *clinical reasoning* as "thinking through the various aspects of patient care to arrive at a reasonable decision regarding the prevention, diagnosis, or treatment of a clinical problem in a specific patient" (p. 3). Furthermore, Schell (2009) implores occupational therapy practitioners to think of clinical reasoning more as the ability to professionally reason. Professional reasoning is a broader concept than clinical reasoning, which is used more often in a medical model. Occupational therapy practitioners work in community, educational, and consultative models, as well as in the medical model; thus, it is important to take a more thorough look at the type of reasoning that occupational therapy practitioners perform. As a newer term, *professional reasoning* is distinct from clinical reasoning and defined as "the process that practitioners use to plan, direct, perform, and reflect on client care" (Schell, 2009, p. 314). Many of the same skill sets are involved in both clinical and professional reasoning, whether one is trying to become more seasoned in either type of reasoning.

It is important to understand the various methods of reasoning to begin to understand how to clinically reason.

Narrative Reasoning

Narrative reasoning provides a way to learn about a person's life story. Developing an occupational profile on a client is an example of narrative reasoning. In learning to reason through a narrative approach, a student or novice practitioner must begin by building rapport and obtaining a true understanding of the circumstances that put the client in the care of an occupational therapy practitioner. The practitioner must go beyond gathering the basics of an occupational profile and determine how the information gathered will affect the client's present and future (Schell, 2009). Mattingly and Fleming (1994) suggest that narrative reasoning is the method by which occupational therapy practitioners attempt to figure out how the client's life story will develop moving forward from the injury, illness, or life change given the client's specific circumstances.

Procedural Reasoning

Procedural reasoning involves thinking about the client's performance (Fleming, 1991). Occupational therapy practitioners and students use procedural reasoning to think about the disability level or diagnosis. Using this type of reasoning, the occupational therapy practitioner must identify the client's problems and select specific treatment to help remediate or compensate for the deficits identified (Mattingly & Fleming, 1994). When seen in practice, procedural reasoning is often the use of protocols or specific therapeutic procedures deemed appropriate due to the client's disability or diagnosis. The use of standardized assessments to determine deficits and strengths of a client can also be a part of procedural reasoning. On one hand, this can be detached from the client-centered practice that is at the heart of occupational therapy; however, even within science-driven procedural reasoning, an occupational therapy practitioner can utilize parts of narrative reasoning to obtain a client-centered focus.

INTERACTIVE REASONING

Interactive reasoning is used to individualize the therapeutic approach and to understand the client as a human being. This type of reasoning suggests how occupational therapy practitioners may interpret and use verbal and nonverbal cues to engage the client (Crepeau, 1991). Therapeutic use of self is an important aspect of interactive reasoning and is imperative in developing a therapy plan that takes into account the client as an integral part of the therapy process. Students and novice occupational therapy practitioners should practice this skill often, especially during fieldwork experiences.

PRAGMATIC REASONING

Pragmatic reasoning is used to understand the practical issues that may have an impact on the situation with the client and his or her family (Schell, 2009). This type of reasoning enables occupational therapy practitioners to incorporate ideas into the situation that the client and family is enduring, allowing one to identify practical strategies for intervention. Examples can include the following: What are the family, caregiver, and community resources available to support intervention and equipment recommendations? What materials and interprofessional support is available for intervention? These issues are usually not client centered and take into account the intangibles that surround and influence the therapy the client is receiving. Schell (2008) lists several issues that may be part of pragmatic reasoning, including teamwork, scheduling, space, equipment, caseload, insurance coverage, discharge options, and occupational therapy practitioners' ability.

ETHICAL REASONING

Ethical reasoning is used to make sure one selects the morally justifiable choices. Ethical reasoning introduces the consideration of what "should" be done in the best interest of the person and family. Ethical reasoning utilizes the Occupational Therapy Code of Ethics as well as the mission of the facility where one is employed. The moral conflict that may come into play when making decisions about client care and treatment can be weighed against the risks and benefits of each ethical principle. Having a good understanding and working knowledge of the Occupational Therapy Code of Ethics gives the novice occupational therapy practitioner or student an edge in this type of reasoning.

SCIENTIFIC REASONING

Scientific reasoning is used to understand the condition that may be affecting the person and family. Schell (2009) described scientific reasoning as the logical thinking about the nature of the client's problems and the optimal course of action in intervention. Scientific reasoning requires the clinician to consider the background knowledge that might help one to understand the characteristics of the condition better. Evidence-based practice assists in guiding scientific reasoning; therefore, this type of reasoning is sometimes not considered client centered.

DIAGNOSTIC REASONING

Diagnostic reasoning may be considered a part of scientific reasoning; however, this type of reasoning takes into account the client-based information in addition to the evidence-based information available (Schell, 2009).

CONDITIONAL REASONING

According to Schell (2009), conditional reasoning is often seen in proficient to expert occupational therapy practitioners. This type of reasoning is a combination of the other types of reasoning in that the practitioner can combine the reasoning to respond to the ever-changing environment and client and the context or experience of the disability.

The Use of Reasoning in Clinical Practice

The various types of reasoning involved in clinical reasoning require various levels of skill. Even a novice occupational therapy practitioner or student may be able to make decisions based on identifying basic ethical issues, following protocols, identifying outside forces that may impact therapy, and completing an occupational profile. Students and new graduates may even be more skilled than some expert occupational therapy practitioners at utilizing research to make clinical decisions supported by evidence. However, a skilled and experienced expert occupational therapy practitioner may be better able to utilize interactive and conditional reasoning, as well as eclectically joining and switching between the many different types of reasoning. In addition, skilled occupational therapy practitioners spend time in reflection to gain insight into the client in order to clinically reason.

Reflection is an important component of clinical reasoning. Being able to critically analyze one's own actions and experiences as a occupational therapy practitioner is vital to clinical reasoning. Reflection should include comparing experiences; utilizing personal and professional beliefs, values, and ethics; and critically analyzing the actions taken. Atkins and Murphy (1993) advocate that self-awareness, description, critical analysis, synthesis, and evaluation are essential skills for reflection. Bannigan and Moores (2009) suggest that the skills of reflection and evidence-based practice be integrated into occupational therapy education to assist students in learning these vital skill sets. Practice in the skill of reflection is vital to becoming well rounded in the use of clinical reasoning.

Hawkins, Elder, and Paul (2010) offer concepts and structure to the clinical reasoning process. The elements of this structure include the "purpose of clinical reasoning, clinical question at issue, clinical information, clinical interpretation and influence, clinical concepts, clinical assumptions, clinical implications and consequences, and clinical point of view" (p. 5). To begin, there should be a goal or objective to your clinical reasoning. The occupational therapy practitioner is attempting to provide optimal care to the client. Next, there should be a problem or issue at hand for the occupational therapy practitioner to address. In occupational therapy practice, this is usually related to how to best treat the client or which treatment method is appropriate for the client given the specific circumstances. Clinical information must then be gathered through various methods, such as chart review, client interview, assessment, and evaluation using narrative, interactive, and scientific reasoning. Evidence-based practice information can be brought in at this stage as well.

In applying Hawkins, Elder, and Paul's (2010) clinical reasoning model to occupational therapy, the occupational therapy practitioner next draws conclusions from the information and personal experiences. The clinical concepts element has the practitioner draw on theories, models of practice, or frames of reference to assist in moving the clinical issue forward. Subsequently, any assumptions that the occupational therapy practitioner can make based on client diagnosis or presumptions can be taken into account using procedural and scientific reasoning. These assumptions need to be sound and grounded in clinical knowledge.

The occupational therapy practitioner can then decide clinical implications and consequences based on the information gained and gathered through the previous steps grounded in conditional reasoning. These implications should flow logically from the previously gathered information. One must take into account the consequences that may happen based on the decisions made for treatment and look at the ethical reasoning of the situation. Finally, the clinician can use conditional reasoning to derive a clinical point of view on the best plan of action to take for the particular client and clinical question at hand. Pragmatic reasoning would be beneficial to keep in mind throughout the process.

Hawkins, Elder, and Paul (2010) also advocate for determining the type of clinical question that one is trying to answer. In occupational therapy practice, most clinical questions are a question of judgment. These types of clinical questions related to occupational therapy treatment and practice may have more than one answer; however, there is usually a best answer or treatment to select. This type of question and the clinical reasoning that goes along with answering these questions is imperative to occupational therapy practice. In addition, for an occupational therapy student, this is the type of questioning that is utilized on the certification examination. Thinking clinically and using clinical reasoning to come to the best possible solution is paramount in being a successful occupational therapy practitioner.

The occupational therapy process is an "ongoing interaction among evaluation, intervention, and outcomes" (AOTA, 2008, p. 648). These components of the occupational therapy process are a fluid process that is continually adapted based on client need, changes in the client's performance, and the clinician's clinical reasoning. It is important to use clinical reasoning skills throughout the occupational therapy process of evaluation, intervention, and outcomes. Utilization of the Occupational Therapy Practice Framework (OTPF) can assist students and occupational therapy practitioners in becoming better at clinical reasoning. As part of evaluation, occupational therapy practitioners should create an occupational profile (narrative and interactive reasoning). Intervention is an ever-evolving process of planning, implementing, and reviewing treatment and requires clinical reasoning to be effective. Self-reflection and scientific, pragmatic, procedural, and conditional reasoning are used interchangeably and throughout this process. Keeping in mind the outcome that is "supporting health and participation in life through engagement in occupation" (AOTA, 2008, p. 626) can help practitioners with the first step of Hawkins, Elder, and Paul's (2010) concept of clinical reasoning. Many actions must be taken when working with a client, and these actions require clinical reasoning skills. Some examples are outlined in Table 13-1. The OTPF provides practitioners with a foundation and scaffold upon which to build evaluation, treatment, and outcomes for the client.

Knecht-Sabres (2010) conducted a pilot study on the use of experiential learning opportunities and clinical reasoning. In 2010, Coker also studied the effects of experiential learning on clinical reasoning and critical thinking skills. The experiential learning component consisted of students evaluating and treating older adults living in the community with oversight by faculty and pre/post meetings with faculty to reflect and plan for further treatment sessions (Knecht-Sabres, 2010). In the Coker (2010) study, a week-long day camp was held for children with cerebral palsy. Both studies used a convenience sample of occupational therapy students who integrated and taught various aspects of clinical reasoning as part of the experience. The findings of the first study, although preliminary, strongly suggest that student perceptions of their

Table 13-1.

QUESTIONS TO GUIDE CLINICAL REASONING

Clinical reasoning example for selecting the best piece of assistive technology (AT) for a client:
- Isolate and list the client's strengths and deficits from the case.
- Determine the client's most important challenge that you could address using AT.
- Find possible AT that might work to address the most important challenge of the client.
- List the pros and cons for each device. This should include those inherent to the device and list the client's skills, abilities, and deficits in relation to the use of the device.
- Clinically reason the best option for the specific client in each of the following case studies.

Example 1 of Clinical Reasoning Worksheets

Background
- Provide a short summary of the case.
- List five deficits noted based on the diagnosis and case.

Frames of Reference (FOR)/Model of Practice (MOP) to use with this case:
- Justification for FOR/MOP based on deficits/diagnosis/setting.
- List two assessments that you would use.
- What information will you get from the assessments?
- Justify how the assessments link to the FOR/MOP and the listed deficits.

Treatment
- Describe the treatment session in detail, including the order in which activities should be done and why.
- What outcome, according to the OTPF, are you working toward? Explain why this outcome is the best for this client.
- Will you include family and/or caregivers in the treatment session? Why?
- What are the skills/client factors that you are working on during treatment?
- What is the overall goal of the treatment session?
- Address how long the treatment session will last and why.
- What intervention strategies, according to the occupational therapy practice framework (OTPF), are you utilizing in the treatment session?
- What outcomes are you working toward in the treatment session?

Reflection
- Take time away from the case (at least 24 hours) to reflect on the following:
  - ✳ Determine how this case is similar to others you have seen (in practice or fieldwork).
  - ✳ Evaluate the treatment session. List both positive and critical aspects of the session (or plan).
  - ✳ Describe what you would do differently given a similar case.

Example 2 of Clinical Reasoning Worksheets

- List the five most important deficits noted based on the diagnoses and case.
- What psychosocial issues need to be addressed based on your case? List at least three and describe the importance of addressing these issues as part of treatment.
- Discuss the FOR/MOP that you would use and why it meets the needs of this client.
- List one standardized assessment (1 point) and one nonstandardized assessment that should be completed prior to the treatment session you developed. Why would you pick each assessment to complete prior to this specific treatment session?
- Justify how the assessments link to the FOR/MOP and the listed deficits.
- Cite and summarize at least one peer-reviewed article showing evidence that this treatment session meets best practice standards.
- Write one long-term goal and two short-term goals for this client.

(continued)

Table 13-1 (continued).

QUESTIONS TO GUIDE CLINICAL REASONING

Example 3 of Clinical Reasoning Worksheets

- Design a treatment session for your client. Include all activities, equipment, training, and persons involved.
  - ✴ How long would the treatment session last and why?
  - ✴ What is the specific goal of the treatment session?
- Answer the following questions about the treatment session you designed/created.
  - ✴ What are two client factors or skills you are working on, and what is the justification in using these for the client/diagnosis, setting, and FOR/MOP?
  - ✴ What is one outcome from the OTPF you are working toward, and how does this outcome fit with your treatment, FOR/MOP, and assessment?
  - ✴ Pick one intervention strategy from the OTPF and justify how you are using it in this treatment session.
- List preparatory, purposeful, and occupation-based activities you could do with your client. These do not necessarily have to relate to the treatment session you created earlier; however, they must fit the diagnosis and occupational profile information you have on the client. Describe why each activity is appropriate for the client.

clinical reasoning skills are enhanced through experiential learning activities (Knecht-Sabres, 2010). Similarly, Coker (2010) found that overall scores of the students who participated in the experiential learning opportunity were statistically improved. With the use of experiential learning activities, students moved from utilizing scientific and procedural reasoning to more narrative, pragmatic, interactive, and conditional reasoning (Knecht-Sabres, 2010). Likewise, students statistically improved in the subscales of evaluation, inductive reasoning, and deductive reasoning during the Coker (2010) study. Some methods that novice occupational therapy practitioners or students might need based on this study to improve their clinical reasoning are to use an inquiry approach in the classroom or clinical setting, seek out resources to address personal growth needs, give and receive constructive feedback, and engage in self-reflection. Coker (2010) noted that students improved statistically in the ability to complete the following skills: questioning treatment techniques, utilizing protocols, using a frame of reference to structure intervention, and using data and experience to make decisions about treatment. Although these studies show promise in experiential learning activities to improve clinical reasoning skills, caution must be used due to the possible confounding factors and small convenience samples.

Kielhofner, Forsyth, Kramer, Melton, and Dobson (2009) describe a method for using the Model of Human Occupation (MOHO) in therapeutic reasoning. This method may be helpful to novice occupational therapy practitioners and students as clinical reasoning skills are being further developed. The process involves generating questions, gathering information, using this material to describe the client within the MOHO framework,

developing therapy goals and intervention strategies, implementing and monitoring treatment, and assessing outcomes (Kielhofner et al., 2009). The method, while outlined for use with MOHO, could be implemented with other models of practice and frames of reference. Several other examples of an explicit thought process are located in Table 13-1. These examples may help novice occupational therapy practitioners and students as clinical reasoning skills are being established. As the novice gains more experience and knowledge, the worksheets and methods will become more natural and second nature to the occupational therapy practitioner. Table 13-2 lists concrete skills that a novice or student occupational therapy practitioner may want to develop or continue to develop to improve clinical reasoning skills.

Students should assess their clinical reasoning skills while on all levels of fieldwork affiliations and during coursework. Novice occupational therapy practitioners should continue to develop clinical reasoning skills throughout their career. McKay and Ryan (1995) suggest that students share personal therapeutic stories (narrative reasoning) with peers and supervisor(s) in a confidential manner. Buchanan, Moore, and van Niekerk (1998) proposed using a revised case study guide format and reflective writing to improve reasoning. Journaling or reflective writing is commonly used by supervisors to observe just how much students have expanded their scope of practice and decision-making processes. Sladyk and Sheckley (2000) found seven activities that enhanced students' clinical reasoning skill development. These activities included journal writing, videotaping, reviewing case studies, and probing questions; working with a consistent population; role modeling; and listening to supervisor stories.

Table 13-2.

HOW CLINICAL REASONING IS APPLIED IN PRACTICE

Therapist/Student Action	Critical Reasoning Utilized
Choice of frame of reference	Ethical
Use of pool for intervention	Interactive
Observation of the client's environment	Interactive
Consultation with family and caregivers	Narrative, interactive
Use of the framework to guide decisions	Procedural
Choice of intervention approaches	Interactive
Sensory stimulation as an intervention modality	Interactive
Family/caregiver training activities	Pragmatic
Reflection	Conditional
Use of evidence-based practice in guiding intervention planning	Scientific, ethical

EVIDENCE-BASED RESEARCH CHART

Topic	Evidence
Clinical reasoning	Carrier et al., 2010; Kuipers & Grice, 2009; Mu et al., 2010; Yancosek & Howell, 2010
Reflection	Bannigan & Moores, 2009; Dunn & Musolino, 2011; Plack & Santasier, 2004
Experiential learning	Coker, 2010; Knecht-Sabres, 2010

Summary

Clinical reasoning is a complex and multifaceted cognitive process that requires skill and practice. By becoming proficient in clinical reasoning, an occupational therapy practitioner can provide the best possible therapy for clients. Becoming an expert clinical reasoner is difficult for many occupational therapy practitioners. However, the examples, skills, and methods outlined in this chapter may assist practitioners in developing and enhancing clinical reasoning skills. Occupational therapy practitioners should strive to make the best decisions during the therapeutic process, and good clinical reasoning skills can help make these decisions clearer. In fact, in the simplest terms, these clinical decisions regarding best practice and the processes by which one makes the decisions can be referred to as clinical reasoning.

Electronic Resources

- AOTA Evidence-Based Practice and Research: www.aota.org/Educate/Research.aspx
- Critically appraised topics related to occupational therapy: www.otcats.com
- Evidence-Based Practice Research Group: www.srsmcmaster.ca
- National Board for Certification in Occupational Therapy (NBCOT), Competency Resources: www.nbcot.org
- OT Seeker—evidence-based practice briefs related to occupational therapy: www.otseeker.com
- PubMed search engine from the National Library of Medicine and the National Institutes of Health: www.ncbi.nlm.nih.gov/entrez/query.fcgi

References

American Occupational Therapy Association. (2008). Occupational therapy practice framework: Domain and process (2nd ed.). *American Journal of Occupational Therapy, 62,* 625-683.

Atkins, S., & Murphy, K. (1993). Reflection: A review of the literature. *Journal of Advanced Nursing, 18,* 1188-1192.

Bannigan, K., & Moores, A. (2009). A model of professional thinking: Integrating reflective practice and evidence based practice. *Canadian Journal of Occupational Therapy, 76*(5), 342-350.

Buchanan, H., Moore, R., & van Niekerk, L. (1998). The fieldwork case study: Writing for clinical reasoning. *American Journal of Occupational Therapy, 52*(4), 291-295.

Carrier, A., Levasseur, M., Bedard, D., & Desrosiers, J. (2010). Community occupational therapists' clinical reasoning: Identifying tacit knowledge. *Australian Occupational Therapy Journal, 57,* 356-365. doi: 10.1111/j.1440-1630.2010.00875.x

Coker, P. (2010). Effects of an experiential learning program on the clinical reasoning and critical thinking skills of occupational therapy students. *Journal of Allied Health, 39*(4), 280-286.

Crepeau, E. B. (1991). Achieving intersubjective understanding: Examples from an occupational therapy treatment session. *American Journal of Occupational Therapy, 45*(11), 1016-1025.

Dunn, L., & Musolino, G. M. (2011). Assessing reflective thinking and approaches to learning. *Journal of Allied Health, 40*(3), 128-136.

Fleming, M. H. (1991). The therapist with the three-track mind. *American Journal of Occupational Therapy, 45*(11), 1007-1014.

Hawkins, D., Elder, L., & Paul, R. (2010). *The thinker's guide to clinical reasoning.* Dillon Beach, CA: Foundation for Critical Thinking.

Kielhofner, G., Forsyth, K., Kramer, J. M., Melton, J., & Dobson, E. (2009) The model of human occupation. In E. B. Crepeau, E. S. Cohn, & B. A. B. Schell (Eds.), *Willard & Spackman's occupational therapy* (11th ed., pp. 446-461). Philadelphia, PA: Lippincott Williams & Wilkins.

Knecht-Sabres, L. J. (2010). The use of experiential learning in an occupational therapy program: Can it foster skills for clinical practice? *Occupational Therapy in Health Care, 24*(4), 320-334. doi:10.3109/07380577.2010.514382

Kuipers, K., & Grice, J. W. (2009). The structure of novice and expert occupational therapists' clinical reasoning before and after exposure to a domain-specific protocol. *Australian Occupational Therapy Journal, 56,* 418-427. doi: 10.1111/j.1440-1630.2009.00793.x

Mattingly, C. (1991). What is clinical reasoning? *American Journal of Occupational Therapy, 45*(11), 979-986.

Mattingly, C., & Fleming, M. H. (1994). *Clinical reasoning: Forms of inquiry in a therapeutic practice.* Philadelphia, PA: F.A. Davis Company.

McKay, E. A., & Ryan, S. (1995). Clinical reasoning through story telling: Examining a student's case story on a fieldwork placement. *British Journal of Occupational Therapy, 58*(6), 234-238.

Mu, K., Coppard, B. M., Bracciano, A., Doll, J., & Matthews, A. (2010). Fostering cultural competency, clinical reasoning, and leadership through international outreach. *Occupational Therapy in Health Care, 24*(1), 74-85. doi: 10.3109/07380570903329628

Neistadt, M. E. (1998). Teaching clinical reasoning as a thinking frame. *American Journal of Occupational Therapy, 52*(3), 221-229.

Plack, M. M., & Santasier, A. (2004). Reflective practice: A model for facilitating critical thinking skills within an integrative case study classroom experience. *Journal of Physical Therapy Education, 18,* 4-12.

Schell, B. A. B. (2008). Pragmatic reasoning. In B. A. B. Schell & J. W. Schell (Eds.), *Clinical and professional reasoning in occupational therapy* (pp. 169-187). Philadelphia, PA: Lippincott Williams & Wilkins.

Schell, B. A. B. (2009). Professional reasoning in practice. In E. B. Crepeau, E. S. Cohn, & B. A. B. Schell (Eds.), *Willard & Spackman's occupational therapy* (11th ed., pp. 314-327). Philadelphia, PA: Lippincott Williams & Wilkins.

Sladyk, K., & Sheckley, B. (2000). Clinical reasoning and reflective practice: Implications of fieldwork activities. *Occupational Therapy in Health Care, 13*(1), 11-22.

Yancosek, K. E., & Howell, D. (2010). Integrating the dynamical systems theory, the task-oriented approach, and the practice framework for clinical reasoning. *Occupational Therapy in Health Care, 24*(3), 223-238. doi:10.3109/07380577.2010.496824

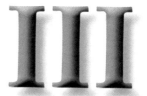

OCCUPATIONAL THERAPY
THEORETICAL PERSPECTIVES

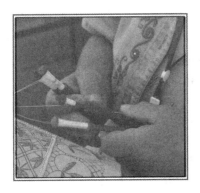

14

OCCUPATIONAL THERAPY THEORY DEVELOPMENT AND ORGANIZATION

Marilyn B. Cole, MS, OTR/L, FAOTA

ACOTE STANDARDS EXPLORED IN THIS CHAPTER
B.3.1, B.3.2, B.3.4, B.3.6 for master's and doctoral OT programs
B.3.1, B.3.3 for COTA programs

KEY VOCABULARY

- **Applied research:** Research addressing problems of practical interest.

- **Applied theory:** The results of applied research, intended to address problems of practical interest.

- **Assumptions:** Broad general statements that are taken for granted for the sake of argument.

- **Basic research:** Research addressing general phenomenon.

- **Concept:** An idea or notion formed by mentally combining characteristics (Reed, 1999).

- **Conceptual models in OT:** Graphic or schematic representations of concepts and assumptions that explain why the profession works as it does (Reed & Sanderson, 1999).

- **Construct:** Invented names for variables that cannot be seen directly, but are inferred by measuring relevant or correlated observable behavior (Portney & Watkins, 2000).

- **Epistemology:** The dynamics of knowing (Hooper, 2006); how we know what we know.

- **Frame of reference:** System of compatible concepts from theory that guides a plan of action within a specific occupational therapy domain of concern (adapted from Mosey, 1986).

- **Holistic approach:** Taking a broader view of a person as a unified whole, including the many contexts and systems within which a person exists and interacts.

(continued)

Jacobs, K., MacRae, N., & Sladyk, K. (Eds.).
Occupational Therapy Essentials for
Clinical Competence, Second Edition (pp. 169-184).
© 2014 SLACK Incorporated.

KEY VOCABULARY (CONTINUED)

- **Humanism:** Dedication to the betterment of the human condition and the right of each person to respect, dignity, and a meaningful and productive role in society.
- **Model:** A simplified representation of structure and content…that describes or explains complex relationships between concepts (Creek, 1992).

- **Nonlinear science in OT:** "According to nonlinear dynamics systems theory, human beings are conceptualized as self-organizing complex dynamical systems who interact with the environment through their occupations for the purpose of creating, changing, and adapting to achieve optimal performance" (Lazzarini, 2005).
- **Paradigm:** A shared vision encompassing fundamental assumptions and beliefs, which serves as the cultural core of the profession (Kielhofner, 1997).

Introduction

Most occupational therapy students and practitioners regard theory as the concern of academia and science, not practice. Although we know that all assessments and interventions have their base in theory, practice focuses on the application of these tools with clients. Theory is elusive, influencing our behaviors, but often without our awareness. Most of us would be surprised at how often we use theory in our daily lives. For decisions as simple as what we eat for breakfast, most of us consider theories about healthy lifestyles. We may feel like eating eggs, bacon, and buttered biscuits, but we may decide on whole grain cereal or yogurt with granola and fresh fruit instead, assuming this to be better for our health long term. Or, we may eat what we want anyway, reasoning that we only live once, so we may as well enjoy it.

Our theories also affect how we react to unexpected situations in life. For example, when Hurricane Sandy headed for the northeastern shores of the United States, news reports used sophisticated weather instruments to predict the trajectory of the storm, estimate its time of arrival, and suggest its likely effect on the people living along the shore. Citizens reacted differently according to their theoretical assumptions. Some assumed that news reports usually exaggerate, and did nothing to prepare. Others dashed out to stores to stock up on supplies. They reasoned that hurricanes generate high winds that knock down power lines and thought about how they might survive without power. They bought foods that do not require cooking or refrigeration, and bought candles, fuel for generators, and batteries to power flashlights and radios and communication devices. Some even filled bottles and tubs with water for drinking or washing in case the water supply became contaminated. But many people failed to predict the effects of Sandy on the tides, or the volumes of water that high winds could blow into narrow water areas such as the Hudson River or Long Island Sound. Because people in the northeast do not encounter hurricanes very often, they could not rely on past experience. They needed to carry the theory further in order to imagine the effects of the 12- to 15-foot storm surge that ultimately did most of the damage.

Whenever we make a decision or form an opinion on something, we are using theory in the reasoning process to justify or validate our thoughts and actions. Only through reflection can we become aware of the assumptions we are making—the theories behind our behavior. It is the same with the practice of occupational therapy. In the beginning of the 20th century, occupational therapists learned techniques and applied them without giving much thought to the theories or assumptions upon which they were based. However, current trends compel us to raise our awareness of frames of reference, to reflect on the outcomes of our tools and techniques, and to read research studies that provide evidence that the theories behind our actions in practice are valid. These are the requirements of evidence-based occupational therapy practice in the 21st century.

In this chapter, we will define theory as it relates to occupational therapy, trace the evolution of theory from occupational therapy's founding in 1917 to the present, and discuss the paradigm shifts in health care within the context of historical events and trends. Finally, we will propose an organizational model for understanding and applying the various levels of theory in occupational therapy practice.

Table 14-1.		
PURPOSES SERVED BY THEORY AND EXAMPLES		
Purpose	**Question Addressed (Theory)**	**Examples**
Define a concept	What is figure-ground perception? (Sensory integration theory)	Ability to recognize shapes of objects in a cluttered line drawing. Ability to find two matching black socks in a cluttered drawer.
Describe	What is good time management? (Cognitive behavioral theory)	Ability to plan and execute daily activities to meet one's needs and obligations in an efficient and satisfying manner.
Correlate	How does exercise relate to successful aging? (Biomechanical theory)	Studies show that 30 minutes of moderate exercise each day maintains both mental and physical fitness for older adults.
Explain why	What causes stress at work? (Person-environment-occupational performance model)	Stress is produced when a worker's occupational performance does not match the demands or cultural/social expectations of the workplace.
Predict	What activities prevent cognitive decline in aging? (Cognitive behavioral theory and cognitive theories of aging)	Practicing mentally challenging tasks (i.e., crossword puzzles), and participating socially with others, (i.e., playing cards or chess), helps to maintain an aging brain.
Evaluate	How does volunteering with the homeless help adolescents develop empathy and compassion? (Attachment theory and social participation)	Informal personal interactions with persons different from one's self increases the likelihood of finding common ground and developing cultural awareness and sensitivity.

What Is Theory?

Kerlinger defined theory as "a set of interrelated constructs (variables), definitions, and propositions that presents a systematic view of phenomena by specifying relations among variables, with the purpose of explaining natural phenomena" (1979, p. 64). In occupational therapy, this "scientific" view of theory assumes that knowledge is derived from systematic, controlled, and empirical study of some aspect of human occupational behavior (Table 14-1).

Some well-known theories, such as Newton's gravitational theory and Einstein's theory of relativity, are examples of scientific theories validated through basic research; Skinner's theory of operant conditioning and Bandura's social learning theory are examples of applied research. This distinction parallels the difference between occupational science and occupational therapy. Occupational science is an academic discipline that is aligned with basic research. Occupational scientists study the form, function, and meaning of occupation without regard to the practical use of the theories generated. Occupational therapists are mainly concerned with the application of theories in practice. While we may borrow from the theories of occupational science, occupational therapists look for ways to relate them to our understanding of occupational dysfunction, deprivation, restoration, and adaptation for the clients and populations we serve.

The practice framework of the American Occupational Therapy Association ([AOTA] 2008, pp. 656-659) defines the following five occupational intervention approaches:

1. Create/promote (health promotion; e.g., arranging sensory environments to promote emotion regulation and self-organization for at-risk adolescents)

2. Establish/restore (remediation, restoration; e.g., constraint-induced functional movement for stroke survivors)

3. Maintain (e.g., engaging in challenging mental activities to maintain cognition)

4. Modify (compensation, adaptation; e.g., ergonomic modification of workstations to prevent musculoskeletal discomfort)

5. Prevent (disability prevention; e.g., fall prevention in well elderly)

Within the existing literature, occupational therapy practitioners can find evidence supporting each of these approaches with specific populations using a wide range of theories. Occupational therapists need to develop and test theories that give us evidence about the best ways to enable occupational performance for our clients.

How Are Theories Developed?

A theory begins with asking a question. Applied theories represent attempts to solve practical problems. Why do children misbehave in school? What causes people to get stressed out with their jobs? How do some elders manage to stay healthy and fit well into old age while others do not? The researcher next forms a hypothesis, a possible explanation for something observed. For example, A. Jean Ayres hypothesized that some school children misbehave because they cannot integrate sensory input, resulting in their inability to sit still and pay attention to the teacher. She tested this hypothesis by creating a method to measure the way children process different types of sensory input, mainly vestibular, proprioceptive, and tactile, but also incorporating auditory and visual systems. By evaluating many children, Ayres identified several patterns of sensory dysfunction. When she applied carefully graded sensory input through play activities, she found that some children integrated sensations more effectively, resulting in dramatic improvement of both their classroom behavior and academic learning (Ayres, 1979). Her research resulted in the theory of sensory integration, a frame of reference used widely by occupational therapists working in school systems today.

Experimental research, such as the study just described, uses the scientific method to collect data according to specific criteria, ideally including a random selection of subjects, control of extraneous influences, and some form of manipulation such as an occupational therapy intervention. When a theory has been developed to a certain point, a good way to test the theory is to do an experiment. Two groups of subjects are randomly selected: one group is treated in a designated way (experimental group) while the other group is not (control group). In order to control for bias or unanticipated influences on the outcome, both groups should be the same in every aspect, except for the intervention being tested. Both groups are evaluated before and after the intervention interval in order to determine whether the experimental group has changed in a way that is different from the control group. Ayres studied a randomly selected sample of school-age children representative of the normal population, and developed age-equivalent norms for each sensory subtest in her sensory integration battery. This is called a *norm-referenced assessment*, which generated a theory of normal sensory integrative development (Ayres, 1979). Many occupational therapy researchers have tested different parts of Ayres's theory by using specific interventions such as scooter board play and spinning on a tire swing with groups of children who have sensory deficits (Bundy, Lane, & Murray, 2002; Royeen & Luebben, 2009).

When the subjects are not randomly selected but are chosen because of their disability status, this type of research is called *quasi-experimental*. Most clinical research falls into this category. The results give occupational therapists useful evidence about how well certain interventions work with disabled populations.

Qualitative research is the preferred method when a theory is not well developed. Qualitative research begins with a different question, one that is more descriptive rather than cause and effect. For example, a group of occupational therapists wondered how they could become better time managers. They designed a qualitative study, which involved in-depth interviews with six people they had identified as good time managers—women who successfully juggled marriage, child care, gainful employment, community involvement, and home maintenance. This is called a purposive sample. Their interviews included many questions about how the women planned their time, what tools they used, what motivated them, and what made them successful time managers. The results described the nature of good time management and identified some themes that helped us to better understand the concepts involved. Occupational therapy intervention suggestions include the practice of routines, the development of social networks that combine or exchange obligations, and the building of short-term memory and self-management strategies. If taken further, this research could form the basis for a theory of "time mastery" (Cole, 1998).

In occupational science, qualitative research has been cited as the preferred method for studying the form, function, and meaning of human occupation. When building theories of occupation's role in maintaining and restoring health and functional abilities, qualitative methods have been most useful in determining the outcomes related to client satisfaction and well-being. In general, qualitative methods relate best to theory development, while experimental research works best for theory testing. This description of research has been simplified for clarification purposes. In fact, there are many categories and variations of research not included in this textbook. Table 14-2 compares experimental and qualitative research methods in relation to theory in occupational therapy.

Evolution of Theory in Science and Occupational Therapy

Occupational therapy theory did not develop in isolation. Historical trends and events have shaped the development of professional theory and practice from the beginning. Some of the trends of the early 1900s included industrialization, economic growth and prosperity, reconstruction after World War I, and a recognition of the need to preserve skilled craftsmanship. Humanism

Table 14-2.

EXPERIMENTAL VERSUS QUALITATIVE RESEARCH IN OCCUPATIONAL THERAPY

Experimental Research	Qualitative Research
Includes manipulation, randomization, and control	Includes single cases, in-depth interviews, detailed descriptions
Theory testing	Theory development
Objective reality, correlation, cause and effect, use of quantitative statistics	Subjective reality, personal narratives and perceptions, multiple truths
Many subjects	Fewer participants
Standardized tests for dependent variables, surveys, controlled observations	Self-reports, attitudes and beliefs, the lived body, the illness experience

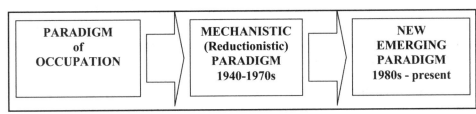

Figure 14-1. Paradigm shifts identified by Kielhofner and Burke. (Adapted from Kielhofner, G. [2004]. *Conceptual foundations of occupational therapy* (3rd ed.). Philadelphia, PA: F.A. Davis Company.)

and pragmatism were the predominant philosophical trends influencing the profession's founding and early years. Breines (1987) recognized the predominance of pragmatism at the time of occupational therapy's founding, citing philosophers William James, George Herbert Meade, and John Dewey at the University of Chicago, colleagues of Adolph Meyer and William Dunton (1919), who later applied pragmatic principles to occupational therapy. Pragmatism, based in part on Darwin's theory of evolution, stresses the growth of knowledge and science through adaptation. The Hull House, in association with the University of Chicago, demonstrated pragmatic principles through the practice of arts and crafts and other activities, which served the needs of both individuals and the community. Occupational therapy founder Eleanor Clarke Slagle trained and later taught arts and crafts at the Hull House. Cofounders Susan Tracy and Susan Johnson, both from a nursing background, devoted most of their lives to practicing and teaching the application of occupations such as arts and crafts, work, and self-care tasks to the healing, rehabilitation, and adaptation of persons with disabilities. Although the assumptions of pragmatism were not clearly defined by occupational therapy founders, they were apparent in the focus on learning by doing, mind/body unity, and building health through engagement in occupation. Tracy is the only occupational therapy founder to publish the applied principles of pragmatism in occupational therapy (1918). Most occupational therapy professionals today take a pragmatic approach.

Knowledge, ideas, and methods are valued according to their practical usefulness. When we read research studies, we look for ways we can use or apply the results in our own lives and in those of our clients. In doing so, we are using the theory of pragmatism. Perhaps the reason the concept of occupation as therapy has withstood the test of time is because of its pragmatic nature. Occupation continues to unify time and space, mind, and body as well as facilitate the growth and development of individuals and societies.

Kielhofner and Burke (1977) traced the history of epistemological changes that took place in occupational therapy and identified two distinct shifts in occupational therapy's professional paradigm (Figure 14-1). Epistemology is the nature of knowledge and the way it is developed and used. Occupational therapy knowledge through the 1930s was based on humanism and pragmatism. Humanism fueled the profession through its dedication to the betterment of the human condition and the right of each person to respect, dignity, and a meaningful and productive role in society. Professionals learned and collected knowledge about the use of occupations in therapy through extensive apprenticeship and practice of its practical (pragmatic) application with a variety of disabilities: mental illness, long-term infectious diseases such as polio and tuberculosis, and injuries due to industrial accidents or war. Kielhofner and Burke identified this period as the "Paradigm of Occupation" (1977, p. 679). Paradigms reflect the theoretical base, views of phenomena, range and nature of problems addressed, problem-solving methods, and goals of a scientific discipline (Kuhn, 1970). According to Kuhn, paradigm shifts occur by revolution, not evolution. When new problems that cannot be solved with the old paradigm emerge, a crisis occurs within the discipline, which calls for fundamental and sweeping changes in both theoretical perspectives and methodology.

Paralleling Kuhn's model of theoretical development in basic science, Kielhofner and Burke (1977) identify a crisis period in occupational therapy toward the end of the 1930s when the profession was challenged to become more scientific. Advances in technology and the predominance of the scientific method in basic science, social sciences, and in medicine challenged the philosophical validations of morality and social responsibility for the medical and allied medical professions, occupational therapy among them. The scientific method, viewed as the only way to discover basic truths and to substantiate theory, calls for the reduction of the focus of study into its component parts for the purpose of more precise examination and understanding. Reductionism directly opposes the holistic and systems perspective of the original paradigm of occupation. In the mid-20th century, occupational therapy resolved this crisis by becoming more closely aligned with the medical profession. Courses in anatomy and physiology, neurology, psychiatry, and medical conditions were added to the requirements for occupational therapy education. Concurrently, a reductionistic view of illness and disability led to a focus on component parts, the diagnosis of specific problems, and the prescription of specific intervention strategies or methods. This approach views man and the world as machines; when they stop working, the method for restoring them is to locate the part that is broken (diagnosis) and fix or replace it (prescription, intervention). Later, Kielhofner renamed this reductionistic approach the "mechanistic paradigm" (2004, p. 56). According to Kielhofner and Burke (1977), the reductionistic paradigm generated three major theoretical models in occupational therapy: kinesiology (biomechanical, rehabilitative), psychoanalytic (psychodynamic), and sensory integrative (neuroscience, motor control).

Occupational therapy enjoyed a period of stability and growth in the 1950s and 1960s. The discipline benefited from its alliance with medicine, with gains in respectability and status within the medical community; membership on health care teams; and inclusion in legislation, reimbursement, and social policy. For example, the passing of Public Law 94-142 (Education for All Handicapped Children Act) in 1975, requiring children with disabilities to be educated in the least restrictive environment, opened up a whole new area of practice for occupational therapists treating children in public schools. Many useful assessment and intervention techniques were developed in occupational therapy

throughout these decades in collaboration with other scientists and medical professionals (e.g., Bobath's [1990] neurodevelopmental treatment [NDT]). However, by the late 1970s, signs of the inadequacy of the mechanistic paradigm became apparent.

In occupational therapy, reductionism had resulted in many extremes of specialization, leading some occupational therapy scholars to view this era as the profession's "identity crisis." The effects of the crisis identified by Kielhofner and Burke in 1977 continue to haunt us in the new millennium, especially in the areas of documentation and reimbursement. The medical profession, which once gave needed recognition to the occupational therapy profession, is itself suffering from cost-cutting measures, both public (Medicare Reform and the Omnibus Budget Reconciliation Act [OBRA] of 1987), and private (managed care, malpractice, and health insurance costs; Evanofski, 2003). Although many state licensure laws still require a doctor's prescription for occupational therapy intervention, doctors and other referral sources must choose between several competing service providers (nursing, physical therapy, speech/language therapy, home health aides) for a piece of the ever-shrinking reimbursement pie. Within the profession, the AOTA initiated some remedial measures to resolve the identity crisis, beginning in 1979 with the publication of uniform terminology (AOTA, 1979), giving the profession a common language and defining the scope of practice. The AOTA further unified the profession by providing standards for the different areas of practice and by establishing the American Occupational Therapy Foundation (AOTF) dedicated to the support of research initiatives. Theory took the form of "frames of reference" in the 1970s (Mosey, 1970), "clinical reasoning" (Mattingly & Fleming, 1994; Rogers, 1983) in the 1980s, and "occupational performance models" in the 1990s (Baum & Christiansen, 2005; Christiansen & Baum, 1997; Dunn, Brown, & McGuigan, 1994; Schkade & Schultz, 1992a, 1992b).

Professional Trends in the New Millennium

The major trends of the profession may be summarized as holistic, client centered, and systems oriented (Cole & Tufano, 2008). In becoming more holistic, occupational therapy must move away from a reductionistic medical model and instead partner with community organizations in the service of public health. Occupational therapy's method of reimbursement will remain under the umbrella of medicine unless we can demonstrate the value of our services in the broader spectrum of wellness and prevention. The client-centered focus gives occupational therapy a structure for making the transition from clinic to community, with an increased focus on collaborating with clients and establishing stronger therapeutic relationships. From the client-centered perspective, occupational therapists apply theoretical knowledge and evidence in partnership with clients to assist them in making informed choices and solving occupational problems and to enable occupational performance. During this decade, client-centered occupational therapy practice has a new focus: enabling occupation (Townsend & Polatajko, 2007). These Canadian authors offer the following updated definition of occupational therapy:

> "Occupational therapy is the art and science of enabling engagement in everyday living through occupation; of enabling people to perform the occupations that foster health and well-being; and of enabling a just and inclusive society so that all people may participate to their potential in the daily occupations of life" (p. xxi).

The trend toward a systems orientation is evident at many levels. Dynamical systems theories have impacted the basic and social sciences; they are evident in the latest revisions of many occupational therapy frames of reference, providing evidence of the importance of environmental factors in facilitating or creating barriers to occupational performance. Occupational therapists need to help clients navigate the vast bureaucracy of the health care system, make use of community resources, and remove barriers to their inclusion in their life occupations. On a practice level, the client's social participation—the performance of roles and occupations in social groups such as families, classrooms, work teams, and the community—must become a part of occupational therapy services if we are to enable our clients to find and perform meaningful roles in society (Cole & Donohue, 2011). These trends have helped to define the current professional paradigm. The shift away from reductionism has occurred across many disciplines and professions. Evidence of this may be seen in the changes in the systems of health care, both nationally and globally.

POLITICS AND HEALTH CARE: MEDICAL VERSUS CLIENT-CENTERED MODELS

The client-centered model, defined for occupational therapists by the Canadian Occupational Therapy Association in conjunction with Canadian national health care, gained prominence in the United States during the 1990s. For health care professionals, the term *client centered* refers to the nature of the therapeutic relationship and implies roles for both the professional and the client that are clearly different from those of the medical model (Table 14-3). As occupational therapy moves away from the medical model, the client-centered model serves the purpose of structuring and clarifying our interactions with clients and gives greater importance to our therapeutic use of self. When clients seek occupational therapy

services directly or through community agencies rather than being referred by a doctor, their satisfaction with the outcome surpasses the need for precise measurement of functional performance. Ideally, clients' progress in the performance of preferred occupations will lead to greater client satisfaction and will validate the value of occupational therapy in many new areas of practice.

THE INTERNATIONAL CLASSIFICATION OF FUNCTIONING, DISABILITY AND HEALTH MODEL OF GLOBAL HEALTH AND WELLNESS

The World Health Organization (WHO) made significant revisions to its classification system that reflect the shift to a holistic and systems perspective of global health care. The International Classification of Functioning, Disability and Health (ICF) encompasses all aspects of human health and some health-relevant components of well-being. Its intent is as a companion classification system for the 10th edition of the International Classification of Disease (ICD-10), which classifies all known diseases, both mental and physical. The stated purposes of ICF are as follows:

- To provide a scientific basis for studying health and health determinants.

- To establish a common language.

- To allow comparison across countries, disciplines, and time.

- To provide systematic coding for purposes of record keeping and research.

Given the global nature of health care today, the fact that this international guideline confirms the central role of occupation (activity) in health has important implications for occupational therapy. ICF places "activity" at the center of its model and defines the goal of health care efforts as "participation in life" (WHO, 2001).

HOLISTIC PERSPECTIVE

The initial publication was entitled International Classification of Impairments, Disabilities, and Handicaps (ICIDH; WHO, 1980). Each of these terms has been replaced to reflect the shift to a holistic perspective:

- *Handicap* is changed to *participation restriction*.

- *Disability* is changed to *activity limitation*.

- *Impairment* is changed to *health condition*, an umbrella term for not only disease, disorder, injury, and trauma, but also for conditions such as pregnancy, aging, stress, congenital anomaly, and genetic predisposition.

In its 2001 revision, the WHO broadens the horizons of health-related research, service provision, and

Table 14-3.	
MEDICAL AND CLIENT-CENTERED MODEL COMPARISON	
Medical Model	**Client-Centered Model**
Patient: Passive recipient of treatment; implies a sick role and a lack of participation or responsibility, requires compliance with doctor's orders.	Client: Actively seeks assistance from medical and other professionals or experts; shifts responsibility for solving health problems onto the client.
Health: Absence of disease. Mental and physical fitness and a sense of well-being. Disease: Illness or injury affecting ability to perform activities of daily living (ADL).	Health condition: Any circumstance that interferes with full participation in life.
Diagnosis: Identification of disease through analysis of signs, symptoms, and syndromes, which allows the doctor to predict the course of illness and to prescribe remedies.	Disability: Experienced by the person, sometimes determined by the person's experience of illness; that which prevents the person from participating in life.
Prescription: Medications or specific techniques or instructions intended to cure disease and/or manage symptoms.	Enablement: Sharing expertise, which empowers the client to set reasonable goals and make informed choices regarding interventions to remove barriers to participation in life.
Objective methods of study, based on experimental research, data gathering, and norms.	Subjective methods of study based on qualitative research, looking at each individual's culture, perceptions, and situation.
Progress is measured by objective measures applied by the medical professional.	Outcome includes both objective measures and client satisfaction with results.
Treatment: Specific medical or surgical procedures prescribed by a doctor or specialist in order to heal or cure a disease.	Intervention: Procedures and strategies created by collaboration between client and professional to overcome barriers to occupational performance.
Occupational therapy applies expertise to focus on using activities to relieve symptoms, to adapt task demands, or to compensate for disability. Rehabilitation ends when the patient has met functional goals established by the therapist and/or medical treatment team.	Occupational therapist collaborates with client to identify occupational problems and priorities, to set goals, and to enable client participation through supporting skill development, as well as taking preventive actions and/or through adaptation of tasks and environments.

policymaking beyond the constraints of the medical model. It states, "There is a widely held misunderstanding that ICF is only about people with disability; in fact, it is about all people" (WHO, 2001, p. 7).

SYSTEMS ORIENTATION

ICF conceives a person's functioning and/or disability as a "dynamic interaction" between a health condition and contextual factors. Contextual factors are those external factors, "features of the physical, social, and attitudinal world," that facilitate or hinder participation (WHO, 2001, p. 8). Accordingly, ICF is divided into two parts. The first lists the components of human functioning and disability, including both body systems and structures as well as activities and participation, denoting both an individual and a societal perspective. The systems of the human body and the activities represented closely resemble occupational therapy's domain of concern according to the framework (AOTA, 2008).

The second half of ICF lists and classifies contexts in the following categories:

- *Products and technology.* Includes foods, consumable goods, money, and the systems for distributing these, as well as objects and tools for other systems such as education, sports and recreation, and the practice of religion.

- *Natural and human-made environments.* Includes land and water, climate, population, light, noise, vibration, natural events such as an earthquake or tsunami, human-made events such as war, and time-related changes such as seasons.

- *Support and relationships.* Includes immediate and extended family, friends, acquaintances, authority figures, subordinates, care providers, domesticated animals, strangers, health care providers, and other professionals.

- *Attitudes.* Includes individual and societal views, biases, and stigmas, as well as norms, practices, and ideologies.

- *Services, systems, and policies.* Includes a vast range of systems such as economic; educational; media; transportation; housing; utilities; communication; legal; labor; and employment, political, and civil protection systems. This category includes the system of health care as well as general social support.

The inclusion of so many external or environmental factors reflects the system's view of occupational performance as a product of the interaction between the person, the task, and the environment. The basic language of ICF is compatible with occupational therapy in this regard, stating, "improvement of participation [can be encouraged] by removing or mitigating societal hindrances and encouraging the provision of social supports and facilitators" (WHO, 2001, p. 6). The model of functioning and disability also describes the interaction of ICF components: health conditions, body structures and functions, personal factors, contexts, activities, and participation in life. One can easily see the parallels with the AOTA practice framework, which uses similar terminology and an equally broad perspective of health (AOTA, 2008).

Occupational therapy's "identity crisis" in the 1970s and 1980s precipitated a search for theories to address common threads and unify occupational therapy practice. While many diverse frames of reference in the profession have been identified, we now needed to develop a systematic theoretical and scientific basis for occupation itself as intervention. Ironically, this is the same goal proposed by our founders (Dunton, 1919; Quiroga, 1995). By the 1990s, scholars had reflected on the problem of professional identity considerably and had come to understand that the unifying concept for all of the areas of specialization within occupational therapy practice was, quite simply, occupation.

Interpreting Theoretical Transformations in Occupational Therapy

While the focus on the broader concepts of occupation seems simple and logical in retrospect, its implications for theory development are quite complex. The collective occupational therapy professional community—practitioners, researchers, scholars, and educators who participated in the process of resolving the 1970s crisis—may recognize the fundamental nature of the recent theoretical shifts only through reflection. At first, we thought all that was needed was to articulate our frames of reference. In doing so, we moved from Mosey's three frames of reference to hundreds (Reed & Sanderson, 1999) with no more professional unity than we had before. We failed to recognize the true nature of the Model of Human Occupation (Kielhofner & Burke, 1980) as an occupation-based model, trying instead to define it as one more frame of reference. This worked as well as fitting the proverbial square peg into a round hole.

Then in the 1980s, Joan Rogers (1983) got us thinking about the clinical reasoning process; this approach to unity proved to be a better fit. If occupational therapists did not all share a common frame of reference, at least they could share a common reasoning process. Mattingly and Fleming (1994) further defined the process of reasoning in occupational therapy, citing three tracks: procedural, interactive, and conditional. Herein lies the beginning of the real transformation—not in the theories of occupational therapy themselves, but in the way we develop these theories. Procedural reasoning applies objective scientific knowledge; interactive reasoning combines objective scientific knowledge with the subjective reality of the individual client's experience (the lived experience); and conditional reasoning considers all of the contexts or systems within which persons exist, live, and perform occupations. Our professional understanding of the process of occupational therapy changed fundamentally as a result of these revelations. We had moved from an exclusively scientific view (procedures such as assessment and intervention) to one that also considered the personal perspective of the client (interactive or client centered) and the contexts (conditional, systems) of occupational performance.

The 1990s focused on two major theoretical trends in occupational therapy: the development of occupation-based models and the movement toward client-centered practice. Occupation-based models moved occupational therapy away from the study of components of occupational performance, which viewed physical, sensory, psychosocial, emotional, and cognitive processes separately. Instead, they refocused our attention on occupation itself. Hooper (2006) explained it as an epistemological transformation, or a shift in the way we define knowledge and in the methods by which we acquire it. The mid-century reductionistic approach led occupational therapists to develop and research many specific techniques, such as sensory integration for the intervention of children with learning disabilities, biomechanical strategies for the intervention of hand injuries, and cognitive rehabilitation for the intervention of traumatic brain injuries. These applied theories, while useful and valid, represented fragments of occupation developed in isolation of each other. Broader theories of occupation, such as the model of human occupation (Kielhofner & Burke, 1980) and subsequent occupation-based models, served the purpose of defining the interconnections between the fragments or components of occupation. Furthermore, the application of dynamical systems theories influenced the newer occupation-based models in synthesizing much of the specific knowledge developed earlier within the multiple dimensions of occupation (Hooper, 2006). The move toward client-centered practice represents a similar change in focus—one that questions the nature of reality itself. Creek put it simply as "… the truth is no longer out there" (1997, p. 50), suggesting that truth is not objective, but subjective, and therefore dependent on personal perspectives and specific contexts. The scientific view of truth relies on accurate and objective observations inherent in the scientific method and without regard for human activity. Mosey identifies this view as "rational empiricism," which can serve as a way of thinking about practice, as well as a context for action (1992, p. 42). According to this view of truth, prominent in mid-20th century reductionism, theories are best tested through experimental research, such as the randomized controlled trials typical of medical research. As late as 1999, Holm (2000) referred to the randomized controlled trial as the most valid form of evidence supporting the theories occupational therapists use in practice. If we compare our research with that of other professions, such as medicine, occupational therapy scholars must recognize that we have a lot of catching up to do. Citing a postmodernist perspective that is shared with science generally, Creek concluded that "truth is not external, universal, and eternal, but is personal, local, and ephemeral. Occupational therapists, with their concern for the personal experiences of individuals as they live their everyday lives, understand this" (p. 52). Using a subjective view of truth, theories should not be tested using quantitative, experimental research methods, large samples, or statistical analysis. Rather, theories are built through qualitative or ethnographic methodology. While this method has been cited as the least valid from a scientific perspective (Holm, 2000), it has also been viewed as the most relevant method for occupational therapy (Clark, 1993; Zemke, 2004). Mosey (1992) has called this method "phenomenological" (p. 42), seeking knowledge through individual experiences (of clients and ourselves) and reflection. Within this approach, "knowledge is not used but rather created anew in the process of assisting each client" (Mosey, p. 42). If we accept this view of reality, using a client-centered approach is more than a new technique. It is the only valid way to build theory in practice. While occupational therapy practitioners may have knowledge of many scientific theories and evidence, they use this expertise differently in client-centered practice, recognizing that the client's perspective is paramount. Theories are only relevant as they relate to specific individuals in specific situations, and the tools and techniques they generate are only valid if they result in positive

changes in occupational performance and client satisfaction. Without this historical background, new students and graduates cannot possibly appreciate the enormity of what has occurred in the occupational therapy profession. Over the past 25 to 30 years, we have witnessed the elevation of occupational therapy from an "allied medical profession" to a profession in its own right, complete with its own body of knowledge and research, its unique theories of occupation, and with a master's degree entry level, the community of scholars needed to continue the quest for prominence as a profession.

The Current Theoretical Challenge: Standing on the Edge of Chaos

Chaos theory came originally from the fields of mathematics and physics in the 1970s. It has expanded to include a wide range of applications such as the analysis of traffic flow, global weather, group dynamics, health epidemics, and economic trends. For example, in the popular TV series *Numbers,* character Charlie Epp, a mathematics professor, used chaos theory to help his FBI brother narrow down suspects when solving a crime. The theory has challenged traditional scientific knowledge and methodology at nearly every level. Because of its extreme complexity, chaos theory is not well understood generally, but at the simplest level, it changes the way one views cause and effect, as it renders long-term predictions impossible. A central concept to chaos theory is sensitivity to initial conditions, widely known as the "butterfly effect." The phrase comes from a presentation given by Edward Lorenz to the American Association for the Advancement of Science in Washington, DC, entitled "Predictability: Does the flap of a butterfly's wings in Brazil set off a tornado in Texas?" (Lorenz, 1972). In other words, even very small changes have the potential to produce large effects, and they do so in ways that are exceedingly complex and unpredictable (Figure 14-2).

Some related terms for chaos are *complexity theory* and *nonlinear science*. The traditional scientific method, implying A + B = C, can be understood as a linear relationship: for example "if you get a flu shot, you will not get the flu." Proponents of chaos theory believe this type of linear prediction is impossible, because we cannot measure all of the initial conditions; even small mistakes could affect vastly different outcomes. The actual outcome depends on too many factors because human systems are extremely complex. The term *chaos* implies a state of disorder, but chaos theory takes us beyond that point—the study of seemingly chaotic systems often leads to self-organization and pattern formation. For this reason, *complexity theory* might be a more accurate term when applied to human systems.

Occupational therapists have only begun to understand how complexity theory applies to our profession. Some occupational therapists have used complexity theory to better understand cognition in the workings of the human brain (Haltiwanger, Lazzarini, & Nazeran, 2007; Lazzarini, 2004, 2005; Loukas, 2010; Royeen, 2003). Zemke and Clark introduce some similar ideas as dynamical systems theory, a central concept in the study of occupational science (1996). Most of us can accept the idea that the brain is highly influenced by initial conditions, that even small stimuli (called *perturbations* in chaos theory) can produce dramatic and unexpected responses. Lazzarini first used the term *neuro-occupation* to describe more fully how occupation influences and is influenced by brain activity (2005). She believes that the "nonlinear dynamics of brain activity" help us better understand human intention, perception, and meaning in performing occupations, thus providing a link between occupational therapy and occupational science (2004).

When Royeen first introduced us to "Charlotte's web of chaos" during her 2003 Slagle Lecture, most of her audience failed to appreciate the theoretical implications of her paper, "Chaotic occupational therapy: Collective wisdom for a complex profession" (2003). Eleven years later, our profession is still not ready to embrace chaos, with its perturbations, bifurcations, basins of attraction, topological mixing, and dense periodic orbits (Lorenz, 1996). Yet perhaps we can begin to appreciate occupational therapy as a complex intervention that integrates five interactive levels, which Creek (2003) defined as follows:

1. The occupational therapist as an independent self-organizing system, with all the beliefs, values, skills, tools, knowledge, abilities and culture that he or she brings to the interaction

2. The client, also as an independent self-organizing system, with all of his or her history, experience at all levels, and contexts, coupled with values, health care beliefs, needs, problems, issues, personal goals, occupations, abilities, skills, attitudes, and interest

3. The context

4. The environment

5. The occupational therapist's actions

Creek acknowledges the dynamic interactive process that occurs between these levels throughout each treatment session, reflecting the active interchanges that occur within the client-centered partnership, ultimately facilitating new self-organized patterns within the client's occupational life. According to this approach, the real key to positive therapeutic outcomes does not only come from evidence-based practice, nor does it come only from an

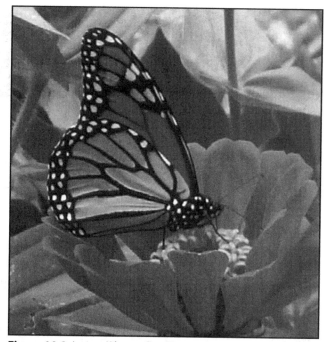

Figure 14-2. Lorenz's butterfly effect in chaos theory represents sensitivity to initial conditions contributing to vastly diverse and unpredictable outcomes. (Reprinted with permission from Marilyn B. Cole, 2009).

effective therapeutic relationship, although these remain critical parts of the process. The key lies in finding that place at the edge of chaos, when the system that is the client—surrounded by all the right initial conditions—stands ready to jump in and reorganize itself into a more adaptive being, enabled and empowered to more effectively engage in the occupations that give meaning to life for both the client and the community.

In another attempt to publicly embrace the complex nature of occupation in life and in occupational therapy practice, Florence Clark coined the phrase "high-definition occupational therapy (HDOT)" in her inaugural address as President of the AOTA (Clark, 2010). In a high-definition photograph, one can "zoom in" to read the license plate on a speeding car, or "zoom out" to appreciate the surrounding situations and circumstances. Applying this metaphor to occupational therapy theory, we can zoom in to use biomechanical principles (a reductionistic approach) to help a client strengthen weakened muscles from a stroke and at the same time zoom out to assess and modify the contexts within which the client needs to use those muscles for self-care, mobility, work, and leisure (a holistic perspective). In other words, in the process of occupational therapy treatment, many levels of interactions among variables might be happening simultaneously, with the therapist intervening at critical points to increase the probability of a positive therapeutic outcome (see Table 14-4 for updated levels of clinical/

Table 14-4.

EXPANDED LEVELS OF CLINICAL/PROFESSIONAL REASONING IN OCCUPATIONAL THERAPY

Type of Reasoning	Description	Example
Scientific	Using logic in systematic ways to make objective decisions.	Daily stretching exercise will increase range of motion.
Procedural	Using evaluation tools and specified intervention strategies.	Following hip replacement, the client should not exceed 90 degrees of hip flexion.
Narrative	Incorporating life history and stories when making occupational choices.	As the oldest of four children, Mary has always identified herself as a caregiver.
Pragmatic	Attending to the practical aspects of service delivery and the best application of one's own skills.	When the client expressed extreme fatigue, we did the evaluation seated rather than standing.
Ethical	Based on beliefs about the right thing to do, acting in the client's best interests.	Although Margaret's vision is poor, she wants to continue driving. Yet doing so would not be safe for her or others.
Interactive	Interpersonal aspects of the therapeutic process, therapeutic use of self.	Listening to clients, communicating empathy, and gaining their trust.
Conditional	Considering contexts and situations, responding to changing circumstances, and anticipating possible outcomes.	Using cooking activities as a step toward returning to the role of mother, helping client to envision the process of change.

Adapted from Schell, B. B., & Schell, J. (2008). *Clinical and professional reasoning in occupational therapy.* Philadelphia, PA: Lippincott Williams & Wilkins.

professional reasoning). Perhaps this conception of occupational therapy brings our profession as a whole one step closer to the proverbial edge of chaos.

Organizing Occupational Therapy Knowledge

Currently, occupational therapy practitioners need both occupation-based models, using a top-down or occupation-first approach (Trombly Latham, 2008), and frames of reference, which address the components of performance using a bottom-up approach. Components such as range of motion or cognition can be targeted for assessment and intervention when these "client factors" are identified as barriers to engagement in occupation. It is comforting to learn that occupation-based models are not going to replace all of the collected wisdom of occupational therapy's more traditional frames of reference. However, as practitioners, occupational therapists will be expected to use specific techniques within the context of the broader occupation-based models, which requires an understanding of both levels. In fact, occupational therapy students and practitioners need to develop an appreciation of all levels of theory as necessary within our new paradigm of client-centered, holistic, and

systems-oriented occupational therapy practice. Mosey (1992) identifies three levels of applied theory in occupational therapy as it had progressed to that point in time:

1. A fundamental body of knowledge including philosophical assumptions, an ethical code, a theoretical foundation of both theories and empirical data, a domain of concern, and legitimate tools. Occupational therapy's professional paradigm and framework fall into this category in our proposed taxonomy because these are common to all practice.

2. An applied body of knowledge that includes sets of guidelines for practice. The occupation-based models addressing the interrelationships of person, environment, and occupation fall into this category in our taxonomy.

3. Practice, which includes action sequences, use of applied knowledge, the clinical reasoning process, and the art of practice. Frames of reference, the most concrete level of theory, fall into this category by providing specific techniques and evidence for specific disabilities.

Taking these distinctions into account, we will clarify some different levels of theory as they currently appear to be understood by our scholars and/or defined by the AOTA. Our proposed organization of theory for occupational therapy appears in Figure 14-3. It includes three

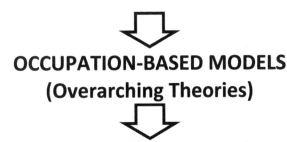

PARADIGM
(Philosophy, Values & Ethics, Knowledge, Domain of Concern, Therapeutic Process & Roles)

⇩

OCCUPATION-BASED MODELS
(Overarching Theories)

⇩

FRAMES of REFERENCE
(Practice guidelines in specific domains)

Figure 14-3. Proposed taxonomy for the occupational therapy profession. (Adapted from Cole, M. B., & Tufano, R. (2008). *Applied theories in occupational therapy.* Thorofare, NJ: SLACK Incorporated.)

levels: occupational therapy paradigm, occupation-based models, and frames of reference. Each of these terms will be defined. Previously we said that the paradigm in health care has shifted to one that is holistic, client centered, and systems oriented. These broad concepts represent the most general levels of theory. In an attempt to both broaden and unify today's practice, the framework has redefined some of the fundamental concepts of occupational therapy practice and has incorporated many of the concepts from occupation-based models as well. For example, patients are now called "clients," treatment is redefined as "intervention," and disease or illness has been replaced by "health condition" (AOTA, 2008). These changes in terminology reflect the shift in focus toward wellness and prevention of disability and imply fundamental changes in the way occupational therapists will practice in the 21st century.

The next level includes the occupation-based models, which have been called *overarching frames of reference* (Dunn, 2000), *conceptual models* (Reed & Sanderson, 1999), or *occupation-based frameworks* (Baum & Christiansen, 2005). In occupational therapy, occupation-based models help explain the relationship between the person, the environment, and occupational performance, forming the foundation for the profession's focus on occupation. However, they do not provide guidelines for application with specific populations or disability areas. For example, the Canadian Model of Occupational Performance-Enablement (CMOP-E; Townsend & Polatajko, 2007) defines the interactions of person, occupation, and environment, with each of these concepts further defined as the following:

- *Person.* Spirituality as the source of the affective, cognitive, and physical self.

- *Occupation.* Consisting of productivity, self-care, and leisure.

- *Environment.* Including physical, institutional, cultural, and societal systems.

The Canadian model has generated a holistic, client-centered assessment tool, the Canadian Occupational Performance Measure, which can be applied in all areas of occupational therapy practice (Law et al., 2005; Townsend, 1997). This may be understood as a top-down approach, beginning with a client's occupational priorities and goals, and working backward to identify barriers to achieving them. Theories that explain how therapy works in practice have been called *practice models* (Kielhofner, 2004; Reed & Sanderson, 1999) or frames of reference (Mosey, 1986, 1992). Frames of reference address specific areas of occupation and help occupational therapists to apply theory with individual clients in specific situations. Most frames of reference were developed to address particular areas of disability. For example, the sensory integration frame of reference was originally developed for the intervention of children with learning disabilities. This frame of reference has produced many specific assessment tools for measuring sensory systems and their motor and cognitive outcomes, as well as tools and techniques for providing specific types of sensory input. The assessment of specific sensory systems and application of remedial strategies demonstrates a bottom-up approach, beginning with foundation skills and working upward toward using these skills during occupational performance. Frames of reference represent the most concrete level of occupational therapy theory.

Certified occupational therapy assistants, as well as master's level therapists, need to have a basic understanding of how the theories used in practice are developed and

Case Example: Jeanette

Jeanette is a 75-year-old woman living alone who had a knee replacement and must learn to use a walker. Her apartment is all one level, but she has a flight of stairs to get from her garage up to her back door. She is able to drive but unable to climb the stairs without assistance. Although her husband died a decade ago and her son and daughter both have families and homes of their own, Jeanette still spends each morning cleaning her 3-room apartment and feels frustrated that she cannot continue to do this as before. Jeanette loves to cook but cannot easily reach the items she needs in her cramped kitchenette. Fatigue sets in quickly, preventing her from completing tasks. Although she had participated in several social activities prior to her surgery, she has avoided attending these events following surgery because of her physical issues. She has no problems with toileting or dressing but fears she will fall while getting in and out of the bathtub. Jeanette's daughter and son-in-law live in the next town. Her daughter, Gail, calls several times each day and visits often, even though she works full time. Her grandson, Rob, a college student, has offered to help Jeanette do her shopping on Saturdays.

- Using the medical model, list five client factors to be addressed in occupational therapy.

- Using a client-centered approach with Jeanette, write 10 questions you would ask the client or her family members in order to gain a "holistic" understanding of her occupational problems.

- Identify three barriers to occupational performance and do an Internet search to learn what theories and applications might be helpful to this case. For example, fear of falling, fatigue, and home adaptation might be relevant areas for Jeanette.

why. The knowledge gained from more traditional frames of reference—such as biomechanical, rehabilitative, sensory integrative, or psychodynamic—is still relevant and useful, but it needs to be applied within occupation-based models of practice. In particular, the client-centered approach has changed the way we perform evaluation and intervention, giving greater importance to therapeutic use of self in the therapeutic relationship. Therapeutic interventions become most meaningful when their relationship to the client's important life roles is outwardly discussed and appreciated by the individuals and groups receiving service.

Chapter 9 reviews some of the more prominent occupation-based models and frames of reference and describes how they are used in practice.

Summary

Theory development has been addressed in this chapter on two levels—general and specific. Generally, theory begins with a desire to better understand something in our own experience and develop the theory through a continuum of qualitative (ethnographic), descriptive, and quantitative (experimental) research. In occupational therapy specifically, theories have evolved over the history of the profession in response to (or in tandem with) the changing nature of client problems with occupational performance resulting from illness, injury, or another cause, requiring occupational therapy intervention, together with occupational therapy's changing role in the overall system of health care service delivery. From occupational therapy's philosophical roots in humanism and pragmatism, the profession has developed many scientific theories to substantiate its unique focus and methods and has broadened into the holistic, client-centered, and systems-oriented practice of the 21st century. Complexity theory (HDOT) compels occupational therapy practitioners to embrace and use all of the collective levels of theory. This includes application of frames of reference, which guide occupational therapy's interventions with specific client occupational issues and priorities within the context of occupation-based models that consider the interrelationships of the client's personal strengths and limitations; the environmental facilitators and barriers to social participation; and the social, cultural, physical, and spiritual nature of human occupation.

Student Self-Assessment

1. How does theory help therapists make decisions? Give an example.

2. Explain how theory in occupational therapy differs from theory in occupational science.

3. What problems occurred in the occupational therapy profession in the 1930s that caused the paradigm to shift? What problems occurred in the 1970s that caused the professional paradigm to shift again?

4. What are two philosophical schools that influenced the founding of occupational therapy in the early 1900s? Explain each and give an example.

5. What is the purpose of theory? How does it help us with practical problems?

6. Describe two types of research that are used to develop and validate theory.

7. Using the medical model, describe the steps you would follow if you fell and broke your ankle.

8. Using the client-centered model in the broken-ankle scenario, what areas of occupational performance

would you evaluate in order to determine what theories should be applied?

9. How does the ICF relate to the professional paradigm of occupational therapy? Name three concepts that are similar.

10. What does the CMOP contribute to occupational therapy's current paradigm in the United States?

11. How is an occupation-based model in occupational therapy different from a frame of reference?

12. What three theoretical trends make up occupational therapy's current paradigm? Describe each briefly.

13. Describe the difference between a "top-down" approach and a "bottom-up" approach to the application of theory in occupational therapy practice.

14. How does a client's social participation impact the occupations that are addressed in therapy, and why is this important to consider?

15. What is complexity theory and how does it change the way occupational therapists apply theoretical principles in practice?

16. What is the meaning of the phrase "standing on the edge of chaos" and how might it apply to the process of occupational therapy practice?

References

American Occupational Therapy Association. (1979). Uniform terminology for reporting occupational therapy services. *Occupational Therapy News, 35*(11), 1-8.

American Occupational Therapy Association. (2008). Occupational therapy practice framework: Domain and process (2nd ed.). *American Journal of Occupational Therapy, 62,* 625-683.

Ayres, A. J. (1979). *Sensory integration and the child.* Los Angeles, CA: Western Psychological Services.

Baum, C., & Christiansen, C. (2005). Person-environment-occupation-performance. In C. Christiansen, C. Baum, & J. B. Haugen (Eds.), *Occupational therapy: Performance, participation, and well-being* (pp. 242-267). Thorofare, NJ: SLACK Incorporated.

Bobath, B. (1990). *Adult hemiplegia: Evaluation and treatment* (3rd ed.). London, England: Butterworth-Heinemann.

Breines, E. (1987). Pragmatism as a foundation for occupational therapy curricula. *American Journal of Occupational Therapy, 41*(8), 522-525.

Bundy, A., Lane, S., & Murray, E. (2002). Sensory integration: theory and practice (2nd ed.) Philadelphia, PA: F.A. Davis Company.

Christiansen, C., & Baum, C. (1997). Person-environment occupational performance. In C. Christiansen & C. Baum (Eds.), *Occupational therapy: Enabling function and well-being* (pp. 46-71). Thorofare, NJ: SLACK Incorporated.

Clark, F. (1993). Occupation embedded in a real life: Interweaving occupational science and occupational therapy. 1993 Eleanor Clarke Slagle Lecture. *American Journal of Occupational Therapy, 47*(12), 1067-1077.

Clark, F. (2010). High definition occupational therapy: HDOT. *American Journal of Occupational Therapy, 64,* 848-854.

Cole, M. B. (1998). Time mastery in business and occupational therapy. *WORK: A Journal of Prevention, Assessment & Rehabilitation, 10*(2), 119-127.

Cole, M. B., & Donohue, M. V. (2011). *Social participation in occupational contexts: In schools, clinics, and communities.* Thorofare, NJ: SLACK Incorporated.

Cole, M. B., & Tufano, R. (2008). *Applied theories in occupational therapy.* Thorofare, NJ: SLACK Incorporated.

Creek, J. (1997). The truth is no longer out there. *British Journal of Occupational Therapy, 60*(2), 50-52.

Creek, J. (2003). *Occupational therapy defined as a complex intervention.* London: College of Occupational Therapists, p. 17.

Dunn, W. (2000). *Best practice occupational therapy: In community service with children and families.* Thorofare, NJ: SLACK Incorporated.

Dunn, W., Brown, C., & McGuigan, A. (1994). The ecology of human performance: A framework for considering the effect of context. *American Journal of Occupational Therapy, 48*(7), 595-607.

Dunton, W. R. (1919). *Reconstruction therapy.* Philadelphia, PA: W. B. Saunders Company.

Evanofski, M. (2003). Occupational therapy reimbursement, regulation, and the evolving scope of practice. In E. B. Crepeau, E. S. Cohn, & B. A. B. Schell (Eds.), *Willard & Spackman's occupational therapy* (10th ed., pp. 887-905). Philadelphia, PA: Lippincott Williams & Wilkins.

Haltiwanger, E., Lazzarini, I., & Nazeran, H. (2007). Application of nonlinear dynamics theory to neuro-occupation: A case study of alcoholism. *British Journal of Occupational Therapy, 70,* 349-357.

Holm, M. B. (2000). The 2000 Eleanor Clarke Slagle Lecture. Our mandate for the new millennium: Evidence-based practice. *American Journal of Occupational Therapy, 54*(6), 575-585.

Hooper, B. (2006). Epistemological transformation in occupational therapy: Educational implications and challenges. *OTJR: Occupation, Participation and Health, 26*(1), 15-24.

Kerlinger, F. N. (1979). *Behavioral research: A conceptual approach.* New York, NY: Holt McDougal.

Kielhofner, G. (2004). *Conceptual foundations of occupational therapy* (3rd ed.). Philadelphia, PA: F.A. Davis Company.

Kielhofner, G., & Burke, J. P. (1977). Occupational therapy after 60 years: An account of changing identity and knowledge. *American Journal of Occupational Therapy, 31*(10), 675-689.

Kielhofner, G., & Burke, J. P. (1980). A model of human occupation, part 1. Conceptual framework and content. *American Journal of Occupational Therapy, 34*(9), 572-581.

Kuhn, T. S. (1970). *The structure of scientific revolutions* (2nd ed.). Chicago, IL: University of Chicago Press.

Law, M., Baptiste, S., Carswell, A., McColl, M., Polatajko, H., & Pollick, N. (2005). Canadian occupational performance measure (4th ed.) Ottawa, ON: CAOT Publications ACE.

Lazzarini, I. (2004). Neuro-occupation: The nonlinear dynamics of intention, meaning and perception. *British Journal of Occupational Therapy, 67,* 342-352.

Lazzarini, I. (2005). A nonlinear approach to cognition: A web of ability and disability. In N. Katz (Ed.), *Cognition and occupation across the life span* (2nd ed., pp. 211-233). Bethesda, MD: AOTA Press.

Lorenz, E. (1972). *Predictability: Does the flap of a butterfly's wings in Brazil set off a tornado in Texas?* Retrieved from http://voluntaryboundaries.blogsome.com/2011/02/03/predictability-does-the-flap-of-a-butterflys-wings-in-brazil-set-off-a-tornado-in-texas

Lorenz, E. (1996). *The essence of chaos*. Seattle, WA: University of Washington Press.

Loukas, K. (2010). Use of the natural environment. In K. Sladyk, K. Jacobs, & N. MacRae (Eds.), *Occupational therapy essentials for clinical competence* (pp. 199-206). Thorofare, NJ: SLACK Incorporated.

Mattingly, C., & Fleming, M. H. (1994). *Clinical reasoning: Forms of inquiry in a therapeutic practice*. Philadelphia, PA: F.A. Davis Company.

Mosey, A. C. (1970). *Three frames of reference for mental health*. Thorofare, NJ: SLACK Incorporated.

Mosey, A. C. (1986). *Psychosocial components of occupational therapy*. New York, NY: Raven Press.

Mosey, A. C. (1992). *Applied scientific inquiry in the health professions: An epistemological orientation*. Rockville, MD: AOTA Press.

Portney, L. G. & Watkins, M. P. (2000) Foundations of clinical research: Applications to practice (2nd ed.) Upper Saddle River, NJ: Prentice-Hall Health.

Quiroga, V. A. M. (1995). *Occupational therapy: The first 30 years 1900-1930*. Bethesda, MD: AOTA Press.

Reed, K. L., & Sanderson, S. N. (1999). *Concepts of occupational therapy* (4th ed.). Philadelphia, PA: Lippincott Williams & Wilkins.

Rogers, J. C. (1983). The 1983 Eleanor Clarke Slagle Lectureship. Clinical reasoning: The ethics, science, and art. *American Journal of Occupational Therapy, 37*(9), 601-616.

Royeen, C. (2003). Chaotic occupational therapy: Collective wisdom for a complex profession. *American Journal of Occupational Therapy, 57,* 609-624.

Royeen, C., & Luebben, A. (Eds.). (2009). *Sensory integration: A compendium of leading scholarship*. Bethesda, MD: American Occupational Therapy Association.

Schell, B. B., & Schell, J. (2008). *Clinical and professional reasoning in occupational therapy*. Philadelphia, PA: Lippincott Williams & Williams.

Schkade, J. K., & Schultz, S. (1992a). Occupational adaptation: Toward a holistic approach to contemporary practice, part 1. *American Journal of Occupational Therapy, 46*(9), 829-837.

Schkade, J. K., & Schultz, S. (1992b). Occupational adaptation: Toward a holistic approach to contemporary practice, part 2. *American Journal of Occupational Therapy, 46*(10), 917-925.

Townsend, E. (1997). *Enabling occupation: An occupational therapy perspective*. Ottawa, Ontario: Canadian Association of Occupational Therapy Publications.

Townsend, E., & Polatajko, H. (2007). *Enabling occupation II: Advancing an occupational therapy vision for health and well-being, and justice through occupation*. Ottawa, CA: Canadian Association of Occupational Therapy Publications.

Tracy, S. E. (1918). *Studies in invalid occupation: A manual for nurses and attendants*. Boston, MA: Whitcomb & Barrows.

Trombly Latham, C. A. (2008). Occupation: Philosophy and concepts. In M. V. Radomski & C. A. Trombly Latham (Eds.), *Occupational therapy for physical dysfunction* (6th ed., pp. 339-357). Philadelphia, PA: Lippincott Williams & Wilkins.

World Health Organization. (1980). *International classification of impairments, disabilities, and handicaps*. Geneva, Switzerland: Author.

World Health Organization. (2001). *International classification of functioning, disability and health*. Geneva, Switzerland: Author.

Zemke, R. (2004). The 2004 Eleanor Clarke Slagle Lecture—Time, space, and the kaleidoscopes of occupation. *American Journal of Occupational Therapy, 58*(6), 608-620.

Zemke, R., & Clark, F. (Eds.). (1996). *Occupational science: The evolving discipline*. Philadelphia, PA: F.A. Davis Company.

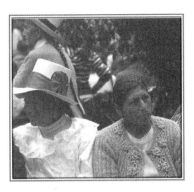

15

OCCUPATIONAL THERAPY THEORY USE IN THE PROCESS OF EVALUATION AND INTERVENTION

Roseanna Tufano, LMFT, OTR/L

ACOTE STANDARDS EXPLORED IN THIS CHAPTER
B.3.1–B.3.3

KEY VOCABULARY

- **Frames of reference:** System of compatible concepts from theory that guides a plan of action within a specific occupational therapy domain of concern (Mosey, 1986).

- **Intervention plan:** A collaborative listing of client-oriented actions meant to enhance occupational performance, with specific targeted outcomes, that is based on select models, frames of reference, and evidence.

- **Occupation-based models:** Proposed interaction of person, environment, and occupation that guide the organization of occupational therapy practice (Cole & Tufano, 2008).

- **Occupational profile:** An initial interview process that may be formal or informal. It is meant to reveal the client's personal history, daily living patterns, interests, values, and needs while highlighting problems from the client's perspective concerning the performance of occupations and daily living activities. The client is asked to prioritize goals for intervention.

(continued)

185

Jacobs, K., MacRae, N., & Sladyk, K. (Eds.).
*Occupational Therapy Essentials for
Clinical Competence, Second Edition* (pp. 185-198).
© 2014 SLACK Incorporated.

KEY VOCABULARY (CONTINUED)

- **Occupational therapy process:** A multistep approach conducted by the practitioner. Based on a select model and/or frame(s) of reference, the occupational therapist analyzes the occupational profile in conjunction with assessments to formulate an intervention plan regarding what factors encourage as well as disrupt the client's successful engagement in occupations within activities of daily living. Occupational therapists conduct ongoing review of the evaluation and intervention process and modify adjustments to this plan in efforts to promote best-practice outcomes.

- **Theoretical constructs:** Visible and nonvisible ideas and explanations that form into a concept and contribute to a theory.
- **Therapeutic use of self:** A practitioner's intuitive nature that derives from one's personality traits, self-awareness and personal experiences, understanding of human behavior, and observations through the use of the five senses. The practitioner makes conscious use of this nature to engage and impact a therapeutic relationship, and foster a meaningful experience for the client.

Introduction

Occupational therapy is a unique profession with its own therapeutic process. Occupational therapists influence a person's health and well-being through positive engagement in occupations (American Occupational Therapy Association [AOTA], 2008). The Occupational Therapy Practice Framework document (2008) outlines a multiphase process for service delivery. Practitioners implement a series of steps in a collaborative manner to attain the best functional outcome for their clients. A brief review of these steps follow.

During the evaluation phase, an occupational therapist's focus is to collect data about a client's occupational preferences, abilities, and skills; contexts and environments that influence engagement; features and demands of activities; and a client's personal health factors. These data are analyzed to formulate a problem list for intervention planning. The intervention plan is designed in collaboration with the client to promote enhancement of occupational performance and overall function. Intervention implementation can now begin. Occupational therapists need to have the knowledge and skills to provide a variety of modalities to best meet the functional and therapeutic needs of clients across the lifespan (AOTA, 2008). Likewise, the practitioner must also monitor the client's response to these intervention strategies and modify approaches accordingly. An occupational therapist constantly re-evaluates the effectiveness of the selected interventions. This analysis includes the review of a client's initial evaluation data to determine if outcomes have been met. It is expected that a client will show some positive change in occupational functioning as a result of service delivery. Plans for discontinuation or ongoing therapy are then determined by the practitioner.

The occupational therapy process, as just summarized, is highly complex and dynamic. It is driven by theory. In an academic curriculum, students are introduced to the many theories that influence practice. Following graduation, it remains the professional responsibility of every practitioner to keep current with new theories and practice approaches as they continue to emerge over time. Understanding the abstract concepts of theory and subsequently applying theoretical principles to practice is a challenge particularly for students or novice therapists. Clinical observation and experience help us to see the connection between theory and practice in a more direct manner.

Our educational standards of practice require that occupational therapists understand theories, models, and frames of reference used in our profession as well as apply theoretical approaches to clients across the lifespan and within different practice environments. Joan Rogers was among the first to study the clinical reasoning of occupational therapists and speak to the complex mind of an occupational therapist (Rogers, 1983). Since her Slagle lecture in the 1980s, many expert practitioners have written about the unique nature of reasoning and thinking that is commonplace to our profession. As we fast forward to our Centennial Vision almost four decades later, we are called on to become a powerful, widely known, science-driven, and evidence-based profession (AOTA,

Table 15-1.

EVIDENCE-BASED STUDIES THAT PROMOTE PROCESS AND SUCCESSFUL OUTCOMES

Theoretical Foundation	Evaluation and/or Intervention Focus	Evidence
Occupational performance	Both	Humphry & Wakeford, 2006; Rebeiro, 2001; Rebeiro & Polgar, 1999; Trombly, 1995
Therapeutic use of self	Both	Goulet, Rousseau, & Fortier, 2007; Maitra & Erway, 2006; Restall, Ripat, & Stern, 2003; Wilkins et al., 2001
Person,-environment-occupation performance model	Both	Letts et al., 1994; Strong et al., 1999
Model of human occupation	Both	Boisvert, 2004; Lee et al., 2008
Occupational adaptation	Both	Schkade & Schultz, 1992; Schultz & Schkade, 1992
Ecology of human performance	Both	Dunn, Brown, & McGuigan, 1994; Lund & Nygard, 2004
Frames of reference	Intervention	Capasso, Gorman, & Blick, 2010; Cicerone et al, 2000; Diller, 2005; Hart & Evans, 2006; Henderson, 1999; Jarus & Ratzon, 2005; Johnson, & Schkade, 2001; Laatsch et al., 2007; Leichsenring et al. 2006; Mastos et al., 2007; Roley et al., 2003; Schaaf & Miller, 2005; Teasell et al. 2003; Watling & Dietz, 2007; Whedon, 2000

Reprinted with permission from Cole, M. B., & Tufano, R. (2008). *Applied theories in occupational therapy*. Thorofare, NJ: SLACK Incorporated.

2006). This mission can only be reached if we remain a theory-driven profession and further research about best-practice evaluations and intervention outcomes.

In this chapter, the reader will be introduced to several common occupational therapy models and frames of reference used for practice across the lifespan with different populations. Learning strategies meant to assist the reader in gaining knowledge for theoretical application will also be highlighted. Table 15-1 lists various levels of evidence-based studies that promote process and successful outcomes.

Understanding Occupation-Based Models and Frames of Reference

How does one begin to learn and understand theories that influence the practice of occupational therapy when there are so many to choose from? This question has been asked by many a student and practitioner. As our occupational therapy scope of practice broadens to include new emerging practice areas and address the complexities of health care, practitioners will need a diverse repertoire of theories, models, and frames of reference from which to base clinical decisions.

Clinical reasoning includes the occupational therapist's ability to plan, direct, perform, and reflect on client care (Schell & Schell, 2008, p. 131). The first step in developing clinical reasoning is to study and comprehend the models and frames of reference that are instrumental to this practice. Occupational therapy students and novice practitioners characteristically rely heavily on theory to guide practice, often applying a rule-based procedural reasoning style for professional decision making to compensate for their limited clinical experience (Crepeau & Schell, 2003).

The key terms that are used among the Accreditation Council for Occupational Therapy Education (ACOTE) standards associated with this chapter need to be defined. Establishing a common set of definitions or terms for theory has been one of the profession's greatest challenges. Terms are often used interchangeably in occupational therapy literature. Scholars have agreed to disagree about how to best label terms that compose our organization of knowledge (Hagedorn, 2001). The following terms and definitions are found in a proposed taxonomy, or classification system, of theories in occupational therapy as proposed by Cole and Tufano (2008).

Theory describes, explains, and predicts behavior; it helps us to understand the relationship between concepts or events. There are varying degrees and levels of theory. At first, all theories start out as hypothetical guesses. A well-founded theory includes the systematic gathering of data with observation and experimental testing.

Occupation-based models are also referred to as overarching theories (Dunn, 2000), conceptual models (Reed & Sanderson, 1999) or occupation-based frameworks (Baum & Christiansen, 2005). These models help to explain the relationship among the person, the environment, and occupational engagement. Occupation-based models help to define the unique role of occupational therapists and explain how to enhance and promote health and well-being as related to occupational performance. These models also provide the practitioner with guidelines on how to prevent occupational disruptions from occurring across the lifespan.

Frame of reference, another type of theory, is based on a system of compatible concepts that guide a plan of action for a specific occupational therapy domain of concern (Mosey, 1986). Frames of reference can be directly applied to treat client factors and enhance related performance areas, patterns, and skills. This group of theories tends to have more of a disability or problem-based focus. Frames of reference are not suited for all clients and have a limited focus or scope for application.

Commonly used occupation-based models and frames of reference found in practice will be highlighted in this chapter. Continued reading and study will undoubtedly be needed to promote further depth of understanding and analysis of these theories.

Summary of Occupation-Based Models

As discussed in the previous chapter, occupation-based models are designed to focus the attention of practitioners on occupations and the interdependent relationship that ensues among person, occupation, and environment. They are often depicted in flow charts that help us to visually see the interdependent nature of various components and theoretical constructs. Common features among these overarching theories include the following:

- All are founded by occupational therapists
- All have their roots in broader theories including humanism, holism, general systems, normal development, behavioral and social psychology, and anthropology
- All are client centered
- All provide guidelines for the evaluation and intervention process
- All emphasize the promotion of health and well-being through occupational performance

Table 15-2 represents an inventory of five such models in chronological order. The first occupation-based model was founded by Mary Reilly. She has been credited by

many proponents in our profession as the catalyst for the paradigm shift back to occupation during a decade when practice was much more medical-model focused and reductionistic (Kielhofner, 1997). Reilly is famous for her quote: "Man through the use of his hands as they are energized by his mind and will, can influence the state of his own health" (Reilly, 1962, p. 2). This statement became a consistent premise among all the occupation-based models that were to follow. Reilly also emphasized that the practice of occupational therapy should be guided by theory. She invited practitioners to base their clinical reasoning on organized knowledge (Reilly, 1958). In 1969, Reilly introduced her theory model called *occupational behavior*. This was the first attempt of our profession to promote a general theory for occupational therapy practice. Kielhofner and Burke, originally two students of Mary Reilly, expanded upon the concepts of occupational behavior through further study. These efforts led to the *model of human occupation*, or *MOHO* for short.

Kielhofner and his colleagues published MOHO for the first time in 1980 (Kielhofner, 1980a, 1980b; Kielhofner & Burke, 1980; Kielhofner, Burke, & Heard, 1980). MOHO has continued to flourish as a practice model for occupational therapy through the collaborative efforts and substantial studies that have emerged over 30 years. In a recent randomized survey sent to 1,000 occupational therapists, it was determined that over 80% of therapists use MOHO as their theoretical base for practice (Lee, Taylor, & Kielhofner, 2009). MOHO uniquely proposes a systems view of occupational performance, including the interdependent effect among a person's internal variables and external environmental contexts. This model explains how a person's internal motivation, routines and habits, performance capacity, and the external feedback from one's physical and social context impacts overall occupational performance. A person's occupational identity and occupational competency are formed from this interactive and complex relationship among internal and external variables. In summary, MOHO attempts to show the complexities that exist within each person and the role of the environment in shaping one's occupational performance throughout the lifespan. "Through participation in therapeutic occupations, persons transform themselves into more adaptive and healthy beings" (Kielhofner & Barrett, 1997, pp. 204-205).

Mary Reilly also identified another significant construct that influenced the future development of occupation-based models. She believed that as a person faces the challenges in dealing with everyday tasks in life, there is a natural opportunity for persons to adapt. The adaptation process has had a long history of interest among occupational therapists. Schkade and Schultz first published their *occupational adaptation model* in 1992, reflecting a comprehensive systems view on the complexity of the adaptation process within occupational therapy. A central

Table 15-2. LIST OF OCCUPATION-BASED MODELS		
Model	**Author**	**Focus of Concern for Occupational Therapy Practice**
Occupational behavior	Reilly, 1969	To prevent and reduce the disruptions and incapacities in occupational behavior that result from injury and illness. Health and well-being is represented by a balance of occupational behavior in self-care, work, and play/leisure.
Model of human occupation	Kielhofner & Burke, 1980	Conceptualized the interactive and cyclical nature of human interaction with one's environment; interplay between person and environment is critical to one's source of motivation, patterns of behavior, and performance.
Occupational adaptation	Schkade & Schultz, 1992	A framework that describes a normal human phenomenon, called adaptation, and its impact on the interactive process between a person and his or her occupational environment
Ecology of human performance	Dunn, Brown, & McGuigan, 1994	A focused area of concern is the role of context in task performance within the areas of ADL, work and productive activities, education, leisure/play, and social participation.
Person-environment-occupation-performance	Christiansen & Baum, 1997	The model views the interdependent relationship among person, occupations (consisting of valued roles, tasks, and activities), and performance. These occupations, in turn, influence one's life roles.

premise to this model is the assumption that as persons become more adaptive, they will become more functional (Schkade & Shultz, 1992). Persons with disrupted or inadequate occupational performance are believed to have a faulty adaptation process at the core. This model focuses on two important phenomena within a complex cycle. Occupational adaptation starts by explaining the normal human experience called *adaptation*. The second phenomenon speaks to the relationship between occupational performance and adaptation. Occupational therapists can plan, guide, and implement interventions for persons in this state of transition (Schkade & McClung, 2001). Occupation is the tool for impacting one's adaptive nature. Occupational adaptation is different from the other models in how it defines functional outcomes. Emphasis is on improving adaptation of the individual; a change in adaptability will ultimately lead to a change in overall occupational performance.

Dunn, Brown, and McGuigan (1994) further identified several issues of concern among the current models of practice. These authors believed that there was not enough attention given to the role of context in occupational therapy practice. Dunn et al. (1994) also drew attention to the benefits of an interdisciplinary relationship among occupational therapy practitioners, educators within school systems, and rehabilitation specialists. *The Ecology of Human Performance* (1994) was published by Dunn and colleagues as a model that could be used not only by occupational therapists but by rehabilitation

specialists as well. Its central focus is on the role of a person's context as it impacts functioning. This emphasis on how context impacts both person variables and task performance provided a unique perspective among the existing occupation-based models. Dunn et al. (1994) identified five intervention strategies for occupational therapy application. These strategies have since been integrated into the framework document (2008). The five intervention strategies include the following:

1. Creating and fostering health promotion.
2. Establishing, remediating, and restoring skills or abilities.
3. Maintaining performance capacities to meet occupational needs.
4. Modifying contexts and/or activity demands as a form of compensation or adaptation.
5. Preventing disability in persons who are at risk for occupational performance problems.

The most recent occupation-based model to be published is the Person-Environment-Occupation Performance Model. It was developed in 1985 and published for the first time in 1991 by Charles Christiansen and Carolyn Baum. It has since been updated in 1997 (Christiansen & Baum, 1997). The Person-Environment-Occupation Performance Model highlights the complexity of person–occupation–environment relationships. Both authors were also greatly influenced by the Canadian guidelines for client-centered practice. In 1983, the Canadian Association of Occupational Therapists with the Department of Health and Welfare published the Model of Occupational Performance and Client-Centered Practice, two critical models that have significantly influenced the Person-Environment-Occupation Performance Model and our current paradigm of practice today. These two Canadian therapeutic approaches both emphasized the reciprocal nature of persons and their occupations within social, cultural, and physical environments. Further study led to the development of the Canadian Occupational Performance Measure (COPM) in 1994, which is a well-accepted assessment tool for gathering data about a client's occupational profile. One of the unique features of Person-Environment-Occupation Performance Model is that it represents a top-down approach, which means that the client's view of the problem is of primary concern when designing an intervention plan. Person-Environment-Occupation Performance Model also complements the current global health care trends that emphasize health and well-being as defined in the revised International Classification of Functioning, Disability, and Health (ICF) system (World Health Organization, 2001).

Summary of Frames of Reference

A frame of reference is defined as "a set of interrelated, internally consistent concepts, definitions, and postulates derived from or compatible with empirical data (theory) that provides a systematic description of or prescription for particular designs of the environment for the purpose of facilitating evaluation and effecting change relative to a specified part of the profession's domain of concern" (Mosey, 1986, p. 12). All frames of reference include the following:

- A clearly defined domain or focus of concern for occupational therapy application.

- A listing of compatible concepts derived from broad or meta theories that explain possible causes and/or contributing factors for function and dysfunction patterns.

- A definition of how persons demonstrate traits, behaviors, attitudes, and emotions that reflect function and dysfunction according to each theoretical perspective.

- A listing of assumptions about how occupational therapy might assist clients in promoting therapeutic change as well as enhancing motivation for engagement in meaningful occupations.

- A plan of action meant to guide occupational therapists in the evaluation and intervention process.

- Evidence gathered by researchers about the validity of the theoretical concepts outlined and the effectiveness of the techniques used by practitioners according to its guidelines.

A brief summary of common frames of reference used in occupational therapy practice is provided below. This list may not be all inclusive, as there are many useful and legitimate frames of reference that may we have omitted. It is recommended that the reader further explore each of the frames of reference for a more comprehensive understanding by consulting Cole and Tufano (2008) as well as other original publications cited at the end of this chapter.

The *psychodynamic frame of reference* in occupational therapy encompasses concepts from object relations, ego psychology, humanism, and human spirituality (Bruce & Borg, 2002). Psychodynamic theory has shaped our professional identity, which is based on the humanistic philosophy, as well as provided a theoretical foundation for mental health practice. Since its inception in the early 1900s, occupational therapy has had a long-standing relationship with psychiatry and psychodynamic theories. Eleanor Clark Slagle's first role as an "occupation therapist" began with persons who had a mental illness. Many occupational therapy scholars have created assessments and intervention groups based on psychodynamic theories. The Azimas (1959) first recognized the therapeutic value of creative activities such as art, music, poetry, drama, dance, and clay/sculpting, also known as *projective techniques*. Gail Fidler (1963) who designed the first task group, emphasized the role of the unconscious in task completion and viewed activities as a means to effectively gratify instinctual needs. Lela Llorens (1966) designed a group program to enhance ego-adaptive skills for children who had experienced trauma. Anne Mosey (1986) founded the analytical frame of reference, which she defined as a "structure for linking psychoanalytic theories, the symbolic potential and reality aspects of activities, and the process of altering intrapsychic content in the direction of providing a more adaptive basis for interaction with the environment." Many facets of psychodynamic theory continue to be currently researched. One example of a modern intervention based on object relations theory is pet therapy. The study of attachment theory continues to be another area of heightened interest in the practice of mental health.

Behavioral frames of reference are represented by a continuum of theories beginning with behavior modification and ending with cognitive behavioral therapy. This group of theories applies the scientific method to human behavior, focusing on the external features of human functioning that can be observed and measured. Significant theorists and contributors to this theory group include Skinner (operant conditioning), Pavlov (classical conditioning), and Bandura (social learning theory). Ann Mosey (1970, 1986) adapted behavioral principles for occupational therapy in her acquisitional frame of reference. The inclusion of behavioral principles are readily found in our practice and often applied for populations with developmental disabilities, school-based populations, autism, various mental disorders, and brain injury. Examples of intervention approaches include applied behavioral analysis, skills training, psychoeducational groups, relaxation training, biofeedback, and systematic desensitization. The common use of reinforcement to increase desired behaviors is a behavioral principle often used in conjunction with other theoretical approaches. Occupational therapy intervention plans include the use of behavioral goals and objectives that are observable and measurable. Royeen and Duncan (1999) have also noted a recent resurgence in behavioral principles to facilitate motor and cognitive skills for children based on Mosey's acquisitional theory.

The biomechanical frame of reference applies the principles of physics to human movement and posture with respect to the forces of gravity. It is a popular theoretical framework for many practitioners who work in rehabilitation and can be applied to both children and adults. It is commonly used with musculoskeletal disorders, cumulative trauma such as back injuries or carpal tunnel syndrome, hand injuries, work hardening, and ergonomics. Intervention focus includes remediation and improvements in strength, range of motion, or endurance. Biomechanical principles guide the design of splints, adaptive seating, and the design and use of prosthetic devices. An example of how this theory can be applied to practice includes positioning of children with motor and postural difficulties to promote engagement in activities and increase occupational functioning (Colangelo, 1999).

Toglia's dynamic interactional model to cognitive rehabilitation (2005) has its foundation in neuroscience and its application guidelines within the theory of occupation. Occupational therapists apply this theoretical approach for persons with brain injury to promote restoration of functional performance. It is based on the central premise that cognitive function is dynamic and context dependent and, therefore, modifiable. The dynamic interactional model is a complex, systems-based theory with two primary goals for intervention: to remediate skills and to compensate for loss of functioning. Cognitive change depends on the client's ability to learn and generalize information. Enhancing a person's self-awareness about that person's disability and promoting processing strategies are inherent in the therapy process.

Allen's cognitive disabilities frame of reference has been updated by Levy (2005) and renamed the *cognitive disabilities reconsidered model* (Levy, 2005; Levy & Burns, 2006). The six clinically defined cognitive levels and 52 cognitive modes, originally designed by Allen, offer occupational therapists some of the best detailed guidelines for assessing, assisting, and adapting environments for persons with cognitive disabilities. This frame of reference focuses on the role of cognition (a process skill), the role of habits and routines, the effect of physical and social contexts, and the analysis of activity demand. It is often applied for persons with developmental disabilities, dementias, and chronic mental illness such as schizophrenia.

The developmental frames of reference are concerned with establishing or restoring client-chosen, age-appropriate occupations for promotion of meaningful life roles. The occupational therapy profession has continuously been influenced by many developmental theories reflecting childhood (Erikson & Erikson, 1997; Gesell & Armatruda, 1967; Kohlberg, 1973; Piaget, 1972), adulthood (Gilligan, 1982; Levinson, 1978) and aging (Atchley, 1976; Havighurst, 1961; Laslett, 1991). Theories based on neuromaturation include the works of Ayres (1974), King (1974), and the Bobaths (1990), while more generalist views were defined by Llorens (1966) and Mosey (1986). Health conditions and injuries often impact normal development. A practitioner using this approach is concerned with providing a growth-facilitating environment for the stimulation of age-appropriate behavior and skill learning. It is most important to consider the client's view when establishing an intervention plan.

Sensory motor frames of reference in occupational therapy have been applied to children, adults with mental health conditions, and older adults. Commonly used approaches include Ayres's *sensory* integration (Bundy, Lane, & Murray, 2002), Dunn's sensory processing (Dunn, 2001), sensory defensiveness (Wilbarger & Wilbarger, 2002) and Ross's five-stage group (Ross & Bachner, 2004). Neuroscientists define sensory integration as the brain's ability to organize sensory information from the body and environment and to produce an adaptive response. Within each of these approaches, interventions are provided by occupational therapists through guided sensory input on a one-on-one or group activity basis.

The next grouping of theories is referred to as *motor control* and *motor learning frames of reference* (Cole & Tufano, 2008). Traditional examples of motor control theories include Bobath's (1990) neurodevelopmental therapy (NDT), Rood's (1954) sensorimotor approach, Knott and Voss's (1968) proprioceptive neuromuscular facilitation (PNF), and Brunnstrom's (1970) movement therapy. Principles of normal neurological development are considered in a reflex-hierarchical or neuromaturational sequence for establishing or restoring functional movement. More recent models have emerged with updated evidence, including the task-oriented frame of reference described by Horak (1991). Motor learning theories currently provide guidelines for restoring functional movement with clients having a broad range of health conditions. Task accomplishment is the ultimate goal. Occupational therapy intervention focuses on assisting clients in developing the optimal motor and cognitive strategies for achieving functional goals (Cole & Tufano, 2008).

How to Use Models and Frames of Reference for Occupational Therapy Evaluation and Intervention Process

The process of service delivery is challenging for anyone working in health care today. Most practitioners implement a variety of assessment tools and intervention strategies within their practice. What do theoretical models and frames of reference have to do with the day-to-day delivery of service? Is it OK to rely on more than one theoretical perspective at the same time? While it may appear comfortable for practitioners to rely on familiar therapeutic approaches one may have used over and over again, new research data continue to provide evidence for best-practice approaches. An eclectic practitioner would select "... a method or approach that is composed of elements drawn from various sources" (Merriam-Webster, n.d.). Imagine if you only had five outfits in your closet to wear every day, regardless of weather conditions in the environment, your internal mood, your external body shape, or the dress occasion. Would you describe your choices as "familiar and comfortable" or "limiting and outdated"? While specializing in one theory approach may seem initially comfortable, like wearing an old pair of shoes, it can also limit the practitioner's ability to be most effective within today's complex health care demands. Not every theory is an appropriate fit for every client; rather, theory should be considered on an individual basis. In like manner, not every theory may be a good match for every occupational therapist. Allowing oneself more choices from a theoretical repertoire, rather than less, in the selection of evaluation and intervention options will increase the likelihood of reaching the end goal of mutual and desired outcomes. As practitioners, we can look to the Framework document (AOTA, 2008) for guidance on how to select and apply theory to practice.

The Framework (2008) serves as our professional guide, describing how practitioners can integrate theory into the scope of occupational therapy practice. Occupational therapy educational standards of practice likewise emphasize that students must learn how theory serves as the foundation for the evaluation and intervention process. The bridge to applying knowledge to practice is not an easy path of discovery. It must be a deliberate and conscious effort. The following statements represent a summary of suggestions based on both the framework document and this author's practical experience for how to use occupation-based models and frames of reference for best-practice outcomes.

Occupation-based models and frames of reference can assist the practitioner in the following ways:

- To understand data and formulate hypotheses about a client's occupational performance issues gathered initially from an occupational profile interview process.
- To guide the practitioner in selecting relevant assessments for further data collection.
- To create a therapeutic framework for interpreting data and forming initial conclusions about a person's occupational performance within this perspective.
- To create collaborative goals with specific outcome measures that are based on sound and rational constructs from theory rather than one's opinion.
- To develop an intervention plan for the client utilizing interventions based on best practice and evidence as supported by various models and frames of reference.

In summary, the application of theory is a reasoning process that can frame a client's occupational needs and wants as determined from the occupational profile along with the practitioner's analysis of a client's occupational performance (AOTA, 2008). While these two components are significant aspects of a collaborative therapeutic process, there are also other factors that will influence the quality of occupational therapy outcomes. The delivery of occupational therapy services is as much an art as it is a science. It is the practitioner's personality, insights, perceptions, and judgments, also defined as *therapeutic use of self* (AOTA, 2008, p. 628), that allow the therapist to form a healthy relationship with clients and affect positive outcomes.

How to Apply Theoretical Constructs in the Evaluation and Intervention Process

So far, we have identified and introduced five common occupation-based models and eight classifications of frames of reference. As previously noted, the process of integrating theory into practice is a multistep process. Each of the theories is complex, with interdependent levels of ideas and its own set of terminology. It is common for students to struggle with such abstract concepts; after all, a theory cannot be seen, only understood.

Table 15-3.

TEMPLATE FOR ANALYSIS OF OCCUPATION-BASED MODELS AND FRAMES OF REFERENCE

Model or Frame of Reference	Analysis
Focus Includes the population suited for and domains of practice according to occupational therapy practice framework.	
Theorists Includes authors and related theorists who have contributed to this body of knowledge.	
Theoretical base Includes defined compatible constructs that explain possible causes and/or contributing factors for function and dysfunction.	
Function How does this theory define healthy or optimal functioning?	
Dysfunction How does this theory define incapacities or barriers to functioning?	
Change What are the concepts that define how change is likely to occur according to this theory?	
Motivation What motivates a client to change according to this theory?	
Assessment What formal or informal assessments are specifically created or recommended according to this theory?	
Intervention guidelines What specific therapeutic techniques or strategies have been developed and/or recommended based on this theory?)	
Research To what extent has this theory been validated through research?)	

Adapted from Cole, M., & Tufano, R. (2008). *Applied theories in occupational therapy*. Thorofare, NJ: SLACK Incorporated.

The first step within this clinical reasoning process is to learn each of the models and/or frames of reference individually. A template designed by Cole and Tufano (2008) is provided to assist the reader in gathering key concepts about each model and frame of reference (Table 15-3). The template is based on Mosey's original definition of a frame of reference and how knowledge is organized within this body of knowledge. Categories listed on the left side of the template reflect the various related parts, or constructs, commonly found in each theory. The student is encouraged to complete this template on each model and/or frame of reference by filling in one section at a time. Further reading and study from references cited at the end of this chapter may be needed to fully complete the template. Students should initially gather and identify the many concepts that compose each theory as identified by each section of the template. A completed template can serve as a study guide and assist the student at a glance to view the overall picture of the theory.

The second learning step is to be able to compare and contrast each model and/or frame of reference to another. The process of distinguishing one theory from another simulates what practitioners are required to do in daily practice. Every practitioner must use clinical judgment in determining best-practice interventions. This reasoning process begins by gathering client data and relying on theoretical explanations to form hypotheses about a client's occupational performance.

Crepeau and Boyt Schell (2003) point out that the major theories in our profession differ in purpose, scope, complexity, extent of development and validation through research, and usefulness in practice (p. 204). In fact, practitioners apply the various levels of theory at different stages of the evaluation, intervention, and outcomes continuum. The occupation-based models help practitioners to develop a perspective on how the client, who engages within a particular environment, is participating in occupations. Constructs from these models relate well to aspects of the framework document and the occupational profile because of their holistic and client-centered orientation. Constructs are also rooted in occupational therapy language and theory because each model is authored by an occupational therapist. These models help to identify the range of possibilities when setting collaborative goals for client engagement in occupations as well as identifying barriers to participation. In addition, occupation-based models help us determine ways in which our clients can find meaningful roles in society.

Frames of reference enter the clinical reasoning process as the occupational therapist thinks about problem areas identified by a client. They specifically target select components of the framework such as performance areas, skills patterns, and, most often, client factors. For example, Allen's cognitive disability frame of reference specifically addresses the following aspects within the framework document: ADL performance areas; process performance skills; the performance patterns of habits, routines, and roles; and client factors defined as mental functions.

Crepeau and Boyt Schell (2003) describe how advanced practitioners tend to incorporate theory into their reasoning process in ways that allow them to use it automatically (i.e., without conscious awareness). Thus, expert occupational therapists may not always be able to articulate the model or frame of reference that they are using. This does not mean that they are not using theory, but rather that its use has become habitual and integrated into their professional reasoning. On the other hand, students who are in the beginning stages of clinical reasoning development. As novices, it is important to consciously think about procedures and make clinical choices based on

objective information deduced from various theoretical approaches (Cole & Tufano, 2008).

Occupational therapy assistants (OTAs) are expected to know about the various occupation-based models and frames of reference used in occupational therapy practice. Understanding these theories will enhance the ability of OTAs to have a more comprehensive view of working with a client. As part of their role delineation, OTAs are not required to apply the theoretical constructs to practice. Rather, OTAs will take direction from the registered occupational therapist (OTR) on what model and/or frame of reference to employ when providing intervention strategies.

Summary

The process of understanding relevant occupational therapy theories is often a challenge for students, academicians, and practitioners alike. This chapter attempts to demystify the process for learning about various theories by highlighting common occupation-based models and popular frames of reference found in current practice. The five occupational therapy models mentioned here represent a holistic, client-centered, and universal application to persons across the lifespan and across all domains of practice. These models support the current health care trend toward prevention of disease and promotion of health, with emphasis on occupational performance. Each model provides a list of guidelines for the occupational therapy practitioner within the evaluation and intervention process. They pose a direct contrast to the frames of reference that are much more prescriptive and specific in nature. Generally speaking, frames of reference are oriented toward restoring, adapting, and/or compensating for the loss of occupational functioning. In their own unique way, these theories are limited in their application scope, each targeting a specific focus of concern within practice. Unlike the occupation-based models, specific assessments, techniques, and strategies are prescribed by each frame of reference for use in the evaluation and intervention process.

As a profession, we look to the framework document for guidance on how these models and frames of reference assist the practitioner in the therapeutic process. The art and science of occupational therapy practice includes a two-prong evaluative approach. First, we assess a client's occupational needs while we also consider the practitioner's objective analyses of a client's performance. The delivery of occupational therapy service is an evolving interactive process impacted by both the practitioner's therapeutic use of self and the personality traits of the client. Practitioners need to balance their professional knowledge with the desires and needs of their clients in a collaborative relationship.

Case Example: John

John is a 58-year-old divorced male with two adult children. He is employed at a naval base where he works as a chief engineer. He lives alone in a nearby apartment and reports that his favorite pastime is "hanging out" with his old naval buddies at the local pub. "We look out for each other," John tells the occupational therapist, who notices missing teeth as he laughs out loud.

The client has been diagnosed with peripheral neuropathy due to chronic alcohol abuse. Recently hospitalized because he reported difficulty walking over a period of 4 months, John thought his "weak legs" were a result of a motorcycle fall that he sustained last year. "I never would have thought that a few beers a day would have given me sea legs!"

John is presently in a rehabilitation center. He is referred to occupational therapy for evaluation of ADL, instrumental ADL (IADL), work, and social/leisure participation. Due to the recent health concerns, John has decided to pursue retirement. He wants to return to his second floor apartment but worries about his ability to climb stairs and care for himself. "What am I going to do all day long?" he questions. John tells the occupational therapist, "My mind is not as sharp as it used to be. Last week, I left the oven on all night long."

Learning Activities

- After reading the case, fill in as much information as you can gather about John's personal characteristics, his engagement in various occupations, and his present living environment. Make a point to identify both strengths and problem areas in each of the three categories. Based on your knowledge so far about the five occupation-based models, which one would you possibly consider as a theoretical base for evaluation and intervention for John? Briefly explain why.

PERSON   OCCUPATIONS   ENVIRONMENT

_____   _____   _____

- Refer to the case of John and identify practice concerns by completing the following chart. Consult the framework document for the definitions of each category as needed. Based on your knowledge so far about the different types of frames of reference, which ones would you select for occupational therapy evaluation and intervention for John? Briefly explain your reasons.

Performance areas (ADL, IADL, work, education, sleep/rest, leisure, social participation)	
Performance skills (motor, process, communication)	
Performance patterns (habits, routines, roles)	
Contexts	
Client factors (body functions, structures)	

It is common for professions such as occupational therapy to develop and consider multiple and often contrasting ideas about best practice. There are many theories from which to choose. For students, academicians, and practitioners inclusively, the process of becoming proficient at understanding and applying the various theoretical constructs for evaluation and intervention purposes takes time and effort. The process begins with learning the basics of each theory and understanding its intended therapeutic purpose. The ability to analyze and select the best theory option for a client requires that a practitioner have a repertoire of models and frames of reference to choose from. This decision-making process encompasses clinical reasoning—a process that is based on knowing what a theory says and how to use it. Understanding theoretical constructs, combined with applying these principles to simulated or real practical experience, fosters the development of clinical synthesis. As stated in our Centennial Vision, we have a professional responsibility to become more science driven. This includes conducting more research studies and basing our clinical decisions on evidence. The integration of theory must drive practice in order to validate our scope and sustain our unique role as occupational therapists within the professional world.

Student Self-Assessment

1. How do today's complex health concerns impact a practitioner's need for theoretical knowledge?

2. How do occupation-based models support the trend toward health promotion and prevention of illness?

3. What are the pros and cons to practicing within a specialty area of occupational therapy versus practicing as a generalist?

4. What is your opinion about the following statements: "theory drives practice" and "practice drives theory"?

5. State some similarities and differences among the two theoretical classifications of practice discussed in this chapter: occupation-based models and frames of reference.

6. How has Mary Reilly influenced the profession of occupational therapy? Consider her quote, "Man through the use of his hands as they are energized by his mind and will, can influence the state of his own health."

7. When is it appropriate to use more than one theoretical perspective for a given client in occupational therapy practice? Give a specific example.

References

American Occupational Therapy Association. (2006). *Centennial vision*. Retrieved from http://www.aota.org/News/Centennial/Background/36516.aspx

American Occupational Therapy Association. (2008). Occupational therapy practice framework: Domain and process (2nd ed.). *American Journal of Occupational Therapy, 62,* 625-683.

Atchley, R. C. (1076). *The sociology of retirement.* New York, NY: Halsted.

Ayers, A. J. (1974). *The development of sensory integrative theory and practice.* Dubuque, IA: Kendall Hunt.

Azima, H., & Azima, F. (1959). The therapeutic use of self. *American Journal of Occupational Therapy, 12,* 215-225.

Baum, C. M., & Christiansen, C. H. (2005). *Person-environment-occupation-performance: An occupation based framework for practice.* In C. H. Cristiansen, C. M. Baum, & J. Bass-Haugen (Eds.), *Occupational therapy: Performance, participation, and well-being* (3rd ed.). Thorofare, NJ: SLACK Incorporated.

Bobath, B. (1990). *Adult hemiplegia: Evaluation and treatment* (3rd ed.). London, UK: Heinemann.

Boisvert, R. A. (2004). Enhancing substance dependence intervention. *Occupational Therapy Practice, 9*(10), 11-16.

Bruce, M. G., & Borg, B. (2002). Psychosocial frames of reference: Core for occupation-based practice (3rd ed.) Thorofare, NJ: SLACK Incorporated.

Bundy, A. C., Lane, S. J., & Murray, E. A. (2002). *Sensory integration: Theory and practice* (2nd ed.). Philadelphia, PA: F.A. Davis Company.

Canadian Association of Occupational Therapists. (1991). *Client-centered guidelines for the practice of occupational therapy.* Toronto, Ontario, Canada: Author.

Capasso, N., Gorman, A., & Blick, C. (2010). Breakfast group in an acute rehabilitation setting: A restorative program for incorporating client's hemiparetic upper extremities for function. *Occupational Therapy Practice, 5*(8), 14-18.

Christiansen, C. H., & Baum, C. M. (1991). *Occupational therapy: Overcoming human performance deficits.* Thorofare, NJ: SLACK Incorporated.

Christiansen, C. H., & Baum, C. M. (1997). *Occupational therapy: Enabling function and well-being* (2nd ed.). Thorofare, NJ: SLACK, Incorporated.

Cicerone, K. D., Dahlberg, C., Kalmar, K., Langenbahn, D. M., Malec, J. F., Bergquist, T. F., ... Morse, P. A. (2000). Evidence-based cognitive rehabilitation: Recommendations for clinical practice. *Archive Physical Medicine Rehabilitation, 81*(12), 159-615.

Colangelo, C. (1999). Biomechanical frame of reference. In P. Kramer & J. Hinojosa (Eds.), *Frames of reference for pediatric occupational therapy* (2nd ed., pp. 377-400). Philadelphia, PA: Lippincott Williams & Wilkins.

Cole, M., & Tufano, R. (2008). *Applied theories in occupational therapy.* Thorofare, NJ: SLACK Incorporated.

Crepeau, E., & Boyt Schell, B. (2003). Theory and practice in occupational therapy. In E. Crepeau, E. Cohn, & B. Schell (Eds.), *Willard & Spackman's occupational therapy* (10th ed.). Philadelphia, PA: Lippincott Williams & Wilkins.

Diasio, K. (1968). Psychiatric occupational therapy: Search for a conceptual framework in light of psychoanalytic ego psychology and learning theory. *American Journal of Occupational Therapy, XXII*(5), 50-57.

Diller, L. (2005). Pushing the frames of reference in traumatic brain injury rehabilitation. *Archive Physical Medicine Rehabilitation, 86*(6), 1075-1080.

Dunn, W. (2000). *Best practice occupational therapy: In community service with children and families.* Thorofare, NJ: SLACK Incorporated.

Dunn, W. (2001). The 2001 Eleanor Clarke Slagle lecture: The sensations of everyday life: Empirical, theoretical, and pragmatic considerations. *American Journal of Occupational Therapy, 55,* 608-620.

Dunn, W., Brown, C. & McGuigan, A. (1994). The ecology of human performance: A framework for considering the effect of context. *American Journal of Occupational Therapy, 48,* 595-607.

Eclectic. (n.d.). Merriam-Webster Online Dictionary. Retrieved from http://www.merriam-webster.com/dictionary/eclectic

Erikson, E. H., & Erikson, J. M. (1997) *The life cycle completed.* New York, NY: Norton

Fidler G. (1969). The task-oriented group as a context for treatment. *American Journal of Occupational Therapy, XXIII, 1,* 43-48.

Gesell, A., & Armatruda, C. (1967). *Developmental diagnosis.* New York, NY: Harper & Row.

Gilligan, C. (1982). *A different voice.* Cambridge, MA: Harvard University Press.

Goulet, C., Rousseau, J., & Fortier, P. (2007). A literature review on perception of the providers and clients regarding the use of the client centered approach in psychiatry. *Canadian Journal of Occupational Therapy, 74*(3), 172-182.

Hagedorn, R. (2001). Foundations for practice in occupational therapy (3rd ed.) London, UK: Churchill Livingstone.

Hart, T., & Evans, J. (2006). Self-regulation and goal theories in brain injury rehabilitation. *Journal Head Trauma Rehabilitation, 21*(2), 142-155.

Havighurst, R. (1961). Successful aging. *The Gerontologist*, 1, 8-13.

Henderson, S. (1999). Frames of reference utilized in the rehabilitation of individuals with eating disorders. *Canadian Journal of Occupational Therapy, 66*(1), 43-51.

Horak, F. B. (1991). Assumptions underlying motor control for neurologic rehabilitation. In M. J. Lister (Ed.), *Contemporary management of motor control problems: Proceedings of the II STEP conference* (pp. 11-27). Alexandria, VA: Foundation for Physical Therapy.

Humphry, R., & Wakeford, L. (2006). An occupation-centered discussion of development and implications for practice. *American Journal of Occupational Therapy, 60*(3), 258-267.

Jarus, T., & Ratzon, N. Z. (2005). The implementation of motor learning principles in designing prevention programs at work. *WORK: A Journal of Prevention, Assessment & Rehabilitation, 24*, 171-182.

Johnson, J., & Schkade, J. K. (2001). Effects of occupation-based intervention on mobility problems following a cerebral vascular accident. *Journal of Applied Gerontology, 20*(1), 91-110.

Kielhofner, G. (1980a). A model of human occupation, part two. Ontogenesis from the perspective of temporal adaptation. *American Journal of Occupational Therapy, 34*, 657-663.

Kielhofner, G. (1980b). A model of human occupation, part three: Benign and vicious cycles. *American Journal of Occupational Therapy, 34*, 731-737.

Kielhofner, G. (1997). *Conceptual foundations of occupational therapy.* (2nd ed.). Baltimore, MD: Williams & Wilkins.

Kielhofner, G., & Barrett, L. (1997). An overview of occupational behavior. In H. Hopkins & H. Smith (Eds.), *Willard & Spackman's Occupational Therapy.* Philadelphia, PA: J. B. Lippincott.

Kielhofner, G., & Burke, J. (1980). A model of human occupation, part one: Conceptual framework and content. *American Journal of Occupational Therapy, 34*, 572-581.

Kielhofner, G., Burke, J., & Heard, I. C. (1980). A model of human occupation, part four: Assessment and intervention. *American Journal of Occupational Therapy, 34*, 777-788.

King, L. J. (1974). A sensory integrative approach to schizophrenia. *American Journal of Occupational Therapy, 28*, 529-536.

Knott, M., & Voss, D. E. (1968). *Proprioceptive neuromuscular facilitation* (2nd ed.). New York, NY: Harper & Row.

Kohlberg, L. (1973). Stages and aging in moral development: Some speculations. *Gerontologist, 1*(3), 497-502.

Laatsch, L., Harrington, D., Hotz, G., Marcantuono, J., Mozzoni, M. P., Walsh, V., & Hersey, K. P. (2007). An evidence based review of cognitive and behavioral rehabilitation treatment studies in children with acquired brain injury. *Journal Head Trauma Rehabilitation, 22*(4), 248-256.

Laslett, P. (1991). *A fresh map of life: The emergence of the third age.* Cambridge, MA: Harvard University Press.

Lee, S. W., Taylor, R. R., & Kielhofner, G. (2009). Choice, knowledge, and utilization of a practice theory: A national study of occupational therapists who use the Model of Human Occupation. *Occupational Therapy in Health Care, 23*(1), 60-71.

Lee, S. W., Taylor, R., Kielhofner, G. & Fisher, G. (2008). Theory use in practice: A national survey of therapists who use the Model of Human Occupation. *American Journal of Occupational Therapy, 62*(1), 106-117.

Leichsenring, F., Hiller, W., Weissberg, M., & Leibing, E. (2006). Cognitive-behavioral therapy and psychodynamic psychotherapy: Techniques, efficacy, and indications. *American Journal of Psychotherapy, 60*(3), 233-259.

Letts, L., Law, M., Rigby, P., Cooper, B., Stewart, D., & Strong, S. (1994). Person-environment assessments in occupational therapy. *American Journal of Occupational Therapy, 48*(7), 608-618.

Levinson, D. (1973). *The seasons of a man's life.* New York, NY: Ballentine Books.

Levy, L. L. (2005). Cognitive disabilities reconsidered: Rehabilitation of older adults with dementia. In N. Katz (Ed.), *Cognition & occupation across the life span: Models for intervention in occupational therapy.* Bethesda, MD: AOTA Press.

Levy, L. L., & Burns, T. (2006). Neurocognitive practice essentials in dementia: Cognitive disabilities-reconsidered model. *OT Practice, 11*(3), CE1-CE8.

Llorens, L. (1966). Occupational therapy in an ego-oriented milieu. *American Journal of Occupational Therapy, 20*, 178-181.

Lund, M. L., & Nygard, L. (2004). Occupational life in the home environment: The experience of people with disabilities. *Canadian Journal of Occupational Therapy, 71*, 243-252.

Maitra, K. K., & Erway, F. (2006). Perception of client-centered practice in occupational therapists and their clients. *American Journal of Occupational Therapy, 60*, 298-310.

Mastos, M., Miller, K., Eliasson, A. C., & Imms, C. (2007). Goal-directed training: Linking theories of treatment to clinical practice for improved functional activities in daily life. *Clinical Rehabilitation, 21*(1), 47-55.

Mosey, A. (1970). Three frames of reference for mental health. Thorofare, NJ: SLACK Incorporated.

Mosey, A. (1986). *Psychosocial components of occupational Therapy.* New York, NY: Raven Press.

Piaget, J. (1973). *The psychology of the child.* New York, NY: Basic Books.

Rebeiro, K. L. (2001). Enabling occupation: the importance of an affirming environment. *Canadian Journal of Occupational Therapy, 68*(2), 80-89.

Rebeiro, K. L., & Polgar, J. M. (1999). Enabling occupational performance: Optimal experiences in therapy. *Canadian Journal of Occupational Therapy, 66*(1), 14-22.

Reed, K. L, & Sanderson, S. N. (1999). *Concepts of occupational therapy* (4th ed.). Philadelphia, PA: Lippincott Williams & Wilkins.

Reilly, M. (1958). An occupational therapy curriculum for 1965. *American Journal of Occupational Therapy, 12*, 293-299.

Reilly, M. (1962). Occupational therapy can be one of the great ideas of 20th century medicine. *American Journal of Occupational Therapy, 16*, 1-9.

Restall, G., Ripat, J., & Stern, M. (2003). A framework of strategies for client-centered practice. *Canadian Journal of Occupational Therapy, 70*(2), 103-112.

Rogers, J. C. (1983). The Eleanor Clarke Slagle lecture: Clinical reasoning: The ethics, science and art. *American Journal of Occupational Therapy, 37,* 601-616.

Roley, S. S., Clark, G. F., Bissell, J., & Brayman, S. J., Commission on Practice. (2003). Applying sensory integration framework in educationally related occupational therapy practice. *American Journal of Occupational Therapy, 57*(6), 652-659.

Ross, M., & Bachner, S. (2004). *Adults with developmental disabilities: Current approaches in occupational therapy* (2nd ed.). Bethesda, MD: AOTA Press.

Royeen, C., & Duncan, M. (1999). Acquisitional frame of reference. In P. Kramer & J. Hinojosa (Eds.), *Frames of reference for pediatric occupational therapy* (2nd ed., pp. 377-400). Philadelphia, PA: Lippincott Williams & Wilkins.

Schaaf, R. C., & Miller, L. J. (2005). Occupational therapy using a sensory integrative approach for children with developmental disabilities. *American Journal of Occupational Therapy, 11*(2), 143-148.

Schell, B. A., & Schell, J. W. (2008). *Clinical and professional reasoning in occupational therapy.* Baltimore, MD: Lippincott Williams & Wilkins.

Schkade, J. K., & McClung, M. (2001). *Occupational adaptation in practice: Concepts and cases.* Thorofare, NJ: SLACK Incorporated.

Schkade, J. K., & Schultz, S. (1992). Occupational adaptation: Toward a holistic approach to contemporary practice, part 1. *American Journal of Occupational Therapy, 46,* 829-837.

Schultz, S., & Schkade, J. K. (1992). Occupational adaptation: Toward a holistic approach to contemporary practice, part 2. *American Journal of Occupational Therapy, 46,* 917-926.

Stein, F., & Cutler, S. (2002). *Psychosocial occupational therapy: A holistic approach,* (2nd ed.) Canada: Delmar, Thompson.

Strong, S., Rigby, P., Stewart, D., Law, M., Letts, L., & Cooper, B. (1999). Application of the person-environment-occupation model: A practical tool. *Canadian Journal of Occupational Therapy, 66*(3), 122-133.

Teasell, R. W., Foley, N. C., Bhogal, S. K. & Speechley, M. R. (2003). An evidence-based review of stroke rehabilitation. *Top Stroke Rehabilitation, 10*(1), 29-58.

Toglia, J. (2005). A dynamic interactional approach to cognitive rehabilitation. In N. Katz (Ed.), *Cognition and occupation in rehabilitation: Cognitive models for intervention in occupational therapy.* Bethesda, MD: AOTA Press.

Trombly, C. A. (1995). Occupation: Purposefulness and meaningfulness as therapeutic mechanisms. 1995 Eleanor Clarke Slagle lecture. *American Journal of Occupational Therapy, 49*(10), 960-972.

Watling, R. L., & Dietz, J. (2007). Immediate effect of Ayres's sensory integration-based occupational therapy intervention on children with autism spectrum disorders. *American Journal of Occupational Therapy, 61*(5), 574-583.

Whedon, C. A. (2000). Frames of reference that address the impact of physical environments on occupational performance. *WORK: A Journal of Prevention, Assessment & Rehabilitation, 14*(2), 165-174.

Wilbarger, J., & Wilbarger, P. (2002). The Wilbarger approach to treating sensory defensiveness. In A. Bundy, S. Lane, & E. Murray (Eds.), *Sensory integration: Theory and practice* (2nd ed.). Philadelphia, PA: F.A. Davis Company.

Wilkins, S., Pollock, N., Rochon, S., & Law, M. (2001). Implementing client-centered practice: Why is it so difficult to do? *Canadian Journal of Occupational Therapy, 68*(2), 70-79.

Williamson, G. G., & Szczepanski, M. (1999). Coping frame of reference. In P. Kramer & J. Hinojosa, (Eds.), *Frames of reference for pediatric occupational therapy* (2nd ed.). Philadelphia, PA: Lippincott Williams & Wilkins.

World Health Organization. (2001). *International classification of function, disability, and health.* Geneva, Switzerland: Author.

IV

SCREENING, EVALUATION, AND REFERRAL

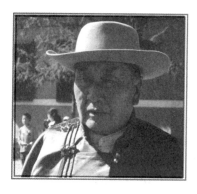

16

SCREENING, EVALUATION, AND REFERRAL

Jessica J. Bolduc, DrOT, MS, OTR/L

ACOTE STANDARDS EXPLORED IN THIS CHAPTER
B.4.1–B.4.3, B.4.5–B.4.10

KEY VOCABULARY

- **Assessment:** Tools, instruments, procedures or interactions used during the evaluation process.
- **Client:** The OTPF defines *client* as "Persons, including families, caregivers, teachers, employers, and relevant others; Organizations, such as businesses, industries, or agencies; and populations within a community, such as refugees, veterans who are homeless, and people with chronic health disabling conditions" (Moyers & Dale, 2007 from AOTA, 2008).

- **Criterion referenced:** A score from an assessment that can be compared to the skills or performance of a group rather than compared to a normative group (i.e., an assessment designed for children with cerebral palsy about motor performance is criterion referenced when compared to children who also have cerebral palsy rather than the general population of children).
- **Documentation:** A permanent legal record that records the client's occupational therapy service (i.e., evaluation, daily notes, progress notes, discharge).
- **Evaluation:** The process of obtaining and interpreting data necessary to understand the client and initiate treatment.

(continued)

Jacobs, K., MacRae, N., & Sladyk, K. (Eds.).
Occupational Therapy Essentials for
Clinical Competence, Second Edition (pp. 201-214).
© 2014 SLACK Incorporated.

KEY VOCABULARY (CONTINUED)

- **Norm referenced:** A score from an assessment that can be compared to the skills or performance of a "normative" group (e.g., adult grip strength).

- **Referral:** Recommendation for a client to receive occupational therapy; often required to initiate an occupational therapy evaluation.
- **Screening:** The process of gathering information to determine the client's skilled need for occupational therapy.

Introduction

The last decade has seen significant changes in the implementation and documentation of occupational therapy services. A variety of factors, both within and outside of our profession, have contributed to these changes. These factors include the view of health and disability in the International Classification of Functioning, Disability and Health (ICF) by the World Health Organization (WHO, 2001), the need for evidence-based practice (American Occupational Therapy Association [AOTA], 2007a; Holm, 2000), the health care system's mandate for efficiency, the implementation of the electronic medical record, and the publication and implementation of the Practice Framework (AOTA, 2008).

With regard to the evaluation process specifically, what is considered to be best practice has led to dramatic improvement in the assessment tools available to practitioners in order to meet the current responsibilities of an occupational therapy evaluation. In addition to the previously available performance, skill, client-centered, and daily living assessments, our profession now has assessments with focused attention related to occupation, social participation, work, activities of daily living (ADL), instrumental activities of daily living (IADL), environment/context, educational performance, and play/leisure. This section serves to identify important concepts related to the occupational therapy evaluation process, including information related to each of the aforementioned assessment areas.

Terms and Definitions

This section is designed to familiarize occupational therapy practitioners with the terms and components of the evaluation process as currently understood within the occupational therapy profession. It is important, however, for clinicians to realize that other professions might use the terms interchangeably or might define them differently. In fact, older occupational therapy texts have offered differing definitions than those described in this chapter because the occupational therapy profession has revised and clarified its understanding of these components over the years. It is important to clarify the occupational therapy perspective when case conferencing, when sharing your occupational therapy evaluation results with other professions, or when (as occurs in some instances) preparing a comprehensive evaluation report that includes the work of several disciplines. Screening, assessment, evaluation, and documentation are discussed next.

Screening

Basically stated, a screening is a process by which the occupational therapy practitioner determines if further assessment is needed (AOTA, 2010b). Therefore, intervention planning can never occur with screening information alone. Screening methods can be formal (i.e., a standardized screening instrument or an organization's intake form) or informal (e.g., chart review, interview of a teacher, or the observation of a client). Please refer to *A Reason to Screen* and to screening examples on the following page.

Although the framework does not specifically discuss the screening process, it is an important component in many institutions. Whereas the more experienced therapist might easily observe a client (informal screen) and determine if additional testing is required, the novice therapist might need more formalized methods to help determine if a potential difficulty in occupational performance is present. In fact, some might argue that when formalized methods of screening are utilized, the results factor into the therapist's clinical decision-making process and form the basis of the occupational therapy evaluation. Screening results are included in the evaluation report as one of the processes utilized for obtaining information.

Assessment

Once the need for a comprehensive evaluation is determined, specific assessment tools can be used based on the information deemed necessary and the environment in

A Reason to Screen

Mrs. Johnson, a second-grade teacher, ran into the occupational therapist in the teacher's lounge and indicated there were concerns about Mary's performance in the classroom. Mrs. Johnson asked if the occupational therapist could "just take a look" at Mary. Since the school district had a pre-referral program to assist children within the general education system prior to referral for special education services, the therapist asked Mrs. Johnson to complete the paperwork that would allow her to review Mary's educational history, observe Mary in the classroom, and send a questionnaire home to Mary's parents.

Upon record review, Mary has been having difficulty since preschool with her fine motor skills and how she organizes educational materials. This was also confirmed via the parent questionnaire. Within the classroom, Mary was observed to sit under her desk with her hands over her ears during morning announcements over the PA system, watch how other children were completing assignments before beginning herself, and rarely finished her workbook assignments within the allotted time. This screening information was sufficient for recommending a complete evaluation to determine Mary's specific difficulties so that an effective intervention plan might be developed. The evaluation report ultimately included these occupational difficulties as examples of the client and contextual factors that interfered with Mary's successful engagement in school-related tasks.

Sample Screening Tools

Name	Target
The Model of Human Occupation Screening Tool (MOHOST) (Parkinson, Forsyth, & Kielhofner, 2006)	Screen uses MOHO concepts of volition, habituation, skills, and environment to screen the client's occupational functioning.
Occupational Therapy Adult Perceptual Screening Test (OT-APST) (Cooke, McKenna, & Fleming, 2005)	Screens adults with agnosia and visual perceptual skills deficits, such as body scheme neglect, apraxia, and acalculia.
Screening Test for Evaluating Preschoolers (FirstSTEP) (Miller, 1993)	Screen detects mild developmental delays in grade school students.

which the client's occupational performance is limited. If a formalized screening was not completed, the informal methods of chart review and interview (e.g., client profile) would be an appropriate starting point in the evaluation process. Appropriate assessment tools can be identified and implemented by the occupational therapist or the occupational therapy assistant. While the occupational therapist directs and initiates the evaluation process, the two practitioners can collaboratively determine which assessment(s) can be administered by the occupational therapy assistant based on professional experience, training, establishment of competency, and level of supervision provided. Per the Guidelines for Supervision, Roles, and Responsibilities During the Delivery of Occupational Therapy Services (AOTA, 2009) and AOTA's Standards of Practice (2010b), the occupational therapy assistant "contributes to the screening, evaluation and re-evaluation process by implementing delegated assessments and by providing verbal and written reports of observations and client capacities to the occupational therapist" (p. S110) so the occupational therapist can interpret and integrate the information into the evaluation and decision-making process. While these are our professional guidelines, licensure regulations for each state have specific requirements with regard to service providers and supervision, which should be investigated prior to the implementation of service by the occupational therapy assistant. Additionally, relevant principles in the Code of Ethics and Ethic Standards (AOTA, 2010a) speak to appropriate delegation of tasks and supervision of occupational therapy assistants.

Assessments are the specific tests, tools, or methods used to collect the data needed for a comprehensive evaluation. Appendix B provides information related to commonly used assessment tools. Each assessment manual provides instructions for implementation, application, and interpretation, and it is each clinician's responsibility to be familiar and competent with each assessment tool that is used as part of his or her practice. Some assessment tools require advanced training and/or certification to implement, whereas some are only applicable to certain populations or age groups. In these cases, it is each professional's responsibility to meet the parameters set forth in the manual to assure ethical implementation in accordance with the test author's guidelines. Novice therapists can include the acquiring of these skills in their annual professional development plans and request time and financial resources to gain these skills.

There are times when an expert clinical decision is made to implement an assessment outside the boundaries set forth in the manual's implementation guidelines (e.g., not the intended population, procedures modified for language or physical limitations). This practice is frowned upon and should only occur when there are no other means of obtaining data to assist with intervention planning. With regard to reporting the assessment results, however, the data collected in these instances can only be used and reported informally, and scores cannot be reported as they are no longer valid or reliable as reported in the assessment manual. This should be made clear in documentation.

As previously stated, significant changes have occurred in available assessment tools during the past decade. If, however, the setting within which you work requires standardized, client factor-focused assessments, it is the occupational therapist's role to determine how these specific pieces of information integrate with a more comprehensive, occupation-based perspective. For it is only with this clinical process that appropriate and effective interventions can be planned so that occupational engagement, which is part of the continuum of care, will eventually be achieved.

STANDARDIZED

An assessment tool manual can maximize consistency of professional implementation by outlining a formalized procedure to be followed. The formalized, or standardized, implementation and interpretation methods designed for best practice do not make a tool "standardized." Clinicians need to be clear: A standardized test requires rigorous research and analysis utilizing accepted psychometric procedures.

Psychometric Properties

- **Reliability, Test-Retest Reliability.** Consistency of a measure, score obtained reflects a true measure rather than an error.

- **Validity.** The assessment measures what it is intended to measure.

- **Precision.** Exactness of a measure.

- **Sensitivity or responsiveness.** Measure's ability to detect the presence of a problem or condition.

- **Clinically important difference.** The smallest change in a test score that is perceived significant by client or therapist.

- **Minimal detectable change.** Minimal amount of change that occurs without error that reflects true change in a test score.

(Adapted from Kielhofner, 2006; StrokEngine, 2013.)

Standardization guarantees an assessment has psychometric characteristics including a statistical review of reliability and validity, established norms, standard error of measurement, and standardized administration (Cohen, Hinojosa, & Kramer, 2005). Understanding the psychometric properties of each assessment tool utilized allows the occupational therapist to have confidence in the fairness and consistency of the results. Verifying the assessment tool's reliability (accuracy and stability of the test; get the same test scores each time the test is given under the same conditions) and validity (measures the constructs, traits, or behaviors it says it will measure) via the test manual and professional literature allows the occupational therapist to speak with authority concerning professional recommendations.

Therapists sometimes determine that only portions of a standardized assessment are appropriate, or busy therapists sometimes try to focus on only certain sections of a standardized assessment. You cannot, however, administer a portion of the assessment tool and still consider the scores valid or reliable. If an assessment tool has several subtests implemented in a particular order or sequence during the standardization process and the therapist only implements some of those subtests, those scores cannot be fairly compared to the standardized population who completed all subtests in the same sequence. Therefore, if the therapist has broken the rules of the assessment administration, then the client is denied the full exploration of his or her issues, resulting in a biased assessment of his or her performance.

Among standardized and nonstandardized assessments, there is also a subcategory of assessments encompassing performance-based versus occupation-based assessments. Performance-based assessments, sometimes referred to as *impairment-based*, measure specific units of performance, such as cognition or dexterity (Coster, 2013). This information may be helpful to aid in treatment planning; however, clinicians should be aware that improvement in impairment does not always equate to an improvement in occupation (Hocking, 2011). Occupation-centered assessments help keep clinicians focused on the client and their occupations rather than specific deficits (Hocking). Some refer to these assessments as *function-based assessments*.

Example of Assessments

Performance-Based	*Occupation-Based*
- Nine Hold Peg Test	- Canadian Occupational Performance Measure (COPM)
- Range of Motion or Strength Testing	- Occupational Self-Assessment
- Test of Visual Motor Skills	- Assessment of Occupational Functioning (AOF)

Although one might argue that standardized assessments are preferred given the evidence-based practice environment we are now in, this is not necessarily an accurate statement. Occupational therapy leaders have long argued the merits of using a variety of assessment tools in order to gain the most comprehensive view of client preferences, habits, routines, skills, and occupational performance levels. To improve on the value of obtaining standardized assessment scores, the therapist's clinical reasoning, professional judgment, and review of evidence-based practice may lead to incorporating non-standardized alternatives. Hinojosa, Kramer, and Crist (2005) argued that clinicians should question how best to get the needed information rather than what information is needed. Therefore, if nonstandardized methods (e.g., skilled observations, interviews, facility-designed questionnaires, checklists, histories, and/or data collection on the frequency and duration of the identified behavior) are deemed necessary to assessing a client's performance, each therapist must know his or her own skill level for implementation and interpretation in order to minimize subjectivity and personal bias.

Norm Referenced

Most tests are developed using a sample from the "normal" population. As a result, each client's scores can be compared to this "normal population." There are times when a test is developed from a group of persons with similar characteristics (i.e., age, gender, diagnosis). If this "normative" group matches your client's profile, the tool would be appropriate for implementation.

Criterion Referenced

A criterion-referenced assessment tool outlines a set of objective criteria or skill components used to document what the client is and is not able to master. In this type of assessment, the client's score is then compared to the set of expected criteria rather than to the performance of other people in a normative group. For example, the components of eating with a fork would be the following: (1) visually locates fork on table, (2) reaches for fork, (3) grasps fork, (4) brings fork to plate, (5) scoops or spears food, (6) brings fork to mouth, (7) opens mouth, (8) inserts fork in mouth, (9) closes lips around fork, (10) removes food from fork, and removes fork from mouth. In this scenario, a client's skill level could be documented and future skills requiring intervention can be identified. These tools are particularly helpful for children with physical or mental difficulties where standardized assessment tools that compare a child to a typically developing child's scores are inappropriate or inapplicable.

Culturally Sensitive Assessments

As previously stated, it is important for the occupational therapy practitioner to use assessment tools in the manner in which they were intended. If the standardization pool utilized during test development was homogeneous, the results for a client with differing characteristics will be limited and inadequate. For example, if the population sample included 500 men and 52 women, the results would be biased with regard to gender. Although many standardized tests are based on the demographic profile provided by the U.S. Census Bureau and the tool's manual should identify the scope of the

population sample used for standardization purposes, it is the clinician's responsibility to interpret the assessment results based on the cultural or ethnic differences of each specific client. For example, if the assessment requires a client to put pictures of his bedtime routine in order and he places "brush his teeth" after he is in bed, this would be clinical data for the therapist. However, if he did not include the brushing the teeth picture, this might be cultural versus clinical. Taugher (2000) identified this cultural bias in our assessment tools as a primary issue as health care shifts from hospital- or institution-based to community-based, and he posed several scenarios where decreased understanding of a client's cultural patterns might lead to inaccurate assessment of a person's skill level. The following examples could be culturally related or consistent with a diagnostic category:

- Talking fast (as with flight of ideas)
- Slow and laborious talk (as in depression and unable to pull thoughts together)
- Illogical syntax and thought (as in schizophrenia)

Lyons (2000) went on to include other examples, such as not sharing during an interview, not following through on home programming, and that clutter in the house yields an unsafe walking environment. Additionally, some cultures have specific gender roles, specific clothing or religious practices, or regard self-care practices in a different light (Black, 2011). A multitude of cultural differences can affect the evaluation process. Wells and Black (2000) defined cultural competency as "lifelong learning designed to foster understanding, acceptance, knowledge, and constructive relations between persons of various cultures and differences" (p. 147). With this definition in mind, it is each clinician's responsibility to seek out the research information necessary to be efficient, effective, and ethical for the variety of cultural influences on one's specific caseload.

Cultural sensitivity is the last point to be discussed and perhaps the most important. Historically, health care workers have the motto, "Treat the client as I would want to be treated." Salimbene (2000) argued just the opposite in her *10 Tips for Successful Caregiver/Client Interaction*. The premise of how "you" want to be treated is based on your cultural background and experiences. If this is not your client's background and you do not recognize that your interactions need to change based on the client's background, then you are not being culturally sensitive. Culturally competent care encompasses understanding the client's "culture and how it impacts health beliefs, health decisions, and activity choices" (Black, 2011, p. 104). With regard to the evaluation process, if you have not educated yourself on the routines, habits, traditions, and practices of a specific client's background, you are not practicing culturally competent care or being culturally sensitive. This is more than simply an insult; this leads to ineffective and inefficient information and inappropriate planning and is professionally unethical (Reitz et al., 2005).

REASSESSMENT

In addition to the professional requirements of reassessment for discharge planning purposes, which includes documenting current performance level and planning for additional or follow-up intervention, the documentation of intervention outcomes itself often requires a reassessment. In today's health care environment of accountability, an assessment tool might be utilized pre- and post-intervention as a mechanism to provide evidence of intervention outcomes, to measure change from the initial evaluation period, request further authorization of therapy visits, and/or to plan for discharge. Additionally, some insurances or payers require reassessment at certain time periods during intervention to support the skilled need of services (Centers for Medicare and Medicare Services, 2013). Using the same assessment tool would be the easiest method to detect change (i.e., by comparing the reassessment score with the initial assessment score and noting any change in score), but many assessment tools are not designed to be reimplemented (test–retest reliability). For example, if retested with the same standardized tool, the client might know what to expect, be comfortable with the format because he or she has been through it before (which is a difference from the first implementation), or become familiar with the test items from the first implementation. Additionally, different observers, testers, and raters should be factored into the reassessment process (termed *interrater reliability* in the test manual). Each factor would influence the reassessment score. Therefore, familiarity with the assessment tool manual is important in order for the clinician to fully understand the strengths and limitations of the assessment tool prior to reimplementation.

Once the assessment tool has been deemed appropriate to readminister, there are additional professional benefits to utilizing a pre- and post-administration of the tool. For example, utilizing pre- and post-assessment data for specific client groups allows the information to be used to compare or evaluate the outcomes for the client group as a whole, as well as provides the ability to compare each client's outcomes to the results found in more rigorous research studies completed on the same client group (Mandich, Miller, & Law, 2002).

A point of consideration, however, is the type and purpose of the reassessment. For example, administering a standardized tool before, during, and after intervention might not yield the information needed to alter or redefine a specific client-centered intervention plan. In fact, these tools might miss personal or environmental factors that need to be considered throughout the intervention process. However, ongoing measurements such as rating scales (criterion-referenced tools that identify objectively observable actions or behaviors) or skilled observations related to targeted goal areas would provide immediate feedback. This immediacy allows the clinician and client to determine if a change in plan is warranted to meet the specific goals for the individual client (Mandich et al., 2002).

SUMMARY

There is a wide variety of assessment tools available, and picking the appropriate tool for each specific client's profile requires individual consideration. The following list will help the practitioner pick the most appropriate tool while meeting professional standards:

- What is the credibility of the assessment tool, and is it commonly used in the profession?
- Does the occupational therapy literature support the use of this assessment tool as appropriate and applicable to occupational therapy practice?
- Is this tool appropriate, useful, and the best method to obtain the information I need?
- Am I adequately prepared and trained to implement and interpret this assessment?
- Are there any cultural (including education level, English as a first language, etc.) limitations for applicability?
- Does the tool have acceptable psychometric qualities (including reliability, validity, adequate specificity, and sensitivity) for my needs?

After choosing the assessment tool, the practitioner must be prepared to do the following:

- Follow the parameters outlined.
- Administer in the manner and for the population which the tool was intended (i.e., if intended for clients with dementia, do not use with clients diagnosed with schizophrenia).
- Interpret as intended and outlined in the manual.
- Provide a clinical rationale for any variance in established procedures, and provide a statement indicating that the results were not gained in the manner intended or outlined in the manual.
- Utilize all necessary assessment tools to gather the needed data within the evaluation process in order to provide the most comprehensive picture of the facilitators of and barriers to participation occupations.

Evaluation

In order to determine which assessment tools will best yield the necessary information and which pieces of information obtained are most important in understanding

---

Ms. Ana

After the physician referral for occupational therapy to see 89-year-old Ana for difficulties with feeding, the occupational therapist chose two assessment tools that focused on strength and cognition. Upon seeing the client at bedside in a skilled nursing facility, the occupational therapist noted that Ana was unable to sit up in the bed. This information prompted the occupational therapist to alter the formal assessment tools originally planned for the evaluation session. Rather, the therapist needed to investigate the client factors and performance skills that impact trunk stability prior to addressing feeding issues.

---

the client's needs, one cannot forget that evaluation is a fluid process. See Ms. Ana example.

To obtain a comprehensive picture of the client, the evaluation process requires ongoing clinical reasoning and a combination of both standardized and non-standardized assessment tools (Strickland, 2005). To complete an evaluation, the therapist must understand the strengths and limitations of each assessment tool, identify information that must be obtained outside of standardized or formal methods of the assessment tools previously mentioned, and make effective decisions about how the evaluation needs to be adjusted based on the findings during the evaluation process.

Evaluation Factors to Consider

In preparation for the evaluation process, several underlying issues need to be considered. Specifically, the influence of professional parameters and initiatives (AOTA, 2007a, 2008, 2010a, 2010b), evidence-based practice mandates (AOTA, 2007a; Holm, 2000), and reimbursement constraints. Additionally, depending on the context in which the evaluation must occur, various factors might be more pertinent than others, while some factors are universal across domains and contexts. This section will discuss considerations that the occupational therapy practitioner must be aware of during the evaluation process.

PROFESSIONAL

The Practice Framework (AOTA, 2008) provides parameters in which the occupational therapist and occupational therapy assistant must function. Specific information related to the components of this document related to evaluation will be presented in the following section, where the evaluation process is discussed. However, the influence of the ICF (WHO, 2001), from

which the framework was created, has greatly changed how the evaluative process is implemented. Specifically, the focus on function, participation, and context have contributed to the development of the framework and are consistent with the longstanding philosophy of occupational therapy to identify the facilitators of and barriers to functional participation in meaningful occupations.

EVIDENCE-BASED PRACTICE

An underlying premise of practice, specifically evaluation, is that decisions need to be made based on evidence. Effective decisions made within the evaluation process yield valuable information that, in turn, leads to appropriate intervention plans and, ultimately, improved outcomes. Muir Gray's (2004) "Doing the Right Things Right" outline for evidence-based medicine also applies to the occupational therapy evaluation process (Table 16-1). Additionally, evidence-based clinical decision models emphasize clinical expertise and client preference as equally important to research/evidence within the clinical process. This triad allows for the clinician to utilize his or her expertise and understanding of client preferences to determine the applicability and appropriateness of the external research evidence. Implementing a client-centered evaluation process, as recommended in occupational therapy literature, fits within this more global model of evidence-based clinical/medical practice. In order to make these decisions correctly, the occupational therapy practitioner needs to understand the design, rationale, strengths, and limitations of various assessment tools and interface this information with client preferences and clinical reasoning for various client populations.

ORGANIZATIONAL

While the unique perspective on occupational engagement should always guide our evaluative choices, the scope of evaluative responsibilities and procedures is determined by each specific setting. Organizations focusing primarily on client factors or performance skills (e.g., acute rehabilitation, hand therapy) literally set the stage for engagement in meaningful occupations later in the continuum of care. Additionally, each practice setting has its own philosophy, and ensuring a match with your own personal philosophy, including your own values and beliefs, is important because it will factor into the evaluative decisions made. Understanding your scope of practice as defined within a specific organization and ensuring it meets the scope of practice outlined by the professional credentialing body and state licensure laws is imperative prior to the implementation of any occupational therapy service.

The financial constraints of an organization will also influence the evaluative process. The assessment resources available; the time available in your schedule

Table 16-1.		
EVIDENCE-BASED EVALUATION PROCESS		
Performance	**Outcome**	**Evaluation Implications**
Doing the right things	Increasing effectiveness	• Choose appropriate evaluation methods and procedures to obtain the information critical to intervention planning and referral to others internal and external to the profession.
		• Ask: How can I best obtain the needed information?
Doing things right	Efficiency; cost effectiveness	• Adhere to the established professional standards related to the role of the occupational therapist and occupational therapy assistant.
		• Focus on occupational engagement throughout the process.
		• Familiarity with, and knowledge of, specific evaluation methods and procedures yields efficient utilization of time and resources.
Doing the right things right	Best; quality improvement	• Thorough documentation of the evaluative process results and plan of intervention.
		• Make effective decisions pertaining to the methods necessary to yield the best information for the evaluative purpose and determine the best or most efficient means of obtaining the needed information is both clinically appropriate and fiscally responsible

to complete the evaluation including implementation, processing information, and documentation; and the requirements of the funding source(s) greatly influence the methods chosen to obtain the necessary information. Therefore, it would be prudent for the practitioner to understand the unique attributes and limitations of the assessment methods within this section, develop a mentoring system to improve clinical reasoning skills related to evaluation implementation, and continually examine personal patterns of performance in order to meet the demands of current practice.

FUNDING SOURCE AND REFERRAL

Understanding the system in which you are working, and thus having specific knowledge of the funding source(s) or referral options, will also help to determine the appropriate assessment tool(s) to be used. First, the therapist needs to be sure the funding source's evaluation requirements to approve payment can be met. If there are requirements that cannot be completed (i.e., standardized scores are required but there is no tool available given the client's physical limitations), the therapist needs to contact the funding agency to clearly explain the limitations of the requirements and gain approval to continue in an alternative manner. Second, if the client has expressed concerns during the client profile that do not fall under the domain of the funding agency or the intervention site, this needs to be discussed and alternative or additional arrangements need to be explored with the organization's administration. It may be necessary to refer the client to another discipline or intervention facility.

It is also important to remember that each funding source has rules on who can refer a patient to occupational therapy. Typically for third-party payers, it is from a physician. Therefore, if the referral is not generated from the physician, as it is often from another professional, self-initiated by the client, or the client's parent after speaking to others in similar circumstances, having the client contact his or her physician for a prescription for occupational therapy would be necessary to ensure proper and timely payment (see Table 16-1).

Evaluation Components

With regard to an occupational therapy evaluation, AOTA (2007b) emphasizes the need to include client information, reason for referral, an occupational profile, the assessments utilized, the assessment results, summary and analysis, and recommendations. The first area, client information, will be dependent on the system in which the practitioner works, but it generally includes name, medical record number, age, insurance provider, referring doctor, diagnoses, medical history, medications, precautions, contraindications, and reason for referral (Figure 16-1). There are instances, however, where the client is an organization, population, or community that supports the engagement of individuals in functional activities. In those instances, the client information would include demographics of the group and any other information that would influence the evaluative process necessary to develop an intervention, support, consultation, or education plan for the group. The subsequent components of the evaluation process are as follows with additional information related to specific assessments, assessment results, and assessment analysis presented in the following chapters (Tables 16-2 and 16-3).

Center for Rehabilitation Excellence
1 Maine Street, Portland, Maine 04123
(888) 207-1234

Occupational Therapy Intake/Client Referral

Name:	DOB:
Address:	Phone:
Insurance/ ID Number:	
Date of Referral:	Referring Physician:
Diagnosis/Code:	
Date of Evaluation:	Name of Therapist:
Precautions:	
Past Medical History:	
Reason for Referral:	
Employer/Employment:	
Goals for Therapy:	
Notes:	

Figure 16-1. Sample intake/client profile form.

> The hospital in which you work has a standard procedure for a referral to occupational therapy if the admitted client has any injury to the head. In this case, you would have access to files with intake information related to the personal and medical histories, initial medical findings by your organization, reports written by the professionals who have already evaluated the client, and so on. In this scenario, your evaluation would focus on the identification of facilitators of and/or barriers to participation in the client's chosen occupations. In essence, are there occupational performance issues secondary to the diagnostic information warranting occupational therapy services?

> A parent calls your clinic to say her neighbor said to call as her baby is colicky and not eating well. In this case, with no other formal documentation available, and the parent potentially not even understanding what occupational therapy can offer, the clinician must obtain as much information as possible to help guide the decision-making process for the evaluation session. Equally important, however, is to remember that the therapeutic relationship begins during this initial conversation.

Reason for Referral

First and foremost, it is imperative to understand the reason for referral so that appropriate assessment methods can be identified. Although this may seem to be a basic concept, it is often overlooked. An occupational therapy evaluation referral can come from many sources, with varying levels of information for you to review and/or with specific outcomes expected. The examples in the boxes illustrate the diverse nature of referral information. If the referral does not have the required information, it would be the therapist's responsibility to obtain the required documentation. This lack of information can range from no age on the referral form to the lack of written documentation of medical clearance for the evaluation of a client with a neck injury. Regardless of what information is missing, the importance of complete information is clear.

These types of "systems" referrals often have specific evaluative procedures, outlined via departmental or organizational review, that need to be followed in order for "eligibility" for occupational therapy services to be determined. Other systems might utilize this type of procedure, including federal or state programs (i.e., Birth-to-Three and Boards of Education). As a point of clarification, these types of eligibility evaluations were previously termed *diagnostic evaluations* but should not be interpreted to indicate that a simple medical or rehabilitative diagnosis alone would determine eligibility. Rather, identifying the unique, client-specific facilitators of and barriers to functional participation in meaningful activities, which might include a qualifying test/assessment score if mandated, would be the information that determines eligibility. See *Reason for Referral* on p. 210 for an example.

The conversation must be a forum to respond to, respect, and empathize with the parent who is now fearful there is something wrong with his or her child; educate the parent on the types of issues that could be impacting the child's patterns; and provide reassurance that the parent is doing the right thing by investigating any support he or she believes would make his or her child's interactions with the world more calm and joyful. While this may be nonbillable therapeutic time, a full discussion with the parent/client at the time of the intake call would be critical for the process to move forward successfully. In fact, this is the beginning of the therapeutic relationship, and the implications of this concept should

Table 16-2.

ENGAGEMENT IN OCCUPATION TO SUPPORT PARTICIPATION IN CONTEXT OR CONTEXTS

• Performance in areas of occupation
  * Activities of daily living (ADL)
  * Instrumental activities of daily living (IADL)
  * Education
  * Work
  * Play
  * Leisure
  * Social participation
	• Context
	  * Cultural
	  * Physical
	  * Social
	  * Personal
	  * Spiritual
	  * Temporal
	  * Virtual

• Performance skills
  * Motor skills/habits
  * Process skills/routines
  * Communication/interaction skills/roles
	• Activity demands
	  * Objects used and their properties
	  * Space demands
	  * Social demands
	  * Sequencing and timing
	  * Required actions
	  * Required body functions
	  * Required body structures

• Performance patterns
  * Habits
  * Routines
  * Roles
	• Client factors
	  * Body functions
	  * Body structures

Adapted from American Occupational Therapy Association. (2008). Occupational therapy practice framework: Domain and process (2nd ed.). *American Journal of Occupational Therapy, 62*, 625-683.

Reason for Referral

The local psychologist has been working with an agitated client for the past 3 months. As the agitation has diminished, the psychologist realizes there are underlying difficulties related to home management, life skills, and ongoing issues with holding a job. While you may now have the psychologist's referral and report, which outlines some of the occupational challenges for the client, the underlying reason for these challenges needs to be investigated. This type of evaluation is intended to determine the most appropriate intervention plan rather than eligibility. In this case, the evaluation report might be more descriptive in nature versus simply stating scores from a standardized assessment tool. Stating that a client requires maximum assistance with a task does not delineate specific enough information; rather, describing the client's function, as with Ana and self-feeding, can facilitate an understanding of barriers and strengths for occupational performance and support the need for continued occupational therapy services.

not be overlooked. The bottom section of the intake/profile form provided in Figure 16-1 provides a framework for beginning this conversation.

It is important to recognize how these preliminary findings help you form an initial picture of the client in your mind. While this assists with designing your approach to the evaluation process, it should not limit your expectations of the client or eliminate the possibility of shifting your preliminary plans to accommodate for your own observations of performance with the unique perspective of occupation. Additionally, once the client's priorities and preferences are communicated—either by the client or by other significant persons if the client is unable—alternative assessment tools may need to be incorporated.

OCCUPATIONAL PROFILE

The occupational profile, defined in the framework as "information that describes the client's occupational history and experiences, patterns of daily living, interests, values, and needs" (AOTA, 2008), identifies and guides our understanding of the occupational issues that are important and meaningful to the client. Beginning the evaluation process with an occupational profile also

Table 16-3.	
COMPONENTS OF AN OCCUPATIONAL THERAPY EVALUATION	
Category	**Description**
Client profile	For recordkeeping purposes: Name; parent name if appropriate; age; client number if needed; funding identification number; contact information. For planning purposes: Pertinent diagnoses; relevant medical history; medications; precautions; limitations; contraindications.
Reason for referral	Generated by whom; for what reason; what information is being requested and for what purpose; include date of request on documentation.
Occupational profile	The framework mandates clinicians utilize a client-centered approach; obtain information that allows the practitioner to understand what is meaningful for the client; client's desired outcomes; past experiences and history contributing to the client's desired outcomes; client priorities and preferences; factors influencing meaningful engagement in occupations.
Assessments methods/tools utilized	Per the framework, the evaluation considers performance skills, performance patterns, context, activity demands, and client factors; an evaluation often requires the implementation of multiple assessment tools when possible; minimum expectations are to have sufficient data to plan interventions; document which tools have been utilized (standardized, norm referenced, criterion referenced, formal, informal, etc.), why implemented, why and how established protocols were not followed if applicable, and how these tools contributed to a full understanding of the client's needs; chosen assessment tools are bias free with regard to cultural (in the broadest sense) issues; therapists must have required level of skill and knowledge to implement the assessment tool; occupational therapist and occupational therapy assistant mutually determine which tools can be administered by the occupational therapy assistant based on level of expertise, training, supervision, and pertinent regulations.
Assessment tool(s) results	Score and report all formalized assessment results according to the procedures outlined in the test manual; identify limitations with information obtained if exact testing protocols were unable to be followed; indicate if you believe the assessment results to be accurate or inaccurate for any external reason; make no other assumptions on the data at this time; include skilled clinical observations and other informal findings.
Analysis and summary	Interpret the assessment findings, summarize strengths and vulnerabilities, and identify the supports and barriers to successful engagement or performance; synthesize the information in a manner consistent with the presenting concerns identified in the referral and the client's life and environment; incorporate information from formal and informal tools, observations, clinical judgment, and how these findings interface with the client's goals, interests, and preferences; do not overinterpret the data—report what you know from your clinical expertise and you can continue to investigate any unsubstantiated hypotheses during the intervention period; provide summary statement of findings.
Recommendation	Use clinical judgment to determine if services are warranted or additional referrals are necessary; these decisions must relate to the initial referral request, client preferences and priorities, potential intervention approach(es) based on best practice and evidence, and the feasibility of the intervention's success given the evaluative findings; identify the types of service that address the presenting concerns (i.e., education, consultation, direct, monitor); depending on the organization's funding source, this section may include goals, objectives, and specifics about the intervention recommended (i.e., frequency, duration)—otherwise, this information would belong in a plan of care.

supports the top-down approach to an occupational therapy evaluation as it begins with the client perspective of occupational performance and then works downward to investigate the factors (client specific or contextual) that contribute to occupational limitations.

ASSESSMENTS UTILIZED AND ASSESSMENT ANALYSIS

As stated earlier and as illustrated in Appendix B, there are many assessment tools available. Although the following chapters in this section will discuss specific assessment tools that focus on occupational performance components, it is clear that the choice of assessment tool(s) needs to be guided by the occupational profile. Therefore, the occupational therapy evaluation report needs to identify which tools were utilized to obtain the data, the rationale for the decision, any alterations to the assessment's procedures required, and how each of these choices contribute to the overarching view of occupation being evaluated. Within the analysis section of the occupational therapy evaluation report, it is important to discuss information from different assessment methods

Table 16-4.	DOCUMENTATION REQUIREMENTS
Professional	• Identify and meet agency/organization expectations and ensure these expectations match professional guidelines, licensure, and ethical responsibilities. • Write for the reader (target audience). • Differentiate direct observations from opinions regarding the performance (i.e., client stated she is the mother of 13 children versus client is delusional as she believes she is the mother of 13 children).
Legal	• Information for referral to another specialist should be prompt and comprehensive. • If using hard-copy format versus computerized, documentation should be legible and well organized. • Complete required documentation in a timely manner. • Remember, every piece of documentation is considered a legal document that can be subpoenaed. • All documentation should meet employer, accrediting body, and funding sources requirements. • All documentation should be complete and accurate (including dates of service and date of documentation of service if required). • If hardcopy format is utilized, do not change, remove, or alter your documentation with erasers or correction fluid. Simply cross out the error with a single line and initial to indicate it was you who deleted the piece of information. Put a line through unused lines or spaces on any forms. • Include only first hand information of what you see or hear versus what the client told you (i.e., client stated he completed the home program once per day versus client completed home program as designed). • Avoid negative statements because, aside from being unprofessional, they can be interpreted as though you disliked the client, then other information would be subject to interpretation. • The treating therapist must sign all documentation, including cosigning as the supervising therapist as required with name, professional credentials, and date. • Client name and identifying information should be on each page of documentation in case pages become separated.

that support the evaluator's analysis as well as information considered to be a contradiction.

Documentation

Documentation is necessary whenever professional services are provided to a client. Occupational therapists and occupational therapy assistants under the supervision of an occupational therapist determine the appropriate type of documentation and document the services provided with their scope of practice (AOTA, 2007b, p. 197).

Documentation is an important legal and professional component for all occupational therapy services, and it has an important function within the evaluation process. An evaluation report, which clearly, accurately, and comprehensively outlines the current level of functioning and concerns to be supported by occupational therapy, not only guides entrance into the health care arena but also offers a framework for communication with the client and other professionals. The evaluation also forms the basis for referral to specialists both internal and external to occupational therapy, establishes the rationale for financial support for services, and provides a mechanism to plan interventions moving forward, which will be

compared to this original baseline of performance. Sames (2005) argued that the report of the initial evaluation is the most important document the occupational therapist will write. Components of documentation requirements can be found in Table 16-4, and additional information can be found in Chapter 22.

PROFESSIONAL

As one begins the evaluation report, understanding the target audience or stakeholder will guide the presentation of results. For example, a report for a child's family for program planning purposes might look very different from a report for a third-party payer. Asking who needs the information and why (i.e., funding source, organization, external accrediting agency requirements) will assist the therapist in producing a report reflective of the practice setting. Despite the nuances, every occupational therapy report should have established components (see Table 16-2).

REIMBURSEMENT

Although documentation is important for the continuity of care and therapeutic intervention planning, it is also intricately linked to payment. Regardless of the payment source, documentation is a mechanism to obtain approval for payment through objective client measures. The type and frequency of documentation is generally determined by the payment source (e.g., federal or state programs, third-party payers, grant funding). Thus, in order to minimize the possibility of claim denial, the therapist needs to be fully aware of the rules and requirements, including any updates or revisions, prior to report completion. Additionally, effectively communicating this information from the perspective of occupational engagement will help distinguish occupational therapy from other therapeutic services also requesting payment for services, as occupational therapy reports on performance skill deficit and its impact on the client's daily occupations.

LEGAL REQUIREMENTS

Any written communication produced by occupational therapy personnel with regard to a client's care is considered a legal document and should be kept confidential in adherence to professional standards, state laws, and the Health Insurance Portability and Accountability Act (HIPAA; United States Department of Health and Human Services, 2002). Not only does the paperwork substantiate that the services were delivered, but it also serves to provide a history of what actually happened on behalf of the client. Even the screening, which led to a full evaluation, should be documented as a client contact in the chart; if it is not documented, it did not happen in the eyes of the law. Therefore, any errors, inconsistencies, or omissions can be used against you in a court of law. It is imperative for each clinician to understand the legal requirements of the funding source and the legal implications for the agency in which you work. Most employers will set the rules of how their staff should perform in terms of documentation, and once the practitioner is aware of the employer's expectations, it is important to be sure the expectations meet professional licensure, guidelines, and ethical expectations. It is the responsibility of the individual practitioner to ensure all of these requirements are met and communicate any disparities to the employer.

Each agency/organization has its own rules on the types of documentation required, as well as its own system of recording the information. If the system is computerized, thorough training for all occupational therapy personnel should be completed, and no other clinician should enter information into the client files of other therapists. If there are hard copy files, there may be one formal/official/legal file where all pertinent information needs to be recorded. Thereafter, there may be a clinical file by each clinician for information related to intervention planning, copies of performance measures, and day-to-day information the therapist needs to monitor and track. Although notes/documents/performance samples

are not in the "official" file, they are still considered legal documents, should be kept in a locked file cabinet, and can be subpoenaed in a court of law.

Summary

The occupational therapy evaluation process is a complicated procedure from a clinical perspective and an administrative process. As the initial evaluation is the entry into occupational therapy services, evaluation from an occupational perspective, competence in administration and interpretation of the assessment tools utilized, and efficient, accurate, and timely documentation are all necessary. Using the evidence-based medicine model previously discussed (Muir Gray, 2004), Table 16-1 provides a synopsis of this concept with regard to the evaluation process. The remainder of this section discusses specific assessment tools and their use in practice.

Student Self-Assessment

1. From the information provided on Mary's case study on p. 203, which assessment tools would be appropriate to administer and why? Which frame of reference do the chosen assessments follow? Identify a part of the assessment process an occupational therapy assistant might be able to complete.

2. Complete the Assessment Tool Grid in Appendix B with additional assessment tools from your coursework.

3. Identify various state, federal, and private funding sources that might influence the evaluative processes within a given practice setting.

4. Discuss how funding source limitations might influence the documentation of the full scope of your occupational therapy services.

5. Examine your own personal values and beliefs regarding service delivery, and identify how these might influence your approach to an occupational therapy evaluation.

6. Identify the assessment tools appropriate for Ana's case study given her inability to sit up in bed and its impact on self-feeding.

7. Based on one occupational therapy setting you have observed, create an intake form you believe would be appropriate in that environment.

8. Based on one occupational therapy client you observed this semester, assume the observed session was the evaluation session and complete the information requested in Table 16-2.

9. Referring to Table 16-4, create a list of situations that you have observed throughout your education

that might be in conflict with the rules provided. Be prepared to discuss these observations in class.

Electronic Resources

- The American Occupational Therapy Association for compliance with Standards of Practice: www. aota.org
- Department of Health and Human Services, Centers for Medicare & Medicaid Services: www.cms.hhs. gov

References

American Occupational Therapy Association. (2007a). *The Centennial Vision*. Bethesda, MD: Author. Retrieved from http://www.aota.org/News/Centennial.aspx

American Occupational Therapy Association. (2007b). Guidelines for documentation of occupational therapy. In *American Occupational Therapy Association. The reference manual of the official documents of the American Occupational Therapy Association* (12th ed., pp. 197-201). Bethesda, MD: AOTA Press.

American Occupational Therapy Association. (2008). Occupational therapy practice framework: Domain and process (2nd ed.). *American Journal of Occupational Therapy, 62*, 625-683.

American Occupational Therapy Association. (2009). Guidelines for supervision, roles, and responsibilities during the delivery of occupational therapy services. *American Journal of Occupational Therapy,63*(6), 797-803.

American Occupational Therapy Association. (2010a). Occupational therapy code of ethics and ethics standards. *American Journal of Occupational Therapy, 64*(6 Suppl.), S17-S26.

American Occupational Therapy Association. (2010b). Standards of practice for occupational therapy. *American Journal of Occupational Therapy, 64*(6 Suppl.), S106-S111.

Black, R. M., (2011). Cultural considerations of hand use. *Journal of Hand Therapy, 24*(2), 104-111. doi:10.1016/j.jht.2010.09.067.

Centers for Medicare and Medicare Services. (2013). *Therapy questions and answers*. Retrieved from http://www.cms.gov/Medicare/Medicare-Fee-for-Service-Payment/HomeHealthPPS/downloads/therapy_questions_and_answers.pdf

Cohen, M. E., Hinojosa, J., & Kramer, P. (2005). Administration of evaluation and assessments. In J. Hinojosa, P. Kramer, & P. Crist (Eds.), *Evaluation: Obtaining and interpreting data* (2nd ed., pp. 81-99). Bethesda, MD: AOTA Press.

Cooke, D. M., McKenna, K., & Fleming, J. (2005). Development of a standardized occupational therapy screening tool for visual perception in adults. *Scandinavian Journal of Occupational Therapy, 12*(2), 59-71.

Coster, W. J. (2013). Making the best match: Selecting outcome measures for clinical trials and outcome studies. *American Journal of Occupational Therapy, 67*(2), 162–170. doi: 10.5014/ajot.2013.006015

Hinojosa, J., Kramer, P., & Crist, P. (Eds.). (2005). *Evaluation: Obtaining and interpreting data*. Bethesda, MD: AOTA Press.

Hocking, C. (2001). Implementing occupation-based assessment. *American Journal of Occupational Therapy, 55*(4), 463-469.

Holm, M. B. (2000). The 2000 Eleanor Clarke Slagle lecture. Our mandate for the new millennium: Evidence-based practice. *American Journal of Occupational Therapy, 54*(6), 575-585.

Kielhofner, G. (2006). *Research in occupational therapy: Methods of inquiry for enhancing practice*. Philadelphia, PA: F. A. Davis Company.

Lyons, A. (2000). Cultural competence in occupational therapy practice. *Home & Community Health Special Interest Section Quarterly, 7*, 1-2.

Mandich, A., Miller, L., & Law, M. (2002). Outcomes in evidence-based practice. In M. Law (Ed.), *Evidence-based rehabilitation: A guide to practice* (pp. 49-69). Thorofare, NJ: SLACK Incorporated.

Miller, L. J. (1993). *First STEP screening test for evaluating preschoolers*. San Antonio, TX: Psychological Corp.

Muir Gray, J. A. (2004). *Evidence-based healthcare: How to make health policy and management decisions*. Upper Saddle River, NJ: Pearson Prentice Hall.

Parkinson, S., Forsyth, K., & Kielfhofner, G. (2006). *The model of human occupation screening tool*. Retrieved from http://www.uic.edu/depts/moho/assess/mohost.html

Reitz, S. M., Arnold, M., Franck, L. G., Austin, D. J, Hill, D., McQuade, L. J., et al. (2005). Occupational Therapy Code of Ethics (2005). *American Journal of Occupational Therapy, 59*(6), 639-642.

Salimbene, S. (2000). *What language does your patient hurt in? A practical guide to culturally competent patient care*. Amherst, MA: Diversity Resources.

Sames, K. M. (2005). *Documenting occupational therapy practice*. Upper Saddle River, NJ: Prentice Hall.

Strickland, L. S. (2005). Evaluation issues in today's practice. In J. Hinojosa, P. Kramer, & P. Crist (Eds.), *Evaluation: Obtaining and interpreting data* (2nd ed., pp. 51-58). Bethesda, MD: AOTA Press.

StrokEngine. (2013). *Glossary of terms*. Retrieved from http://strokengine.ca/assess/definitions-en.html

Taugher, M. (2000). Persons with limited English proficiency: A challenge for home and community practitioners. *Home & Community Health Special Interest Section Quarterly, 7*, 2-4.

U.S. Department of Health and Human Services. (2002). *Standards for privacy of individually identifiable health information*. Retrieved from http://www.hhs.gov/ocr/privacy/hipaa/news/2002/combinedregtext02.pdf

Wells, S. A., & Black, R. M. (2000). *Cultural competency for health professionals*. Bethesda, MD: AOTA Press.

World Health Organization. (2001). *International classification of functioning, disability and health*. Geneva, Switzerland: Author.

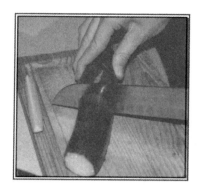

17

EVALUATION OF ACTIVITIES OF DAILY LIVING AND INSTRUMENTAL ACTIVITIES OF DAILY LIVING

Lisa J. Knecht-Sabres, DHS, OTR/L

ACOTE STANDARDS EXPLORED IN THIS CHAPTER
B.2.2, B.4.1, B.4.2, B.4.4, B.4.5

KEY VOCABULARY

- **Activities:** A class of human actions that are goal directed (AOTA, 2008).
- **Activities of daily living (ADL):** Activities that are oriented toward taking care of one's own body (AOTA, 2008).
- **Client-centered approach:** An approach to therapy that fosters a partnership with clients to enable them to identify their needs and individualize the services they perceive they will need in order to accomplish their goals (Law, Baum, & Dunn, 2005).
- **Instrumental activities of daily living (IADL):** Complex or domestic activities of daily living such as meal preparation, homemaking, and laundry (Fisher, 2003).

- **Occupational profile:** The initial step in the evaluation process that provides an understanding of the client's occupational history and experiences, patterns of daily living, interests, values, and needs. The client's problems and concerns about performing occupations and daily life activities are identified, and the client's priorities are determined (AOTA, 2002).
- **Occupations:** Activities that have unique meaning and purpose in a person's life. Occupations are central to a person's identity and competence, and they influence how one spends time and makes decisions (AOTA, 2002).

(continued)

215

Jacobs, K., MacRae, N., & Sladyk, K. (Eds.).
Occupational Therapy Essentials for
Clinical Competence, Second Edition (pp. 215-229).
© 2014 SLACK Incorporated.

KEY TERMS (CONTINUED)

- **Performance patterns:** The habits, routines, and roles that are adopted by an individual as he or she carries out occupations or daily life activities (AOTA, 2002).

- **Performance skills:** The goal-directed actions enacted in the context of occupational performance. They are the actions performed as one interacts with task objects in the context of enacting a task performance that is meaningful, purposeful, and relevant to the person who is performing the task (Fisher, 2005).

Introduction

Occupational therapy practitioners have a unique perspective of their clients. That is, the expertise of an occupational therapy practitioner lies in his or her ability to appreciate the broad range of human occupations and activities that make up peoples' lives (American Occupational Therapy Association [AOTA], 2008). Since occupational therapy practitioners focus on enabling people to engage (or re-engage) in the everyday activities that bring meaning and purpose to their lives, the occupational therapy practitioner's evaluation process must include an assessment of the daily activities the person either needs or wants to perform. According to the Occupational Therapy Practice Framework (OTPF) (AOTA, 2008), the types of activities people engage in each day consist of activities of daily living (ADL), instrumental activities of daily living (IADL), education, work, play, leisure, and social participation.

The OTPF defines occupations as activities that have unique meaning and purpose in one's life, are central to one's identity, and influence how one spends time and makes decisions.

Similarly, Fisher, Bryze, and Hume (2002) defined occupations as the purposeful and meaningful task performances people engage in that support the social and personal roles that define each person. In contrast, the OTPF asserted that activities are the tasks or actions in which an individual may participate in order to achieve a goal. Thus, one of the key differences between occupations and activities is that, even though certain activities may be vital to the completion of an occupation, activities do not hold a place of central importance or meaning to the individual. For instance, even though a person may highly value his or her role as a parent, and despite the fact that this role is central to his or her identity and influences how he or she spends her time, it may entail numerous activities that are not particularly important or meaningful to this person. Another way to look at the difference between an occupation and an activity is with

an example related to cooking. For instance, one person may view cooking as a mandatory activity that needs to be done on a daily basis to sustain life. However, another person may view cooking as an occupation, whether it is because the person is the head chef in an Italian restaurant or because the person finds enormous pleasure and a sense of fulfillment from making gourmet meals for family and friends.

This chapter focuses on how occupational therapy practitioners should approach the evaluation of ADL and IADL with their clients (Table 17-1). The OTPF (AOTA, 2008) defines ADL as the activities that are oriented toward taking care of one's own body. They include the following (AOTA, 2008):

- Bathing/showering
- Bowel and bladder management
- Dressing
- Eating
- Feeding
- Functional mobility
- Personal device care
- Personal hygiene and grooming
- Sexual activity
- Sleep/rest
- Toilet hygiene

The OTPF defines IADL as activities that are oriented toward interacting with the environment and often complex. IADL include the following (AOTA, 2008):

- Care of others
- Care of pets
- Child rearing
- Use of communication devices
- Community mobility
- Financial management

Table 17-1.

ROLE OF THE OCCUPATIONAL THERAPIST VERSUS ROLE OF THE OCCUPATIONAL THERAPY ASSISTANT WITH ACTIVITIES OF DAILY LIVING AND INSTRUMENTAL ACTIVITIES OF DAILY LIVING EVALUATION

Occupational Therapist	Occupational Therapy Assistant
Administer standardized and nonstandardized screening and assessment tools to determine the need for occupational therapy intervention including but limited to (1) specific screening tools; (2) assessments; (3) skilled observation; (4) checklists; (5) histories; (6) interviews with the client, family, and significant others; and (7) consultations with other professionals.	Gather and share data for the purposes of screening and evaluation by implementing delegated assessments including but not limited to (1) specific screening tools; (2) assessments; (3) skilled observation; (4) checklists; (5) histories; (6) interviews with the client, family, and significant others; and (7) consultations with other professionals.
Select appropriate assessment tools based on client need, contextual factors, and psychometric properties of tests. The assessment tools must be relevant to the individual client, based on available evidence, and incorporate occupational performance in the assessment process. Use appropriate procedures and protocols when administering assessments.	Administer selected assessments using appropriate procedures and protocols including standardized formats and use of occupation for the purpose of assessment.
Evaluate client's occupational performance in ADL, IADL, education, work, play, leisure, and social participation, including: • Client factors • Performance patterns • Contextual factors • Activity demands affecting performance • Performance skills	Gather and share data for the purposes of evaluating client's occupational performance in ADL, IADL, education, work, play, leisure, and social participation, including: • Client factors • Performance patterns • Contextual factors • Activity demands affecting performance • Performance skills
Determine the client's goals and priorities. Establish intervention priorities. Determine additional assessment needs. Determine specific assessment tasks that can be delegated to the occupational therapy assistant.	
Interpret criterion-referenced and norm-referenced standardized test scores based on an understanding of sampling, normative data, standard and criterion scores, reliability, and validity.	
Consider factors that might bias assessment results such as culture, disability status, and situational variables related to the individual and context.	
Interpret the evaluation data in relation to accepted terminology of the profession and relevant theoretical frameworks.	
Evaluate the appropriateness and discuss mechanisms for referring clients for additional evaluation to specialists internal and external to the profession.	Identify when to recommend to the occupational therapist the need for referring clients for additional evaluation.
Document occupational therapy services to ensure accountability of service provision and to meet standards for reimbursement of services, adhering to applicable facility, local, state, federal, and reimbursement agencies. Documentation must effectively communicate the need and rationale for occupational therapy services.	Document occupational therapy services to ensure accountability of service provision and to meet standards for reimbursement of services, adhering to applicable facility and local, state, federal, and reimbursement agencies. Documentation must effectively communicate the need and rationale for services.
In Summary	
The occupational therapist initiates and directs the evaluation process.	The occupational therapy assistant contributes to the evaluation process by implementing delegated assessments and sharing the findings with the occupational therapist.
The occupational therapist interprets the data, including information provided by occupational therapy assistant, and develops the intervention plan.	

- Health management and maintenance
- Home establishment and maintenance
- Meal preparation and clean-up
- Safety procedures and emergency responses
- Shopping

Each ADL and IADL activity listed is individually defined in the OTPF. The first critical step in any occupational therapy evaluation is to obtain an understanding of the client's occupational profile (AOTA, 2008). In other words, it is imperative for the occupational therapy practitioner to gain a deep understanding of the person's occupational history and experiences, patterns of daily living, interests, values, and needs. Furthermore, it is essential to ascertain the person's concerns about performing his or her occupations and daily life activities, as well as his or her priorities for occupational performance. After obtaining the occupational profile, the next vital step in the evaluation process is the analysis of occupational performance, which requires the therapist to observe the person's occupational performance, ideally within the natural context, in order to determine what supports and hinders performance (AOTA, 2008).

Obtaining the Client's Occupational Profile

Since the first essential step in the occupational therapy evaluation process is to obtain an understanding of the person's occupational profile, the occupational therapy practitioner needs to decide how he or she is going to gather this vital information. Using a client-centered approach to evaluate one's ADL and IADL provides a natural means for the client to identify his or her own unique occupational performance problems that are pertinent to his or her unique circumstances and context (Law et al., 2005). There are a few occupational therapy evaluations that evaluate occupational performance in a client-centered manner. The Canadian Occupational Performance Measure (COPM) (Law, Baptiste, et al., 2005) appears to be a widely used and clinically sound client-centered occupational therapy evaluation tool. The COPM is a semistructured interview designed to have the client do the following (Law, Baptiste, et al., 2005):

- Identify concerns regarding his or her performance during self-care, productivity, and leisure activities.
- Evaluate his or her performance and satisfaction relative to the identified problematic occupational performance areas.
- Prioritize his or her problems in occupational performance.

- Measure changes in his or her perception of his or her occupational performance over the course of occupational therapy intervention.

The COPM can be used with virtually any client regardless of his or her age or diagnosis because this tool can be administered to a family member or caregiver if the client is unable to participate in the interview. Not only is the COPM an excellent tool to gain critical information about the client's occupational profile, but equally important is the plethora of research on the COPM, which has repeatedly demonstrated the reliability and validity of this tool, as well as the usefulness of this tool as an outcome measure (Carswell et al., 2004; Dedding, Cardol, Eyssen, Dekker, & Beelen, 2004; Gilbertson & Langhorne, 2000; Harper, Stalker, & Templeton, 2006; Kjeken et al., 2005; Pan, Chung, & Hsin-Hwei, 2003; Persson, Rivano-Fischer, & Eklund, 2004; Verkerk, Wolf, Louwers, Meester-Delver, & Nollet, 2006; Wressle, Lindstrand, Neher, Marcusson, & Henricksson, 2003).

Other occupational therapy evaluation tools that measure occupational performance and capture the client's perspective regarding his or her performance include, but are not limited to, the Occupational Self-Assessment (OSA; Ay-Woan, Sarah, Lyinn, Tsyr-Jang, & Ping-Chuan, 2006; Baron, Kielhofner, Ienger, Goldhammer, & Wolenski, 2002; Kielhofner & Forsyth, 2001), the Child Occupational Self-Assessment (COSA; Keller, Kafkes, Basu, Federico, & Kielhofner, 2004; Keller & Kielhofner, 2005), and the Occupational Performance History Interview: Version 2.0 (Kielhofner et al., 1998).

The OSA, like the COPM, was developed to capture the client's perceptions of his or her own occupational competence. However, in addition to enabling the client to identify and prioritize his or her problems in occupational performance, it was also designed to assess the impact of the environment on the client's occupational adaptation. More specifically, the client is asked to respond to a series of statements about his or her occupational competence by labeling each as an area of strength, adequate functioning, or weakness, and then indicate the level of importance of each item. Likewise, the client is asked to respond to a series of questions related to his or her environment by identifying components of the environment that either support or hinder occupational competence. Similarly, the client is asked to identify the level of importance of each item related to the environment. The last step in the OSA entails having the client identify specific items from both the occupational and environmental assessment forms that he or she would like to change/focus on in therapy. Comparable to the OSA, the COSA was developed to provide an assessment tool in which a child can be actively involved in the occupational therapy evaluation and intervention process. Similar to the OSA, the COSA has the child identify and prioritize his or her problems in occupational performance on a child-friendly 4-point scale.

Observation of Performance

After determining the person's occupational profile, the next essential step in the evaluation process, according to the OTPF, is to observe the client's occupational performance, ideally within the natural context, in order to determine what supports and hinders performance (AOTA, 2008). Observation of occupational performance is vital to the assessment process, especially because information from an interview alone may be inaccurate. For instance, a client may overestimate his or her functional abilities out of fear of being admitted to a nursing home. Or, perhaps the client may overestimate or underestimate his or her abilities because he or she has not even had the opportunity to perform his or her ADL or IADL since the onset of his or her accident, injury, or illness.

Because there are numerous standardized and nonstandardized methods available, the shrewd therapist will base his or her decision to use a particular ADL/IADL assessment tool on sound critical-thinking skills. That is, the astute occupational therapist should ask him- or herself a series of questions before selecting an assessment tool. For example, the therapist should ask him- or herself the following:

- Which specific ADL and/or IADL needs to be evaluated for each individual client?

- What are the advantages and disadvantages of the particular evaluation tools available to assess the explicit needs of each individual client?

- Is the purpose of the evaluation to determine why the client is having difficulty performing his or her ADL and/or IADL, or is the purpose of the evaluation to determine if a client is able to perform his or her ADL and IADL safely and/or independently? Or, perhaps, is the purpose of the evaluation to demonstrate the extent of improvement or the effectiveness of intervention?

- Is the selected method an efficient use of time?

- Is there evidence to support the soundness of the selected evaluation tool?

Needless to say, the therapist who takes time to ensure best practice in every step of the evaluation process is very different from the therapist who decides to use an evaluation tool just because "it's the tool that all of the therapists in the facility use" or because "I've always done it this way."

After completing the occupational profile, the occupational therapist should have a clear understanding of which specific ADL and/or IADL need to be observed for each individual. The specific ADL and/or IADL to be assessed should relate directly to the client's unique desires, choices, and needs. For example, the types of activities to be assessed for a client who lives alone, was previously independent in all ADL and IADL, does not have any support systems, plans on returning to his or her previous environment, and wants and needs to be independent in almost all ADL and IADL should be very different from the types of activities to be assessed for a client who lives with a spouse; participated in very few IADL previously; and has no desire or need to cook, clean, do laundry, or pay the bills. Likewise, the types of ADL and IADL to be assessed throughout the lifespan (e.g., a very young child versus an adolescent versus a young adult versus an older adult) will differ as well.

Furthermore, since occupational performance involves a transaction between the individual, the task, and the environment (Law et al., 1996), it is essential that the therapist not only consider selecting a specific ADL and/or IADL assessment based on the type of activities it evaluates, but also select a tool that provides the occupational therapy practitioner with critical information regarding the individual and the environment. Likewise, the OTPF (AOTA, 2008) asserted that the execution of a performance skill occurs when the performer, the context, and the demands of the activity unite in the performance of an activity. In other words, each factor (the individual, the task, and the environment) influences the execution of a skill and may support or hinder performance skills and, ultimately, one's occupational performance. Thus, the most accurate means to assess one's ability to perform his or her ADL and/or IADL is to observe the client's performance within its natural context. Not only does the literature suggest that observation of occupational performance within the natural context is a more accurate means of assessment, but researchers have also indicated that it is a better predictor of safety and independence as well (Doble, Fisk, Fisher, Ritvo, & Murray, 1994; Linden, Boschian, Eker, Schalen, & Nordstrom, 2005; McNulty & Fisher, 2001; Park, Fisher, & Velozo, 1994). Lastly, observation of occupational performance in its natural context, as well as the identification of performance skill deficits, should provide the skilled therapist with the necessary information to determine the method of intervention (i.e., if the intervention will focus on remediation of performance skills, compensation, or a combination of remediation and compensation).

While there are a plethora of instruments to assess one's ability to perform his or her ADL and IADL, most standardized ADL and IADL assessments tools have the following characteristics:

- Are not designed to be flexible (i.e., meet the distinct needs of each individual client).

- Do not assess the individual's performance skills in the context of one's occupational performance.

- Do not consider the impact of the environment on occupational performance.

- Do not provide the therapist with information related to why the individual is having problems with his or her performance.

These factors have probably led to the popularity of many "homegrown evaluation tools," which have little (if any) evidence to support their use.

As indicated previously, an occupational therapy practitioner needs to consider the individual's skills underlying occupational performance when observing and assessing ADL and IADL. The performance skills are the goal-directed actions enacted in the context of occupational performance and consist of the individual's motor, process, and social/interaction skills (Fisher, 2005). To date, the Assessment of Motor and Process Skills (AMPS) (Fisher & Jones, 2012) is the only client-centered, performance-based, standardized occupational therapy ADL/IADL evaluation tool available to the occupational therapy practitioner. AMPS is unique for several reasons (Bernspang, 1999; Bernspang & Fisher, 1995; Dickerson & Fisher, 1995; Doble, Fisk, Lewis, & Rockwood, 1999; Ellison, Fisher, & Duran, 2001; Fisher, Liu, Velozo, Pan, 1992; Goldman & Fisher, 1997; Goto, Fisher, & Mayberry, 1996; Magalhães, Fisher, Bernspång, & Linacre, 1996; McNulty & Fisher, 2001; Sellers, Fisher, & Duran, 2001; Stauffer, Fisher, & Duran, 2000):

The client is able to self-select which ADL and/or IADL he or she wants to perform.

- It contains over 10 standardized ADL tasks and over 75 standardized IADL tasks.

- It emphasizes the importance of the client performing each task in his or her usual manner.

- It measures the quality of a person's performance in terms of effort, efficiency, safety, and independence.

- It assesses the motor and process skills (not the person's underlying functions or capacities).

- It can be used with all persons above 3 years of age, regardless of the client's diagnosis or reason for his or her disability.

- It provides information to the occupational therapy practitioner that aids in the planning of effective interventions.

- It is a sensitive evaluation tool that can be used to document change and outcomes.

- There is strong evidence of its reliability and validity both internationally and cross-culturally.

Thus, in other words, AMPS is currently the only standardized assessment tool available to occupational therapists that evaluates the individual's performance skills during the performance of client-centered ADL and/or IADL occurring within its natural context.

Much like the AMPS evaluates performance skills during the natural context of ADL and IADL, the School AMPS evaluates performance skills during the natural context of schoolwork. When evaluating a child, adolescent, or young adult (if applicable), it is imperative that the occupational therapy practitioner assess that individual's ability to fulfill his or her role as a student. Since an individual is able to assume the role of student only to the extent that he or she can effectively perform those tasks integral to defining that role, it is vital that the occupational therapy practitioner observe and determine which of the student's activities support and/or hinder performance (Fisher et al., 2002). The School AMPS (Fisher et al., 2005) is a tool that enables a true top-down (Trombly, 1993), client-centered, and occupationally based approach to the assessment and intervention of the student's role performance within the classroom environment. However, the School AMPS addresses schoolwork performance only and not the ADL or IADL related to student role performance (e.g., getting on/off a bus, dressing for gym class, using communication devices).

On the other hand, the School Function Assessment (SFA) (Coster, Deeny, Haltiwanger, & Haley, 1998) is a criterion-referenced assessment that measures the student's ability to participate in most of the tasks expected of a student in the school setting. The SFA is a judgment-based questionnaire designed to measure the student's performance in a wide variety of functional tasks that support the student's participation in the academic and social aspects of elementary education. The SFA contains three scales. The student's teacher or other knowledgeable professional within the school environment rates the following:

- Level of participation in a variety of school settings (e.g., in the classroom, on the playground or at recess, during lunch/snack time, during transportation, in the bathroom, and while moving from one location in the school to another).

- Type or amount of task support needed with a wide variety of physical and cognitive/behavioral tasks (e.g., using classroom materials, managing clothes and personal hygiene, ability to access the school environment).

- Performance on very specific physical and cognitive/behavioral tasks (e.g., using writing utensils, wiping or cleaning self after toileting, washing hands, opening and closing doors).

Thus, even though the SFA does assess the child's ability to perform a variety of ADL and IADL in the school setting and considers the environmental modifications and/or lack thereof, unfortunately it does not formally assess the student's performance skills as defined by the framework (AOTA, 2008). Furthermore, the SFA does not provide the therapist with any information regarding the student's opinion of his or her performance, the student's level of satisfaction, or which specific activities the student would prefer to address. Thus, if the SFA is administered, the occupational therapy practitioner will need to use his or her keen observational skills to determine why the client is unable to perform the various tasks in the school environment and, perhaps, may want to also consider using a client-centered assessment like the school setting interview (Hemmingsson, Egilson, Hoffman, & Kielhofner, 2005; Hemmingsson, Kottorp, & Bernspang, 2004) or the COPM (Law, Baptiste, et al., 2005) in order to gain a better appreciation of the student's opinion regarding his or her own level of satisfaction with his or her own performance in the school setting.

The Functional Independence Measure (FIM) (Uniform Data System for Medical Rehabilitation [UDSMR], 1999) and the WeeFIM (UDSMR, 2000) are two tools that are commonly used in rehabilitation settings and have a substantial amount of evidence to support their use as outcome measures (Cohen & Marino, 2000; Cottir, Burgio, Stevens, Roth, & Gitlin, 2002; Dickson & Köhler, 1995; Dodds, Martin, Stolov, & Deyo, 1993; Granger & Hamilton, 1992; Lundgren-Nilsson et al., 2005; Ottenbacher et al., 2000; Stineman, Ross, Fiedler, Granger, & Maislin, 2003). However, the therapist must keep in mind the purpose of these instruments and what type of information is gained through their administration. That is, the FIM and WeeFIM are part of the UDSMR and were developed to measure the effectiveness of medical rehabilitation services and programs. In other words, the FIM was not developed to specifically aid occupational therapists in their assessment and intervention process (i.e., it does not assess the person's performance skills and it does not provide the therapist with any information as to why the person is having difficulty with the observed tasks). However, since the FIM and WeeFIM are discipline-free assessments, they can be administered by any health care professional (e.g., nurse, physical therapist, speech therapist) and have the potential to create a common language that can be used across disciplines. In addition, the FIM and WeeFIM measure functional ability/degree of disability and were designed to detect change over time by rating the client's performance across three different domains (self-care, motor, and cognitive) on a 7-point scale (7 = complete independence and 1 = complete assistance).

Summary

The purpose of this chapter was to introduce the occupational therapy practitioner to the general process of evaluating a person's ability to perform his or her ADL and IADL. As previously indicated, the first critical step in any occupational therapy evaluation is to obtain an understanding of the person's occupational profile (AOTA, 2008). After obtaining the occupational profile, it is vital that the occupational therapy practitioner observe the person's occupational performance in order to determine what supports and hinders performance

(AOTA, 2008). Since occupational performance involves a transaction between the individual, the task, and the environment (Law et al., 1996), it is essential the therapist not only consider selecting a specific ADL and/or IADL assessment based on the type of activities it evaluates, but he or she should also consider selecting a tool that provides him or her with critical information regarding the individual and the environment. There are a plethora of ADL and IADL tools available to the occupational therapy practitioner. However, best practice entails selecting a specific evaluation tool based on sound critical-thinking skills, as well as the evidence available to support its use. This chapter introduces the occupational therapy practitioner to a few of the ADL/IADL evaluation tools available (Table 17-2). Since there are an abundance of other tools available to the occupational therapy practitioner, it is imperative that he or she takes the time to go through the clinical reasoning process outlined in this chapter to ensure that whatever tool is chosen, it meets not only the needs of the therapist, but also the unique aspects of the client and his or her environment.

Student Self-Assessment

1. Define the terms *occupation* and *activity*. Provide an example from your own life that demonstrates that you are able to differentiate the two terms.

2. Define the terms *activities of daily living* and *instrumental activities of daily living*. Provide at least five examples of each term.

3. What is an occupational profile? Describe how an occupational therapy practitioner can best obtain information related to his or her client's occupational profile.

4. After obtaining the client's occupational profile, what is the next vital step in the evaluation process of one's ADL and IADL?

5. What is the ultimate purpose of observing the client's occupational performance?

6. Name at least two evaluation tools that capture the client's perception of his or her occupational performance and have the client identify the level of importance of each identified ADL and/or IADL.

7. What is the name of the client-centered, performance-based ADL/IADL evaluation tool that was designed to assist the occupational therapy practitioner in the intervention planning process?

8. Describe some of the principles that a therapist should consider before selecting which specific evaluation tool he or she should use to assess performance in ADL and IADL.

9. Become familiar with the assessment tools discussed in this chapter. Compare and contrast them.

Table 17-2. SUMMARY OF SELECTED ACTIVITIES OF DAILY LIVING AND INSTRUMENTAL ACTIVITIES OF DAILY LIVING EVALUATION TOOLS			
Name of Assessment	**Areas of Assessment**	**Type of Client**	**Format of Assessment**
Assessment of Motor and Process Skills (AMPS)	Quality of motor and process skills in the performance of 11 possible ADL and/or 73 possible IADL	3 years and older Any diagnosis or disability	Client self-selects one to three ADL/IADL items. Therapist observes the client's motor and process skills concurrently with the observation of occupational performance and rates each motor and process skill item on a 4-point scale. The calibrated AMPS rater is able to input data into computer scoring software. Results of AMPS data can be used to answer: (1) Why is the client experiencing difficulty? (2) What level of task challenge can the client manage? (3) Is the client a candidate for restorative interventions via the use of therapeutic occupation or compensatory interventions via the use of adaptive occupations? and (4) Has the client's ADL/IADL performance improved?
Canadian Occupational Performance Measure (COPM)	Client's self-perception of his or her performance in self-care, productivity, and leisure	Any age Any diagnosis or disability	Semi-structured interview. The client: (1) identifies concerns regarding his or her performance during self-care, productivity, and leisure activities; (2) evaluates his or her performance and satisfaction relative to the identified problematic occupational performance areas; and (3) prioritizes his or her problems in occupational performance. The COPM is able to measure changes in the client's perception of his or her occupational performance over the course of occupational therapy intervention.
Child Occupational Self-Assessment (COSA)	The client's self-perception of sense of competence and level of importance in everyday activities in his or her home, school, and community	Any child able to self-report	Self-report assessment is composed of 24 statements related to everyday activities in the client's home, school, and community. Child rates each item in terms of personal competence and level of importance on a 4-point child-friendly scale. There are two different formats to choose from: the card sort method or the checklist format.
Functional Independence Measure (FIM)	Level of independence/disability on a total of 18 items related to: (1) self-care (eating, grooming, bathing, dressing, and toileting), (2) sphincter control (bowel and bladder management), (3) transfers (bed/chair/wheelchair, toilet, and tub/shower), (4) locomotion (walk/wheelchair and stairs), (5) communication (comprehension and expression), and (6) social cognition (social interaction, problem solving, and memory)	Adults with various physical disabilities	Therapist observes client's performance and rates each item on a 7-point scale (7 = complete independence, 1 = total assistance). Scores are intended to reflect the impact of the disability on the individual and on the human and economic resources in the community.

(continued)

Table 17-2 (continued).

SUMMARY OF SELECTED ACTIVITIES OF DAILY LIVING AND INSTRUMENTAL ACTIVITIES OF DAILY LIVING EVALUATION TOOLS

Name of Assessment	Areas of Assessment	Type of Client	Format of Assessment
Occupational Self-Assessment (OSA)	Measures (1) client's perceptions of his or her competence in occupational performance, using the Model of Human Occupation as a framework and (2) the impact of the environment on the client's occupational adaptation	All occupational therapy clients who can self-report	Self-rated occupational performance. On a 4-point scale, the client labels: (1) each statement about his or her occupational performance as an area of strength, adequate functioning, or weakness; (2) components of the environment that either support or hinder occupational competence; (3) the level of importance of each item; and (4) specific items from both the occupational and environmental assessment forms that he or she would like to change/focus on in therapy.
Occupational Performance History Interview (OPHI-II)	Explores a client's life history in the areas of work, self-care, and play Assesses the impact of disability on occupational performance Identifies the direction in which the client would like to take in his or her life	Any client capable of responding to a life history interview	Semistructured interview. After the interview, the therapist fills out rating forms related to occupational identity, occupational competence, and occupational settings.
Pediatric Evaluation of Disability (PEDI)	Describes a child's functional status as it relates to self-care, mobility, and social function Monitors change in individuals or groups of children with functional disabilities Can be used for program evaluation of inpatient, outpatient, or school-based programs	Children 6 months to 7.5 years old (or older if their functional development is delayed)	Parents or professionals fill out a 3-part form related to: (1) functional skills, (2) caregiver assistance, and (3) modifications. Each of these three parts is further divided into a self-care domain, a mobility domain, and a social function domain. Items on Part I: Functional Skills are rated on a 2-point scale (able or unable to perform). Items on Part II: Caregiver Assistance are rated on a 6-point scale ranging from total assistance to independent. Items on Part III: Modification are rated on a 4-point scale ranging from extensive modifications to no modifications. Scores can be put into a computer program or it can be scored manually. Raw scores, normative standard scores, or scaled scores can be used.
School Function Assessment (SFA)	Measures and monitors a student's ability to participate in most of the tasks expected of a student in elementary school	Students in elementary school, grades kindergarten through 6th grade	A criterion-referenced assessment. Teacher or other professional in the school setting fills out 3-part evaluation form. Part I evaluates the student's level of participation in various school settings on a 6-point scale (1 = extremely limited participation; 6 = full participation). Part II assesses the student's need for assistance or modifications on various physical and cognitive/behavioral tasks. Items are rated on a 4-point scale (1 = extensive assistance/modification; 4 = no assistance/modification). Part III assesses the student's functional performance on specific activities in the school setting. Items are rated on a 4-point scale (1 = does not perform; 4 = consistent performance).

(continued)

Table 17-2 (continued).

SUMMARY OF SELECTED ACTIVITIES OF DAILY LIVING AND INSTRUMENTAL ACTIVITIES OF DAILY LIVING EVALUATION TOOLS

| School Setting Interview | Allows the child/adolescent with a disability to describe the impact of the environment on his or her functioning in the school setting | Students 10 years old through high school with some type of motor dysfunction | A semistructured interview containing 16 items regarding everyday school activities that provide the occupational therapy practitioner with information about the child's functioning and need for adjustments in the school setting. Each item is rated on a 4-point scale related to the student-environment fit (1 = unfit/needs new adjustments; 4 = perfect fit/no need for adjustments). |

EVIDENCE-BASED RESEARCH CHART

Evaluation Tool	Evidence
The Assessment of Motor and Process Skills (AMPS)	Bernspang, 1999; Bernspang & Fisher, 1995; Dickerson & Fisher, 1995; Doble et al., 1999; Ellison et al., 2001; Fisher et al., 1992; Goldman & Fisher, 1997; Goto et al., 1996; Magalhães et al., 1996; McNulty & Fisher, 2001; Sellers et al., 2001; Stauffer et al., 2000
The School Assessment of Motor and Process Skills (School AMPS)	Atchison, Fisher, & Bryze, 1998; Fisher, Bryze, & Atchison, 2000; Fisher, Bryze, Hume, & Griswold, 2005
The Barthel Index	Gauggel et al., 2004; Houlden, Edwards, McNeil, & Greenwood, 2006; Hsueh, Lin, Jeng, & Hsieh, 2006; Nicholl, Hobart, Dunwoody, Cramp, & Lowe-Strong, 2004; Sangha et al., 2005; van Exel, Scholte op Reimer, & Koopmanschap, 2004
The Child Occupational Self-Assessment (COSA)	Keller et al., 2004; Keller, Kafkes, & Keilhofner, 2005; Keller & Kielhofner, 2005
The Canadian Occupational Performance Measure (COPM)	Carswell et al., 2004; Dedding et al., 2004; Gilbertson & Langhorne, 2000; Harper et al., 2006; Kjeken et al., 2005; Pan et al., 2003; Persson et al., 2004; Verkerk et al., 2006; Wressel et al., 2003
The Functional Independent Measure (FIM) and Wee FIM	Cohen & Marino, 2000; Cottir et al., 2002; Dickson & Köhler, 1995; Dodds et al., 1993; Granger & Hamilton, 1992; Lundgren-Nilsson et al., 2005; Ottenbacher et al., 2000; Stineman et al., 2003
The Kohlman Evaluation of Living Skills (KELS)	Pickens et al., 2007; Thomson, 1992; Zimnavoda, Weinblatt, & Katz, 2002
The Occupational Self-Assessment (OSA)	Ay-Woan et al., 2006; Baron et al., 2006; Kielhofner & Forsyth, 2001
The Occupational Performance History Interview (OPHI-II)	Kielhofner, Dobria, Forsyth, & Basu, 2005; Kielhofner, Mallinson, Forsyth, & Lai, 2001; Mallinson, Mahaffey, & Kielhofner, 1998
The Nottingham Extended Activities of Daily Living Scale	Green, Forster, & Young, 2001; Harwood & Ebrahim, 2002; Nicholl, Lincoln, & Playford, 2002
The Pediatric Evaluation of Disability (PEDI)	Berg, Frøslie, & Hussain, 2003; Berg, Jahnsen, Frøslie, & Hussain, 2004; Haley, Coster, Ludlow, Haltiwanger, & Andrellos, 1992; Ho, Curtis, & Clarke, 2006; Iyer, Haley, Watkins, & Dumas, 2003; Kothari, Haley, Gill-Body, & Dumas, 2003; Vos-Vromans, Ketelaar, & Gorter, 2005; Wassenberg-Severijnen, Custers, Hox, Vermeer, & Helders, 2003
The School Function Assessment (SFA)	Coster et al., 1998; Davies, Lee Soon, Young, & Clausen-Yamaki, 2004; Egilson & Costner, 2004; Hwang, Nochajski, Linn, & Wu, 2004
The School Setting Interview	Hemmingsson et al., 2004, 2005

What do they assess? What are their strengths? Limitations?

10. Differentiate the role of the occupational therapist and the occupational therapy assistant.

Electronic Resources

- The American Occupational Therapy Association: www.aota.org
- The Assessment of Motor and Process Skills (AMPS): http://ampsintl.com
- The Model of Human Occupation Clearinghouse: www.moho.uic.edu
- Occupational Therapy: Systematic Evaluation of Evidence: www.otseeker.com
- Evidence-Based Occupational Therapy: www.otevidence.info

References

American Occupational Therapy Association. (2004). *The reference manual of the official documents of the American Occupational Therapy Association* (10th ed.). Bethesda, MD: AOTA Press.

American Occupational Therapy Association. (2006a). *Accreditation standards for a master's-degree level educational program for the occupational therapist.* Bethesda, MD: AOTA Press.

American Occupational Therapy Association. (2006b). *Accreditation standards for an educational program for the occupational therapy assistant.* Bethesda, MD: AOTA Press.

American Occupational Therapy Association. (2008). Occupational therapy practice framework: Domain and process, second edition. *American Journal of Occupational Therapy, 62,* 625-683.

Asgari, A., & Kramer, J. (2008). Construct validity and factor structure of the Persian Occupational Self-Assessment (OSA) with Iranian students. *Occupational Therapy in Health Care, 22,* 187-200.

Atchison, B. T., Fisher, A. G., & Bryze, K. (1998). Rater reliability and internal scale and person response validity of the School Assessment of Motor and Process Skills. *American Journal of Occupational Therapy, 52,* 843-850.

Ay-Woan, P., Sarah, C. P., Lyinn, C., Tsyr-Jang, C., & Ping-Chuan, H. (2006). Quality of life in depression: Predictive models. *Quality of Life Research, 15*(1), 39-48.

Baron, K., Kielhofner, G., Iyenger, A., Goldhammer, V., & Wolenski, J. (2006). *Occupational self-assessment: Version 2.2.* Chicago, IL: Model of Human Occupation Clearinghouse, Department of Occupational Therapy, College of Applied Health Sciences..

Berg, M., Aamodt, G., Stanghelle, J., Krumlinde-Sundholm, L., & Hussain, A. (2008). Cross-cultural validation of the pediatric evaluation of disability inventory (PEDI) norms in a randomized Norwegian population. *Scandinavian Journal of Occupational Therapy, 15,* 143-152.

Berg, M., Frøslie, K. F., & Hussain, A. (2003). Applicability of the pediatric evaluation of disability inventory in Norway. *Scandinavian Journal of Occupational Therapy, 10*(3), 118-126.

Berg, M., Jahnsen, R., Frøslie, K. F., & Hussain, A. (2004). Reliability of the pediatric evaluation of disability inventory (PEDI). *Physical and Occupational Therapy in Pediatrics, 24*(3), 61-77.

Bernspang, B. (1999). Rater calibration stability for the Assessment of Motor and Process Skills. *Scandinavian Journal of Occupational Therapy, 6*(3), 101-109.

Bernspang, B., & Fisher, A. G. (1995). Validation of the Assessment of Motor and Process Skills for use in Sweden. *Scandinavian Journal of Occupational Therapy, 2*(1), 3-9.

Bouwens, S., Van Heugten, C., Aalten, P., Wolfs, C., Baarends, E., Van Mexel, D., & Verhey, F. (2008). Relationship between measurement of dementia severity and observation of daily life functioning as measured with the Assessment of Motor and Process Skills (AMPS). *Dementia and Geriatric Cognitive Disorders, 25,* 81-87.

Burnett, J., Dyer, C., & Naik, A. (2009). Convergent validation of the Kohlman Evaluation of Living Skills as a screening tool of older adults' ability to live safely and independently in the community. *Archives of Physical Medicine and Rehabilitation, 90,* 1948-1952.

Carswell, A., McColl, M. A., Baptise, S., Law, M., Polatajko, H., & Pollock, N. (2004). The Canadian Occupational Performance Measure: A research and clinical literature review. *Canadian Journal of Occupational Therapy, 71*(4), 210-222.

Chatfield, J., & Beckett, D. (2007). The Canadian Occupational Performance Measure: Use in an independent living centre. *International Journal of Therapy and Rehabilitation, 14,* 280-283.

Chen, K., Tseng, M., Hu, F., & Koh, C. (2010). Pediatric Evaluation of Disability Inventory: A cross-cultural comparison of daily function between Taiwanese and American children. *Research in Developmental Disabilities, 31,* 1590-1600.

Chen, K., Hsieh, C., Sheu, C., Hu, F., & Tseng, M. (2009). Reliability and validity of a Chinese version of the Pediatric Evaluation of Disability Inventory in children with cerebral palsy. *Journal of Rehabilitation Medicine, 41,* 273-278.

Chumney, D., Nollinger, K., Shesko, K., Skop, K., Spencer, M., Newton, R. (2010). Ability of the Functional Independence Measure to accurately predict functional outcome of stroke-specific population: Systematic review. *Journal of Rehabilitation Research and Development, 47,* 17-29.

Cohen, J., Marino, R., Sacco, P., & Terrin, N. (2012). Association between the Functional Independence Measure following spinal cord injury and long term outcomes. *Spinal Cord, 50,* 728-733.

Cohen, M. E., & Marino, R. J. (2000). The tools of disability outcomes research functional status measures. *Archives of Physical Medicine and Rehabilitation, 81*(12 suppl 2), S21-S29.

Colquhoun, H., Letts, L., Law, M., MacDermid, J., & Missiuna, C. (2012). Administration of the Canadian Occupational Performance Measure: Effect on Practice. *Canadian Journal of Occupational Therapy, 79,* 120-128.

Cournan, M. (2011). Use of the Functional Independence Measure for outcome measurement in acute inpatient rehabilitation. *Rehabilitation Nursing, 36,* 111-117.

Coster, W. J., Deeny, T., Haltiwanger, J., & Haley, S. (1998). *School Function Assessment.* San Antonio, TX: The Psychological Corporation.

Coster, W., Haley, S., Ni, P., Dumas, H., & Fragala-Pinkham, M. (2008). Assessing self-care and social function using a computer adaptive testing version of Pediatric Evaluation of Disability Inventory. *Archives of Physical Medicine and Rehabilitation, 89,* 622-629.

Cottir, E. M., Burgio, L. D., Stevens, A. B., Roth, D. L., & Gitlin, L. N. (2002). Correspondence of the Functional Independence Measure (FIM) self-care subscale with real-time observations of dementia patients' ADL performance in the home. *Clinical Rehabilitation, 16*(1), 36-45.

Das Nair, R., Moreton, B. & Lincoln, N. (2011). Rasch analysis of the Nottingham Extended Activities of Daily Living Scale. *Journal of Rehabilitation Medicine: Official Journal of the UEMS European Board of Physical Medicine and Rehabilitation Medicine, 43,* 944-950.

Davies, P. L., Soon, P. L., Young, M., & Clausen-Yamaki, A. (2004). Validity and reliability of the School Function Assessment in elementary school students with disabilities. *Physical and Occupational Therapy in Pediatrics, 24*(3), 23-43.

Dedding, C., Cardol, M., Eyssen, I. C., Dekker, J., & Beelen, A. (2004). Validity of the Canadian Occupational Performance Measure: A client-centered outcome measure. *Clinical Rehabilitation, 18*(6), 660-667.

Della Pietra, G., Savio, K., Oddone, E., Reggiani, M., Monaco, F., & Leone, M. (2011). Validity and reliability of the Barthel Index administered by telephone. *Stroke: A Journal of Cerebral Circulation, 42,* 2077-2079.

Dickerson, A. E., & Fisher, A. G. (1995). Culture-relevant functional performance assessment of the Hispanic elderly. *Occupational Therapy Journal of Research, 15*(1), 50-68.

Dickson, H., & Köhler, F. (1995). Interrater reliability of the 7-Level Functional Independence Measure. *Scandinavian Journal of Rehabilitation Medicine, 27*(4), 253-256.

Doble, S. E., Fisk, J. D., Fisher, A. G., Ritvo, P. G., & Murray, T. J. (1994). Functional competence of community-dwelling persons with multiple sclerosis using the Assessment of Motor and Process Skills. *Archives of Physical Medicine and Rehabilitation, 75*(8), 843-851.

Doble, S. E., Fisk, J. D., Lewis, N., & Rockwood, K. (1999). Test-retest reliability of the Assessment of Motor and Process Skills in elderly adults. *Occupational Therapy Journal of Research, 19*(3), 203-215.

Dodds, T. A., Martin, D. P., Stolov, W. C., & Deyo, R. A. (1993). A validation of the Functional Independence Measurement and its performance among rehabilitation patients. *Archives of Physical Medicine and Rehabilitation, 74*(5), 531-536.

Dumas, H., Fragala-Pinkham, M., & Haley, S. (2010). Development of a postacute hospital item bank for the new Pediatric Evaluation of Disability Inventory-Computer Adaptive Test. *International Journal of Rehabilitation Research, 33,* 332-338.

Dumas, H., Fragala-Pinkham, M., Haley, S., Coster, W., Kramer, J., Kao, Y., & Moed, R. (2010). Item bank development for a revised Pediatric Evaluation of Disability Inventory (PEDI). *Physical and Occupational Therapy in Pediatrics, 30,* 168-184.

Egilson, S. T., & Coster, W. J. (2004). School Function Assessment: Performance of Icelandic students with special needs. *Scandinavian Journal of Occupational Therapy, 11*(4), 163-170.

Eichhorn-Kissel, J., Dassen, T., & Lohrmann, C. (2011). Comparison of the responsiveness of the Care Dependency Scale for rehabilitation and the Barthel Index. *Clinical Rehabilitation, 25,* 760-767.

Elad, D., Barak, S., Eisenstein, E., Bar, O., Herzberg, O., & Brezner, A. (2012). Reliability and validity of Hebrew Pediatric Evaluation of Disability Inventory (PEDI) in children with cerebral palsy—health care professionals vs. mothers. *Journal of Pediatric Rehabilitation Medicine, 5,* 107-115.

Ellison, S., Fisher, A. G., & Duran, L. (2001). The alternate forms reliability of the new tasks added to the Assessment of Motor and Process Skills. *Journal of Applied Measurement, 2*(2), 121-134.

Enemark Larsen, A., & Carlsson, G. (2012). Utility of the Canadian Occupational Performance Measure as an admission and outcome measure in interdisciplinary community-based geriatric rehabilitation. *Scandinavian Journal of Occupational Therapy, 19,* 204-213.

Ennels, P., & Fossey, E. (2007). The Occupational Performance History Interview in community mental health case management: Consumer and occupational therapist perspectives. *Australian Occupational Therapy Journal, 54,* 11-21.

Ennels, P., & Fossey, E. (2009). Using the OPHI-II to support people with mental illness in their recovery: The Occupational Performance History Interview (OPHI-II). *Occupational Therapy in Mental Health, 25,* 138-150.

Eyssen, I., Steultjens, M., Oud, T., Bolt, E., Maasdam, A., & Dekker, J. (2011). Responsiveness of the Canadian Occupational Performance Measure. *Journal of Rehabilitation Research and Development, 48,* 517-528.

Fioavanti, A., Bordignon, C., Petti, S., Woodhouse, L., & Ansley, B. (2012). Comparing the responsiveness of the Assessment of Motor and Process Skills and the Functional Independence Measure. *Canadian Journal of Occupational Therapy, 79,* 167-174.

Fisher, A. & Jones, K. (2012). *Assessment of Motor and Process Skills, Vol. 1: Development, standardization, and administration manual* (7th ed.). Fort Collins, CO: Three Star Press.

Fisher, A. G., Bryze, K., & Atchison, B. T. (2000). Naturalistic Assessment of functional performance in school settings: Reliability and validity of the School AMPS. In R. M. Smith (Ed.), *Objective outcome measurement: Examples in physical medicine and rehabilitation* (Vol. 1). Chicago, IL: MESA Press.

Fisher, A. G., Bryze, K., & Hume, V. (2002). *School AMPS: School version of the Assessment of Motor and Process Skills.* Fort Collins, CO: Three Star Press.

Fisher, A. G., Bryze, K., Hume, V., & Griswold, L. A. (2005). *School AMPS: School version of the Assessment of Motor and Process Skills* (2nd ed.). Fort Collins, CO: Three Star Press.

Fisher, A. G., Liu, Y., Velozo, C. A., & Pan, A. W. (1992). Cross-cultural assessment of process skills. *American Journal of Occupational Therapy, 46*(10), 876-885.

Gantsching, B., Page, J., & Fisher, A. (2012). Cross-regional validity of the Assessment of Motor and Process Skills for use in middle Europe. *Journal of Rehabilitation Medicine: Official Journal of the European Board of Physical and Rehabilitation Medicine, 44,* 151-157.

Gauggel, S., Heinemann, A. W., Bocker, M., Lammler, G., Borchelt, M., & Steinhagen-Thiessen, E. (2004). Patient-staff agreement on Barthel Index scores at admission and discharge in a sample of elderly stroke patients. *Rehabilitation Psychology, 49*(1), 21-27.

Gilbertson, L., & Langhorne, P. (2000). Home-based occupational therapy: Stroke patients' satisfaction with occupational performance and service provision. *British Journal of Occupational Therapy, 63*(10), 464-468.

Goldman, S., & Fisher, A. G. (1997). Cross-cultural validation of the Assessment of Motor and Process Skills (AMPS). *British Journal of Occupational Therapy, 60,* 77-85.

Goto, S., Fisher, A. G., & Mayberry, W. L. (1996). The assessment of motor and process skills applied cross-culturally to the Japanese. *American Journal of Occupational Therapy, 50*(10), 798-806.

Granger, C. V., & Hamilton, B. B. (1992). UDS Report: The uniform data system for medical rehabilitation report of first admissions for 1990. *American Journal of Physical Medicine and Rehabilitation, 71*(2), 108-113.

Green, J., Forster, A., & Young, J. (2001). A test-retest reliability study of the Barthel Index, the Rivermead Mobility Index, the Nottingham extended Activities of Daily Living Scale and the Frenchay Activities Index in stroke patients. *Disability and Rehabilitation, 23*(15), 670-676.

Haley, S., Coster, W., Dumas, H., Fragala-Pinkham, M., Kramer, J., Ni, P., Tian, F., Kao, Y., Moed, R., & Ludlow, L. (2011). Accuracy and precision of the Pediatric Evaluation of Disability Inventory Computer-Adaptive Tests (PEDI-CAT). *Developmental Medicine and Child Neurology, 53,* 1100-1106.

Haley, S., Coster, W., Kao, Y., Dumas, H., Fragala-Pinkham, M., Kramer, J., Ludlow, L., & Moed, R. (2010). Lessons from use of the Pediatric Evaluation of Disability Inventory: Where do we go from here? *Pediatric Physical Therapy, 22,* 69-75.

Haley, S. M., Coster, W. J., Ludlow, L. H., Haltiwanger, J. T., & Andrellos, P. J. (1992). *Pediatric Evaluation of Disability Inventory: Development, standardization and administration manual, version 1.0.* Boston, MA: Trustees of Boston University, Health and Disability Institute.

Harper, K., Stalker, C. A., & Templeton, G. (2006). The use and validity of the Canadian Occupational Performance Measure in a posttraumatic stress program. *OTJR: Occupation, Participation, and Health, 26*(2), 45-55.

Hartigen, I., & O'Mahony, D. (2011). The Barthel Index: comparing inter-rater reliability between nurses and doctors in an older adult rehabilitation unit. *Applied Nursing Research, 24,* 1-7.

Harwood, R. H., & Ebrahim, S. (2002). The validity, reliability and responsiveness of the Nottingham Extended Activities of Daily Living scale in patients undergoing total hip replacement. *Disability and Rehabilitation, 24*(7), 371-377.

Haslam, J., Pepin, G., Bourbonnais, R., & Grignon, S. (2010). Processes of task performance as measured by the Assessment of Motor and Process Skills (AMPS): A predictor of work-related outcomes for adults with Schizophrenia? *Australian Occupational Therapy Journal, 37,* 53-64.

Hemmingsson, H., Egilson, S., Hoffman, O., & Kielhofner, G. (2005). *A User's Manual for the School Setting Interview (SSI)* (Version 3.0). Chicago, IL: Model of Human Occupation Clearinghouse, University of Illinois at Chicago and Swedish Association of Occupational Therapists.

Hemmingsson, H., Kottorp, A., & Bernspang, B. (2004). Validity of the School Setting Interview: An assessment of the student-environment fit. *Scandinavian Journal of Occupational Therapy, 11*(4), 171-178.

Hemmingsson, H., & Penman, M. (2010). Making children´s voices visible: The School Setting Interview (SSI). *Kairaranga, 11,* 45-49.

Hill, D. (2006). A discharge planning tool for older adults: The Kohlman Evaluation of Living Skills. *Gerontology Special Interest Section Quarterly, 29,* 3-8.

Ho, E. S., Curtis, C. G., & Clarke, H. M. (2006). Pediatric Evaluation of Disability Inventory: Its application to children with obstetric brachial plexus palsy. *Journal of Hand Surgery, 31*(2), 197-202.

Houlden, H., Edwards, M., McNeil, J., & Greenwood, R. (2006). Use of the Barthel Index and the Functional Independence Measure during early inpatient rehabilitation after single incident brain injury. *Clinical Rehabilitation, 20*(2), 153-159.

Hsueh, I. P., Lin, J. H., Jeng, J. S., & Hsieh, C. L. (2006). Comparison of the psychometric characteristics of the Functional Independence Measure, 5 Item Barthel Index, and 10 Item Barthel Index in patients with stroke. *Journal of Neurosurgery Psychiatry, 73*(2), 188-190.

Hwang, J. (2005). The reliability and validity of the School Function Assessment-Chinese version. *OTJR: Occupation, Participation, and Health, 25,* 44-54.

Hwang, J., & Davies, P. (2009). Rasch analysis of the School Function Assessment provides additional evidence for the internal validity of the activity performance scales. *American Journal of Occupational Therapy, 63,* 369-373.

Hwang, J. L., Nochajski, S. M., Linn, R. T., & Wu, Y. W. (2004). The development of the School Function Assessment-Chinese version for cross-cultural use in Taiwan. *Occupational Therapy International, 11*(1), 26-39.

Iyer, L. V., Haley, S. M., Watkins, M. P., & Dumas, H. M. (2003). Establishing minimal clinically important differences for scores on the Pediatric Evaluation of Disability Inventory for inpatient rehabilitation. *Physical Therapy, 83*(10), 888-898.

Johnson, S., & Nelson, D. (2010). Convergent validity of three Occupational Self-Assessments. *Physical and Occupational Therapy in Geriatrics, 28,* 13-21.

Kao, Y., Kramer, J., Liljenquist, K., Tian, F., & Coster, W. (2012). Comparing the functional performance of children and youths with autism, developmental disabilities, and no disability using the revised Pediatric Evaluation of Disability inventory item banks. *American Journal of Occupational Therapy, 66,* 607-616.

Keller, J., Kafkes, A., Basu, S., Federico, J., & Kielhofner, G. (2005). *Children's occupational self-assessment, version 2.1.* Chicago, IL: Model of Human Occupation Clearinghouse.

Keller, J., Kafkes, A., & Kielhofner, G. (2005). Psychometric characteristics of the Child Occupational Self-Assessment (COSA), part one: An initial examination of psychometric properties. *Scandinavian Journal of Occupational Therapy, 12*(3), 118-127.

Keller, J., & Kielhofner, G. (2005). Psychometric characteristics of the Child Occupational Self-Assessment (COSA), part two: Refining the psychometric properties. *Scandinavian Journal of Occupational Therapy, 12*(4), 147-158.

Kielhofner, G., Dobria, L., Forsyth, K., & Basu, S. (2005). The construction of key forms for obtaining instantaneous measures from the Occupational Performance History Interview rating scales. *OTJR: Occupation, Participation and Health, 25*(1), 23-32.

Kielhofner, G., Dobria, L., Forsyth, K., & Kramer, J. (2010). The Occupational Self-Assessment: Stability and the ability to detect change over time. *Occupational Therapy Journal of Research: Occupation, Participation, and Health, 30,* 11-19.

Kielhofner, G., & Forsyth, K. (2001). Measurement properties of a client self-report for treatment planning and documenting therapy outcomes. *Scandinavian Journal of Occupational Therapy, 8*(3), 131-139.

Keilhofner, G., Mallinson, T., Forsyth, K., & Lai, J. S. (2001). Psychometric properties of the second version of the Occupational Performance History Interview (OPHI-II). *American Journal of Occupational Therapy, 55*(3), 260-267.

Kielhofner, G., Mallinson, T., Crawford, C., Nowak, M., Rigby, M., Henry, A., et al. (1998). *The Occupational Performance History Interview* (Version 2.0) OPHI-II. Chicago, IL: Model of Human Occupation Clearinghouse.

Kjeken, I., Dagfinrud, H., Uhlig, T., Mowinckel, P., Kvien, T., & Finset, A. (2005). Reliability of the Canadian Occupational Performance Measure in patients with ankylosing spondylitis. *Journal of Rheumatology, 32*(8), 1503-1509.

Kothari, D. H., Haley, S. M., Gill-Body, K. M., & Dumas, H. M. (2003). Measuring functional change in children with acquired brain injury (ABI): Comparison of generic and ABI-specific scales using the Pediatric Evaluation of Disability Inventory (PEDI). *Physical Therapy, 83*(9), 776-785.

Kottorp, A. (2008). The use of the Assessment of Motor and Process Skills (AMPS) in predicting need of assistance for adults with mental retardation. *OTJR: Occupation, Participation, and Health, 28,* 72-80.

Kramer, J. (2009). Using mixed methods to establish the social validity of a self-report assessment: An illustration using the Child Occupational Self-Assessment (COSA). *Journal of Mixed Methods, 5,* 52-76.

Kramer, J., Kielhofner, G., & Smith, E. (2010). Validity evidence for the Child Occupational Self Assessment. *American Journal of Occupational Therapy, 64,* 621-632.

Kwakkel, G., Veerbeek, J. M., Harmeling-van der Wel, B. C., van Wegen, E., & Kollen, B. (2011). Diagnostic accuracy of the Barthel Index for measuring activities of daily living outcome after ischemic stroke: Does early poststroke timing of assessment matter? *Stroke: A Journal of Cerebral Circulation, 42,* 342-346.

Lange, B., Spagnolo, K., & Fowler, B. (2009). Using the Assessment of Motor and Process Skills to measure functional change in adults with severe traumatic brain injury: A pilot study. *Australian Occupational Therapy Journal, 56,* 89-96.

Law, M., Baptise, S., Carsweel, A., McColl, M., Polatajko, H., & Pollock, N. (2005). *Canadian occupational performance measure* (4th ed.). Ottawa, Ontario: CAOT Publications.

Law, M., Baum, C., & Dunn, W. (2005). *Measuring occupational performance: Supporting best practice in occupational therapy.* Thorofare, NJ: SLACK Incorporated.

Law, M., Cooper, B. A., Strong, S., Stewart, D., Rigby, P., & Letts, L. (1996). The person-environment-occupation model: A transactive approach to occupational performance. *Canadian Journal of Occupational Therapy, 63*(1), 9-23.

Lekamwassam, S., Karunatilake, K., Kankanamge, S., & Lekamwasam, V. (2011). Physical dependency of elderly and physically disabled; measurement concordance between 10-item Barthel Index and 5-item shorter version. *The Ceylon Medical Journal, 56,* 114-118.

Linden, A., Boschian, K., Eker, C., Schalen, W., & Nordstrom, C. H. (2005). Assessment of Motor and Process Skills reflects brain-injured patients' ability to resume independent living better than neurological tests. *ACTA Neurologica Scandinavica, 111*(1), 48-53.

Lundgren-Nilsson, A., Grimby, G., Ring, H., Tesio, L., Lawton, G., Slade, A., et al. (2005). Cross-cultural validity of Functional Independence Measure items in stroke: A study using Rasch Analysis. *Journal of Rehabilitation Medicine, 37*(1), 23-31.

Magalhães, L., Fisher, A. G., Bernspang, B., & Linåcre, J. M. (1996). Cross-cultural assessment of functional mobility. *Occupational Therapy Journal of Research, 16,* 45-63.

Mallinson, T., Mahaffey, L., & Kielhofner, G. (1998). The Occupational Performance History Interview: Evidence for three underlying constructs of occupational adaptation. *Canadian Journal of Occupational Therapy, 65*(4), 219-228.

McNulty, M. C., & Fisher, A. G. (2001). Validity of using the Assessment of Motor and Process Skills to estimate overall home safety in person with psychiatric conditions. *American Journal of Occupational Therapy, 55*(6), 649-655.

Merritt, B. (2011). Validity of using the Assessment of Motor and Process Skills to determine the need for assistance. *American Journal of Occupational Therapy, 65,* 643-650.

Munkholm, M., Berg, B., Lofgren, B., & Fisher, A. (2010). Cross-regional validation of the School Version of the Assessment of Motor and Process Skills. *American Journal of Occupational Therapy, 64,* 768-775.

Munkholm, M., & Fisher, A. (2008). Differences in schoolwork performance between typically developing students and students with mild disabilities. *OTJR: Occupation, Participation, and Health, 28,* 121-132.

Murad, M., Farnsworth, L., & O'Brien, L. (2011). Reliability and validation properties of the Malaysian language version of the Occupational Self-Assessment Version 2.2 for injured workers with musculoskeletal disorders. *British Journal of Occupational Therapy, 74,* 226-232.

Nicholl, L., Hobart, J., Dunwoody, L., Cramp, F., & Lowe-Strong, A. (2004). Measuring disability in multiple sclerosis: Is the Community Dependency Index an improvement on the Barthel Index? *Multiple Sclerosis, 10*(4), 447-450.

Nicholl, C. R., Lincoln, N. B., & Playford, E. D. (2002). The reliability and validity of the Nottingham Extended Activities of Daily Living Scale in patients with multiple sclerosis. *Multiple Sclerosis, 8*(5), 372-376.

Ohura, T., Ishizaki, T., Higashi, T., Konishi, K., Ishiguro, R., Nakanishi, K., Shah, S., Nakayama, T. (2011). Reliability and validity tests of an evaluation tool based on the modified Barthel Index. *International Journal of Therapy and Rehabilitation, 18,* 422-428.

Ottenbacher, K. J., Msall, M. E., Lyon, N., Duffy, L. C., Ziviani, J., Granger, C. V., et al. (2000). The WeeFIM Instrument: Its utility in detecting change in children with developmental disabilities. *Archives of Physical Medicine and Rehabilitation, 81*(10), 1317-1326.

Pan, A. W., Chung, L., & Hsin-Hwei, G. (2003). Reliability and validity of the Canadian Occupational Performance Measure for clients with psychiatric disorders in Taiwan. *Occupational Therapy International, 10*(4), 269-277.

Padankatti, S. M., Macaden, A. S., Cherian, S. M., Thirumugam, M., Pazani, D., Kalaiselvan, M.,...Srivastava, A. (2011). A patient-prioritized ability assessment in hemophilia: The Canadian Occupational Performance Measure. *Hemophilia, 17,* 605-611.

Park, S., Fisher, A. G., & Velozo, C. A. (1994). Using the Assessment of Motor and Process Skills to compare occupational performance between clinic and home settings. *American Journal of Occupational Therapy, 48*(8), 697-709.

Peny-Dahlstrand, M., Gosman-Hedstrom, G., & Krumlinde-Sundholm, L. (2012). Are there cross-cultural differences of ADL ability in children measured with the Assessment of Motor and Process Skills (AMPS)? *Scandinavian Journal of Occupational Therapy, 19,* 26-32.

Persson, E., Rivano-Fischer, M., & Eklund, M. (2004). Evaluation of changes in occupational performance among patients in a pain management program. *Journal of Rehabilitation Medicine, 36*(2), 85-91.

Pickens, S., Naik, A. D., Burnett, J., Kelly, P. A., Gleason, M., & Dyer, C. B. (2007). The utility of the Kohlman Evaluation of Living Skills test is associated with substantiated cases of elder self-neglect. *Journal of the American Academy of Nurse Practitioners, 19*(3), 137-142.

Quinn, T., Langhorne, P., & Stott, D. (2011). Barthel Index for stroke trials: Development, properties, and application. *Stroke: A Journal of Cerebral Circulation, 42,* 1146-1151.

Rollnik, J. (2011). The Early Rehabilitation Barthel Index. *Rehabilitation, 50,* 408-411.

Sahin, F., Yilmaz, F., Ozmaden, A., Kotevoglu, N., Sahin, T., & Kuran, B. (2008). Reliability and validity of the Turkish version of the Nottingham Extended Activities of Daily Living Scale. *Aging Clinical and Experimental Research, 20,* 400-405.

Sangha, H., Lipson, D., Foley, N., Salter, K., Bhogal, S., Pohani, G., et al. (2005). A comparison of the Barthel Index and the Functional Independence Measure as outcome measures in stroke rehabilitation: Patterns of disability scale usage in clinical trials. *International Journal of Rehabilitation Research, 28*(2), 135-139.

Sarker, S., Rudd, A., Douiri, A., & Wolfe, C. (2012). Comparison of 2 extended activities of daily living scales with the Barthel Index and predictors of their outcomes: Cohort study within the South London Stroke Register (SLSR). *Stroke: A Journal of Cerebral Circulation, 43,* 1362-1369.

Schlote, A., Kruger, J., Topp, H., & Wallesch, C. (2004). Inter-rater reliability of the Barthel Index, the Activity Index, and the Nottingham Extended Activities of Daily Living: The use of ADL instruments in stroke rehabilitation by medical and non-medical personnel. *Rehabilitation, 43,* 75-82.

Sellers, S. W., Fisher, A. G., & Duran, L. J. (2001). Validity of the Assessment of Motor and Process Skills with students who are visually impaired. *Journal of Visual Impairment and Blindness, 95*(3), 164-167.

Shin Liu, Y., Fujimoto, M., Hase, M., Tsuji, K., Fujiwara, T., & Okajima, Y. (2009). Identification of quasi-in-need-of-care state (QUINOCS) among community dwelling elderly people using a seven-item subset of the Functional Independence Measure (FIM). *An International, Multidisciplinary Journal, 31,* 381-386.

Silverman, M., & Smith, R. (2006). Consequential validity of an assistive technology supplement for the School Function Assessment. *Assistive Technology, 18,* 155-165.

Stauffer, L. M., Fisher, A. G., & Duran, L. (2000). ADL performance of Black Americans and White Americans on the Assessment of Motor and Process Skills. *American Journal of Occupational Therapy, 54*(6), 607-613.

Stineman, M. G., Ross, R. N., Fiedler, R., Granger, C. V., & Maislin, G. (2003). Functional Independence staging: Conceptual foundation, face validity, and empirical derivation. *Archives of Physical Medicine and Rehabilitation, 84*(1), 29-37.

Taylor, R., Lee, S., Kramer, J., Shirashi, Y., & Kielhofner, G. (2011). Psychometric study of the Occupational Self-Assessment with adolescents after infectious mononucleosis. *American Journal of Occupational Therapy, 65,* 20-28.

Thomson, L. K. (1992). *The Kohlman Evaluation of Living Skills* (3rd ed.). Bethesda, MD: AOTA Press.

Toneman, M., Brayshaw, J., Lange, B., & Trimboli, C. (2010). Examination of the change in the Assessment of Motor and Process Skills performance in patients with acquired brain injury between the hospital and home environment. *Australian Occupational Therapy Journal, 57,* 246-252.

Trombly, C. (1993). Anticipating the future: Assessment of occupational function. *American Journal of Occupational Therapy, 47*(3), 253-257.

Turner-Stokes, L., Williams, H., Rose, H., Harris, S., & Jackson, D. (2010). Deriving a Barthel Index from the Northwick Park Dependency Scale and the Functional Independence Measure: Are they equivalent? *Clinical Rehabilitation, 24,* 1121-1126.

Uniform Data System for Medical Rehabilitation. (1999). *The Functional Independence Measure (FIM) user guide and self-guided training manual, version 5.20.* Buffalo, NY: Author.

Uniform Data System for Medical Rehabilitation. (2000). *The WeeFIM system clinical guide, version 5.01.* Buffalo, NY: Author.

van Exel, N. J., Scholte op Reimer, W. J., & Koopmanschap, M. A. (2004). Assessment of post-stroke quality of life in cost-effectiveness studies: The usefulness of the Barthel Index and the EuroQoL-5D. *Quality of Life Research, 13*(2), 427-433.

Verkerk, G. J., Wolf, M. J., Louwers, A. M., Meester-Delver, A., & Nollet, F. (2006). The reproducibility and validity of the Canadian Occupational Performance Measure in parents of children with disabilities. *Clinical Rehabilitation, 20*(11), 980-988.

Vos-Vromans, D. C., Ketelaar, M., & Gorter, J. W. (2005). Responsiveness of evaluation measures for children with cerebral palsy: The Gross Motor Function Measure and the Pediatric Evaluation of Disability Inventory. *Disability and Rehabilitation, 27*(20), 1245-1252.

Wassenberg-Severijnen, J. E., Custers, J. W., Hox, J. J., Vermeer, A., & Helders, P. J. (2003). Reliabilty of the Dutch Pediatric Evaluation of Disability Inventory (PEDI). *Clinical Rehabilitation, 17*(4), 457-462.

Wressle, E., Lindstrand, J., Neher, M., Marcusson, J., & Henricksson, C. (2003). The Canadian Occupation Performance Measure as an outcome measure and team tool in a day treatment programme. *Disability and Rehabilitation, 25*(10), 497-506.

Wu, C., Chaung, L., Lin, K., Lee, S., & Hong, W. (2011). Responsiveness, minimal detectable change, and minimal clinically important difference of the Nottingham Extended Activities of Daily Living Scale in patients with improved performance after stroke rehabilitation. *Archives of Physical Medicine and Rehabilitation, 92,* 1281-1287.

Young, Y., Fan, M., Hebel, J., & Boult, C. (2009). Concurrent validity of administering the Functional Independence Measure (FIM) instrument by interview. *Journal of Physical Medicine and Rehabilitation, 88,* 766-770.

Zimnavoda, T., Weinblatt, N., & Katz, N. (2002). Validity of the Kohlman Evaluation of Living Skills (KELS) with Israeli elderly individuals living in the community. *Occupational Therapy International, 9*(4), 312-325.

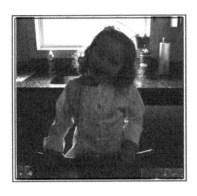

18

EVALUATION OF EDUCATION AND WORK

Barbara Larson, MA, OTR/L, FAOTA

ACOTE STANDARDS EXPLORED IN THIS CHAPTER
B.4.4

KEY VOCABULARY

- **Client:** Entity that receives occupational therapy services.
- **Client-centered evaluation:** Focus is on the client's priorities; client is an active participant in the evaluation process.
- **Context:** Conditions that exist in and around the person; may influence the client's performance, and the process of service delivery.
- **Education:** Occupational performance area that includes activities for being a student and participating in learning activities.
- **Environment:** The external factors—physical, social, and attitudinal—that have an effect on how people live their lives.

- **Evaluation:** Includes the occupational profile and the analysis of occupational performance.
- **Occupational performance:** The ability to perform in life activities.
- **Occupational profile:** Information on the client's occupational history and experiences, patterns of daily living, interests, values, and needs.
- **Work:** Occupational performance area that includes activities needed for engaging in paid employment or volunteer activities.

Jacobs, K., MacRae, N., & Sladyk, K. (Eds.).
*Occupational Therapy Essentials for
Clinical Competence, Second Edition* (pp. 231-240).
© 2014 SLACK Incorporated.

Introduction

The health, productivity, and efficiency of individuals, organizations, or populations can be greatly impacted by illness, injury, or incidences that interrupt the ability to engage in meaningful occupational performance. Central to occupational therapy practice is an understanding of the value and use of occupation (LaVesser, Aird, & Lieberman, 2004). This chapter focuses on the components and factors involved in the evaluation of education and work as occupational performance areas. The practice framework (American Occupational Therapy Association [AOTA], 2008), provides definition to occupational therapy practice and guidance to practitioners in evaluation and as intervention decisions are made. The important task demands and performance factors that might need to be assessed in order to plan effective interventions will be discussed.

Education

Education is both a primary therapeutic tool and a primary occupational performance area. When the therapist is planning the educational experiences, education is a primary therapeutic tool. For a child in a classroom or for a college student, education is a primary occupational performance area. In other cases, education might be a more casual experience, such as participating in a continuing education experience or otherwise learning a new skill. In each case, there are relevant barriers to learning.

Education has been described as the work of children (Larson, 2004). The barriers to a child being able to perform as a student may include sensory processing disorder, development delays, physical disabilities, and psychosocial deficits such as autism, behavioral problems, and those things that interfere with the ability of a child to take advantage of a learning experience (Case-Smith, 2005). The occupational therapist must determine the most appropriate assessment for the identified problems. One example of a highly sophisticated assessment for limitations in sensory integration is the Sensory Integration and Praxis Tests (SIPT; Bodison & Mailloux, 2006). Another assessment is the Sensory Profile, which measures sensory processing abilities in young children with autism (Watling, Deitz, & White, 2001).

Besides carefully selecting the accurate assessment, the occupational therapist must consider the environment and context in which the assessment takes place. The child's positioning, proximal distal stability (Smith-Zuzovsky & Exner, 2004), as well as the furniture the child sits on related to the testing activity are important and could influence test performance and outcomes (Naider-Steinhart & Katz-Leurer, 2007). In a study of children's work, the author's findings indicated that kindergarten, first, and second graders view handwriting as

work. The author thus cautions therapists to view this activity in a work context, "promoting quiet and concentration, setting standards, and encouraging students to achieve them through persistent effort" (Larson, 2004, p. 377).

In like manner, there are numerous straightforward sensorimotor, cognitive, and psychosocial deficits (Law, Baum, & Dunn, 2005) that can interfere with the adult's occupational performance and, subsequently, the individual's ability to participate in educational experiences. Interviews, observations, a review of medical records, and client history information provide the necessary data to allow the therapist to gain an understanding of the individual's life activities. The occupational therapy practitioner uses standardized or nonstandardized assessments to determine how the occupational performance in those life activities is affected (Law et al., 2005).

Determining an individual's priorities during the assessment phase allows the occupational therapy practitioner to carefully and selectively design education programs that address the needs and wants of the adult. The importance of doing this is illustrated in a study involving the development of a health education program for an elderly population with macular degeneration (Dahlin Ivanoff, Sonn, & Svensson, 2002). The authors concluded that to maintain a sense of security in daily occupations, health education programs should be founded on the needs and problems of the elderly age group (Dahlin Ivanoff et al., 2002). In another study on fall prevention education for older adults, the authors described the importance of using individual assessment information to develop the educational message (Schepens, Panzer, & Goldberg, 2011).

In selecting assessment tools, the Canadian Occupational Performance Measure (COPM) can be used to identify client priorities and determine individual needs and wants. The COPM assesses self-perception of performance and satisfaction of daily occupations over time (McColl & Pollock, 2001). Problems in occupational performance areas are identified and weighted in terms of importance to the client. The therapist sets client-centered goals for the education program based on those identified priorities (Law et al., 2005). Along with identifying problems carefully and selecting the appropriate assessment, the occupational therapist must interpret findings accurately and cautiously. It is important to understand the purpose and outcome of each assessment used in order to plan appropriate interventions. The contexts and activity demands must be taken into consideration when conducting assessments.

Changing behavior is an important outcome of client education. Whether looking at the occupation of children, the voluntary or educational occupations of adults, or the occupational therapy practitioner using learning as a therapeutic approach, there are, as previously discussed, a host of barriers that can interfere with the educational process. These barriers must be evaluated in the context of relevant educational theories and models. Multiple educational theories and models will be presented next.

The Health Belief Model

The Health Belief Model, which focuses on individual health behavior, supports that, in general, individuals will take action to ward off, screen for, or control ill health under certain circumstances (Rosenstock & Strecher, 1997). For behavior change to succeed, people must feel threatened by their current situation and believe that change of a specific kind will be beneficial and result in a valued outcome at an acceptable cost (Rosenstock, 1990; Rosenstock & Strecher, 1997). People must also feel competent to implement that change. As clients move toward goal attainment, the occupational therapy practitioner should reinforce their successes verbally, while behavior problems should be treated as opportunities to analyze and control the factors that cause the problem.

Value Expectancy Theory

Value expectancy theories, reasoned action, and multiattribute utility provide a method for operationally defining and systematically assessing the elements of a decision to perform a specific behavior. These theories do not attempt to describe how individuals make decisions. The theory of reasoned action predicts an individual's intention to perform a given behavior in a specifically defined setting. This action is influenced by the individual's attitude toward the behavior and the influence of the social environment on the desired behavior (Carter, 1990).

Multiattribute Utility Theory

Multiattribute utility theory predicts behavior directly from an individual's evaluation of the consequences or outcomes associated with the performance and nonperformance of the behavior in question. For both theories, the individuals who perform the behavior are the ones who identify the most important issues or barriers to behavioral performance (Carter, 1990). Designing any health education program requires a thorough understanding of the behavioral consequences or outcomes most important to the intended population (Carter, 1990).

Attribution Theory

Lewis and Daltroy (1990) discussed attribution theory related to health behavior. They defined attributions as "the causes individuals generate to make sense of their world" (p. 92).

Determining how a person attributes causes to the state of his or her current health is often a first step in the development of a therapeutic relationship (Lewis & Daltroy, 1990). What is critical is that clients attribute potential effectiveness to their own behavior. Once this happens, clients can work through failures, initiate difficult tasks, and proceed in the face of obstacles (Lewis & Daltroy, 1990). Health-related skills will not be abandoned in the face of failure, difficult tasks will be initiated, and task persistence will occur even in the face of obstacles. The most potent attributions center on controllability and locus of causation of disease. Personal change needs to be reinforced to be sustained. Both environmental and personal changes are important, and both should be addressed by health promotions efforts (Lewis & Daltroy, 1990).

Social Learning Theory

Social learning theory addresses both the methods of promoting behavior change and the psychosocial dynamics underlying health behavior (Perry, Barnowski, & Parcel, 1990, 1997). From a cognitive viewpoint, social learning theory emphasizes what people think. According to social learning theory, individuals with an internal locus of control are more likely to initiate change, whereas those who are externally controlled are more likely to be influenced by others. The literature provides evidence that giving people control over their lives improves their health outcomes (Perry et al., 1990).

Self-efficacy is the most important prerequisite for behavior change (Perry et al., 1990, 1997). Self-efficacy relates to the confidence a person feels about performing a given activity and affects the amount of effort invested in a given task and the levels of performance that are attained. Goal setting is important in self-efficacy (Perry et al., 1990, 1997). To make use of self-efficacy in promoting self-control of performance, goals should be set in increments similar to a given behavior, possible to achieve, and meaningful and relevant to the client.

Bandura (as cited in Perry et al., 1990) suggested that excessive emotional arousal inhibits learning and performance. Fearful thoughts produce emotional arousal and trigger defensive behaviors. When individuals experience heightened anxiety, it becomes difficult to attend to the health messages being sent by health professionals. Before health care professionals can help clients change their behavior, they must learn methods to aid people in their ability to minimize emotional arousal. If heightened anxiety cannot be minimized, education efforts should be postponed until anxiety has subsided. The health professional must plan interventions that will take into consideration the exploration of multiple relevant concepts.

The application of these models and theories supports clinical reasoning and helps the occupational therapist build therapeutic relationships with clients and caregivers, which are so vital to affecting behavior change.

Current theorists of client–provider relationships blend social and psychological perspectives and interpersonal influences to explain how the characteristics and behaviors of others affect a person's attitudes, feelings, and behavior. Joos and Hickam (1990) indicated that theories of cognition point to a number of factors that may interfere with clients' understanding and recall of information in the health care setting. Jargon and vocabulary that are too complex for the majority of clients are often present in verbal and written information, situational influences affect a client's ability to attend to and recall information, and the different backgrounds between provider and client often hamper their communication. Research on cognition and learning shows that providers can enhance the client's ability to understand written and verbal information by using shorter words and sentences, presenting and stressing the most important information first, using clear categories, giving specific rather than general instruction, and being aware of and checking for comprehension of major points (Joos & Hickam, 1990). There is strong evidence in patient outcomes to show the connection between patient satisfaction and patient–provider communication (Roter & Hall, 1997). Communication that is timely, meaningful, and presented in a thoughtful manner can influence patients' compliance and strengthen their ability to recall information (Roter & Hall, 1997).

Clients have certain cultural expectations based on their social roles as group members and their behavior is influenced by the process of communication (Joos & Hickam, 1990). It is important for the health care provider to use culturally appropriate tools that match the client's educational and literacy levels (Pasick, 1997).

Rogers (as cited in Joos & Hickman, 1990) stated, "Empathy, genuineness, and acceptance of the client are the core conditions necessary for positive therapeutic change" (p. 221). A client-centered, rather than provider-centered, approach to care should be promoted.

Occupational behavior is influenced by the client's physiological, cognitive, and psychological conditions. These conditions also affect the client's ability to learn (Berkeland & Flinn, 2005). The occupational therapy practitioner needs to create a comfortable, safe environment in which the client can benefit from the educational experience. Client education is important in the practice of occupational therapy. Written materials, while most commonly used in client education, need to reflect the reading level and comprehensibility of the reader to be effective (Griffin, McKenna, & Tooth, 2006). A survey of 147 Australian occupational therapists working with adults in physical disabilities found that 74% of therapists used client education often or most of the time (McEneany, McKenna, & Summerville, 2002).

Teaching and learning provide clients with a way to take action, explore possibilities, and engage in occupation, and they are fundamental to the occupational therapy process (Berkeland & Flinn, 2005). "In designing teaching and learning experiences, practitioners consider models or frameworks for client education, principles of adult learning, and the mechanics of constructing education programs" (Berkeland & Flinn, 2005, p. 421). Client education is a vital link between the occupational therapy practitioner and those individuals under their care (Griffin et al., 2006).

Work

Work is important socially and economically and it often defines our place in a community. Work has been an integral part of occupational therapy since the early 1900s (Hanson & Walker, 1992). Occupational therapy grew out of the moral treatment movement. Employment, recreation, and self-care came to be important components in the intervention of those with mental illness as the handling of those in asylums became more humane (Hanson & Walker, 1997; Harvey-Krefting, 1985). The development of the veterans hospital in 1922 provided occupational therapy for "therapeutic, economic and diversional reasons" (Hanson & Walker, 1992, p. 57). Work programs were developed to treat those with chronic illnesses and were held in or near sanatoriums. The industrial era of the mid-1930s saw the introduction of curative workshops serving workers who were injured in industrial accidents (Hanson & Walker, 1992). In the 1950s, the focus of the injured worker became return to gainful employment (Harvey-Krefting, 1985). The 1970s brought the first Work Hardening programs, with the ultimate goal of return to work (Wyrick, Ogden Niemayer, Ellexson, Jacobs, & Taylor, 1991). As practice evolves and the needs of those individuals we serve change, assisting individuals to participate in meaningful work roles continues to be the goal of the occupational therapy practitioner in work practice (Larson, Ellexson, & Commission on Practice, 2005). "Work provides structure for people's lives" (Matheson, 2001, p. 103). In the event of chronic disease or disability, an individual's ability to work is often compromised. In the rehabilitation process, the evaluation of the worker, development of work skills, and maintaining worker behaviors are an important part of occupational therapy practice (Matheson, 2001).

In the evaluation of work, occupational therapists must consider the multiple contexts and activity demands that affect performance. According to Sandqvist and Henriksson (2004), work function assessment includes participation in work as it relates to society, work performance as it relates to the client, and the client's capacity as it relates to physical and psychological functioning. A client's deficits in the occupational performance area of work may be both physical and psychological. When work is interrupted, or when the individual is not able to continue working, the public recognition and identity as a worker is missing. The individual may lose the sense of being a productive member of society (Dickie, 2003). The order and expectations of work can provide the stability an individual needs to move forward with overall life activities.

Understanding the psychosocial aspects of disability is as important as having knowledge of those injuries and illnesses that affect the workers' abilities to perform essential job functions. Psychological events could be triggered by family or work stress. Sociocultural issues such as age discrimination could displace a worker (Rice & Luster, 2002). Neurological, sensory, or other changes related to aging could affect a worker's safety and productivity (Larson, 2001). The occupational therapist works with other professionals in addressing issues affecting an individual's ability to work. These professionals may include employers, human resource departments, safety personnel, or case managers. In the past, physical illnesses or injuries have been the primary focus of the employer. There is a definite need in the workplace for occupational therapists to address the performance deficits in those individuals who suffer the effects of mental illness. Competitive work has been shown to be valuable to integrating individuals with schizophrenia into the community. A study in Japan demonstrated how important competitive work, along with clinical support and occupational and vocational rehabilitation services, was in providing individuals with schizophrenia the motivation, income, and stability to move into the community (Oka et al., 2004).

Following a lack of acknowledgment, the recognition of anxiety and depressive disorders in the workplace and the employer costs associated with these illnesses are now being documented (Langlieb & Kahn, 2005). "Research, improved treatment options, and a gradual lessening of the stigma associated with mental illness have created an environment in which their importance to the employer community is more apparent" (Langlieb & Kahn, 2005, p. 1099). In the evaluation of work, the ability to analyze job tasks is critical. Identifying the physical job requirements allows the occupational therapy practitioner to determine job adaptations or modifications or to assist an employer to make reasonable accommodations for a qualified individual with a disability (Americans with Disabilities Act [ADA], 1990; ADA Amendments of 2008). Knowing the physical job requirements is necessary to identify the potential for ergonomic changes, determine options for transitional work, write functional job descriptions, and design post-offer tests.

A comprehensive evaluation looks at the physical requirements of the work, the worker, and the workplace to gain an understanding of factors affecting participation in work. Consideration is given to the activity demands of the work such as the forces, angles, weights, distances, and repetitions the job requires; the design or layout of the work area; organization of the work; and the tools and equipment used to perform the job. Knowledge of gender, age, skill level, and general health of an individual worker or worker population is an important factor in identifying both strengths and limitations in performance skills and patterns (Larson et al., 2005).

Functional capacity evaluation (FCE), a comprehensive tool used to evaluate an individual's physical capacities related to work abilities, has been around since the 1980s (Isernhagen, 1995). FCE provides an objective measure of an individual's physical abilities related to specific work tasks. Cheng and Cheng (2011) studied the predictive ability of the FCE in return to work following a radial wrist fracture. The authors determined that, on the basis of standard testing items in a given FCE protocol, a job-specific FCE could be developed. They determined that a job-specific FCE could have better predictive validity in relation to the work ability status of patients with a specific injury than of patients with a nonspecific injury (Cheng & Cheng, 2011).

The complexities involved in assessing work performance require observing and testing worker skills and abilities in the context of the job and workplace in which the worker intends to work. Based on a review of FCE literature (Gouttebarge, Wind, Kuijer, Sluiter, & Frings-Dressen, 2010), a three-step procedure was proposed to select specific tests from an FCE to address functional limitations in individuals with musculoskeletal complaints (MSC):

- Step 1: Establishing the medical condition of the worker with MSC and related functional limitations.

- Step 2: Assigning the activities limited by the medical condition.

- Step 3: Selecting the functional tests from the full FCE method measuring the limited activities (Gouttenbarge et al., 2010, p. 113).

Environmental and psychosocial factors must also be considered (Sandqvist & Henriksson, 2004). After analyzing the assessment data, the occupational therapist draws conclusions on which to base clinical decisions that will guide workers toward engagement in meaningful, purposeful work activities.

Occupational therapy practitioners use education as a therapeutic tool, designing education programs for clients based on the needs and wants identified in the assessment. The programs could include injury prevention, stress management, safety, proper body mechanics, postural awareness, pain management strategies, joint protection, and symptom awareness (AOTA, 2008).

To be effective in the role of educator, the occupational therapy practitioner must create an environment for learning, becoming aware of the persons or populations being served, understanding the principles of how individuals learn, and selecting the most appropriate teaching approach. As stated earlier, it is important for occupational therapists to be aware of the reading level and comprehensibility of the education materials, as well as the individual client's or population's reading ability and comprehension level. Material should be written at a fifth- to sixth-grade reading level, have a clear purpose, and be meaningful and relevant to the audience (Griffin et al., 2006; Sharry, McKenna, & Tooth, 2002).

A clinical example illustrates this point. A client arrived at an outpatient facility for a scheduled functional capacity assessment. Prior to beginning the test, the client was given medical forms to read and sign. He completed the required paperwork and the occupational therapist began the assessment. As the test progressed, the client followed directions but appeared frustrated and was not engaged in the process. The therapist decided to stop the test and talk with the client. The client confided that he was upset because of the paperwork he was given to fill out when he came into the clinic. He signed the forms but did not know what he was signing. He said he was a poor reader and embarrassed to ask for assistance. Once the therapist was made aware of the situation, she carefully and thoughtfully reviewed the forms to make sure he understood what he had signed. The client's attitude changed. He was now able to fully participate in the functional assessment.

This issue raised the following concerns. First, the client's uncooperative behavior was a result of his inability to read and understand the forms, not because he did not want to fully participate in the functional assessment. Second, the facility had not created an environment in which the client felt comfortable to ask for assistance. The occupational therapist's ability to recognize and address the needs and wants of the client allowed him to fully participate in and benefit from the functional assessment. The results, in turn, will provide the occupational therapist with vital information in intervention planning. With the engagement of the client in the process, the outcome is directed toward increasing the individual's health and well-being for participation in the occupational performance area of work (Law, 2002).

Role of the Occupational Therapy Assistant

The occupational therapy assistant shares a collaborative role with the occupational therapist in the performance areas of work and education. The occupational therapist evaluates, while the occupational therapy assistant, working under the supervision of the occupational therapist, assists in the evaluation process by gathering and sharing data (Accreditation Council for Occupational Therapy Education [ACOTE], 2011).

Case Example

The client is a 54-year-old female who works in a light manufacturing industry that specializes in die cutting. Her job responsibilities include the production line and product inspection. The client has worked for the company for 15 years. She has been treated for thoracic outlet syndrome and continues to complain of left shoulder and neck pain. She has frequent doctor visits and has been on light duty for several years, stating that she cannot do her regular job. Table 18-1 illustrates both worker and employer issues that, in the past, have impeded the return-to-work process for this individual. The occupational therapist has been asked to evaluate the individual's current functional level related to her essential job functions. The human resources department at the company is working on case resolution and plans to use the functional assessment findings along with vocational data in the company's final placement decision.

The occupational therapist focuses on problem identification, problem analysis, and the planning required for problem solution. The occupational therapy assistant focuses on delivering direct services and documenting client response and progress (Larson, 2005). The occupational therapy assistant collects and reports selected information during the evaluation process. The occupational therapy assistant may be asked to participate in the interview process, assist in the development of an education program, or facilitate education and training sessions.

The occupational therapy assistant, having successfully completed an accredited occupational therapy assistant program, has the knowledge, skills, and abilities required to be part of a work rehabilitation team (Moyers, 1999). Assisting with job analysis, providing continuity in a work-hardening or work-conditioning program, and reporting client physical and behavior changes to the occupational therapist are important occupational therapy assistant roles. Specializing in work allows the occupational therapy assistant to gain a depth of skill and knowledge in this area (James & Kehrhahn, 2005). This valued experience enhances what the occupational therapy assistant brings to the team and benefits the therapeutic process for all occupational therapy practitioners. While it is the responsibility of the occupational therapist to delegate responsibilities to the occupational therapy assistant, service competency is the responsibility of the occupational therapy assistant (AOTA, 2009). The occupational therapist and the occupational therapy assistant demonstrate and document service competency for clinical reasoning and judgment during the service delivery process as well as for the performance of specific techniques, assessments, and intervention methods used (AOTA, 2009, p. 799).

Table 18-1.	
ISSUES IMPEDING RETURN TO WORK	
Worker Issues	**Employer Issues**
• Bad body schema	• Chronically absent from work
• No responsibility for own health and well-being (i.e., poor shoes, footwear) • Multiple physical complaints • Poor work habits	• Employee was not performing the essential job functions on a full-time basis • Employee was frequently late, and needed reminders to keep on task
• Various work restrictions • Unhappy with job	• Employee had various work restrictions over the years that were never re-evaluated
• Personal issues outside of work affecting her job satisfaction • Husband on disability	• Performance issues were never addressed • Employee had heavy use of workers' compensation, medical, and disability systems

Summary

To facilitate meaningful participation in the evaluation of education or work, the occupational therapy practitioner needs to create an environment in which clients can focus on and attend to tasks, have a sense of choice or control over the activity, and experience a sense of mastery (Law, 2002). In both the evaluation of the performance areas of work and education, identifying both the physical and psychosocial needs of the client is a crucial step in addressing problems manifested by those needs.

Student Self-Assessment

1. Locate and review client education materials of your choice. Evaluate the clarity, reading level, and appropriateness for the intended population. Document positive findings as well as any changes you would make to improve the materials for the intended population.

2. Identify what contextual and environmental issues you need to consider when teaching handwriting skills to young children with sensory processing deficits.

3. Review the educational theories and models discussed in the chapter and identify the common themes.

4. Research the ADA Web site (www.ada.gov) to review cases involving rulings on mental health issues in the workplace.

5. List the 3 components of work function assessment described by Sandqvist and Henriksson (2004).

6. Access the Job Accommodation Network (www.jan.wvu.edu) on the Internet and determine how it can be used to address the client's need for reasonable accommodations.

7. Explain why both physical and psychological issues must be considered when evaluating a client's deficits in the occupational performance area of work.

8. Describe how the principles from the educational theories and models discussed in the chapter are useful in establishing therapeutic relationships.

9. Working with a peer, identify the occupational therapy assistant's role in the evaluation of an individual with deficits affecting work performance.

10. Describe how education is both a primary therapeutic tool and a primary occupational performance area.

Electronic Resources

- Job Accommodation Network (JAN): www.jan.wvu.edu
- Americans with Disabilities Act: www.ada.gov
- National Institute on Aging: www.nia.nih.gov
- National Institute for Occupational Safety and Health: www.cdc.gov/niosh

EVIDENCE-BASED RESEARCH CHART

Issue	Subject/Activity	Evidence
Educational theories and models	Behavior change; self-efficacy	Carter, 1990; Lewis & Daltroy, 1990; Perry et al., 1990, 1997; Rosenstock & Strecher, 1997
Health education	Needs and problems	Dahlin Ivanoff et al., 2002; Schepans, Panzer, & Goldberg, 2011
	Comprehension, reading level; communication	Griffin et al., 2006; Joos & Hickam, 1990; McEneany, McKenna, & Summerville, 2002
Sensory deficits	Assessments	Bodison & Mailloux, 2006; Watling, Deitz, & White, 2001
Handwriting	Positioning	Naider-Steinhart & Katz-Leurer, 2007
Client centered	Self-perception	Joos & Hickam, 1990; Law, 2002; Law, Baum, & Dunn, 2005; McColl & Pollock, 2001;
Children's work	Education; classroom	Larson, 2004
Work	Psychological issues	Dickie, 2003; Langlieb & Kahn, 2005; Oka et al., 2004; Rice & Luster, 2008; Sandqvist & Henriksson, 2004
	History	Hanson & Walker, 1992; Harvey-Krefting, 1985; Wyrick, Ogden Niemeyer, Ellexson, Jacobs, & Taylor, 1991
Work assessment	Functional capacity evaluation	Cheng & Cheng, 2011; Gouttebarge, Wind, Kuijer, Sluiter, & Frings-Dressen, 2010; Isernhagen, 1995
Essential job functions	Reasonable accommodations	Americans with Disabilities Act, 1990; Americans with Disabilities Act Amendments, 2008
Work performance	Measurement	Matheson, 2001

References

Accreditation Council for Occupational Therapy Education. (2011). *Accreditation Council for Occupational Therapy Education (ACOTE) Standards and Interpretive Guide* (effective July 31, 2013) August 2012 Interpretive Guide Version. Retrieved from http://www.aota.org/Educate/Accredit/DraftStandards/50146.aspx?FT=.pdf

Americans with Disabilities Act of 1990, Pub. L. No. 101-336, §2, 104 Stat. 328 (1991).

Americans with Disabilities Act Amendments of 2008, Pub. L. No. 110-325, 42 USCA § 12101,(2008).

American Occupational Therapy Association. (2008). Occupational therapy practice framework: Domain and process (2nd ed.). *American Journal of Occupational Therapy, 62,* 625-683.

American Occupational Therapy Association. (2009). Guidelines for supervision, roles, and responsibilities during the delivery of occupational therapy services. *American Journal of Occupational Therapy, 63,* 797-803.

Berkeland, R., & Flinn, N. (2005). Therapy as learning. In C. H. Christiansen, C. M. Baum, & J. Bass Haugen (Eds.), *Occupational therapy: Performance, participation, and well-being* (3rd ed., pp. 420-448.). Thorofare, NJ: SLACK Incorporated.

Bodison, S., & Mailloux, Z. (2006). The Sensory Integration and Praxis Tests: Illuminating struggles and strengths in participation at school. *OT Practice, 11*(17), CE1-CE8.

Carter, W. B. (1990). Health behavior as a rational process: Theory of reasoned action and multiattribute utility theory. In K. Glanz, F. M. Lewis, & B. K. Rimer (Eds.), *Health behavior and health education: Theory, research and practice* (pp. 39-62). San Francisco, CA: Jossey-Bass.

Case-Smith, J. (2005). *Occupational therapy for children* (5th ed.). St. Louis, MO: Mosby.

Cheng, A. S. K., & Cheng, S. W. C. (2011). Use of job-specific functional capacity evaluation to predict the return to work of patients with a distal radius fracture. *American Journal of Occupational Therapy, 65,* 445-452.

Dahlin Ivanoff, S., Sonn, U., & Svensson, E. (2002). A health education program for elderly persons with visual impairments and perceived security in the performance of daily occupations: A randomized study. *American Journal of Occupational Therapy, 56*(3), 322-330.

Dickie, V. A. (2003). Establishing worker identity: A study of people in craft work. *American Journal of Occupational Therapy, 57*(3), 250-261.

Griffin, J., McKenna, K., & Tooth, L. (2006). Discrepancy between older clients' ability to read and comprehend and the reading level of written educational materials used by occupational therapists. *American Journal of Occupational Therapy, 60*(1), 70-80.

Gouttebarge, V., Wind, H., Kuijer, P. P. F. M., Sluiter, J. K., & Frings-Dressen, M. H. W. (2010). How to assess physical work-ability with functional capacity evaluation methods in a more specific and efficient way? *WORK, 37,* 111-115.

Hanson, C. S., & Walker, K. F. (1992). The history of work in physical dysfunction. *American Journal of Occupational Therapy, 46*(1), 56-62.

Harvey-Krefting, L. H. (1985). The concept of work in occupational therapy: A historical review. *American Journal of Occupational Therapy, 39*(5), 301-307.

Isernhagen, S. J. (1995) Contemparary Issues in Functional Capacity Evaluation. In S. J. Isernhagen (Ed.) Comprehensive guide to work injury management (pp. 410-429). Gaithersburg, MD: Aspen.

James A. B., & Kehrhahn, M. T. (2005). Professional development. In S. Ryan & K. Sladyk (Eds.), *Ryan's occupational therapy assistant: Principles, practice issues, and techniques* (4th ed., pp. 560-570). Thorofare, NJ: SLACK Incorporated.

Joos, S. K., & Hickam, D. H. (1990). How health professionals influence health behavior: Patient-provider interaction and health outcomes. In K. Glanz, F. M. Lewis, & B. K. Rimer (Eds.), *Health behavior and health education: Theory, research and practice* (pp. 39-62). San Francisco, CA: Jossey-Bass.

Langlieb, A. M., & Kahn, J. P. (2005). How much does quality mental health care profit employers? *Journal of Occupational and Environmental Medicine, 47*(10), 1099-1109.

Larson, B. (2001). The aging worker. *WORK, 16*(1), 67-68.

Larson, B. (2005). Work injury activities. In S. Ryan & K. Sladyk (Eds.), *Ryan's occupational therapy assistant: Principles, practice issues, and techniques* (4th ed., pp. 462-469.). Thorofare, NJ: SLACK Incorporated.

Larson, B., Ellexson, M., & Commission on Practice. (2005). Occupational therapy services in facilitating work performance. *American Journal of Occupational Therapy, 59*(6), 676-679.

Larson, E. A. (2004). Children's work: The less-considered childhood occupation. *American Journal of Occupational Therapy, 58*(4), 369-379.

LaVesser, P. D., Aird, L., & Lieberman, D. (2004). Scope of practice. *American Journal of Occupational Therapy, 58*(6), 673-677.

Law, M. (2002). Participation in the occupations of everyday life. *American Journal of Occupational Therapy, 56*(6), 640-649.

Law, M., Baum, C. M., & Dunn, W. (2005). Occupational performance assessment. In C. H. Christiansen, C. M. Baum, & J. Bass Haugen (Eds.), *Occupational therapy: Performance, participation, and wellbeing* (3rd ed., pp. 338-370). Thorofare, NJ: SLACK Incorporated.

Lewis, F. M., & Daltroy, L. H. (1990). How causal explanations influence health behavior: Attribution theory. In K. Glanz, F. M. Lewis, & B. K. Rimer (Eds.), *Health behavior and health education: Theory, research and practice* (pp. 39-62). San Francisco, CA: Jossey-Bass.

Matheson, L. N. (2001). Measuring work performance from an occupational performance perspective. In M. Law, C. M. Baum, & W. Dunn (Eds.), *Measuring occupational performance, supporting best practice in occupational therapy* (pp. 103-120). Thorofare, NJ: SLACK Incorporated.

McColl, M. A., & Pollock, N. (2001). Measuring occupational performance using a client-centered approach. In M. Law, C. M. Baum, & W. Dunn (Eds.), *Measuring occupational performance: Supporting best practice in occupational therapy* (pp. 81-91). Thorofare, NJ: SLACK Incorporated.

McEneany, J., McKenna, K., & Summerville, P. (2002). Australian occupational therapists working in adult physical dysfunction settings: What treatment media do they use? *Australian Occupational Therapy Journal, 49*(3), 115-127.

Moyers, P. A. (1999.) The guide to occupational therapy practice. American Occupational Therapy Association. *American Journal of Occupational Therapy, 53*(3), 247-322.

Naider-Steinhart, S., & Katz-Leurer, M. (2007). Analysis of proximal and distal muscle activity during handwriting tasks. *American Journal of Occupational Therapy, 61*(4), 392-398.

Oka, M., Otsuka, K., Yokoyama, N., Mintz, J., Hoshino, K., Niwa, S., et al. (2004). An evaluation of a hybrid occupational therapy and supported employment program in Japan for persons with schizophrenia. *American Journal of Occupational Therapy, 58*(4), 466-475.

Pasick, R. J. (1997). Socioeconomic and cultural factors in the development and use of theory. In K. Glanz, F. M. Lewis, & B. K. Rimer (Eds.), *Health behavior and health education: Theory and research* (pp. 425-440.). San Francisco, CA: Jossey-Bass.

Perry, C. L., Barnowski, T., & Parcel, S. (1990). How individuals, environments, and health behaviors interact: Social learning theory. In K. Glanz, F. M. Lewis, & B. K. Rimer (Eds.), *Health behavior and health education: Theory, research and practice* (pp. 162-186). San Francisco, CA: Jossey-Bass.

Perry, C. L., Barnowski, T., & Parcel, S. (1997). How individuals, environments, and health behavior interact: Social cognitive theory. In K. Glanz, F. M. Lewis, & B. K. Rimer (Eds.), *Health behavior and health education: Theory, research, and practice* (2nd ed., pp. 153-178). San Francisco, CA: Jossey-Bass.

Rice, V. J., & Luster, S. (2008). Restoring competence for the worker role. In C. A. Trombley & M. V. Radomski (Eds.), *Occupational therapy for physical dysfunction* (6th ed., pp. 875-908). Baltimore, MD: Lippincott Williams & Wilkins.

Rosenstock, I. M. (1990). The health belief model: Explaining health behavior through expectancies. In K. Glanz, F. M. Lewis, & B. K. Rimer (Eds.), *Health behavior and health education: Theory, research and practice* (pp. 39-62). San Francisco, CA: Jossey-Bass.

Rosenstock, I. M., & Strecher, R. J. (1997). The health belief model. In K. Glanz, F. M. Lewis, & B. K. Rimer (Eds.), *Health behavior and health education: Theory, research, and practice* (2nd ed., pp. 41-59). San Francisco, CA: Jossey-Bass.

Roter, D. L., & Hall, J. A. (1997). Patient-provider education. In K. Glanz, F. M. Lewis, & B. K. Rimer (Eds.), *Health behavior and health education: Theory, research, and practice.* (pp. 206-226). San Francisco, CA: Jossey-Bass.

Sandqvist, J. L., & Henriksson, C. M. (2004). Work functioning: A conceptual framework. *WORK, 23*(2), 147-157.

Schepans, S. L., Panzer, V., & Goldberg, A. (2011). Randomized controlled trial comparing tailoring methods of multimedia-based fall prevention education for community-dwelling older adults. *American Journal of Occupational Therapy, 65*(6), 702-709.

Sharry, R., McKenna, K., & Tooth, L. (2002). Occupational therapists' use and perceptions of written client educational materials. *American Journal of Occupational Therapy, 56*(5), 573-576.

Smith-Zuzovsky, N., & Exner, C. E. (2004). The effect of seated positioning quality on typical 6- and 7-year-old children's object manipulation skills. *American Journal of Occupational Therapy, 58*(4), 380-388.

Watling, R. L., Deitz, J., & White, O. (2001). Comparison of sensory profile scores of young children with and without autism spectrum disorders. *American Journal of Occupational Therapy, 55*(4), 416-423.

Wyrick, J. M., Ogden Niemeyer, L., Ellexson, M., Jacobs, K., & Taylor, S. (1991). Occupational therapy work-hardening programs: A demographic study. *American Journal of Occupational Therapy, 45*(2), 109-112.

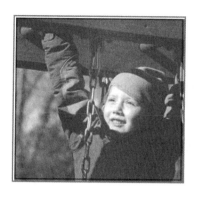

19

EVALUATION OF PLAY AND LEISURE

Lori Vaughn, OTD, OTR/L

ACOTE STANDARDS EXPLORED IN THIS CHAPTER
B.4.1, B.4.4, B.4.5

KEY VOCABULARY

- **Framing:** Cues that a player offers regarding how her or she wants to be treated (Bateson, 1972).
- **Freedom to suspend reality:** A child's ability to defer ther restrictions of realistic play and use his or her imaginatio to take on new roles and identities and tus sue objects in a creative way (Bundy, 1997).
- **Internal control:** The individual is the mechanism that drives play. The player is in control of the materials, the play interactions, and some aspects of the outcome (Bundy, 1997; Connor, Williamson & Siepp, 1978)

- **Intrinsic motivation:** Children are actively engaged in the process of play and are able to continue participation despite barriers and obstacles experienced during the activity (Bundy, 1997; Primeau & Ferguson, 1999).
- **Leisure activities:** Those activitess in which people engage that are non-obligatotory, stress free,n and guild free (Sellar & Boshoff, 2006).
- **Play activities:** Diversionary activities that promote pleasure and amusement (AOTA, 2010).
- **Playfulness:** Describes how an individual approaches any task (not just play or leisure); incorporates intrinisic motivation, internal control, and freedom to suspend realitty. It is a characteristic of the person rather than the task (Barnett, 1990; Bundy, 1993).

Jacobs, K., MacRae, N., & Sladyk, K. (Eds.).
*Occupational Therapy Essentials for
Clinical Competence, Second Edition* (pp. 241-258).
© 2014 SLACK Incorporated.

Introduction

THE OCCUPATIONAL THERAPY PRACTITIONER'S SCOPE OF PRACTICE IN THE EVALUATION OF PLAY AND LEISURE

The American Occupational Therapy Association (AOTA) Scope of Practice (AOTA, 2010), the core of occupational therapy practice, values the understanding and use of occupations. The domain of occupational therapy is the occupations that people find purposeful and meaningful, enabling individuals to participate in everyday life activities and situations, desired roles, and contexts (AOTA, 2010). Play activities are defined as "spontaneous and organized activities that promote pleasure, amusement, and diversion" (AOTA, 2010, p. 573) and leisure activities are described as "non-obligatory, discretionary, and intrinsically rewarding activities" (AOTA, p. 572). In practice, occupational therapy practitioners must consider several factors including the client's repertoire of occupations, performance skills and patterns utilized, the influence of contexts on participation, activity demands, and the structures and functions of the client's body (AOTA). The AOTA recognizes play as an essential domain of occupational therapy practice for people across the lifespan and the role of practitioners in supporting, enhancing, facilitating, and defending the right of all individuals to engage in this important occupation (Primeau, 2008).

THE ROLE OF THE OCCUPATIONAL THERAPIST AND OCCUPATIONAL THERAPY ASSISTANT IN THE EVALUATION OF PLAY AND LEISURE

Evaluations are directed by occupational therapists and include the following: determination of service need, problem identification and definition; establishment of priorities, goals, and interventions; determination of additional assessment; interpretation of the data; and integration of information. The occupational therapy assistant contributes to the process of evaluation by the implementation of assigned assessments if service competency has been established, provision of verbal and/or written reports based on observations and experience, and dissemination of other pertinent information necessary for the occupational therapist for interpretation and decision making (Brayman et al., 2004). Throughout the evaluation process, the occupational therapist develops a client's occupational profile, assesses the client's ability to participate in everyday activities, and works with the client to determine areas of need and priorities for intervention to support engagements in meaningful occupations (AOTA, 2010).

Evaluation includes several factors that can impact basic and instrumental activities of daily living (BADL, IADL), education, work, play, leisure, and social participation (AOTA).

Evaluation of Play

You can discover more about a person in an hour of play than in a year of conversation.
—*Plato, Greek philosopher (427 B.C. to 347 B.C.)*

Play is a concept familiar to everyone. Just the mention of the word can evoke thoughts and emotions. However, the feelings induced are subjective to each individual. A child can be observed while engaged in a variety of play activities such as playing dress-up or chasing a friend on the playground. An adolescent can be engrossed in playing a video game, or a little leaguer can play baseball. Play is individual to the player and possesses meaning an outside observer can only assume. While the activities themselves can be labeled or defined, a clear understanding remains elusive, and a child's motivation a mystery. Contributing to the difficulty with conceptualization are the divergent cultural and societal norms, beliefs, and values associated with play. While play is difficult to understand, it is an inherent part of who children are, how they learn and develop, and how they interact with people and objects in the environment. The first section of this chapter focuses on theories contributing to the concept of play and specific assessment tools used to evaluate play.

WHAT IS PLAY?

Despite an inherent personal concept of play subject to individual interpretations, theorists have long struggled to conceive of, develop, and concur on a definitive definition (Parham & Primeau, 1997; Takata, 1969). While observers might easily label the previous examples as play, the ability to determine what intrinsic value a task holds for the player and what elements of the task constitute a playful experience is much more complex. While lacking an operational definition may seem inconsequential, the inability to operationalize the term impacts the ability to develop appropriate assessment instruments (Parham & Primeau, 1997). Scholars have long attempted to form a consensus on a definition in an attempt to ensure that they were talking about the same thing (Garvey, 1990); however, play remains an elusive concept (Bundy, 2010). Without the ability to find a common language, scholars are unable to adequately evaluate and research all of the intricacies of play (Parham & Primeau, 1997) and are unable to distinguish it from non-play (Bundy, 1993; Rubin, Fein, & Vandenberg, 1983). Labeling what constitutes play is much more challenging than determining what it is not (Takata, 1969), as it is easy to identify but difficult to define (Johnson, Christie, & Yawkey, 1987). What scholars can agree on is that play is the primary occupation of children (Bundy, 1993; Heard, 1977; Knox, 1997; Muys, Rodger, & Bundy, 2006), one in which people engage throughout their lifespan (Christiansen, 1991; Kielhofner, 1995; Lautamo & Heikkila, 2011; Primeau, Clark, & Pierce, 1989; Yerxa et al., 1989), and something in which they want to engage, rather than are obliged to engage (Lautamo & Heikkila, 2011). Children are less concerned with how to define play, but describe their purpose for persistent engagement as "fun" and an escape from "boredom" (Miller & Kuhaneck, 2008). Some of the prevailing operational concepts are found within the constructs of occupational science (Clark et al., 1991), which focus on the study of occupation (Parham & Primeau, 1997). Under this theory, in order to understand the occupation of play, scholars must study play rather than focus on the performance skills and client factors that can impact play (Parham & Primeau, 1997). In occupational science, play is open ended, limitless, and a completely pleasurable experience (Burke, 1996). Yerxa et al. (1989) stressed the importance of understanding what the process of engagement means to the individual. Another view involves the belief that play is more than a method to achieve a therapeutic end but is an end in and of itself because of its intrinsic value and its ability to promote health. It is inappropriate to view play simply as a therapeutic tool but rather as an entity that should not be reduced to its individual components (Miller & Kuhaneck, 2008). Play has also been linked to the development of creativity, curiosity, humor, imagination, and communication skills (Caplan & Caplan, 1973; McCune-Nicolich & Bruskin, 1982; Russ, 2003; Saltz & Brodie, 1982; Singer & Singer, 1992). While engaged in play, children are at, or close to, their optimal level of development (Vygotsky, 1967, cited in Linder, 1993). It exists for the intrinsic pleasure of the player, and there is no correct or incorrect way to play (Olsen, 1999). It is also highly dependent on the attitudes and beliefs of the player (Takata, 1974). For this reason, defining play is not the only challenge that is presented—evaluating play is equally difficult.

Theories of Play

Occupational therapists have recognized the value of play as a role and as a method of health promotion. However, not until the work of Mary Reilly (1974) and her students did the profession contribute to the knowledge base of play. While there exists an extensive body of knowledge regarding play theories, much of that knowledge was acquired through other disciplines, especially education and psychology. Still, efforts to develop an occupational therapy theory of play have been limited (Parham & Primeau, 1997). Because much of the knowledge is derived from other disciplines, and because of the unique foci and perspectives of these other disciplines, the ability to develop a comprehensive occupational therapy taxonomy regarding the occupational components of play is challenging (Parham & Primeau, 1997). With the lack of an appropriate taxonomy, therapists often apply other models of practice to play, which may or may not appropriately address the deficits (Bryze, 1997). Despite the challenges, these disciplines provide a basis on which occupational therapy can build. According to Reilly (1974), an interdisciplinary explanation is necessary because of the complexity of play.

Historical Perspectives

History provides several play perspectives. In the research, these theories are typically labeled either classical or modern theories, with World War I as the marker between the two periods (Gilmore, 1971; Mellou, 1994). Classical theories attempted to identify why play existed and define its purpose. These theories were based on philosophical principles rather than scientific research (Ellis, 1973, cited in Parham & Primeau, 1997). Four classical theories were identified (Gilmore, 1971; Mellou, 1994) and are briefly described in the following examples:

1. **Surplus Energy Theory.** Hypothesized that every organism has a fixed quantity of energy available, which must be expended. When the energy is not required for self-preservation, it is manifested in non–goal-directed ways. Because children are typically cared for and do not expend a great deal of energy in these endeavors, they have excess energy and play occurs as a result (Gilmore, 1971; Lieberman, 1977; Mellou, 1994; Parham & Primeau, 1997; Rubin, 1982; Stagnitti, 2004; Tsao, 2002). Remnants of this theory persist today. Consider parents directing their children to "go outside and play" to burn off some energy.

2. **Recreation/Relaxation Theory.** Proposed that play was a result of a lack of energy and occurred to replenish depleted energy. Because children are always busy learning and acquiring new skills, a great deal of energy is utilized. Play is relaxing and rejuvenating because there are no cognitive demands (Gilmore, 1971; Lieberman, 1977; Mellou, 1994; Parham & Primeau, 1997; Stagnitti, 2004). Remnants of this theory can be found in the "rejuvenating" outings that occur in the business world and the newfound "energy" a young adult finds after a long day of work when a friend calls to make plans for the evening.

3. **Pre-Exercise Theory.** Hypothesized that play is instinctive and is preparatory for mature adult behavior in the future. As species become

increasingly complex on the evolutionary scale, organisms are not born with the required skills to survive in adulthood. For this reason, periods of time during which adaptive skills are acquired are necessary and play is a method of acquiring these skills. Play is utilized as rehearsal for adult roles and for the acquisition of skills necessary for survival and adaptation (Parham, 1996; Reilly, 1974; Saracho & Spodek, 1995; Stagnitti, 2004; Tsao, 2002). Remnants of this theory can be found in the preponderance of gender-based toys that are marketed to children to "play house" or to "play pretend" in various life roles.

4. **Recapitulation Theory.** Postulated that play is part of an evolutionary process. Human development follows an evolutionary path, and the development of play is no exception. For example, children swing and climb trees during an "animal" phase of development (Mellou, 1994; Rubin et al., 1983; Stagnitti, 2004). This theory may also be found in how play behaviors are often described, such as how a person "acts like an animal" and even play equipment, such as the monkey bars.

Modern theories developed after World War I and were based on classical theories. These theorists were more interested in addressing play and how it relates to human development (Parham & Primeau, 1997). Parham and Primeau grouped modern theories into 4 categories—arousal modulation, psychodynamic, cognitive developmental, and sociocultural theories. These are briefly described as follows:

- **Arousal Modulation Theories.** Hypothesized that novelty and uncertainty increase arousal levels, and when aroused, organisms enter an exploratory state. When children are presented with a novel toy or are in a new environment, play is limited because they enter the discovery state, which is cognitively based and requires focused attention. Play is more relaxed as a child experiments with a familiar toy in a known environment (Mellou, 1994; Parham & Primeau, 1997).

- **Psychodynamic Theories.** Based on the works of Freud and Erikson (1959), these theories hypothesized that children develop coping strategies through play. These strategies are "acted out" through play to rehearse for situations that might occur in reality later in life. This allows them to actively mediate stressful events rather than falling prey to anxiety and helplessness (Gilmore, 1971; Parham & Primeau, 1997; Rubin et al., 1983).

- **Cognitive Developmental Theories.** Postulated that play is volitional and contributes to the development of cognitive skills, symbolism, adaptation, flexibility, and a repertoire of skills necessary for later life

(Bruner, 1972; Mellou, 1994; Parham & Primeau, 1997; Rubin et al., 1983; Sutton-Smith, 1967). These theories further postulate that creativity develops through play. Children also learn the consequences of their actions and self-expression (Gardner, 1982).

- **Sociocultural Theories.** Hypothesized that children learn social and cultural norms and behaviors through play, with both play and culture reciprocally influencing each other. Children also learn the rules of social conduct and the concept of self-identity through playful activities. Empathy and the ability to function as a member of society are learned through game play and games with rules (Mead, 1934, cited in Parham & Primeau, 1997; Roopnarine & Johnson, 1994; Sutton-Smith, 1980).

While many of the classical and modern theories were based in philosophy, psychology, and education, the field of occupational therapy has also been interested in play throughout its history. The early founders stressed the importance of finding a balance between work, rest, play, and sleep (Parham & Primeau, 1997). Play developed as a primary tool when treating children and became synonymous with occupational therapy (Granoff, 1995, as cited in Parham & Primeau, 1997). Economic factors influenced the use of play as a therapeutic tool in the early 20th century. Individuals deemed able to work were placed in work programs, and those unable to work participated in recreational programs (Inch, 1936, cited in Parham & Primeau, 1997). The differentiation between work and play became less defined as practitioners learned that both could exist within a given activity (Parham & Primeau, 1997). Through Mary Reilly's work (1974), play was once again brought to the forefront of occupational therapy and utilized as a valuable therapeutic and research tool. Reilly recognized the complexity of play, which she described as a "cobweb" through which children learn mastery of their environment and gain the skills and competency required for adulthood. Many of Reilly's students continued her work and have added substantial information to the field, inspiring a new generation of scholars and practitioners.

Why Evaluate Play?

Researchers have stressed the importance of embracing play as a valid occupational therapy area of practice (Bundy, 1991; Couch, Deitz, & Kanny, 1998; Florey, 1981; Lautamo & Heikkila, 2011). While play is acknowledged as the primary occupation of children and one that lasts throughout the lifetime, it is rarely evaluated (Bundy, 1997; Lawlor & Henderson, 1989). The reasons for this are varied but are likely related to the lack of assessment tools that truly evaluate play (Bundy, 1993; Bundy, Nelson, Metzger, & Bingaman, 2001; Morrison & Metzger, 2001; Sturgess, 1997). Further, it is acknowledged that observation of a child's play skills in natural environments is important; observation alone does not provide enough objective information with regard to a child's play abilities in the absence of objective assessment tools (Sturgess, 1997). Because play and the components that compose play are difficult to define, the ability to quantify and standardize these components can be even more challenging (Kalverboer, 1977). Other constraints diminishing the use of play as a therapeutic tool include negativity regarding play with an emphasis on non–play-based skill development, intervention based on site-specific roles, and reimbursement issues (Couch et al., 1998). Assessments exist, but they tend to focus more on play-related skills such as fine motor, gross motor, and cognitive abilities (Bundy, 1997). While these assessments assist in identifying a child's underlying capabilities and capacity to engage in play, they do not assess play as an occupation (Wallen & Walker, 1995). Assessing the occupation of play provides the therapist with valuable information regarding developmental levels across several domains including socialization, preacademic, motor, communication, and self-awareness (Fewell & Glick, 1993; Florey, 1971; Michelman, 1974; Schaaf, 1990; Takata, 1974), and has been called the "window to development" (Stagnitti, Unsworth, & Rodger, 2000, p. 292). Further, the evaluation of play provides valuable information relative to a child's ability to interact within the environment (Lautamo & Heikkila, 2011).

To effectively evaluate play, it is important to look at the entire occupation of play rather than simply evaluating the related client factors. Play is essential to healthy development as well as a sense of meaning and purpose in life (Kolehmainen, Francis, Ramsay, Owen, McKee, Ketelaar, & Rosenbaum, 2011). Children who cannot play or who have difficulty engaging in play do not develop the skills necessary for typical development. This difficulty can precipitate lifelong difficulties including decreased participation and satisfaction in occupational roles (Bledsoe & Shepherd, 1982; O'Brien & Shirley, 2001; Stagnitti & Unsworth, 2000), as well as social and emotional well-being (Kolehmainen et al., 2011). Effective assessment of play serves multiple purposes. Play assessments can be used diagnostically to assess development across domains, as well as therapeutically for intervention planning and to determine the effectiveness of intervention (Kelly-Vance & Ryalls, 2005; Miller & Kuhaneck, 2008). Lack of empirically researched assessment tools may also be related to the cultural value that has been placed on play as an occupation. Cultural and societal beliefs have impacted the prioritization of areas of focus within the profession, and play has historically been viewed as a volitional rather than compulsory activity such as self-care, work, and education (Bundy, 2005). This lack of tools often leads to the use of informal observation-based evaluation. While this can be a valuable and informative method of obtaining information, there are many factors that can impact the quality of such

an evaluation including the knowledge and experience of the practitioner and his or her ability to adequately interpret the information (Bundy, 2005).

This is further compounded by the lack of culturally appropriate assessment tools. The majority of standardized assessment tools used in pediatric occupational therapy practice were normed on typically developing children from North America and England using items and materials culturally appropriate for those populations, yet they are used to evaluate children from other cultures without consideration of their cultural relevance (Dender & Stagnitti, 2011; Pfeifer, Queiroz, Santos, & Stagnitti, 2011; Thorley & Lim, 2011). This can lead to difficulties in both developing a culturally appropriate intervention plan and an over- or under-identification of children as "delayed" (Dender & Stagnitti, 2011) and place children from other cultures at a disadvantage (Pfeifer et al.).

In addition, there is a paucity of tools that adequately measure play in children with disabilities because of the inherent difficulty in determining and measuring participation (Coster & Khetani, 2008; Hoogsteen & Woodgate, 2010; McConachi, Colver, Forsyth, Jarvis, & Parkinson, 2006). Despite this, difficulty in play has been identified in children with a variety of diagnoses, including developmental, emotional, learning, and movement/coordination disorders (Cordier, Bundy, Hocking, & Enfield, 2010; McDonald & Vigen, 2012; Muys, Rodger, & Bundy, 2006; Poulsen, Ziviani, Cuskelly, & Smith, 2007). Because play is central in the lives of children, and practitioners are ethically bound to utilize a client-centered approach with children and families, it is incumbent on practitioners to evaluate it as an occupation when play is a concern, using culturally and developmentally appropriate assessment tools. Evaluation of play should include the family and caregivers in the process, and whenever possible, it should occur within the child's natural settings of home, school, and community (Townsend, 1997, cited in Primeau, 2003).

Using this top-down, collaborative approach to evaluation, the client and practitioner are able to identify the occupations that children want, need, and have to do and the factors that impact their ability to fully participate in these areas (Coster, 1998; Law et al., 1990; Trombly, 1993). According to Anita Bundy (1997), a comprehensive evaluation of play should include the following five factors:

1. What the player does.
2. Why the player enjoys the chosen activity.
3. How the player approaches play.
4. The player's capacity to play.
5. Relative supportiveness of the environment.

What the Player Does

Regardless of the words used to define play, theorists agree that play is activity for its own sake and not one that is based on external factors (Parham & Primeau,

1997; Rubin et al., 1983). In play, it is the process of *doing* rather than the end product that is rewarding (Rubin et al.). There are three factors that researchers have identified of which play is composed: intrinsic motivation, internal control, and freedom to suspend reality (Bundy, 2002; Morrison, Bundy, & Fisher, 1991; Neuman, 1971). Intrinsic motivation is what drives a child to participate in an activity for pleasure rather than for extrinsic reward (Bundy, 1993). However, it is difficult to assess, as children do not always demonstrate outward expressions of pleasure while engaged in play activities (Morrison et al., 1991). With intrinsic motivation, children are actively engaged in the process of play and are able to continue participation despite barriers and obstacles experienced during the activity (Bundy, 1997; Primeau & Ferguson, 1999). Intrinsic motivation involves pleasure, which differentiates play from work (West, 1990). With internal control, the individual is the mechanism that drives the play. The player is in control of the materials, the play interactions, and some aspects of the outcome (Bundy, 1997; Connor, Williamson, & Siepp, 1978). The child is motivated, is able to modify his or her approach despite challenges, is willing to share materials and equipment, and seeks play opportunities with peers (Bundy, 1997). With the freedom to suspend reality, the child is able to defer the restrictions of realistic play and use his or her imagination to take on new roles and identities and to use objects in a creative way (Bundy, 1997; Rubin et al., 1983). With the ability to suspend reality, the child is able to be mischievous, playful, joking, teasing, and imaginative (Bundy, 1997). This is recognized as important for the acquisition and development of cognitive, social, and language skills (McCune-Nicholich & Fenson, 1984, as cited in Rodger & Ziviani, 1999).

Why the Player Enjoys the Chosen Activity

As an observer, it can be difficult to understand why an individual chooses a specific activity and what value participation holds for the individual. Theorists have struggled over this concept, attempting to deconstruct the value and purpose ascribed to one activity over another that appears equally enticing (Lawlor, 2003). According to Rubin et al. (1983), play involves self-imposed goals that are subject to change according to the wishes and desires of the player, making it spontaneous. Understanding why a person selects a particular activity and the intrinsic pleasure derived from it is difficult and equally challenging for the player to articulate. Intrinsic motivation is difficult to assess but important to understand if we are to consider play as an important occupation (Bundy, 1997). According to Bruner (1986), it is impossible to understand what an individual is experiencing while engaged in any activity. However, through observation, clues are emitted on which inferences can be drawn. Although motivation is difficult to assess, information can be obtained through the observation of play patterns. Activities in which the child derives pleasure and engages in regularly can provide clues as to the player's motivation (Bundy, 1997). Pleasure is subjective, with each individual deriving something personal from any given activity. Evaluating personal meaning, while difficult, is important if intervention is aimed at building and improving an individual's repertoire of play skills and interests (Bundy, 2001).

How the Player Approaches Play

It is important to consider not just what a player does, but also how the child approaches play (Bundy, 1993), which has been termed *playfulness* (Barnett, 1990; Bundy, 1993; Lieberman, 1977). Playfulness incorporates intrinsic motivation, internal control, and freedom to suspend reality, but it is not limited to play and may be seen in any activity (Bundy, 1993). In addition to the three factors of which play is composed, Bateson (1972) described a fourth factor—framing—that he identified as essential for playfulness. He likened play to a frame through which players offer cues about how they want to be treated. For success, players must be able to give and receive these social cues (Bateson, 1972; Bundy, 1997). With playfulness, the outcome is not as important as the process. It is the individual who determines whether a task is playful, rather than the activity itself (Bryze, 1997; Bundy, 1997). Assessing playfulness may provide therapists with greater and more valuable information than assessing the play activities themselves (Bundy, 1997). Anita Bundy (1991) recognized the importance of incorporating several factors into the evaluation of play and developed a model of playfulness and a complementary assessment, the Test of Playfulness (ToP), which is included in the evidence based chart on page 251.

The Player's Capacity to Play

The player's capacity to play relates to active participation in a play activity (Rubin et al., 1983). Play assessments have historically focused on evaluating the skills necessary to participate in play activities (Bundy, 1997). Fine and gross motor, sensory, and neurological deficits may play a role in play deficits. While it is important to evaluate these skills to determine how skill performance impacts an individual's ability to play, it is not the only area that should be evaluated. The best information will result from an evaluation of these skills within the context of play rather than in isolation (Bundy, 1997). Including a variety of recognizable toys in a familiar environment with minimal intrusion will aid in obtaining the most accurate information of play skills (Rubin et al., 1983).

The Relative Supportiveness of the Environment

Play represents an interaction of players and the environment in which they play, and a complete evaluation of play must include how the environment supports participation (Bundy, 1997). This environmental assessment should include the caregivers and other individuals, objects, space, safety, comfort, and sensory input relative to their support of play (Bundy, 1997; Olsen, 1999; Parham & Primeau, 1997). A child's daily routines and interactions become incorporated into play experiences and are drawn upon for imagination (Harris, 2000). Children who are deemed "playful" exhibit a decrease in playfulness in a less supportive environment, and conversely, less playful children exhibit an increase in playfulness in a more supportive environment (Bronson & Bundy, 2001; Lieberman, 1977). If environmental factors impede an individual's ability to play, the development of required skills and behaviors may be inhibited (Bryze, 1997; Burke, 1993; Reilly, 1974). Theorists have espoused the benefits of a supportive environment and have advocated the benefits of the reciprocal person–environment interaction, with each influencing the other (Bronson & Bundy, 2001; Kielhofner, 1995; Wicker, 1987). Both physical and social aspects of the environment can influence the development of play skills. The "fit" between the environment and the person is considered positive when the environment is able to meet the individual's needs and when the individual's abilities match the demands imposed by the environment (Pervin, 1968, as cited in Bronson & Bundy, 2001; Rodger & Ziviani, 2006). Boredom or anxiety can exist if the demands of the environment are too low or too high relative to the abilities of the child (Bronson & Bundy, 2001). Play can occur when the child feels comfortable and safe within his or her environment (Hamm, 2006).

PLAY ASSESSMENTS

As indicated earlier in this chapter, play is complex. A thorough evaluation is necessary to determine which factors relate to deficits in this multifaceted occupation. A variety of assessment tools are available; however, they are not inclusive of all potential deficit areas, nor are they wholly occupationally focused. The selection of a play assessment should be carefully considered. Inclusion of the word *play* in the name of the tool does not necessarily mean that play is being assessed. Therefore, consideration of various tools and options is recommended for an accurate evaluation (Bundy, 1997). Play assessments generally consist of an observation of the child within the context of play to evaluate the child's abilities across all areas when compared to typically developing peers (Kelly-Vance & Ryalls, 2005). These assessments can provide a wealth of information related to a child's areas of strength and areas of need (Fewell, 1991; Kelly-Vance & Ryalls, 2005; Linder, 1993). Neisworth and Bagnato (1988) outlined a continuum of assessment approaches that are typically utilized by multidisciplinary assessment teams. Norm-based

assessments evaluate a child's developmental level to a similar cohort group. Curriculum-based assessments involve following an individual's achievement along a "developmentally sequenced curriculum" (Neisworth & Bagnato, 1988, p. 27). Adaptive-to-disability assessments allow for altered presentation and response modes and modified responses on test items by a child with sensory impairments to minimize incorrect or false failure on test items. Process assessments examine the changes in a child's reaction to changes in stimuli and can be indicative of a child's cognitive functioning. This includes changes in behavior and can have an effect on the response to the presentation of different stimuli. Judgment-based assessments quantify the impressions and observations of individuals familiar with the child, including parents, caregivers, teachers, and other professionals. This assessment approach is typically used for traits not easily evaluated through other means, including temperament, muscle tone, motivation, and impulse control (Linder, 1993). Ecological assessment examines the child's social, physical, and psychological contexts. Interactive assessment is considered a component of ecological assessment (Linder, 1993) and involves the examination of the social synchronicity of the infant and caregiver. Systematic observation occurs in a child's natural environment of home, school, or community. It may also occur through simulations and/or role playing and involves measurable, observed aspects of behavior such as frequency, duration, and intensity (Neisworth & Bagnato, 1988). A brief description of play assessments is included in Appendix C to assist the practitioner in selecting the appropriate tool.

Evaluation of Leisure

To be able to fill leisure intelligently is the last product of civilization, and at present, very few people have reached this level.

—Bertrand Russell,
British author and philosopher (1930)

According to Mary Reilly (1974), play possesses both social and biological components. Socially, children learn to interact with both physical and nonphysical aspects of the environment and adapt their responses based on those experiences. Biologically, living things engage in play, which lends to the assumption that, as beings become increasingly complex, the activities in which they engage also become more physically and cognitively complex (Gilfoyle, Grady, & Moore, 1990). As individuals mature beyond childhood, play transforms to leisure, encompassing both social and solitary activities as they continue to refine their understanding of the world and the roles in which they participate (Gilfoyle et al., 1990). While the theoretical beliefs related to leisure have changed throughout history, there is no disputing that, like play, leisure is an important occupation in which we engage and a core concept in the Occupational Therapy Practice Framework (AOTA, 2008).

WHAT IS LEISURE?

Similar to play, theorists have long contemplated the characteristics and value of leisure. The definition of leisure has changed throughout history, adding new elements with each revision. Although each definition added a new dimension to leisure conceptualization, empirical research lagged behind (Esteve, San Martin, & Lopez, 1999). Research indicated that leisure participation, satisfaction, and attitude are positively correlated with satisfaction and quality of life (Caldwell & Witt, 2011; Hawkins, 1994; Hawkins, Ardovino, & Hsieh, 1998; Lloyd & Auld, 2002) and has been associated with contributing to promoting and maintaining mental and physical health (Caldwell & Smith, 1988; Coleman & Iso-Ahola, 1993; Passmore, 2003; Tinsley & Tinsley, 1986), as well as positive social functioning (Caldwell & Witt, 2011) and improved academic performance (Mahone, 2000). Some research also indicated that leisure impacts development by providing opportunities for skill acquisition (Evans & Poole, 1991), social competency, self-awareness, and self-control (Silbereisen, Noack, & Eyferth, 1986, as cited in Passmore, 2003). There have been many terms that have become synonymous with leisure such as relaxation, stress free, freedom from "necessaries," and guilt free (Sellar & Boshoff, 2006). Work is often considered obligatory, whereas leisure is the freedom from obligation (Kelly, 1987; Kleiber, 1999; Sellar & Boshoff, 2006). Historically, work has been more highly regarded than leisure, causing the work–leisure dichotomy to exist. Occupational choices were made out of financial necessity and responsibility, creating a barrier to leisure participation and a sense of guilt over what a person can do and what he or she should do (Sellar & Boshoff, 2006). By removing or minimizing the barriers of obligatory tasks, the meaning and experience of leisure is enhanced (Kelly, 1987; Sellar & Boshoff, 2006). Like play in children, leisure has been linked to playfulness (Guitard, Ferland, & Dutil, 2005). The benefits of playfulness in everyday life have been linked to increased creativity, improved ability to heal, increased motivation, and enhanced affect and morale (Auerhahn & Laub, 1987; Etienne, 1982, as cited in Guitard et al., 2005; Lyons, 1987; Tegano, 1990). Despite the benefits, the components of playfulness are different in adults than in children, with adults expressing decreases in spontaneity and tolerance for joy and humor (Guitard et al., 2005; Lieberman, 1977). Guitard et al. (2005) found that playfulness in adults is composed of five components: creativity, curiosity, sense of humor, pleasure, and spontaneity. They further found that playfulness, as defined by the aforementioned components,

is helpful in enhancing an individual's occupational performance. Leisure is also similar to play, in that cultural values of leisure time vary. The meaning of "free time" holds different values and beliefs in different societies and cultures (Godbey & Jung, 1991). In English-speaking countries, leisure is equated with free time and can hold a negative value because of its contrast with the concept of work and the value therein (Goodale & Cooper, 1991). There are several factors that impact time use including work beliefs and values, socioeconomic status, politics, gender roles, and weather (Godbey & Jung, 1991). Regardless of the conceptual framework from which leisure is viewed, its intrinsic motivation cannot be denied (Caldwell & Witt, 2011).

PAST AND PRESENT THEORIES OF LEISURE

Theories related to leisure and the use of discretionary time have been in a continuous state of evolution for centuries. It was first defined by Aristotle as being in a state in which an individual was free from the need to toil in laborious tasks and dedicated to more virtuous tasks of self-discovery, self-development, and the pursuit of pleasure (Dare, Welton, & Coe, 1987; Goodale & Cooper, 1991; Sellar & Boshoff, 2006; Veal & Lynch, 2001). These beliefs continued until the period of industrialization and the prevalence of the Protestant work ethic dichotomizing the concepts of work and leisure (Goodale & Cooper, 1991; Primeau, 1996; Sellar & Boshoff, 2006; Veal & Lynch, 2001). Leisure time became that which was left over after domestic and vocational tasks were complete (Veal & Lynch, 2001). It was viewed as a time for consumption, whereas work was a time for production (Goodale & Cooper, 1991). Focus on the concept of leisure as a component of residual time persisted until approximately 20 years ago, when a shift in thinking occurred. The focus became less of a concept of time and more a concept of the subjective experience of the individual (Primeau, 1996; Suto, 1998; Veal & Lynch, 2001). The perception of the individual became the prevailing determinant in the classification of an activity as leisurely, existing within the individual's consciousness (Kelly, 2000; McDowell, 1984).

WHY EVALUATE LEISURE?

Like play, leisure is a primary occupation and an important component of well-being (Turner, Chapman, McSherry, Krishnagiri, & Watts, 2000). Technological advancements, improved health care services, and increased awareness of wellness and prevention have led to an increased number of active, older adults (Stanley, 1995). This number is expected to continue to increase, highlighting the need to ensure that people are able to maintain healthy, active, satisfying existences throughout the lifespan (Sellar & Boshoff, 2006; Stanley, 1995). It is important for health care providers, especially occupational therapy practitioners, to enhance their understanding of the meaning of roles and occupations. Leisure is an important area of practice and is related to improved quality of life, overall health, successful aging, and functional capacity (Charters & Murray, 2006; Easton & Herge, 2011; Law, 2002; Lloyd & Auld, 2002; Sellar & Boshoff, 2006). Like play, leisure can also be viewed as a means to an end and a beneficial area for intervention (Caldwell & Witt, 2011). As such, the necessity to incorporate the evaluation of leisure in occupational therapy is undeniable. However, until recently, the concept of including the subjective experience of the individual in the evaluation was minimal, with a greater focus on more objective factors including the actual activity and time utilization. This led to the implication that the act of participation was more important than the meaning (Sellar & Boshoff, 2006; Suto, 1998). Understanding the meaning behind participation in certain activities can help therapists utilize leisure as a therapeutic activity and enhance the identification of specific barriers that preclude participation (Sellar & Boshoff, 2006; Suto, 1998). To do so effectively, it is important to explore common conceptual factors of leisure including the temporal, activity, and experiential components. It is also important to consider the role of culture in leisure participation and the concept of leisure as a "flow" experience (Csikszentmihalyi & Kleiber, 1991).

Leisure as Time

There are certain obligatory activities that everyone engages in to occupy their time. Once these activities are completed, certain discretionary time remains. This discretionary time has fluctuated throughout history depending on the prevailing cultural and societal work demands (Csikszentmihalyi & Kleiber, 1991). Despite the existence of this discretionary time, family responsibilities, religious obligations, and personal ambition may drive a person to engage in externally driven projects rather than intrinsically motivating pursuits (Csikszentmihalyi & Kleiber, 1991). The distinction between work and nonwork time in defining leisure leads to identifying leisure not as what it is, but rather as what it is not (Henderson et al., 2001). Even when the workday ends, leftover time is not necessarily "free." Long drives are often associated with getting to and from work, and the end of one work day is often the beginning of a second shift of both paid and unpaid labor (Csikszentmihalyi & Kleiber, 1991). Time demands and time use vary from person to person, which is an important consideration in leisure assessment.

Leisure as Activity

Leisure is identified as activity when engagement occurs for fun and enjoyment, and the activities are categorized according to similar characteristics such as sports, games, outdoor and cultural activities, and socializing (Henderson et al., 2001). Despite the tendency to identify leisure by the activities in which people engage, it is difficult to identify the intrinsic pleasure derived by these activities (Csikszentmihalyi & Kleiber, 1991). This makes it unclear which activities constitute leisure to which individuals. When business executives play golf while discussing business, is this considered work or leisure? Do professional athletes who earn a living playing baseball or football actually work? Is gardening considered work or leisure to a retired person versus a farmer? It is difficult to determine which activities are considered work and which ones are considered leisure and by whom. Researchers tend to identify leisure as those activities that culture identifies as recreational and not engaged in for productive purposes (Csikszentmihalyi & Kleiber, 1991). Csikszentmihalyi (1981) argued that it is more than participation in an activity that constitutes leisure. A single meaningful leisure experience is more significant within a person's life than participation in mundane obligatory experiences over time. For example, participation in a one-time event, such as attendance at a World Series game, may hold greater relevance to an individual than an activity requiring participation over time. However, the frequency of participation in an activity does not determine importance, but perhaps it is the quality of the experience that determines relevance (Csikszentmihalyi & Kleiber, 1991). The activity is less important than the satisfaction derived from engagement (Brown, Frankel, & Fennell, 1991).

Leisure as Experience

A trend has occurred over the past few decades to shift from the view of leisure as culturally defined, discretionary versus obligatory time, and the subjective experience of the individual (Csikszentmihalyi & Kleiber, 1991). Freedom and intrinsic motivation are essential features of the leisure experience—when an activity is freely selected and engaged in for intrinsic pleasure, it should be considered leisure (Csikszentmihalyi & Kleiber, 1991; Henderson et al., 2001; Neulinger, 1981; Parr & Lashua, 2004). It is a state of mind, and the value of the experience means different things to different people (Estes, 2003; Parr & Lashua, 2005). However, cultural norms and mores cannot be separated from this definition. Some delinquent and vandalistic acts can fall into that definition. Youth gang members who steal and vandalize do so out of free choice and some form of intrinsic pleasure (Csikszentmihalyi & Larson, 1978). Watching television can be considered leisure, but research indicated that it can lead to feelings of apathy and depression (Kubey & Csikszentmihalyi, 1990). To avoid the problem of defining leisure as experience based on these dichotomous viewpoints, two rationalizations can be drawn. First is the admission that leisure can be depressing, tiresome, and even criminal. Second is the idea that an activity cannot be deemed leisure unless it leads to increased positive and culturally accepted experiences in addition to possessing intrinsic motivation and free choice (Csikszentmihalyi & Kleiber, 1991).

Leisure as a Construct of Culture

Each society identifies certain activities as work and others as leisure (Henderson et al., 2001). How an individual experiences leisure is often dependent on external factors such as the societal value of work (Parker, 1971, as cited in Henderson et al., 2001). Leisure is encumbered by the influence of social norms, mores, beliefs, and values (Henderson et al., 2001) and cannot occur without consideration of historically conditioned political, economic, and social contexts (Parr & Lashua, 2004). Social influences and peer pressure impact the meaning an individual places on both specific activities as well as the use of discretionary time. Preferences, behaviors, and expectations are dependent, at least in part, on the influence of cultural customs (Henderson et al., 2001).

Leisure and the Flow Experience

Because of the incongruence of theory related to leisure, the theory of leisure as a "flow experience" was developed and inspired by the work of Abraham Maslow (Csikszentmihalyi & Kleiber, 1991). The research on this theory indicated that when people enjoy what they are doing, the experiential states that they report are similar across cultural, gender, and age boundaries (Csikszentmihalyi, 1990; Csikszentmihalyi & Kleiber, 1991). According to this theory, there is a change in the state of consciousness with the pleasure of the experience. The pleasurable state experienced envelopes the individual, creating a feeling likened to being engulfed in a current or flow. There is a melding of play and player into a single entity devoid of the "duality of consciousness" typically present in ordinary life—the player becomes the play, able to enjoy new experiences without repercussion (Csikszentmihalyi & Kleiber, 1991, p. 95).

LEISURE ASSESSMENTS

A variety of leisure assessments are available to measure several domains of the leisure experience. Because leisure is subjective, many of the assessments are self-report or interviewer-guided questionnaires (Ben-Arieh & Ofir, 2002; Rosenblum, Sachs, & Schreuer, 2010). Several assessments are described in Appendix C.

Theories of play and leisure have changed over time. However, both are valuable occupations in which people engage throughout the lifespan. Benefits have been linked to physical, social, and psychological well-being, as well as improved quality of life, self-esteem, and self-identity. As such, assessment of play and leisure through a variety of standardized and nonstandardized assessment tools, interviews, and observation in a variety of contexts is an essential component to developing a complete occupational profile and developing holistic, client-centered intervention.

Summary

After our basic needs of food and shelter are addressed, play and leisure become a significant foundation for how we define ourselves as human beings. Play is so important in childhood because of its importance in early learning. Leisure provides adults with healthy outlets to the stresses of a fast-paced life. Even adults with strong and meaningful work relationships know the significance of play and leisure for forming important relationships in life. As play and leisure are so individualized, the occupational therapy practitioner must address the meaning of these activities to the client if the client is to return to a rich and full life.

Student Self-Assessment

1. Observe a child at play. Take note of the following: What is the child playing with? Is the child intrinsically motivated? What evidence do you have to support your answer? Is the child demonstrating internal control? What evidence do you have to support your answer? Is the child free to suspend reality? What evidence do you have to support your answer?

2. If possible, observe the child playing with a peer. Does the child demonstrate the same level of intrinsic motivation, internal control, and freedom to suspend reality?

3. Attend a child or youth sporting event. Are all of the children demonstrating the same level of playfulness? Why or why not?

4. Interview people at different stages of life, such as a high school or college student, new parents, a still-working baby boomer, and a recent retiree. What differences and similarities do these individuals describe in their leisure pursuits? What about their leisure satisfaction? How does each describe his or her quality of life?

5. Make a play assessment kit. Pediatric therapists are often itinerant staff, traveling from site to site. This makes it necessary to travel with all of the items that you need for evaluation and intervention. Because you can only use what you can carry, develop a play assessment kit that you can carry in one bag. What toys/activities would you include? Why would you select these toys? Would you carry different items to assess a preschooler and a second grader?

EVIDENCE-BASED RESEARCH CHART

Leisure Assesment	Evidence
Assessment of Preschool Children's Participation (APCP)	Law, King, Petrenchik, Kertoy, & Anaby, 2012
Child Initiated Pretend Play Assessment (ChIPPA)	Dender & Stagnitti, 2011; Pfeifer, Pacciulio, Santos, Santos, & Stagnitti, 2011; Pfeifer, Queiroz, Santos, & Stagnitti, 2011; Stagnitti, 2002 as cited in Swindells & Stagnitti, 2006; Stagnitti & Unsworth, 2000, 2004; Stagnitti, Unsworth, & Rodger, 2000; Swindells & Stagnitti, 2006; Uren & Stagnitti, 2009
Children's Playfulness Scale	Barnett, 1990, 1991; Bundy & Clifton, 1998; Muys, Rodger, & Bundy, 2006
Child Occupational Self Assessment	Keller, Kafkes, Basu, Frederico, & Kielhofner, 2005; Keller, Kafkes, & Kielhofner, 2005; Keller & Kielhofner, 2005; Kramer, Kielhofner, & Smith, 2010
Knox Play Scale (now Preschool Play Scale or Revised Knox Preschool Play Scale)	Bundy, 1989; Clifford & Bundy, 1989; Harrison & Kielhofner, 1986; Knox, 1974, 1997; Pacciulio, Pfeifer, & Santos, 2010; Rodger & Ziviani, 1999
McDonald Play Inventory:	McDonald & Vigen, 2012
Play Assessment for Group Settings	Lautamo, Kottorp, & Salminen, 2005; Lautamo, Laakso, Aro, Ahonen, & Tormakangas, 2011; Lautamo & Heikkila, 2011
Play History	Behnke & Fetkovich, 1984; Rodger & Ziviani, 1999; Stagnitti et al., 2000; Takata, 1969
Play in Early Childhood Evaluation System (PIECES)	Cherney, Kelly-Vance, Gill, Ruane, & Ryalls, 2003; Gill-Glover, McCaslin, Kelly-Vance, & Ryalls, 2001, as cited in Kelly-Vance & Ryalls, 2005; Kelly-Vance & Gill-Glover, 2002, as cited in Kelly-Vance & Ryalls, 2005; Kelly-Vance, Gill, Ruane, Cherney, & Ryalls, 1999, as cited in Kelly-Vance & Ryalls, 2005; Kelly-Vance, Needelman, Troia, & Ryalls, 1999; Kelly-Vance, Gill, Schoneboom, Cherney, Ryan, Cunningham, & Ryalls, 2000, as cited in Kelly-Vance & Ryalls, 2005; Kelly-Vance, Ryalls, & Glover, 2002; King, McCaslin, Kelly-Vance, & Ryalls, 2003, as cited in Kelly-Vance & Ryalls, 2005; McCaslin, King, Kelly-Vance, & Ryalls, 2003, as cited in Kelly-Vance & Ryalls, 2005; Ryalls, Gill, Ruane, Cherney, Schoneboom, Cunningham, & Ryan, 2000, as cited in Kelly-Vance & Ryalls, 2005; Kelly-Vance & Ryalls, 2005
Preschool Play Scale	Bledsoe & Shepherd, 1982; Bundy, 1987, as cited in Bundy et al., 2001; Bundy, 1989; Clifford & Bundy, 1989; Couch, 1996; Harrison & Kielhofner, 1986; Kielhofner, Barris, Bauer, Shoestock, & Walker, 1983; Knox, 1974, 1997; O'Brien et al., 2000; Restall & Magill-Evans, 1994; Shepherd, Brollier, & Dandrow, 1994; Tanta, Deitz, White, & Billingsley, 2005; von Zuben, Crist, & Mayberry, 1991
Symbolic Play Test	Casby, 1997; Cunningham, Glenn, Wilkinson, & Sloper, 1985; Gould, 1986; Lowe & Costello, 1988; Power & Radcliffe, 1989
Test of Playfulness	Bretnall, Bundy, & Kays, 2008; Bundy, 1997, 2003; Bundy, 2001; Cameron et al., 2001; Gaik & Rigby, 1994, as cited in Cameron et al., 2001; Hamm, 2006; Harkness & Bundy, 2001; Hess & Bundy, 2003; Liepold & Bundy, 2000; Muys et al., 2006; O'Brien et al., 2000; O'Brien & Shirley, 2001; Okimoto, Bundy, & Hanzlik, 2000; Reed, Dunbar, & Bundy, 2000; Rodger & Ziviani, 2006; Rogers Bronson & Bundy, 2001
Transdisciplinary Play-Based Assessment	Friedli, 1994; Kelly-Vance & Ryalls, 2005; Kelly-Vance et al., 1999; Myers, McBride, & Peterson, 1996; Rodger & Ziviani, 1999
Penn Interactive Peer Play Scale (PIPPS)	Castro, Mendez, & Fantuzzo, 2002; Coolahan, Fantuzzo, Mendez, & McDermott, 2000; Fantuzzo, Coolahan, Mendez, McDermott, & Sutton-Smith, 1998; Fantuzzo, Mendez, & Tighe, 1998; Fantuzzo et al., 1995; Mendez, Fantuzzo, & Cicchetti, 2002; Mendez, McDermott, & Fantuzzo, 2002
Leisure Assessment	Evidence
Activity Card Sort (ACS)	Katz, Karpin, Lak, Furman, & Hartman-Maeir, 2003; Sachs & Josman, 2003
Children's Assessment of Participation and Enjoyment (CAPE)	King et al., 2003, 2007; Law et al., 2006

(continued)

EVIDENCE-BASED RESEARCH CHART (CONTINUTED)

Leisure Assessment	Evidence
Children's Assessment of Participation and Enjoyment (CAPE)	King et al., 2003, 2007; Law et al., 2006
Interest Checklist/ Activity Checklist	Katz, 1988; Klyczek, Bauer-Yox, & Fiedler, 1997; Matsutsuyu, 1967, 1969; Rogers, Weinstein, & Figone, 1978
Leisure Activity Profile (LAP)	Mann & Talty, 1991
Leisure Assessment Inventory	Hawkins, 1993, 1994; Hawkins, Ardovino, & Hsieh, 1998; Hawkins & Freeman, 1993
Leisure Attitude Scale	Ragheb & Beard, 1982; Ragheb & Tate, 1993; Siegenthaler & O'Dell, 2000
Leisure Boredom Scale	Gordon & Caltabiano, 1996; Iso-Ahola & Weissinger, 1990; Wegner, Flisher, Muller, & Lombard, 2002
Leisure Competence Measure	Kloseck, Crilly, Ellis, & Lammers, 1996; Kloseck, Crilly, & Hutchinson-Troyer, 2001
Leisure Diagnostic Battery (1)	Beard & Ragheb, 1983; Trottier, Brown, Hobson, & Miller, 2002
Leisure Diagnostic Battery (2)	Chang & Card, 1994; Ellis & Witt, 1986; Peebles, McWilliams, Norris, & Park, 1999; Thomas, 1999; Witt & Ellis, 1984
Leisure Satisfaction Scale	Beard & Ragheb, 1980; DiBona, 2000; Lysyk, Brown, Rodrigues, McNally, & Loo, 2002; Ragheb & Griffith, 1982; Ragheb & Tate, 1993; Raj, Manigandan, & Jacobs, 2006; Siegenthaler & O'Dell, 2000; Trottier et al., 2002
Preferences for Activities of Children (PAC)	King et al., 2003, 2007
Victoria Longitudinal Study Activity Questionnaire	Jopp & Hertzog, 2010

References

American Occupational Therapy Association. (2010). Scope of practice. *American Journal of Occupational Therapy, 64*(Suppl.), S70-S77. doi: 10.5014/ajot.2010.64S70-64S77

Auerhahn, N., & Laub, D. (1987). Play and playfulness in Holocaust survivors. *Psychoanalytic Study of the Child, 42*, 45-58.

Barnett, L. A. (1990). Playfulness: Definition, design, and measurement. *Play and Culture, 3*(4), 319-336.

Barnett, L. A. (1991). The playful child: Measurement of a disposition to play. *Play and Culture, 4*(1), 51-74.

Bateson, G. (1972). Toward a theory of play and fantasy. In G. Bateson (Ed.), *Steps to an ecology of the mind* (pp. 14-20). New York, NY: Bantam.

Beard, J. G., & Ragheb, M. G. (1980). Measuring leisure satisfaction. *Journal of Leisure Research, 12*(1), 20-33.

Beard, J. G., & Ragheb, M. G. (1983). Measuring leisure motivation. *Journal of Leisure Research, 15*(3), 219-228.

Behnke, C. J., & Fetkovich, M. M. (1984). Examining the reliability and validity of the play history. *American Journal of Occupational Therapy, 38*(2), 94-100.

Ben-Arieh, A., & Ofir, A. (2002). Time for (more) time-use studies: Studying the daily activities of children. *Childhood, 9,* 225-248. doi: 10.1177/0907568202009002805

Bledsoe, N. P., & Shepherd, J. T. (1982). A study of reliability and validity of a preschool play scale. *American Journal of Occupational Therapy, 36*(12), 783-788.

Brayman, S. J., Clark, G. F., DeLany, J. V., Garza, E. R., Radomski, M. V., Ramsey, R., American Occupational Therapy Association, Commission on Practice. (2004). Guidelines for supervision, roles, and responsibilities during the delivery of occupational therapy services. *American Journal of Occupational Therapy, 58*(6), 663-667.

Bretnall, J., Bundy, A. C., & Kay, F. C. S. (2008). The effect of the length of observation on Test of Playfulness scores. *OTJR: Occupation, Participation, and Health, 28*(3), 13-140.

Bronson, M. R., & Bundy, A. C. (2001) A correlational study of a test of playfulness and a test of environmental supportiveness for play. *Occupational Therapy Journal of Research, 21*(4), 241-259.

Brown, B. A., Frankel, B. G., & Fennell, M. (1991). Happiness through leisure: The impact of type of leisure activity, age, gender, and leisure satisfaction on psychological well-being. *Journal of Applied Recreation Research, 16*(4), 368-392.

Bruner, E. M. (1986). Experience and its expressions. In V. W. Turner & E. M. Bruner (Eds.), *The anthropology of experience* (pp. 3-30). Urbana, IL: University of Illinois.

Bruner, J. S. (1972). Nature and uses of immaturity. *American Psychologist, 27*(8), 687-708.

Bryze, K. (1997). Narrative contributions to the play history. In L. D. Parham & L. S. Fazio (Eds.), *Play in occupational therapy for children* (pp. 23-34). St. Louis, MO: Mosby.

Bundy, A. (2010). Evidence to practice commentary: Beware the traps of play assessment. *Physical and Occupational Therapy in Pediatrics, 30*(2), 98-100.

Bundy, A. C. (1989). A comparison of the play skills of normal boys and boys with sensory integrative dysfunction. *Occupational Therapy Journal of Research, 9,* 84-100.

Bundy, A. C. (1991). Play theory and sensory integration. In A. G. Fisher, E. A. Murray, & A. C. Bundy (Eds.), *Sensory integration: Theory and practice* (pp. 46-68). Philadelphia, PA: F. A. Davis Company.

Bundy, A. C. (1993). Assessment of play and leisure: Delineation of the problem. *American Journal of Occupational Therapy, 47*(3), 217-222.

Bundy, A. C. (1997). Play and playfulness: What to look for. In L. D. Parham & L. S. Fazio (Eds.), *Play in occupational therapy for children* (pp. 52-66). St. Louis, MO: Mosby.

Bundy, A. C. (2001). Measuring play performance. In M. Law, C. M. Baum, & W. Dunn (Eds.), *Measuring occupational performance: Supporting best practice in occupational therapy* (pp. 89-102). Thorofare, NJ: SLACK Incorporated.

Bundy, A. C. (2002). Play theory and sensory integration. In A. C. Bundy, S. J. Lane, & E. A. Murray (Eds.), *Sensory integration: Theory and practice* (2nd ed.). Philadelphia, PA: F. A. Davis Company.

Bundy, A. C. (2003). *Test of playfulness (ToP), version 4.* Sydney, Australia: School of Occupation and Leisure Sciences, The University of Sydney.

Bundy, A. C. (2005). Measuring play performance. In M. Law, C. M. Baum, & W. Dunn (Eds.), *Measuring occupational performance: Supporting best practice in occupational therapy* (2nd ed., pp. 128-149). Thorofare, NJ: SLACK Incorporated.

Bundy, A. C., & Clifton, J. (1998). Construct validity of the children's playfulness scale. In M. C. Duncan, G. Chick, & A. Aycock, *Play & culture studies, volume 1: Diversions and divergences in fields of play* (pp. 37-47). New York, NY: Ablex Publishing.

Bundy, A. C., Nelson, L., Metzger, M., & Bingaman, K. (2001). Validity and reliability of a test of playfulness. *Occupational Therapy Journal of Research, 21*(4), 276-292.

Burke, J. P. (1993). Play: The life role of the infant and young child. In J. Case-Smith (Ed.), *Pediatric occupational therapy and early intervention* (pp. 198-224). Boston, MA: Andover Medical Publishers.

Burke, J. P. (1996). Variations in childhood occupations: Play in the presence of chronic disability. In R. Zemke & F. Clark (Eds.), *Occupational science: The evolving discipline* (pp. 413-418). Philadelphia, PA: F. A. Davis Company.

Caldwell, L. L., & Smith, E. A. (1988). Leisure: An overlooked component of health promotion. *Canadian Journal of Public Health, 79*(2), S44-S48.

Caldwell, L. L., & Witt, P. A. (2011). Leisure, recreation, and play from a developmental context. *New Directions for Youth Development, 130,* 13-27. doi: 10.1002/yd.394

Cameron, D., Leslie, M., Teplicky, R., Pollock, N., Steward, D., Toal, C., & Gaik, S. (2001). The clinical utility of the Test of Playfulness. *Canadian Journal of Occupational Therapy, 68*(2), 104-111.

Caplan, F., & Caplan, T. (1973). *The power of play.* New York, NY: Doubleday.

Casby, M. W. (1997). Symbolic play of children with language impairments: A critical review. *Journal of Speech, Language, and Hearing Research, 40*(3), 468-479.

Castro, M., Mendez, J. L., & Fantuzzo, J. (2002). A validation study of the Penn interactive peer play scale with urban Hispanic and African American preschool children. *School Psychology Quarterly, 17*(2), 109-127.

Chang, Y. S., & Card, J. A. (1994). The reliability of the Leisure Diagnostic Battery Short Form Version B in assessing healthy, older individuals: A preliminary study. *Therapeutic Recreation Journal, 28*(3), 163-167.

Charters, J., & Murray, S. B. (2006). Design and evaluation of a leisure educational program for caregivers of institutionalized care recipients. *Topics in Geriatric Rehabilitation, 22,* 334-347.

Cherney, I. C., Kelly-Vance, L., Gill, K., Ruane, A., & Ryalls, B. O. (2003). The effects of stereotyped toys and gender on play-based assessment in children aged 18-47 months. *Educational Psychology, 22*(5), 95-106.

Christiansen, C. H. (1991). Occupational therapy: Intervention for life performance. In C. H. Christiansen & C. M. Baum (Eds.), *Occupational therapy: Overcoming human performance deficits* (pp. 4-43). Thorofare, NJ: SLACK Incorporated.

Clark, F. A., Parham, D., Carlson, M. E., Frank, G., Jackson, J., Pierce, D. ... Zemke, R. (1991). Occupational science: Academic innovation in the service of occupational therapy's future. *American Journal of Occupational Therapy, 45*(4), 300-310.

Clifford, J. M., & Bundy, A. C. (1989). Play preference and play performance in normal boys and boys with sensory integrative dysfunction. *Occupational Therapy Journal of Research, 9*(4), 202-217.

Coleman, D., & Iso-Ahola, S. E. (1993). Leisure and health: The role of social support and self-determination. *Journal of Leisure Research, 25*(2), 111-128.

Connor, F. P., Williamson, G. G., & Siepp, J. M. (Eds.). (1978). *Program guide for infants and toddlers with neuromotor and other developmental disabilities.* New York, NY: Teachers College Press.

Coolahan, K., Fantuzzo, J., Mendez, J., & McDermott, P. (2000). Preschool peer interactions and readiness to learn: Relationships between classroom peer play and learning behaviors and conduct. *Journal of Educational Psychology, 92*(3), 458-465.

Cordier, R., Bundy, A., Hocking, C., & Einfeld, S. (2010). Empathy in the play of children with attention deficit hyperactivity disorder. *OTJR: Occupation, Participation, and Health, 30,* 122-132.

Coster, W. (1998). Occupation-centered assessment of children. *American Journal of Occupational Therapy, 52*(5), 337-344.

Coster, W., & Khetani, M. A. (2008). Measuring participation of children with disabilities: Issues and challenges. *Disability and Rehabilitation, 30*(8), 639-648.

Couch, K. J. (1996). The use of the preschool play scale in published research. *Physical and Occupational Therapy in Pediatrics, 16*(4), 77-84.

Couch, K. J., Deitz, J. C., & Kanny, E. M. (1998). The role of play in pediatric occupational therapy. *American Journal of Occupational Therapy, 52*(2), 111-117.

Csikszentmihalyi, M. (1981). Some paradoxes in the definition of play. In A. T. Cheska (Ed.), *Play as context* (pp. 14-26). West Point, NY: Leisure Press.

Csikszentmihalyi, M. (1990). *Beyond boredom and anxiety: The experience of play in work and games.* San Francisco, CA: Jossey-Bass.

Csikszetmihalyi, M., & Kleiber, D. A. (1991). Leisure as self actualization. In P. J. Brown, B. L. Driver, & G. L. Peterson (Eds.), Benefits of leisure (pp. 91-102). State College, PA: Venture Publishing.

Csikszentmihalyi, M., & Larson, R. (1978). Intrinsic rewards in school crime. *Crime and Delinquency, 24*(3), 322-335.

Cunningham, C. C., Glenn, S. M., Wilkinson, P., & Sloper, P. (1985). Mental ability, symbolic play and receptive and expressive language of young children with Down's Syndrome. *Journal of Child Psychology and Psychiatry and Allied Disciplines, 26*(2), 255-265.

Dare, B., Welton, G., & Coe, W. (1987). *Concepts of leisure in western thought: A critical and historical analysis.* Dubuque, IA: Kendall/Hunt.

Dender, A., & Stagnitti, K. (2011). Development of the indigenous child initiated pretend play assessment: Selection of play materials and administration. *Australian Occupational Therapy Journal, 58,* 34-42.

DiBona, L. (2000). What are the benefits of leisure? An exploration using the leisure satisfaction scale. *British Journal of Occupational Therapy, 63*(2), 50-58.

Easton, L., & Herge, E. A. (2011). Adult day care: Promoting meaningful and purposeful leisure. *OT Practice, 1,* 20-23, 26.

Ellis, G. D., & Witt, P. A. (1986). The leisure diagnostic battery: Past, present, and future. *Therapeutic Recreation Journal, 20*(4), 31-47.

Erikson, E. H. (1959). Identity and the life cycle. *Psychology Issues, 1*(Monograph 1). New York, NY: International Universities Press.

Estes, C. (2003). Knowing something about leisure: Building a bridge between leisure philosophy and recreation practice. *SCHOLE: A Journal of Leisure Studies & Recreation Education, 18,* 51-66.

Esteve, R., San Martin, J., & Lopez, A. E. (1999). Grasping the meaning of leisure: Developing a self-report measurement tool. *Leisure Studies, 18*(2), 79-91.

Evans, G., & Poole, M. E. (1991). *Young adults: Self perceptions and life contexts.* London, England: Falmer Press.

Fantuzzo, J., Coolahan, K., Mendez, J., McDermott, P., & Sutton-Smith, B. (1998). Contextually relevant validation of peer play constructs with African-American head start children: Penn interactive peer play scale. *Early Childhood Research Quarterly, 13*(3), 411-431.

Fantuzzo, J., Mendez, J., & Tighe, E. (1998). Parental assessment of peer play: Development and validation of the parent version of the Penn interactive peer play scale. *Early Childhood Research Quarterly, 13*(4), 659-676.

Fantuzzo, J., Sutton-Smith, B., Coolahan, K. C., Manz, P. H., Canning, S., & Debnam, D. (1995). Assessment of preschool play interaction behaviors in young low-income children: Penn interactive peer play scale. *Early Childhood Research Quarterly, 10*(1), 105-120.

Fewell, R. R. (1991). Trends in the assessment of infants and toddlers with disabilities. *Exceptional Children, 58*(2), 166-173.

Fewell, R. R., & Glick, M. P. (1993). Observing play: An appropriate process for learning and assessment. *Infants and Young Children, 5*(4), 35-43.

Florey, L. L. (1971). An approach to play and play development. *American Journal of Occupational Therapy, 25*(6), 275-280.

Florey, L. L. (1981). Studies of play: Implications for growth, development, and for clinical practice. *American Journal of Occupational Therapy, 35*(8), 519-524.

Friedli, C. (1994). *Transdisciplinary play-based assessment: A study of reliability and validity.* Unpublished doctoral dissertation, University of Colorado at Boulder.

Gardner, H. (1982). *Art, mind, and brain: A cognitive approach to creativity.* New York, NY: Basic Books.

Garvey, C. (1990). *Play.* Cambridge, MA: Harvard University Press.

Gilfoyle, E. M., Grady, A. P., & Moore, J. C. (1990). *Children adapt: A theory of sensorimotor-sensory development* (2nd ed.). Thorofare, NJ: SLACK Incorporated.

Gilmore, J. B. (1971). Play: A special behavior. In R. E. Herron & B. Sutton-Smith (Eds.), *Child's play* (pp. 311-325). New York, NY: John Wiley and Sons.

Godbey, G. C., & Jung, B. (1991). Relations between the development of culture and philosophies of leisure. In B. L. Driver, P. J. Brown, & G. L. Peterson (Eds.), *Benefits of leisure* (pp. 37-45). State College, PA: Venture Publishing.

Goodale, T. L., & Cooper, W. (1991). Philosophical perspectives on leisure in English-speaking countries. In B. L. Driver, P. J. Brown, & G. L. Peterson (Eds.), *Benefits of leisure* (pp. 25-35). State College, PA: Venture Publishing.

Gordon, W. R., & Caltabiano, M. L. (1996). Urban-rural differences in adolescent self-esteem, leisure boredom, and sensation-seeking as predictors of leisure-time usage and satisfaction. *Adolescence, 31*(124), 883-901.

Gould, J. (1986). The Lowe and Costello Symbolic Play Test in socially impaired children. *Journal of Autism and Developmental Disorders, 16*(2), 199-213.

Guitard, P., Ferland, F., & Dutil, E. (2005). Toward a better understanding of playfulness in adults. *OTJR: Occupation, Participation, and Health, 25*(1), 9-22.

Hamm, E. M. (2006). Playfulness and the environmental support of play in children with and without developmental disabilities. *OTJR: Occupation, Participation, and Health, 26*(3), 88-96.

Harkness, L., & Bundy, A. C. (2001). The test of playfulness and children with physical disabilities. *OTJR: Occupation, Participation, and Health, 21*(2), 73-89.

Harris, P. L. (2000). *The work of the imagination.* Oxford, England: Wiley-Blackwell.

Harrison, H., & Kielhofner, G. (1986). Examining reliability and validity of the preschool play scale with handicapped children. *American Journal of Occupational Therapy, 40*(3), 167-173.

Hawkins, B. A. (1993). An exploratory analysis of leisure and life satisfaction of aging adults with mental retardation. *Therapeutic Recreation Journal, 27*(2), 98-109.

Hawkins, B. A. (1994). Leisure as an adaptive skill area. *AAMR News & Notes, 7*(1), 5-6.

Hawkins, B. A., Ardovino, P., & Hsieh, C. M. (1998). Validity and reliability of the leisure assessment inventory. *Mental Retardation, 36*(4), 303-313.

Hawkins, B. A., & Freeman, P. A. (1993). Correlates of self-reported leisure among adults with mental retardation. *Leisure Sciences, 15,* 131-147.

Heard, C. (1977). Occupational role acquisition: A perspective on the chronically disabled. *American Journal of Occupational Therapy, 31,* 243-247.

Henderson, K. A., Bialeschki, M. D., Hemingway, J. L., Hodges, J. S., Kivel, B. D., & Sessoms, H. D. (2001). *Introduction to recreation and leisure services* (8th ed.). State College, PA: Venture Publishing.

Hess, L. M., & Bundy, A. C. (2003). The association between playfulness and coping in adolescents. *Physical and Occupational Therapy in Pediatrics, 23*(2), 5-17.

Hoogsteen, L., & Woodgate, R. L. (2010). Can I play? A concept analysis of participation in children with disabilities. *Physical and Occupational Therapy in Pediatrics, 30*(4), 325-339.

Iso-Ahola, S. E., & Weissinger, E. (1990). Perceptions of boredom in leisure: Conceptualization, reliability, and validity of the Leisure Boredom Scale. *Journal of Leisure Research, 22*(1), 1-17.

Johnson, J. E., Christie, J. F., & Yawkey, T. D. (1987). *Play and early childhood development.* Glenview, IL: Scott Foresman.

Jopp, D. S., & Hertzog, C. (2010). Assessing adult leisure activities: An extension of a self-report activity questionnaire. *Psychological Assessment, 22*(1), 108-120.

Kalverboer, A. F. (1977). Measurement of play: Clinical application. In B. Tizard & D. Harvey (Eds.), *Biology of play* (pp. 100-122). Philadelphia, PA: J. B. Lippincott.

Katz, N. (1988). Interest checklist: A factor analytical study. *Occupational Therapy in Mental Health, 8*(1), 45-55.

Katz, N., Karpin, H., Lak, A., Furman, T., & Hartman-Maeir, A. (2003). Participation in occupational performance: Reliability and validity of the activity card sort. *OTJR: Occupation, Participation, and Health, 23*(1), 10-17.

Keller, J., Kafkes, A., Basu, S., Federico, J., & Kielhofner, G. (2005). *The Child Occupational Self Assessment (COSA)* (version 2.1). Chicago: University of Illinois, College of Allied Health Sciences, Department of Occupational Therapy, Model of Human Occupation Clearinghouse.

Keller, J., Kafkes, A., & Kielhofner, G. (2005). Psychometric characteristics of Child Occupational Self Assessment (COSA), part one: An initial examination of psychometric properties. *Scandinavian Journal of Occupational Therapy, 12,* 147-158.

Keller, J., & Kielhofner, G. (2005). Psychometric characteristics of the Child Occupational Self Assessment (COSA), part two: Refining the psychometric properties. *Scandinavian Journal of Occupational Therapy, 12,* 147-158. doi:10.1080/11038120510031761

Kelly, J. R. (1987). *Freedom to be: A new sociology of leisure.* New York, NY: Macmillan.

Kelly, J. R. (2000). Leisure, play, and recreation. In J. R. Kelly & V. J. Freysinger (Eds.), *21st century leisure: Current issues* (pp. 14-24). San Francisco, CA: Benjamin-Cummings Publishing Company.

Kelly-Vance, L., Needelman, H., Troia, K., & Ryalls, B. O. (1999). Early childhood assessment: A comparison of the Bayley Scales of Infant Development and a play-based assessment in two-year-old at-risk children. *Developmental Disabilities Bulletin, 27*(1), 1-15.

Kelly-Vance, L., & Ryalls, B. O. (2005). A systematic, reliable approach to play assessment in preschoolers. *School Psychology International, 26*(4), 398-412.

Kelly-Vance, L., Ryalls, B. O., & Glover, K. G. (2002). The use of play assessment to evaluate the cognitive skills of two- and three-year-old children. *School Psychology International, 23*(2), 169-185.

Kielhofner, G. (1995). Environmental influences on occupational behavior. In G. Kielhofner, *A model of human occupation: Theory and application* (pp. 91-111). Baltimore, MD: Lippincott-Raven.

Kielhofner, G., Barris, R., Bauer, D., Shoestock, B., & Walker, L. (1983). A comparison of play behavior in nonhospitalized and hospitalized children. *American Journal of Occupational Therapy, 37*(5), 305-312.

King, G. A., Law, M., King, S., Hurley, P., Hanna, S., Kertoy, M., & Rosenbaum, P. (2007). Measuring children's participation in recreation and leisure activities: Construct validation of the CAPE and PAC. *Child: Care, Health and Development, 33*(1), 28-39.

King, G., Law, M., King, S., Rosenbaum, P., Kertoy, M. K., & Young, N. L. (2003). A conceptual model of the factors affecting the recreation and leisure participation of children with disabilities. *Physical and Occupational Therapy in Pediatrics, 23*(1), 63-90.

Kleiber, D. A. (1999). *Leisure experience and human development: A dialectical interpretation.* New York, NY: Basic Books.

Kloseck, M., Crilly, R. G., Ellis, G. D., & Lammers, E. (1996). Leisure competence measure: Development and reliability testing of a scale to measure functional outcomes in therapeutic recreation. *Therapeutic Recreation Journal, 30*(1), 13-26.

Kloseck, M., Crilly, R. G., & Hutchinson-Troyer, L. (2001). Measuring therapeutic recreation outcomes in rehabilitation: Further testing of the leisure competence measure. *Therapeutic Recreation Journal, 35*(1), 31-42.

Klyczek, J. P., Bauer-Yox, N., & Fiedler, R. C. (1997). The interest checklist: A factor analysis. *American Journal of Occupational Therapy, 51*(10), 815-823.

Knox, S. (1974). A play scale. In M. Reilly (Ed.), *Play as exploratory learning: Studies of curiosity behavior* (pp. 247-266). Thousand Oaks, CA: Sage Publications.

Knox, S. (1997). Development and current use of the Knox Preschool Play Scale. In L. D. Parham & L. S. Fazio (Eds.), *Play in occupational therapy for children* (pp. 35-51). St. Louis, MO: Mosby.

Kolehmainen, N., Francis, J. J., Ramsay, C. R., Owen, C., McKee, L., Ketelaar, M., & Rosenbaum, P. (2011). Participation in physical play and leisure: Developing a theory and evidence based intervention for children with motor impairments. *BMC Pediatrics, 11,* 100-107.

Kramer, J. M., Kielhofner, G., & Smith, E. V., Jr. (2010). Validity evidence for the child occupational self assessment. *American Journal of Occupational Therapy, 64,* 621-632. doi:10.5014/ajot.2010.08142

Kubey, R., & Csikszentmihalyi, M. (1990). *Leisure and the benefits of television.* New Brunswick, NJ: L. Erlbaum.

Lautamo, T., & Heikkila, M. (2011). Inter-rater reliability of the play assessment for group settings. *Scandinavian Journal of Occupational Therapy, 18,* 3-10.

Lautamo, T., Kottorp, A., & Salminen, A. L. (2005). Play assessment for group settings: A pilot study to construct an assessment tool. *Scandinavian Journal of Occupational Therapy, 12,* 136-144.

Lautamo, T., Laakso, M., Aro, T., Ahonen, T., & Tormakangas, K. (2011). Validity of the Play Assessment for Group Settings: An evaluation of differential item functioning between children with specific language impairment and typically developing peers. *Australian Occupational Therapy Journal, 58,* 222-230.

Law, M. (2002). Participation in the occupations of everyday life. *American Journal of Occupational Therapy, 56,* 640-649.

Law, M., Baptiste, S., McColl, M., Opzoomer, A., Polatajko, H., & Pollock, N. (1990). The Canadian Occupational Performance Measure: An outcome measure for occupational therapy. *Canadian Journal of Occupational Therapy, 57*(2), 82-87.

Law, M., King, G., King, S., Kertoy, M., Hurley, P., Rosenbaum, P., et al. (2006). Patterns of participation in recreational and leisure activities among children with complex physical disabilities. *Developmental Medicine and Child Neurology, 48*(5), 337-342.

Law, M., King, G., Petrenchik, T., Kertoy, M., & Anaby, D. (2012). The assessment of preschool children's participation: Internal consistency and construct validity. *Physical and Occupational Therapy in Pediatrics, 32*(3), 272-287.

Lawlor, M. C. (2003). The significance of being occupied: The social construction of childhood occupations. *American Journal of Occupational Therapy, 57*(4), 424-434.

Lawlor, M. C., & Henderson, A. (1989). A descriptive study of the clinical practice patterns of occupational therapists working with infants and young children. *American Journal of Occupational Therapy, 43*(11), 755-764.

Lieberman, J. N. (1977). *Playfulness: Its relationship to imagination and creativity.* New York, NY: Academic Press.

Liepold, E. E., & Bundy, A. C. (2000). Playfulness in children with attention deficit hyperactivity disorder. *OTJR: Occupation, Participation, and Health, 20*(1), 61-82.

Linder, T. W. (1993). *Transdisciplinary Play-Based Assessment: A functional approach to working with young children* (2nd ed.). Baltimore, MD: Paul H. Brookes.

Lloyd, K. M., & Auld, C. J. (2002). The role of leisure in determining quality of life: Issues of content and measurement. *Social Indicators Research, 57*(1), 43-71.

Lowe, M., & Costello, A. J. (1988). *Symbolic play test* (2nd ed.). Windsor, Berkshire, England: NFER-Nelson.

Lyons, M. (1987). A taxonomy of playfulness for use in occupational therapy. *Australian Journal of Occupational Therapy, 34*(4), 152-156.

Lysyk, M., Brown, G. T., Rodrigues, E., McNally, J., & Loo, K. (2002). Translation of the Leisure Satisfaction Scale into French: A validation study. *Occupational Therapy International, 9*(1), 76-89.

Mahoney, J. L. (2000). Participation in school extracurricular activities as a moderator in the development of antisocial patterns. *Child Development, 71,* 502-516.

Mann, W. C., & Talty, P. (1991). Leisure activity profile: Measuring use of leisure time by persons with alcoholism. *Occupational Therapy in Mental Health, 10*(4), 31-41.

Matsutsuyu, J. S. (1967). The interest checklist. *American Journal of Occupational Therapy, 11,* 179-181.

Matsutsuyu, J. S. (1969). The interest checklist. *American Journal of Occupational Therapy, 23*(4), 323-328.

McConachie, H., Colver, A. F., Forsyth, R. J., Jarvis, S. N., & Parkinson, K. N. (2006). Participation of disabled children: How should it be characterized and measured? *Disability and Rehabilitation, 28*(18), 1157-1164.

McCune-Nicholich, L., & Bruskin, C. (1982). Combinatorial competency in symbolic play and language. In D. J. Pepler & K. H. Rubin (Eds.), *The play of children: Current theory and research* (Vol. 6, pp. 30-45). New York, NY: Karger.

McDonald, A. E., & Vigen, C. (2012). Reliability and validity of the McDonald play inventory. *American Journal of Occupational Therapy, 66,* e52-e60. http://dx.doi.org/10.5014/ajot.2012.002493

McDowell, C. F. (1984). An evolving theory of leisure consciousness. *Society and Leisure, 7,* 53-87.

Mellou, E. (1994). Play theories: A contemporary review. *Early Child Development and Care, 102,* 91-100.

Mendez, J. L., Fantuzzo, J., & Cicchetti, D. (2002). Profiles of social competence among low-income African American preschool children. *Child Development, 73*(4), 1085-1100.

Mendez, J. L., McDermott, P., & Fantuzzo, J. (2002). Identifying and promoting social competence with African American preschool children: Developmental and contextual considerations. *Psychology in the Schools, 39*(1), 111-123.

Michelman, S. (1974). Play and the deficit child. In M. Reilly (Ed.), *Play as exploratory learning* (pp. 157-207). Thousand Oaks, CA: Sage Publications.

Miller, E., & Kuhaneck, H. (2008). Children's perceptions of lay experiences and play preferences: A qualitative study. *American Journal of Occupational Therapy, 62*(4), 407-415.

Morrison, C. D., Bundy, A. C., & Fisher, A. G. (1991). The contribution of motor skills and playfulness to the play performance of preschoolers. *American Journal of Occupational Therapy, 45*(8), 687-694.

Morrison, C., & Metzger, P. (2001). Play. In J. Case-Smith, A. S. Allen, & P. N. Pratt (Eds.), *Occupational therapy for children* (pp. 528-544). St. Louis, MO: Mosby.

Muys, V., Rodger, S., & Bundy, A. C. (2006). Assessment of playfulness in children with autistic disorder: A comparison of the children's playfulness scale and the test of playfulness. *OTJR: Occupation, Participation, and Health, 26*(4), 159-170.

Myers, C. L., McBride, S. L., & Peterson, C. (1996). Transdisciplinary, play-based assessment in early childhood special education: An examination of social validity. *Topics in Early Childhood Special Education, 16,* 102-127.

Neisworth, J. T., & Bagnato, S. J. (1988). Assessment in early childhood special education: A typology for independent measures. In S. L. Odom & M. B. Karnes (Eds.), *Early intervention for infants and children with handicaps: An empirical base* (pp. 23-49). Baltimore, MD: Paul H. Brookes Publishing Co.

Neulinger, J. (1981). *To leisure: An introduction.* Boston, MA: Allyn & Bacon.

Neuman, E. A. (1971). *The elements of play.* New York, NY: MSS Information Corporation.

O'Brien, J., Coker, P., Lynn, R., Suppinger, R., Pearigen, T., Rabon, S., et al. (2000). The impact of occupational therapy on a child's playfulness. *Occupational Therapy in Health Care, 12*(2), 39-51.

O'Brien, J. C., & Shirley, R. J. (2001). Does playfulness change over time? A preliminary look using the test of playfulness. *Occupational Therapy Journal of Research, 21*(2), 132-139.

Okimoto, A. M., Bundy, A., & Hanzlik, J. (2000). Playfulness in children with and without disability: Measurement and intervention. *American Journal of Occupational Therapy, 54*(1), 73-82.

Olsen, L. J. (1999). Psychosocial frame of reference. In P. Kramer & J. Hinojosa (Eds.), *Frames of reference for pediatric occupational therapy* (2nd ed., pp. 323-375). Baltimore, MD: Lippincott Williams & Wilkins.

Pacciulio, A. M., Pfeifer, L. I., & Santos, J. L. (2010). Preliminary reliability and repeatability of the Brazilian version of the revised Knox preschool play scale. *Occupational Therapy International, 17*(2), 74-80. doi: 10.1002/oti.289

Parham, L. D. (1996). Perspectives on play. In R. Zemke & F. Clark (Eds.), *Occupational science: The evolving discipline* (pp. 71-80). Philadelphia, PA: F.A. Davis Company.

Parham, L. D., & Primeau, L. A. (1997). Play and occupational therapy. In L. D. Parham & L. S. Fazio (Eds.), *Play in occupational therapy for children* (pp. 2-21). St. Louis, MO: Mosby.

Parr, M. G., & Lashua, B. D. (2004). What is leisure? The perceptions of recreation practitioners and others. *Leisure Sciences, 26*(1), 1-17.

Parr, M. G., & Lashua, B. D. (2005). Students' perceptions of leisure, leisure professionals and the professional body of knowledge. *Journal of Hospitality, Leisure, Sport, and Tourism Education, 4*(2), 16-26.

Passmore, A. (2003). The occupation of leisure: Three typologies and their influence on mental health in adolescence. *OTJR: Occupation, Participation, and Health, 23*(2), 76-83.

Peebles, J., McWilliams, L., Norris, L. H., & Park, K. (1999). Population-specific norms and reliability of the leisure diagnostic battery in a sample of patients with chronic pain. *Therapeutic Recreation Journal, 33*(3), 135-141.

Pfeifer, L. I., Pacciulio, A. M., dos Santos, C. A., dos Santos, J. L., & Stagnitti, K. E. (2011). Pretend play of children with cerebral palsy. *Physical and Occupational Therapy in Pediatrics, 31*(4), 390-402.

Pfeifer, L. I., Queiroz, M. A., Santos, J. L. F., & Stagnitti, K. E. (2011). Cross-cultural adaptation and reliability of child initiated pretend play assessment (ChIPPA). *Canadian Journal of Occupational Therapy, 78*(3), 187-195.

Poulsen, A. A., Ziviani, J. M., Cuskelly, M., & Smith, R. (2007). Boys with developmental coordination disorder: Loneliness and team sports participation. *American Journal of Occupational Therapy, 61*, 451-462. http://dx.doi.org/10.5014/ajot.61.4.451

Power, T. J., & Radcliffe, J. (1989). The relationship of play behavior to cognitive ability in developmentally disabled preschoolers. *Journal of Autism and Developmental Disorders, 19*(1), 97-107.

Primeau, L. (2003). Play and leisure. In E. B. Crepeau, E. S. Cohn, & B. A. Boyt Schell (Eds.), *Willard & Spackman's occupational therapy* (10th ed., pp. 354-363). Philadelphia, PA: Lippincott Williams & Wilkins.

Primeau, L. A. (2008). AOTA's societal statement on play. *American Journal of Occupational Therapy, 62*(6), 707-708.

Primeau, L. A., Clark, F., & Pierce, D. (1989). Occupational therapy alone has looked upon occupation: Future applications of occupational science to pediatric occupational therapy. *Occupational Therapy in Health Care, 6*, 19-32.

Primeau, L. A., & Ferguson, J. F. (1999). Occupational frame of reference. In P. Kramer & J. Hinojosa (Eds.), *Frames of reference for pediatric occupational therapy* (2nd ed., pp. 469-516). Philadelphia, PA: Lippincott Williams & Wilkins.

Ragheb, M. G., & Beard, J. G. (1982). Measuring leisure attitude. *Journal of Leisure Research, 14*(2), 155-167.

Ragheb, M. G., & Griffith, C. A. (1982). The contribution of leisure participation and leisure satisfaction to life satisfaction of older persons. *Journal of Leisure Research, 14*(4), 295-306.

Ragheb, M. G., & Tate, R. L. (1993). A behavioral model of leisure participation, based on leisure attitude, motivation and satisfaction. *Leisure Studies, 12*(1), 61-70.

Raj, J. T., Manigandan, C., & Jacob, K. S. (2006). Leisure satisfaction and psychiatric morbidity among informal carers of people with spinal cord injury. *Spinal Cord, 44*(11), 676-679.

Reed, C. N., Dunbar, S. B., & Bundy, A. C. (2000). The effects of an inclusive preschool experience on the playfulness of children with and without autism. *Physical & Occupational Therapy in Pediatrics, 19*(3), 73-89.

Reilly, M. (1974). *Play as exploratory learning*. Thousand Oaks, CA: Sage Publications.

Restall, G., & Magill-Evans, J. (1994). Play and preschool children with autism. *American Journal of Occupational Therapy, 48*(2), 113-120.

Rodger, S., & Ziviani, J. (1999). Play-based occupational therapy. *International Journal of Disability, Development and Education, 46*(3), 337-365.

Rodger, S., & Ziviani, J. (Eds.). (2006). *Occupational therapy with children: Understanding children's occupations and enabling participation*. Malden, MA: Wiley-Blackwell.

Rogers, J. C., Weinstein, J. M., & Figone, J. J. (1978). The interest check list: An empirical assessment. *American Journal of Occupational Therapy, 32*(10), 628-630.

Roopnarine, J. L., & Johnson, J. E. (1994). The need to look at play in diverse cultural settings. In J. L. Roopnarine, J. E. Johnson, & F. H. Hooper (Eds.), *Children's play in diverse cultures* (pp. 1-8). Albany, NY: State University of New York Press.

Rosenblum, S., Sachs, D., & Schreuer, N. (2010). Reliability and validity of the children's leisure assessment scale. *American Journal of Occupational Therapy, 64*, 633-641. doi: 10.5014/ajot.2010.08173

Rubin, K. H. (1982). Early play theories revisited: Contributions to contemporary research and theory. In D. J. Pepler & K. H. Rubin (Eds.), *Play of children: Current theory and research* (Vol. 6, pp. 4-14). New York, NY: Karger.

Rubin, K. H., Fein, G. G., & Vandenberg, B. (1983). Play. In P. Mussen & E. M. Hetherington (Eds.), *Handbook of child psychology, socialization, personality and social development* (Vol. 4, 4th ed., pp. 693-774). New York, NY: Wiley.

Russ, S. W. (2003). Play and creativity: Developmental issues. *Scandinavian Journal of Educational Research, 47*(3), 291-303.

Sachs, D., & Josman, N. (2003). The activity card sort: A factor analysis. *OTJR: Occupation, Participation, and Health, 23*(4), 165-174.

Saltz, E., & Brodie, J. (1982). Pretend play training in childhood: A review and critique. In D. J. Pepler & K. H. Rubin (Eds.), *Play of children: Current theory and research* (Vol. 6, pp. 97-113). New York, NY: Karger.

Saracho, O. N., & Spodek, B. (1995). Children's play and early childhood education: Insights from history and theory. *Journal of Education, 177*(3), 129-148.

Schaaf, R. C. (1990). Play behavior and occupational therapy. *American Journal of Occupational Therapy, 44*(1), 68-75.

Sellar, B., & Boshoff, K. (2006). Subjective leisure experiences of older Australians. *Australian Occupational Therapy Journal, 53*(3), 211-219.

Shepherd, J., Brollier, C., & Dandrow, R. (1994). Play skills of pre-school children with speech and language delays. *Physical and Occupational Therapy in Pediatrics, 14*(2), 1-20.

Siegenthaler, K. L., & O'Dell, I. (2000). Leisure attitude, leisure satisfaction, and perceived freedom in leisure within family dyads. *Leisure Sciences, 22*(4), 281-296.

Singer, D. G., & Singer, J. L. (1992). *The house of make-believe: Children's play and the developing imagination.* Cambridge, MA: Harvard University Press.

Stagnitti, K. (2004). Understanding play: The implications for play assessment. *Australian Occupational Therapy Journal, 51*(1), 3-12.

Stagnitti, K., & Unsworth, C. (2000). The importance of pretend play in child development: An occupational therapy perspective. *British Journal of Occupational Therapy, 63*(3), 121-127.

Stagnitti, K., & Unsworth, C. (2004). The test-retest reliability of the child-initiated pretend play assessment. *American Journal of Occupational Therapy, 58*(1), 93-99.

Stagnitti, K., Unsworth, C., & Rodger, S. (2000). Development of an assessment to identify play behaviors that discriminate between the play of typical preschoolers and preschoolers with pre-academic problems. *Canadian Journal of Occupational Therapy, 67*(5), 291-303.

Stanley, M. (1995). An investigation into the relationship between engagement in valued occupations and life satisfaction for elderly South Australians. *Journal of Occupational Science, 2*(3), 100-114.

Sturgess, J. L. (1997). Current trend in assessing children's play. *British Journal of Occupational Therapy, 60*(9), 410-414.

Suto, M. (1998). Leisure in occupational therapy. *Canadian Journal of Occupational Therapy, 65*(5), 271-278.

Sutton-Smith, B. (1967). The role of play in cognitive development. *Young Children, 22,* 361-370.

Sutton-Smith, B. (1980). A sportive theory of play. In H. B. Schwartzman (Ed.), *Play and culture* (pp. 10-19). West Point, NY: Leisure Press.

Swindells, D., & Stagnitti, K. (2006). Pretend play and parents' view of social competence: The construct validity of the Child-Initiated Pretend Play Assessment. *Australian Occupational Therapy Journal, 53*(4), 314-324.

Takata, N. (1969). The play history. *American Journal of Occupational Therapy, 23*(4), 314-318.

Takata, N. (1974). Play as prescription. In M. Reilly (Ed.), *Play as exploratory learning* (pp. 209-246). Thousand Oaks, CA: Sage Publications.

Tanta, K. J., Deitz, J. C., White, O., & Billingsley, F. (2005). The effects of peer-play level on initiations and responses of preschool children with delayed play skills. *American Journal of Occupational Therapy, 59*(4), 437-445.

Tegano, D. W. (1990). Relationship of tolerance ambiguity and playfulness to creativity. *Psychological Reports, 66,* 1047-1056.

Thomas, D. W. (1999). Evaluating the relationship between pre-morbid leisure preferences and wandering among patients with dementia. *Activities, Adapting and Aging, 23*(4), 33-48.

Thorley, M., & Lim, S. M. (2011). Considerations for occupational therapy assessment for indigenous children in Australia. *Australian Occupational Therapy Journal, 58,* 3-10.

Tinsley, H. A., & Tinsley, D. J. (1986). A theory of attributes, benefits, and causes of the leisure experience. *Leisure Sciences, 8,* 1-45.

Trombly, C. (1993). Anticipating the future: Assessment of occupational function. *American Journal of Occupational Therapy, 47*(3), 253-257.

Trottier, A. N., Brown, G. T., Hobson, S. J., & Miller, W. (2002). Reliability and validity of the leisure satisfaction scale (LSS—short form) and the adolescent leisure interest profile (ALIP). *Occupational Therapy International, 9*(2), 131-144.

Tsao, L. (2002). How much do we know about the importance of play in child development? Review of research. *Childhood Education, 78*(4), 230-234.

Turner, H., Chapman, S., McSherry, A., Krishnagiri, S., & Watts, J. (2000). Leisure assessment in occupational therapy: An exploratory study. *Occupational Therapy in Health Care, 12*(2/3), 73-85.

Uren, N., & Stagnitti, K. (2009). Pretend play, social competence and involvement in children aged 5-7 years: The concurrent validity of the child initiated pretend play assessment. *Australian Occupational Therapy Journal, 56,* 33-40.

Veal, A. J., & Lynch, R. (2001). *Australian leisure* (2nd ed.). Frenchs Forest, New South Wales, Australia: Longman.

Von Zuben, M. V., Crist, P. A., & Mayberry, W. (1991). A pilot study of differences in play behavior between children of low and middle socioeconomic status. *American Journal of Occupational Therapy, 45*(2), 113-118.

Wallen, M., & Walker, R. (1995). Occupational therapy practice with children with perceptual motor dysfunction: Findings of a literature review and survey. *Australian Occupational Therapy Journal, 42,* 15-25.

Wegner, L., Flisher, A. J., Muller, M., & Lombard, C. (2002). Reliability of the leisure boredom scale for use with high school learners in Cape Town, South Africa. *Journal of Leisure Research, 34*(3), 340-351.

West, J. (1990). Play, work, and play therapy: Distinctions and definitions. *Adoption and Fostering, 14*(4), 31-37.

Wicker, A. W. (1987). Behavior settings reconsidered: Temporal stages, resources, internal dynamics, context. In D. Stokols & I. Altman (Eds.), *Handbook of environmental psychology* (pp. 613-653). New York, NY: Wiley.

Witt, P. A., & Ellis, G. D. (1984). The leisure diagnostic battery: Measuring perceived freedom in leisure. *Society and Leisure, 7*(1), 109-124.

Yerxa, E. J., Clark, F., Jackson, J., Parham, D., Pierce, D., Stein, C., & Zemke, R. (1989). An introduction to occupational science: A foundation for occupational therapy in the 21st century. *Occupational Therapy in Health Care, 6*(4), 1-17.

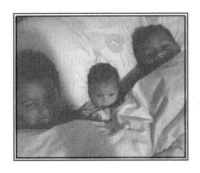

20

EVALUATION OF OCCUPATIONAL PERFORMANCE IN REST AND SLEEP

Michelle Goulet, MS, OTR/L; Courtney S. Shufelt, MS, OTR/L; and Briana Youland, MS, OTR/L

ACOTE STANDARDS EXPLORED IN THIS CHAPTER
B.1.4, B.4.1–B.4.4

KEY VOCABULARY

- **Central sleep apnea:** A breathing-related sleep disorder caused by the brain not sending signals to the diaphragm or other muscles of the respiratory system.
- **Circadian process:** The process within our body that uses environmental cues (light/dark cycle) to train the body to have the ability of knowing when to sleep even if there are no environmental cues present at a given time.
- **Efficiency:** The ratio of total sleep time to time spent in bed.
- **Hypersomnia:** Excessive sleep, usually occurring during the day or at times when sleeping would normally not be considered appropriate.

- **Insomnia:** The inability or great difficulty falling asleep, maintaining sleep, or not feeling refreshed upon waking.
- **Latency:** The duration of time between going to bed and falling asleep.
- **Mental rest:** Freeing one's mind of anything that exhausts or drains the mind while obtaining peace and calmness.
- **Narcolepsy:** Excessive sleepiness accompanying frequent daytime attacks of sleep. There is usually a bilateral loss of muscle tone during these sudden sleep attacks, known as *cataplexy,* and can be connected with feelings of intense emotion.
- **Obstructive sleep apnea:** A breathing-related sleep disorder caused by a hindrance in the airway.

(continued)

Jacobs, K., MacRae, N., & Sladyk, K. (Eds.).
Occupational Therapy Essentials for Clinical Competence, Second Edition (pp. 259-269).
© 2014 SLACK Incorporated.

KEY VOCABULARY (CONTINUED)

- **Periodic limb movements:** Repetitive, twitching leg jerks that occur every 20 to 60 seconds during sleep onset, decreasing as one falls into a deeper sleep.
- **Physical rest:** Cessation of taxing physical activity and relaxing one's body.
- **Rapid eye movement (REM) behavior disorder:** Nerve conduction is not inhibited like normal REM sleep where there is a cease of transmission with muscle activity. Persons may violently thrash around during sleep, acting out a dream they are having and potentially causing injury or harm to either themselves or their bed partner.
- **Rest:** A way to restore energy through easy or effortless acts that provide a break from mental and physical activities. There are three components of rest: physical, mental, and spiritual.
- **Restless leg syndrome:** A feeling of discomfort and the desire to move, more commonly the legs, but sometimes also the arms, while falling asleep or waking during the night. The uncomfortable feeling is described as a creeping, crawling, tingling, burning, or itching feeling.

- **Sleep:** A sequence of activities resulting in going to sleep, staying asleep, and maintaining health through participating in sleep.
- **Sleep adequacy:** The feeling of being rested and refreshed after a night of sleep.
- **Sleep debt:** The amount of time an individual is awake. Therefore, the longer an individual stays awake, the more sleep debt he or she accumulates.
- **Sleep diary:** Journals that are kept for a period of a couple weeks to a month or more so that practitioners can identify patterns and discrepancies from what bed partners report and potential reasons why a client may be experiencing sleeping difficulties.
- **Sleep hygiene:** The overall term as to how a client combines aspects of both sleep preparation and sleep participation to create quality and quantity within nighttime sleep.
- **Sleep participation:** The act of engaging in restful sleep.
- **Sleep preparation:** Routines that prepare the client for a comfortable rest.
- **Spiritual rest:** Freeing one's mind of any burdens through relaxation.

Introduction

One of occupational therapy's original founders, Adolf Meyer, established four occupational performance areas, including work, play, rest, and sleep. Meyer (1922) concluded that a balance must be established between the four performance areas in order to promote healthy living. Even though our founders emphasized the importance of rest and sleep for a balanced life, the majority of occupational therapy research and practice is still primarily on work, education, play, self-care, and leisure (Nurit & Michal, 2003).

Occupational therapy practitioners must remain conscious of the profession's theoretical basis and be sure to establish a balance between all occupational performance areas, including rest and sleep.

This chapter will focus on those frequently neglected areas of occupation, rest and sleep. It will explore what exactly constitutes rest and sleep according to the occupational therapy profession and the medical field. It will touch on improving clients' sleep hygiene as well as the preparation of their sleep. Common sleep disorders across the lifespan will also be identified. Lastly, evaluations and assessments that may be used in the occupational therapy process will be suggested.

Rest

Rest is an area of occupation that was established during the beginning years of the occupational therapy profession and has since been apparent in occupational therapy literature. Meyer (1922) was the first to classify human occupations and established work, play, rest, and sleep as primary performance areas. In addition to establishing the performance areas, Meyer (1922) focused on a balance between the four for healthy living. In later years, Mosey (1981) supported Meyer's theory by addressing the need for balance between work, play, and rest in his philosophical assumptions. Along with Meyer and Mosey, Llorens (1991) revised her original perception of occupational performance from work, education, play, self-care, and leisure to include rest and relaxation. Many pioneers within the occupational therapy profession have included rest and relaxation as a performance area throughout time. As a result, rest is currently an important part of the occupational therapy practice framework.

Rest is described as "effortless actions that interrupt physical and mental activity resulting in a relaxed state" (American Occupational Therapy Association [AOTA], 2008, p. 632). When individuals engage in a restful activity, they are restoring energy and renewing interest in engagement (AOTA, 2008). Although different for each individual, restful activities can include listening to relaxing music, reading, walking, sitting quietly, or lying down, but not engaging in sleep.

There are three components of rest: physical rest, mental rest, and spiritual rest (Nurit & Michal, 2003). Physical rest includes cessation of taxing physical activity and relaxing one's body. An example of physical rest could be when an individual who is engaging in a tiring game of soccer retreats to the sideline in order to give his or her body a break from the strenuous physical activity. Mental rest is freeing one's mind of anything that exhausts or drains and obtaining peace and calm. An example of mental rest would be taking a break from studying for an important exam by taking a walk or listening to relaxing music. Spiritual rest includes establishing inner peace, harmony, nirvana, and calm, and it is often obtained by many people through meditation.

Although physical and mental rest are the two types of rest primarily incorporated throughout daily routines, the idea of "rest" has been tied to spirituality and various religions throughout history. Tibetan Buddhism describes meditation as rest. Meditation is a state of relaxation; its purpose is to free an individual's mind of any burdens. Also, within the Christian, Jewish, and Muslim religions, specific times and places are dedicated to rest and prayer (Nurit & Michal, 2003). There is a strong link between spirituality and rest and relaxation. There is also a strong link between meaningful occupations and spirituality. There are many ways that an individual can find spirituality through everyday activities. Simple activities such as reading, listening to music, writing, walking, being in nature, and gardening can be turned into meaningful and spiritual activities. Most all of the activities listed are also nontaxing and relaxing. According to Christiansen (1997), "any occupation can be spiritual if attention is given to its style and context" (p. 170). Therefore, similarly to incorporating spirituality into certain activities, most activities have the potential to be restful and relaxing. Spirituality and rest are closely related for some individuals; it is crucial for practitioners to address spirituality within the realm of rest.

A balance between rest and performance areas allows individuals to maintain energy and power to continue with leisure pursuits, work, and play, as well as other activities of daily living (ADL). The amount of rest an individual has incorporated into the daily routine will affect that individual's ability to perform daily activities. As an occupational therapy practitioner, it is important to educate clients about incorporating rest into one's routine and establishing a balance between activities and time for rest. Also, more important than educating individuals about balanced routines and how to include rest, practitioners must demonstrate this practice by allowing clients ample time for rest during therapy. Whether the client needs mental, physical, or spiritual rest, the practitioner should organize therapy in a way that this performance area is included. In addition, when helping a client establish a balance between activities and a time for rest, practitioners must also take into consideration that a balance between performance areas and other ADL is individualized; a balanced routine to one client may not be a balanced routine to another.

Sleep

Sleep is a sequence of activities resulting in going to sleep, staying asleep, and maintaining health through participating in sleep (AOTA, 2008). Like "rest," sleep was also one of the four major performance areas determined by Meyer (1922). In the English language, rest and sleep are often used interchangeably. Even though it is a common misconception that *rest* and *sleep* hold the same meaning, studies show that being asleep and resting are not the same. Resting takes place when one is awake and engages in a calm, relaxing activity. Sleep is a state of unconsciousness with special restorative functions (Nurit & Michal, 2003).

A typical adult falls asleep within 10 minutes and goes through a series of four sleep stages. The stages consist of three nonrapid eye movement stages (NREM) and one rapid eye movement (REM) stage. A typical adult will go through the series of sleep stages three to five times during a night. On average, the sleep cycle repeats every 90 minutes, with REM sleep occupying the majority, of the cycle, about 80 percent (Tolbaldini, et al, 2013; Valenza, Rodenstein, & Ferández-de-las-Peñas, 2011). When sleep is recorded via brain waves, eye movements, and muscle movements, the five sleep stages can be identified. During stage one, the eyelids may begin to close and eyes may move laterally, known as *slow eye movements* (SEMs), and the pupils become smaller. People describe this stage as being half awake and half asleep. When an individual progresses to stage two, short bursts of bilateral parietal area waves, also known as *sleep spindles*, appear. Individuals occasionally exhibit small, jerky muscle movements and one's heart rate and respiratory rate begin to slow. During stage three, which is considered to be the deeper stage of sleep, there is an increase in high-amplitude delta waves. Muscle tone begins to decrease with the exception of the diaphragm (Izac, 2006; Tobaldini et al, 2013; Valenza et al., 2011; Wilson, 2008). Restorative functions within the body take place during this deep sleep. If woken during the third sleep stage, individuals feel tired for a while after being woken. The last stage is REM sleep, which includes decreased muscle tone, inhibition of postural muscles, twitching seen with distal flexor muscles, and rapid eye movements (Izac, 2006). This is the stage during which most dreams occur (Wilson, 2008).

There is no specific number of hours of sleep a person needs per night. The amount of sleep an individual needs for optimal functioning varies from person to person. Even though there is no magic number, sleep duration can be specified to different populations, such as infants, adolescents, and adults, but even within these groups sleep needs are still individual. According to the National Sleep Foundation (2011), general recommended sleep durations are as follows:

- Newborns (0 to 2 months) need 12 to 18 hours
- Infants (3 to 11 months) need 14 to 15 hours
- Toddlers (1 to 3 years) need 12 to 14 hours
- Preschoolers (3 to 5 years) need 11 to 13 hours
- School-aged children (5 to 10 years) need 10 to 11 hours
- Teens (10 to 17 years) need 8.5 to 9.25 hours
- Adults need 7 to 9 hours

Sleep is a homeostatic process. An individual's need to sleep and the amount of sleep required depends on the time elapsed since the last time that individual slept and how many hours of sleep was achieved during that time. While individuals are awake, sleep debt accumulates. The longer an individual stays awake, the more sleep debt he or she accrues. If an individual has a large amount of sleep debt, the body will add extra hours onto future sleep periods or it will engage in short sleep bursts, known as *microsleeps* (for 3 to 30 minutes) until the sleep debt has been restored (Luyster, Strollo, Zee, & Walsh, 2012).

Another process involved in controlling an individual's need to sleep is the circadian process. The circadian process is controlled within the suprachiasmatic nucleus in the hypothalamus and repeats about once every 24 hours. The suprachiasmatic nucleus is responsible for hormone release, regulating body temperature, melatonin, and the sleep–wake cycle. There are three components to the circadian process. The first component is the pathways that correspond with environmental cues, such as the light–dark cycle, that indicate the need for our bodies to sleep. The second component is a circadian pacemaker that is responsible for specific rhythms that cycle through a 24-hour period. The circadian pacemaker helps our body know when sleep is needed when environmental cues, such as the light–dark cycle, are absent. Lastly, the third component is the output pathways controlled by the circadian pacemaker (Luyster et al., 2012).

Sleep is programmed into the human brain for a good reason—it is essential for survival and our bodies require adequate sleep in order to properly function. Even though no human studies have been conducted, research suggests that sleep deprivation along with longer sleep durations may be associated with cardiovascular disease, diabetes, and obesity. According to the Centers for Disease Control and Prevention ([CDC] 2012), about 30% of employed adults reported sleeping equal to or less than 6 hours per day. The National Sleep Foundation (2011) suggests that adults need 7 to 9 hours of sleep per night. Based on this information, 30% of adults in the United States may not be receiving the optimal number of hours of sleep. Even though research suggests 7 to 9 hours of sleep, it is important to keep in mind that sleep is individualized and not every adult requires that same amount. Therefore, even though 30% of people report receiving equal to or less than 6 hours of sleep, these individuals are not necessarily sleep deprived. Optimal sleep has been achieved when an individual wakes feeling rested and energized. Multiple factors contribute to maintaining a consistent and optimal sleep duration on a nightly basis. In order to engage in healthy sleep routines and habits, there are two components to sleep that must be incorporated. These components are sleep preparation and sleep participation.

Sleep Preparation

The Occupational Therapy Practice Framework (AOTA, 2008) describes sleep preparation as engaging in routines that prepare the client for a comfortable rest. These routines may include tasks such as grooming, dressing/undressing, calming activities (reading or listening to music, etc.) to help the client fall asleep, spiritual or religious routines, establishing sleep patterns that support growth and health, and preparing the physical environment. Tasks of sleep preparation are often associated with a client's nighttime or sleep routine.

Nighttime/Sleep Routines

Routines are patterns of behavior that are observable, regular, repetitive, and that provide structure for daily life. Healthy routines play an important role in client's sleep participation because they assist in preparing the client for nighttime and letting the body know that it is time to go to sleep. Each client's routine is different from another and may include many aspects such as engaging in calming activities (reading, yoga, knitting, listening to music), hygiene (brushing teeth, bathing, changing clothes), meditation, prayer, or going to bed at a consistent time (AOTA, 2008). There are also tasks that would be considered unhealthy to include in a client's routine including drinking caffeine or alcohol, which will cause one's body to wake up once metabolized, eating too much or too little, watching television, or viewing information on a computer or cellular phone (Vinson et al., 2010).

Practicing healthy sleep routines has been found to reduce sleep loss while improving clients' physical and emotional health (Morin et al., 1999). Therefore, it is important that the clients feel comfortable in their environment where they can practice familiar routines, have the materials needed to complete tasks of routines, and the means to complete routines at a reasonable time and pace set by themselves. As occupational therapy practitioners, it is our domain to assess our clients' nighttime routines and determine factors that may be hindering their sleep. Once the client has been assessed, intervention includes assisting clients to identify health patterns/routines for bedtime, recommending strategies or adaptive equipment if needed to improve the quantity/quality of their sleep, and possible referral to specialists or testing if indicated.

Sleep Participation and Sleep Hygiene

Sleep participation involves taking care of a personal need for sleep which includes cessation of activities to ensure onset of sleep, napping, sustaining a sleep state without disruption, nighttime care of toileting needs, hydration, etc. (AOTA, 2008). Disruption in a client's sleep routine will have an effect on the client's sleep adequacy and the feeling of being rested and refreshed after a night of sleep. This can be disrupted in three different ways. One is sleep latency, the duration of time between going to bed and falling asleep; another is sleep efficiency, or the ratio of total sleep time to time spent in bed; and last is the client's duration of sleep, which is the total number of minutes spent sleeping (Morin & Espie, 2003). For adequate sleep, a client should fall asleep within 15 minutes of lying down and stay asleep for at least 85% of the time in bed (Sateia, Doghramji, Hauri, & Morin, 2000). Sleep hygiene involves the aspects of both sleep preparation and sleep participation to create

quality and quantity within nighttime sleep. Involving poor hygiene in one's nighttime routine may be the cause of sleeplessness, interrupted sleep, or the onset of sleep disorders.

Healthy sleep hygiene practices may include the following:

- Avoid napping during the day; it can disturb the normal pattern of sleep and wakefulness.

- Avoid stimulants such as caffeine, nicotine, and alcohol too close to bedtime. While alcohol is well known to speed the onset of sleep, it disrupts sleep in the second half as the body begins to metabolize the alcohol, causing arousal.

- Exercise can promote good sleep. Vigorous exercise should be performed in the morning or late afternoon. A relaxing exercise, like yoga, can be done before bed to help initiate a restful night's sleep.

- Food can be disruptive right before sleep; stay away from large meals close to bedtime. Dietary changes can also cause sleep problems; if someone is struggling with a sleep problem, it is not a good time to start experimenting with spicy dishes. And, remember, chocolate has caffeine.

- Ensure adequate exposure to natural light. This is particularly important for older people who may not venture outside as frequently as children and adults. Light exposure helps maintain a healthy sleep–wake cycle.

- Establish a regular relaxing bedtime routine. Try to avoid emotionally upsetting conversations and activities before trying to go to sleep. Do not dwell or bring your problems to bed.

- Associate your bed with sleep. It is not a good idea to use your bed to watch TV, listen to the radio, or read.

- Make sure that the sleep environment is pleasant and relaxing. The bed should be comfortable, the room should not be too hot, too cold, or too bright (National Sleep Foundation, 2011).

Sleep Disorders

There are many reasons why clients' sleep may be disrupted across the lifespan. More often than not, sleeping difficulties are the result of other underlying medical conditions or the side effects of medications. This is one of the reasons why sleep disorders tend to be more common in older adults. With age also comes an increase in medical conditions or problems that may affect sleep on their own and an increase in the use of medication that may have effects on sleep (Westley, 2004). According to the American Psychiatric Association's (APA) Diagnostic

Criteria Manual (2000), sleep disorders fall into one of many different categories.

Insomnia affects many people, more so in the older population. It is the inability or great difficulty falling asleep, maintaining sleep (APA, 2000; Rajki, 2011) or not feeling refreshed upon waking (Subramanian & Surani, 2007). The degree to which insomnia affects someone falls into three categories: transient, acute, and chronic. Transient insomnia occurs no more than a few nights a week. Acute insomnia is less than 3 or 4 weeks of sleeping difficulty, and chronic insomnia is when the sleeping difficulty lasts beyond 1 month (Rajki, 2011). Insomnia may also be characterized based on its causes. For instance, when insomnia cannot be linked to a health condition, it is considered primary insomnia; when it can be attributed to a particular health problem, it is known as *secondary insomnia* (Subramanian & Surani, 2007).

The opposite of insomnia, hypersomnia, is characterized by excessive sleep, usually occurring during the day or at times when sleeping might not be considered appropriate (Westley, 2004). Hypersomnia may cause "clinically significant distress" in functioning for patients within social, occupational, and/or other important areas of daily living (APA, 2000).

Narcolepsy is much less common but can also cause significant distress within patients' lives. It presents as excessive sleepiness accompanying frequent daytime attacks of sleep. There is usually a bilateral loss of muscle tone during these sudden sleep attacks, known as *cataplexy*, and can be connected with feelings of intense emotion (APA, 2000). The difficulty of performing everyday tasks is not hard to imagine when one must be aware of the risk of falling asleep at any given moment.

Sleep may also be affected by breathing-related sleep disorders such as obstructive sleep apnea caused by a hindrance in the airway, or central sleep apnea in which the brain does not send signals to the diaphragm or other muscles of the respiratory system (Rajki, 2011; Westley, 2004). In both cases, clients often complain of increased sleepiness during the day with headaches occurring in the morning and a decrease in functioning during daytime activities. During the night when the client is sleeping, breathing will periodically cease for periods of 10 seconds or greater. The breathing cessation causes the person to wake because the brain recognizes the decrease in oxygen. These episodes of ceased breathing may even occur up to or more than 20 times within one night (Rajki, 2011; Vitiello, 2000; Westley, 2004). Snoring is also a characteristic of obstructive sleep apnea, often more noticed by bed partners than the actual patients themselves (Rajki, 2011). Sleep apnea is more common in men and also more common with older populations (Vitiello, 2000).

Circadian rhythm sleep disorders affect many people regardless of age; these disorders disrupt one's usual sleep–wake cycle. These disruptions in the usual circadian sleep–wake pattern cause excessive sleepiness and sometimes insomnia, both of which have a profound effect on a patient's ability to perform everyday tasks effectively. There are four types: jet lag type, shift work type, an unspecific type, and a delayed sleep phase type, in which one may go to bed late or get up late with an inability to fall asleep or get up at a preferred earlier time (APA, 2000).

Restless leg syndrome presents as discomfort and the desire to move, more commonly the legs, but sometimes also the arms, while falling asleep or waking during the night. The uncomfortable feeling is described as a creeping, crawling, tingling, burning, or itching feeling. Movements of the legs relieve the uncomfortable sensations, but delay falling asleep and often wake the person during the night, both of which lead to daytime sleepiness. This sleep disorder is more common in women and older adults, affecting 10% to 30% of those older than 65 years of age (APA, 2000; Rajki, 2011).

Often occurring hand-in-hand with restless leg syndrome, but more common on its own, is periodic limb movements. These are repetitive, twitching leg jerks that occur every 20 to 60 seconds during sleep onset, decreasing as one falls into a deeper sleep. The limb movements cause affected individuals to wake frequently, but they may not be aware of what actually woke them; bed partners are commonly the ones to provide such information. These frequent awakenings cause increased daytime sleepiness, thus also have a profound effect on the performance of everyday occupations (APA, 2000; Rajki, 2011).

Sleep can also be affected by dreams. Nightmare disorder is characterized by one waking from a deep sleep caused by extremely frightening dreams that commonly involve death or other threats to survival or one's security. Upon waking, one is able to orient oneself to reality, contrary to sleep terror disorder. Sleep terror disorder is related in that it also involves the sleeper waking from a frightening dream. The abrupt waking of the person is usually accompanied by a panicky scream, tachycardia, rapid breathing, and sweating. Although incapable of recalling the dream, the affected individual is unable to be consoled by others and often wakes disoriented and confused (APA, 2000).

During REM sleep, usually there is a cease of transmission with muscle activity. REM behavior disorder is just the opposite, in which nerve conduction is not inhibited. Persons may violently thrash around during sleep, acting out a dream they are having and potentially causing injury or harm to either themselves or their bed partner (APA, 2000; Rajki, 2011). These episodes are more common in males and usually occur later into the sleep cycle, as opposed to sleepwalking disorder, which tends to occur during the beginning third of a sleep cycle. During sleepwalking disorder, individuals may get out of bed and walk around. Their expression is blank and they are unresponsive to others who may attempt to communicate with them. While sleepwalking, arousal is very difficult, and if the person does wake, there is usually no recollection of the episode (APA, 2000).

As mentioned previously, sleep disorders are more commonly caused by an underlying medical condition or can be attributed to a side effect of certain medications. Diagnoses that have an increased chance of affecting sleep are the following (Misra & Malow, 2008):

- Arthritis causes sleep interruption secondary to pain and an increased chance of having restless leg syndrome.

- Gastroesophageal reflux disease (GERD) has a two-way relationship with sleep, as lying down increases the chance of reflux and reflux often results in the person wakening.

- Congestive heart failure has been linked with the inability to maintain sleep, resulting in daytime sleepiness.

- Diabetic patients have an increased chance of comorbidities with restless leg syndrome, periodic limb movement disorder, or obstructive sleep apnea.

- Patients with dementia struggle with the ability to regulate sleep and sleep patterns; this is known as *sundowning*. The severity of a client's dementia parallels the severity of sleep disturbance. These changes in sleep often do not cause distress to the client, but instead more so to the caregiver, as the client's sleep rhythm does not match up with routine daily activities (Westley, 2004).

- Chronic pain can be a factor in difficulty falling asleep, frequent awakenings during the night, and not having restful sleep. In addition, sleep deprivation can decrease pain tolerance and thus exacerbate pain symptoms (Gooneratne et al., 2011).

- Depression and anxiety often cause an increase in the number of times a person wakes during the night, how early a person may rise, and difficulty falling asleep caused by racing thoughts or too much on one's mind (Rajki, 2011).

Side effects of medications vary greatly; it is not uncommon for medications to disrupt the ability to maintain, begin, or have restful sleep. Specific medications affecting sleep include the following (Misra & Malow, 2008; Rajki, 2011; Subramanian & Surani, 2007):

- Beta blockers have been known to disrupt sleep by causing vivid dreams or nightmares, general increased waking during the night, or insomnia.

- Decongestants may contain a specific ingredient that heavily contributes to insomnia, known as *nonselective alpha-adrenoceptor agonists*.

- Antihypertensives can have stimulating affects on clients, disrupting the ability to fall asleep.

- Corticosteroids also contain simulating ingredients affecting one's ability to fall asleep.

- Bronchodilators' stimulating ingredients inhibit the ability to fall asleep.

- Antidepressants, like many other medications, contain ingredients that stimulate a client physically and mentally, making it difficult to fall asleep. These may also exacerbate periodic limb movements or restless leg syndrome.

- Diuretics increase urine output; clients may wake to void more often during the night.

- Beta agonist inhalants and selective serotonin reuptake inhibitors (SSRIs) both have been found to affect sleep efficiency, delay the onset of sleep, and increase the amount of times a client wakes during the night.

- Nicotine and alcohol use have been found to decrease a client's sleep continuity throughout the night.

Evaluation and Assessment

Evaluation and assessment of clients is a crucial part of the occupational therapy process. Often these words are used interchangeably, but they are two different, though related, terms. The evaluation of a client can be thought of as a whole process, whereas the assessment of a client is a piece of the evaluation process (Moyers, 1999).

This process can be thought of as a "top-down" approach (Coster, 1998), in which evaluation begins by focusing on what the client needs and wants to be able to do, as well as what the client can currently do or has done in the past. Lastly, the evaluation identifies the barriers hindering not only the client's performance with occupations but also the client's health in general (AOTA, 2008; Fisher & Short-DeGraff, 1993). This top-down approach supports a more client-centered evaluation versus a disability-centered evaluation. This results in better communication between the practitioner and the client about occupational therapy and ensures that the evaluation process is supporting an occupation-centered intervention (Fisher & Short-DeGraff, 1993). The evaluation process should contain four specific items (Smith, 2006):

1. Personal client information such as name, date of birth, gender, diagnoses, and precautions.

2. Referral information that includes the services requested, by whom they were requested, the client's source of funding, and the length of time that the therapist believes services will be provided.

3. The occupational profile should include information about a client's daily activities, values, beliefs, needs, interests, and past history. Most important, it should also collect information on the contexts

that are causing the most problems and the patient's goals for therapy.

4. Assessments are the tools that therapists use to gather information that contribute to the evaluation process. These could be standardized or nonstandardized tests, checklists, or even interviews and skilled observations by the therapist.

REST

When performing an occupational profile with a client, it is always important to ask about quiet leisure activities the client performs and considers "restful." Asking specific questions surrounding the occupation of rest can give you a good idea about whether clients are providing themselves an adequate amount or too much rest. Examples of these kinds of questions follow:

- Can you describe a typical weekday/weekend day?
- Do you feel like you get enough rest? If not, what do you think stands in the way of you getting enough rest (work, school, family, or illness)?
- What restful activities do you enjoy?
- What helps you relax?
- Do have any difficulty doing the things that help you rest and relax? If so, what do you have difficulty with?

Rest is most commonly evaluated through the use of interviews with a client. However, there are some assessments that specifically ask about rest and relaxation. For instance, the Canadian Occupational Performance Measure (COPM; Law et al., 1991) looks at clients' satisfaction with their performance in categories of everyday activities. One of the categories that should be asked about is "quiet recreation," which may include knitting, reading, listening to the radio, and arts and crafts. This category not only provides a practitioner with ideas of what clients enjoy but also gives a clinical picture of how satisfied they are or difficulties they may be having. An Interest Checklist (Katz, 1988; Matsutsuyu, 1969) could also be helpful. This assessment allows a client to individually, or together with a practitioner, check off activities that the client has done in the past year, in the past 10 years, is currently participating in, or would like to pursue in the future. This provides the practitioner with information regarding whether the client has healthy rest/relaxation activities and which ones the client may be experiencing difficulty with. These are only a few examples of assessments available to occupational therapy practitioners.

SLEEP

Typically, sleep is not the reason that clients seek out or are referred to occupational therapy services. Commonly, clients are referred for another reason that may be affecting their sleep or difficulty with sleep is something that is discovered during the evaluation process. During evaluation, it is important to ask about sleep because about half of people who experience sleep difficulties do not talk with a health care provider about their sleep complaints (Gooneratne et al., 2011). If a practitioner feels like there may be some underlying sleep problems, the evaluation may be tailored to provide more focus on this. If a spouse or bed partner is available, that individual may also provide key information about the client's sleeping habits because clients are often unaware of what they do when they are sleeping (Rajki, 2011). Some important questions to ask during an evaluation about sleep may include the following (Misra & Malow, 2008; Vitiello, 2000; Westley, 2004):

- What is your normal bedtime routine?
- Do you have difficulties falling or staying asleep? If so:
  ◊ How long have you been having trouble sleeping?
  ◊ How long would you say it takes you to fall asleep?
  ◊ How many times per night do you wake up and for how long?
  ◊ How does it affect your performance during the day?
  ◊ Do you feel that you are excessively drowsy during the day?
  ◊ Do you take naps during the day? If so, for how long and how many per day?
  ◊ What time do you fall asleep at night and get up in the morning? On average, how many hours of sleep do you get per night?
  ◊ Do you use prescription drugs, over-the-counter drugs, or alcohol to help you fall asleep?
  ◊ How much caffeine or alcohol do you consume per day?
  ◊ Do you exercise? If so, how much do you get per day?
  ◊ Questions about snoring, cessation of breathing, or leg movements.
  ◊ Questions about narcoleptic symptoms.

Assessments for the disruption of sleep mainly focus on validating data the practitioner gathered in the extended occupational profile. One of the ways a practitioner can do this is by asking the client to keep a sleep log or sleep diary. The journals are usually kept for a period of 2 weeks to a month or more so that practitioners can identify patterns, discrepancies from what bed partners report, and potential reasons why a client may be experiencing sleeping difficulties (Davidson,

Waisberg, Brundage, & Maclean, 2001). Occupational therapy practitioners ask patients to pay special attention to and record information regarding the following (Davidson et al., 2001; Vitiello, Rybarczyk, Von Korff, & Stephanski, 2009):

- How much time clients spent in their bed when they were not sleeping.

- If the client took a nap; if so, for how long?

- If the client performed any physical activity that day; if so, for how long and at what time?

- If the client consumed any coffee or alcohol that day; if so, how much and at what time?

- If the client took any medications to aid in falling asleep.

- What time the client went to bed and woke up.

- The perceived quality of the sleep or how restful the client felt.

- If the client woke up during the night; if so, why and for how long? If waking during the night, what did the client do?

The profession of occupational therapy has not adopted or created an assessment that may be used for sleep specifically. However, there are a few sleep assessments created by other professionals within the health care field that occupational therapy practitioners have the clinical knowledge to administer. There are four well-known self-assessments that occupational therapists can either have the patient fill out individually or can fill out with the patient collaboratively.

The Pittsburgh Sleep Quality Index (Buysse, Reynolds, Monk, Berman, & Kupfer, 1989) could be very easily administered by an occupational therapy practitioner, but it is important to know that this assessment requires permission by the creator in order to be used. It is a 19-item questionnaire that assesses a month-long period of sleep. The assessment has three main focus areas: the client's sleep habits, the effects of the client's sleep disorder, and the potential cause of nighttime sleep disruption (Gooneratne et al., 2011). These focus areas create seven component scores: personal sleep quality, sleep latency, sleep duration, how effective the client's sleep is on a consistent basis, what is causing the sleep disturbance, whether the patient uses sleep medication, and how it affects daytime activities (Misra & Malow, 2008). Scores can range from 0 to 21; anything greater than a score of 5 indicates poor sleep quality (Gooneratne et al., 2011).

There are also more basic assessments that an occupational therapy practitioner would have the clinical knowledge to administer, including the Stanford Sleepiness Scale, the Epworth Sleepiness Scale, and the Sleep Impairment Index. All of these are quick and easy to use

---

Case Example: Evaluation of Sleep Habits and Routines

Jane is a 21-year-old woman who is currently finishing her last semester in college. Jane is constantly busy with school. She is writing many final papers and studying for her final exams. On top of completing her schoolwork, Jane is also involved in intramural soccer and is the president of the Sustainability Club. Her involvement in both of these programs, along with attending classes, forces Jane to stay up late at night in order to complete her schoolwork. Jane reports that after she finishes studying or writing papers at 1:00 AM, she does not feel tired right away and needs to watch television or use her computer for about an hour before she can fall asleep. Jane reports drinking coffee to help her through the day. On the weekends, Jane reports napping when she has time. Jane likes to go out with friends on Friday and Saturday nights, partaking in a few alcoholic drinks. Jane reports that drinking usually helps her to fall asleep immediately when she returns home. Jane reports feeling constantly tired and run down.

Consider the following questions:

- What would be the first step in evaluating Jane?

- Is there a specific assessment you would choose to evaluate Jane?

- What questions are important to ask during the evaluation?

- What sleep habits may be interfering with Jane's quality of sleep?

- Based on the information provided during the evaluation, develop an intervention plan for Jane.

---

self-assessments that take a close look at different specific topics (Davidson et al., 2001; Misra & Malow, 2008).

The Stanford Sleepiness Scale is a quick way to test how alert someone is feeling at a given time. The scale ranges from 1 (feeling active, vital, alert, or wide awake) to a 7 (no longer fighting sleep, sleep onset soon; having dream-like thoughts), and after a score of 7, would be sleeping. Assessing a client's degree of alertness throughout the day can give a good idea as to whether the client may not be getting an adequate amount of sleep (Misra & Malow, 2008).

The Epworth Sleepiness Scale assesses the likelihood of a client falling asleep on a 0 (would never doze) to 3 (high chance of dozing) scale during specific given activities. Everyday activities are rated such as sitting and reading, sitting and talking with someone, or being

EVIDENCE-BASED RESEARCH CHART

Topic	Evidence
The occupational therapy process	Moyers, 1999
Definition of rest and its components	Christiansen, 1997; Nurit & Michal, 2003
Stages of sleep	Izac, 2006; Valenza, Rodenstein, & Ferández-de-las-Peñas, 2011; Wilson, 2008
Amount of sleep required for specific populations	National Sleep Foundation, 2011
The process of sleep debt and how it affects an individual	Luyster et al., 2012
Circadian process	Luyster et al., 2012
Sleep preparation/routines	AOTA, 2008; Morin et al., 1999
Sleep participation/hygiene	Morin & Epsie, 2003; Sateia, Doghramji, Hauri, & Morin, 2000
Sleep disorders	APA, 2000; Rajki, 2011; Subramanian & Surani, 2007; Vitiello, 2000; Westley, 2004
Medical conditions that affect sleep	Gooneratne et al., 2011; Misra & Malow, 2008; Rajki, 2011; Westley, 2004
Medications that affect sleep	Misra & Malow, 2008; Rajki, 2011; Subramanian & Surani, 2007

in a car while stopped in traffic. A score of 10 or higher provides reason to check with a health care professional about the possibility of a sleep disorder (Misra & Malow, 2008).

The Sleep Impairment Index asks seven questions that create a score providing information about the severity of a patient's insomnia. Each item is rated on a 5-point scale for a total score between 7 and 35; the higher the score, the more severe the insomnia is considered to be (Pallesen et al., 2003).

References

American Occupational Therapy Association. (2008). Occupational therapy practice framework: Domain and process (2nd ed.). *American Journal of Occupational Therapy, 62*(6), 625-688.

American Psychiatric Association. (2000). *Sleep disorders. In Diagnostic and Statistical Manual of Mental Disorders* (4th ed.). Washington, DC: Author.

Buysse, D. J., Reynolds, C. F., Monk, T. H., Berman, S. R., & Kupfer, D. J. (1989). The Pittsburgh Sleep Quality Index (PSQI): A new instrument for psychiatric research and practice. *Psychiatry Research, 28*(2), 193-213.

Centers for Disease Control and Prevention. (2012). Short sleep duration among workers—United States, 2010. *Morbidity and Mortality Weekly Report, 61*(16), 281-285.

Christiansen, C. (1997). Acknowledging a spiritual dimension in occupational therapy practice. *American Journal of Occupational Therapy, 51*(3), 169-173.

Coster, W. (1998). Occupation-centered assessment of children. *American Journal of Occupational Therapy, 52*(5), 337-344.

Davidson, J. R., Waisberg, J. L., Brundage, M. D., & Maclean, A. W. (2001). Nonpharmacologic group treatment of insomnia: A preliminary study with cancer survivors. *Psycho-Oncology, 10,* 389-397. doi: 10.1002pon.525

Fisher, A. G., & Short-DeGraff, M. (1993). Improving functional assessment in occupational therapy: Recommendations and philosophy for change. *American Journal of Occupational Therapy, 47*(3), 199-201.

Gooneratne, N. S., Tavaria, A., Patel, N., Madhusudan, L., Nadaraja, D., Onen, F., & Richards, K. C. (2011). Perceived effectiveness of diverse sleep treatments in older adults. *Journal of the American Geriatrics Society, 59*(2), 297-303.

Izac, S. M. (2006). Basic anatomy and physiology of sleep. *American Journal of Electroneurodiagnostic Technology, 46*(1), 18-38.

Katz, N. (1988). Interest checklist: A factor analytical study. *Occupational Therapy in Mental Health, 8*(1), 45-55.

Law, M., Baptiste, S., Carswell-Opzoomer, A., McColl, M., Polatajko, H., & Pollock, N. (1991). *Canadian Occupational Performance Measure Manual.* Toronto, Ontario, Canada: CAOT Publications.

Llorens, L. (1991). Performance tasks and roles throughout the life span. In C. Christiansen, C. Baum (Eds.), *Occupational therapy: Overcoming human performance deficits* (pp. 45-68). Thorofare, NJ: SLACK Incorporated.

Luyster, F. S., Strollo, P. J., Zee, P. C., & Walsh, J. K. (2012). Sleep: A health imperative. SLEEP, 35(6), 727-734.

Matsutsuyu, J. S. (1969). The Interest Checklist. *American Journal of Occupational Therapy, 23,* 323-328.

Meyer, A. (1922). The philosophy of occupational therapy. *Archives of Occupational Therapy, 1,* 1-10.

Misra, S., & Malow, B. A. (2008). Evaluation of sleep disturbances in older adults. *Clinics in Geriatric Medicine, 24*(1), 15-26.

Morin, C., & Espie C. (2003). *Insomnia: A clinical guide to assessment and treatment.* New York, NY: Kluwer Academic/Plenum Publishers.

Morin, C. M., Hauri, P. J., Espie, C. A., Spielman, A. J., Buysse, D. J., Bootzin, R. R. (1999). Nonpharmacologic treatment of chronic insomnia. *SLEEP, 22,* 1134-1156.

Mosey, A. C. (1981). *Occupational therapy: Configuration of a profession.* New York, NY: Raven Press.

Moyers, P. A. (1999). The guide to occupational therapy practice. *American Journal of Occupational Therapy, 53*(3), 247-322.

National Sleep Foundation. (2011). *How much sleep do we really need?* Retrieved from http://www.sleepfoundation.org/article/how-sleep-works/how-much-sleep-do-we-really-need

Nurit, W., & Michal, A. (2003). Rest: A qualitative exploration of the phenomenon. *Occupational Therapy International, 10*(4), 227-238.

Pallesen, S., Nordhus, I. H., Kvale, G., Nielsen, G. H., Havik, O. E., Johnsen, B. H., & Skjotskift, S. (2003). Behavioral treatment of insomnia in older adults: An open clinical trial comparing two interventions. *Behaviour Research and Therapy, 41,* 31-48.

Rajki, M. (2011). Sleep problems in older adults. *ADVANCE for NP & PAs, 2*(12), 16-22.

Sateia, M. J., Doghramji, K., Hauri, P. J., & Morin, C. M. (2000). Evaluation of chronic insomnia. *American Academy of Sleep Medicine, 23,* 243-308.

Smith, J. (2006). Documentation of occupational therapy services. In H. Pendleton & W. Schultz-Krohn (Eds.), *Pedretti's occupational therapy: Practice skills for physical dysfunction* (6th ed., pp. 110-129). St. Louis, MO: Mosby Elsevier.

Subramanian, S., & Surani, S. (2007). Sleep disorders in the elderly. *Geriatrics, 62*(12), 10-32.

Tobaldini, E., Nobili, L., Strada, S., Casali, K., Braghiroli, A., & Montano, N. (2014). Heart rate variability in normal and pathological sleep. *Frontiers in Physiology, 4,* 294.

Valenza, M. C., Rodenstein, D. O., & Ferández-de-las-Peñas, C. (2011). Consideration of sleep dysfunction in rehabilitation. *Journal of Bodywork & Movement Therapies, 15,* 262-267.

Vinson, D. C., Manning, B. K., Galliber, J. M., Dickinson, L. M., Pace, W. D., & Turner, B. J. (2010). Alcohol and sleep problems in primary care patients: A report from the AAFP National Research Network. *Annals of Family Medicine* (8)6, 484-492.

Vitiello, M. V. (2000). Effective treatment of sleep disturbances in older adults. *Clinical Cornerstone, 2*(5), 16-24.

Vitiello, M. V., Rybarczyk, B., Von Korff, M., & Stepanski, E. J. (2009). Cognitive behavioral therapy for insomnia improves sleep and decreases pain in older adults with co-morbid insomnia and osteoarthritis. *Journal of Clinical Sleep Medicine, 5*(4), 355-362.

Westley, C. (2004). Sleep: Geriatric self-learning module. *MEDSURGE Nursing, 13*(5), 291-295.

Wilson, S. (2008). A good night's sleep, part one: Normal sleep. *Nursing & Residential Care, 10*(11), 543-547.

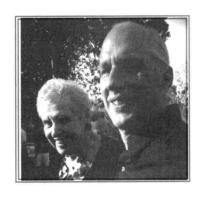

21

EVALUATION OF OCCUPATIONAL PERFORMANCE IN SOCIAL PARTICIPATION

Danielle J. Cropley, MSOT Student; Jan Froehlich, MS, OTR/L; and Mary V. Donohue, PhD, OTL, FAOTA

ACOTE STANDARDS EXPLORED IN THIS CHAPTER
B.4.4, B.5.1

KEY VOCABULARY

- **Associative or project participation:** The second most basic level of social participation, in which members of a group work on a task together and incorporate some sharing and competition.
- **Behavioral response:** Ability to express oneself in a social situation using independently generated verbal and nonverbal cues.
- **Cooperative participation:** Level of engagement in which a group works homogeneously and cooperatively to achieve a task and meet each other's needs while the practitioner or group leader advises rather than participates.
- **Egocentric-cooperative participation:** Engagement in a shared group interest or task with long-term participation aimed at group members meeting the needs of others.

- **Mature participation:** Level of engagement in which group roles and tasks are divided among group members in order to achieve success, practice flexibility, and develop leaders within the group.
- **Parallel participation:** The most basic level of social participation in which individuals work side by side in a group with little to no interaction.
- **Social cognition:** Ability to analyze, integrate, and plan responses to a continuing social situation.
- **Social participation:** Active engagement in the norms and behaviors of an individual within his or her social system.
- **Social perception:** Ability to receive input from others' social cues.

Jacobs, K., MacRae, N., & Sladyk, K. (Eds.).
*Occupational Therapy Essentials for
Clinical Competence, Second Edition* (pp. 271-282).
© 2014 SLACK Incorporated.

Introduction

The term *social participation* aims to outline the specific norms and behaviors of an individual in the individual's unique social system (American Occupational Therapy Association [AOTA], 2008, adapted from Mosey, 1996, p. 340). As one of the eight primary areas of occupation, social participation is a fundamental part of a person's occupational identity as it defines one's ability to engage with family, peers, friends, coworkers, and the community. A positive correlation can be drawn between several of the basic tenets of occupational therapy and the principles of interpersonal interactions and relationships needed for proper social participation. Since AOTA's Accreditation Council for Occupational Therapy Education (ACOTE, 2011) not only identifies two standards on evaluation and intervention for social participation (B.4.4. & B.5.1.), but also requires that occupational therapists "express support for the quality of life, well-being, and occupation of the individual, group, or population to promote physical and mental health and prevention of injury and disease considering the context (e.g. , cultural, personal, temporal, virtual and environment" (B.2.9.), it is essential that occupational therapists address the complex interrelationship between social participation and well-being.

The International Classification of Functioning, Disability, and Health (ICF) of the World Health Organization (WHO) emphasizes the importance of all relationships in its section on activities and participation (WHO, 2001), as well as the influence occupational therapy can have on improving one's independence in this area. The guidelines provided by the ICF help to outline each level of relationship that is composed of an individual's social system from how to relate appropriately to strangers to the complexities of the formal and informal, familial, and intimate relationships one encounters in one's lifetime (WHO, 2001). Each type of relationship and the dynamics found within these relationships can apply to occupational therapy and practitioners' intervention focus on social performance.

Every person's occupational identity is in some way supported and shaped by that person's social system and ability to engage and interact with others. The Accreditation Council for Occupational Therapy Education (ACOTE) expects occupational therapy practitioners to understand how vital social performance is in relation to occupational balance and one's overall health, wellness, and quality of life. The ACOTE tenets echo the ICF expectations of becoming part of organized social life outside of the family by developing community and civic relationships (WHO, 2001). Appropriate evaluation of social participation is necessary to integrate this area of occupation into therapy effectively. Therefore, various evaluation processes have been established as a means of preparation for designing interventions for both individual and group interactions.

A social approach, such as the therapeutic use of self, provides the most effective means of observing clients' abilities, skills, and behaviors in the area of social participation. These same perceptions developed in observing individuals and groups of clients and in designing interventions prepare the practitioner to consider social aspects of the larger community for an understanding of contextual factors in the management of service delivery. Overall, the evaluation of social participation provides a glimpse into the social supports available to the client before, during, and after therapy, allowing the practitioner to understand each client's strengths and areas for improvement.

Integration of Social Participation Concepts

Many people perceive the evaluation of social participation as abstract, complex, and subjective in nature. Because the assessment of social cues is not a hard science, this poses a challenge as to how practitioners can accurately evaluate an individual's level of functioning in the social context. Ultimately, practitioners must break down the situational social demands of the environment and context as well as the required actions and performance skills of the client in order to assess the client's social abilities adequately (AOTA, 2008).

In occupational therapy, practitioners are most often evaluating clients' functioning during "social activity participation," yet this chapter needs to distinguish between the conceptual parts of this term. Throughout occupational therapy intervention, activity participation is planned for and incorporated as its basis. In group settings of intervention, the type of participation designed and expected is social activity participation. This distinction is necessary because many mechanical or physical types of intervention may employ activity participation for individuals but not social activity participation (Isaksson, Lexell, & Skär, 2007). Social activity participation can be defined as consisting of verbal and interpersonal activity interactions among people; however, further explanation of the social skills and subskills of group interaction are needed.

In her seminal work, Parten designed a study to evaluate activity group participation of preschool children using the concepts of parallel, associative, and cooperative play. Parten's theoretical base was developmental across children's ages, with the expectation that children would function at higher levels of participation as they advanced in age. She observed 30 children—six children

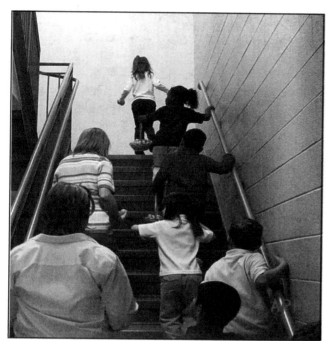

Figure 21-1. Parallel level participation: School-aged children transition from one classroom to another, side by side with little to no interaction.

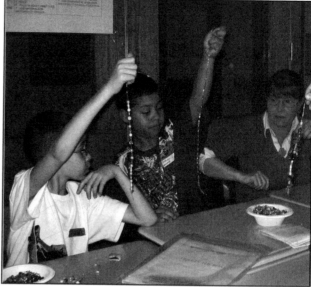

Figure 21-2. Associative or project participation. Young boys use crafts as an icebreaker to begin the early stages of interaction.

in each of five preschool ages. Collecting 360 data points, Parten reported an association between ages and the three developmental group concept levels. Parten first defined the three levels of social participation as follows:

- Parallel participation: Playing, activities, or working side by side with little to no interaction or sharing. Observable examples include children playing in a sandbox without talking, and older adults doing movement to music at an adult day care program (Figure 21-1).

- Associative participation: Approaching others briefly in verbal or nonverbal interactions as needed. Observable examples include children's games such as "Simon Says" and "Musical Chairs" with brief interactions, and young adults using a name game, such as a parachute, to learn each other's names during high school or college orientation (Figure 21-2).

- Basic cooperative participation: Selecting longer activities or tasks for building on mutual self-interest. Observable examples include children dressing up in costumes to role play and adults choosing to play charades with two teams of people competing against one another.

Parten's concepts have been used most commonly when evaluating the social participation of children; many child psychologists have evaluated children's groups using these concepts. More recently, *Parten's schema*, or construct of group participation, has been used to evaluate outdoor play, symbolic play, block play, cooperative play, day care centers, and free play programs

(Aureli & Colecchia, 1996; Fantuzzo et al., 1996; Field, 1984; Garnier & Latour, 1994; Guralnick, 1990; Howes, 1988; Petrakos & Howe, 1996; Saracho, 1993). All but one study confirmed the association of the children's ages with their level of participation delineated by Parten's three concepts.

Mosey's developmental frame of reference (1968, 1986) took Parten's work a step further when she incorporated the original concepts of social participation and added levels of performance for adolescents and adults. She separated Parten's cooperative level into two parts—an egocentric cooperative level and a cooperative level—and added a mature level. Mosey also included the typical age range when each social skill should emerge as a means of gauging an individual's social abilities in relation to those developing normally. Mosey's modified social participation concepts are as follows, with the parallel group remaining the most basic level (emerging at age 18 months to 2 years):

- Project participation (similar to Parten's associative participation; emerging at age 2 to 4 years): Interacting on a task-based level, in which members work individually with some sharing, cooperation, and competition. Observable examples include children in an arts and crafts group and young adults in a cooking class with everyone preparing the same recipe as independently as possible.

- Egocentric-cooperative participation (emerging at age 4 to 7 years): Selecting and engaging in a shared interest together on a long-term task that yields group members meeting each other's needs. Observable examples include children in a reading

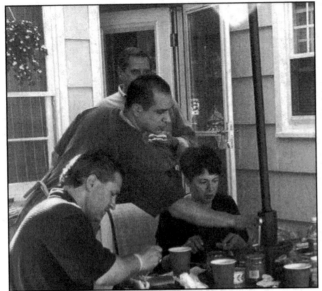

Figure 21-3. Egocentric-cooperative participation. Group members coordinate a longer, structured task of picnic preparation and eating together.

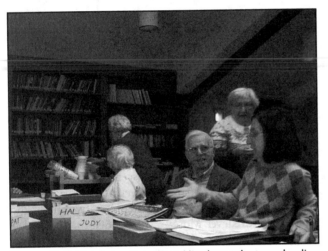

Figure 21-5. Mature participation. Members take turns leading a book club, making sure that the task is as important as the group interaction and emotions.

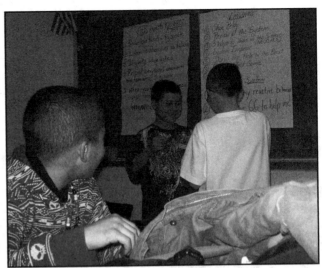

Figure 21-4. Cooperative participation. Young boys express emotion in role-playing scenarios in class.

a group outing, and older adults leading their own exercise class (Figure 21-5).

While Mosey's interaction skills appeared to have clinical face validity, they were not tested empirically until recently. However, the concepts of Mosey's five levels of social interactive skills have appealed to many occupational therapy practitioners who continue to publish them in recent textbooks (Cole, 2012; Moyer & O'Brien, 2013; Stoffel & Tomlinson, 2011) and use them in activity group process therapy. These five level concepts have formatted the perceptual observations and interventions of occupational therapy practitioners working on social participation in mental health, pediatric, rehabilitation medicine, and geriatric settings.

In conjunction with Parten and Mosey's developmental models, the social skills model provides a basis for understanding the social functions and dysfunctions that practitioners may encounter (Tenhula & Bellack, 2008). Often used with patients diagnosed with schizophrenia, this model breaks down the idea of social competence into three client factors: social perception, social cognition, and behavioral response. Social perception, or one's receiving skills, enable the individual to read both verbal and nonverbal social cues. Building on this, social cognition, or one's processing skills, involves the analysis of the perceived cues, the integration of current and past interactions with an individual, and the planning of an appropriate response to continue participation in a social event. Finally, the behavioral response, or one's expressive skills, allow an individual to provide the social partner with adequate verbal and nonverbal feedback to the previous statement. Ideally, a seamless integration of these three skills is required for functional social participation; failure to achieve one or more of these skills suggests that a social dysfunction is present (Tenhula & Bellack, 2008). To evaluate social participation effectively, identifying

circle, and young adults working together on a community art mural (Figure 21-3).

- Cooperative participation (emerging at age 9 to 12 years): Fulfilling mutual needs of homogenous and compatible group; the leader or practitioner acts as an advisor rather than a member. Observable examples include adolescents working on leadership or trust exercises, and adults in a support group for dealing with grief and loss (Figure 21-4).

- Mature participation (emerging at age 15 to 18 years): Varying roles and tasks taken on by members who share leadership and act flexibly when completing tasks and meeting member needs. Observable examples include young adults planning and organizing the level of some or all of these skills will provide the best understanding of the client's abilities in varying social situations.

Understanding Observation and Context

Some people are "naturals" at keen observation of others' social participation in terms of verbal and nonverbal cues. Many have acquired expertise through experience working with individuals and groups of people in formal and informal settings. However, others may need guidance or structure to learn what to discern as functional and dysfunctional social skills. For some occupational therapy practitioners, one or more assessment tools can provide the structure needed to guide therapy sessions and develop the necessary observation skills. In whichever of these categories practitioners find themselves, professional development demands that the prospective observer review the available guidelines, manual, or training opportunities before beginning to use a tool.

Some of the methods employed to prepare students and therapists to use the various tools available are training workshops, in-service presentations, seminars, individual coaching, videotapes, worksheets, and discussion. Of these methods, discussion with others who are knowledgeable about the tool and familiar with the developmental model of social participation has been shown to be most helpful (Smith, 1986). If an observer is at the beginning of the process of developing observation skills, the use of a general observation worksheet during 30 minutes in groups is recommended. Factors such as cooperation, goals, roles, activity involvement, power, attraction, norms, and interaction are valuable to begin with as a focus of interpersonal aspects of function (Borg & Bruce, 1991; Cole, 2005; Howe & Schwartzberg, 2001; Johnson & Johnson, 2000; Posthuma, 2002). Establishing familiarity with these general components of activity group process before undertaking observations with a specific tool for measuring social participation adds to the validity and reliability of the results.

While assessment in the field of occupational therapy is the prerogative of the registered therapist, certified occupational therapy assistants may report and discuss behavioral observations from groups with their occupational therapist supervisor. Therefore, working to establish these skills in all practitioners is just as important as properly administering a social assessment.

Observation within the proper setting and context will also add to the overall quality of the evaluation of one's social participation. As identified in the framework (AOTA, 2008), access to and using one's natural environments and contexts during the entire occupational therapy process is key to best practice. As compared to a clinical setting, observing a client perform socially in environments in which they would typically participate will provide a more accurate and thorough understanding of the individual's skills. Depending on the client, an evaluation should combine the right assessment tool with the client's natural context in order to properly assess for successful intervention planning that will strengthen and adapt the client's current social abilities.

Social Skill Tools

As identified previously, several tools for assessing occupational performance in social participation and social skills functioning are available for use by occupational therapy practitioners. Each tool addresses various issues related to social interaction and can be used in a variety of settings. Two types of assessments are presented in this chapter: those that were made specifically for occupational therapy practitioners and those found from other fields that are also applicable in occupational therapy (see Evidence-Based Research Chart on p. 279). In general, many of these assessments have been found to be particularly useful when working with schizophrenics.

Occupational Therapy Assessments for Evaluating Social Participation Performance Patterns and Skills

Several of the occupational therapy tools that partially or fully address social issues are reviewed here. They are further broken down into those tools that establish performance patterns in the form of an occupational profile and those that look at specific skill sets needed for social participation. The first set of assessments that incorporate the structure of an occupational profile include the Model of Human Occupation Screening Tool (MOHOST), the Occupational Circumstances Assessment Interview and Rating Scale (OCAIRS), and the Role Checklist. Following these tools is a second section looking at the various skills needed in a client's natural context. These include the Assessment and Communication of Interaction Skills (ACIS), the Bay Area Functional Performance Evaluation (BaFPE), the Comprehensive Occupational Therapy Evaluation (COTE), the Evaluation of Social Interaction (ESI), the Role Activity Performance Scale (RAPS), the Social Profile, and a Conceptual Framework for Work-Related Social Skills (WSS).

Tools for Establishing an Occupational Profile

Both the MOHOST (Kielhofner et al., 2009) and the OCAIRS (Forsyth et al., 2005) were developed as tools for gathering an occupational profile under the Model of Human Occupation. The MOHOST includes a section on communication and interaction skills that assesses behavioral categories of nonverbal cues, conversation, vocal expression, and relationships (Kielhofner et al., 2009). In conjunction with this primary section on social functioning, the MOHOST also looks to identify motivation for occupation, patterns of occupation, process skills, and environment—all of which are influenced by social participation. The OCAIRS also looks at the specific set of communication and interaction skills as well as the social environment of the client (Forsyth et al, 2005). Furthermore, this tool assesses a variety of areas impacted by social functioning, especially with regard to interpreting past experiences and defining long- and short-term goals. Both of these tools have been widely used to structure occupational interviews such that intervention planning and treatment is based on a well-rounded assessment of an individual's strengths and areas of improvement.

The Role Checklist is an additional tool that can be used during an occupational profile, but not as the only basis for evaluation. This tool was developed to be used by an individual independently or with an occupational therapist to identify major roles in the individual's life (Oakley, Kielhofner, Barris, & Reichter, 1986). Broken down into three parts, the Role Checklist identifies social roles that have been or will be performed in the past, present, and future, as well as the value of each of these roles. This tool is meant to meet the individual needs of each client, specifically identifying the social occupations that have been and will continue to be important. When used in conjunction with an assessment or evaluation, the Role Checklist will help structure intervention planning and rapport building between the client and the occupational therapy practitioner.

Tools for Identifying Performance Skills

The ACIS (Forsyth, Salamy, Simon, & Kielhofner, 1998) also focuses on individuals and the skills they use to accomplish occupations of daily living. The behavioral categories of the ACIS include an examination of physicality, information exchange, and relations with others. Specifically, as examples, the ACIS looks at gestures, focus of attention, and respect for others as items of assessment. See Evidence-Based Research Chart (p. 279)

for a list of citations of studies used to provide evidence of the value of the ACIS.

The BaFPE (Bloomer & Williams, 1979) was developed as a comprehensive tool with two parts; Part A is a Task-Oriented Scale and Part B is called the Social Interaction Scale. This assessment examines people through interviews, at mealtime, and in unstructured and structured oral and activity groups. It examines their verbal communications, psychomotor behaviors, social appropriateness, response to authority, independence, ability to work with others, and participation in groups and programs. The BaFPE evaluates individuals, but not a group as a whole. See Evidence-Based Research Chart (p. 279) for research carried out to provide evidence of the BaFPE's usefulness. For further research on the BaFPE, refer to Hemphill-Pearson's book on mental health assessment tools (1999).

The COTE is defined as an instrument practitioners use to identify the client factors, performance skills, and patterns of behavior that impede engagement in the occupation of social participation, and is one of the original social skills tools (Brayman, 2008). Originally developed in 1975, the COTE focuses on traditional occupational therapy behaviors (as established by Ayres in 1954) such as punctuality, organization, initiative, responsibility, dependability, attention to detail, neatness, interest, and concentration (Brayman, 2008). The COTE developed into an instrument that uses a checklist format to assess 26 behaviors related to social participation under the categories of general behaviors, interpersonal behaviors, and task behaviors. Various research studies have been established to evaluate the validity and reliability of this tool, yielding evidence to suggest that it is highly effective in structuring skills to assess during intervention for both the client and practitioner.

The ESI was initially designed for practitioners to assess an individual's social abilities when engaging in the natural context with client-centered goals and persons the individual would interact with on a regular basis (Fisher & Griswold, 2010). This tool includes an interview to determine the types of social interactions the individual has concerns about participating in, even though wanting or needing to engage in those social situations. In total, the ESI has 27 different social interaction items, or skills, that are standardized based on social competency to determine the client's strengths, social dysfunctions, establish a baseline, and plan interventions for improvement (Fisher & Griswold, 2010). Similar to MOHOST, the ESI uses the Rasch measurement model to appropriately assess an individual's quality of social participation and acts as a very sensitive tool. The ESI can also be used for all persons age 2 and older with high rater reliability and person response validity.

The Social Profile was developed in 2009 to empirically evaluate the concepts of social participation as valid and reliable, and then evaluate the level of performance of individuals and group members (Donohue, 2009). A tool of a developmental nature, the Social Profile uses the five levels of social participation concepts (parallel, associative/project, basic cooperative/cooperative-egocentric, supportive cooperative/cooperative, and mature) assembled in an ordinal manner and rated using a Likert scale of 0 to 5. Forty items drawn from various literary sources (Borg & Bruce, 1991; Cole, 2005; Howe & Schwartzberg, 2001; Johnson & Johnson, 2000; Lisina, 1985; Mosey, 1986; Parten, 1932) spread across the five levels were arranged under three topics of activity participation, social interaction, and group membership/roles. These three topics provide an analysis of group participation skill levels designed for practitioners to understand the meaning and dynamics of evaluation of interactive occupation in an appropriate context. Activity participation items evaluate social performance contexts of interaction fostered by the activity. Social interaction items evaluate performance components of a psychosocial nature. Finally, group membership/roles items evaluate performance areas of application to the family and society.

Tests of content, construct, and criterion validity were carried out, along with an exploratory factor analysis, to study the validity of the social profile. Item analysis, internal consistency, and interrater reliability statistical analyses were also undertaken (Donohue, 2003, 2005, 2007).

Several populations—children, seniors, psychiatric, and drug-abusing adults—were observed by pairs of students and clinician and student pairs using the Social Profile. The groups were located in inpatient psychiatric services, schools, and senior centers.

The RAPS has an interview-based structure that incorporates a social role component in several of the 12 sections that compose this tool (Good-Ellis, Fine, Spencer, & DiVittis, 1987). Each of the 12 sections aims to address an individual's level of functioning and impact of occupational therapy on individuals with mental illness. Specifically, the RAPS examines varied social relationships and how illness impedes social and role functioning. As social functioning is one of the primary occupations impacted by mental illness, the RAPS has been designed to be used in the process of evaluating, intervention planning, and implementing occupational therapy to guide clients back to a functional level of social participation.

The WSS is a conceptual framework of social skills used in psychiatric rehabilitation to delineate the basic skills, core skills, and behaviors needed to guide training for work-related situations (Tsang & Pearson, 1996). This model uses a three-tier hierarchy and showcases several variables seen in the typical workplace environment, such as basic social skills, skills needed to interact with older adults, skills needed to interact with coworkers and subordinates, and skills for handling work-related scenarios.

Using this tool will allow practitioners to assess a client's task-related and personal-social competence using this systemic model, although more research is needed in this area for it to be directly applied to the rehabilitation setting (Tsang & Pearson, 1996).

Other Relevant Assessments for Evaluating Areas of Performance in Social Participation

Various other tools developed outside of the field of occupational therapy, but are still very relevant, are now examined. These include the Communication Skills Questionnaire (CSQ), the Independent Living Skills Survey (ILSS), the Maryland Assessment of Social Competence (MASC), the Social-Adaptive Functioning Evaluation (SAFE), the Social Functioning Interview (SFI), the Social Functioning Scale (SFS), and the Social Occupational Functioning Scale (SOFS).

COMMUNICATION SKILLS QUESTIONNAIRE

The CSQ (Takahashi, Tanaka, & Miyaoka, 2006) evaluates the differences in the same social skill when applied to different interpersonal relationships. Because communication skills are essential to other social participation skills, such as social recognition, the CSQ acts as an easy and convenient tool for evaluating interpersonal communication. Unlike other tools discussed that rely on the observations of the occupational therapy practitioner, the CSQ has fewer limitations in that it can be administered by other medical staff, family members of the client, or self-administered. Containing 29 items, the CSQ looks at three categories of cooperative skills, assertive skills, and general communication skills, which include verbal and nonverbal skills. Results of studies of the reliability and validity of the CSQ indicate that this tool could be used as an initial assessment for social skills training for a variety of mental illnesses, although further studies need to be conducted (Takahashi et al, 2006).

INDEPENDENT LIVING SKILLS SURVEY

The ILSS was developed as a comprehensive and objective performance measure to assess basic functional living skills, especially for individuals with severe and persistent mental illness (Wallace, Liberman, Tauber, & Wallace, 2000). There are two versions of the ILSS that have been established, one for informants (ILSS-I) and another for self-reporting (ILSS-SR). Each questionnaire aims to establish the view of an individual's community adjustment or the performed tasks needed to live a satisfying, independent life within a community (Wallace et al., 2000). Both forms of the ILSS address a number of areas of self-care, including appearance and clothing, personal hygiene, care of personal possessions, food preparation and storage, health maintenance, money management, transportation, leisure and community, job seeking, and job maintenance; the ILSS-I also includes sections on eating and social relations. Although the ILSS is not directly related to social participation, addressing the number of times an individual participates in each of these areas enables practitioners to get a better understanding of an individual's strengths for independent living.

MARYLAND ASSESSMENT OF SOCIAL COMPETENCE

Occupational therapy practitioners and other professionals working with the mental health population, specifically persons with schizophrenia, have found role playing to be a helpful tool when assessing social abilities. The MASC was a measure designed to evaluate social skills present in simulated social and behavioral situations, as role playing has been so widely used and recognized as a valid assessment to aid the formation of social skills intervention (Bellack, Brown, & Thomas-Lohrman, 2006). The psychometric properties of the MASC indicate that it is a good tool for measuring social skills abilities, especially between different diagnoses in the chronic psychiatric populations (Bellack et al., 2006). Based on the population being assessed, the MASC uses a number of 3-minute scenes to evaluate general social skills and specific skills needed for interpersonal problem solving. This tool is very sensitive; research shows it works best when the scenarios are planned specifically for the individual or population being examined (Bellack et al., 2006).

SOCIAL-ADAPTIVE FUNCTIONING EVALUATION

The SAFE (Harvey et al., 1997) was constructed to address the adaptive life functioning deficits faced by older adults living as chronic psychiatric inpatients. This scale is used to measure social-interpersonal, instrumental, and life skills based on the observations of the practitioner, contact with the caregiver, and subject interview, if available. Using a 17-item scale, the SAFE establishes the severity of an individual's impairment concerning the diagnosis, usually schizophrenia, in relation to instrumental and self-care, impulse control, and social functions. Overall, the SAFE yields good internal consistency, interrater reliability, and test–retest reliability (Harvey et al., 1997).

SOCIAL FUNCTIONING INTERVIEW

The SFI is a tool that uses interviewing to gain information on an individual's role functioning, problematic social situations, personal goals, and social skill strengths and weaknesses (Bellack, Mueser, Gingerich, & Agresta, 2004). As a structured social functioning tool, the SFI is a key tool used for interventions such as social skills training, particularly for persons living with schizophrenia. It uses subcategories under each general category that provide guiding questions for discussion in order to get to know the individual and prevent simple one-word replies (Bellack et al., 2004). The SFI can be used individually or in conjunction with other tools, such as the SFS or MASC.

SOCIAL FUNCTIONING SCALE

The SFS was constructed to address the areas of social functioning necessary to community maintenance and engagement, particularly for those individuals diagnosed with schizophrenia (Birchwood, Smith, Cochrane, Wetton, & Copestake, 1990). It addresses seven areas of social function, including social engagement and withdrawal, interpersonal behavior, pro-social activities, recreation, independence competence, independence performance, and employment and occupation. Similar to other tools listed previously, the SFS aims to first assess an individual's social strengths and limitations in order to design a treatment plan with client-centered goals and interventions. Overall, this tool is reliable, valid, and sensitive in measuring an individual's social functioning, specifically impairments, and identifying needs (Birchwood et al., 1990).

SOCIAL OCCUPATIONAL FUNCTIONING SCALE

The SOFS was also designed to measure the functional status of persons living with schizophrenia. It uses a three-factor structure to address adaptive living skills, social appropriateness, and interpersonal skills with regard to social and occupational functioning (Saraswat, Rao, Subbakrishna, & Gangadhar, 2006). Identified as "simple and easy to administer," the SOFS can be used in inpatient, outpatient, and rehabilitation settings and can be administered by medical practitioners as well as family members (Saraswat et al., 2006). Unlike other tools, the SOFS does not require any formal training and can be used repeatedly throughout treatment.

For further references to assessment tools used in occupational therapy, see *Occupational Therapy Assessment Tools: An Annotated Index*, a comprehensive volume that includes tools from psychology (Asher, 2007).

All of these tools examining the dimensions of social participation focus on detailed interaction skills by

EVIDENCE-BASED RESEARCH CHART

Tool Focus	Categories for Observation	Research
Assessment and Communication of Interaction Skills (ACIS; 1998): Individuals Used to accomplish activities of daily living (i.e., gesturing, respecting others, focusing, etc.)	Physicality Information exchange Relations with others	Forsyth, Lai, & Kielhofner, 1999; Helfrich & Aviles, 2001; Keller & Forsyth, 2004
Bay Area Functional Performance Evaluation (BaFPE; 1979): Individuals Part B: Social Interaction Scale (SIS) during interview of the individual, mealtime, unstructured group situation, structured activity group, and structured oral group	Verbal communications Psychomotor behaviors Socially appropriate Response to authority Independence/dependence Ability to work with others Participation in group and program activities	Klyczek, Bloomer, & Fiedler, 1999; Klyczek & Mann, 1990; Mann & Klyczek, 1991
Comprehensive Occupational Therapy Evaluation (COTE; 1975): Individuals Evaluates client factors, performance skills, and behavior patterns affecting occupation	General behaviors (8 sub-behaviors) Interpersonal behaviors (6 sub-behaviors) Task behaviors (12 sub-behaviors)	Brayman, 2008
Communication Skills Questionnaire (CSQ; 2006): Individuals Identifies differences of the same social skill when applied to various relationships	General communication (6 items) Interpersonal communication (23 items)	Takahashi, Tanaka, & Miyaoka, 2006
Evaluation of Social Interaction (ESI; 1992): Individuals Quality of social interaction and desired level of participation in their natural context	Initiation and termination Producing Physical support Shaping content Maintaining flow Verbal support Adaptation	Asplund & Forsberg, 2006; Englund, Bernspång, & Fisher, 1995; Fisher, 2002, 2006; Fisher & Griswold, 2010; Simmons, Griswold, & Berg, 2010
Independent Living Skills Survey (ILSS; 2000): Individuals Basic functional living skills of individuals with severe and persistent mental illness	Community adjustment	Wallace et al., 2000
Maryland Assessment of Social Competence (MASC; 1991): Individuals Representative role-playing scenarios that are behaviorally coded	Conversational content Nonverbal content Overall effectiveness	Bellack, Brown, & Thomas-Lohrman, 2006
Model of Human Occupation Screening Tool (MOHOST; 2006): Individuals Section on communication and interaction skills	Nonverbal cues Conversation Vocal expression Relationships	Parkinson, Forsyth, & Kielhofner, 2006; G. Kielhofner, personal communication, November 3, 2006
Role Activity Performance Scale (RAPS) (1987): Individuals Components of social roles	Quality and quantity of social performance	Good-Ellis, Fine, Spencer, & DeVittis, 1987
Social-Adaptive Functioning Evaluation (SAFE; 1997): Individuals Adaptive changes associated with aging and chronic mental illness	Social-interpersonal Instrumental activities of daily living Life skills functioning	Harvey et al., 1997

(continued)

EVIDENCE-BASED RESEARCH CHART (CONTINUTED)

Tool Focus	Categories for Observation	Evidence
Social Functioning Interview (SFI; 2004): Individuals Structured social functioning interview	Role functioning Problematic social situations Personal goals Social skills strengths and weaknesses	Bellack et al., 2004
Social Functioning Scale (SFS; 1990): Groups or Individuals Areas of functioning needed for community maintenance of individuals with schizophrenia	Social engagement/withdrawal Interpersonal behavior Pro-social behaviors Recreation Independence-competence Independence-performance Employment/occupation	Birchwood et al., 1990
Social Profile (unpublished): Groups or Individuals Parallel level, associate level, basic cooperative, and supportive cooperative	Activity participation Social interaction Group membership and roles	Donohue, 2003, 2005, 2007, 2009
Social Occupational Functioning Scale (SOFS; 2005): Individuals Social functioning and ability to live in a community for persons with schizophrenia	Adaptive living skills Social appropriateness Interpersonal skills	Saraswat et al., 2006
Work-Related Social Skills (WSS) (1996): Groups or Individuals Conceptual framework for work-related skills	Basic social skills Basic social survival skills Job-securing social skills Job-retaining social skills	Tsang & Pearson, 1996

individuals and groups. Because most treatment of social skills in occupational therapy is carried out in activity groups, it is important to assess the larger issues of levels of interaction in groups and of individuals in groups. Therefore, careful selection of the tool(s) used for each client or group of clients is essential for proper evaluation and subsequent intervention.

Summary

Identifying the skills needed to achieve proper social functioning and participation is key to the evaluation of this occupation in therapy. The various theories and skills provide the structure needed to evaluate individual and group social interactions accurately. Research has also been conducted to demonstrate how the evaluation of social participation is an evidence-based practice.

Several assessment tools have also been published to include items and sections examining the area of social participation. While some have been developed specifically for occupational therapy practitioners, all are devoted to measuring the varying levels of social functioning around activities and roles that group members assume during group interaction for clinical, educational, and well populations. ACOTE (2006) and AOTA (2008) remind occupational therapy students and practitioners of the importance of social and behavioral foundations of intervention across the lifespan and in each context. There is at least one tool available for each level of social function found in children, adolescents, adults, and older adults.

When emphasizing the need for standardized and nonstandardized screening and assessment tools, ACOTE Standards (2006) provide opportunity for both occupational therapists and assistants to begin with their informal observations of human social behavior in social settings. Occupational therapy assistants can report and discuss their observations of social participation during therapy groups with their occupational therapy supervisors and other team professionals. The occupational therapists may then validate and record these social participation behaviors using occupational therapy assessment tools described in this chapter. Ideally, observations, assessments, and analyses will determine the therapeutic levels used during interventions for the individuals and groups treated.

Student Self-Assessment

1. Are my observation skills adequate to use a social skills assessment?

2. Do I need training or practice to strengthen my skills of observing group interaction?

3. Would I like to study some aspect of social participation in a research study during my student program in occupational therapy?

4. Should Internet sites, exchanges, or chat room interaction be considered social participation?

5. As a student educated on the different aspects of social participation, am I capable of evaluating my own skills?

Electronic Resources

- National Alliance of the Mentally Ill: www.nami.org
- Suicide Prevention: www.save.org
- AOTA Special Interest Section—Mental Health: www.aota.org (see http://www1.aota.org/SISQuarterlies/MHSIS-Dec-2012.pdf)
- National Organization on Disability: www.nod.org
- American Speech-Language-Hearing Association: http://asha.org (see study on "The Role of Social Participation Intervention")

References

Accreditation Council for Occupational Therapy Education. (2006). *ACOTE Standards*. Bethesda, MD: AOTA Press.

Accreditation Council for Occupational Therapy Education. (2011). Accreditation council for occupational therapy education (ACOTE) standards and interpretive guide (effective July 31, 2013.) Retrieved from: http://www.aota.org/-/media/Corporate/Files/EducationaCareers/Accredit/DraftStandards/2011%20Standards-and-Interpretive-Guide-August-2013.ashx.

American Occupational Therapy Association. (2008). Occupational therapy practice framework: Domain and Process (2nd ed.). *American Journal of Occupational Therapy, 62*, 625-683.

Asher, I. E. (Ed.). (2007). *Occupational therapy assessment tools. An annotated index* (3rd ed.). Bethesda, MD: AOTA Press.

Asplund, M., & Forsberg, E. (2006). *Bedömning av sociala interaktionsfärdigheter hos personer med generellt god social förmåga – ett steg mot att fastställa användbarheten av BSI-II* [Evaluation of social interaction skills of persons with good overall social ability: One step towards establishing the usability of the BSI-II]. Unpublished bachelor thesis, Department of Occupational Therapy, Umeå University, Umeå, Sweden.

Aureli, T., & Colecchia, N. (1996). Day care experience and free play behavior in preschool children. *Journal of Applied Developmental Psychology, 17*(1), 1-17.

Bellack, A. S., Brown, C. H., & Thomas-Lohrman, S. (2006). Psychometric characteristics of role-play assessments of social skill in schizophrenia. *Behavior Therapy, 37*, 339-352.

Bellack, A. S., Mueser, K. T., Gingerich, S., & Agresta, J. (2004). *Social skills training for schizophrenia: A step-by-step guide* (2nd ed.). New York, NY: Guilford Press.

Birchwood, M., Smith, J., Cochrane, R., Wetton, S., & Copestake, S. (1990). The Social Functioning Scale: The development and validation of a new scale of social adjustment for use in family intervention programmes with schizophrenic patients. *British Journal of Psychiatry, 157*, 853-859.

Bloomer, J., & Williams, S. (1979). *The Bay Area Functional Performance Evaluation (BaFPE)*. Palo Alto, CA: Consulting Psychologists Press.

Borg, B., & Bruce, M. A. G. (1991). *The group system: The therapeutic activity group in occupational therapy*. Thorofare, NJ: SLACK Incorporated.

Brayman, S. J. (2008). The Comprehensive Occupational Therapy Evaluation (COTE). In B. J. Hemphill-Pearson (Ed.), *Assessments in occupational therapy mental health: An integrative approach* (pp. 113-126). Thorofare, NJ: SLACK Incorporated.

Cole, M. B. (2005). *Group dynamics in occupational therapy: The theoretical basis and practice application of group treatment* (3rd ed.). Thorofare, NJ: SLACK Incorporated.

Cole M. B. (2012). *Group dynamics in occupational therapy, (4th ed.)*. Thorofare, NJ: SLACK Incorporated.

Donohue, M. V. (2003). Group Profile Studies with children: Validity measures and item analysis. *Occupational Therapy in Mental Health, 19*(1), 1-23.

Donohue, M. V. (2005). Social Profile: Assessment of validity and reliability with preschool children. *Canadian Journal of Occupational Therapy, 72*(3), 164-175.

Donohue, M. V. (2007). Interrater reliability of the Social Profile: Assessment of community and psychiatric group participation. *Australian Occupational Therapy Journal, 54*(1), 49-58.

Donohue, M. V. (2009). Social Profile. Unpublished assessment tool. Retrieved July 28, 2009, from http://www.Social-Profile.com

Englund, B., Bernspång, B., Fisher, A.G. (1995). Development of an instrument for assessment of social interaction skills in occupational therapy. *Scandinavian Journal of Occupational Therapy, 2*, 17-23.

Fantuzzo, J., Sutton-Smith, B., Atkins, M., Meyers, R., Stevenson, H., Coolahan, K. . . . Manz P. (1996). Community-based resilient peer treatment of withdrawn maltreated preschool children. *Journal of Consulting and Clinical Psychology, 64*(6), 1377-1386.

Field, T. (1984). Play behaviors of handicapped children who have friends. In T. Field, J. L. Roopnarine, & M. Segal (Eds.), *Friendships in normal and handicapped children*. Santa Barbara, CA: Greenwood Publishing Group.

Fisher, A. G. (2002). Cellular identity and lineage choice. *Nature Reviews Immunology, 2*, 977–982.

Fisher, A. G. (2006). Overview of performance skills and client factors. In H. M. Pendleton, & W. Schultz-Krohn (Eds.), *Pedretti's occupational therapy: Practice skills for physical dysfunction* (6th ed., pp. 372-402). St. Louis, MO: Mosby Elsevier.

Fisher, A. G., & Griswold, L. A. (2010). *Evaluation of social interaction (ESI)* (2nd ed.). Fort Collins, CO: Three Star Press.

Forsyth, K., Deshpande, S., Kielhofner, G., Henriksson, C., Haglund, L., Olson, L.... Kulkarni, S. (2005). *A User's Manual for the Occupational Circumstances Assessment Interview and Rating Scale (version 4.0) OCAIRS.* Model of Human Occupation Clearinghouse, Department of Occupational Therapy, College of Applied Health Sciences, University of Illinois at Chicago.

Forsyth, K., Lai, J., & Kielhofner, G. (1999). The assessment of communication and interaction skills (ACIS): Measurement properties. *British Journal of Occupational Therapy, 62*(2), 69-74.

Forsyth, K., Salamy, M., Simon, S., & Kielhofner, G. (1998). *The Assessment of Communciation and Interaction Skill (ACIS), version 4.0.* Chicago, IL: MOHO Clearinghouse.

Garnier, C., & Latour, A. (1994). Analysis of group process: Cooperation of preschool children. *Canadian Journal of Behavioural Science, 26*(3), 365-384.

Good-Ellis, M. A., Fine, S. B., Spencer, J. H., & DiVittis, A. (1987). Developing a role activity performance scale. *The American Journal of Occupational Therapy, 41*(4), 232-241.

Guralnick, M. J. (1990). Peer interactions and the development of handicappd children's social and communicative competence. In H.C. Foot, M. J. Morgan, & R. H. Shute (Eds.), *Children helping children.* London, England: Wiley.

Harvey, P. D., Davidson, M., Mueser, K. T., Parrella, M., White, L., & Powchik, P. (1997). Social-Adaptive Functioning Evaluation (SAFE): A rating scale for geriatric psychiatric patients. *Schizophrenia Bulletin, 23,* 131-145.

Helfrich, C., & Aviles, A. (2001). Occupational therapy's role with victims of domestic violence: Assessment and intervention. *Occupational Therapy in Mental Health, 16*(3/4), 53-70.

Hemphill-Pearson, B. J. (Ed.). (1999). *Assessments in occupational therapy mental health. An integrative approach.* Thorofare, NJ: SLACK Incorporated.

Howe, M. C., & Schwartzberg, S. L. (2001). *A functional approach to group work in occupational therapy* (3rd ed.). Philadelphia, PA: Lippincott Williams & Wilkins.

Howes, C. (1988). Peer interaction of young children. *Monographs of the Society for Research in Child Development, 53*(1), 1-88.

Isaksson, G., Lexell, J., & Skär. (2007) Social support provides motivation and ability to participate in occupation. *OTJR: Occupation, Participation and Health, 27*(1), 23-30.

Johnson, D. W., & Johnson, F. P. (2000). *Joining together: Group theory and group skills* (7th ed.). Upper Saddle River, NJ: Prentice Hall.

Keller, J., & Forsyth, K. (2004). The model of human occupation in practice. *Israel Journal of Occupational Therapy, 13,* E99-E106.

Kielhofner, G., Fogg, L., Braveman, B., Forsyth, K., Kramer, J., & Duncan, E. (2009). A factor analytic study of the Model of Human Occupation Screening Tool of hypothesized variables. *Occupational Therapy in Mental Health, 25,* 127-137.

Klyczek, J., Bloomer, J., & Fiedler, R. (1999). *Analysis of a shortened BaFPE: Task oriented assessment.* Buffalo, NY: D'Youville College.

Klyczek, J. P., & Mann, W. C. (1990). Concurrent validity of the Task-Oriented Assessment component of the Bay Area Functional Performance Evaluation with the American Association on Mental Deficiency Adaptive Behavior Scale. *American Journal of Occupational Therapy, 44*(10), 907-912.

Lisina, M. I. (1985). *Child-adults-peers: Patterns of communication.* Moscow, Russia: Progress Publishers.

Mann, W. C., & Klyczek, J. P. (1991). Standard scores for the Bay Area Functional Performance Evaluation Task Oriented Assessment. *Occupational Therapy in Mental Health, 11*(1), 13-24.

Mosey, A. C. (1968). Recapitulation of ontogenesis: A theory for practice of occupational therapy. *American Journal of Occupational Therapy, 22*(5), 426-438.

Mosey, A. C. (1986). *Psychosocial components of occupational therapy.* New York, NY: Raven Press.

Moyer, E. A. & O'Brien, J. C. (2013). Occupational and group analysis: adults. In J. C. O'Brien & J. W. Solomon (Eds.), *Occupational analysis and group process.* St. Louis, MO: Elsevier.

Oakley, F., Kielhofner, G., Barris, R., & Reichler, R. K. (1986). The Role Checklist: Development and empirical assessment of reliability. *Occupational Therapy Journal of Research.*

Parkinson, S., Forsyth, K., & Kielhofner, G. (2006). *The Model of Human Occupation Screening Tool (MOHOST), version 2.0.* Chicago, IL: MOHO Clearinghouse.

Parten, M. B. (1932). Social participation among pre-school children. *Journal of Abnormal and Social Psychology, 27,* 243-269.

Petrakos, H., & Howe, N. (1996). The influence of the physical design of the dramatic play center on children's play. *Early Childhood Research Quarterly, 11*(1), 63-77.

Posthuma, B. W. (2002). *Small groups in counseling and therapy: Process and leadership* (4th ed.). Columbus, OH: Allyn & Bacon.

Saracho, O. N. (1993). A factor analysis of young children's play. *Early Childhood Development and Care, 84*(1), 91-102.

Saraswat, N., Rao, K., Subbakrishna, D. K., & Gangadhar, B. N. (2006). The Social Occupational Functioning Scale (SOFS): A brief measure of functional status in persons with schizophrenia. *Schizophrenia Research, 81,* 301-309.

Simmons, D.,Griswold, L .A., & Berg, B. (2010). Evaluation of social interaction during occupational engagement. *Amercian Journal of Occupaitonal Therapy, 64,* 10-17. doi:10.5014/ajot.64.1.10

Smith, D. E. (1986). Training programs for performance appraisal: A review. *Academy of Management Review, 11*(1), 22-40.

Stoffel,V. C. & Tomlinson, J. (2011). Communication and social skills. In C. Brown & V. C. Stossel (Eds.), Occupational therapy in mental health: A vision for participation. (298-312). Philadelphia: FA Davis Company.

Takahashi, M., Tanaka, K., & Miyaoka, H. (2006). Reliability and validity of Communication Skills Questionnaire (CSQ). *Psychiatry and Clinical Neurosciences, 60,* 211-218.

Tenhula, W. N., & Bellack, A. S. (2008). Social skills training. In K. T. Mueser & D. V. Jeste (Eds.), *Clinical handbook of schizophrenia* (pp. 240-248). New York, NY: Guilford Press.

Tsang, H. W. H., & Pearson, V. (1996). A conceptual framework for work-related social skills in psychiatric rehabilitation. *Journal of Rehabilitation, July/August/September,* 61-66.

Wallace, C. J., Liberman, R. P., Tauber, R., & Wallace, J. (2000). The Independent Living Skills Survey: A comprehensive measure of the community functioning of severely and persistently mentally ill individuals. *Schizophrenia Bulletin, 26*(3), 631.

World Health Organization. (2001). *International classification of functioning disability and health (ICF).* Geneva, Switzerland: Author.

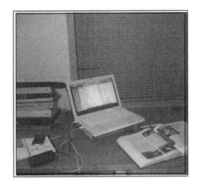

DOCUMENTATION OF
OCCUPATIONAL THERAPY SERVICES

William R. Croninger, MA, OTR/L and Nancy MacRae, MS, OTR/L, FAOTA

ACOTE STANDARDS EXPLORED IN THIS CHAPTER
B.4.10, B.5.20, B.5.30, B.5.32

KEY VOCABULARY

- **DAP:** A documentation format that combines the subjective and objective portions into "D"; "A" is the assessment or summary portion; and "P" is for the plan.
- **Discontinuation note:** Documentation that summarizes the course of therapy and makes recommendations.

- **Documentation:** A written account of a therapy session.
- **SOAP note format:** The basic skeletal format for documentation that includes subjective, objective, assessment, and plan portions.

Introduction

Documentation is an important part of the communication process in occupational therapy and serves a number of goals.

Documentation provides a record of interventions and a client's reaction to those interventions. Documentation is an important means to verify that an intervention session has occurred. It is also crucial for stating the goals of intervention, listing baseline data, a description of the plan and the implementation, and a detailing of the outcomes. Complete documentation provides a view of intervention and can be used for retrospective research, comparing the course and outcomes of similar cases.

Documentation promotes communication across the disciplines charged with a single client's care. Occupational therapy documentation provides a tool for communicating with other disciplines. It notifies the referring physician about the progress of intervention and other disciplines about what goals are being pursued and what specific techniques and media are being used. Reinforcement of these can occur in other disciplines'

Jacobs, K., MacRae, N., & Sladyk, K. (Eds.).
*Occupational Therapy Essentials for
Clinical Competence, Second Edition* (pp. 283-292).
© 2014 SLACK Incorporated.

Figure 22-1. The occupational therapy process.

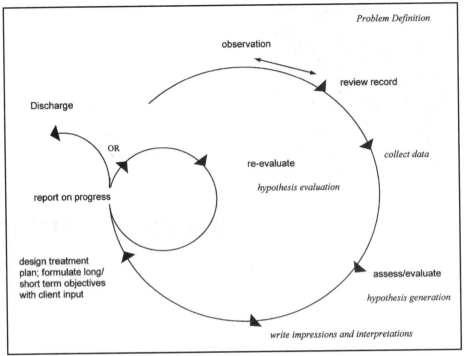

sessions as a way to promote the transfer of learning and the ability to generalize. Documentation can also specify and validate the times a splint or adaptive device needs to be worn or used.

Documentation provides a record of care and is thus a legal document that can be and often is used in court. If an intervention session is not documented, it did not occur from the viewpoint of the reimbursor, the administration, and the legal system. Because a client note is part of the client record, it is also a legal document. If a client becomes involved in a legal case and needs practitioner testimony, documentation is essential for such testimony to be reliable. Because the time span between intervention and a legal case may be long, documentation also provides a memory reference to the testifying practitioner. Documentation is part of the clinical reasoning process. It can also be fodder for prospective research, providing data for the success or failure of certain intervention approaches. Additionally, it helps the therapist recall what transpired during the last session, can promote reflection on the course of intervention, and can encourage adaptations to sessions. Thus, client notes can be a part of professional growth in improving the clarity of what is written, assessing the intervention's effectiveness, and refining clinical reasoning skills.

The documentation process is a reflection of the clinical reasoning process. It is represented by a circular diagram (Figure 22-1). During the occupational therapy process, there are various needs for documentation.

An initial note documents the first meeting and interview of a client. The progress note details the continuing and changing status of a client. A discontinuation note summarizes the course of intervention, model of practice, frames of reference, strategies and activities used, participation of the client, outcomes realized, and recommendations for the future. The latter kind of documentation becomes particularly important to the next practitioner. A discontinuation note needs to provide a history of intervention with the client, detailing what has occurred and providing recommendations for future intervention to make for a smooth transition for continuing therapy.

Documentation can take a number of other forms depending on the setting, such as an educational, business, or industrial setting and area of practice (e.g., industrial rehabilitation and ergonomics). The individual education plan (IEP) is found in an educational setting along with a report written to a parent, teacher, special education administrator, principal, superintendent, etc. In the area of industrial rehabilitation and ergonomics, documentation can take other forms, such as a written job site analysis. In a community setting, it often takes the form of a report of findings to include recommendations. In any context, a commonality is that all documentation, when done properly, promotes and justifies the value of occupational therapy.

The "Language" of Documentation

Formats may vary in different settings and practice areas, but components of good documentation remain the same: documentation needs to be clear, accurate, relevant, and it needs to list exceptions. Additionally, documentation should be succinct, written simply and in an active voice. The writer needs to consider the audience for whom a document is being written. Particularly, when written for nonmedically trained readers, documentation needs to make sense for the designated readers, and it must contain specificity in goals and directions to make it useful. Thus, an official client note in a client chart would likely differ from a progress note sent home to a parent or family member. The content might be similar, but the way it is expressed would differ.

- *Example of note in chart:* Rose was able to tolerate a 20-minute session in the kitchen. She demonstrated a 15-degree increase in shoulder flexion, allowing her to access items in cabinets above eye level. She was able to gather supplies to make a light lunch.
- *Example of note sent to family:* Rose is showing improvement in her ability to independently prepare a light lunch for herself.

Another example is a home program written for an outpatient client with deficits in fine motor control of the hand. The program could include suggestions for using everyday activities (e.g., folding clothes, washing and drying dishes) to help improve functional use.

Process of Documentation

Documentation could be thought of as taking three general forms: initial notes; intervention notes; and discontinuation notes such as discharge, reports, or letters to physicians.

BASICS

Basics need to be included in any client note. Many are common sense, but reminders are needed to ensure inclusion. The basics are as follows:

- Include the following:
  - ◊ Name of client
  - ◊ Date of session
  - ◊ Diagnoses of concern for intervention
  - ◊ How goals have been addressed, with progress or difficulty noted
  - ◊ Any unusual happenings during the session
- Use ink (with appropriate color when designated by site) when writing notes
- Use acceptable terminology and abbreviations (American Occupational Therapy Association [AOTA], 2008a)
- Remember to sign name with appropriate initials included
- Most sites do not allow erasures. If you need to correct an error, draw a single line through the mistake

and write the correction above and then initial the correction
- Write note as soon after the session as possible
- Be accurate, clear, and relevant
- If extra space remains at the end of the note, draw a line to the end of the section so no one else can add to your documentation

INITIAL NOTES

Initial notes are essentially evaluation notes with the specific form varying among entities: general medical, mental health, home health, public education, etc. The initial documentation process can be divided into three stages: actions before meeting the client, the client interview, and actions after the interview.

Actions Before Meeting the Client

Data collection begins before the client interview. Table 22-1 provides an overview of what and where a therapist working in an acute care physical disabilities setting would look to gather data during an initial assessment from a chart review. The clinician begins by examining medical records, reports of previous assessments, results of educational testing, and other pertinent documents. At this stage, the therapist needs to form a mental "picture" of the client and an idea of what the therapist is being asked to do. Practitioners should note the following:

- Who is the referral agent (e.g., a physician, a parent, a classroom teacher, another therapist)?
- What is being asked of the therapist (e.g., a splint, a safety evaluation, a fine motor writing evaluation)?

Using the Occupational Therapy Practice Framework (OTPF; AOTA, 2008b), the therapist gathers data related to the individual's highest level of performance on each of the following domains: activities of daily living (ADL) and instrumental activities of daily living (IADL), education and work, play and leisure, and social participation. If a problem exists, the therapist then looks for any information on the client's performance skills or performance patterns. The therapist also looks for information on the client's contexts and any pertinent client factors. He or she continues to review documents, looking for information about diagnoses, any precautions, the client's support systems, and the suspected disposition of the client (e.g., return to home, discharge to skilled nursing facility, or unknown).

An experienced therapist also looks for information concerning the client's history, interests, and experiences. Although not absolutely necessary, sharing this information with the client often helps build rapport and trust during the next stage.

Table 22-1.	
CHART REVIEW	
Criteria	**Components**
Basic information to be retrieved from a chart review	• Date of onset • Admitting diagnosis • Medical history (pertinent medical problems, procedures, preexisting conditions that may affect the evaluation or intervention) • Current medical intervention (medications, procedures, rehabilitation efforts, and progress) • Current medical status (client getting better or deteriorating, intervention plan, discharge plan, results of recent tests, and DNR status; information can be found in nursing and medical notes) • Personal information (age, marital status, family configuration, residence, work history, financial information) • Medication lists (will any medications affect intervention?)
Components pertinent to occupational therapy (where you will find the information)	• Medical section (physician notes, pertinent past medical history, general information on social situation, response to intervention, course of intervention, referrals to specialists, upcoming surgeries or procedures, precautions, complications during acute phase that might affect recovery [e.g., infection, hydrocephalus, respiratory distress, seizures]) • Nursing section (day-to-day status, response to intervention or disability, often report response to splinting, positioning, activities of daily living, and mobility performances) • Test section (laboratory reports, radiography, computed tomography, magnetic resonance imaging) • Medication lists (sometimes grouped in this section are vital signs, weights, calorie counts) • Professionals section (Physical Therapy, Speech Pathology, Social Work, Therapeutic Recreation, neuropsychology, Vocational Rehabilitation evaluations, and progress notes); some institutions have continuous problem-oriented records, and these reports are within the body of the medical section
Reprinted with permission from York, C. D., & MacRae, N. (1993). *Class handout*. Biddeford, ME: Occupational Therapy Department, University of New England.	

The Client Interview

Two "interviews" take place during the first meeting. The therapist is interviewing and assessing the client. At the same time, the client is conducting a silent interview, determining whether the therapist is competent and able to be trusted and whether the client can or even wants to work with the therapist. Not all clients will want to work with you. It may be pain, nausea, fear, or simply a mismatch of personalities. However, in those first few minutes, the weight is on the therapist to demonstrate competency and approachability and to develop trust.

Data collection in the client interview begins "at the door," with the therapist noting performance factors such as posture, balance, body symmetry, eye contact, bilateral upper extremity use, and cognition. Following the protocol of the hosting agency, the therapist records the client's responses to questions and assessments related to occupational therapy domains and performs an occupational history and profile. Performing the latter can help build rapport and provides points where client and practitioner can connect. Of equal importance is the client's perception of strengths, problems, and his or her goals. Before leaving the client, the therapist usually discusses findings and any anticipated occupational therapy interventions. In other settings, the therapist may not discuss the

findings with the involved individual because the "client" may be a disability insurance company, an organization such as a school system, or another professional.

Actions After the Interview

The therapist now has a clear view of the reasons for referral, the desired outcomes, and the expected outcomes, as well as the client's strengths and problem areas. The therapist must now summarize findings, develop a list of strengths and problem areas, and develop appropriate goals and activities that will help the client achieve those goals and collaboratively determine goals and activities that meet the client's needs.

PROGRESS NOTES

Usually, each intervention session requires a progress note, also called a "contact" note. It is much shorter than the initial note and commonly details only the date, duration, therapeutic activities used, client reactions, and plan of the next intervention.

DISCONTINUATION NOTES

Known also as "discharge notes," this type of note represents a melding of both the initial and progress note. Included is the background information that provides an overview of the reason for referral as well as expected outcomes. Next, a synopsis of problem areas and goals, along with progress, is detailed. It is also informative to include models and methodologies used to inform a subsequent occupational therapy practitioner (Jack & Estes, 2011). The therapist ends by noting any ongoing problems and recommendations for addressing them.

Documentation Formats

Initial, progress, and discontinuation are types of documentation, but there are other documentation formats. The types of notes occur across all areas of specialization with formats simply providing different methods of organizing data.

SOAP

A universally accepted format that organizes findings from each of the note types is the SOAP, or problem-oriented format (Weed, 1969) for the problem-oriented medical record system (Borcherding, 2000). The SOAP format has become the preferred format in many facilities (Sames, 2010). This format is composed of the following four sections, each with specific areas that need to be addressed and included to have a complete document:

- "S," or the subjective portion, includes the reason for referral and any of the following information given to the practitioner by the client or a designated member of the family.
  ◊ History, including prior level of functioning
  ◊ Lifestyle or home situation
  ◊ Emotions or attitudes
  ◊ Client's goals
  ◊ Client's complaints
  ◊ Client's response to intervention
  ◊ Any other information relevant to case or present condition(s)
- "O," or the objective portion, includes measurable or observable information.
  ◊ Objective measurements or observations
  ◊ Part of intervention already given to client
  ◊ Relevant client history taken from medical charts (may be setting dependent)
- "A," or the assessment portion, includes five sections that together provide the reader with the practitioner's clinical reasoning for goals and intervention. These sections are as follows:
  ◊ Assets: The strengths of the client and any areas without normal limits. This is an incredibly important section because the identification of the client's strengths facilitates viewing the client as a whole person, not just as one with problems

and deficits. Strengths can then be used to assist in intervention.
  ◊ Problem list: Listing of areas of deficit for occupational performance with a goal to address prioritized problem areas.
  ◊ Long-term goals: Goals that address the functional outcome of the client, worded "in order to..."
  ◊ Short-term goals: Behavioral objectives with a listing of specific methods and activities used.
  ◊ Summary of intervention: Impressions with a succinct correlation between all of the parts; the reader should be able to determine quickly what the course of intervention has been and what outcomes have been achieved just by reading the summary.
- "P," or the plan for the future, includes a number of items such as the following:
  ◊ Frequency and amount of time a client needs to be seen by the occupational therapist
  ◊ Location of intervention session
  ◊ Intervention progression
  ◊ Client and family education
  ◊ Equipment needs and equipment ordered/sold to client
  ◊ Plans for future assessment or reassessment
  ◊ Plans for discharge
  ◊ Referral to other services

The original SOAP format includes goals in the "A" section; other authors (Kettenbach, 2009; Sames, 2010) now place goals in the "P" section.

Description, Assessment, Plan Notes and Findings, Interpretation, and Plan Notes

These other forms vary somewhat from the SOAP version, but they all incorporate the skeletal underpinnings of the SOAP version. The DAP notes combine the subjective and objective portions into the "D" portion, or the description, of the client. The "A" section is the assessment or summary portion, and the "P" part is for the plan. A variation of this type of note is the FIP note, standing for findings (both subjective and objective), interpretation (similar to the summary or assessment), and plan.

Individual Education Plan

The IEP is a standardized format that documents the information determined at an IEP meeting for a specific student. The IEP is a formal process to plan what services and programs are needed for the child

Table 22-2.			
SAMPLE CHECKLIST FORMAT			
Intervention	**Date: 9/1**	**9/2**	**9/3**
Minutes taken to complete dressing (upper and lower body)	30	28	27
Verbal cues needed to don shoes	10	9	8

to meet educational goals. Guidelines of Individuals with Disabilities Education Act (IDEA; United States Department of Justice, 2005) establish the format. Elements of an IEP are as follows (Case-Smith, Roger, & Johnson, 2004):

- Present health status
- Present levels of educational performance
- Annual goals and short-term objectives (usually 3 months in length)
- Special education and related services
- Explanation of nonparticipation
- Participation in assessments
- Dates, frequency, location, and duration of services
- Transition services—begin at age 14 years and annually after that
- Measuring and reporting student progress

Practitioners need to use sound assessment instruments that are nondiscriminatory. Evaluations determine the current ability of the child to perform ADL and IADL; his or her ability to access education, work, and play activities; and his or her ability for social participation. Deficit areas are identified, and goals and objectives focus on improving these areas so the child is better able to access the educational process (Sames, 2010). Whereas IDEA requires evaluations every 3 years, IEP goals are set annually, usually meeting four times a year to check on the status of the child in reaching outcomes of intervention. An example of an IEP is found in Appendix E.

The Documentation of Occupational Therapy Session during Intervention (D.O.T.S.I.) has recently been developed and validated for use in pediatrics. It also allows documentation in a unified and professional manner and stimulates clinical reasoning (Bart, Avrech Bar, Rosenberg, Hamudot, & Janus, 2011).

CHECKLISTS

This format allows for a quick recording of a client's problems and progress using preselected categories. The organization makes it easy for a second therapist to "step in" if the primary therapist is not available. There are, however, disadvantages in that often there is little room to record observations. Some checklists do not allow the therapist to add problems to the prescribed list (Sames, 2010; Table 22-2).

NARRATIVE

As implied, this format has data written directly into the client record as soon after intervention as possible. Narrative notes are commonly free form because there is no universally accepted structure or model for writing them. Although preferred by many therapists, the result is all too often a wordy and poorly organized note. The lack of organization makes it extremely hard for a therapist unfamiliar with the client to step in and provide therapy. It is time consuming and often inefficient to trace back through prior notes in an effort to learn of the client's problems, progress, and clinician's goals. If the organizational sequence provided by the SOAP note structure is used as a guide, this format can be informative and effective.

ELECTRONIC HEALTH RECORDS

Electronic health records (EHRs), also known as *electronic medical records* (EMRs), have made slow but steady progress as a means of documentation. They will become even more pervasive by 2015 because they are mandated as part of the Health Information Technology for Economic and Clinical Health (HITECH) Act, a component of the American Recovery and Reinvestment Act of 2009. To encourage hospitals, clinics, and physicians to adopt EHRs, a number of incentives and penalties were set in place (United States Department of Health and Human Services for Medicare and Medicaid, Final Rule). In a client's EMR, data are generally entered via computer workstations or handheld devices. Individuals involved in a client's care including medical staff, nursing, and allied health personnel, contribute from evaluations, assessments, and interactions in the respective sections of the document. Data entry is often standardized by being entered via built-in "drop-down menus." Narrative can be entered but may be discouraged. The software allows health care workers to examine information entered by other medical personnel; however, data can only be entered into the area of an individual's responsibility. Hospital-based occupational therapy sections often include evaluation, recommendations, and intervention sections. Some systems have a "copy forward" feature that allows one health care worker to bring data entered by another into an assessment or intervention note. Another feature is that laboratory test values, medical images, and consultation reports are readily available to authorized personnel.

EHRs bring with them both promise and problems. Advocates argue that moving to electronic records will reduce costs and potentially decrease the incidence of medical errors caused by poor handwriting. They should also lead to a standardization of medical terminology as well as abbreviations. Countering potential gains are arguments that EHR systems are often very expensive to implement both in terms of the initial purchase as well as the need to increase information technology staff to maintain the system. At least initially, productivity may decrease as medical and allied health personnel struggle to learn the system. Finally, there is the question of security with EHRs being vulnerable to intrusion both from the outside (hacking) and from within (unauthorized access by medical personnel not involved in a specific client's care).

PROFESSIONAL LETTERS

Letters are also often required in the occupational therapy process. The practitioner may need to write a letter to a physician, documenting the progress of a client or requesting an extension of a prescription for continued therapy. A letter of referral to a professional colleague may be considered good protocol for getting the kind of information requested. Providing the specifics and detailing concerns help the other professional do a better and more thorough job. A letter may be necessary to a reimbursing agency to document the reasons for a piece of adapted equipment. Photographs of a client with that specified piece of adapted equipment can graphically help demonstrate the difference that piece of equipment will make in the client's life (Figure 22-2). Another reason for a professional letter may be to ask for a donation or to thank a donor.

Letters of reference are requested by new professionals and colleagues who are changing practice sites, jobs, or applying for licensure. Being able to clearly and accurately reflect on a colleague's job performance provides the prospective hiring agency with the information needed to make a good decision. Elements that should be included are the dates you have worked with the colleague or student, examples of work with clients and team members, personal characteristics, ethical behavior, potential for growth and strengths, and areas in need of improvement in job performance. A grading of your endorsement or lack thereof should end the letter.

Medical Abbreviations

Knowing how information should be reported in a medical record is as important as knowing what information to include. Historically, health care professionals have used medical abbreviations as a means to shorten the length of time spent writing notes while maintaining thorough client care records. However, there is no universally accepted set of medical abbreviations; therefore, abbreviations accepted at one facility may not be accepted by another. More important, an abbreviation may not have the same meaning at different facilities. In 2001, the Joint Commission on Accreditation of Health care Organizations (JCAHO; now called The Joint Commission) issued an alert related to dangerous medical abbreviations. This was followed in 2005 by the creation of a "do not use" list by the JCAHO. The use of medical abbreviations by health care professionals continues to be both common and controversial. It is, therefore, imperative that clinicians use only the abbreviations accepted at their worksite.

Goal Writing

Effective goal writing is a vital part of documentation. It is also one of the more difficult skills for new therapists to perfect. Occupational therapy values a collaborative relationship between the therapist and client. Therefore, the goals should be developed collaboratively by the client and therapist working together. Goals help prioritize intervention, measure the effectiveness of intervention, and assist with keeping health care costs in line.

Goals are composed of a number of components. An easy way to understand the components is by use of an "A-B-C-D" approach (Kettenbach, 2009, p. 138).

- A represents the *who,* or the audience; is always client oriented.

- B represents the *what,* or the functional behavior; action words need to be used in this portion of the goal.

- C represents the *how,* with a description of the situation and the circumstances under which the behavior will be accomplished.

- D is represented by some form of measurement, such as percentage, number, or time (i.e., how the outcome will be measured).

An example of each portion of a goal follows:

- Observing hip precautions 100%, the client will don her socks using a sock aide within two intervention sessions.

- Observing hip precautions 100% (measurement), the client (who) will don her socks (what) using a sock-aide (how) within two intervention sessions.

7 August 2013

To: Eleanor Small, D.O.
               Hand Surgical Associates
               Anywhere, USA

From: Daniel Williams, OTR/L
               Regional Hospital
               Anywhere, USA

Re: Splint fabrication for Rita Newman

Mrs. Newman was seen in occupational therapy on this date following her recent skiing accident in which she injured the ulnar collateral ligament of her dominant hand. Per your order, a thumb-based, carpo-metacarpal (CMC) immobilization splint was fabricated. The client was provided with written wear and care information.

She was able to perform a simulated housekeeping task with report that the splint fit well and that she experienced a decrease in pain while performing these activities.

I will continue to monitor her comfort and document decrease in pain via telephone for one month. She has been advised to call with any incidence of increased pain or loss in motion. For your review, we have enclosed a picture of the splint that you ordered.

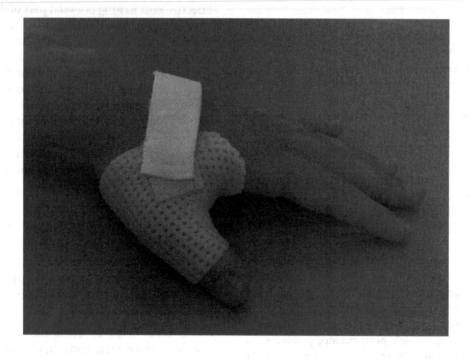

Figure 22-2. Sample physician's letter.

Another helpful acronym for effective goal writing is RUMBA, a goal-writing method developed by the AOTA in the 1970s (Sames, 2010):

- Relevant: The goal must be relevant to the client.
- Understandable: The goal must be easily understood.
- Measurable: The goal must be able to be measured; you must be able to know when and how well the goal has been met.
- Behavioral: The goal must be observable.
- Achievable: The goal must be able to be accomplished by the client.

If these descriptors are used as references by the goal writer, goals have a much better chance of being clear and concise.

Functional Outcomes

Outcomes identify what the client will be able to do functionally as a result of the intervention. They have resulted from the managed care push for accountability in our health care system, with managed care companies scrutinizing costs to make sure they are receiving value for their expenditures. Outcomes also notify the third-party reimbursor of the functional reason behind the goal formation. More importantly, particularly to reflect the framework (AOTA, 2008b), a functional outcome should be seen as contributing to an improved occupational performance that promotes social participation by the client. This exemplifies a shift from focusing on improved strength or range of motion, or components, as the goal of intervention to a more top-down, holistic approach that aims for improved occupational performance. An example of a functional outcome is improved upper extremity functioning to assist in the independence in the ADL of dressing.

Administrative Outcomes

Documentation of clients' functional outcomes can also be used to gather administrative outcome data to support research and quality assurance activities of the department.

Occupational Therapist–Occupational Therapy Assistant Differentiation

Occupational therapy assistants collaborate with occupational therapists throughout the occupational therapy process, from screening and evaluation to discontinuation of services. Assistance is always done under the supervision of the occupational therapist. The same is true of documentation. Depending on the site, the occupational therapy assistant may contribute to the documentation note or may write the entire note. If the latter is the case, it is most often a progress note, and an occupational therapist's signature is usually required by reimbursors. Because both practitioners contribute to the documentation process, both need to understand what is entailed in the process and how to do it effectively and efficiently.

Summary

For many practitioners, new and experienced, being able to write well-organized and concise documentation is a major challenge. Well-crafted assessments and notes help practitioners organize, deliver, assess, and demonstrate occupation-centered interventions. This skill is at the core of clinical reasoning. Effective documentation enhances client care and protects both the practitioner and agency if litigation occurs. Finally, effective documentation allows a "trail" of thinking and actions that can be later analyzed to demonstrate the efficacy of the profession by research that supports our evidence-based practices. The rewards, therefore, are worth the effort needed to learn this skill.

Student Self-Assessment

1. Place the following into its proper location in a SOAP note:
   ◊ Activities to include active assistive range of motion (AAROM) and ADL concentrating on dressing
   ◊ AROM R UE 0-150 flexion
   ◊ Using a rolling walker, was close supervision from bed to bathroom and return.
   ◊ Nursing reports patient spent a "restless night."
   ◊ Client seen x 30 minutes in room to concentrate on lower body dressing.
   ◊ Ability to perform dressing independently continues to be decreased secondary to inability to remember sequence.
   ◊ "I hate this."
   ◊ With distant supervision, client will be able to gather and don all clothing (I) within 20 minutes.
   ◊ Client has been seen in occupational therapy x 20 since admission and has met all goals; no further occupational therapy intervention warranted at this time.

2. Reorganize and reformat the following narrative note, shortening it while being concise and

EVIDENCE-BASED RESEARCH CHART

Topic	Evidence
Forms of documentation	Bart, Avrech Bar, Rosenberg, Hamudot, & Janus, 2011; Jack & Estes, 2010
Guidelines for documentation	AOTA, 2008a; Kettenbach, 2009; Sames, 2010

thorough. Use approved abbreviations and medical terminology where appropriate.

◊ "Mr. Jones is a 35-year-old married man who was involved in a motor vehicle accident 24 hours ago. He is complaining of quite a bit of pain in both legs. His car was struck in the driver's side. He broke his left leg and has quite a few bruises and abrasions on the right. He broke his left arm. He has some facial cuts and a concussion. I saw him in his room for about 30 minutes to start the evaluation, but he did not know where he was or what day it was. He does remember his name and what happened to him. I think my goals are to make him independent in dressing by discharge. He should also be independent in mobility during ADL using the walker that physical therapy provided. He can only put as much pressure on the left leg so as to not break an eggshell at this time. The nurse also said he was in a lot of pain. He rates it as an 8 on a scale of 10. In the memory assessment, he can remember five numbers forward and three numbers backward. I think he will eventually be able to go home, but I'm not sure if he will need rehab first."

3. From the scenario in Question 2, create two properly formatted goals for Mr. Jones.

4. Write a letter to the attending physician, assuming goals have been met and that Mr. Jones is ready for discontinuation from occupational services.

Electronic Resource

- For further clarification of documentation for occupational therapy, see www.aota.org/pubs/otp/1997-2007/columns/capital briefing/2004/cb-071204.aspx.

References

American Occupational Therapy Association. (2008a). Guidelines for documentation of occupational therapy. *American Journal of Occupational Therapy, 62*(Suppl. 6).

American Occupational Therapy Association. (2008b). Occupational therapy practice framework: Domain and process (2nd ed.). *American Journal of Occupational Therapy, 62,* 625-683.

Bart, O., Avrech Bar, M., Rosenberg, L., Hamudot, V., & Jarus, T. (2011). Development and validation of the Documentation of Occupational Therapy Session during Intervention (D.O.T.S.I.). *Research in Developmental Disabilities, 32,* 719-726.

Borcherding, S. (2000). *Documentation manual for writing soap notes in occupational therapy.* Thorofare, NJ: SLACK Incorporated.

Case-Smith, J., Roger, J., & Johnson, J. (2004). School-based occupational therapy. In J. Case-Smith (Ed.), *OT for children* (5th ed., pp. 758-709). St. Louis, MO: Elsevier Mosby.

Jack, J., & Estes, R. I. (2010). Documenting progress: Hand therapy treatment shift from biomechanical to occupational adaptation. *American Journal of Occupational Therapy, 64*(1), 82-87.

Joint Commission on Accreditation of Health Care Organizations. (2005). *Do not use list.* Retrieved from http://www.jointcommission.org/PatientSafety/DoNotUseList

Kettenbach, G. (2009). *Writing patient/client notes: Ensuring accuracy on documentation* (4th ed.). Philadelphia, PA: F. A. Davis Company.

Sames, K. (2010). *Documenting occupational therapy practice* (2nd ed.). Boston, MA: Pearson.

U.S. Department of Health and Human Services for Medicare & Medicaid Services 42 CFR Parts 4512, 413, 412 et al. *Medicare and Medicaid Programs: Electronic Health Record Incentive Program: Final rule.* Retrieved from http://www.gpo.gov/fdsys/pkg/FR-2010-07-28/pdf/2010-17207.pdf

U.S. Department of Justice. (2005). *A guide to disability rights laws.* Retrieved from http://www.usdoj.gov/crt/ada/cguide.pdf

Weed, L. L. (1969). *Medical records, medical education and patient care: The problem-oriented record as a basic tool.* Cleveland, OH: Case Western Reserve University Press.

York, C. D., & MacRae, N. (1993). *Class handout.* Biddeford, ME: Occupational Therapy Department, University of New England.

V

INTERVENTION PLAN
FORMULATION AND IMPLEMENTATION

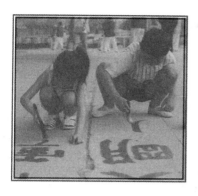

23

INTERVENTION PLANNING

Jane O'Brien, PhD, OTR/L

ACOTE STANDARDS EXPLORED IN THIS CHAPTER
B.5.1–B.5.3

KEY TERMS

- **Adapting:** Activities involving changing the actual task to make it easier or more difficult for the clien. Adapting may involve the use of assistive technology.
- **Contexts:** Refers to cultural, physical, social, personal, temporal and virtual considerations (AOTA, 2008).
- **Frames of reference (FOR):** Helps the occupational therapy practitioner develop an intervention plan and provides specific intervention techniques.

- **Grading:** Refers to making an activities easier or harder for the client.
- **Models of practice:** Provide an overview of how to look at the client; as such, models of practice help clinicians organize their thinking (MacRae, 2001).
- **Occupation based activity:** Involves doing the actual occupation, which provides meaning and is part of one's identity (Fisher, 1998).

Introduction

Occupational therapy practitioners work with a variety of clients who have a wide range of abilities and disabilities. A crucial skill in the development of effective intervention planning is the ability to interpret, develop, and use evidence to support practice. Occupational therapy practitioners must be able to analyze activity so that they may adjust (i.e., grade or adapt) intervention according to a client's needs. Importantly, clinicians must be aware of safety issues throughout the process and ensure that clients are safe after being

Jacobs, K., MacRae, N., & Sladyk, K. (Eds.).
Occupational Therapy Essentials for
Clinical Competence, Second Edition (pp. 295-307).
© 2014 SLACK Incorporated.

discharged from services. Occupational therapy practitioners use activity to help clients return to engagement in the things they find meaningful. This chapter provides an overview of the intervention process by examining how models of practice and frames of reference guide practitioners in their decision making for activity selection. A description of the role of the occupational therapist and occupational therapy assistant in intervention is provided. A discussion of how to develop occupational-based intervention plans reflective of the client's needs is followed by suggestions in how to select and provide occupational therapy intervention. Finally, this chapter provides guidelines on how to grade and adapt activities to meet the client's needs.

Overview of the Intervention Process

Intervention plans provide a map for the occupational therapy process. The plan requires that the occupational therapy practitioner problem solve, reason, and make decisions based on current evidence, knowledge, past experiences, and the setting in which the intervention takes place. Intervention planning requires creativity, knowledge of available resources, and practice. The plan includes the goals of the intervention; who will perform the intervention; and where, when, how often, and how long the intervention will take place. The plan includes a rationale for the type of intervention with desired outcomes. Intervention plans clarify the role of the occupational therapy practitioner and specify the team members (see Appendix D for an outline of an intervention plan). Occupational therapy students and novice practitioners learn from carefully describing each part of the intervention plan with a well-developed rationale. As practitioners gain experience, the rationale may not necessarily be written in the plan. However, experienced practitioners should always be able to articulate the rationale for interventions and be aware of current research evidence to support the plan.

The occupational therapist is ultimately responsible for the intervention plan, but he or she receives input from the occupational therapy assistant. The occupational therapy assistant assists in the plan by providing data, updates, and information about the client. After the plan is developed, the occupational therapy assistant and occupational therapist work toward the selected goals (American Occupational Therapy Association [AOTA], 1990, 1994, 2008). The occupational therapist provides supervision to the occupational therapy assistant, as needed, depending on the occupational therapy assistant's experience. Both the occupational therapy assistant and occupational therapist design activities to meet the plan.

Models of Practice

Occupational therapy is based on the premise that engagement in activity (i.e., meaningful to the client) is beneficial to clients and will help them recover, relearn, or reengage in life's activities (AOTA, 2008). A model of practice provides an overview of how to look at the client; as such, models of practice help clinicians organize their thinking (MacRae, 2001). Occupational therapy models of practice include occupation and describe how, in a holistic manner, factors influence an individual's engagement in occupation. Occupational therapy models of practice include the Model of Human Occupation (MOHO; Kielhofner, 1985, 2002), Person-Environment-Occupation Performance model (Law, Cooper, Strong, Stewart, Rigby, & Letts, 1996), Canadian Occupational Performance Measure (Townsend, Brintnell, & Staisey, 1990), and Occupational Adaptation (Schkade & Schultz, 1992). Table 23-1 provides a description of these occupational therapy models of practice. Readers are encouraged to explore these models and choose the one that will be of greatest help to the client. Occupational therapy practitioners use the model of practice to organize their thinking of clients and their abilities (see Chapter 16 for more information on evaluation).

Frame of Reference

The frame of reference (FOR) helps the occupational therapy practitioner develop an intervention plan and provides specific intervention techniques. It should be noted that some models (e.g., the MOHO and Canadian Occupational Performance Measure) are both models of practice and frames of reference. Frames of reference include a description of the theory, population, principles surrounding the intervention, description of function and dysfunction, role of the clinician, intervention process, and techniques (Mosey, 1981). Frames of reference also include assessment and measurement tools (Table 23-2).

Commonly used occupational therapy frames of reference include the MOHO, sensory integration, biomechanical, motor control, neurodevelopmental (NDT) treatment, cognitive disabilities, and developmental. See Table 23-3 for a description of selected frames of reference. Students and occupational therapy practitioners commonly ask, "Why do we need to use a frame of reference or theory?" Although expert practitioners may rely on experience and prior knowledge to determine what to do with certain clients, novice practitioners and students rely on the research of others to determine the most effective intervention techniques. The model of practice frames the evaluation and intervention session because it provides parameters for viewing the client. The FOR

Table 23-1.
MODELS OF PRACTICE

Model	Author(s)	Components	Premises
Model of Human Occupation (MOHO)	Kielhofner, 1985, 2008	Volition Habituation Performance Environment	The human is an open system. The clinician's role is to understand the client in terms of these systems (and subsystems) and intervene to facilitate engagement in occupation.
Canadian Occupational Performance Measure(COPM)	Canadian Occupational Therapy Association (Townsend et al., 1990)	Spirituality Occupation Context (institutional included)	The worth of the individual is central to this model. Spirituality is the core of a person. Thus, occupational therapy practitioners must understand the client's spirituality to facilitate engagement in occupations. Performance of occupations takes place within social, physical, and cultural environments.
Occupational Adaptation (OA)	Schkade & Schultz, 1992	Occupations Physical and emotional strengths and weaknesses Examination of available support systems (physical and emotional)	Help people participate in their desired occupations by adapting or modifying the occupation or using other methods to perform the occupation.
Person-Environment-Occupation-Performance (PEOP)	Christiansen & Baum, 1997; Law et al., 1996	Person Environment Occupation Performance	Occupations are the everyday things people do. PEOP looks at the person in terms of physical, social, and emotional factors. The environment (context) influences the person and occupations. Performance is influenced by person, environment, and occupation factors. The environment includes culture and political institutions.

Adapted with permission from O'Brien, J. C., & Solomon, J. W. (2006). Scope of practice. In J. W. Solomon & J. C. O'Brien (Eds.), *Pediatric skills for occupational therapy assistants* (2nd ed.). St. Louis, MO: Mosby. Copyright Elsevier Mosby, 2006.

Table 23-2.
FRAMES OF REFERENCE

Description of theory	The FOR begins with a description of the thought process and reasoning for addressing change. The author provides a detailed background of the intentions of the FOR based on research evidence.
Population	A description of who will benefit from the strategies provided by the FOR, including the rationale for the use with a specific population.
Principles for intervention	The foundation for the intervention includes the specific principles that help practitioners make therapeutic decisions. This section should include research evidence to support each claim.
Description of function and dysfunction	A description of the continuum of function and dysfunction as described by the FOR helps practitioners understand the scope of the FOR.
Role of the practitioner	A clear description of the practitioner's role when using this intervention is provided. The FOR outlines the strategies and techniques the practitioner uses in therapy.
Intervention process and techniques	The author provides a description of how intervention proceeds using the given techniques. This allows practitioners to observe, assess, and intervene accordingly.
Assessment tools	Assessment tools designed specifically for the FOR allow practitioners to operationalize concepts and follow specific guidelines provided. Assessment tools are needed to evaluate clients accordingly.
Measurement	Descriptions of how to measure change are required.
Research evidence	Evidence to support the methodology and theoretical premises of the FOR.

Table 23-3.			
PEDIATRIC FRAMES OF REFERENCE			
Frame of Reference	**Author(s)**	**Principles**	**Treatment Modalities**
Developmental	Llorens, 1976	Development occurs over time and between skills (e.g., gross and fine motor). Some children experience a "gap" in their development because of physical, emotional, or social trauma. The occupational therapist's role is to "fill in the gap."	Identify current level of functioning. Work on the next step to achieve the skill. Intervention includes practice, repetition, education, and modeling of skills.
Biomechanical	Pedretti & Paszuinielli, 1990	Improve strength, endurance, and range of motion.	Strength: Increase weight of toys or repetitive use of objects. Endurance: Increase time engaged in occupation. Range of motion: Repetitively provide slow, sustained stretch to increase end range.
Sensory integration	Ayres, 1979	Children with sensory integration dysfunction have difficulty processing sensory information (vestibular, proprioceptive, tactile). Improvements in sensory processing lead to improved engagement in occupations.	Provide controlled sensory input to improve the child's ability to process sensory stimuli. Use of suspended equipment and the "just-right challenge." Activities are child directed.
Motor control	Shumway-Cook & Woollacott, 2007	Acquisition of motor skills is based on dynamical systems theory (all systems work on each other for movement to occur, including sensory, motor, and cognitive).	Task-oriented approach: Clients learn motor skills best by repeating the occupations in the most natural setting, varying the requirements.
Neurodevelopmental	Bobath, 1975; Schoen & Anderson, 1993	Clients learn motor patterns when they "feel" normal movement patterns.	Clinician uses handling techniques and key points of control to inhibit abnormal muscle tone and facilitate normal movement patterns.
Sensorimotor	Trombly, 1994	Sensory input to change the muscle tone or promote a muscle contraction.	Icing techniques, neutral warmth, slow stroking, and vibration are all techniques used in this approach.

Adapted with permission from O'Brien, J. C., & Solomon, J. W. (2006). Scope of practice. In J. W. Solomon & J. C. O'Brien (Eds.), *Pediatric skills for occupational therapy assistants* (2nd ed.). St. Louis, MO: Mosby. Copyright Elsevier Mosby, 2006.

provides a systematic manner by which to conduct intervention. Together, the model of practice and FOR help the occupational therapy practitioner define and observe factors influencing function. Occupational therapy practitioners who do not use a model of practice or FOR may waste time and energy organizing intervention.

Those who say they do not use a FOR or theory may, in fact, not be able to articulate the FOR or theory ("It is just what we do."). For example, NDT approaches are based on the theories of brain plasticity. An NDT approach relies on repeating activities so that the client learns them and is more able to perform the activity because of improved brain plasticity.

Because frames of reference change as new research becomes available, occupational therapy practitioners must become consumers of research if they want to provide the best care to their clients. For example, changes have been made in the NDT approaches with the realization that children learn motorically through mistakes and that children with cerebral palsy may need to make some motor mistakes to be functional (Howle, 2005; Nichols, 2005; Schoen & Anderson, 1999). Therefore, the best compromise might be to allow the child to perform the movement and help him or her perform it in the best way for him or her. The goal does not have to be a perfect movement pattern, as was previously implied by

Table 23-4.

GUIDING QUESTIONS TO CONSIDER WHEN DECIDING ON A MODEL OF PRACTICE OR FRAME OF REFERENCE

Setting	Does this model of practice or FOR fit within the setting?
Population	Does this model of practice or FOR address the needs of the population being treated?
Basic principles	What is the theory of this model of practice or FOR, and does it make sense for the population being treated? Is this model of practice or FOR congruent with occupational therapy practice? Is there adequate research to support the theory and principles?
Evidence	Has the research supported the use of this model of practice or FOR and, if so, with which population? Does this model of practice or FOR support cost-effective intervention? Are the assessment tools associated with this model of practice or FOR well designed and clinically relevant? Is there documentation that this model of practice or FOR can improve the occupations of clients? Is this model of practice or FOR congruent with occupational therapy core values and beliefs?
Assessment and evaluation	What assessments or tests are compatible with the model of practice or FOR? Are the assessments standardized, reliable, and valid? Does the model of practice or FOR provide reliable measures for assessment and evaluation?
Practical considerations	Does the clinic or site have the equipment necessary to competently use this model of practice or FOR?
Clinical expertise	Is the practitioner adequately trained to use the associated techniques or assessment tools? How much training is necessary?

this FOR. The newest models for NDT include functional movement throughout the therapy session.

Practitioners evaluate whether the intervention strategies associated with the FORs are working. If the client is not making the desired progress, a closer review of the techniques, principles, and assessment tools described in the FOR may provide an alternative plan. A closer inspection of the research or protocols associated with the FOR may promote success. Alternatively, the occupational therapy practitioner may decide to try another FOR altogether. Informed practitioners benefit from the knowledge of many frames of reference in that they are able to treat diverse client issues. When practitioners understand the principles and theory guiding the FOR, they are better able to adapt techniques for clients for whom the FOR was not originally intended. Occupational therapy practitioners evaluate many factors when choosing a model of practice or FOR. See Table 23-4 for guiding questions to consider when selecting a model of practice or FOR.

Occupational-Based Intervention Plans

After the occupational therapist has evaluated the client and determined the client's needs through interpretation of the data, the occupational therapist develops the intervention plan. After establishing service competency (ensuring that two practitioners will obtain the same results [AOTA, 1990]) in administering standardized tests, the occupational therapy assistant may assist by providing information and administering standardized tests as requested by the occupational therapist. The occupational therapy assistant is not responsible for interpreting the data. The first step in developing the intervention plan is to collaborate with the client on the goals for the intervention.

The goals are based on helping clients re-engage in their occupations, the everyday things we do that provide us with meaning (AOTA, 2008). Occupations vary from person to person. The occupational therapy practitioner collaborates with the client, family, and team members to develop appropriate goals that reflect the client's occupations. Intervention is based on these occupationally based goals developed with the client and family. Therapy goals are designed to create or promote, establish or restore, maintain, modify, and prevent, according to the practice framework (AOTA, 2008).

Collaboration With Clients

Collaborating with clients and family members on developing goals for occupational therapy services helps occupational therapists gain trust from clients. Clients who collaborate in goal setting are motivated to participate in therapy and home programs, and they make better gains (Maurer, Smith, & Armetta, 1989; Melchert-McKearnan, Dietz, Engel, & White, 2000; Steinbeck, 1986). Therapists use their awareness of the client's strengths and weaknesses, occupational desires, and contextual support to develop goals. Collaborating with clients on goal setting requires skill in interviewing, and, until a client is ready to participate in the process, the therapist may need to look for nonverbal clues, work with family, and investigate possible alternative goals. However, the time taken to really understand clients and develop an intervention plan that meets their needs makes for a more successful session (AOTA, 2008; Kielhofner, 2008; Law et al., 1996).

The mechanics of goal writing are described in Chapter 22. Occupational therapists developing occupational-based goals may be successful by using the documentation guidelines. Goals must be meaningful and relevant to the person, measurable, achievable, and written clearly. As a general rule, successful practitioners write goals that clients hope to achieve. The short-term goals are steps toward the long-term goals. The steps are not so challenging as to discourage the client. Furthermore, goals must be written so that all who read them can determine how they will be met. People are more likely to achieve things that they can see and understand.

Intervention plans and strategies depend on the context in which the goal must be achieved. The framework (AOTA, 2008) lists contexts or environments as including cultural, physical, social, personal, temporal, and virtual (see the sidebar for a description of each). The following examples describe important issues showing how contexts may impact the intervention plan.

CULTURAL

Culture is reflected in everyday events such as feeding, dressing, grooming, and hygiene. The goal of occupational therapy is to help the person regain function within his or her culture. Thus, practitioners must be sensitive to how the person and culture views the occupation. Goals and subsequent intervention plans are designed around the cultural expectations and beliefs for the occupation.

Because occupational therapy practitioners work with clients who have experienced some form of disability, an awareness of the client's cultural view of disability may prove insightful. For example, it may not be the wish of every disabled client to "fit in." In fact, disability scholars argue that the disability is part of the person's identity and that rehabilitation professionals may reinforce the idea that the client is "abnormal" (Giangreco, 1995 as cited in Kielhofner, 2005). Kielhofner and colleagues propose that occupational therapy practitioners rethink how they view disability (Kielhofner, 2005; McColl, 2005; Neville-Jan, 2005; Taylor, 2005; Thibodaux, 2005). Black and Wells (2007) proposed that occupational therapy

practitioners become first aware of their own culture and be open to other cultures through experience and discussion (see Chapter 2).

Questions to ask when collaborating on goal setting include the following:

- What would you like to do?
- What is causing you trouble?
- When you leave, what would you like to be doing?
- What is your favorite thing to do?
- Can you list three things that you would like to do again?
- What types of things do you enjoy doing?
- Describe a typical day.

PHYSICAL

Occupations are performed in many different physical settings. Occupational therapy practitioners consider all of the physical factors required for success. For example, although a client may be successful cooking in the occupational therapy clinic with all materials readily available, the same client may not be able to maneuver around his or her own kitchen. Intervention may need to include making the kitchen accessible to the client. In another case, a child with juvenile rheumatoid arthritis was provided with an electronic wheelchair. This worked well at school, and the teachers, parents, and child were happy. The chair fit well. However, the client's mother complained of a sore back and upon further discussion revealed that she had to lift the wheelchair up the stairs into the child's home. In this situation, the child was successful in the school but not at home. These examples show the importance of understanding all of the physical contexts in which the occupations occur.

SOCIAL

Social demands change the interpersonal and sometimes physical demands of occupations. Therefore, occupational therapy practitioners planning intervention need to consider the social expectations and demands of a given occupation. For example, going to lunch with one's sister requires very different social skills than attending a large formal dinner party. Occupational therapy practitioners provide interventions aimed at helping clients function in both of these situations as well as in many different scenarios. For clients to successfully engage in occupations, they must be prepared for the social expectations. This may require education to those in the support system (e.g., teachers sometimes ask children to discuss differences within a supportive environment with their classmates). Caregivers may not understand the social differences observed in their loved one. Occupational therapy practitioners can play an important role in helping others understand so they may support intervention plans.

PERSONAL

Occupational therapy practitioners develop activities and intervention plans based on a person's age, gender, socioeconomic status, and educational status. For example, elderly clients typically do not wish to engage in the same type of activities as adolescents or young children. Age-related and gender differences are easily identified. However, practitioners must also be open to differences in terms of other cultures and individual preferences (see Chapter 2). For example, many elderly people engage in activities that may be considered limited to young people (e.g., snowboarding, lifting weights, surfing).

TEMPORAL

People participate in different activities at certain stages of life. The temporal aspects of occupations also include time of day, time of year, and duration of the activity. For example, some activities depend on the season (e.g., snowboarding, skiing). Some activities are part of a morning routine (e.g., breakfast, dressing, grooming), but others may be more suitable for afternoon (e.g., lunch). For some clients, performing activities in their natural temporal context allows them to be more successful.

VIRTUAL

Many driving simulator programs use virtual context to help retrain individuals to drive. The virtual context of this activity may help prepare the individual for driving. Occupational therapy practitioners analyze the virtual nature of activities and may address how a person accesses the virtual environment.

Activity Analysis

The importance of finding activities that are motivating and purposeful to clients is a key assumption of occupational therapy practice. Occupational therapy practitioners examine individual motivations and desires as essential to the intervention process. After goals and objectives have been established for clients, practitioners design intervention activities to reach these goals. Before performing the actual occupation, clients may have to engage in preparatory activities.

Preparatory Activities

Preparatory activities may include exercise, stretching, range of motion, postural preparation, and positioning

Contexts

Cultural: Customs, beliefs, activity patterns, behavior standards, and expectations accepted by the society of which the individual is a member. Includes ethnicity and values as well as political aspects, such as law that affect access to resources and affirm personal rights. Also includes opportunities for education, employment, and economic support.

Physical: Natural, nonhuman, and built and the objects in them. Includes the accessibility to and performance within environments having natural terrain, plants, animals, buildings, furniture, objects, tools, or devices.

Social: Constructed by the presence, relationships, and expectations of persons, organizations, and populations. Availability and expectations of significant individuals, such as spouse, friends, and caregivers. Also includes relationships with individual groups or organizations and systems.

Personal: Features of the individual that are not part of the health conditions or health status (World Health Organization, 2001, p. 17). Personal context includes age, gender, socioeconomic status, and educational status.

Temporal: Location of occupational performance in time (Neistadt & Crepeau, 1998, p. 292).

Virtual: Environment in which communication occurs by means of airways or computers and an absence of physical contact.

Reproduced with permission from American Occupational Therapy Association. (2008). Occupational therapy practice framework: Domain and process (2nd ed.). *American Journal of Occupational Therapy, 62,* 625-683.

(Fisher, 1998). These activities are designed to provide the person with the necessary prerequisite skills. For example, runners stretch before running long distances. In this case, stretching is considered a preparatory activity. Children may participate in hand warm-up exercises before completing handwriting in school (Figure 23-1). After preparatory work is completed, the occupational therapy practitioner may engage the client in some purposeful activities.

Purposeful Activities

Purposeful activities are ones that are meaningful to the person or may help the client reach his or her goals (Fisher, 1998). Purposeful activities are chosen by the client, have an end goal, and involve many separate skills and abilities. In the case of running, purposeful activities

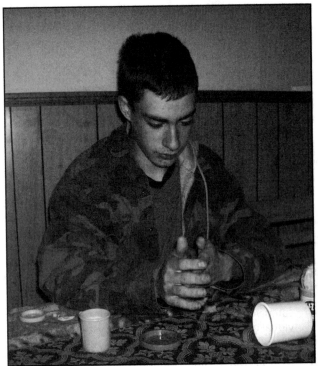

Figure 23-1. Preparatory activity—Scott performs some hand exercises to get ready for writing.

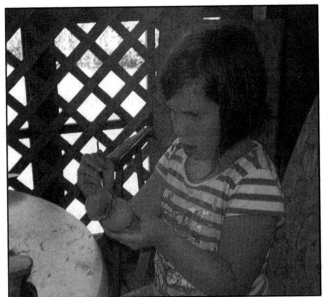

Figure 23-2. Purposeful activity—Alison paints a clay vase as a way to improve her hand skills for writing.

may include doing some speed work to get faster. In this case, the activity relates to the occupation but is not performed in the same context as the actual occupation. In the case of the child, purposeful activity may include practicing letter formation or painting (Figure 23-2).

Occupation-Based Activities

The goal of occupational therapy intervention is that the client engages in the chosen occupation. Occupation-based activity involves doing the actual occupation, which provides meaning and is part of one's identity (Fisher, 1998). Using occupation-based activity requires the person use the actual materials and context in which the activity is performed (e.g., running along the road for a distance runner or a child writing a story in school) (Figure 23-3). Occupations are personal and thus depend on the client. A skilled occupational therapist takes the time to find out what occupations are most vital to the person's identity and targets intervention on those. A person who enjoys gardening may identify him- or herself as a gardener. This may provide him or her with pleasure, a sense of being, and accomplishment. For this person, returning to gardening is important and a part of his or her identity (AOTA, 2008). For others, gardening may be a task they accomplish every year because it makes the home look better, and for them, being a homemaker is

important. In this case, gardening is an activity associated with taking care of the home. Still other people may find gardening a chore that comes along with owning a home, but it is not enjoyable and not important to their identity. Occupational therapy practitioners use all types of activity in practice. However, intervention should be made up mostly of occupation-based activity (AOTA, 2008; Fisher, 1998). Occupational therapy practitioners believe that engaging in occupations is therapeutic and will lead to larger gains. Furthermore, participating in the actual occupation in the actual context promotes adaptation, generalization, and transfer of learning.

Safety

Throughout the intervention process, the occupational therapy practitioner considers safety issues and addresses the ability of the client to return to occupations in a safe manner. The occupational therapy practitioner carefully watches clients as they perform occupations to determine if judgment, cognition, and physical abilities allow them to be safe. Frequently, the occupational therapist will perform a home evaluation before discharge to assure the client and team that the environment is safe. It may be the occupational therapy practitioner's role to adapt and modify equipment so the client is able to use safety devices (e.g., phone, grab bars). Prevention of accidents may be achieved with analysis of the environment (e.g., getting rid of throw rugs). Creating a safe environment by teaching safety skills (e.g., locking doors) may be the occupational therapist's role.

Grading and Adapting

The ability to analyze activities is learned early in occupational therapy curricula with activity analysis coursework. These skills are refined and enhanced, leading to improved observational skills. Entry-level occupational therapy practitioners are successful at analyzing activities and using activities to improve function. Grading refers to making an activity easier or harder for the client. Providing clients with the "just-right challenge" (a challenge that is neither too hard nor too easy) is motivating and therapeutic. If the activity is too difficult or too easy, clients become discouraged or bored and do not want to continue. Thus, occupational therapy practitioners work to challenge clients toward their goals without overwhelming or boring them. Activities may be graded by the following:

- Providing more or less direction (consider the type of direction: verbal, demonstrative, written, one-step, two-step)
- Providing more or less physical assistance
- Increasing or decreasing the time requirements
- Adding or subtracting the following:
  ◊ Steps
  ◊ Environmental demands
  ◊ Choices
  ◊ Cognitive or psychological demands
  ◊ Physical demands
  ◊ Required details

Adapting activities involves changing the actual task to make it easier or more difficult for the client. Adapting may involve the use of assistive technology. For example, providing clients with a built-up handled spoon makes gripping easier. Other adaptations may include teaching a person to dress using one-hand techniques. Adaptations may include the following:

- Technology to change tasks (e.g., cooking food using a microwave instead of an oven)
- Eliminating steps or performing activities differently (e.g., buying fruit that has already been cut up)
- Providing adaptive equipment (e.g., picking things up using a reacher)
- Changing the physical demands of the task (e.g., sitting while dressing)

All activities can be graded and adapted to meet the needs of the client. Occupational therapy practitioners may change activities by examining the client factors required to perform or by changing the contextual aspects of the tasks. Suggestions to change the contextual aspects of the task include the following:

- Cultural: Increase or decrease the cultural nature of the activity. Discuss the cultural aspects.

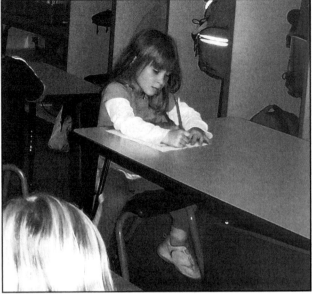

Figure 23-3. Occupation-based activity—Molly writes a story about her dog during writing time at school.

- Physical: Increase the distance required for walking; change the terrain. Conduct the activity in a familiar or unfamiliar setting. Make the materials larger or smaller. Change the lighting of the room. Increase or decrease the size of the space.
- Social: Increase or decrease the number of people in the activity. Involve familiar or unfamiliar people. Require the client to organize an event or attend only. Vary the time of the interactions or the intensity of the exchanges. Provide varying degrees of structure to the interactions.
- Personal: Consider gender and age when selecting activities.
- Spiritual: Change the intensity, focus, and meaning of the activity. Ask the individual to discuss the meaning of the activity or reflect on the event.
- Temporal: Perform the activity at the same time. Vary the length of time for the activity or change time expectations.
- Virtual: Require the client to use more or less familiar or unfamiliar technology.

Environmental Modifications and Adaptations

Occupational therapists analyze context (cultural, physical, social, personal, spiritual, temporal, and virtual) and the client factors required for success to determine the activity demands on the person. The goal of therapy is for the client to engage in the occupation in its most natural context. Thus, if the person comes from a large social

Table 23-5.

SUGGESTED ACTIVITIES

Activity	Description	Goals	Comments
Treasure hunt	Ask a child to follow the written steps to find a "treasure." Reinforce the concept of the list. Ask the child to write the steps for an activity to reinforce organization skills.	Increase organization for school.	Children will do better if they come up with the system for organizing their work. Be sure to include them in the process and be flexible with the outcome.
Lunch group	Have a regular lunch group requiring each client to prepare a part of the meal, depending on his or her ability. When clients are able, require one client to make the entire lunch for the group. Praise the success and have the clients enjoy a lunch break.	Increase ability to prepare meals. Increase ability to plan and follow sequential steps. Increase hand function.	Asking family members, friends, or even other staff members to lunch may help the person feel special and proud of his or her accomplishments.
Picture frame	Glue beads on a wooden or cardboard picture frame to decorate it. Place a picture inside the frame upon completion.	Increase hand function. Increase activity endurance.	Providing a variety of beads, stickers, and paint changes the complexity of the project.

and/or talkative family, the therapist's job is to help him or her return to this social context. Intervention aimed at having the person return to this environment differs from that in which the client may be returning home with minimal visitors.

TOOLS

The tools used in occupational therapy intervention include therapeutic use of self (see Chapter 9), therapeutic use of occupations or activities, consultation (see Chapter 36), and education (see Chapter 21). The tools used when conducting therapeutic use of occupations and activities include the following:

- Materials (e.g., arts and crafts, self-care, work, leisure, communication)
- Social (e.g., role playing, acting, dance, sports)
- Animal assisted (e.g., dogs, pet care, hippotherapy)
- Specialized setting (e.g., aquatic therapy, vocational rehabilitation)
- Personal reflections (e.g., writing, singing, meditation, artwork)

MATERIALS

The materials used in occupational therapy intervention include any materials used for self-care, work, education, leisure, and social participation. In the clinical setting, occupational therapists may use craft activities, computer-based cognitive activities, or simulators to ensure that clients are ready for the actual occupation. The occupational therapist must analyze the materials used and help the client be successful through adapting

the materials. Table 23-5 provides a description of some of the activities that may be used in practice.

Summary

Planning intervention involves determining occupational-based goals, adapting and grading activities, and being mindful of the impact the context has on the success of the activity. Intervention planning requires a clear evaluation of the clients' strengths and weaknesses and collaboration on occupational-based goals. The occupational therapy practitioner bases intervention on a well-developed FOR. The materials, activities, and techniques used vary with clients and goals. Practice and experience with reflection make the process of activity analysis creative and meaningful, which benefits clients.

Student Self-Assessment

1. Develop an activity. Decide on the age, client population, goals, and purpose of the activity. Describe how the activity can be adapted or modified to meet various clients' needs.

2. Examine an activity using Appendix D as your guide. Describe the contextual aspects of the activity, the client factors involved, and the performance habits required. Present the activity to the class as a teaching and learning experience.

3. Conduct an activity with classmates role playing different client issues. Discuss how to intervene and change the activity so that all are successful.

Case Example: Intervention Plan Using Model of Practice

Evidence exists to support the use of the Model of Human Occupation (Kielhofner, 2008) in practice (Forsyth, Mann, & Kielhofner, 2005; Keller & Forsyth, 2004; Lee, Taylor, Kielhofner, & Fisher, 2008). The Model of Human Occupation provides occupational therapy practitioners with a framework for viewing occupational performance. The following case example provides an overview of how one might use this model for intervention planning.

Mabel is a 75-year-old woman who experiences health issues of diabetes, heart disease, and arthritis. Recently, Mabel fell and fractured her hip. Mabel has difficulty walking up the stairs and is unable to lift heavy objects. She has recently lost her husband and lives on her own in the country. Her daughter lives 1 hour away from her; she is concerned about her mother's ability to live on her own. The occupational therapy practitioner working in acute care received a referral to evaluate and treat Mabel.

- Volition: Mabel loves to cook. She enjoys watching soap operas and talking to family and friends. Mabel has two dogs. She used to love to do puzzles with her husband. She will not do puzzles now.

- Habituation: Mabel reported that recently she has no desire to watch television or talk to friends. Mabel stated she gets up "whenever," "sort of eats," and takes a shower. Mabel stated she spent her day "hanging out at home." She has a few friends who come to visit. Her daughter visits at least once a week.

- Performance: Mabel moved slowly and has made little contact with the therapist. She followed simple verbal directions and answered questions in complete sentences. Mabel had difficulty moving from her bed to the chair. She has a right hip fracture.

- Environment: Mabel lives in the country in a cold climate. She has a few friends nearby who visit her weekly. Her daughter also visits her weekly. Mabel lives in a two-storey house. She does not drive, and there is no bus available.

- Intervention plan: The occupational therapy practitioner considers Mabel's volition, habituation, performance, and environment when selecting activities and designing the intervention plan. The practitioner decides (with Mabel's input) that they will work to help her revisit her joy of cooking. Because the practitioner is working in an acute care setting, the goal of the intervention is to provide Mabel with right hip precautions for healing. Thus, the practitioner is able to determine if Mabel is capable of safely living at home while evaluating her kitchen skills. Furthermore, the practitioner considers Mabel's environment and works with the physical therapist to be sure that Mabel is mobile in her home. Because winter is approaching, the practitioner meets with the daughter and Mabel to develop strategies for home safety concerning snow shoveling and emergency preparedness in case of power outages. Intervention also includes goals to improve Mabel's habits and routines so that she can reengage in occupations such as cooking, visiting with friends, watching television, and doing puzzles.

Case Sample: Intervention Plan Using Frame of Reference

The developmental FOR (Llorens, 1976) is frequently used to facilitate learning and development in children. This FOR relies on identifying the child's level of ability and providing activity to promote the next step. Thus, a developmental approach uses practice in a variety of activities. The central principle underlying the developmental approach is that through practice, improved neural synapses occur, resulting in improved performance and improved motor patterns. The following example illustrates the use of the developmental FOR to structure intervention.

Trevor is a 2-year-old boy diagnosed with global developmental delays. Trevor lives at home with his mother, father, and 4-year-old brother in the city. The occupational therapy practitioner begins intervention planning by conducting a developmental assessment to determine the level at which Trevor is functioning in terms of feeding, dressing, bathing, and play. After completing the Hawaii Early Learning Profile (HELP), a developmental checklist, the practitioner determines a level of functioning for Trevor for gross motor, fine motor, social participation, feeding, dressing, and play. After age levels for these systems are established, the practitioner is able to design intervention to address the next logical step in development. For example, Trevor will pick up a variety of foods and feed himself (9-to 12-month skill), but he will not bring a spoon to his mouth (12- to 15-month skill) or hold a cup handle (12- to 15.5-month skill). The practitioner works on a variety of developmental skills through play each session and provides parents with a home program to reinforce the concepts. This approach relies on practice to teach the child.

4. Cultural considerations. Interview a person from a culture different from your own. Discuss occupations of importance to them and the activities involved. Present the activity to the class, discussing the importance of this to the culture. Provide directions for each class member.

5. Compile a notebook of activities that you may use in clinical settings. Include Web site references and handouts that may be helpful. Organize the activities so that you can readily find an appropriate one for a client.

6. Examine an occupation prevalent in your area (e.g., lobsterman, basket weaver). What are the skills, client factors, habits, and contextual aspects of this activity? How could you adapt or grade the activity?

7. Find a local resource that may help a client (e.g., recreational center, therapeutic horseback riding center). Find out the cost, benefits, times, and services provided. Share these with your classmates.

References

American Occupational Therapy Association. (1990). Entry-level role delineation for registered occupational therapists (OTRs) and certified occupational therapy assistants (COTAs). *American Journal of Occupational Therapy, 44*(12), 1091-1102.

American Occupational Therapy Association. (1994). Guide for supervision of occupational therapy personnel. *American Journal of Occupation Therapy, 48*(11), 1045-1046.

American Occupational Therapy Association. (2008). Occupational therapy practice framework: Domain and process (2nd ed.). *American Journal of Occupational Therapy, 62,* 625-683.

Ayres, A. J. (1979). *Sensory integration and the child.* Los Angeles, CA: Western Psychological Services.

Black, R. M., & Wells, S. A. (2007). *Culture and occupation: A model of empowerment in occupational therapy.* Baltimore, MD: AOTA Press.

Bobath, B. (1975). Sensorimotor development. *NDT Newsletter, 7,* 1.

Christiansen, C., & Baum, C. M. (1997). Person-environment occupational performance: A conceptual model for practice. In C. Christiansen & C Baum (Eds.), *Occupational therapy: Enabling function & wellbeing* (2nd ed.). Thorofare, NJ: SLACK Incorporated.

Fisher, A. G. (1998). Uniting practice and theory in an occupational framework. 1998 Eleanor Clarke Slagle lecture. *American Journal of Occupational Therapy, 52*(7), 509-521.

Forsyth, K., Mann, L. S., & Kielhofner, G. (2005). Scholarship of practice: Making occupation-focused, theory-driven, evidence-based practice a reality. *British Journal of Occupational Therapy, 68*(6), 260-268.

Howle, J. (2005). Neuro-developmental treatment approach: Theoretical foundations and principles of clinical practice. In J. Case-Smith (Ed.), *Occupational therapy for children* (5th ed., p. 296). St. Louis, MO: Mosby.

Keller, J., & Forsyth, K. (2004). The model of human occupation in practice. *Israel Journal of Occupational Therapy, 13*(3), E99-E106.

Kielhofner, G. (1985). *A model of human occupation: Theory and application* (2nd ed.). Philadelphia, PA: Lippincott Williams & Wilkins.

Kielhofner, G. (2002). Dimensions of doing. In G. Kielhofner (Ed.), *A model of human occupation: Theory and application* (3rd ed.). Philadelphia, PA: Lippincott Williams & Wilkins.

Kielhofner, G. (2005). Rethinking disability and what to do about it: Disability studies and its implications for occupational therapy. *American Journal of Occupational Therapy, 59*(5), 487-496.

Kielhofner, G. (2008). *A model of human occupation: Theory and application* (4th ed.). Baltimore, MD: Lippincott Williams & Wilkins.

Law, M., Cooper, B. A., Strong, S., Stewart, D., Rigby, P., & Letts, L. (1996). The person-environment-occupation model: A transactive approach to occupational performance. *Canadian Journal of Occupational Therapy, 63*(1), 9-23.

Lee, S. W., Taylor, R., Kielhofner, G., & Fisher, G. (2008). Theory use in practice: A national survey of therapists who use the Model of Human Occupation. *American Journal of Occupational Therapy, 62*(1), 106-117.

Llorens, L. A. (1976). Application of a developmental theory for health and rehabilitation. Rockville, MD: AOTA Press.

MacRae, N. (2001). *Unpublished lecture notes: OT 301 foundations of occupational therapy.* Biddeford, ME: University of New England.

Maurer, T., Smith, D., & Armetta, C. (1989). Purposeful activity as exercise. *Occupational Therapy in Mental Health, 9,* 9-20.

McColl, M. A. (2005). Disability studies at the population level: Issues of health service utilization. *American Journal of Occupational Therapy, 59*(5), 516-526.

Melchert-McKearnan, K., Dietz, J., Engel, J. M., & White, O. (2000). Children with burn injuries: Purposeful activity versus rote exercise. *American Journal of Occupational Therapy, 54*(4), 381-390.

Mosey, A. C. (1981). *Occupational therapy: Configuration of a profession.* New York, NY: Raven Press.

Neistadt, M., & Crepeau, E. B. (1998). *Willard & Spackman's occupational therapy* (9th ed.). Philadelphia, PA: Lippincott Williams & Wilkins.

Neville-Jan, A. (2005). The problem with prevention: The case of spina bifida. *American Journal of Occupational Therapy, 59*(5), 527-539.

Nichols, D. (2005). Development of postural control. In J. Case-Smith. *Occupational therapy for children* (5th ed.). St. Louis, MO: Mosby.

Pedretti, L. W., & Paszuinielli, S. (1990). A frame of reference for occupational therapy in physical dysfunction. In L. W. Pedretti & B. Zoltan (Eds.), *Occupational therapy: Practice skills for physical dysfunction* (3rd ed., pp. 1-17) St. Louis, MO: Mosby.

Schkade, J. K., & Schultz, S. (1992). Occupational adaptation: Toward a holistic approach in contemporary practice, Part I. *American Journal of Occupational Therapy, 46*(9), 829-837.

Schoen, S., & Anderson, J. (1993). Neurodevelopmental treatment frame of reference. In P. Kramer & J. Hinojosa (Eds.), *Frames of reference for pediatric occupational therapy.* Baltimore, MD: Lippincott Williams & Wilkins.

Schoen, S., & Anderson, J. (1999). Neurodevelopmental treatment frame of reference. In P. Kramer & J. Hinojosa (Eds.), *Frames of reference for pediatric occupational therapy* (2nd ed.). Philadelphia, PA: Lippincott Williams & Wilkins.

Shumway-Cook, A., & Woollacott, M. (2007). *Motor control: Theory and practical applications.* Philadelphia, PA: Lippincott Williams & Wilkins.

Solomon, J. W., & O'Brien, J. C. (2006). Scope of practice. In J. W. Solomon & J. C. O'Brien (Eds.), *Pediatric skills for occupational therapy assistants* (2nd ed.). St. Louis, MO: Mosby.

Steinbeck, T. M. (1986). Purposeful activity and performance. *American Journal of Occupational Therapy, 40*(8), 529-534.

Taylor, R. R. (2005). Can the social model explain all of disability experience? Perspectives of persons with chronic fatigue syndrome. *American Journal of Occupational Therapy, 59*(5), 497-506.

Thibodaux, L. R. (2005). Habitus and the embodiment of disability through lifestyle. *American Journal of Occupational Therapy, 59*(5), 507-515.

Townsend, E., Brintnell, S., & Staisey, N. (1990). Developing guidelines for client-centered occupational therapy practice. *Canadian Journal of Occupational Therapy, 57*(2), 69-76.

Trombly, C. A. (1994). Rood approach. In C. Trombly (Ed.), *Occupational therapy for physical dysfunction* (4th ed.). Baltimore, MD: Williams & Wilkins.

World Health Organization. (2001). *International classification of functioning, disability and health* (ICF). Geneva, Switzerland: Author.

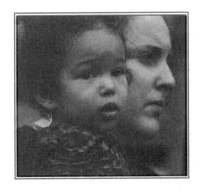

24

CLIENT FACTORS IN OCCUPATIONAL PERFORMANCE FUNCTIONING

Regula H. Robnett, PhD, OTR/L and Tara Kaminski, MSOT Student

---

ACOTE STANDARDS EXPLORED IN THIS CHAPTER
B.5.6

KEY VOCABULARY

- **Anosmia:** Lack of sense of smell.
- **Decubitus ulcers:** Pressure sores due to excessive pressure on or shearing of the skin.
- **Errorless learning:** Learning a skill without making mistakes in performance during the learning process.
- **Executive skills:** Complex cognitive skills (e.g., weighing options, problem solving, multi-task planning, and self-monitoring).
- **Ideational apraxia:** Loss of skilled movement patterns that make up task performance, based on the loss of the conceptual idea of performing the task (not on sensorimotor dysfunction).

- **Ideomotor apraxia:** Loss of skilled movement patterns that make up task performance, based on "the loss of access to kinesthetic memory patterns" (Gillen, 2009, p. 112).
- **Isometric contractions:** Muscle contraction during which the muscle maintains a constant muscle length.
- **Isotonic contractions:** Muscle contraction during which the muscle belly shortens while activated.
- **Kinesthesia:** Perception of the direction and movement of one's body and limbs in space.
- **Proprioception:** Perception of a joint's position in space.
- **Task-specific training:** Direct training in tasks without the expectation of generalization of learning.

Jacobs, K., MacRae, N., & Sladyk, K. (Eds.).
Occupational Therapy Essentials for
Clinical Competence, Second Edition (pp. 309-331).
© 2014 SLACK Incorporated.

Introduction

Occupational therapy practitioners work with people who have a variety of impairments. While these impairments are rarely seen in isolation, this chapter divides some of the major categories of impairments into separate sections to more clearly and succinctly explain each one at a fundamental level. However, in occupational therapy intervention, combinations of techniques are usually used simultaneously to promote occupational functioning. This chapter presents an overview of occupational therapy interventions focused on providing development, remediation, and/or compensatory measures to promote optimal performance in the realms of physical (including neuromuscular), cognitive (including mental and perceptual), and behavioral skills. Sensory functions (e.g., vision, tactile, auditory, gustatory, olfactory, pain, temperature, pressure, vestibular, proprioception) are also considered. Each section provides a definition and overview of the specific aspect and reviews some of the more common occupational therapy interventions currently in use. Brief overviews of evidence-based practice are included whenever possible.

Certified Occupational Therapy Assistants

Throughout this chapter, clinicians involved in the intervention process are referred to as *occupational therapy practitioners*. This is done intentionally because the Accreditation Council for Occupational Therapy Education (ACOTE) standard on which this chapter is based is exactly the same for both the registered occupational therapist and the certified occupational therapy assistant. Both professionals carry out interventions using clinical reasoning, evidence-based practice (to the extent available), and occupational therapy principles. However, the title *occupational therapist* is used when referring to the practitioner with a professional role as an evaluator.

Intervention Within the Occupational Therapy Practice Framework

The occupational therapy process, as described in the American Occupational Therapy Association (AOTA) Practice Framework (AOTA, 2008), involves intervention planning, implementation, and follow-up. Although intervention is the core of the occupational therapy process, to be intentionally effective, the intervention phase needs to be based on a comprehensive occupational therapy evaluation appropriate for the setting and the client.

The process of intervention planning should incorporate solid theoretical underpinnings and relevant practice-based research to the extent available. The process, which involves the practitioner working with one or more clients, includes the following types of interventions: creating or promoting, establishing or restoring, maintaining, modifying or preventing, establishing, remediating or developing, and compensating. The ultimate goal of occupational therapy intervention is "engagement in occupation" or successful participation in those areas of occupation that have personal meaning for the client. Intervention techniques can follow a more functional, real-life "top-down" approach (Trombly, 1993), which includes engagement in occupational tasks as primary aspects of each intervention session, or a "bottom-up" approach, in which therapeutic sessions focus more on the underlying client performance skills or factors (with the intention of transferring these skills to broader occupations outside of the session). Performance skills include motor skills and process skills, whereas client factors include mental functions, sensory functions, neuromuscular and movement-related functions, and bodily functions (AOTA, 2008).

The framework (AOTA, 2008, p. 640) outlines aspects of performance skills to include motor and praxis, sensory perceptual, emotional regulation, and cognitive skills. Each of these skill areas involves actions and behaviors of the client that promote occupational performance. For example, praxis involves planned and sequential motor acts (of any body part that moves) to carry out the motoric aspects of an occupational task. These performance skills are as varied as our personal occupations and are imbedded in all areas of occupation. This chapter includes performance skill areas, but we use the language of the ACOTE standard.

Intervention Related to Physical Performance

Physical performance generally relies on the supervisory control exerted by the brain. Intact neurological connections within the brain plan and send efferent messages distally to execute the movement in question. The brain provides the control center for motor performance, but the person also needs intact musculature in order to complete movement and manipulation tasks. The aspects of physical performance of primary concern in occupational therapy intervention at the impairment level are range of motion (ROM), strength, balance, coordination, and functional mobility. Completing occupational tasks successfully requires at least minimal levels of ability in these client factors, or the use of adaptations or compensatory measures. The occupational therapist can complete an in-depth activity analysis to determine the specific physical demands of any task under consideration. Ideally, based on the results of the analysis, the practitioner can then determine how to assist the person by adapting the task or the environment, if the task currently exceeds the client's capabilities. The physical factors described are applicable for all age groups, but not all people need to be equally capable in all areas to be successful and to feel fulfilled occupationally. For example, lumberjacks need to have excellent strength and gross motor coordination in order to be successful at their chosen profession. On the other hand, a computer programmer is likely to need less upper body ROM and strength, though intact fine motor coordination is a prerequisite for using a computer the way it is intended to be used. Fortunately, technology has advanced to the point that much of the programmer's job can be done without the stated prerequisites, if necessary (e.g., through voice activation or head pointing devices).

With regard to the physical aspects of the client, an evaluation is followed by mutual goal setting. Occupational therapy intervention then takes place to move the client toward the agreed-upon meaningful occupational goals. The process may involve remediation to improve physical performance in one or more physical realms for the purpose of improving occupational performance (e.g., not to just improve movement), compensation (also for improved occupational outcomes), or a combination of both, always depending on the needs of the client. A crucial element of any intervention plan also involves client and/or family education related to safe and effective occupational performance. Although this section focuses on the physical aspects of intervention, it should be noted that simple physical outcome goals such as improved strength, ROM, and balance are never sufficient; occupational therapy must always include functional aspects of goals following on the heels of improved physical performance. For example, in occupational therapy, a client may work on improving ROM, but the ultimate goal is improved ability in the activity of daily living (ADL) or home management skills.

Occupational therapy sessions often involve providing physically based interventions both in individual and group settings. These interventions may be component- or client factor–based, such as an upper-extremity exercise group, balance training, or motor control practice. These would be considered bottom-up sessions. On the other hand, intervention sessions may use either purposeful activities (such as practicing important tasks) or be occupation based, which involves direct engagement in personally meaningful daily tasks (AOTA, 2008). The preferred method is to strive toward occupation, since that is the crux of meaning for our profession. However, since the areas of occupation that include physical aspects are covered in other chapters, relevant intervention at the physical client-factor level is addressed briefly.

Biomechanical Frame of Reference

As discussed in more detail in other chapters, frames of reference help occupational therapists guide the way that they structure intervention plans. The biomechanical frame of reference is a bottom-up approach to therapy that works well under many different models of practice. The principles that compose the frame of reference, as explained by Cole and Tufano (2008), include ROM, strength, endurance, kinematics, and torque. This frame of reference requires therapists to look at the underlying musculoskeletal structures when creating the intervention plan for a client. Although this may be a useful tool when trying to understand the biomechanics of a movement, it is a somewhat limited frame of reference in that it does not include the more holistic psychosocial aspects of human motor performance.

RANGE OF MOTION AND STRENGTH

As part of a therapeutic evaluation, the occupational therapist needs to at least screen for dysfunction in the realms of ROM and strength. The human body has over 430 voluntary muscles that move all moveable body parts. For the extremities to be considered "normal," that is, within normal limits (WNL), people need to be able to move their limbs through full ROM and be able to withstand the application of a maximal amount of resistance during manual muscle testing. Before being able to lift additional weight beyond the weight of the limb or before being able to resist outside pressure, the limb must be able to move through full ROM (unless ROM is compromised by a joint obstruction). As learned through the study of kinesiology, every joint in the human body has a normal or usual ROM. If the joint is compromised in some way through injury, disease, or disuse, then performance on life tasks could be impacted, and ROM needs to be addressed as a part of therapeutic intervention. Depending on the cause of the decrease, it may be appropriate to attempt to improve joint mobility through ROM exercises, joint mobilization, and stretching.

When exercises are used in occupational therapy, the use of active ROM is preferred to passive ROM whenever possible. If the client is incapacitated (for example, if the client is in a coma), active ROM on command is not an option. Those who cannot move limbs on one side of the body (as in hemiparesis secondary to acquired brain injury) may be able to learn to complete a self-ROM program, giving them a degree of control over their movement patterns. Engaging the client in a ROM program (either through exercise or functional activity) is necessary to avoid contractures of the joints caused by immobilization, as well as to provide the person with some degree of normal proprioceptive input, which may enhance personal awareness of the body and the environment.

When ROM is compromised, strength is generally impaired as well. After a client has obtained the maximum ROM for a joint, strength training usually begins. Strength is the "degree of muscle power when movement is resisted as with objects or gravity" (Stedman's, 1997, p. 832) and "is the result of complex interactions of neurologic, biomechanical, and cognitive systems" (Hall & Brody, 2005, p. 58). As with ROM, strength can be compromised with the onset of injury, disease, or disuse. Examples include, but are not limited to, spinal cord injury, acquired brain injury, a physical injury to a muscle or joint, or a sedentary lifestyle. Compromised ROM and strength can impact functioning in every area of occupation. Therefore, physical performance involving ROM and building strength is an important aspect of intervention for many clients.

To increase the strength of a muscle, it needs to contract repeatedly at near maximal capacity. Muscle strengthening involves the utilization of different types of contractions. An isotonic contraction occurs when a muscle shortens in length "against a constant load," such as when a weight is lifted against gravity (Stedman's, 1997, p. 457). An isometric contraction, in comparison, involves holding a muscle contraction at an increased tension point in the muscle. During this type of contraction, the muscle is not shortening while contracting, but rather staying the same length for the duration of the tightening. Exercise groups or individual exercise sessions in occupational therapy often use repeated isotonic contractions with weights and resistance bands. Isometric contractions are used when the limb is immobile, but resisting either an immovable or potentially movable force (e.g., the former may be a wall, while the latter may be a challenging opponent, as in sports). While muscles do need to fatigue to gain strength, over-fatiguing muscles can be more damaging than beneficial. Soreness can result after one engages in an exercise program, but significant pain should not. Throughout the therapy session, pain should be periodically monitored because it can affect the client's recovery as well as the client's quality of movement. The therapist must communicate with the client to ensure that pain is not interfering with overall performance. Pain is considered as an aspect of intervention in a separate section in this chapter.

Making a direct connection between the client's interests, hobbies, or daily activities and the exercise program has shown better adherence rates compared to rote exercise alone. This contention is supported by research such as the Nelson et al. study (1999), which found that the group involved in an occupationally based exercise program significantly outperformed a rote exercise group in a randomized control trial of 26 clients post-stroke. In an interesting aside to usual exercise training, one study compared an exercise program including a virtual reality bicycle exercise tour with a control program just involving the physical exercises. Grealy, Johnson, and Rushton (1999) found that the addition of virtual reality exercise was associated not only with more significantly improved strength but also with enhanced reaction times and cognitive performance. This finding highlights, once again, the interconnectedness of the physical and the cognitive client factors. Strength training has been shown to decrease heart rate, normalize blood pressure, increase cardiac output, and it may lower bad cholesterol levels (Hall & Brody, 2005). Proper diaphragmatic breathing techniques should be incorporated into all strength and ROM exercise programs. Not breathing deeply enough or holding one's breath during exertion can be dangerous, especially for those with compromised cardiac systems (such as when one engages in the Valsalva maneuver).

Resistance training for healthy adults is recommended by the American Heart Association, the American College of Sports Medicine, and the Surgeon General's 1996 report (as cited in Feigenbaum, 2001). The exercise program should be rhythmical, performed at a slow-to-moderate rate of speed, completed at minimum level 2 or 3 days per week, and include 8 to 10 exercises with 1 to 2 sets of 8 to 15 repetitions. The Physical Activity Guidelines (Department of Health and Human Services, 2008) recommend 1 hour of aerobic physical activity each day for those who are 6 to 17 years old and a half-hour daily (or 150 minutes per week minimum) for those who are 18 to 64. Although discomfort can be acceptable as tolerated, a high level of pain should be avoided, especially if any movement used causes the level of pain to escalate. Any exercise program should be geared to the individual (e.g., physical and health status, personal goals) and can be beneficial even if the recommended parameters for repetitions and frequency cannot be met (Garber et al., 2011).

The sources mentioned previously also recommend strength training for populations who have physical impairments. However, the program would be expected to start at a lower intensity level and the progression would be expected to be slower. Feigenbaum (2001) recommended a slow and temperate start in order to avoid an overambitious beginning with a subsequent higher dropout rate. Progression to more resistance should occur every week or two if possible, when the person can lift the current weight comfortably a dozen times but still perceives the intensity to be difficult. These guidelines apply to all adult age groups. Sedentary older people, however, may need to start with weights of 1 kilo or even less, take more care in stabilizing at the hip, and may do better on machines not requiring the exerciser to have normal postural control (Feigenbaum, 2001). Few guidelines for specific client populations are available, highlighting the need for further empirical research. Interesting, creative, and occupationally based research projects could involve comparing rote ROM and strength training to the use of repetitive functional tasks such as leisure sports, hobbies, or home management skills.

ENDURANCE

Endurance as a physical component of occupational therapy intervention is included here only as an adjunct to the other physical aspects of intervention. Decreased endurance manifests itself as an inability to carry through repetitive motions or sustained resistance over time. It results in a decreased ability to complete daily tasks because the person lacks energy. Clients are not likely to be referred to occupational therapy intervention for impaired endurance alone. However, decreased strength is often coupled with lowered endurance. Each contraction of a weakened muscle uses a larger proportion of the overall performance capacity, resulting in the muscle fatiguing more quickly. When aiming to build muscle strength, a high-load regimen with a lower number of repetitions is preferred, but when the focus is on building endurance, a lower amount of resistance or weight over a greater number of repetitions has been determined to be more effective (Breines, 2006).

BALANCE/POSTURAL CONTROL

Intact balance or postural control is a prerequisite for safe, ambulatory, functional mobility. Since many of our daily occupations involve ambulating or moving from one place to another, postural control is an important consideration for the occupational therapy practitioner. This is especially true for practitioners working with those who have sustained acquired brain injuries or who have diagnoses associated with impaired balance such as multiple sclerosis or cerebral palsy. According to Peterson and Clemson (2008), occupational therapy practitioners are well suited to working with elders on fall prevention and rehabilitation due to our in-depth understanding of physical functioning and the contextual and intrinsic factors impacting balance, as well as our ability to implement multifactorial, evidence-based interventions. Falls are common among the elderly, with about 1 out of 3 community-living elders falling annually (Gillespie et al., 2003). One direct cause of falls is decreased postural control. Balance training can occur in groups, on an individual basis by providing balance exercises and education, or through occupational therapy–related interventions such as virtual reality or Tai Chi courses. In their systematic review, Gillespie et al. (2003) determined that fall prevention interventions are often effective. A number of studies have now been completed on Tai Chi as an intervention to improve balance and strength with overall positive results (e.g., Han et al., 2004; Li et al., 2005; Taylor-Piliae, Haskell, Stotts, & Froehlicher, 2006). Hsieh, Nelson, Smith, and Peterson (1996), in an occupation-based study, found that small groups of stroke survivors who participated in real or simulated functional activities in addition to rote exercise had better outcomes related to dynamic standing balance. In two recent studies, both mental practice (Hosseini, Fallahpour, Sayadi, Gharib, & Haghgoo, 2012) and virtual reality balance training (Cho, Lee, & Song, 2012) were shown to improve dynamic balance in older adults post-stroke. A more general community-based course intended to improve balance is called "Stepping On," a 7-week program offered to people 70 years of age and older in Australia. Clemson et al. (2004) reported that the "Stepping On" program resulted in a 31% reduction in falls ($P=0.025$), and that the program was particularly effective for men. A "Matter of Balance," designed by rehabilitation scientists at Boston University, is a similar 8-week program that uses volunteer instructors with occupational therapy and physical therapy consultants or visiting instructors. In their 2009 replication report, the Partnership for Healthy Aging reported that overall participants of the "Matter of Balance" program tended to demonstrate increased efficacy in the realm of balance, improved strength, improved ability to manage stairs, and increased exercise levels.

In a systematic review of 19 randomized control trials of interventions to decrease fear of falling, Zijlstra et al. (2007) found overwhelming support for the effectiveness of interventions (including Tai Chi, "Matter of Balance," "Stepping On," and other multifactorial balance programs). Along with a decreased fear of falling, Zijlstra and colleagues also recommended looking at functional outcomes for balance programs (e.g., decreased incidence of falling and increased safe engagement in meaningful activities). Besides remediating balance through the interventions mentioned, occupational therapy practitioners play a significant role in ensuring safety by helping the client to compensate when balance is impaired. Compensatory safety measures can involve removing clutter from the home and improving organization in the living space. Adaptive equipment such as safety bars, bath seats, and long-handled dustpans can facilitate successful occupational performance in the client's customary daily tasks. Education on fall prevention is a crucial component of occupational therapy in this realm as well. For example, if older people understand the factors impacting balance and the ways to make the environment safer, they are more likely to feel a higher degree of efficacy related to balance and to complete mobility tasks with more awareness of proper body mechanics.

Intervention Related to Neuromuscular Disorders

Neuromuscular disorders are a combination of cognitive and physical impairments, often with accompanying sensory dysfunction. This discussion will focus on motor control, which encompasses coordination and movement in general. According to Shumway-Cook and Woollacott (2007), motor control is "the ability to regulate or direct the mechanisms essential to movement" (p. 4). Movement is the result of neuromuscular interactions involving sensory input to the brain. The central nervous system (CNS) organizes and interprets this input and then directs subsequent physical actions. When functioning at an adequate level, motor control allows the person to complete essential and optional daily tasks. Intact perceptual and cognitive processes are necessary to carry through purposeful and efficient movement. For example, tossing and catching a ball, feeding oneself, and writing numbers and letters all represent skills that require a high degree of coordination or motor control. The reader should be aware that there are several theories of motor control (reflex, hierarchical, systems, dynamic action, and ecological) and that entire textbooks have been written about this subject. Shumway-Cook and Woollacott (2007) provide a comprehensive resource for those seeking more detail.

MOTOR CONTROL

Motor control is the term used to explain how the different body systems interact in order to perform skilled motor movement. Through practice or experience, motor control can be improved. Motor learning has occurred when practice or experience has made a change in the performance of a motor movement (Tse & Spaulding, 1998). Although motor control covers the entire lifespan, the focus for occupational therapy practitioners using motor control models of intervention is on initial motor learning in the young and in relearning movement patterns in adults, specifically those with a diagnosis or condition that impairs normal movement.

Cerebral palsy and developmental coordination disorder are two common diagnoses causing movement impairments in children, whereas acquired brain injuries, multiple sclerosis, and Parkinson's disease are common diagnoses interfering with normal movement in adults. The ultimate goal of the intervention is to improve occupational performance through the use of the most effective movement patterns possible. While evidence-based practice exists within this realm, it is lacking in its scope. Much has been written in occupational therapy and physical therapy literature about different aspects of motor control intervention, including assessment of motor control, types of learning, types of practice, practice schedules, instructions, and the parameters surrounding feedback. In guiding intervention, O'Brien and Savoyski (2006) contend that optimal motor learning is best achieved through occupational therapy intervention that is both individualized and allows for active experimentation, as well as being occupation based in the client's natural environment.

Research conducted on motor control and motor learning focuses on the different intervention strategies that occupational therapists can utilize in order to increase motor control. More occupation-based research projects in this intervention area, as well in other intervention areas, need to be undertaken. In the following studies, the Functional Independence Measure (FIM) was used as an outcome measure to show the gains in motor control in stroke survivors' hemiparetic limbs with the use of constraint-induced movement therapy. Lin, Wu, Wei, Lee, and Liu (2007) used modified constraint-induced movement therapy with their clients at an average of 6.2 hours per day, hypothesizing that it would increase motor control of the hemiparetic limb. The results from the randomized controlled study showed that clients in the experimental group had increased motor control with reach-to-grasp movements and better performance of daily activities compared to those treated with traditional approaches. A study conducted by Wu, Lin, Chen, Chen, and Hong (2007), focused on unilateral and bilateral upper-extremity functional tasks also to evaluate the effects of modified constraint-induced movement therapy. The results from this study showed more specifically that the clients treated with modified constraint-induced movement therapy had better bimanual motor control following intervention when compared to those treated with traditional approaches. They also found that unilateral movement improved, but the results were not as significant as the bimanual motor control improvements.

A few research-based articles specifically address the effectiveness of techniques designed to promote the development or relearning of motor skills. They generally compare one type of motor control intervention to another. The following research projects are worth noting, especially for those wishing to expand their knowledge in this realm. DeGangi, Wietlisbach, Goodin, and Scheiner (1993) compared two methods of motor control intervention in 12 preschoolers with sensorimotor deficits and found no order effect of the structured sensorimotor versus child-centered approaches, with all of the children in the project gaining in motor skills. The structured sensorimotor approach promoted gross motor skills better, while the child-centered approach promoted the more rapid development of fine motor coordination. Miyahara and Wafer (2004) also found general support for the motor control approaches of a skill theme program and a movement concepts program in a group of 7 children with developmental coordination disorder, with the former focusing more on targeted skills training and the latter focusing more on self-esteem building and creativity. Similarly, Thorpe and Valvano (2002) examined three different practice protocols in a group of 13 children with cerebral palsy. They found that the majority of children improved no matter what strategy was used. However, they did conclude that some children especially benefited from using cognitive strategies to augment practice in motor tasks. In a physiotherapy review that focused on intervention of postural control for those who had sustained a stroke, Pollock, Baer, Pomeroy, and Langhorne (2007) compared orthopedic, neurophysiologic, and motor learning approaches. They determined that one approach was not significantly more effective than the others for improving balance. Since occupational therapy practitioners also work in the realm of postural control, this finding, imprecise as it is, still has meaning for the profession and highlights—once again—the need for more occupation-based research projects in this intervention area and beyond.

INTERVENTION INVOLVING FUNCTIONAL ACTIVITIES

While specific types of motor control intervention approaches may not be overwhelmingly better than others based on the research available thus far, a few studies did come to a conclusion that greatly impacts the practice of occupational therapy. In her study, Neistadt (1994) demonstrated that the 45 adult males with brain injuries performed significantly better in fine motor coordination tasks when the intervention involved functional activities, such as meal preparation, as compared to when the intervention involved the contrived remedial task of parquetry puzzle construction. In quite a different study with yet a similar outcome, Wu, Trombly, Lin, and Tickle-Degnen (2000) found that using real-life objects elicited better kinematic reaching performance than having the person simulate reaching for objects without the objects being present. To occupational therapy practitioners, the conclusion that occupation-based rather than contrived intervention activity promotes better functioning is self-evident. Yet the need for additional empirical research to substantiate this claim using various daily living tasks that involve motor control remains paramount.

Intervention Related to Sensory Dysfunction

Occupational therapy intervention in the realm of sensory dysfunction is often compensatory and concerns primarily the sensory system of vision, since the majority of sensory input to the brain comes through this modality for those with normally functioning visual systems. Other sensory systems can sometimes be the focus of occupational therapy intervention, and these will be considered first. In general terms, sensory functioning is considered as it impacts safe and successful occupational performance.

SMELL AND TASTE

Olfaction and gustation are closely related sensory systems. Olfaction has the distinct characteristic of being the only sensory system that does not digress through the thalamus before progressing to the specific sensory processing area in the cortex. Because of the direct linkage of the sense of smell to sensory processing, using scents might be most effective in eliciting a response when stimulating a person in a coma. Olfaction can be impacted by disease processes such as sinus infections and acquired brain injuries. It tends to be significantly impacted by the aging process, often without awareness of its decline. Gaines (2010) reported that olfaction decreases significantly with age, with over 50% of older people (65 and over) having an impaired sense of smell. There is also a discrepancy between reported decreased sense of smell and empirically based assessments. For example, Nordin, Monsch, and Murphy (1995) found that while the majority of their older subjects had a decreased sense of olfaction, most of these respondents nonetheless reported that their sense of smell was intact. The insidious nature of decline in olfaction sense necessitates that the occupational therapist include the impact of this potential loss in evaluation and intervention, especially for older people. Problems secondary to anosmia (or the loss of smell sensation) beyond being disconcerting or annoying (e.g., not being able to notice if one is wearing too much perfume) can also impact safety for independent living. Someone with a normal sense of smell can readily detect spoiled food in the refrigerator, burning food in the oven, or a natural gas leak. Utility companies may have "scratch and sniff" cards available for easy detection of olfaction sensory loss. Occupational therapy intervention following smell loss can involve labeling food in the refrigerator with dates and teaching the client and family about the need for additional caution during cooking tasks. Being unaware of this deficit or being unable to learn compensatory techniques would require the client to be monitored regularly.

Since the sense of smell is a backdrop for the sense of taste, similar issues arise with decreased gustation. Heckmann et al. (2005) reported that taste dysfunction following stroke is common. Gustatory sense losses were exhibited by 30% of their 102 clients, while others had distortions in their sense of taste. The impairment may be caused by acquired brain injuries, medications, or the aging process. People with decreased gustatory sense may have difficulty following a healthy diet. In addition to perhaps ingesting spoiled food, they may eat foods that are too salty and consume too many sweets. As people age, their sense of salty and bitter naturally decreases, while sensation for sweet and sour is maintained (Hayflick, 1994). Besides making sure that a client can either prepare or attain proper meals, a dietary consultation might be in order.

Tactile, Pain, Temperature, Pressure, Proprioception, and Kinesthesia

The somatosensory system manages incoming sensation that is superficial (e.g., touch, pressure, and sharp/dull pain sensation). Proprioception is the awareness of a joint's position in space (Cooper & Canyock, 2013) while kinesthesia is "the ability to perceive extent, direction, and weight of movement" of the appendage in space (Tabor's, 2001, p. 1178). People rarely give much conscious thought to the sensory systems of touch, proprioception, and kinesthesia unless there is a problem. Perhaps the most common condition impacting touch sensation is acquired brain injury, which often impacts sensory functioning on the contralateral (opposite) side of the body to where the lesion occurred. Diabetes is another common diagnosis impacting distal sensation. Diabetic peripheral neuropathy involves a decrease or loss of touch sensation, especially distally (lower extremities being impacted more than the upper extremities). Loss of sensation can result in significant safety concerns in nearly every daily task. Even if movement is normal, the person must take extra care in doing tasks to ensure that the limbs are maintained in safe positions and protected from excess pressure. Whereas sharp items could puncture the skin without the person being aware, sustained pressure brought about by not moving enough or by something pressing against the skin can also cause skin damage. In the worst case scenario, the sustained pressure can cause decubitus ulcers, which are very serious single- to multi-layered skin lesions that heal extremely slowly and only with the utmost of care. Skin breakdown can occur within hours of sustained pressure and may eventually penetrate to the level of bone. With proper initial positioning, frequent repositioning, and other protective measures, decubitus ulcers should never or only rarely occur. Compensatory measures for decreased touch sense and proprioception/kinesthesia include using one's sense of vision to carefully watch what one is doing, the removal of sharp items from the environment, and client and family education to ensure safety.

Since acquired brain injury and other conditions can lead to sensory losses or distortions, occupational therapy practitioners may be involved in retraining sensory discrimination if sensation is present but not accurate in the affected limb(s). Cooper and Canyock (2013) describe occupational therapy desensitization program parameters for those with hypersensitivity, and protective and discriminatory sensory re-education programs for those who have impairments in these realms. Protective sensation must be intact before undertaking discriminatory retraining. In a quasi-experimental research project using graded sensory discrimination tasks, sensory exploratory tasks without the use of vision, and specific feedback, Carey, Matyas, and Oke (1993) found long-term clinically significant improvements in the ability to distinguish sensory stimuli in a small group of stroke survivors in Australia.

Pain

Pain has many aspects, both physical and psychosocial. While physical pain, primarily due to unpleasant or hurtful touch sensations, is the aspect of pain primarily covered in this chapter, Engle (2011), in her chapter on "Pain Regulation," describes the multifaceted nature of pain, including assessment of and intervention for chronic pain management. Her comprehensive chapter provides the level of detail needed for the occupational therapy practitioner to address the global issue of pain management effectively and holistically.

The touch sense of pain is protective because it typically causes us to remove any impacted body part from the painful stimulus. This sense of touch is more likely to be lost due to brain injury, not simple aging. Occupational therapy practitioners need to include education when pain sense is absent, such as after a cerebrovascular accident, which might cause the contralateral side to be affected. Loss of pain sense could have dire consequences, for example, if the affected limb is neglected and gets damaged due to this neglect.

Pain can impact all aspects of life. As people age they are more likely to have one or more painful conditions such as arthritis, stroke, and heart disease. Effective movement patterns and concentration can be negatively impacted by pain. Szafron (2011) provides a concise overview of occupational therapy's role in the realm of pain control for older adults. She suggests using a biopsychosocial approach to pain management involving both traditional and complementary or alternative interventions. For example, occupational therapy practitioners may use breathing techniques, icing, and heat as preparatory methods; educate the client on work simplification, energy conservation, body mechanics, and the use of adaptive equipment; and engage the client in purposeful activities and occupations of interest while taking precautions to minimize pain. The occupational therapy practitioner can play an important role on a pain management team, helping those with chronic pain to "live life to the fullest."

Hearing

Although the sense of hearing is not an area for which occupational therapy practitioners are primarily responsible, the consideration of one's ability to hear is still a crucial element in promoting successful occupational performance. If one cannot hear, then compensatory measures need to be taken for safety. For example, using a vibrating alarm to alert one to wake up or a light to signal that the doorbell just rang could be ways to adapt the home environment. Hearing is a sensory modality that also decreases with age, thus impairments in this realm are encountered frequently in the field of rehabilitation.

An occupational therapy practitioner may be called upon to work with the client on the ADL of hearing aid care and insertion after the loss of these skills (i.e., due to disease or injury). When working with clients who have a decreased sense of hearing, optimal intervention depends on appropriate communication techniques. Therapeutic use of self includes an awareness of and ability to modify verbal interactions, such as speaking more clearly and deliberately, making face-to-face contact, lowering pitch, and eliminating background noise whenever possible. Ensuring the use and working order of assistive devices is necessary as well (Robnett, 2010).

Vision

Vision is often a focus of occupational therapy intervention either as a primary or secondary diagnosis. An estimated 1 of every 2 clients in a rehabilitation hospital has visual impairments that impact functioning, and an estimated 1 of every 4 children has visual impairments. Specialists in the field of vision, including rehabilitation teachers and orientation and mobility specialists, work on a full-time basis with those who have visual losses. While occupational therapy practitioners and physical therapists undertake similar jobs in these realms, respectively, the previously mentioned two types of professionals have much more specialized education and training exclusively in the field of vision. Occupational therapy practitioners are considered qualified providers of intervention for visual impairments under the Medicare system.

Vision is a complex sensory system involving many different pathways and components. Deficits can therefore be extremely varied. Warren (1993) describes the visual system as a hierarchy. The basic skills of visual acuity, oculomotor control, visual fields, and visual attention are foundational skills providing the backdrop for the more complex visual and perceptual skills such as scanning, pattern recognition, visual memory, and visuocognition. Interested readers are directed to two comprehensive occupational therapy textbooks on the topic of intervention for those with decreased vision: *Functional Visual Behavior in Adults, Second Edition* (Gentile, 2005) and *Vision, Perception, and Cognition, Fourth Edition* (Zoltan, 2007).

Occupational therapy intervention in the area of vision often involves starting with a functional visual assessment and following up with compensation for decreased visual skills. Occasionally, however, development or remediation of visual skills occurs in occupational therapy. For example, after an acquired brain injury, intervention may involve training and the use of functional tasks to promote better scanning and attention, especially to any quadrant or area of space that tends to get neglected.

Occupational therapy practitioners may sometimes work with behavioral optometrists in helping clients follow through with eye exercises for the purpose of restoring visual functioning in the realm of scanning, attention, and binocular visual skills. Occupational therapy practitioners may also be involved in teaching eccentric viewing, a special viewing technique for those who have macular degeneration. In addition, occupational therapy was shown to be effective, along with other disciplines, in assisting those with low vision to attain their functional goals, as demonstrated by the results of an experimental visual rehabilitation program for older adults in the mid-west (Pankow, Luchins, Studebaker, & Chettleburgh, 2004).

Visual skills tend to decrease as people age, already starting in the third decade of life. Common diagnoses more prevalent in older clients include age-related macular degeneration, glaucoma, diabetic retinopathy, cataracts, and visual losses secondary to stroke. Completing a functional visual assessment will aid the occupational therapist in determining how to structure the environment to promote optimal visual functioning. Besides corrective lenses (including making sure that they are worn when needed and that they are clean), some of the more common compensatory and adaptive measures include the following (Robnett, 2010):

- Increasing the size of the object to be viewed (e.g., printed material, images, signs).
- Using magnifying glasses or closed circuit television when using larger objects is not possible.
- Using protective lenses to reduce glare and shield out bright sunlight.
- Increasing the contrast of items to one another (e.g., plate and placement, black print on white paper, safety strips on the edges of stairs).
- Improving lighting (e.g., effective spot lighting for work area, nightlights, shielding glare from bright light bulbs).
- Avoiding tasks that can no longer be completed safely due to decreased vision (e.g., driving at night; use of sharp items).
- Making sure that the home environment is as safe as possible (e.g., well-organized, clutter-free, removal of loose rugs).

Intervention Related to Mental and Cognitive Skills

Human cognition includes all "mental activities associated with thinking, learning, and memory" (Stedman's, 1997, p. 174). All purposeful activity is regulated or supervised by one's brain. Therefore, the successful completion of mental activities is based on the foundation of adequate cognition. However, while intact task-specific cognitive functioning is essential, it is not singularly adequate for successful occupational performance. For example, even if a person has the cognitive skills to understand the motions and rules of a specific sport, the individual still may not have the physical performance capabilities to carry through these skilled motions in order to be a successful player. Cognitive dysfunction can occur due to genetics, developmental delays, trauma, or disease processes such as cerebral palsy, acquired brain injury, mental illness, or dementia at any age (Giles et al., 2013). The Occupational Therapy Practice Framework (AOTA, 2008, p. 635) divides mental functions into the specific mental functions of higher level cognitive, attention, memory, perception, and thought; mental functions related to sequencing complex movement, emotional regulation, and experience of self and time; and global cognitive functions of consciousness, orientation, temperament and personality, energy and drive, and the physiological process of sleep.

Occupational therapists need to evaluate cognition, or mental abilities, especially as these relate to their clients' daily functional performance. The complex interaction of cognitive capabilities and volition, general behavioral performance in occupational areas of concern, and the multifactorial contextual factors impacting performance need to be thoroughly investigated. Based on the assessment outcomes, joint client-centered goal setting is vital to ensure meaningful intervention, whether the ensuing therapy is intended to enhance or maintain performance, to provide education, and/or to offer/design compensatory and adaptive measures.

Occupational therapy services in the realm of cognition are often multimodal and fall into the following broad categories:

- Remediation (rehabilitation) or development (habilitation) of cognitive skills and training in specific tasks.
- Maintaining cognitive skills for those who are at risk of losing skills.
- Compensating for decreased cognitive skills.
- Providing education on cognitive performance in relation to safety, independent living, and/or life quality for the client and the family.

The AOTA Commission on Practice statement on Cognition, Cognitive Rehabilitation, and Occupational Performance (2013) lists several occupation-based cognitive theorists who have furthered the realm of cognitive rehabilitation, including Allen, Earhart, and Blue (1992; the Cognitive Disabilities Model); Toglia (2005; the Dynamic Interactional Model); Averbuch and Katz (2011; the Cognitive Rehabilitation Model; Polatajko and Mandich (2004; the Cognitive Orientation to Daily Occupational Performance [CO-OP] Model); and Giles (2011; the Neurofunctional Approach).

Performance skill deficits generally impact activities across different areas of occupation. For example, decreases in short-term memory will impact ADL as well as work tasks. Rather than focusing on the individual client factor components (such as short-term memory or attention) for a review of cognitive interventions, the following list from the AOTA practice statement (2013) spotlights the key features of the models for occupation-based intervention. The approaches include the following:

- Global (across areas of occupation) and domain- or task-specific strategy training
- Awareness training
- Cognitive retraining using functional activities
- Task-specific training
- Environmental modification
- Use of technology

GLOBAL AND DOMAIN- OR TASK-SPECIFIC STRATEGY TRAINING

Toglia, Rodger, and Polatajko (2012) have developed a detailed framework of cognitive strategy intervention. They describe the use of strategies to promote improved occupational engagement in-depth. Cognitive strategies can be mental or self-verbalization, or specific to the task to be accomplished. For example, rehearsal, the use of imagery, and self-coaching are examples of mental cognitive strategies; stimuli reduction, task reorganization, and task simplification are examples of task-specific modification. The authors have also identified the dimensions of cognitive strategies such as source (external or internal), orientation (person or task), purpose, level of visibility, and scope or range (Toglia et al., 2012, p. 229). By helping clients of all ages use cognitive strategies effectively, the occupational therapy practitioner is promoting learning (or relearning) and best occupational performance.

AWARENESS TRAINING

An aspect of higher-level cognition is self-awareness. In the framework (Giles et al., 2013) self-awareness of one's own cognitive abilities is defined as *metacognition*. The awareness of self, including the ability to self-monitor and being able to assess one's own strengths and weaknesses, is generally necessary for successful occupational performance. A systematic review of self-awareness training following brain injury (Schmidt, Lannin, Fleming, & Ownsworth, 2011) included 12 studies, three of which were randomized control studies. The overall consensus was that awareness training tended to have a modest but positive effect on improving self-awareness and a large effect on the participants' level of satisfaction with their performance. Not surprisingly, more research in this realm is advised.

Fleming, Lucas, and Lightbody (2006) conducted a pilot study on four adult males with acquired brain injury who demonstrated decreased self-awareness. They determined that an occupation-based program to improve awareness was effective in all four cases, but increased self-awareness was accompanied by increased anxiety across the board. This result highlights the necessity of considering psychosocial aspects of intervention along with the cognitive factors (as well as the physical) at all times.

COGNITIVE RETRAINING USING FUNCTIONAL TASKS

Occupational therapy practitioners have a long history of using functional tasks to improve performance, by presenting the "just right challenge" for their clients to promote successful engagement. According to the AOTA statement (2013), this approach uses functional activities to improve cognitive performance. The training is "context specific," based on the transfer appropriate processing hypothesis (p. S12) originally put forth by Craik and Lockhart (1972). This processing hypothesis is often related to memory performance, in which memory processing and retrieval is described as being enhanced when the tasks engaged in during initial processing (e.g., training) are also engaged in during retrieval.

TASK-SPECIFIC TRAINING

Task-specific training, as the name implies, involves training of specific meaningful tasks that then get incorporated into the client's daily routines. Repeated engagement in basic ADL routines and other real-world, meaningful tasks for the client are used. Hubbard, Parsons, Neilson, and Carey (2009) suggest that the practitioner "deconstruct" the task to determine the problematic components interfering with performance and then work to have the client "reconstruct" the entire task. Other recommendations include ensuring task variability to generalize learning and using positive reinforcement given in a timely manner to promote learning. Tasks may be taught in a step-by-step, broken-down process, often using errorless learning (not allowing the person to make mistakes along the way), until the entire routine is incorporated into the client's daily repertoire. This training method is described in AOTA (2012) based on the work of Giles (Giles, 2011; Giles & Shore, 1989).

ENVIRONMENTAL MODIFICATION

Occupational therapy practitioners consider the global idea of context (AOTA, 2008) throughout the intervention process. Since the environment can both support or hinder occupational performance, it becomes the practitioner's role to modify the environment in such a way as to promote optimal functioning while keeping environmental barriers to a minimum. This can be as simple as making sure that lighting is adequate or using high-contrast items. In the realm of cognitive rehabilitation, examples are as varied as the creative mind can envision. Basic examples of environmental adaptations to support improved performance may include limiting distractions in the environment, the use of labels or signs, or designing the workspace to enhance attention.

USE OF TECHNOLOGY

Current technology can be used freely as tools of the trade. The world has seen the exponential rise in technological advances and options available to the public over the past few decades. The use of technological devices is a hit or miss venture; only those devices that fit the client's needs and lifestyle will be helpful. It behooves the occupational therapist to carefully evaluate the desires and needs of the client so that a clinically reasoned decision can be made regarding the potential usefulness of any device or program. The therapist will need to ensure that the client wants and has the capacity to learn to use the technology offered. As an ever-increasing proportion of the population is getting more comfortable with the use of technological gadgets, practitioners who value lifelong learning need to stay up-to-date with the trends so that they can build up their repertoire of potentially helpful technological developments. The possibilities are limitless, but it takes skilled intervention to match the technology to the needs of the client. Nonetheless, the use of technology can open doors heretofore locked for those with certain cognitive impairments.

Specific Cognitive Skills

Next we consider specific cognitive skills involved in the habilitation or rehabilitation process. While it is rare for intervention to focus on one skill exclusively without a more global view toward occupational performance in a complex world, the following brief overview is offered to clarify aspects of intervention in the realm of cognition.

The development of cognitive skills most often takes place in younger clients who have not been exposed to the cognitive task before, whereas remediation implies that the client was once able to do the task but now cannot due to impairments in brain functioning. Diagnoses and conditions related to cognitive dysfunction are extremely varied and may cause slight, moderate, or severe impairments in just one or many areas of cognition. Even the highest performing individuals cannot be expected to perform at an optimal cognitive level at all times. An important consideration for all populations is how cognitive performance can be enhanced by providing both internal and external conditions and environments to promote the highest level of functioning. Performance is context dependent in the ever-changing world. Factors to consider include comfort level, body positioning, amount and type of environmental stimulation, and physical condition (e.g., nutrition, level of fatigue, pain). The client factors under consideration in this section need to be viewed from this broader multidimensional perspective. Remediation of or compensation for decreased cognitive performance generally involves one or more global or specific mental functions such as orientation, attention, memory, and visuospatial perception.

ORIENTATION

Orientation training involves the repetition of basic orienting information in which the client answers pertinent questions about his or her life situation, such as who, where, what, when, and how. Being able to improve orientation skills is based on the theoretical notion that repetition or practice will help the information stick, especially for those who are expected to make improvements, such as those who have sustained a brain injury and are now in the midst of the healing process. Orientation is related to memory in that it involves remembering key information about aspects of one's life. In a study by Arkin (2000) using 30 biographical items, even those with Alzheimer's disease (AD) could improve in basic orientation skills when compared to a control group who had a similar amount of contact but no commensurate orientation training.

ATTENTION

Attention, in its various forms, is mediated by the reticular activating system in the brain. Attention is an important aspect of memory in that it is believed that one must be attending to environmental stimulation in order to remember the information. As might be expected, adequate attention is needed to complete many daily tasks. More difficult tasks such as driving in an unfamiliar city require more focused attention, and automatic tasks such as teeth brushing require less. Attention process training (APT) is a common aspect of the cognitive neurorehabilitation techniques developed by Sohlberg and Mateer (2001) and is sometimes undertaken by occupational therapy practitioners. The system is based on practicing bottom-up cognitive exercises in order to hone in on improving one particular aspect of attention (e.g., sustained, alternating) at a time. A number of studies have found APT to be effective in improving attention (e.g., as cited in Sohlberg & Mateer, 2001, p. 134). A Cochrane database of systematic reviews, in an overview of two trials with 56 participants, found attention training following a stroke was generally effective (Lincoln, Majid, & Weyman, 2000). However, improved attention on retraining exercises may not necessarily correlate with improved functional performance in daily life tasks.

MEMORY

Memory has many different facets, including remembering language and common knowledge (both semantic), events (episodic), how to do tasks (procedural), and remembering to actually do specific tasks at a set time in the future (prospective). Memory can also be classified by duration (e.g., immediate, short term, or long term). Working memory tasks are complex in that the person has to remember information while engaging in a related or unrelated task (e.g., recalling a phone number while dialing the phone or remembering the rules while playing a game). Not all aspects of memory are amenable to improvement and not all people are candidates for memory training.

Strong empirical evidence supporting the improvement of memory ability after memory practice drills is still lacking. Sohlberg and Mateer (2001) suggested that if improvement does occur, it is more likely due to improvements in the foundational skill of attention (which could improve the process of storing information). A Cochrane review of memory training in older adults (Martin, Clare, Altgassen, Cameron, & Zehnder, 2011) reported inconclusive results regarding the efficacy of memory training but did find some improvements in immediate and delayed verbal recall. Again, further research should be done; for the field of occupational therapy, this research should involve testing the efficacy of functionally based interventions to enhance memory performance.

EXECUTIVE SKILLS

Levy and Burns (2005) described cognition as based on a hierarchy in which the base is attention and the tip is executive functioning. Executive skills are defined as high-level cognitive skills that involve planning, problem solving, cognitive flexibility, metacognition, and judgment/insight. Monitoring one's own behavior and adapting one's behavior to fit the current situation are also part of executive skills. These high-level skills develop during adolescence and are easily damaged in common brain injuries involving the frontal and prefrontal lobes. With brain diseases such as AD, the loss of ability in executive skills happens early in the disease process, while more basic skills are lost later (often in a reverse ontogenetic sequence; Levy & Burns, 2005). A number of approaches for the management of executive dysfunction are detailed in Sohlberg and Mateer (2001). All involve repeated engagement in cognitive activities that challenge the person's level of thinking. Improvement is only expected to occur after rigorous and recurring practice.

COGNITIVE PERFORMANCE REMEDIATION OR MAINTENANCE

Remediating cognitive performance often involves drills or repeated engagement in tasks with the intended goal being improved skill level in one or more realms of cognition and the ultimate outcome being improvement in areas of occupation. For example, by improving short-term memory performance, one would likely perform better on classroom testing. Maintaining cognitive performance can also be a goal of occupational therapy rehabilitation, especially for those with neurological conditions expected to worsen over the course of time. Diagnoses such as Alzheimer's disease, Parkinson's disease, and Huntington's chorea are associated with cognitive decline. Therefore, short-term occupational therapy intervention to maintain the current cognitive performance level could be appropriate. Maintaining cognitive skills can involve all of the aforementioned intervention techniques, with the goal being forestalling decline in performance, rather than improvement. Yet even maintaining function can pose significant challenges. Nussbaum (2003) encouraged those who want to improve or maintain brain health into old age to actively engage the brain through lifestyle choices that encourage new learning. In his list of 10 behaviors to foster optimal brain health, he included healthy eating, not smoking, adequate physical activity, socializing, learning to relax, building strong ties to others, engaging in new and novel learning experiences, and finally, the occupational therapy practitioner's favorite: maintaining a role or purpose in life.

COMPENSATION FOR DECREASED COGNITION

When neither improvement nor maintenance of cognitive functioning is the anticipated outcome, therapeutic intervention adjusts its focus to the safe engagement in occupation in spite of persistent cognitive impairments. Compensation for decreased cognition puts the emphasis on changing the actions of others and the context rather than expecting a change in the self (client). This may be true for one aspect of cognition (e.g., memory) even while other aspects are maintained. For example, if the client has decreased safety awareness, then supervision and/or a more constricted environment may be necessary. Certain complex cognitive activities such as driving are simply no longer appropriate, thus other arrangements need to be made. Environments may need to be more structured and simplified. Establishing routines to capitalize on the use of basic overlearned tasks can help those with significant cognitive deficits maintain ADL skills. Studies by Graff, Vernooij-Dassen, Hoefnagels, Dekker, and de Witte (2003), as well as Hällgren and Kottorp (2005) have demonstrated the effectiveness of occupational therapy in improving ADL skills for those with cognitive impairments. Occupational therapy practitioners, through their keen observation skills, use of functional cognitive assessments and activity analyses, and ability to adapt the environment, are often instrumental in assisting the person to continue to live in the least restrictive environment

possible. For example, the simple act of removing the stove knobs or putting a safety bar in a strategic location may be what it takes to keep the home safe for the client.

MODELS RELATED TO COGNITIVE REMEDIATION AND COMPENSATION

Gillen (2009) provides a concise overview of the primary models that guide practice in the realm of cognitive rehabilitation. The Dynamic Interactional Model (Toglia, 2005) emphasizes the dynamic interaction between the person, activity, and environment. Performance is likely to vary based on environmental and personal parameters, as well as the demands of the task. Self-awareness and the use of cognitive strategies play key roles in this approach, which combines both remediation and compensation.

Allen, Earhart, and Blue (1992) developed the Cognitive Disabilities Model, based on Allen's earlier work (1985). In the Cognitive Disabilities Model, the expectation is not that occupational therapy will improve cognition, but rather that intervention will optimize current functioning through the use of environmental cues and adaptations. First, the practitioner must identify the level of functioning through an assessment tool such as the Allen Cognitive Level Screen. The determined cognitive level (1 through 6, with specific modes) guides intervention so that the occupational therapy practitioner can capitalize on the person's cognitive strengths (Levy & Burns, 2005). For example, someone functioning at a level 4 can pay attention to visual cues and may need set-up and reminders to successfully complete daily tasks. People functioning at this level pose a safety risk because if a hazard is out of sight, they are not likely to attend to it.

The Quadraphonic Approach (Abreu, 1997) is a holistic cognitive rehabilitation approach that considers the client from both the macro and micro levels, strongly emphasizing the contextual dimensions of intervention in order to ensure that all of the influential factors on learning are included. This approach, which involves both retraining programs (such as practice drills) and compensatory measures (such as memory aids), was designed specifically for those who exhibit cognitive dysfunction.

Averbuch and Katz (2011) developed the Cognitive Rehabilitation Retraining Model for use with adolescents and adults. This model focuses on first assessing general functioning and then enhancing the clients' retained cognitive abilities. Clients build self-awareness (e.g., metacognition) and learn to use alternative cognitive strategies in helping themselves to perceive, process, and act on incoming information. Through improved self-awareness, clients are better able to assess their own capabilities and learn to respond in appropriate ways, thus improving their cognitive functioning related to everyday tasks. For example, a client who needed to improve his initiation skills in social situations first built awareness of the issue and then was guided in occupational therapy about how to approach others through social interaction training (pp. 287–288).

The Cognitive Orientation to Daily Occupational Performance treatment approach (CO-OP) was developed by Polatajko and Mandich (2004). It focuses on teaching the cognitive strategy "Goal-Plan-Do-Check" to clients to help them with their everyday cognitive performance. In a series of design experiments, McEwen, Polatajko, Huijbregts, and Ryan (2010) used the CO-OP model to determine how well the strategy model improved performance on both trained and untrained tasks, such as cutting with a knife or putting on a coat (p. 551). The practitioner works with the client to learn to use this strategy consistently during engagement in tasks of interest (based on outcomes of the Canadian Occupational Performance Measure). The McEwen study determined that the CO-OP model held promise to improve motor performance not only in trained tasks, but also to transfer beyond the tasks used during the sessions once the client had learned the general strategic approach.

The neurofunctional approach (Giles, 2011) focuses on specific task retraining and compensatory strategies to help people who have sustained severe acquired brain injuries. This approach targets function at the occupation level rather than focusing on the impairments themselves. This top-down approach works on skill development through repetitive engagement and practice in tasks that have meaning for the client. Using habits and routines and environmental adaptations, clients enhance their repertoire of appropriate and well-learned behavioral responses.

EVIDENCE-BASED PRACTICE FINDINGS

Cicerone, Mott, Azulay, and Friel (2004) concluded through a nonrandomized controlled intervention study that intensive, holistic cognitive rehabilitation was an effective form of rehabilitation, especially for community re-entry for those with traumatic brain injury, and an additional positive effect resulted when clients felt satisfied with their level of cognitive functioning. Through a systematic review of the literature from 2003 to 2008, Cicerone et al. (2011) also concluded that there is sufficient evidence to support rehabilitative interventions for attention, memory, social communication skills, and executive functioning for people who have sustained an acquired brain injury. Visuospatial rehabilitation following a lesion to the right brain and interventions to manage apraxia have both been found to be effective, although specific protocols have not been firmly established. Occupational therapy practitioners certainly can be key players in this team of cognitive rehabilitation experts, especially with their level of expertise in wholly functional and individualized client-centered intervention.

Intervention Related to Behavioral Skills

Behavioral impairments are not entirely different from cognitive impairments because neurological or cognitive deficits have behavioral manifestations. Behavioral intervention in the framework (AOTA, 2008) is extremely broad and focuses on changing behavior that is inadequate to support successful occupational engagement. Starting at one end of the age spectrum, an example might be a premature infant who has difficulty regulating environmental stimulation and thereby flails, cries, and becomes easily agitated. On the other end of the age spectrum, an older person with AD may have similar difficulties with related behavioral manifestations. The elder with dementia might lash out and yell instead of cry, but in both cases, the person is not able to respond to the environment appropriately. In these examples, and in a myriad of others involving behavioral dysfunction, occupational therapy intervention can help regulate one's response to the environment.

SENSORY APPROACH TO PRACTICE

Occupational therapists rely on their client evaluations, knowledge of human performance, and activity analysis to design interventions that will assist people who need to develop skills or need adaptations to function. A common behavioral intervention in the field of pediatric occupational therapy is the use of sensory integration (SI) originated by the late Jean Ayres (1979). SI theory explains the brain's ability to filter, organize, and integrate sensory information to promote learning (Walker, 2004). Ayres believed that sensory input to the human nervous system was necessary for it to evolve. SI dysfunction is caused by processing problems in the brain, leading to suboptimal functioning (Ayres, 2005). Ayres's theory explained the relationship between the child's ability to interpret sensations from the body and environment and his or her ability to succeed in academic and motor learning (Bundy & Murray, 2002). SI theory focused on the role of the tactile, proprioceptive, and vestibular systems. Through observation, Ayres identified the following four areas of dysfunctional sensory processing (Walker, 2004):

1. Visual form and space dysfunction

2. Developmental dyspraxia

3. Deficits in vestibular and bilateral integration

4. Tactile defensiveness

An occupational therapist using SI intervention principles designs individualized intervention programs based on the results of a thorough evaluation. One goal of intervention is to control sensory input so that a child's brain is able to reorganize and adapt (Walker, 2004). Through engagement in play, a child is able to form adaptive responses that will either inhibit or facilitate sensory integration. Intervention is based on normal developmental sequences, posture, and the integration of sensory input. Ayres felt strongly that SI treatment needed to include equipment, such as suspension devices (swings, hammocks), scooter boards, balance boards, therapy balls and mats that challenge the senses to develop adaptive responses (Walker, 2004). Each child with SI dysfunction will need an individualized plan. In successful cases, the behavior no longer interferes with their occupational performance.

Related to SI, Sensory Processing Disorder was proposed by Schaaf and Davies (2010). These researchers are turning to neuroscience to explain sensory function/dysfunction into subtypes to enable evidence-based research and the clearer delineation of sensory approaches. Schaff and Miller (2005) proposed the following three distinct patterns:

1. **Sensory modulation disorder:** Inability to regulate a response to sensory stimulation.

2. **Sensory discrimination disorder:** Difficulty interpreting qualities of sensory stimulation.

3. **Sensory-based mood disorder:** Poor postural or volitional movement as a result of sensory problems (James, Miller, Schaff, Nielsene, & Schoen, 2011; Miller, Anzalone, Lane, Cermack, & Osten, 2007).

Behavioral Management Strategies

Behavioral management strategies are often used for children with disruptive behaviors such as aggression, screaming, or self-injurious behaviors that may accompany autism, attention deficit disorder (with or without hyperactivity), as well as SI dysfunction or sensory processing disorder. Strong empirical evidence demonstrating successful outcomes is scant, but anecdotal evidence and single-case studies are more abundant. Rosen and Scott (2003) described the behavioral management techniques that can be used with children with autism who appear to be less aware of others in the environment and more focused on their own needs. The occupational therapy practitioner can use the analysis and interpretation of ongoing behavior to formulate a plan. The goal is successful occupational engagement in learning activities and at home. Primary techniques include the consistent use of rewards for positive behaviors, redirection or natural consequences for negative behaviors, and environmental restructuring. Rosen and Scott wrote about the use of positive reinforcement, natural consequences, and redirection techniques with a client called "Patty" (a pseudonym), a 9 year old with severe self-destructive tendencies. The behavior management strategies allowed Patty to have some choice in selecting tasks, which were introduced slowly with the initial expectation being that she would engage in the task only briefly. The occupational therapy practitioner used edible reinforcements and picture symbol communication since Patty was initially unable to clearly verbalize her needs. Through a rearrangement of the environment to decrease the level of compulsory stimulation to which Patty was exposed and by providing deep sensory input (e.g., joint compression, bear hugs, and deep massage), occupational therapy intervention was able to help Patty relate to her environment more effectively and to tolerate being in a classroom setting without resorting to maladaptive behaviors. Watling and Schwartz (2004) also described the use of applied behavior analysis on children with developmental disabilities, specifically positive reinforcement, based on decades of research.

Making behavioral changes in life is a goal of many adults as well. In rehabilitation, sometimes changes in behavior are required to adapt to new life situations. For example, after having a heart attack, dietary changes are warranted. Often, behavioral changes are focused on habits that no longer are, or never were, productive or healthy. For example, a few of the common behavioral changes sought by people relate to improving diet, exercising, and giving up unhealthy habits such as smoking or substance abuse. Occupational therapy practitioners can be helpful in moving people through the stages of change by collaborating with clients to develop reasonable goals, and by helping them to break down these goals into more distinct and achievable steps or objectives. Based on the Transtheoretical Model of Behavior Change (Prochaska & Velicer, 1997), there are five phases of behavioral change:

1. Precontemplation

2. Contemplation

3. Preparation

4. Action

5. Maintenance

The role of the occupational therapy practitioner is to move the client from one stage to the next, always closer to the ultimate goal of an improved and healthier lifestyle. For example, in the precontemplation phase when the person is not yet thinking about making a change in lifestyle, the occupational therapy practitioner can assist the person in making a list of the benefits and drawbacks of a new behavior, such as adopting a diabetic diet for someone with diabetes. Just by acknowledging that there are pros and cons of making a change, the person is beginning to move into the contemplation phase: acknowledgment that the current diet or situation may not be promoting optimal health.

Visual Perception

Perceptual skills are higher level, top-of-the-pyramid visual skills that require not only intact visual pathways

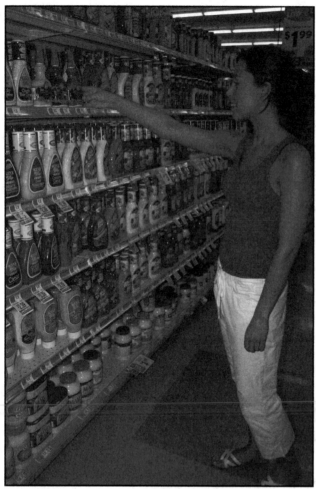

Figure 24-1. Grocery shopping provides wonderful opportunities to work on various cognitive and visual skills.

but also accurate interpretations of the visual information in the right hemispheric occipital and parietal lobes of the brain. Perception also involves the processing and analysis of other types of sensory information in the brain. Due to their complexity, perceptual deficits are some of the most fascinating and difficult problems to treat. They are rarely seen in isolation and are often combined with more general cognitive impairments. Visual perceptual disorders include the inability to recognize common objects (e.g., agnosia), the inability to understand spatial relationships (e.g., figure–ground, right–left, and depth perception impairments), the inability to recognize subtle differences in similar objects and people (e.g., form constancy disorder), the inability to distinguish objects by touch (e.g., astereognosis), and a distortion of body scheme. Included in the realm of perceptual disorders are both *ideomotor* and *ideational apraxias*. These are defined as an inability to carry out common motor tasks due to perceptual impairments rather than because of decreased sensation or motor skills. Ideomotor apraxia is less severe because, although the person has lost the "access to kinesthetic

memory patterns" (Gillen, 2009, p. 112), the individual may be able to do the task automatically but not be able to simulate the task or do it on command. In the case of ideomotor apraxia, one may display inaccurate, imprecise, uncoordinated, or clumsy movements. Ideational apraxia (or conceptual apraxia) is a loss of the "mental representation" (Gillen, 2009, p. 110) of how to even complete the task (including sequencing the steps of a task). The person does not know how to use objects or understand how the objects needed for a task relate to one another. Difficulty with initiation of the task due to the more encompassing loss of the concept and slowed performance is also likely, making ideational apraxia more difficult to remediate. Remediation of perceptual deficits involves repetitive engagement in tasks requiring perceptual skills, starting at the client's level and working up to more complicated tasks as the person is able (Figures 24-1 and 24-2). Gillen offers a protocol for instructing and providing assistance and feedback for people with perceptual deficits. These include individualized cueing and assistance based on the client's needs (Gillen, 2009, p. 126).

In a pivotal study involving occupational therapy, Neistadt (1992) compared 45 men in two intervention groups who had perceptual deficits due to brain injuries. One group completed remedial parquetry block assembly and the other worked on functional meal preparation. The results showed that the functional approach was preferable to the remedial approach, although both groups did show improvements in the realm of perception. A more recent study (Vlok, Smit, & Bester, 2011) presented a framework for a visual perceptual training program for young learners between the ages of 7 and 9 years old (when perceptual skills are developing). The researchers provided a set protocol and recommended including a set of preparatory eye exercises along with activities to enhance general visual skills and to promote higher-level perceptual skills.

Compensation for decreased perceptual skills can involve graded cueing; graded assistance; giving verbal, physical, or video feedback (Gillen, 2009); simplifying the environment; establishing basic daily routines; and making sure that the environment is safe for someone who has decreased awareness of surroundings. Since supervision may be needed for successful physical completion of basic daily tasks, caregiver training may also be an important aspect of occupational therapy intervention (Gillen, 2009).

Frequently, the research completed on the intervention of perceptual disorders has focused on unilateral neglect, which more often accompanies right-sided lesions of the brain. A Cochrane review of cognitive rehabilitation for spatial neglect following stroke (Bowen, Lincoln, & Dewey, 2007) found that cognitive rehabilitation clearly did result in decreased visual neglect at the impairment level as measured by neuropsychological assessments, but additional research in this area was recommended to ensure that these improvements actually transfer to enhanced functioning in day-to-day tasks. Cicerone et al. (2004) recommended "relatively intense (i.e., daily)" (p. 1601) visuospatial training, which includes scanning to decrease the level of visual neglect as a practice standard based on robust evidence of its effectiveness. However, this research group did not recommend the use of isolated computerized exercises as intervention. Warren (1993), who described the hierarchical model of visual functioning, recommended that occupational therapy practitioners focus on restoring basic visual functioning (visual acuity, visual fields, and oculomotor control) because in doing so, a natural consequence may be the spontaneous recovery of higher-level skills.

Summary

All of the interventions described in this chapter have been condensed for the sake of parsimony in a broad-based text. As stated initially, the impairments—though often described individually—are nonetheless rarely seen in isolation. In addition, although the primary impairment may be cognitive, sensory, behavioral, or physical, these typically have accompanying psychosocial implications. Losses in the realm of client factors and/or performance skills can be traumatic and can result in deep emotional responses in the clients and their significant others. These feelings and accompanying responses can certainly have an influence on the rehabilitation process and should not simply be ignored.

Effective occupational therapy intervention is based on a thorough review of the multifactorial biopsychosocial factors pertinent to the individual case, a full and individualized client evaluation, and a strong dose of clinical reasoning to ensure that the subsequent intervention plan is both client centered and based on the best and most accurate empirical knowledge currently available. In this chapter, further references are often cited and should be consulted prior to working with clients in the areas described. We need to strive for excellence in occupational therapy and do our utmost to promote improved quality of life and help clients develop the skills needed to "live life to the fullest," which is, after all, our ultimate goal as professionals within this exhilarating and challenging field.

Student Self-Assessment

1. Many people have a rather superficial level of understanding of disabilities. We can define them, but we do not truly comprehend what it is like to have impairments. Therefore, a valuable learning tool is to simulate life with a disability. This activity can lend insight into the difficulties encountered in everyday life. The activity can be completed

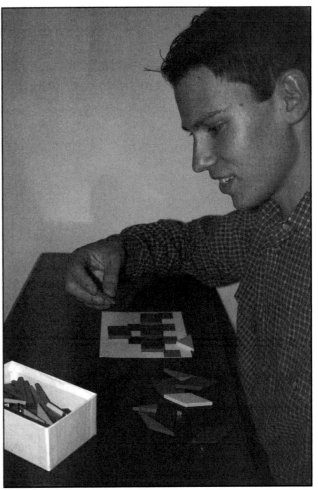

Figure 24-2. Parquetry puzzles are sometimes used to help clients regain skills in perceptual functioning.

in a classroom, lab setting, or in the community (although care should be taken not to offend people with disabilities in the community). All of these exercises should be undertaken only under supervision. The following list is just a few examples of how this exercise can work:

◊ Simulating paralysis of the legs, use a wheelchair to get around. Be sure to go around several buildings and roll on graded surfaces.

◊ Wearing heavy gloves, try to make a peanut butter and crackers snack (or another snack requiring opening containers and using utensils).

◊ Using just one arm, put on a shirt and shoes, including tying them. You are not allowed to move your "affected" arm.

◊ Smear lotion on some old sunglasses and put them on. Then try doing a puzzle or playing a game.

◊ Wearing ear plugs and earmuffs, try to write down the words to a song you are listening to on the radio (if there is static on the radio, that's even better).

EVIDENCE-BASED RESEARCH CHART

Area	Intervention	Evidence
Physical	Range of motion/strength	Andrews & Bohannon, 2003; Grealy, Johnson, & Rushton, 1999; Latham, Anderson, Bennett, & Stretton, 2003; Liu et al., 2011; Mathieux et al., 2009; Xu, Wang, Mai, & He, 2012; Weiss, Suzuki, Bean, & Fielding, 2000
	Endurance	Javier & Montagnini, 2011; Singh, Stewart, Franzsen, & MacKay-Lyons, 2011
	Balance/postural control	Chase, Mann, Wasek, & Arbesman, 2012; Clemson et al., 2004; Davison, Bond, Dawson, Steen, & Kenny, 2005; Garcia, Marciniak, McCune, Smith, & Ramsey, 2012; Gillespie et al., 2003; Han et al., 2004; Hsieh et al., 1996; Leland, Elliott, O'Malley, & Murphy, 2012; Li et al., 2005; Taylor-Piliae et al., 2006; Zijlstra et al., 2007
Neuromuscular	Motor control	Chen, Chen, Wu, Wu, & Chang, 2010; Denton, Cope, & Moser, 2006; Dickson, 2002; Pollock, Baer, Pomeroy, & Langhorne, 2007; Thorpe & Valvano, 2002; Whitall, McCombe Waller, Silver, & Macko, 2000
Sensory	Olfactory and gustatory	Neumann et al., 2012; Zasler, McNeny, & Heywood, 1992
	Touch, proprioception, and kinesthesia	Carey, Matyas, & Oke, 1993; Dannenbaum & Jones, 1993; Imperatore, Reinoso, Chang, & Bodison, 2012; Leanne, Chester, & Jerosch-Herold, 2012; Proto, Pella, Hill, & Gouvier, 2009
	Hearing	Andersson, Green, & Melin, 1997; Sheff, 2010
	Vision	Perlmutter, Bhorade, Gordon, Hollingsworth, & Baum, 2010; Schoessow, 2010; Smallfield, Clem, & Myers, 2013; Weisser-Pike & Kaldenberg, 2010
	Visual perception	Aki & Kayihan, 2003; Bowen et al., 2007; Cicerone et al., 2011; Lin, Cermak, Kinsbourne, & Trombly, 1996; Vlok, Smit, & Bester, 2011
	Sensory stimulation—coma	Mitchell, Bradley, Welch, & Britton, 1990; Oh & Seo, 2003
	Pain	Arbesman & Mosley, 2012; Stanos, 2012
Cognitive	General cognitive rehabilitation	Cicerone et al., 2011; Hayslip, Paggi, Poole, & Pinson, 2009; McHugh & Warren 2009; Rand, Weiss, & Katz, 2009
	Attention training	Akinwuntan et al., 2010; Loetscher & Lincoln, 2013; Sohlberg & Mateer, 2001
	Memory training	Boman, Stenvall, Hemmingsson, & Bartfai, 2010; Cavallini, Pagnin, & Vecchi, 2003; Cicerone et al., 2000
	Self-awareness	Dirette, 2010; Fleming, Lucas, & Lightbody, 2006; Ownsworth, Fleming, Desbois, Strong, & Kuipers, 2006; Schmidt, Fleming, Ownsworth, Lannin, & Khan, 2012
	Cognitive strategies	Thorpe & Valvano 2002; Toglia, Rodger, & Polatajko, 2012
Behavioral	Sensory integration/sensory processing disorder	Arbesman & Lieberman, 2010; Roley et al., 2003; Smith, Press, Koenig, & Kinnealey, 2005
	Behavioral change	Clark, Nigg, Greene, Riebe, & Saunders, 2002; Glasgow, Bull, Gillette, Klesges, & Dzewaltowski, 2002

◊ Try cleaning a kitchen area or dusting while blindfolded.

2. In small groups of two to four, brainstorm intervention ideas for the impairments listed. Be sure to think of ideas that incorporate remediation and ideas that incorporate compensation or adaptation whenever possible. For example, for decreased sense of smell, although remediation is probably

not possible, compensation might involve labeling leftovers with dates, getting a second opinion about perfume (or not wearing any), and making sure that areas are well-ventilated when working with any harmful airborne substances.

Remember that the broad list you devise will not be client centered, but it will stimulate your individualized intervention planning when working with people who have the following impairments:

◊ Decreased vision
◊ Unilateral neglect
◊ Ideational/ideomotor apraxia
◊ Figure–ground deficit
◊ Orientation deficit
◊ Decreased attention
◊ Decreased short-term memory
◊ Decreased endurance
◊ Decreased strength
◊ Impaired self-awareness

References

Abreu, B. C. (1997). *The quadraphonic approach.* Galveston, TX: Unpublished course manual.

Aki, E., & Kayihan, H. (2003). The effect of visual perceptual training on reading, writing, and daily living activities in children with low vision. *Fizyoterapi Rehabilitasyon, 14*(3), 95-99.

Akinwuntan, A. E., Devos, H., Verheyden, G., Baten, G., Kiekens, C., Feys, H., & De Weerdt, W. (2010). Retraining moderately impaired stroke survivors in driving-related visual attention skills. *Topics in Stroke Rehabilitation, 17*(5), 328-336.

Allen, C. K. (1985). *Occupational therapy for psychiatric diseases: Measurement and management of cognitive disabilities.* Boston, MA: Little, Brown, and Company.

Allen, C. K., Earhart, C., & Blue, T. (1992). *Occupational therapy treatment goals for the physically and cognitively disabled.* Rockville, MD: AOTA Press.

American Occupational Therapy Association. (2008). Occupational therapy practice framework: Domain and process (2nd ed.). *American Journal of Occupational Therapy, 62,* 625-683.

American Occupational Therapy Association. (2012). *Commission on Practice statement on Cognition, Cognitive Rehabilitation, and Occupational Performance.*

Andersson, G., Green, M., & Melin, L. (1997). Behavioural hearing tactics: A controlled trial of a short treatment programme. *Behaviour Research and Therapy, 35*(6), 523-530.

Andrews, A. W., & Bohannon, R. W. (2003). Short-term recovery of limb muscle strength after acute stroke. *Archives of Physical Medicine and Rehabilitation, 84*(1), 125-130.

Arbesman, M., & Mosley, L. J. (2012). Systematic review of occupation- and activity-based health management and maintenance interventions for community-dwelling older adults. *American Journal of Occupational Therapy, 66*(3), 277-283.

Arkin, S. M. (2000). Alzheimer memory training: Students replicate learning successes. *American Journal of Alzheimer's Disease and Other Dementias, 15*(3), 152-162.

Averbuch, S., & Katz, N. (2011). Cognitive rehabilitation: A retraining model for clients with neurological disabilities. In N. Katz (Ed.), *Cognition, occupation, and participation across the lifespan* (3rd ed., pp. 277-298). Bethesda, MD: AOTA Press.

Ayres, A. J. (1979). *Sensory integration and the child.* Los Angeles, CA: Western Psychological Services.

Ayres, A. J. (2005). *Sensory integration and the child: understanding hidden sensory challenges.* Los Angeles, CA: Western Psychological Services.

Boman, I., Stenvall, C. L., Hemmingsson, H., & Bartfai, A. (2010). A training apartment with a set of electronic memory aids for patients with cognitive problems. *Scandinavian Journal of Occupational Therapy, 17*(2), 140-148.

Bowen, A., Lincoln, N. B., & Dewey, M. (2007). Cognitive rehabilitation for spatial neglect following stroke. *Cochrane Database for Systemic Reviews, 2,* CD003586.

Breines, E. B. (2006). Therapeutic occupations and modalities. In H. M. Pendleton & W. Schultz-Krohn (Eds.), *Pedretti's occupational therapy: Practice skills for physical dysfunction* (6th ed.). St. Louis, MO: Mosby Elsevier.

Bundy, A. C., & Murray, E. A. (2002). Sensory integration: A. Jean Ayres' theory revisited. In A. C. Bundy, S. J. Lane, & E. A. Murray (Eds.), *Sensory integration: Theory and practice* (pp. 3-33). Philadelphia, PA: F. A. Davis Company.

Carey, L. M., Matyas, T. A., & Oke, L. E. (1993). Sensory loss in stroke patients: Effective training of tactile and proprioceptive discrimination. *Archives of Physical Medicine and Rehabilitation, 74*(6), 602-611.

Cavallini, E., Pagnin, A., & Vecchi, T. (2003). Aging and everyday memory: the beneficial effect of memory training. *Archives of Gerontology and Geriatrics, 37*(3), 241-257.

Chase, C. A., Mann, K., Wasek, S., & Arbesman, M. (2012). Systematic review of the effect of home modification and fall prevention programs on falls and the performance of community-dwelling older adults. *American Journal of Occupational Therapy, 66*(3), 284-291.

Chen, Y., Chen, C., Wu, C., Wu, C., & Chang, Y. (2010). The effects of bilateral arm training on motor control and functional performance in chronic stroke: A randomized controlled study. *Neurorehabilitation and Neural Repair, 24*(1), 42-51.

Cho, K. H., Lee, K. J., & Song, C. H. (2012). Virtual reality balance training with video-game system improves dynamic balance in chronic stroke patients. *Tohoku Journal of Experimental Medicine, 228,* 69-74.

Cicerone, K. D., Langenbahn, D. M., Braden, C., Malec, J. F., Kalmar, K., Fraas, M. … Ashman, T. (2011). Evidence-based cognitive rehabilitation: Updated review of the literature from 2003 through 2008. *Archives of Physical Medicine & Rehabilitation, 92*(4), 519-530.

Cicerone, K. D., Mott, T., Azulay, J., & Friel, J. C. (2004). Community integration and satisfaction with functioning after intensive cognitive rehabilitation for traumatic brain injury. *Archives of Physical Medicine and Rehabilitation, 85*(6), 943-950.

Clark, P. G., Nigg, C. R., Greene, G., Riebe, D., & Saunders, S. D. (2002). The study of exercise and nutrition in older Rhode Islanders (SENIOR): Translating theory into research. *Health Education Research, 17*(5), 552-561.

Clemson, L., Cumming, R. G., Kendig, H., Swann, M., Heard, R., & Taylor, K. (2004). The effectiveness of a community-based program for reducing the incidence of falls in the elderly: A randomized trial. *Journal of the American Geriatrics Society, 52*(9), 1487-1494.

Cole, M. B., & Tufano, R. (2008). *Applied theories in occupational therapy: A practical approach.* Thorofare, NJ: SLACK Incorporated.

Cooper, C., & Canyock, J. D. (2013). Evaluation of sensation and intervention for sensory dysfunction. In H. M. Pendelton & W. Schultz-Krohn (Eds.), *Pedretti's occupational therapy practice skills for physical dysfunction* (7th ed., pp. 575-589). St. Louis, MO: Elsevier Mosby.

Craik, F. I. M., & Lockhart, R. S. (1972). Levels of processing: A framework for memory research. *Journal of Verbal Learning and Verbal Behavior, 11*(6), 671-684.

Dannenbaum, R. M., & Jones, L. A. (1993). The assessment and treatment of patients who have sensory loss following cortical lesions. *Journal of Hand Therapy, 6*(2), 130-138.

Davison, J., Bond, J., Dawson, P., Steen, I. N., & Kenny, R. A. (2005). Patients with recurrent falls attending Accident & Emergency benefit from multifactorial intervention—A randomized controlled trial. *Age and Ageing, 34*(2), 162-168.

DeGangi, G. A., Wietlisbach, S., Goodin, M., & Scheiner, N. (1993). A comparison of structured sensorimotor therapy and child-centered activity in the treatment of preschool children with sensorimotor problems. *American Journal of Occupational Therapy, 47*(9), 777-786.

Denton, P. L., Cope, S., & Moser, C. (2006). The effects of sensorimotor-based intervention versus therapeutic practice on improving handwriting performance in 6- to 11-year-old children. *American Journal of Occupational Therapy, 60*(1), 16-27.

Department of Health and Human Services (2008). *Physical activity guidelines for Americans.* http://www.health.gov.pageguidelines/pdf/paguide.pdf

Dickson, M. (2002). Rehabilitation of motor control following stroke: Searching the evidence. *British Journal of Occupational Therapy, 65*(6), 269-274.

Dirette, D. (2010). Self-awareness enhancement through learning and function (SELF): A theoretically based guideline for practice. *British Journal of Occupational Therapy, 73*(7), 309-318.

Engle, J. M. (2011). Pain regulation. In C. Brown & V. C. Stoffel (Eds.), *Occupational therapy in mental health: A vision for participation.* Philadelphia, PA: F. A. Davis Company.

Feigenbaum, M. S. (2001). Rationale and review of current guidelines. In J. E. Graves & B. A. Franklin (Eds.), *Resistance training for health and rehabilitation.* Leeds, UK: Human Kinetics Publishers.

Fleming, J. M., Lucas, S. E., & Lightbody, S. (2006). Using occupation to facilitate self-awareness in people who have acquired brain injury: A pilot study. *Canadian Journal of Occupational Therapy, 73*(1), 44-55.

Gaines, A. D. (2010). Anosmia and hypnosmia. *Allergy and Asthma Proceedings, 31*, 185-189.

Garber, C. E., Blissmer, B., Deschenes, M. R., Franklin, B. A., Lamonte, M. J., Lee, I. ... Swain, D. P. (2011). Quantity and quality of exercise for developing and maintaining cardio-respiratory, musculoskeletal, and neuromotor fitness in apparently healthy adults: Guidance for prescribing exercise. *Medicine & Science in Sports & Science, 43*(7), 1334-1359.

Garcia, A., Marciniak, D., McCune, L., Smith, E., & Ramsey, R. (2012). Promoting fall self-efficacy and fall risk awareness in older adults. *Physical and Occupational Therapy in Geriatrics, 30*(2), 165-175.

Gentile, M. (2005). *Functional visual behavior in adults: An occupational therapy guide to evaluation and treatment options* (2nd ed.). Bethesda, MD: AOTA Press.

Giles, G. M. (2011). A neurofunctional approach to rehabilitation following brain injury. In N. Katz (Ed.), *Cognition, occupation and participation across the life span* (3rd ed., pp. 351-381). Bethesda, MD: AOTA Press.

Giles, G. M., & Shore, M. (1989). A rapid method for teaching severely brain injured adults how to wash and dress. *Archives of Physical Medicine and Rehabilitation, 70*(2), 156-158.

Giles, G. M., Radomski, M. V., Champagne, T., Corcoran, M. A., Gillen, G., Kuhaneck, H. M. ... Toglia, J. (2013). Cognition, cognitive rehabilitation, and occupational performance. *American Journal of Occupational Therapy, Nov/Dec supplement*, S9-S31.

Gillen, G. (2009). *Cognitive and perceptual rehabilitation: Optimizing function.* St. Louis, MO: Mosby Elsevier.

Gillespie, L. D., Gillespie, W. J., Robertson, M. C., Lamb, S. E., Cumming, R. G., & Rowe, B. H. (2003). Interventions for preventing falls in elderly people. *Cochrane Database for Systematic Reviews, 4*, CD000340.

Glasgow, R. E., Bull, S. S., Gillette, C., Klesges, L. M., & Dzewaltowski, D. A. (2002). Behavior change intervention research in healthcare settings: A review of recent reports with emphasis on external validity. *American Journal of Preventive Medicine, 23*(1), 62-69.

Graff, M. J. L., Vernooij-Dassen, M. J. F. J., Hoefnagels, W. H. L., Dekker, J., & de Witte, L. P. (2003). Occupational therapy at home for older individuals with mild to moderate cognitive impairments and their primary caregivers: A pilot study. *OTJR: Occupation, Participation, and Health, 23*(4), 155-164.

Grealy, M. A., Johnson, D. A., & Rushton, S. K. (1999). Improving cognitive function after brain injury: The use of exercise and virtual reality. *Archives of Physical Medicine and Rehabilitation, 80*(6), 661-667.

Hall, C. M., & Brody, L. T. (2005). Impairment in muscle performance. In C. M. Hall & L. T. Brody (Eds.), *Therapeutic exercise: Moving toward function* (2nd ed.). Philadelphia, PA: Lippincott Williams & Wilkins.

Hällgren, M., & Kottorp, A. (2005). Effects of occupational therapy intervention on activities of daily living and awareness of disability in persons with intellectual disabilities. *Australian Occupational Therapy Journal, 52*(4), 350-359.

Han, A., Robinson, V., Judd, M., Taixiang, W., Wells, G., & Tugwell, P. (2004). Tai Chi for treating rheumatoid arthritis. *Cochrane Database for Systemic Reviews, 3*, CD004849.

Hayflick, L. (1994). *How and why we age.* New York, NY: Ballantine Books.

Hayslip, B., Paggi, K., Poole, M., & Pinson, M. W. (2009). The impact of mental aerobics training on memory impaired older adults. *Clinical Gerontologist, 32*(4), 389-394.

Heckmann, J. G., Stössel, C., Lang, C. J. G., Neundörfer, B., Tomandl, B., & Hummel, T. (2005). Taste disorders in acute stroke: A prospective observational study on taste disorders in 102 stroke patients. *Stroke, 36*(8), 1690-1694.

Hosseini, S. A., Fallahpour, M., Sayadi, M., Gharib, M., & Haghgoo, H. (2012). The impact of mental practice on stroke patients' postural balance. *Journal of Neurological Sciences, 322,* 263-267.

Hsieh, C. L., Nelson, D. L., Smith, D. A., & Peterson, C. Q. (1996). A comparison of performance in added-purpose occupations and rote exercise for dynamic standing balance in persons with hemiplegia. *American Journal of Occupational Therapy, 50*(1), 10-16.

Hubbard, I. J., Parsons, M. W., Neilson, C., & Carey, L. M. (2009). Task-specific training: Evidence for and translation to clinical practice. *Occupational Therapy International, 16*(3-4), 175-189.

Imperatore, B. E., Reinoso, G., Chang, M. C., & Bodison, S. (2012). Proprioceptive processing difficulties among children with autism spectrum disorders and developmental disabilities. *American Journal of Occupational Therapy, 66*(5), 621-624.

James, C., Miller, L. J., Schaaf, R., Nielsene, D. M., & Schoen, S. A. (2011). Phenotypes within sensory modulation dysfunction. *Comprehensive Psychiatry 52,* 715-724.

Javier, N. S. C., & Montagnini, M. L. (2011). Rehabilitation of the hospice and palliative care patient. *Journal of Palliative Medicine, 14*(5), 638-648.

Latham, N., Anderson, C., Bennett, D., & Stretton, C. (2003). Progressive resistance strength training for physical disability in older people. *Cochrane Database of Systematic Reviews, 2,* CD002759.

Leland, N. E., Elliott, S. J., O'Malley, L., & Murphy, S. L. (2012). Occupational therapy in fall prevention: Current evidence and future directions. *The American Journal of Occupational Therapy, 66*(2), 149-160.

Levy, L. L., & Burns, T. (2005). Cognitive disabilities reconsidered. In N. Katz (Ed.), *Cognition and occupation across the lifespan* (2nd ed.). Bethesda, MD: AOTA Press.

Li, F., Harmer, P., Fisher, K. J., McAuley, E., Chaumeton, N., Eckstrom, E., & Wilson N. L. (2005). Tai Chi and fall reductions in older adults: A randomized controlled trial. *Journals of Gerontology Series A, Biological Sciences and Medical Sciences, 60*(2), 187-194.

Lin, K. C., Cermak, S. A., Kinsbourne, M., & Trombly, C. A. (1996). Effects of left-sided movements on line bisection in unilateral neglect. *Journal of the International Neuropsychological Society, 2*(5), 404-411.

Lin, L. C., Wu, C. Y., Wei, T. H., Lee, C. Y., & Liu, J. S. Effects of modified constraint-induced movement therapy on reach-to-grasp movements and functional performance after chronic stroke: A randomized controlled study. *Clinical Rehabilitation, 21*(12), 1075-1086.

Lincoln, N. B., Majid, M. J., & Weyman, N. (2000). Cognitive rehabilitation for attention deficits following stroke. *Cochrane Database of Systematic Reviews, 4,* CD002842.

Liu, C., Becker, J., Ford, S., Heine, K., Scheidt, E., & Wilson, A. (2011) Effects of upper-extremity progressive resistance strength training in older adults: The missing picture. *Physical and Occupational Therapy in Geriatrics, 29*(4), 255-269.

Loetscher, T. and Lincoln, N. B., (2013) Cognitive rehabilitation for attention deficits following stroke. *Cochrane Database of Systematic Reviews,* 5.

Martin, M. C., Clare, M., Altgassen, A. M., Cameron, M. H., & Zehnder, F. (2011). Cognition-based interventions for healthy older people and people with mild cognitive impairment. *Cochrane Review, 1,* CD006220.

Mathieux, R., Marotte, H., Battistini, L., Sarrazin, A., Berthier, M., & Miossec, P. (2009). Early occupational therapy programme increases hand grip strength at 3 months: Results from a randomised, blind, controlled study in early rheumatoid arthritis. *Annals of the Rheumatic Diseases, 68*(3), 400-403.

McEwen, S. E., Polatajko, H. J., Huijbregts, M. P. J., & Ryan, J. D. (2010). Inter-task transfer of meaningful, functional skills following a cognitve-based treatment: Results of three multiple baseline design experiments in adults with chronic stroke. *Neuropsychological Rehabilitation, 20*(4), 541-561.

McHugh, G. & Warren, A. (2009). A report into cognitive intervention strategies with older adults with cognitive impairment: Recommendations for occupational therapy practice. *Irish Journal of Occupational Therapy, 37*(1), 30-37.

Miller, L. J., Anzalone, M. E., Lane, S. J., Cermak, S. A., & Osten, E. T. (2007). Concept evolution in sensory integration: A proposed nosology for diagnosis. *American Journal of Occupational Therapy, 61*(2), 135-140.

Miller, L. K., Chester, R., & Jerosch-Herold, C. (2012). Effects of sensory reeducation programs on functional hand sensibility after median and ulnar repair: A systematic review. *Journal of Hand Therapy, 25* (3), 297-307.

Mitchell, S., Bradley, V. A., Welch, J. L., & Britton, P. G. (1990). Coma arousal procedures: A therapeutic intervention in the treatment of head injury. *Brain Injury, 4*(3), 273-279.

Miyahara, M., & Wafer, A. (2004). Clinical intervention for children with developmental coordination disorder: A multiple case study. *Adapted Physical Activity Quarterly, 21*(3), 281-300.

Neistadt, M. E. (1992). Occupational therapy treatments for constructional deficits. *American Journal of Occupational Therapy, 46*(2), 141-148.

Neistadt, M. E. (1994). The effects of different treatment activities on functional fine motor coordination in adults with brain injury. *American Journal of Occupational Therapy, 48*(10), 877-882.

Nelson, D. L., Konosky, K., Fleharty, K., Webb, R., Newer, K., Hazboun, V. P. ... Licht, B. C. (1999). The effects of an occupationally embedded exercise on bilaterally assisted supination in persons with hemiplegia. *American Journal of Occupational Therapy, 50*(8), 639-646.

Neumann, C., Tsioulos, K., Merkomidis, C., Salam, M., Clark, A., & Philpott, C. (2012), Validation study of the "Sniffin' Sticks" olfactory test in a British population: a preliminary communication. *Clinical Otolaryngology, 37*(1), 23-27.

Nordin, S., Monsch, A. U., & Murphy, C. (1995). Unawareness of smell loss in normal aging and Alzheimer's disease: Discrepancy between self-reported and diagnosed smell sensitivity. *Journals of Gerontology Series B. Psychological Sciences and Social Sciences, 50*(4), P187-P192.

Nussbaum, P. (2003). *Brain health and wellness.* Tarentum, PA: Word Association Publishers.

O'Brien, J., & Savoyski, J. (2006). *Application of motor control and motor learning concepts in pediatric occupational therapy practice.* Charlotte, NC: American Occupational Therapy Association National Conference.

Oh, H., & Seo, W. (2003). Sensory stimulation programme to improve recovery in comatose patients. *Journal of Clinical Nursing, 12*(3), 394-404.

Ownsworth, T., Fleming, J., Desbois, J., Strong, J., & Kuipers, P. (2006). A metacognitive contextual intervention to enhance error awareness and functional outcome following traumatic brain injury: A single case experimental design. *Journal of the International Neuropsychological Society, 12*(1), 54-63.

Pankow, L., Luchins, D., Studebaker, J., & Chettleburgh, D. (2004). Evaluation of a vision rehabilitation program for older adults with visual impairment. *Topics in Geriatric Rehabilitation, 20*(3), 223-232.

Partnership for Healthy Aging (2009). *Replication report: Matter of balance.* Portland, ME: Author.

Perlmutter, M. S., Bhorade, A., Gordon, M., Hollingsworth, H. H., & Baum, M. C. (2010). Cognitive, visual, auditory, and emotional factors that affect participation in older adults. *American Journal of Occupational Therapy, 64*(4), 570-579.

Peterson, E. W., & Clemson, L. (2008). Understanding the role of occupational therapy in fall prevention for community-dwelling older adults. *OT Practice, 13*(3), CE1-CE8.

Polatajko, H. J., & Mandich, A. (2004). *Enabling occupation in children: The cognitive orientation to daily occupational performance.* Ottawa, Ontario, Canada: CAOT Publications.

Pollock, A., Baer, G., Pomeroy, V., & Langhorne, P. (2007). Physiotherapy treatment approaches for the recovery of postural control and lower limb function following stroke. *Cochrane Database of Systemic Reviews, 1,* CD001920.

Prochaska, J. O., & Velicer, W. F. (1997). The transtheoretical model of health behavioral change. *American Journal of Health Promotion, 12*(1), 38-48.

Proto, D., Pella, R. D., Hill, B. D., & Gouvier, W. D. (2009). Assessment and rehabilitation of acquired visuospatial and proprioceptive deficits associated with visuospatial neglect. *NeuroRehabilitation, 24*(2), 145-157.

Rand, D., Weiss, P. L., & Katz, N. (2009). Training multitasking in a virtual supermarket: A novel intervention after stroke. *American Journal of Occupational Therapy, 63,* 535-542. doi: 10.5014/ajot.63.5.535

Robnett, R. H. (2010). The psychological, behavioral, and cognitive aspects of aging. In R. H. Robnett & W. C. Chop (Eds.), *Gerontology for the health care professional* (2nd ed.). Sudbury, MA: Jones and Bartlett.

Roley, S. S., Clark, G. F., Bissell, J., Brayman, S. J., & Commission on Practice. (2003). Applying sensory integration framework in educationally related occupational therapy practice. *American Journal of Occupational Therapy, 57*(6), 652-659.

Rosen, S., & Scott, J. B. (2003). Behavior management strategies for students with autism. *OT Practice, 8*(11), 16-20.

Schaaf, R. C., & Davies, P. L. (2010). Evolution of the sensory integration frame of reference. *American Journal of Occupational Therapy, 64*(3), 363-367.

Sheff, A. (2010). In the clinic: Meeting the needs of clients with hearing impairments. *OT Practice, 15*(8), 7-8, 21.

Szafron, S. H. (2011). Physical, mental, and spiritual approaches to managing pain in older clients. *OT Practice, 16*(3), CE1-CE8.

Schmidt, J., Fleming, J., Ownsworth, T., Lannin, N., & Khan, A. (2012) Feedback interventions for improving self-awareness after brain injury: A protocol for a pragmatic randomised controlled trial. *Australian Occupational Therapy Journal, 59*(2), 138-146.

Schmidt, J., Lannin, N., Fleming, J., & Ownsworth, T. (2011). Feedback interventions for impaired self-awareness following brain injury: A systematic review. *Journal of Rehabilitation Medicine, 43*(8), 673-680.

Schoessow, K., (2010). Shifting from compensation to participation: a model for occupational therapy in low vision. *British Journal of Occupational Therapy, 73*(4),160-169.

Shumway-Cook, A., & Woollacott, M. H. (2007). *Motor control: Translating research into clinical practice* (3rd ed.). Philadelphia, PA: Lippincott Williams & Wilkins.

Singh, A., Stewart, A. Franzsen, d., & MacKay-Lyons, M. (2011). Energy expenditures of dressing in patients with stroke. *International Journal of Therapy & Rehabilitation, 18(12),* 683-693.

Smallfield, S., Clem, K., & Myers, A. (2013) Occupational therapy interventions to improve the reading ability of older adults with low vision: A systematic review. *The American Journal of Occupational Therapy, 67(3),* 288-295.

Smith, S. A., Press, B., Koenig, K. P., & Kinnealey, M. (2005). Effect of sensory integration intervention on self-stimulating and self-injurious behaviors. *American Journal of Occupational Therapy, 59*(4), 418-425.

Sohlberg, M. M., & Mateer, C. A. (2001). *Cognitive rehabilitation: An integrative neuropsychological approach.* New York, NY: Guilford Press.

Stanos, S. (2012). Focused review of interdisciplinary pain rehabilitation programs for chronic pain management. *Current Pain & Headache Reports, 16*(2), 147-152.

Stedman's concise medical dictionary for the health professions (3rd ed.). (1997). Baltimore, MD: Lippincott Williams & Wilkins.

Taber's cyclopedic medical dictionary (20th ed.). (2001). Philadelphia, PA: F.A. Davis Company.

Taylor-Piliae, R. E., Haskell, W. L., Stotts, N. A., & Froehlicher, E. S. (2006). Improvement in balance, strength, and flexibility after 12 weeks of Tai Chi exercise in ethnic Chinese adults with cardiovascular disease risk factors. *Alternative Therapies in Health & Medicine, 12*(2), 50-58.

Thorpe, D. E., & Valvano, J. (2002). The effects of knowledge of performance and cognitive strategies on motor skill learning in children with cerebral palsy. *Pediatric Physical Therapy, 14*(1), 2-15.

Toglia, J. P. (2005). A dynamic interactional approach to cognitive rehabilitation. In N. Katz (Ed.), *Cognition and occupation across the life span* (pp. 29-72). Bethesda, MD: AOTA Press.

Toglia, J. P., Rodger, S. A., & Polatajko, H. J. (2012). Anatomy of cognitive strategies: A therapist's primer for enabling occupational performance. *Canadian Journal of Occupational Therapy, 79,* 225-236.

Trombly, C. (1993). Anticipating the future: Assessment of occupational function. *American Journal of Occupational Therapy, 47*(3), 253-257.

Tse, D. W., & Spaulding, S. J. (1998). Review of motor control and motor learning: Implications for occupational therapy with individuals with Parkinson's disease. *Physical and Occupational Therapy In Geriatrics, 15*(3), 19-38.

Vlok, E. D., Smit, N, E., & Bester, J. (2011). A developmental approach: A framework for the development of an integrated visual perception program. *South African Journal of Occupational Therapy, 41*(3), 25-33.

Walker, K. F. (2004). Jean Ayres. In K. F. Walker & F. M. Ludwig (Eds.), *Perspectives on theory for the practice of occupational therapy* (pp. 145-236). Austin, TX: PRO ED.

Warren, M. (1993). A hierarchical model for evaluation and treatment of visual perception dysfunction in adult acquired brain injury, part 1. *American Journal of Occupational Therapy, 47*(1), 42-54.

Watling, R., & Schwartz, I. S. (2004). Understanding and implementing positive reinforcement as an intervention strategy for children with disabilities. *American Journal of Occupational Therapy, 58*(1), 113-116.

Weiss, A., Suzuki, T., Bean, J., & Fielding, R. A. (2000). High intensity strength training improves strength and functional performance after stroke. *Archives of Physical Medicine and Rehabilitation, 79*(4), 369-376.

Weisser-Pike, O. & Kaldenberg, J. (2010), Occupational therapy approaches to facilitate productive aging for individuals with low vision. *OT Practice, 153*), CE1-CE8.

Whitall, J., McCombe Waller, S., Silver, K. H., & Macko, R. F. (2000). Repetitive bilateral arm training with rhythmic auditory cueing improves motor function in chronic hemiparetic stroke. *Stroke, 31*(10), 2390-2395.

Wu, C. Y., Lin, K. C., Chen, H. C., Chen, I. H., & Hong, W. I. (2007). Effects of modified constraint-induced movement therapy on movement kinematics and daily function in patients with stroke: A kinematic study of motor control mechanisms. *Neurorehabilitation and Neural Repair, 21*(5), 460-466.

Wu, C. Y., Trombly, C. A., Lin. K. C., & Tickle-Degnen, L. (2000). A kinematic study of contextual effects on reaching performance in persons with and without stroke: Influences of object availability. *Archives of Physical Medicine and Rehabilitation, 81*(1), 95-101.

Xu, K., Wang, L., Mai, J., & He, L. (2012). Efficacy of constraint-induced movement therapy and electrical stimulation on hand function of children with hemiplegic cerebral palsy: a controlled clinical trial. *Disability & Rehabilitation, 34*(4), 337-346.

Zasler, N. D., McNeny, R., & Heywood, P. G. (1992). Rehabilitation management of olfactory and gustatory dysfunction following brain injury. *Journal of Head Trauma Rehabilitation, 7*(1), 66-75.

Zijlstra, G. A., van Haastregt, J. C., van Rossum, E., van Eijk, J. T., Yardley, L., & Kempen, G. I. (2007). Interventions to reduce the fear of falling in community-living older people: A systematic review. *Journal of the American Geriatrics Society, 55*(4), 603-615.

Zoltan, B. (2007). *Vision, perception, and cognition: A manual for the evaluation and treatment of the adult with acquired brain injury* (4th ed.). Thorofare, NJ: SLACK Incorporated.

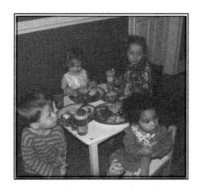

25

INTERVENTIONS TO ENHANCE OCCUPATIONAL PERFORMANCE IN ACTIVITIES OF DAILY LIVING AND INSTRUMENTAL ACTIVITIES OF DAILY LIVING

Michael E. Roberts, MS, OTR/L

ACOTE STANDARDS EXPLORED IN THIS CHAPTER

B.5.1–B.5.6

KEY VOCABULARY

- **Activities of daily living (ADL):** Activities directed toward caring for one's own body; also referred to as basic activities of daily living (BADL) or personal activities of daily living (PADL).
- **Adaptation:** When practitioners decrease the demands of the environment and task to meet the client's expected skill level after remediation.
- **Instrumental activities of daily living (IADL):** Activities that involve interaction with the environment or community, such as pet care, meal preparation, or financial management.

- **Maintenance:** Ensuring continued competency through the use of external devices, templates, or skill retraining despite expectations of potential or eventual declines in occupational performance.
- **Performance context:** Environment in which occupational performance occurs, including the physical environment, available resources, sensory input, temporal and societal influences, or the presence or availability of caregivers.

Jacobs, K., MacRae, N., & Sladyk, K. (Eds.).
*Occupational Therapy Essentials for
Clinical Competence, Second Edition* (pp. 333-346).
© 2014 SLACK Incorporated.

Introduction

Occupational performance in activities of daily living (ADL) and instrumental activities of daily living (IADL) serve as the foundation for expression of meaning and identity for clients of occupational therapy practitioners (American Occupational Therapy Association [AOTA], 2008; Christiansen, 1999). It follows logically, therefore, that evaluation, intervention, and outcomes related to these areas of occupation are of critical importance to effective service delivery. Indeed, this focus on effective self-management of these areas of occupation has served as the defining core of the profession since its earliest days (Meyer, 1922).

Assessment of Activity of Daily Living and Instrumental Activity of Daily Living Performance

Evaluation of ADL and IADL performance is composed of an initial occupational profile and a more focused performance analysis, frequently involving direct observation and standardized assessments (AOTA, 2008). During this first phase of developing and implementing the intervention plan, the frame of reference or model of practice most appropriate for the client is selected, client priorities and perspective are evaluated and incorporated, and the influence of the context of performance is assessed. This process must be ultimately directed by the needs of each client and his or her input. The frame of reference or model of practice must be selected exclusively by an assessment of client needs and capacities, not practitioner preference. Evaluation of client priorities drive treatment selection and goal setting. Accurate assessment of client perspective and context are critical to ensuring the durability and applicability of goals and treatment plans throughout the continuum of care.

The occupational profile frequently includes questions such as "Tell me about your typical day," or "What activities or roles are most important to you?" or "How is your life different because of your disease/trauma/life change?" These questions allow for identification by the client of the most typical patterns of performance, habits, or roles that compose their occupational existence. Follow-up questions or active listening techniques can elicit important information about client priorities, perceived obstacles to effective performance, or adaptive/maladaptive strategies for improving performance. In addition, occupational history, influence of caregivers or other contextual issues, and client goals may be understood more effectively through strategic use of initial interviews with clients. It is important to remember that

effective use of the occupational profile and initial interview period must result in specific, occupation-focused priorities in order to result in an effective intervention plan (Neistadt, 1995). This occupation-directed outcome is important for defining our profession for our clients and continues as a challenge to practitioners in current practice (McAndrew, McDermott, Vitzakovitch, Warunek, & Holm, 1999).

The next step in the evaluation of ADL and IADL performance is to determine more specifically how to focus the practitioner efforts through analysis of occupational performance (AOTA, 2008). Informed by the occupational profile, evidence-based practice strategies, and the frame of reference or model of practice most effective for the client, performance is directly observed in the most appropriate context, using standardized assessments where possible (AOTA, 2008). Ideally, tasks such as meal preparation, laundry management, bathing, or dressing are observed and performance assessed in the environment most commonly used by the client. In certain clinical settings or due to particular medical issues, this is not always possible. In these instances, the alternative context must be specifically documented in order to provide the most complete picture of ADL and IADL performance. Observation of performance in a clinical context rather than a client's usual or home context is preferable to relying exclusively on self-report of function. Research comparing standardized assessments with self-reported IADL status suggests that greater accuracy is obtained through performance-based measures (Hilton, Fricke, & Unsworth, 2001), as practitioners may expect.

The order or priority given to assessment of specific performance skills, performance patterns, or client factors depends on the needs and priorities of the client. Utilization of an occupation-focused, or "top-down" approach, may be effective for certain clients, whereas a "bottom-up," or component-based approach, may be best for other clients (Trombly, 1993, p. 253); yet others may receive the most effective treatment through assessment of the client's context and its impact (Weinstock-Zlotnick & Hinojosa, 2004). For example, in a female client who presents with diabetic peripheral polyneuropathy, an assessment from a top-down approach may identify decreased client satisfaction with her role as an independent grandparent who cooks brunch for her family every Sunday morning. Her occupational therapist may determine from the occupational profile to perform a more focused assessment of safety with sharp items in the kitchen, foot care as part of her morning self-care routine, and functional mobility assessments in the kitchen during meal preparation to directly identify the roles or occupational priorities most important to this client. A bottom-up approach may also be determined to be the best for this client, including standardized assessments of balance, peripheral sensation, safety awareness, or other foundational skills, which when addressed in the intervention plan are expected to result in resolution of the larger occupational performance issues. The client may benefit most from a contextual assessment first, evaluating the effectiveness of resource utilization, impact of caregivers, and influence of the physical, social, cultural, or temporal environments on the client's performance of her Sunday morning brunch routine.

The most effective approach is the one that is most effective in meeting the needs of the client, not the approach with which the practitioner is most comfortable or the one that is routinely used in the setting where assessment occurs. Rather, effectiveness in evaluation depends on the "fit" of the approach to the client (Weinstock-Zlotnick & Hinojosa, 2004) while maintaining the focus on occupation inherent in occupational therapy practice.

Nonstandardized assessments of ADL and IADL performance can provide valuable information for intervention plan development, but selection of a frame of reference or model of practice, or an intention of adherence to evidence-based practice, often necessitates the incorporation of standardized assessments of performance of basic and instrumental ADL. It is important to note that standardized assessments need not be full self-care assessments in order to inform intervention planning. Standardized assessments of client factors may prove predictive of self-care performance, such as deficits in categorization and deductive reasoning logically proving effective predictors of IADL performance (Goverover & Hinojosa, 2002).

The following are a selection of standardized assessments of ADL and IADL performance in current use in occupational therapy clinical practice:

- **Arnadottir OT-ADL Neurobehavioral Evaluation (A-ONE).** The A-ONE is a two-part observational assessment. Part 1 focuses on ADL performance in dressing, grooming/hygiene, transfers/mobility, feeding, and communication. Part 2 correlates 11 areas of impairment with ADL performance to assist the practitioners in identifying the most likely neurological deficit responsible for the observed performance deficits (Arnadottir, 1990).

- **Assessment of Living Skills and Resources (ALSAR).** The ALSAR is an interview-based assessment for IADL that incorporates an appreciation for the impact of available resource utilization as a mitigating or exacerbating factor in determining the true relevance and prioritization of IADL dysfunction (Williams et al., 1991).

- **Assessment of Motor and Process Skills (AMPS).** Fifty-six tasks typical to IADL routines of children, adolescents, or adults have been deconstructed to allow standardized ratings on specific motor and process skills associated with each task. The occupational therapy practitioner assists the client in identifying several typical tasks from the daily IADL routine for the client. Of these, a small number of AMPS components are recommended and observed. Competency in performance is assessed, and prediction of future IADL function is possible (Fisher, 1999).

- **Canadian Occupational Performance Measure (COPM).** This semi-structured interview is used to identify the client's perception of his or her occupational performance in self-care, productive, and leisure tasks. The five areas identified by the client as most important are rated for performance in addition to satisfaction with performance. As a directly client-centered assessment, the COPM can assist the occupational therapy practitioner in tracking perceived effectiveness of the intervention plan (Law et al., 2005).

- **Functional Independence Measure (FIM).** Used widely to assess functional performance in physical dysfunction settings and adapted for use with children as the WeeFIM, the FIM uses a seven-point scale to describe the amount of assistance required for the subject to perform 18 tasks relating to self-care, cognition, and communication. This assessment is multidisciplinary and is part of the Uniform Data System for Medical Rehabilitation (UDSMR, 2000).

- **Klein-Bell Activities of Daily Living Scale (Klein-Bell).** One hundred and seventy subtasks of dressing, elimination, mobility, hygiene and bathing, emergency communication, and eating are rated and weighted according to relative importance and difficulty. Observation and scoring results in a score as a percentage of the potential maximum score. This assessment may be used with children and adults (Klein & Bell, 1979).

- **Kohlman Evaluation of Living Skills (KELS).** Utilized primarily to determine the likelihood of safe, independent function in the community for clients with psychiatric diagnoses and/or cognitive dysfunction, this assessment combines interview and observation to determine the number of 18 assessed self-care areas with which a client requires assistance. The assessment covers self-care, safety/health, work and leisure, money management, transportation, and telephone use (McGourty, 1979).

- **Minimum Data Set (MDS).** Used for residents in long-term care and covering a large and comprehensive view of the client's health and function, occupational therapy practitioners are generally contributing to only a few sections, primarily section G, which relates to mobility and ADL/IADL performance (Nelson & Glass, 1999). Performance of components must be observed, and scores must represent the resident's performance at his or her status of greatest need across all hours within the previous 7 days (Centers for Medicare and Medicaid Services [CMS], 2005). Sections of the MDS are also used in determination of placement of cases in resource utilization groups (RUGs) in skilled nursing facilities, which impacts reimbursement rates for the facility.

- **Occupational Self Assessment (OSA).** Designed to be used within the Model of Human Occupation, the OSA is a self-report assessment that measures client satisfaction in performance of tasks and activities as well as perceived mastery of his or her environment. This data is then used in collaborative intervention planning sessions to identify client factors, activities, and environmental issues of greatest concern for that particular client. Understandably, this assessment requires a requisite level of insight and cognitive function in the subject in order to procure useful information (Kielhofner & Forsyth, 2001).

- **Outcome and Assessment Information Set (OASIS).** Sixteen ADL/IADL performance subtests are included in this very comprehensive home-care assessment. Observation of status is considered best for treatment planning, but assessment strategies are not highly regimented. Questions on this assessment are used to determine reimbursement based on acuity, functional assistance required, complexity, and other factors (Center for Health Services and Policy Research [CHSPR], 1998).

- **Performance Assessment of Self-Care Skills (PASS).** This assessment is used with adults to evaluate performance in functional mobility, home management, and basic ADL, with differing protocols depending on whether assessment occurs at the client's home or in the clinic of the assessing occupational therapy clinician (Rogers & Holm, 1994). Scoring includes subtask breakdown, which is a valuable tool in intervention planning.

- **Routine Task Inventory (RTI).** For practitioners operating within Allen's cognitive disability model, this assessment relates observed or reported self-care performance to Allen's cognitive levels (Allen, Earhart, & Blue, 1992). The RTI also provides expected performance of tasks correlated to each applicable cognitive level. This assessment provides limited directive instructions on administration and recommends not using self-report of status with lower-functioning clients.

- **Safe At Home.** This assessment is specific to safety and safety awareness of clients in the home environment, involving 12 test items related to typical environmental hazards in the home. The Safe At Home assessment is intended for use with adults (Robnett, Hopkins, & Kimball, 2002).

- **Satisfaction With Performance Scaled Questionnaire (SPSQ).** Subjects for this assessment report the percentage of time in the past 6 months that they were satisfied by their performance in 46 ADL/IADL tasks, differentiated into two subscales: home management and social/community function. Community-dwelling adults can use the information in collaboration with their occupational therapy practitioners to identify and prioritize potential areas of IADL intervention (Yerxa, Burnett-Beaulieu, Stocking, & Azen, 1988).

Contextual Issues With Assessment

In the current practice environment, there are a number of factors that can impact or influence assessments and outcomes, and they must be considered in anticipation of developing a treatment plan. A necessary consideration in contemporary practice is reimbursement (see Chapter 39). Whether discussing a prospective payment system (PPS), RUGs, individual education plans (IEPs), health maintenance organizations (HMOs), managed care organizations (MCOs), preferred provider options (PPOs), or any other configuration of reimbursement for occupational therapy services, practitioners must strive for effective outcomes and optimal treatment planning regardless of payer source (AOTA, 2000).

Despite expected adherence to the AOTA Code of Ethics, some discrepancies have surfaced (see Chapter 48). One typical example is research describing functional outcomes for clients with a cerebrovascular accident (CVA) who receive rehabilitation services. Those who utilized a Medicare HMO instead of the traditional fee-for-service plans for their treatment received fewer therapy and medical specialist visits but more home care visits, made less progress in functional performance, and were more likely to be living in a nursing home 1 year after stroke (Kramer et al., 2000). Ideally, practitioners are developing intervention plans as if they were "blind" to reimbursement issues, but incorporating an appreciation of expected utilization limits may help ensure equality of outcomes across payer sources.

Practitioners must also be aware of how they are perceived by their clients and their clients' perceptions of their own function because these may impact the data collected in assessments and thereby impact intervention planning. Mothers who are engaged in the IADL of child rearing report that practitioners who present with a more relaxed and friendly demeanor are perceived as having better insight into the daily routine of child rearing and having a greater capacity to "tailor" services to the specific needs of the family (Thompson, 1998). This fact encourages practitioners to be aware of their interactive styles from the development of the intervention plan and to reassess the effectiveness of their therapeutic use of self through the intervention process.

Practitioners may also be affected by their own prejudices regarding settings, populations, and ADL/IADL function. Misguided generalizations may negatively impact the capacity of an intervention plan to most directly and efficiently enhance the functional independence and quality of life for our clients. Research has identified that residents in long-term care facilities perceived themselves to present with significantly higher levels of function than those documented by practitioners (Atwood, Holm, & James, 1994). Dunford, Missiuna, Street, and Sibert (2005) reported that children with a developmental coordination disorder described concerns regarding limitations in performance of self-care and leisure activities, although these deficits were largely not identified for these children by parents or teachers. Self-awareness regarding preconceptions in assessment of clients becomes a matter of ensuring a professional level of intervention, and this information must be incorporated into the assessment and intervention planning processes.

The environment utilized for assessment and intervention may also affect results of assessment and intervention. As described earlier, assessment in the client's most commonly used performance context is ideal, whereas observation of performance, regardless of setting, is still preferable to relying solely on self-report of status. Some inpatient facilities invest significant resources into replicating, as closely as possible, contextually appropriate environments for their clients, with the expectation that contextually appropriate settings lead to contextually appropriate carryover. This theory, however, has not been borne out. Richardson, Law, Wishart, and Guyatt (2000) demonstrated that no significant functional performance difference was achieved with the use of contextually appropriate intervention settings. Davis, Hoppes, and Chesbro (2005) reported that there is no substitute for assessment in clients' homes (their most personally relevant context), wherein clients with dementia and IADL dysfunction were found to be largely similar in functional profile, except that clients exhibited higher levels of motor skills in their homes.

Intervention

Once evaluation data are obtained, an intervention plan can be developed that includes objectives, expected time frames for goal completion, roles for practitioners, and an evidence-based intervention approach within the chosen model of practice or frame of reference (AOTA, 2008). Throughout implementation of the intervention plan, a constant treatment outcome "feedback loop" informs an evaluation of the plan's efficacy, including not only functional progress with ADL and IADL but also the effectiveness of changes to the available resources, performance context, or therapeutic use of self strategies (AOTA, 2008).

Once the evaluation data has been compiled and the objectives determined in collaboration with the client and other members of the client's health care team, the most appropriate intervention approach must be selected. The practice framework (AOTA, 2008) describes five approaches: create or promote, establish or restore, maintain, modify, and prevent. Each of these approaches is used in combination with some or all of the others, depending on the client's needs.

- **Create or promote.** The *create* or *promote* approach, also described as health promotion, involves interventions that facilitate enhancement of health and function in natural contexts of life (AOTA, 2008). This approach may involve utilization of universal design strategies for living spaces or offering cooking classes to enhance nutrition, socialization, and mobility practice in an assisted living facility.

- **Establish or restore.** The *establish, restore,* or *remediation* approach seeks to ensure acquisition and mastery of skills that are absent, lost, or impaired (AOTA, 2008). This approach may include establishing a well-balanced and effective morning ADL routine for a client with a chronic disease, enhancement of activity tolerance in standing for meal preparation or clean-up, or addressing limitations of fine motor control and hand strength to allow return to independence with grooming and oral care after carpal tunnel release surgery.

- **Maintain.** The *maintenance* approach, although frowned upon in documentation for rehabilitation settings, is also important for ensuring maximal ADL and IADL performance because its implementation is based on an assumption that without these interventions, occupational performance would decrease (AOTA, 2008). For example, practitioners using this approach may use magnifiers and templates to allow clients with low vision to complete budgeting, write checks, or develop grocery lists. Practitioners may teach the use of timers and pillboxes to clients with chronic mental illness to ensure effective medication management once they are discharged from an inpatient clinical setting. This approach may also be used to train clients with amyotrophic lateral sclerosis (ALS) in energy conservation and work simplification to delay the outpacing of ADL demands with declining activity tolerance.

- **Modify.** The *modify* or *adaptation* approach (AOTA, 2008) is used quite frequently in rehabilitation settings. In this setting, practitioners use adaptation to decrease the demands of the environment and task to meet the client's expected skill level after remediation. This approach is evident when practitioners teach the use of a sock aid after a client's hip replacement surgery, modify workspaces to maximize ergonomic fit of the client and task, or train clients with chronic obstructive pulmonary disease (COPD) in the use of tub seats, handheld showers, and long-handled sponges to decrease trunk flexion and conserve energy during bathing. Given this information, it is important to use adaptive equipment and adaptations judiciously because too many changes to the home environment, too many new strategies at once, or too great an expenditure of resources to ensure success with adaptations may defeat the initial purpose. The social, developmental, and cultural impact of adaptations and adaptive equipment must be taken into consideration before time and effort are carved out of the intervention plan for their training and use.

- **Prevent.** *Prevention* is also utilized as an intervention approach in clients and populations determined to be at risk. Teaching communication skills to school-age children to reduce school violence, teaching proper body mechanics during home maintenance and laundry tasks for clients with chronic low back pain, or incorporating effective foot care into the ADL routines of clients with diabetes are all examples of preventative approaches with at-risk clients.

As described previously, these approaches are not necessarily mutually exclusive, and most effective intervention plans incorporate all of the approaches. For instance, a client with rheumatoid arthritis who presents with pain in both hands with grooming tasks, difficulties with lower body ADL due to limited joint range of motion and low back pain, difficulty with food preparation, opening pill bottles, and writing checks due to hand deformities may require all of the approaches in order to achieve ADL and IADL independence and improved quality of life. This client may require joint protection retraining to *prevent* future deterioration of joint function. The client may use an occupational therapy selected or fabricated upper extremity splint to *prevent* further deterioration of joints in his or her hands, as well as to *maintain* range and alignment in the hands at this point. The demands of the client's environment may be *modified* by introducing adaptive equipment that decreases the demands of tasks to meet the client's current status, such as an adapted built-up toothbrush to decrease the pain and coordination demands of oral care tasks or a dressing stick to reduce the trunk range and low back pain demands of lower body dressing. The practitioner may also assist the client in establishing a new daily routine of ADL and IADL to enhance joint protection and energy conservation strategies for daily living tasks that must be completed by the client. Finally, the creation of adaptive equipment or strategies within the client's home

environment may reduce dysfunction and pain and may promote greater participation and engagement in occupations that enhance functional independence, such as money management, medication management, laundry and clothing management, or other potentially difficult IADL tasks.

As shown in the example described previously, a number of instruments are used by the practitioner in conjunction with the client. These instruments have classifications depending on their complexity and intention. Preparatory activities are interventions that help a client prepare for functional performance. These may include splinting, modalities, or joint mobilization. In the arthritis example, a practitioner may don or doff a splint for the client, apply moist heat or paraffin to the client's hands, or perform manual joint distraction to enhance joint range of motion and reduce pain. These are not specifically occupation-based activities; however, if they are completed in advance of meal preparation retraining or grooming retraining and the results of the preparatory activities enhance and improve performance, they therefore have been used effectively and appropriately by the practitioner.

Some activities used in occupational therapy are described as purposeful activities, which achieve movement along therapeutic continua through engagement in goal-directed activities (AOTA, 2008). Practice with durable medical equipment for bathroom mobility, such as grab bars, tub seats, or commodes would qualify as purposeful activities. These practice sessions addressing components of ADL and IADL are intended to enhance functional performance but have the added benefit of additional focus on the most troublesome components leading to dysfunction, or breaking down occupational performance into manageable "pieces," without losing focus on ultimate functional independence for the client and his or her caregivers.

Occupation-based activities involve participation in the specific occupations identified by clients and practitioners as priorities to ensure independence and quality of life. Making a meal in the client's kitchen, training in donning and doffing the client's prosthesis, and practicing wheelchair-level toileting in the client's home bathroom are all examples of occupation-based activities used therapeutically. As expected, progression up the hierarchy of activities to occupation-based activities is often the goal of the intervention plan and an effective strategy for ADL/IADL retraining (Richards et al., 2005; Smallfield & Karges, 2009).

These different types of activities are then directed appropriately to address each of the components of the domain of occupational therapy. Client factors are addressed by adaptive equipment use, upper extremity orthosis construction and use, or preparatory methods such as joint distraction or modalities. Performance patterns are addressed by joint protection and energy conservation training. Contextual issues are addressed when making environmental changes, using adaptive devices, or addressing temporal issues in training with ADL and IADL routines. The use of upper extremity orthoses, adaptive equipment for lower body dressing, or enhancing body mechanics training may all change activity demands. Teaching joint protection strategies, practicing them, and providing informed feedback to the client would impact and improve performance skills. In this way, all components of the domain of occupational therapy may be addressed (AOTA, 2008). In fact, comprehensive interventions of this type, and of joint protection retraining specifically, have been reported to be effective occupational therapy interventions with clients with rheumatoid arthritis (Steultjens et al., 2004).

It is important to remember that these interventions may address several approaches or aspects of occupational therapy's domain at once, and that the goals of effectively selected occupational tasks address as many components of independence and quality of life as possible. For instance, in the previous example, an occupational therapist or occupational therapy assistant may address the client's difficulty with check writing through the use of an adapted writing implement and a more ergonomically correct writing environment. Addressing this relatively small area of the client's occupational performance may accomplish many objectives at once. Joint degradation may be reduced, pain may be reduced, the client's satisfaction with maintaining financial independence may enhance his or her quality of life and mood. Confidence in the occupational therapy team may improve, therefore enhancing the likelihood of carryover and success of other components of the intervention plan. In this way, an elegantly simple "melody" may enhance the overall effect of the occupational therapy intervention "symphony."

The previous example provides a description of ADL and IADL interventions for a client with a chronic disease. The domain remains the same for acute trauma and disease as well. For example, a client diagnosed with a left hemiparesis and left neglect after a stroke will require a number of different interventions from his or her occupational therapy team members. Given that all of the aspects of the occupational therapy domain will be affected in this clinical situation, a wide variety of interventions are possible. Evidence must be utilized to determine which of the interventions will most likely be of benefit to the client and family. Expected ADL and IADL dysfunctions for a client with left hemiparesis are many. Limited motor function will make bilateral self-care tasks (donning socks, tying shoes) very difficult. Clothing management during toileting, meal preparation, grooming, medication management, kitchen and bathroom mobility, transfers in the home environment, sexuality, safety with sharp items in the kitchen and temperatures in the bathroom, learning the use of adaptive equipment or strategies, attention to the left side for functional tasks, balance during functional transfers, and health maintenance of the left side of the body—all of these components of occupational performance may be negatively affected by the onset of the stroke. All of these may have different and changing priorities for the client. All of these may have dozens of different activities that are appropriate for use in intervention by practitioners with this client.

The ADL/IADL retraining process for more acute cases is the same as for chronic cases. The activity selection process depends on the evidence available, the frame of reference or model of practice, the resources available to the client, the client's priorities, and the impact of other contextual issues, such as service delivery issues or family concerns. For this population in particular, recent research describes the following components critical to successful occupational therapy intervention: the use of specific client-identified activities, the use of and training with appropriate adaptations, maximizing the familiarity of the context, providing feedback to improve performance, and providing ample practice with the activities (Guidetti & Ytterberg, 2011; Trombly & Ma, 2002).

To illustrate, a number of client characteristics may impact independence in bathing, which is an important and foundational ADL. The client may highly value the activity and prioritize it for treatment. The client's left hemiparesis, left neglect, and impaired sensation on the left side may negatively affect task completion, safety, and bathroom mobility. Family members may express specific concerns about their ability to use the resources available to them to assist in ensuring the client's independence in this activity. The client may be concerned about the expertise of the occupational therapy team, the efficacy of the bathing retraining plan, or the possibility of institutionalization, all lending expanded meaning to bathing as an occupation-based activity.

The inherent complexity of meaning of the activity within occupational performance for this client in this situation must be seen as an opportunity, not an obstacle, by the practitioners with whom this client works. One effective option for the occupational therapy team would be to incorporate the family members in the bathing retraining therapy sessions in as familiar a context as possible, given the clinical situation. If, for instance, the practitioner demonstrates the use of adaptations such as tub benches, handheld showers, long-handled sponges, long mirrors, or grab bars to the client and family during a bathing retraining session, a number of objectives are addressed. Primarily, the client's functional performance improves. This activity may also reinforce transfer retraining, skin inspection, or other health management strategies, enhancement of activity tolerance, sitting balance, attention to the affected side, problem solving and scanning retraining, or energy conservation strategies. Demonstrated success with occupational therapy retraining may also enhance self-esteem, build confidence in the occupational therapy team and intervention plan, reduce family concerns about functional outcomes, and enhance carryover of other components of the intervention plan. Utilizing self-care retraining to enhance functional performance directly is also borne out as the most effective strategy for enhancing ADL performance (Walker et al., 2004). With effective application of occupational therapy principles and a specific focus of intervention utilizing ADL retraining, positive results can be achieved in this population with dressing tasks (Christie, Bedford, & McCluskey, 2011) or general self-care and functional mobility (Landi et al., 2006; Sackley et al., 2006). A specific focus on intervention for personal ADL after CVA has even been shown in one review to significantly reduce the incidence of "poor outcomes" described as "death, deterioration or dependency in personal activities of daily living" in this population (Legg et al., 2007).

Both of these clinical examples demonstrate the richness of ADL and IADL tasks as modalities within the intervention plan, or as melodies within the occupational therapy intervention symphony. Because so many of these tasks are profoundly meaningful, defining, and personal for the clients, even the simplest of ADL or IADL tasks wield significant power to affect many or all aspects of occupational therapy's domain; therefore, they are invaluable instruments within the occupational therapy orchestra of potential interventions and strategies.

Therapeutic Outcomes

There are a number of different areas for intervention by practitioners in collaboration with their clients. Practitioners can incorporate movement along an adaptation–gradation continuum to match the demands of the retraining activity to the client's performance level and expected goals. An understanding of the performance skills that are intact may be used to enhance the skills that are lacking. Contexts must be understood and incorporated into treatment planning, especially available resources, influence of caregivers, the expected disease or recovery process, and other therapies active with the client. Performance patterns, habits, routines, and roles of the client also may be affected and therefore prioritized for intervention planning (AOTA, 2008). Communication skills, client insight, client goals/priorities, sociocultural and socioeconomic influences, setting, acuity, and developmental level are also important potentially impactful issues to be addressed and utilized in enhancing or focusing the collaboration between clinician and client to maximize the effectiveness of the intervention plan. Currently, new technologies are providing new opportunities for ADL/IADL interventions including neuroprostheses used with ADL retraining

(Hill-Hermann et al., 2008), electronic aids to daily living for clients with acquired brain injuries (Boman, Tham, Granqvist, Bartfai, & Hemmingsson, 2007), and virtual reality for community-based shopping tasks (Rand, Weiss, & Katz, 2009).

Each of these potential intervention-maximizing components has an influence on the effectiveness of the practitioner's efforts to improve the client's quality of life and move with the client toward functional independence. Not all of the components need to be in effect or be actively addressed at all times in all situations; however, it stands to reason that in order to "treat the whole person," practitioners should be utilizing or manipulating as many of these components at once with each intervention.

One way to envision this strategy is to picture each of the potential intervention components or influences as a musical instrument. Just as there are different kinds of music appropriate for different situations in life, different combinations of these components of ADL/IADL function are addressed in whole or in part depending on the client and the context. For instance, a relatively uncomplicated case, such as an otherwise well client status post an elective orthopedic procedure, may require a simpler melody or fewer instruments, like 1950s-style rock-and-roll. The instruments still need to work together in rhythm, tempo, and key, and be adaptable to the demands of the situation, but can match the complexity of the case more directly.

More complex clinical cases, such as a client who is socioeconomically disadvantaged, diagnosed with a chronic disease, and serves as caregiver to a spouse with a progressive neurological syndrome, will require more intricate interweaving of instruments. A highly skilled clinician "conductor" must ensure that all interventions are of one purpose, directing production of one elegant symphonic masterpiece where the varied, unique, and inherently complex components construct a whole greater than the sum of the parts—more Mozart than Buddy Holly. Regardless of situation or complexity, recruiting and effectively utilizing as many of the instruments as possible for each client will enhance the holistic, life-changing potential of each intervention plan and thereby ensure the most effective collaboration with clients in their efforts to achieve success in ADL and IADL performance.

Current Service Delivery Environment

The value of functional independence in self-care is appreciated not only by practitioners and their clients but also by regulators and purchasers of health care services. More outcome measures related to the efficacy of therapy and health care services in general are focused on function and quality of life, which are traditional practice domains of practitioners. For example, MDS data are collected on all residents of long-term care facilities that receive Medicare or Medicaid funding. Ninety percent of occupational therapists responding to a survey reported that they were involved in the MDS data collection in the long-term care facilities where they worked, mostly with subsections related to self-care and changes in ADL function (Nelson & Glass, 1999). Given the need for practitioners with this expertise, it is not surprising, therefore, that the change in Medicare reimbursement from a cost-based system to a patient-specific resource utilization system has been associated with a greater likelihood of receiving occupational therapy services for non-elderly institutional long-term care residents (Wodchis, Fries, & Pollack, 2004).

The value associated with self-care and quality of life is also increasingly appreciated by other clinical professionals with whom practitioners frequently collaborate. Multiple research articles describe how the inclusion of occupational therapy and their focus on ADL, self-care, and IADL interventions into interdisciplinary treatment teams enhance outcomes in function and quality of life (Gitlin et al., 2006; Miyai, 2012; Stark, Landsbaum, Palmer, Somerville, & Morris, 2009; Szanton et al., 2011), reduce caregiver burden (Graff et al., 2006), decrease length of inpatient stays (O'Brien, Bynon, Morarty, & Presness, 2012), and decrease the use of (and inherent cost of) home health aides for community-dwelling clients (Zingmark & Bernspång, 2011).

This appreciation extends beyond the many interdisciplinary collaborations, however. Lysaght & Wright (2005) suggested that in work-related practice settings, physical therapy approaches and interventions closely resembled those of occupational therapy practitioners. A psychiatric pilot study described the efficacy of a combined nursing case management and health management skills training program intended to enhance functional independence, independent living, and social functioning, which utilized caseworkers and nurses, not practitioners (Bartels et al., 2004). In other research, non–occupational therapy psychosocial programs focusing on promoting functional independence through the use of ADL retraining, client-centered practice, "skill elicitation," and group therapies were lauded as "innovations" in the care of residents with dementia in nursing homes (Haitsma & Ruckdeschel, 2001). Perhaps the most direct example is a description of a 1-week retreat for persons with multiple sclerosis staffed by physical therapists, who assessed participants on self-esteem, quality of life, and ADL self-care (Beatus, O'Neill, Townsend, & Robrecht, 2008). The results of their retreat described a significant increase in quality of life related to mental components, but also a lack of significant differences in self-esteem, physical components of quality of life, or functional independence.

These examples are important in that they describe an increased appreciation of professionals with whom practitioners collaborate for the traditional goals of occupational therapy's practice domain—some even attempting to expand their own practice domains to include these traditional occupational therapy goals. Two such examples are physical therapists attempting to expand their scope of practice to include "functional training in self-care and in home, community or work integration" (APTA, 2003) and athletic trainers claiming knowledge about implementation of return-to-work programs (Smith, 2006).

The increased appreciation for functional training in other professions is not a substitute, however, for the unique history, tradition, and skill set of occupational therapy practitioners that has been honed over generations, informed by evidence-based practice, and tempered through a client-centered approach. Current occupational therapy practice has been shown to uniquely enhance occupational functioning in recent research (Alexander, Bugge, & Hagen, 2001; Hagsten, Svensson, & Gardulf, 2004; Hastings, Gowans, & Watson, 2004; Walker et al., 2004). It should be noted, therefore, that appreciation for enhancing quality of life and functional independence among nonoccupational therapy practitioners is not a substitute for occupational therapy practitioners' unequalled expertise in addressing ADL and IADL performance.

Summary

Perhaps the most emblematic interventions utilized by occupational therapy practitioners are those involving basic and instrumental ADL. Effective evaluation and treatment of deficits in these occupational performance areas are critical to a client-centered approach, particularly because of their potential for expression of uniquely personal meaning for clients. Successful assessment and interventions related to these areas include standardized evaluations, clinical reasoning within an appropriate model of practice or frame of reference, effective use of proper strategies and approaches, and judicious application of an appreciation for the impact of contextual issues on occupational performance.

Student Self-Assessment

1.   IADL Group Discussion. Each of the following questions can be asked of students in groups, and then compiled answers can be presented to the rest

Case Study

Veronica, a 42-year-old married mother of two teenage daughters, had suffered from intractable right hip joint pain for many months. She had worked in a state government office for about 8 years but was increasingly unable to work because of the pain. Doctors suspected osteoarthritis despite its solitary presentation in her hip. She agreed to an elective total hip replacement and went in for surgery reluctantly. When the surgeons opened her hip joint for the arthroplasty, they found not arthritic changes, but a stage III osteosarcoma within the joint capsule. She was brought out of the anesthesia and told she instead needed a hemipelvectomy. She underwent the procedure and was admitted to inpatient rehabilitation. She was very tearful and withdrawn for the first 2 weeks of treatment. Later weeks of functional mobility and self-care treatment were hampered by her significant anxiety. She had been assured that it would be very unlikely that the cancer would recur because it was well encapsulated and later scans showed no evidence of recurrence anywhere else in her body.

Consider the following questions:

- What are Veronica's priorities for effective functioning at home?
- Which model of practice and which assessments would you use in intervention planning?
- What impact will her family have on her recovery?
- What potential areas of psychosocial dysfunction could limit her function?
- What would your treatment plan include?
- Which of Veronica's strengths will you utilize to improve her function?

of the class and discussed. Discussion can focus on identifying personal stereotypes or assumptions that may impair treatment planning, enhancing understanding of the client's perspective, expression of personal values, or identity through occupational performance, or the impact of resources on occupational performance, including contextual and caregiver issues.

◊ Which IADL tasks are most important to you?

◊ Do you believe that there are particular client populations less focused on certain components of self-care?

◊ When you are busy or not feeling well, with which ADL and IADL tasks does your performance slip first, either by necessity or choice?

◊ If you were working with a client with advanced Parkinson's disease in home care, how would your ADL retraining differ between your work with the client, the client's spouse, and the home health aide?

2. **Nontraditional Case Study.** This activity encourages thinking about function and personal values as opposed to rigid diagnosis-based reasoning. Additional information may be added to match recent course content, or role-playing may be used to enhance incorporation of a client-centered approach to treatment planning.

3. **Group Activities**

◊ Nontraditional Occupations: This activity can engender discussions about cultural sensitivity, unique challenges to client education or teaching, communication issues, or enhancing the scope of available occupational performance components for use in treatment planning.

* Have students gain an appreciation for ADL or IADL retraining from the client's perspective by teaching each other how to perform tasks not common to their cultural experience, such as learning to roll sushi, wrap a sari, tie a bowtie, or other tasks with or without simulated impairments/disabilities.

◊ "Stump Your Classmates": This activity is a lower-complexity activity that can be fun as well as educational. Teams of students can either ask other groups to guess the function of a device or present three potential uses for the device and have competing groups guess which potential use is correct.

* Have students dig through catalogs of durable medical equipment and medical suppliers to find obscure adaptive equipment, and attempt to "stump" each other in groups as to the purpose and application of the devices.

◊ "Desert Island": This activity can be completed in groups and then each group's results discussed and critiqued by classmates.

* Each group is given a "desert island" scenario where they are assigned a disability, impairment, or limitation and an occupational performance context. They are then asked to select the three most important ADL/IADL in which to be independent and the three most important resources or assistive equipment to enhance function and safety. Examples could include a married client with total hip replacement precautions in a two-storey house, a client with low vision in elderly housing, and a married mother of three with hemiplegia and perceptual difficulties in an urban apartment.

EVIDENCE-BASED RESEARCH CHART

Population	Evidence	References
Cerebrovascular accident (CVA)	Client-specific interventions, particularly ADL-specific retraining, enhance independence of function	Christie et al., 2011; Guidetti & Ytterberg, 2011; Hill-Hermann et al., 2008; Kwan & Sandercock, 2006; Landi et al., 2006; Legg et al., 2007; Rand et al., 2009; Richards et al., 2005; Sackley et al., 2006; Trombly & Ma, 2002; Walker, Gladman, Lincoln, Siemonsma, & Whiteley, 1999; Walker et al., 2004
Chronic obstructive pulmonary disease (COPD)	ADL performance and quality of life improved with a simple program	Bendstrup, Ingemann Jensen, Holm, & Bengtsson, 1997
Alzheimer's disease/dementia	ADL retraining can improve client quality of life and decrease the sense of burden for caregivers	Dooley & Hinojosa, 2004; Graff et al., 2006
Spinal cord injury	Client-centered intervention planning requires a focus on self-care and mobility	Donnelly et al., 2004
Traumatic brain injury	Behavioral observation, task analysis, consistent practice, cue fading, and acclimation to electronic aids to daily living are key to success with ADL/IADL	Boman et al., 2007; Erikson, Karlsson, Soderstrom, & Tham, 2004; Giles, Ridley, Dill, & Frye, 1997
Multiple sclerosis/ataxia	Combination of contextual changes, adaptations, and orthoses increase ADL function; early intervention improves function. Changes sustained up to 24 months	Gillen, 2000; Miyai, 2012
Posttraumatic stress disorder, homeless	Role identified for occupational therapy in addressing IADL, especially financial management	Davis & Kutter, 1998
Intellectual disabilities	ADL performance hierarchy of difficulty for clients with mild and moderate intellectual disability identified; ADL and IADL performance can be improved even in absence of change in insight	Drysdale, Casey, & Porter-Armstrong, 2008; Hallgren & Kottorp, 2005; Kottorp, Bernspang, & Fisher, 2003
Rheumatoid arthritis	Impact of comprehensive occupational therapy, instruction in joint protection, and splints on functional ability	Steultjens et al., 2004
Orthopedics/hip fracture	Individualized occupational therapy training enhances ADL function, likelihood of independent living, and reduces need for care at home	Hagsten et al., 2004
Pediatrics/teens/young adults	Occupational therapy contributes to increased function, cognition, mobility in inpatient setting, increases peer connection, environmental adaptation, independence in 20-day summer program	Chen, Heinemann, Bode, Granger, & Mallinson, 2004; Healy & Rigby, 1999
Cancer/brain tumors	Quality of life improvements may occur later than functional improvements; functional assessments may not sufficiently represent changes in clients	Huang, Wartella, & Kreutzer, 2001; Kasven-Gonzalez, Souverain, & Miale, 2010; Perez de Heredia, Cuadrado, Rodriguez, Lopez, & Miangolarra, 2001
Medical/surgical: Organ transplantation, emergency medicine	Direct correlations between contact with occupational therapy and greater independence with ADL and shorter LOS	Hastings et al., 2004; O'Brien et al., 2012; Patterson & Williams, 2005
Mental health	Evidence for life skills and IADL training is moderate	Gibson, D'Amico, Jaffe, & Arbesman, 2011
Mechanical ventilation	Early intervention with occupational therapy for programs including ADL training are safe and effective from the onset of mechanical ventilation	Pohlman et al., 2010; Schweickert et al., 2009
Community-dwelling elders/home modification	Daily activity performance and health-related quality of life are enhanced by interdisciplinary programs including occupational therapy and home modification	Gitlin et al., 2006; Stark et al., 2009; Szanton et al., 2011; Zingmark & Bernspång, 2011

Electronic Resources

- Adaptive equipment and durable medical equipment:
  - ◊ www.alimed.com
  - ◊ www.sammonspreston.com
  - ◊ www.invacare.com

References

Alexander, H., Bugge, C., & Hagen, S. (2001). What is the association between the different components of stroke rehabilitation and health outcomes? *Clinical Rehabilitation, 15,* 207-215.

Allen, C. K., Earhart, C. A., & Blue, T. (1992). *Occupational therapy treatment goals for the physically and cognitively challenged.* Rockville, MD: AOTA Press.

American Occupational Therapy Association. (2000). Occupational therapy code of ethics. *American Journal of Occupational Therapy, 54,* 614-616.

American Occupational Therapy Association. (2008). Occupational therapy practice framework: Domain and process (2nd ed.). *American Journal of Occupational Therapy, 62,* 625-683.

American Physical Therapy Association. (2003). *Guide to physical therapist practice* (2nd ed.) Alexandria, VA: Author.

Arnadottir, G. (1990). *The brain and behavior: Assessing cortical dysfunction through tasks of daily living.* St. Louis, MO: C. V. Mosby.

Atwood, S. M., Holm, M. B., & James, A. (1994). Activities of daily living capabilities and values of long-term-care facility residents. *American Journal of Occupational Therapy, 48,* 710-716.

Bartels, S. J., Forester, B., Mueser, K., T., Miles, K. M., Dums, A. R., Pratt, S. I., ... Perkins, L. (2004). Enhanced skills training and health care management for older persons with severe mental illness. *Community Mental Health Journal, 40,* 75-90.

Beatus, J., O'Neill, J. K., Townsend, T., & Robrechet, K. (2002). The effect of a one-week retreat on self-esteem, quality of life, and functional ability for persons with multiple sclerosis. *Neurology Report, 26*(3), 154-159.

Boman, I-L., Tham, K., Granqvist, A., Bartfai, A., & Hemmingsson, H. (2007). Using electronic aids to daily living after acquired brain injury: A study of the learning process and the usability. *Disability and Rehabilitation: Assistive Technology, 2*(1), 23-33.

Center for Health Services and Policy Research. (1998). *Outcome and Assessment Information Set (OASIS-BI).* Denver, CO: Author.

Centers for Medicare and Medicaid Services. (2005). *Minimum Data Set, 2.0.* Washington, DC: U.S. Government Printing Office.

Christiansen, C. H. (1999). Defining lives: Occupation as identity: An essay on competence, coherence, and the creation of meaning. *American Journal of Occupational Therapy, 53,* 547-558.

Christie, L., Bedford, R., & McCluskey, A. (2011). Task-specific practice of dressing tasks in a hospital setting improved dressing performance post-stroke: A feasibility study. *Australian Occupational Therapy Journal, 58,* 364-369.

Davis, L. A., Hoppes, S., & Chesbro, S. B. (2005). Cognitive-communicative and independent living skills assessment in individuals with dementia: A pilot study of environmental impact. *Topics in Geriatric Rehabilitation, 21,* 136-143.

Dunford, C., Missiuna, C., Street, E., & Sibert, J. (2005). Childrens' perceptions of the impact of developmental coordination disorder on activities of daily living. *British Journal of Occupational Therapy, 68,* 207-214.

Fisher, A. G. (1999). *Assessment of motor and process skills* (3rd ed.). Fort Collins, CO: Three Star Press.

Gitlin, L. N., Winter, L., Dennis, M. P., Corcoran, M., Schinfeld, S., & Hauck, W. W. (2006). A randomized trial of a multicomponent home intervention to reduce functional difficulties in older adults. *Journal of the American Geriatric Society, 54,* 809-816.

Goverover, Y., & Hinojosa, J. (2002). Categorization and deductive reasoning: Predictors of instrumental activities of daily living performance in adults with brain injury. *American Journal of Occupational Therapy, 56,* 509-516.

Graff, M. J. L., Vernooij-Dassen, M. J. M., Thijssen, M., Dekker, J., Hoefnagels, W. H. L., & Olde Rikkert, M. G. M. (2006). Community based occupational therapy for patients with dementia and their care givers: Randomized controlled trial. *British Medical Journal, 333*(7580), 1196.

Guidetti, S., & Ytterberg, C. (2011). A randomized controlled trial of a client-centred self-care intervention after stroke: A longitudinal pilot study. *Disability and Rehabilitation, 33,* 494-503.

Hagsten, B., Svensson, O., & Gardulf, A. (2004). Early individualized postoperative occupational therapy training in 100 patients improves ADL after hip fracture. *Acta Orthopaedica Scandinavica, 75,* 177-183.

Haitsma, K., V., & Ruckdeschel, K. (2001). Special care for dementia in nursing homes: Overview of innovations in programs and activities. *Alzheimer's Care Quarterly, 2,* 49-56.

Hastings, J., Gowans, S., & Watson, D. E. (2004). Effectiveness of occupational therapy following organ transplantation. *Canadian Journal of Occupational Therapy, 71,* 238-242.

Hill-Hermann, V., Strasser, A., Albers, B., Schofield, K., Dunning, K., Levine, P., & Page, S. J. (2008). Task-specific, patient-driven neuroprosthesis training in chronic stroke: Results of a 3-week clinical study. *American Journal of Occupational Therapy, 61,* 466-472.

Hilton, K., Fricke, J., & Unsworth, C. (2001). A comparison of self-report versus observation of performance using the Assessment of Living Skills and Resources (ALSAR) with an older population. *British Journal of Occupational Therapy, 64,* 135-143.

Kielhofner, G., & Forsyth, K. (2001). Measurement properties of a client self-report for treatment planning and documenting therapy outcomes. *Scandinavian Journal of Occupational Therapy, 8,* 131-139.

Klein, R. M., & Bell, B. (1979). *The Klein-Bell ADL Scale manual.* Seattle, WA: Educational Resources, University of Washington.

Kramer, A. M., Kowalsky, J. C., Lin, M., Grigsby, J., Hughes, R., & Steiner, J. F. (2000). Outcome and utilization differences for older persons with stroke in HMO and fee-for-service systems. *Journal of the American Geriatrics Society, 48,* 726-724.

Landi, F., Cesari, M., Onder, G., Tafani, A., Zamboni, V., & Cocchi. A. (2006). Effects of an occupational therapy program on functional outcomes in older stroke patients. *Gerontology, 52,* 85-91.

Law, M., Baptiste, S., Carswell, A., McColl, M. A., Polatajko, H. J., & Pollack, N. (2005). *Canadian Occupational Performance Measure* (4th ed.). Ottawa, Ontario, Canada: CAOT Publications ACE.

Legg, L., Drummond, A., Leonardi-Bee, J., Gladman, J. R. F., Corr, S., Donkervoort, M., Edmans, J., Gilbertson, L., Jongbloed, L., Logan, P., Sackley, C., Walker, M., & Langhorne, P. (2007). *Occupational therapy for patients with problems in personal activities of daily living after stroke: Systematic review of randomized trials.* Retrieved from www.bmj.com/content/335/7626/922.pdf%2Bhtml

Lysaght, R., & Wright, J. (2005). Professional strategies in work-related practice: An exploration of occupational and physical therapy roles and approaches. *American Journal of Occupational Therapy, 9,* 209-217.

McAndrew, E., McDermott, S. Vitzakovitch, S., Warunek, M., & Holm, M. B. (1999). Therapist and patient perceptions of the occupational therapy goal-setting process: A pilot study. *Physical and Occupational Therapy in Geriatrics, 17,* 55-63.

McGourty, L. K. (1979). *Kohlman Evaluation of Living Skills.* Seattle, WA: KELS Research.

Meyer, A. (1922). The philosophy of occupational therapy. *Archives of Occupational Therapy, 1,* 11-17.

Miyai, I. (2012). Challenge of neurorehabilitation for cerebellar degenerative diseases. *Cerebellum, 11,* 436-437.

Neistadt, M. E. (1995). Methods of assessing clients' priorities: A survey of adult physical dysfunction settings. *American Journal of Occupational Therapy, 49,* 428-436.

Nelson, D. L., & Glass, L. M. (1999). Occupational therapists' involvement with the Minimum Data Set in skilled nursing and intermediate care facilities. *American Journal of Occupational Therapy, 53,* 348-352.

O'Brien, L., Bynon, S., Morarty, J., & Presnell, S. (2012). Improving older trauma patients' outcomes through targeted occupational therapy and functional conditioning. *American Journal of Occupational Therapy, 66,* 431-437.

Rand, D., Weiss, P. L., & Katz, N. (2009). Training multitasking in a virtual supermarket: A novel intervention after stroke. *American Journal of Occupational Therapy, 63*(5), 535-542.

Richards, L. G., Latham, N. K., Jette, D. U., Rosenberg, L., Smout, R. J., & DeJong, G. (2005). Characterizing occupational therapy practice in stroke rehabilitation. *Archives of Physical Medicine and Rehabilitation, 86,* S51-S60.

Richardson, J., Law, M., Wishart, L., & Guyatt, G. (2000). The use of a simulated environment (Easy Street) to retrain independent living skills in elderly persons: A randomized controlled trial. *Journal of Gerontology, 55A,* M578-M584.

Robnett, R. H., Hopkins, V., & Kimball, J. G. (2002). The SAFE AT HOME: A quick home safety assessment. *Physical and Occupational Therapy in Geriatrics, 20,* 77-101.

Rogers, J. C., & Holm, M. B. (1994). *Performance Assessment of Self-Care Skills PASS)* (version 3.1). Unpublished manuscript, University of Pittsburgh at Pittsburgh.

Sackley C., Wade, D. T., Mant, D., Atkinson, J. C., Yudkin, P., Cardoso, K., ... Reel, K. (2006). Cluster randomized pilot controlled trial of an occupational therapy intervention for residents with stroke in UK care homes. *Stroke, 37,* 2336-2341.

Smallfield, S., & Karges, J. (2009). Classification of occupational therapy intervention for inpatient stroke rehabilitation. *American Journal of Occupational Therapy, 63,* 408-413.

Smith, K. (2006). Athletic trainers aim to expand scope. [Electronic version]. *Occupational Therapy Practice, 11*(5), 6.

Stark, S., Landsbaum, A., Palmer, J., Somerville, E. K., & Morris, J. C. (2009). Client-centered home modifications improve daily activity performance of older adults. *Canadian Journal of Occupational Therapy, 76,* 235-245.

Steultjens, E. M., Dekker, J., Bouter, L. M., Schaardenburg, D., van Kuyk, M. A., & van den Ende, C. H. (2004). Occupational therapy for rheumatoid arthritis. *Cochrane Database of Systematic Reviews, 1,* CD003114.

Szanton, S. L., Thorpe, R. J., Boyd, C., Tanner, E. K., Leff, B., Agree, E., ... Gitlin, L. N. (2011). Community aging in place, advancing better living for elders: A bio-behavioral environmental intervention to improve function and health-related quality of life in disabled older adults. *Journal of the American Geriatric Society, 59,* 2314-2320.

Thompson, K. M. (1998). Early intervention services in daily family life: Mothers' perceptions of "ideal" versus "actual" service provision. *Occupational Therapy International, 5,* 206-221.

Trombly, C. (1993). Anticipating the future: Assessment of occupational function. *American Journal of Occupational Therapy, 47,* 253-257.

Trombly, C., & Ma, H. (2002). A synthesis of the effects of occupational therapy for persons with stroke, part 1: Restoration of roles, tasks, and activities. *American Journal of Occupational Therapy, 56,* 250-259.

Uniform Data System for Medical Rehabilitation. (2000). *Guide for the Uniform Data Set for Medical Rehabilitation (including the FIM instrument* (version 5.1). Buffalo, NY: State University of New York.

Walker, M. F., Leonardi-Bee, J., Bath, P., Langhorne, P., Dewey, M., Corr, S., ... Parker, C. (2004). Individual patient data meta-analysis of randomized controlled trials of community occupational therapy for stroke patients. *Stroke, 35,* 2226-2232.

Weinstock-Zlotnick, G., & Hinojosa, J. (2004). The issue is: Bottom-up or top-down evaluation: Is one better than the other? *American Journal of Occupational Therapy, 58,* 594-599.

Williams, J. H., Drinka, T. J. K., Greenburg, J. R., Farrel-Holtan, J., Euhardy, R., & Schram, M. (1991). Development and testing of the Assessment of Living Skills and Resources (ALSAR) in elderly community-dwelling veterans. *Gerontologist, 31,* 84-91.

Wodchis, W. P., Fried, B. E., & Pollack, H. (2004). Payer incentives and physical rehabilitation therapy for nonelderly institutional long-term care residents: Evidence from Michigan and Ontario. *Archives of Physical Medicine Rehabilitation, 85,* 210-217.

Yerxa, E. J., Burnett-Beaulieu, S., Stocking, S., & Azen, S. P. (1988). Development of the satisfaction with scaled performance questionnaire (SPSQ). *American Journal of Occupational Therapy, 42,* 215-222.

Zingmark, M., & Bernspång, B. (2011). Meeting the needs of elderly with bathing disability. *Australian Occupational Therapy Journal, 58,* 164-171.

Suggested Readings

Bendstrup, K. E., Ingemann Jensen, J., Holm, S., & Bengtsson, B. (1997). Out-patient rehabilitation improves activities of daily living, quality of life and exercise tolerance in chronic obstructive pulmonary disease. *European Respiratory Journal, 10,* 2801-2806.

Chen, C. C., Heinemann, A. W., Bode, R. K., Granger, C. V., & Mallinson, T. (2004). Impact of pediatric rehabilitation services on children's functional outcomes. *American Journal of Occupational Therapy, 58,* 44-53.

Davis, J., & Kutter, C. J. (1998). Independent living skills and posttraumatic stress disorder in women who are homeless: Implications for future practice. *American Journal of Occupational Therapy, 52,* 39-44.

Donnelly, C., Eng, J. J., Hall, J., Alford, L., Giachino, R., Norton, K., & Kerr, D. S. (2004). Client-centred assessment and the identification of meaningful treatment goals for individuals with a spinal cord injury. *Spinal Cord, 42,* 302-307.

Dooley, N. R., & Hinojosa, J. (2004). Improving quality of life for persons with Alzheimer's disease and their family caregivers: Brief occupational therapy intervention. *American Journal of Occupational Therapy, 58,* 561-569.

Drysdale, J., Casey, J., & Porter-Armstrong, A. (2008). Effectiveness of training on the community skills of children with intellectual disabilities. *Scandinavian Journal of Occupational Therapy, 15,* 247-255.

Erikson, A., Karlsson, G., Soderstrom, M., & Tham, K. (2004). A training apartment with electronic aids to daily living: Lived experiences of persons with brain damage. *American Journal of Occupational Therapy, 58,* 261-271.

Gibson, R. W., D'Amico, M., Jaffe, L., & Arbesman, M. (2011). Occupational therapy interventions for recovery in the areas of community integration and normative life roles for adults with serious mental illness: A systematic review. *American Journal of Occupational Therapy, 65,* 247-256.

Giles, G. M., Ridley, J. E., Dill, A., & Frye, S. (1997). A consecutive series of adults with brain injury treated with a washing and dressing retraining program. *American Journal of Occupational Therapy, 51,* 256-266.

Gillen, G. (2000). Improving activities of daily living performance in an adult with ataxia. *American Journal of Occupational Therapy, 54,* 89-96.

Hallgren, M., & Kottorp, A. (2005). Effects of occupational therapy intervention on activities of daily living and awareness of disability in persons with intellectual disabilities. *Australian Occupational Therapy Journal, 52,* 350-359.

Healy, H., & Rigby, P. (1999). Promoting independence for teens and young adults with physical disabilities. *Canadian Journal of Occupational Therapy, 66,* 240-249.

Huang, M. E., Wartella, J. E., & Kreutzer, J. S. (2001). Functional outcomes and quality of life in patients with brain tumors: A preliminary report. *Archives of Physical Medicine and Rehabilitation, 82,* 1540-1546.

Kasven-Gonzalez, N., Souverain, R., & Miale, S. (2010). Improving quality of life through rehabilitation in palliative care: Case report. *Palliative and Supportive Care, 8,* 359-369.

Kottorp, A, Bernspang, B., & Fisher, A. (2003). Activities of daily living in persons with intellectual disability: Strengths and limitations in specific motor and process skills. *Australian Occupational Therapy Journal, 50,* 195-204.

Kwan, J., & Sandercock, P. (2006). In-hospital care pathways for stroke. *Cochrane Database of Systematic Reviews, 18*(4), CD002924.

Patterson, S., & Williams, M. (2005). *An occupational therapy consultation provided to older adults presenting to accident and emergency improves ADL functioning and reduces falls and hospital stays.* Retrieved from www.otcats.com/topics/CAT-OT&ADLTownsville12Jan2006.html

Perez de Heredia, M., Cuadrado, M. L., Rodriguez, G., Lopez, S., & Miangolarra, J. C. (2001). Eficacia de la Terapia Ocupacional en adolescentes con neoplasias intracraneales: Estudio piloto. *Rehabilitacion, 35*(3), 140-145.

Pohlman, M. C., Schweickert, W. D., Pohlman, A. S., Nigos, C., Pawlik, A. J., Esbrook, C. L., ... Kress, J. P. (2010). Feasibility of physical and occupational therapy beginning from initiation of mechanical ventilation. *Critical Care Medicine, 38,* 2089-2094.

Walker, M. F., Gladman, J. R. F., Lincoln, N. B., Siemonsma, P., & Whitely, T. (1999). Occupational therapy for stroke patients not admitted to hospital: A randomised controlled trial. *Lancet, 354,* 278-280.

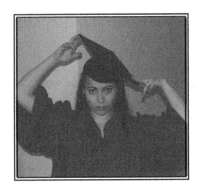

26

INTERVENTIONS TO ENHANCE OCCUPATIONAL PERFORMANCE IN EDUCATION AND WORK

Barbara J. Steva, MS, OTR/L

ACOTE STANDARDS EXPLORED IN THIS CHAPTER

B.5.1–B.5.6, B.5.19–B.5.21

KEY VOCABULARY

- **Consultation:** A type of intervention in which the practitioner uses their knowledge and expertise to collaborate with the client or caregivers. When providing consultation, the practitioner is not directly responsible for the outcome of the intervention.(AOTA, 2011).
- **Educational activities:** Tasks that facilitate learning, such as reading, writing, and math.
- **Exceptional educational need (EEN):** Determination that a student exhibits a disability or handicapping condition that prevents educational progress.
- **Goal:** Outcome measure of progress.
- **Inclusion:** The act of including and providing intervention to students with disabilities in the regular education classroom; adapting the environment for persons with disabilities to be successful in occupations, roles, and activities with others.
- **Individual education plan (IEP):** Written legal document developed by the individual education team that incorporates the student's strengths and need areas as well as goals and objectives for intervention.
- **Least restrictive environment (LRE):** An educational environment most like a regular education classroom; developing a natural environment that enhances a person's occupational performance in as self-structured a format as possible.
- **Objective:** Building blocks needed to achieve a larger goal.

(continued)

Jacobs, K., MacRae, N., & Sladyk, K. (Eds.).
*Occupational Therapy Essentials for
Clinical Competence, Second Edition* (pp. 347-365).

KEY VOCABULARY (CONTINUED)

- **Related service:** Services that may be required for a student to benefit from special education; service providers include, but are not limited to, occupational therapy, physical therapy, social work, and school health services.

- **Response to Intervention (RtI):** A method of systematic academic assistance for students experiencing learning challenges.

Introduction

This chapter addresses client identification, evaluation, and intervention within the educational setting, during the process of transition into the work force or post-secondary education, and within the work force. Models of practice are reviewed and discussed as to how they impact practice. Federal laws and regulations are outlined with the outcome of each on occupational therapy practice. The role of the occupational therapy practitioner is discussed throughout the chapter.

Medical and Educational Models of Service Delivery

Occupational therapy practitioners must have a clear understanding of the medical and educational service delivery models guiding practice in these areas. Within the medical model, occupational therapy is a primary service provider, and services are provided to promote wellness and independence within the individual's daily occupations. In contrast, occupational therapy within the educational model is a related service in which services supplement the educational program, are provided within the educational setting, and are related to the student's success within that environment. As part of the occupational therapy evaluation, the practitioner determines whether or not occupational therapy services are medically necessary or required for successful access to the educational curriculum and setting. Although services may be helpful to the overall function of the student, the therapist evaluates whether the disability or impairment impacts the student's ability to access and benefit from the academic instruction before recommending and implementing services. For example, a student diagnosed with cerebral palsy may be referred for an occupational therapy evaluation and found to have challenges with upper extremity function due to limited range of motion and increased muscle tone. This same student is proficient in the use of assistive technology to complete classroom work and independently uses adaptive devices for eating and dressing. It may be determined that although the

student may benefit from occupational therapy to address management of muscle tone and range of motion, it is not necessary for the student's ability to access the curriculum or educational setting. Therefore, occupational therapy could be justified within the medical model but not the educational model. Practitioners adhere to federal and state mandates by selecting evaluation tools, goals, objectives, and interventions that will address the identified educational needs of the student. Mandates within the Individuals with Disabilities Education Act (IDEA; United States Department of Education, n.d.) require that services be provided within the least restrictive environment (LRE) and support access to the general education or special education curriculum.

Occupational Therapy in the Educational Setting

Occupational therapy services within the public education setting are provided under federal mandates as outlined in Table 26-1. The Rehabilitation Act was enacted in 1973 (United States Department of Education, 2004). This act requires services for all eligible students, enabling them to participate in their regular or special education program. The Education for All Handicapped Children Act (Cengage Learning, n.d.) ensures a free and appropriate public education without discrimination based on disability. This act was amended to become IDEA in 1977, with further amendments made in 1990, 1994 and 2004. Under the original IDEA (1977), students with specific learning disabilities (SLDs) were classified using IQ and individual achievement scores as the primary means of identification. An over-identification of students categorized as having an SLD was suspected when students recognized with SLDs increased 200% (Vaughn, Linan-Thompson, & Hickman, 2003).

The reauthorization of IDEA in 2004 described an additional means of identification, now commonly referred to as Response to Intervention (RtI), to identify students struggling in the classroom. RtI was developed to assist in appropriately recognizing and instructing students before they fail. The role of the occupational therapy

Table 26-1.

PUBLIC SCHOOL LAWS

The Education for All Handicapped Children Act (P.L. 94-142)	• All children, ages 3 to 21, are entitled to a free and appropriate education. • Parent and student rights and legal recourses are outlined in the event that this right is denied.
Individuals with Disabilities Education Act (IDEA) (P.L. 108-446) http://idea.ed.gov	• Services are to be provided to assist the student with a disability to benefit from special education.
Section 504 of the Rehabilitation Act (P.L. 93-112)	• Services are to be provided without discrimination of disability. • Ensures free and appropriate accommodations and services for eligible students and entitles students with chronic diseases or disabling conditions to modifications that will allow them to participate within the regular or special education program.
Assistive Technology Act of 2004 (P.L. 108-364)	• Federally funded program under IDEA that provides access to assistive technology to individuals with disabilities to assist them with access to education, employment, and daily activities.

practitioner within this process varies within states and settings. Occupational therapy consultation and strategies offered to teachers and RtI providers regarding fine motor skill development, visual perception, and sensory processing as it relates to the skills being addressed can be beneficial to the student's success. RtI is a tiered intervention provided within the regular education model that occurs prior to referral to special education. Although models vary in specifics, Berkley, Bender, Peaster, and Saunders (2009) describe a typical model consisting of three tiers. Tier 1 involves large group instruction typically found in a regular education classroom. This may include core instructional interventions provided by the classroom teacher within the context of the regular education classroom. Tier 2 uses small group instruction targeted at specific skill development and guided by evidence-based interventions and close progress monitoring. This instruction is provided in addition to that received within the large group classroom setting. Tier 3, the most intensive tier, provides more concentrated and longer durations of individual instruction with frequent monitoring of progress. If a student progresses through the tiers without meeting specific individualized goals, he or she is referred for a special education evaluation.

INDIVIDUAL EDUCATION PLAN TEAM

Practitioners collaborate with educational staff and support personnel to ensure that services are available in a timely and appropriate manner. An individual education plan team (IEP team) is formed when a student is not benefiting from academic instruction despite RtI

efforts. The team consists of the parent or guardian, the student (when appropriate), at least one regular education teacher, at least one special education teacher, a school administrator, and all other appropriate representatives such as a psychologist, speech and language therapist, occupational therapist, physical therapist, and social worker. Occupational therapy practitioners are related service providers and are included when the team makes a referral stating that the student would benefit from an occupational therapy evaluation.

EVALUATION OF THE STUDENT

Evaluation in the school setting looks at the primary areas of function and uses a problem-solving approach to identify issues impacting the student's academic progress. Table 26-2 lists skill areas assessed and implications for functional performance within the educational setting. For example, the evaluation assesses sensorimotor skills that may limit access to the physical environment, self-care, or participation in daily tasks expected within the academic setting. Fine motor skills are assessed to ensure adequate appropriate function in tasks requiring manipulation of objects or the use of fine motor tools and manipulatives. Visual motor skills are assessed with a focus on spatial organization, directionality, organization of work on a page, and the ability to control the writing tool for legible writing. Visual perception, inclusive of discrimination, figure ground, form constancy, spatial relationships, part or whole concepts, and memory for one or more forms are important aspects of the evaluation. These areas can impact reading ability; multi-step task completion; part or

Table 26-2. PERFORMANCE AREAS AND FUNCTIONAL IMPLICATIONS IN THE EDUCATIONAL SETTING		
Area of Function	**Skills Assessed**	**Potential Impact on Accessing the Educational Curriculum**
Cognitive	Attention	Ability to listen, attend, and benefit from instruction
	Problem solving	Ability to use a variety of strategies (increasingly abstract) to solve a problem
	Visual perception: • Discrimination	Ability to read and identify safety signs, letters, shapes, or pictures for communication
	• Memory	Ability to recall letters, shapes, numbers, and mathematical operations
	• Sequential memory	Ability to remember a series of letters or numbers for tasks such as spelling, copying text, remembering phone numbers, and sequencing visual cues within the environment for vocational activities
	• Form constancy	Ability to mentally manipulate visual information when some attributes (i.e., size or orientation) have been changed; recognize letters or forms in different contexts such as print to cursive; impacts ability to use mental pictures for tasks such as sequencing the alphabet, using the calendar, telling time, reading maps, and applying mathematical concepts; is an important skill for sewing and construction
	• Figure ground	Ability to locate salient information within a busy background such as words, numbers, or mathematical operations on worksheets, text, desk, drawer, bookshelf, or grocery store shelf
	• Visual closure/ part or whole relationships	Ability to recognize forms or objects partially hidden or incomplete letters or words; also related to part–whole integration and the ability to see the overall picture of a situation; impacts ability to tell time, perform mathematical skills, and perform mechanical or constructional tasks
	• Spatial relationships	Ability to recognize the directionality of letters and numbers (i.e., "b" and "d"); spatial organization of work within lines or on the page; also impacts the ability to use mental pictures to perform tasks such as sequencing the alphabet, using the calendar, telling time, reading maps, and applying mathematical concepts
	Visual motor: • Spatial organization	Ability to organize work on a page, space letters and words, set up mathematical operations, complete artwork or projects, conceptualize parts as they relate to the whole
	• Directionality	Ability to correctly orient letters, numbers, and shapes; follow instructions of "up, down, right, left"
Developmental	Core/postural strength and stability	Ability to maintain an upright, stable, and unsupported position during instruction and tabletop/fine motor work
	Fine motor muscle development	Ability to activate the small/intrinsic muscles of the hand with graded controlled force and speed when writing, cutting with scissors, and object manipulation
	Bilateral hand coordination	Ability to use both hands together to manipulate objects and participate in physical education, recess, scissor use, writing, and drawing
	Eye–hand coordination	Ability to participate in play, physical education, recess, scissor use, writing, and drawing.
	Motor planning	Ability to navigate obstacles within the classroom, learn new motor tasks such as letter formations, academic games, participation in physical education, recess, and peer interactions
Functional	Dressing	Clothing management before/after toileting and outdoor play, fasteners, shoe tying
	Mealtime	Utensil use including cutting, spreading, and opening containers
	Toileting	Clothing management, navigation of the bathroom environment, hygiene after toilet use
	Grooming	Hand washing, wiping face after meals, nose care, general appearance

whole concepts; and spatial concepts used in telling time, mathematical operations, and science. Challenges in the area of perceptual skills can also suggest a nonverbal learning disability or assist in excluding this as an identifier if strong perceptual skills are present. Finally, functional self-care skills such as toileting, feeding, grooming, and hygiene are assessed as they relate to the student's ability to participate in the school day (Figure 26-1).

INDIVIDUAL EDUCATION PLAN DEVELOPMENT

The team reviews the evaluation/assessment material collected by all disciplines to determine whether the student meets state eligibility requirements for special education. Eligibility is based on exceptional educational need (EEN). The team determines whether the information from the evaluations indicates a specific disabling or handicapping condition that prevents the student from participating in and benefiting from academic instruction.

Suchomel (2000) lists the following considerations when determining eligibility for occupational therapy services within the school:

- Does the student have an EEN that qualifies him or her for special education services, or does he or she qualify for services under Section 504 of the Rehabilitation Act?

- Does the evaluation indicate a need for occupational therapy services by demonstrating a significant delay in one or more areas of occupational performance that is impacting the student's ability to participate in academic tasks?

- Will occupational therapy assist the student in accessing and benefiting from academic instruction?

- Does the student require the skilled service of an occupational therapist or occupational therapy assistant, or can the tasks and interventions be carried out by other personnel?

ROLE OF THE PRACTITIONER IN THE EVALUATION AND DEVELOPMENT OF INDIVIDUAL EDUCATION PLAN

The occupational therapist establishes the areas and methods that will be used in the evaluation of the student. The occupational therapy assistant collaborates with the occupational therapist by providing observations, collecting data, and administering/scoring assessments within their level of competency. The occupational therapist interprets and reports the information from the assessments. The practitioners collaborate in the development of goals and objectives for intervention. The occupational therapy assistant is a member of the IEP

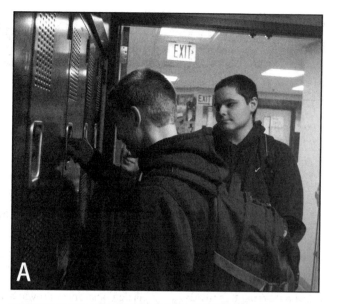

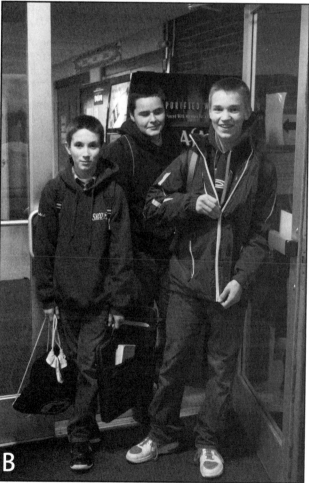

Figure 26-1. Daily occupations within the academic setting often require independence with activities involving visual perception and fine motor skill development. (A) Tasks can include opening a combination locker and (B) managing clothing before/after toileting or when entering/leaving the school. Students may require intervention, accommodations or modification to assist with these skills.

Table 26-3.

REPRESENTATIVE GOAL AND OBJECTIVES

Condition	Behavior	Measurement	Outcome
Under what circumstances you expect the student to perform	What you are expecting the student to do	How you will measure success	Why this area of performance is being addressed
"Given…"	"Joey will…"	"…trials, over a 2-week period" "…% of the time during 3 consecutive intervention sessions"	"for use in…"

Goal

Given therapeutic activities, Joey will demonstrate improved strength, endurance, and control in the trunk and upper extremity 70% of the time, as needed for fine motor, visual motor, and academic occupations by December 2014.

Objectives

Given therapeutic activities, Joey will demonstrate improved trunk strength and control as seen by the ability to maintain an upright sitting position in a chair or on the floor without external support for 5 minutes (first trimester), 10 minutes (second trimester), and 15 minutes (third trimester), 3 times per day on 4 of 5 consecutive school days, for use in daily occupations.

Given therapeutic activities, Joey will demonstrate the ability to use bilateral upper extremities at midline for writing, cutting, and playing while in an unsupported sitting position for 3 minutes (first trimester), 5 minutes (second trimester) and 10 minutes (third trimester), 3 times per day on 4 of 5 consecutive school days, for use in daily occupations.

team and can attend the IEP meeting under the direction and supervision of the occupational therapist to report the findings and review goals and objectives (Solomon, 2000).

The occupational therapist provides supervision to the occupational therapy assistant by overseeing service delivery and assisting in his or her professional growth and competence. Frequency of supervision may vary depending on the knowledge and experience of the occupational therapy assistant and his or her ability to ensure safe, effective intervention. The practitioners collaborate to decide on an appropriate amount and method of supervision. Factors to consider include the practice setting, complexity of client needs, requirements of the practice setting, and skills of both the practitioners. Regulations set forth by state and federal agencies must be followed with completion of clear and appropriate documentation of supervision.

GOALS AND OBJECTIVES

Together, the team determines the student's strength and need areas in order to develop goals and objectives for the IEP. Occupational therapy goals and objectives are individualized and specific to the student, address educational needs, and are measurable. The goal is overarching and less specific than the objectives. The objectives break the goal into specific tasks or skills required to successfully achieve the goal. Each objective defines the conditions in which you expect to see the student perform well,

along with the behavior you wish the student to exhibit, how you are going to measure the behavior, and why you are intervening in this area. The goals and objectives must be directly linked to educational development. Table 26-3 shows a sample goal and objectives.

SERVICE DELIVERY MODELS

The type of practice model that the therapist chooses to employ depends on the educational setting and student needs. Current federal mandates call for instruction to take place in the LRE. This challenges the practitioner to develop an intervention program that can be incorporated into the classroom whenever possible. The model of practice must be determined by carefully examining the classroom environment, the student's needs, and the ability to accomplish the prescribed goals and objectives.

DIRECT SERVICE

Direct service occurs individually or in a small group setting. The therapist decides whether this should take place in a setting outside of the classroom, often referred to as "pullout," or in an inclusive setting within the classroom environment. Pullout services involve removal of the student from the classroom for the duration of the therapy session. Inclusive therapy involves the practitioner providing therapy within the classroom environment in a nonintrusive manner. The inclusive model allows the therapist to gain knowledge regarding skills that the student needs to be successful within the classroom and allows the teacher to observe the therapeutic approach, preparing him or her to assist the student during activities when the practitioner is not present. Services are typically provided on a weekly basis for an amount of time discussed and decided on by the IEP team. Inclusion therapy ensures that the intervention supports the educational process and increases the likelihood of generalization of therapeutic techniques throughout the school day. Direct pullout services require ongoing consultation with educational staff outside of the therapy session to ensure carryover of learned tasks. This service delivery is most effective when a student is working on a skill that is significantly below that of peers and intervention within the classroom would be a distraction to other students.

CONSULTATION

The consultation, or collaboration, model involves the practitioner providing service through direct contact with the teacher or other educational staff working with the student (Figure 26-2). This can be the primary method of service delivery and should always be pursued in addition to the provision of direct services. When providing consultation, the practitioner must have good communication skills and insight to recognize when the tasks being asked of the teaching staff cannot be successfully implemented in the classroom. Teachers provide motivating instruction while implementing modifications and accommodations to students with varying learning styles and speeds. A common mistake of therapists is to overwhelm a teacher with activities, equipment, and specialized programs for one or two children within the classroom. As a result, teachers can become resentful and less receptive to the practitioner's ideas. It is important for the practitioner to be a part of the classroom to which he or she is consulting by observing the environment on an ongoing basis to better understand the inner workings and expectations of the environment and to tailor recommendations to the flow of the classroom schedule.

Dunn (1990) conducted a study of direct service and consultation and the effect of each practice model on student outcomes and adult attitudes. Fourteen preschool- and kindergarten-age children were randomly assigned to either a direct service or a consultation model. Children in both groups achieved nearly 75% of all IEP goals. Teachers in the consultation group, however, reported a 24% greater occupational therapy contribution to goal attainment than the direct service group. Palisano (1989) researched the use of therapist-directed groups and consultation groups. Results revealed statistically higher scores between pre- and post-test scores for the consultation group in the area of motor skills, whereas the therapist-directed group showed clinically higher scores in the area of visual perception. There was no difference in visual motor scores. These findings suggest

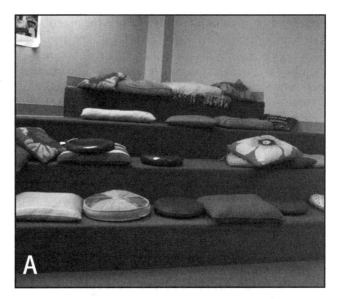

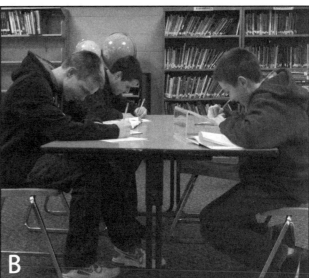

Figure 26-2. Through consultation, students can be provided with adaptations and accommodations that promote success. Here, (A) seating options (wiggle seats) and (B) writing strategies (slant board) can be made available to many students within the classroom setting, rather than isolating the student with challenges.

the need for care in determining the appropriate service delivery model and the need to assess its effectiveness on a regular basis.

TERMINATION OF SERVICES

A recommendation to discontinue services is made by the occupational therapist when the established goals and objectives have been achieved. The IEP team is reconvened to review progress and discuss discontinuation of services. The student's disabilities are not necessarily "cured," but he or she is functioning within the academic setting with supports and strategies acquired through occupational therapy intervention. Through effective collaboration with the student's teacher, the practitioner can identify and address concerns regarding dismissal. There can be a safety net put in place in the event of regression by developing a measurable goal outlining expected performance. The occupational therapist can step back in to provide more consultation or support to the teacher and student if the goal is not being met. The occupational therapist can help the teacher intervene immediately and support the student when challenged. The therapist does not want to promote a situation in which the student and teacher are unable to function without ongoing intervention by the occupational therapist. The practitioner may slowly withdraw from the immediate environment.

Alternative Education Settings

Recommendations for an alternative education setting are often made for students at risk for dropping out of school or failing in the public school. Risk factors include the following:

- Truancy
- Low motivation
- Inability to maintain attention
- Low self-esteem
- Behavioral difficulties

These settings incorporate the student's social, emotional, intellectual, physical, spiritual, and moral development with their education. Classroom size, teaching styles, and methods are commonly different from those seen in public or traditional school settings. Using questionnaires distributed to educational staff, Dirette and Kolak (2004) studied the needs of students within alternative educational settings. The top three areas of student concern included the following:

1. Difficulty with time management.
2. Lack of participation in healthy play and leisure activities.
3. Maintenance of healthy lifestyle behaviors.

Other areas of concern are as follows:

- Cognitive deficits such as multitasking or the ability to follow multistep instructions.
- Higher-level thinking skills such as problem solving and retaining/recalling information.
- Coping skills.
- Anger management.
- Poor self-concept.

Occupational therapy services are provided within this setting as in a public school setting. These settings are often privately funded and are not obligated by the federal and state mandates guiding special education services. The student's public school district is responsible for evaluating, developing, and implementing an IEP for the student regardless of placement.

Transition Planning

Legislation guiding the transition from school to the workplace is defined in Section 602(30) of IDEA (United States Department of Education, n.d.), which describes "transition services" for students with disabilities beginning at age 14 years. By age 16, the IEP should contain a statement regarding services to be provided and designate responsibilities for the student's successful transition into the workplace, higher education, and/or community. Specifically, the mandate is designed as an outcome-oriented process, promoting transition of the student from school to post-school activities. Post-school activities may include post-secondary education, vocational training, supported or unsupported employment, adult services, independent living, or community participation. The transition plan is based on the student's strengths, preferences, and interests. Transition services should include instruction, related services, community experiences, development of employment, post-school adult living objectives, acquisition of daily living skills (as appropriate), and vocational evaluation (United States Department of Education, n.d.). The Americans with Disabilities Act (ADA) (United States Equal Employment Opportunity Commission [EEOC], n.d.) provides individuals with disabilities an opportunity to fulfill typical roles in the community. The act requires reasonable accommodations for the qualified individual with a disability including accessibility, job restructuring, modifications to equipment and training materials, and provision of qualified readers or interpreters. The intention of the School-to-Work Opportunities Act (Fessler State Board of Education Site, n.d.), jointly managed by the Department of Education and the Department of Labor, is to build partnerships between schools and communities and provide school to work programs. This mandate serves to provide opportunities for students to engage in performance-based education and training to prepare them for competitive employment, participation in post-secondary education, and navigation of the workplace. Sanford and colleagues (2011) reported that 55% of individuals with disabilities accessed post-secondary education within 6 years of leaving high school, as compared to 62% of non-disabled peers. Individuals with disabilities were as likely (71%) as their non-disabled counterparts (71%) to be engaged in paid employment outside the home within 6 years of leaving high school.

Occupational therapy practitioners can offer knowledgeable and unique perspectives when preparing for education and employment of the student with special needs

Table 26-4.

FACTORS FOR SUCCESSFUL SCHOOL/WORK TRANSITION

Factor	Evaluation/Assessment Area	Intervention
Accessibility of the work area	Is adaptive equipment required for positioning or accessibility?	Training in appropriate use of the equipment.
Student	Sensory, motor, and cognitive-perceptual skills	Development and training in the use of adaptations.
Task	Analysis of job requirements and components	Preteach the sequence or specific job tasks that may be problematic. Develop supports to assist with successful completion of the tasks.
Skill development	Assessment of job requirements (i.e., standing, finger dexterity)	Develop and implement a program into the school day to work on needed skills..
Personal care	Independence in self-care	Develop and implement a program involving personal hygiene (i.e., grooming, toileting, eating) into the school day.
Communication	Evaluation of the need for assistive technology	Develop and implement assistive technology in conjunction with the speech and language clinician as appropriate to enhance communication.
Job carving	Assessment of the job site to discern any other job possibilities not previously considered	Training in areas required to fulfill other responsibilities within the site.

following high school. It is the practitioner's responsibility to understand the current terminology, laws, trends, and interventions that will best serve this population. Depending on the practitioner's role within the school setting and IEP team, advocacy for involvement along with education of school personnel may be needed to promote recognition of the impact and role of occupational therapy in this process.

Practitioners contribute to the transition from school to post-secondary education or work by offering skills in the assessment, training, and reinforcement of work skills and behavior. Despite the knowledge and expertise that practitioners have to offer in this area, Kardos and White (2005) found a lack of occupational therapy involvement in transitional planning. Barriers to involvement included transition services being handled by other professionals (special education teachers, guidance or transition coordinators), a lack of understanding of the role of occupational therapy in transition planning, a lack of funding within the school budget to utilize occupational therapy as a transitional team member, a lack of knowledge regarding assessment tools for evaluation in this area, and students being dismissed from occupational therapy prior to age 14 when transition planning is initiated. Asher (2003) described factors that potentially impact successful transition from secondary education to community and areas where practitioners

can provide meaningful intervention. These are outlined in Table 26-4.

Work

Work is one of the primary roles in life that is essential to health and wellness. However, there have been several incomplete definitions. Work has been defined as what people do to earn a living (Brief & Nord, 1990); as an activity done in a specific place and time, on a regular basis (Hearnshaw, 1954); and as employment perceived by individuals as their main occupation, by which they are known, and from which they derive their societal role (Shimmin, 1966). Work may mean different things to different individuals. One may see it as obligatory, whereas another may find it enjoyable regardless of whether there is a monetary value attached to it. The American Occupational Therapy Association (AOTA) Occupational Therapy Practice Framework (OTPF) (2011) describes work as having six components addressed by occupational therapy practice. These are employment interests and pursuits, employment seeking and acquisition, job performance, retirement preparation and adjustment, volunteer exploration, and volunteer participation (Ellexson & Larson, 2011).

Individuals participate in work as a means of financially supporting themselves and their families. After retirement from this role, senior citizens and the elderly often continue to contribute to the workforce through volunteering. This provides a fulfilling experience to individuals who have spent most of their lives in the worker role and may ease their transition to retirement. The terms *work* and *occupation* have evolved to be used synonymously, creating confusion. The Merriam-Webster dictionary defines work as "the labor, task, or duty that is one's accustomed means of livelihood," and occupation as "an activity in which one engages" or "the principal business of one's life." Regardless of the reason an individual participates in work-related activities, whether for financial reimbursement or enjoyment, the role of the worker often encompasses the majority of the individual's time each day, making work a primary occupation for him or her.

Before providing any type of intervention within the work environment, a comprehensive evaluation of the worksite and the worker must be completed. A conceptual framework, proposed by Sandqvist and Henriksson (2004), identifies three dimensions for the assessment of work function. These are work participation, work performance, and individual capacity. Work participation refers to the ability of the individual to gain and maintain employment within society. Factors such as public support and the demands on the individual are considered. Work performance refers to the individual's ability to perform the tasks associated with the work activity. Finally, individual capacity refers to the individual's ability to physically and psychologically complete the work activities.

Role of the Practitioner in the Evaluation and Intervention Within the Workplace

Before an individual treatment plan is developed, the occupational therapy practitioner conducts a thorough evaluation of the worker's skills and the workplace. The occupational therapist is responsible for all aspects of the evaluation, planning, and intervention process. The occupational therapy assistant works under direct supervision of the occupational therapist to complete this process. Both practitioners work together to ensure the appropriate level of supervision required based on the complexity of client needs; experience of the practitioners; type of practice setting; and state, agency, and other regulatory requirements. The occupational therapist is responsible for conducting the evaluation process, interpreting the results, defining need areas, and developing a treatment plan based on the client's goals and priorities. The occupational therapy assistant participates in the process by implementing tasks deemed appropriate by the occupational therapist. The assistant is responsible for

understanding evaluation results and intervention goals. The occupational therapy assistant provides ongoing written and verbal reports to the occupational therapist as the process progresses for effective collaboration in the implementation of the intervention plan and achievement of client goals (AOTA, 2009).

Intervention

Performance challenges impacting fulfillment of the worker role can be related to motor, sensory, perceptual, and/or emotional skills. In addition, performance patterns, activity demands, or environmental contexts play a part in the successful participation of the worker. Occupational therapy practitioners are skilled in providing services addressing work hardening or conditioning, pre-work screening, functional capacity assessment and ergonomics, pre-vocational assessment and training, sheltered or supported employment, and transition from school to work (Ellexson & Larson, 2011).

Intervention is required for those individuals with physical, cognitive, and developmental disabilities, as well as those who become injured as a result of work-related stress or other activities such as carpal tunnel injury, chronic back pain, or brain injury. Interventions may include direct service in the form of job training, training to perform a specific task, muscle strengthening, implementation of task modifications, and accommodations such as ergonomic supports to assist with back pain or repetitive use injuries. Occupational therapists may be used as consultants to the employer to ensure that hiring procedures and job descriptions are nondiscriminatory and the workplace is ergonomically safe for workers and meets ADA regulations (AOTA, 2000). Table 26-5 outlines laws and regulations for services for individuals with disabilities. Social Security or Supplemental Security Income (SSI) benefits are granted to individuals unable to work due to disability. If and when the individual is ready to explore employment, the Ticket to Work (TTW) incentive program allows individuals 18 to 64 years of age to receive free employment support services. The program provides incentives to seek or return to work without the threat or fear of losing current health care or cash benefits. Individuals seeking employment have been presented with additional barriers in the areas of employment, vocational rehabilitation, and TTW knowledge and utilization (Hernandez et al., 2007). Employment barriers include negative employer attitudes to individuals with disabilities, limited transportation options, and limited formal education. Consumers reported vocational rehabilitation to offer only low-paying, temporary, and menial positions in addition to unresponsive and non-collaborative counselors. Consumers' response to their knowledge of the TTW program revealed poor knowledge of the

Table 26-5.

WORKPLACE LEGISLATION

Federal Employees Liability (FELA) Act, 1908 (45 U.S.C. 51, et seq.)	• No-fault insurance system • Pays benefits to employees for accidental, work-related injuries and diseases
Vocational Rehabilitation Act Amendments of 1943 (P.L. 78-113)	• Amended Vocational Rehabilitation Act of 1920 • Includes individuals with physical disabilities, blindness, developmental delays, and psychiatric disabilities • Office of Vocational Rehabilitation established • New focus on activities of daily living and adaptation • Removed ceiling on payment
Vocational Rehabilitation Act Amendments (Hill-Burton Act) of 1954 (P.L. 86-565)	• Greater financial support, research and demonstration grants, and professional preparation grants • State agency expansion and improvement grants • Grants to expand rehabilitation facilities
Vocational Rehabilitation Act Amendments of 1965 (P.L. 89-333)	• Expanded services to people with disabilities and social handicaps • Money for construction of rehabilitation centers and workshops made available
Architectural Barriers Act of 1968 (P.L. 90-48)	• Initiated changes in access for people with disabilities
Developmental Disabilities Services and Facilities Construction Act of 1970 (P.L. 91-517)	• States received responsibility for planning and implementing service programs for people with developmental delays, epilepsy, cerebral palsy, and other neurological impairments
Occupational Safety and Health Act of 1970 (P.L. 91-596)	• Mandated employers to provide a work environment free of hazards that were likely to cause death or serious harm to workers
Rehabilitation Act of 1973 (P.L. 93-112)	• Services expanded to include individuals with more severe disabilities • Provided affirmative action in employment (section 503) and non-discrimination in facilities (section 504) by federal contractors and grantees
Rehabilitation Act Amendments of 1986 (P.L. 99-506)	• Clarification to include that evaluation of clients must include recreation, employability, and rehabilitation needs
Education of the Deaf Act (EDA) of 1986 (P.L. 99-371)	• Provided technical training and education to prepare people with hearing impairments for employment
Omnibus Budget Reconciliation Act of 1987 (P.L. 99-371)	• Allowed states to offer prevocational, educational, and supported employment services to individuals deinstitutionalized prior to the waiver program
Americans with Disabilities Act (ADA) of 1990 (P.L. 101-336)	• Prevented discrimination against people with disabilities • Guaranteed equal protection to individuals with disabilities in employment, public accommodations, transportation, state and local government, and telecommunications
Ticket to Work and Work Incentive Improvement Act of 1999 (P.L. 106-170)	• Increased opportunities to recipients of Social Security benefits to obtain employment, vocational rehabilitation, and other support services (from public or private providers, employers, and other organizations)
Americans with Disabilities Act Amendments Act (ADAAA) of 2008 (P.L. 110-325)	• Focused on discrimination rather than the disability • Made changes in the definition of disability

Adapted from Ellexson, M., & Larson, B. (2011). Occupational therapy services in facilitating work performance. *American Journal of Occupational Therapy, 65*, s55-s64.

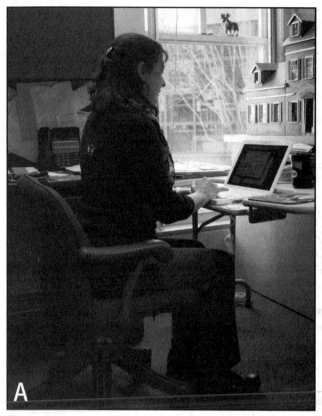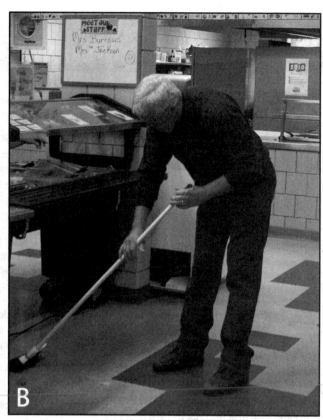

Figure 26-3. Management and prevention of work place injuries can involve consultation to employers and staff regarding ergonomics, body mechanics, and work modification.

benefit, fear of losing medical benefits, and limited utilization of the program.

Traditional vocational rehabilitation efforts have focused on "supply-side" training when working with individuals with disabilities who are seeking employment. Supply-side training involves a comprehensive evaluation of the individual's current skills, function, and individual interests for employment. Specific intervention is then provided to teach needed skills for successful participation in the workplace. "Demand-side" training has more recently become a focus in the employment of individuals with disabilities. The demand-side approach looks at the workplace demands and needs—that is, the employer and workplace involved in hiring and retaining individuals. Chan and colleagues (2010) found barriers to employment of individuals with disabilities to include a lack of the category of disability as part of diversity plans within companies, a lack of resources to recruit and retain persons with disabilities, and inadequate training in the ADA and workplace accommodations.

The practitioner working with individuals with disabilities seeking employment opportunities must work with the clients to develop required physical, cognitive, and social skills. They must also be a resource to potential employers by providing information regarding the needs of the client/worker in addition to providing education and training regarding ADA regulations and accommodations that can be put in place to support both the worker and the employer.

Regardless of the reason for initial referral to occupational therapy, a thorough evaluation of the client's needs and abilities, as well as an analysis of the work task, are required before developing an intervention plan (Figure 26-3). Goals and objectives are developed and written in conjunction with the client and with the employer when appropriate. These are objective, task oriented, and measurable to assist in planning for dismissal from occupational therapy services. Knowledge of universal design, construction guidelines, specialized products, and government guidelines is essential in providing guidance to the employer and solutions for the worker within the workplace.

Pohlman, Poosawtsee, Gerndt, and Lindstrom-Hazel (2001) surveyed workers' compensation carriers to assess how occupational therapy programs can best meet the needs of the carriers. Results showed that carriers consider a rehabilitation program successful if the worker is able to return to any job position. The carriers reported that occupational therapy programs are beneficial for return to work, although it was stated that most carriers did not understand what occupational therapy was or how it could assist in returning an individual to the workforce. This study suggests the need for educating insurance carriers as to the role of the practitioner with the worker who has an injury or disability.

Frames of Reference

A model of practice is used to guide the practitioner's thinking and subsequent intervention plan and activities. The following section summarizes five models of practice used in school and work intervention. Practitioners may use several different models within their practice. Some practitioners choose one model to guide their philosophy and interventions with all students/clients, whereas others may choose to use several different models based on the presentation of the client. It is important to focus on the student/client's occupation and desired outcome when choosing a model of practice.

Neurodevelopmental

The original theory and practice of neurodevelopmental treatment (NDT) was developed from the work of Karel and Berta Bobath's intervention of individuals with brain injury. NDT is a sensorimotor approach focusing on motor and postural aspects that translate to independence in active tasks (Dunn, 1990). The theory has a strong foundation in normal development and the interpretation of motor responses. These include motor control developing from head to foot, midline to the limbs, and large to small movements. The theory progresses through the developmental sequence, integrating primitive reflexes and achieving developmental milestones. Mobility is built on stability and progresses outward as the child begins to explore the environment. The trunk is typically where intervention is initiated, progressing to more advanced movements performed away from the trunk. Because NDT focuses on abnormal movement patterns and attempts to extinguish these in favor of more appropriate or typical motor patterns, this theory may not always be effective in treating children with changes in muscle tone, such as cerebral palsy. These children build motor patterns that are successful for them. By changing their motor pattern, they may become dependent in areas or tasks in which they were previously independent.

Biomechanical

The biomechanical frame of reference is based in physical science such as kinesiology and physics. A balance between stability and mobility is a primary focus, which takes into consideration muscle tone and skeletal alignment (Dunn, 2000). Muscle tone is the amount of tension in a muscle or muscle group at any given time. Muscle tone is not an exact science and exists along a continuum. Many individuals with high or low muscle tone, relative to "typical," lead functional and productive lives with no detriment to themselves or their lifestyle.

An individual with a disorder of the central nervous system may have more severe challenges in regulating the amount of tension present in the muscles during activity or rest. An individual with cerebral palsy may have "high" or "increased" muscle tone resulting from excess tension in the muscles. This leaves the individual at risk for shortened muscle length or contractures due to poor stretch and relaxation. Function is impacted due to the decreased ability to relax and tense the muscle as needed for mobility. An individual exhibiting "low" or "decreased" muscle tone results from an excessive relaxation of the muscles. This leaves the individual at risk for subluxation of joints due to laxity and poor tension in the muscles. Function is impacted by a lack of stability. The underlying goal of the biomechanical frame of reference is improved skeletal alignment by developing postural control for use in functional occupations (Dunn, 2000). This can be done through strengthening exercises and activities or the use of positioning devices. Indicators of poor postural control are a decreased ability to maintain an upright position without external support. This is often seen when the individual leans on a table or desk for support or slouches in a chair. These are often seen in school and work settings and can impact an individual's ability to work effectively and efficiently. The biomechanical approach is most commonly used when assessing and providing wheelchairs or splints to improve positioning and function.

Motor Learning

The motor learning theory focuses on the process of learning rather than a specific task. Approaches of feedback, feed-forward, and event are described in the literature (Breslin, 1996). The feedback approach relies on information from the environment to provide feedback regarding movement. Arguments to this approach include the closed loop system, which does not allow for variability in the routine (Gliner, 1985). The feed-forward approach suggests that a motor plan is created prior to carrying out the motor task and is adapted during future use based on feedback from the environment. This is felt to promote variability, although Croce and DePaepe (1989) argued that a separate motor plan for every motor task would be very complex. Gliner (1989) pointed out that these approaches focus on the learner as the primary component and the environment being a secondary factor. The event approach brings both the learner and the environment together and purposeful activity to the forefront. This approach describes the learner as subconsciously choosing the motor plan for a purposeful task from a learned repertoire. The environment provides the learner with feedback regarding the success of the plan, and movements are adjusted at that time or stored for future use. The therapist provides intervention through the use of feedback regarding the success or failure of a movement, structuring the environment or task while

Table 26-6.

FACTORS IMPACTING SENSORY REGULATION

Type of Input	Relaxing/Calming	Alerting
Vestibular movement of the head through space	• Slow • Rhythmic • Linear—one plane • Movement while on stable ground	• Fast • Jerky • Frequent changes of direction • Angular movement • Suspended equipment
Proprioception—compression or stretch of a joint	• Joint compression • Slow stretch • Heavy and sustained resistance	• Quick/unexpected changes • Jarring/jerking • Abrupt stops and starts
Tactile—any kind of touch	• Firm/deep pressure • Swaddling • Firm stroking over large areas • Smooth texture • Familiar and predictable • Warmth	• Light touch • Poking • Touch on the face • Rough texture • Unexpected touch • Cold
Visual	• Rhythmic • Constant • Blue and green shades • Dim or dark • Familiar and predictable	• Unexpected • Bright colors or lights • Red and yellow shades • Black on white • Changing or moving stimuli
Auditory	• Expected • Familiar • Quiet gentle rhythm • Melodic	• Unexpected • Loud • Complex
Olfactory	• Familiar—associated with comforting experiences	• All odors

the individual engages in a purposeful movement activity (Breslin, 1996). This approach is commonly used within the academic and work settings to address fine motor skill development and skills needed to engage in physical education or playground activities.

SENSORY INTEGRATION

A. Jean Ayres developed sensory integration theory in the early 1970s as she attempted to apply neuroscientific knowledge to her practice with children diagnosed with "minimal brain dysfunction," today known as attention deficit hyperactivity disorder (ADHD). The theory emphasizes the individual's ability to interact with the environment by receiving and organizing sensory information. This information is used to produce an adaptive response and adjust to changes within the environment. Sensory input impacts aspects of physical, cognitive, and emotional responses. An individual exhibiting an extreme response to an otherwise benign input such as a gentle tap on the shoulder by a friend would be displaying over-responsivity. Over-responsivity describes the nervous system's state of hyperarousal, or fright, fight, or flight, where all input is interpreted as a threat. An individual displaying under-responsivity requires excessive input to register sensory stimulation. This may be the case with the child who loves to spin and purposely crashes to the floor or does not cry when injured. Sensory integration theory attempts to normalize sensory input to produce an adaptive response that fits the situation at hand.

Sensory integration theory can be implemented in several ways within the educational or work environment. Many schools and most workplaces do not have the equipment or space to apply optimal intervention using this theory. This approach can be effectively used to develop and implement a sensory diet of activities or strategies to provide individuals with an optimal level of arousal to participate in their academic or work occupations. Table 26-6 reviews the sensory systems and the type of stimulation used to facilitate a calming or alerting response in an individual. These strategies can be used throughout the day to maintain an optimal level of arousal for productive work.

MODEL OF HUMAN OCCUPATION

The Model of Human Occupation (MOHO) as described by Kielhofner (1995) identifies four factors influencing work behavior. Volition describes the manner in which the individual chooses, experiences, anticipates, and interprets the occupational behaviors. Personal causation, interest, and value components all contribute to volition. Habituation describes internal roles and habits that convey a pattern and regularity in daily life. Performance, or the individual's innate abilities, is the foundation for adept function. Finally, the environment always results from the interaction of the previous three factors. In applying this model to practice, the occupational therapist takes the individual and setting into consideration, looking at the four subsystems. The occupational therapist must also attend to how the individual's injury or disability is affecting his or her relationship to the setting (Kielhofner et al., 1999).

The choice of a practice model and frames of reference depends on the practice setting and client's needs. One approach may work with a client in one setting, whereas a different model is most effective in another practice setting. Examples of these are work hardening and ergonomics (see Chapter 30). However, these specialized areas of practice require further training, and the occupational therapy practitioner must be open to all approaches and use the one (or pieces of several) that provides the best care to the client.

Summary

The implementation of occupational therapy services within the education and work models requires teamwork and ongoing collaboration with the members of the IEP team or the employers to ensure that individuals are capable of interacting and participating in the tasks being asked of them. The practitioner assists in the transition from secondary education into the workforce, independent/supported living, or post-secondary education.

Student Self-Assessment

Sam is a 7-year-old boy with cerebral palsy. He is in a regular first-grade classroom with educational support from an educational technician 100% of the day. Sam is independent with ambulation using a rear walker. His upper extremity strength and control are poor, with ataxic movements impacting precision with fine motor tasks. He uses raking finger movements and a lateral pinch to retrieve objects. Release is not always volitional, and he drops many items. Sam is independent in toileting, with the exception of clothing management. At this time, there is a private bathroom within the classroom where Sam's educational technician can assist him as needed. Sam's difficulty in toileting has been an ongoing area of need described by his parents at the IEP meeting. The team agrees that this is an area of need, particularly as he gets older and needs to use one of the public restrooms while at school.

1. Write at least one goal and two objectives to address Sam's independence in self-care while in school.
2. Describe the theoretical model, intervention activities, and potential accommodations or modifications that the occupational therapy practitioner may use in Sam's intervention.

Susan, a receptionist, is referred to occupational therapy due to chronic back and shoulder pain resulting from work-related stress. During your evaluation, you find that her computer desk is above elbow level when she is sitting. The computer is set to her right, at an angle to the keyboard, causing Susan to rotate her upper body while working. She schedules appointments and is frequently using the telephone and computer simultaneously, needing to hold the telephone between her ear and shoulder. Susan enjoys her job and does not want to leave in pursuit of other opportunities.

1. Describe the approach most beneficial in the intervention of Susan's pain.
2. Write a care plan for Susan that includes outcome potential, at least one goal, and two objectives.
3. How can the occupational therapy practitioner work with Susan's employer to provide accommodations to assist her in working pain free? What are those accommodations?

EVIDENCE-BASED RESEARCH: OCCUPATIONAL THERAPY IN THE EDUCATIONAL SETTING

Area Addressed	Reference
Autism	Ashburner, Ziviani, & Rodger, 2008; Bagatell, Mirigliani, Patterson, Reyes, & Test, 2010; Kinnealey, Pfeiffer, Miller, Roan, Shoener, & Ellner, 2012; Koenig, Buckley-Reen, & Garg, 2012
Handwriting	Ratzon, Efraim, & Bart, 2007; Roberts, Siever, & Mair, 2010
Frame of reference	Wuang, Wang, Huang, & Su, 2009
Evaluation	Brown, Unsworth, & Lyons, 2009; Tsai, Lin, Liao, & Hsieh, 2009
Physical disabilities	Egilson & Hemmingsson, 2009; Egilson & Traustadottir, 2009
Inclusion	Bazyk, S., Michaud, P., Goodman, G., Papp, P., Hawkins, E., & Welch, M. A. (2009)

EVIDENCE-BASED RESEARCH: OCCUPATIONAL THERAPY IN THE WORK PLACE

Area Addressed	Reference
Low back injuries/illnesses	Snodgrass, J. (2011). Effective occupational therapy interventions in the rehabilitation of individuals with work-related low back injuries and illnesses: A systematic review. *American Journal of Occupational Therapy, 65,* 37-43.
Shoulder injuries/illnesses	Von der Heyde, R. L. (2011). Occupational therapy interventions for shoulder conditions: A systematic review. *American Journal of Occupational Therapy, 65,* 16-23.
Elbow injuries/illnesses	Bohr, P. C. (2011). Systematic review and analysis for work-related injuries to and conditions of the elbow. *American Journal of Occupational Therapy, 65,* 24-28.
Forearm, wrist, and hand injuries/illnesses	Amini, D. (2011). Occupational therapy interventions for work-related injuries and conditions of the forearm, wrist, and hand: A systematic review. *American Journal of Occupational Therapy, 65,* 29-36.
Mental health	Cook, S., Chambers, E., & Coleman, J. H. (2009). Occupational therapy for people with psychotic conditions in community settings: A pilot randomized controlled trial. *Clinical Rehabilitation, 23,* 40-52. Mcgurk, S. R., Mueser, K. T., Feldman, K., Wolfe, R., & Pascaris, A. (2007). Cognitive training for supported employment: 2-3 year outcomes of a randomized controlled trial. *American Journal of Psychiatry, 164,* 437-441.

Electronic Resources

- Sensory Processing Disorder Foundation Resources: www.spdfoundation.net
- Sensory Integration Resources: www.fhsensory.com

- Work and School Intervention/Practice Resources: www.aota.org
- Education Mandates, Regulations, and Resources: www.ed.gov/index.jhtml
- Model of Human Occupation Clearinghouse: www.moho.uic.edu

EVIDENCE-BASED RESEARCH CHART

Topic	Area Addressed	Evidence
Sensory integration	Effectiveness	Humphries, Wright, McDougall, & Vertes, 1990; Soper & Thorley, 1996; Urwin & Ballinger, 2005; Wilson, Kaplan, Fellowes, Gruchy, & Faris, 1992
Neurodevelopmental intervention	Effectiveness	Brown & Burns, 2001; DeGangi, 1994a, 1994b; Jonsdottir, Fetters, & Kluzik, 1997; Kluzik, Fetters, & Coryell, 1990; Lilly & Powell, 1990; Miles Breslin, 1996; Tsorlakis, Evaggelinou, Grouios, & Tsorbatzoudis, 2004
Motor learning	Effectiveness	Baron & Littleton, 1999; Miles Breslin, 1996
Model of Human Occupation	Effectiveness	Basu, Jacobson, & Keller, 2004; Parrott, 2001
Intervention	Alternative education settings	Dirette & Kolak, 2004
	Transition planning	Spencer et al., 2003
	Fine motor development	Case-Smith, 1996
	Handwriting remediation	Lockhart & Law, 1994
Sensory diet strategies	Effectiveness: Wilbarger brushing and joint compression protocol	Moore & Henry, 2002
	Oral motor activity	Scheerer, 1992
	Weighted vest	Fertel-Daly, Bedell, & Hinojosa, 2001; VandenBerg, 2001

References

American Occupational Therapy Association. (2000). Occupational therapy and the Americans with Disabilities Act (ADA). *American Journal of Occupational Therapy, 54*(6), 622-625.

American Occupational Therapy Association. (2009). Guidelines for supervision, roles, and responsibilities during the delivery of occupational therapy services. *American Journal of Occupational Therapy, 63*, 797-803.

American Occupational Therapy Association. (2011). Occupational therapy practice framework: Domain and process (2nd ed.). *American Journal of Occupational Therapy, 62*, 625-683.

Asher, A. (2003). From student to employee: Helping students with disabilities make the transition. *Developmental Disabilities Special Interest Section Quarterly, 26*(4), 1-4.

Assistive Technology Act of 2004, Pub. L. 108-364, 118 Stat. 1707.

Berkley, S., Bender, W. N., Peaster, L. G., & Saunders, L. (2009). Implementation of Response to Intervention. A snapshot of progress. *Journal of Learning Disabilities, 42*, 85-95.

Breslin, D. (1996). Motor learning theory and the neurodevelopmental treatment approach: A comparative analysis. *Occupational Therapy in Health Care, 10*(1), 25-40.

Brief, A. P., & Nord, W. R. (1990). *The meanings of occupational work: A collection of essays.* Lanham, MD: Lexington Books.

Cengage Learning. (n.d.). *The Education for All Handicapped Children Act (PL 94-142) 1975.* Retrieved from http://college.cengage.com/education/resources/res_prof/students/spec_ed/legislation/pl_94-142.html

Chan, F., Strauser, D., Maher, P., Lee, E., Jones, R., & Johnson, E. T. (2010). Demand-side factors related to employment of people with disabilities: A survey of employers in the midwest region of the United States. *Journal of Occupational Rehabilitation, 20*, 412-419.

Croce, R., & DePaepe, J. (1989). A critique of therapeutic intervention programming with reference to an alternative approach based on motor learning theory. *Physical and Occupational Therapy in Pediatrics, 9*(3), 5-33.

Dirette, D., & Kolak, L. (2004). Occupational performance needs of adolescents in alternative education programs. *American Journal of Occupational Therapy, 58*(3), 337-341.

Dunn, W. (1990). A comparison of service provision models in school-based occupational therapy services: A pilot study. *Occupational Therapy Journal of Research, 10*(5), 300-320.

Dunn, W. (2000). *Best practice occupational therapy: In community service with children and families.* Thorofare, NJ: SLACK Incorporated.

Ellexson, M., & Larson, B. (2011). Occupational therapy services in facilitating work performance. *American Journal of Occupational Therapy, 65*, s55-s64.

Fessler State Board of Education Site. (n.d.). *School-to-Work Opportunities Act of 1994.* Retrieved from http://www.fessler.com/SBE/act.htm

Gliner, J. A. (1985). Purposeful activity in motor learning: An event approach to motor skill acquisition. *American Journal of Occupational Therapy, 39*(1), 28-34.

Hernandez, B., Cometa, M. J., Velcoff, J., Rosen, J., Schober, D., & Luna, R. D. (2007). Perspectives of people with disabilities on employment, vocational rehabilitation, and the Ticket to Work program. *Journal of Vocational Rehabilitation, 27,* 191-201.

Hearnshaw, L. S. (1954). Attitudes of work. *Occupational Psychology, 28,* 129-139.

Kardos, M., & White, B. P. (2005). The role of the school-based occupational therapist in secondary education transition planning: A pilot survey study. *American Journal of Occupational Therapy, 59,* 173-180.

Kielhofner, G. (1995). *A model of human occupation: Theory and application.* Baltimore, MD: Williams & Wilkins.

Kielhofner, G., Braveman, B., Baron, K., Fisher, G., Hammel, J., & Littleton, M. (1999). The model of human occupation: Understanding the worker who is injured or disabled. *WORK, 12*(1), 37-45.

Palisano, R. J. (1989). Comparison of two methods of service delivery for students with learning disabilities. *Physical and Occupational Therapy in Pediatrics, 9*(3), 79-100.

Pohlman, J., Poosawtsee, C., Gerndt, K., & Lindstrom-Hazel, D. (2001). Improving work programs' delivery of information and service to workers' compensation carriers. *Work, 16*(2), 91-100.

Sandqvist, J. L., & Henriksson, C. M. (2004). Work functioning: A conceptual framework. *WORK, 23*(2), 147-157.

Sanford, C., Newman, L., Wagner, M., Cameto, R., Knokey, A.-M., & Shaver, D. (2011). *The post-high school outcomes of young adults with disabilities up to 6 years after high school.* Key findings from the National Longitudinal Transition Study-2 (NLTS2) (NCSER 2011-3004). Menlo Park, CA: SRI International.

Shimmin, S. (1966). Concepts of work. *Occupational Psychology, 40,* 195–201.

Solomon, J. W. (2000). *Pediatric skills for occupational therapy assistants.* St. Louis, MO: Mosby.

Suchomel, S. K. (2000). Educational system. In J. W. Solomon (Ed.), *Pediatric skills for occupational therapy assistants.* St. Louis, MO: Mosby.

United States Department of Education. (n.d.). *Building the legacy: IDEA 2004.* Retrieved July 31, 2009, from http://idea.ed.gov

United States Department of Education. (2004). *The Rehabilitation Act.* Retrieved from http://www.ed.gov/policy/speced/reg/narrative.html

United States Equal Employment Opportunity Commission. (n.d.). *American with Disabilities Act (ADA): 1990–2002.* Retrieved July 31, 2009, from http://www.eeoc.gov/ada

Vaughn, S., Linan-Thompson, S., & Hickman, P. (2003). Response to Instruction as a means of identifying students with reading/learning disabilities. *Exceptional Children, 69,* 391-409.

Suggested Readings

Baker, N. A., & Jacobs, K. (2003). The nature of working in the United States: An occupational therapy perspective. *WORK, 20*(1), 53–61.

Baron, K. B., & Littleton, M. J. (1999). The model of human occupation: A return to work case study. *Work, 12*(1), 3-12.

Barris, R., & Kielhofner G. (1985). Generating and using knowledge in occupational therapy: Implications for professional education. *Occupational Therapy Journal of Research, 5*(2), 113-124.

Basu, S., Jacobson, L., & Keller, J. (2004). Child-centered tools: Using the model of human occupation framework. *School System Special Interest Section Quarterly, 11*(2), 1-3.

Berry, J., & Ryan, S. (2002). Frames of reference: Their use in pediatric occupational therapy. *British Journal of Occupational Therapy, 65*(9), 420-427.

Brayman, S. J., Clark, G. F., DeLany, J. V., Garza, E. R., Radomski, M. V., Ramsey, R., et al. (2004). Guidelines for supervision, roles and responsibilities during the delivery of occupational therapy services. *American Journal of Occupational Therapy, 58*(6), 663-667.

Brown, G. T., & Burns, S. A. (2001). The efficacy of neurodevelopmental treatment in paediatrics: A systematic review. *British Journal of Occupational Therapy, 64*(5), 235-244.

Case-Smith, J. (1996). Fine motor outcomes in preschool children who receive occupational therapy services. *American Journal of Occupational Therapy, 50*(1), 52-61.

Clark, G. F., Jackson, L., & Polichino, J. (2011). Occupational therapy services in early childhood and school-based settings. *American Journal of Occupational Therapy, 65,* s46-s54.

DeGangi, G. A. (1994a). Examining the efficacy of short-term NDT intervention using a case-study design: Part 1. *Physical and Occupational Therapy in Pediatrics, 14*(1), 71-88.

DeGangi, G. A. (1994b). Examining the efficacy of short-term NDT intervention using a case-study design: Part 2. *Physical and Occupational Therapy in Pediatrics, 14*(2), 21-61.

Fertel-Daly, D., Bedell, G., & Hinojosa, J. (2001). Effects of a weighted vest on attention to task and self-stimulatory behaviors in preschoolers with pervasive developmental disorders. *American Journal of Occupational Therapy, 55*(6), 629-640.

Fetters, L., & Kluzik, J. (1996). The effects of neurodevelopmental treatment versus practice on the reaching of children with spastic cerebral palsy. *Physical Therapy, 76*(4), 346-358.

Humphries, T., Wright, M., McDougall, B., & Vertes, J. (1990). The efficacy of sensory integration therapy for children with learning disability. *Physical and Occupational Therapy in Pediatrics, 10*(3), 1-17.

Jonsdottir, J., Fetters, L., & Kluzik, J. (1997). Effects of physical therapy on postural control in children with cerebral palsy. *Pediatric Physical Therapy, 9*(2), 68-75.

Kemmis, B. L., & Dunn, W. (1996). Collaborative consultation: The efficacy of remedial and compensatory interventions in school contexts. *American Journal of Occupational Therapy, 50*(9), 709-717.

King, G. A., McDougall, J., Tucker, M. A., Gritzan, J., Malloy-Miller, T., Alambets, P., et al. (1999). An evaluation of functional, school-based therapy services for children with special needs. *Physical and Occupational Therapy in Pediatrics, 19*(2), 5-29.

Kluzik, J., Fetters, L., & Coryell, J. (1990). Quantification of control: A preliminary study of effects of neurodevelopmental treatment on reaching in children with spastic cerebral palsy. *Physical Therapy, 70*(2), 65-76.

Lilly, L. A., & Powell, N. J. (1990). Measuring the effects of neuro-developmental treatment on the daily living skills of 2 children with cerebral palsy. *American Journal of Occupational Therapy, 44*(2), 139-415.

Lockhart, J., & Law M. (1994). The effectiveness of a multi-sensory writing programme for improving cursive writing in children with sensorimotor difficulties. *Canadian Journal of Occupational Therapy, 61*(4), 206-214.

Miles Breslin, D. M. (1996). Motor-learning theory and the neurodevelopmental treatment approach: A comparative analysis. *Occupational Therapy in Health Care, 10*(1), 25-40.

Moore, K. M., & Henry, A. D. (2002). Treatment of adult psychiatric patients using the Wilbarger protocol. *Occupational Therapy in Mental Health, 18*(1), 43-63.

Parrott, M. (2001). Further research into specific models of practice. *British Journal of Occupational Therapy, 64*(10), 519.

Scheerer, C. R. (1992). Perspectives on an oral motor activity: The use of rubber tubing as a "chewy." *American Journal of Occupational Therapy, 46*(4), 344-352.

Shamberg, S. (2005). Occupational therapy practitioner role in the implementation of worksite accommodations. *WORK, 24*(2), 185-194.

Soper, G., & Thorley, C. R. (1996). Effectiveness of an occupational therapy program based on sensory integration theory for adults with severe learning disabilities. *British Journal of Occupational Therapy, 59*(10), 475-482.

Storch, B. A., & Eskow, K. G. (1996). Theory application by school-based occupational therapists. *American Journal of Occupational Therapy, 50*(8), 662-668.

Tsorlakis, N., Evaggelinou, C., Grouios, G., & Tsorbatzoudis, C. (2004). Effect of intensive neurodevelopmental treatment in gross motor function of children with cerebral palsy. *Developmental Medicine and Child Neurology, 46*(11), 740-745.

Urwin, R., & Ballinger, C. (2005). The effectiveness of sensory integration therapy to improve functional behaviour in adults with learning disabilities: Five single-case experimental designs. *British Journal of Occupational Therapy, 68*(2), 56-66.

VandenBerg, N. L. (2001). The use of a weighted vest to increase on-task behavior in children with attention difficulties. *American Journal of Occupational Therapy, 55*(6), 621-628.

Wilson, B. N., Kaplan, B. J., Fellowes, S., Gruchy, C., & Faris, P. (1992). The efficacy of sensory integration treatment compared to tutoring. *Physical and Occupational Therapy in Pediatrics, 12*(1), 1-36.

World Institute on Disability. (n.d.). *The Ticket to Work and Work Incentives Improvement Act of 1999: Federal fact sheet on Public Law 106-170.* Retrieved from http://www.wid.org/publications/the-ticket-to-work-and-work-incentives-improvement-act-of-1999-federal-fact-sheet-on-public-law-106-170

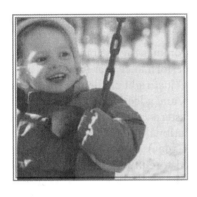

27

INTERVENTIONS OF PLAY AND LEISURE

Kathryn M. Loukas, OTD, MS, OTR/L, FAOTA and Bevin J. Journey, MS, OTR/L

<table>
<tr><td colspan="2" align="center">ACOTE STANDARDS EXPLORED IN THIS CHAPTER
B.5.2</td></tr>
<tr><td colspan="2" align="center">KEY VOCABULARY</td></tr>
<tr><td valign="top">

- **Freedom to suspend reality:** The ability to participate in make-believe activities or pretend play (Bundy, 1997).
- **Fun:** "That which provides mirth and amusement; enjoyment; playfulness" (Parham & Fazio, 1997, p. 250).
- **Internal control:** The extent to which the child is in control of his or her actions and to some aspects of outcome of the activity (Bundy, 1997).
- **Intrinsic motivation:** The self-initiation or drive to action that is rewarded by the activity itself rather than some external reward (Bundy, 1997).

</td><td valign="top">

- **Leisure:** "A nonobligatory activity that is intrinsically motivated and engaged in during discretionary time, that is, time not committed to obligatory occupations such as work, self-care or sleep" (Parham & Fazio, 1997, p. 250).
- **Play:** "Any spontaneous or organized activity that provides enjoyment, entertainment, amusement or diversion" (Parham & Fazio, 1997, p. 252).
- **Playfulness:** "A behavioral or personality trait characterized by flexibility, manifest joy, and spontaneity" (Parham & Fazio, 1997, p. 252).
- **Recreation:** Adult play or activities whose purpose is to "regenerate energy to support the worker role" (Glantz & Richman, 2001, p. 249).

</td></tr>
</table>

Jacobs, K., MacRae, N., & Sladyk, K. (Eds.).
Occupational Therapy Essentials for
Clinical Competence, Second Edition (pp. 367-377).
© 2014 SLACK Incorporated.

Introduction

Play and leisure activities are one part of the important triad of balance in occupational performance areas: work, play, and self-care across the lifespan (American Occupational Therapy Association [AOTA], 2002; Christianson, 1991; Kielhofner, 2008). Occupational therapy practitioners need to employ the use of play and leisure in the process and product of occupations in evaluation, intervention planning, intervention implementation, consultation, and discharge planning. Holistic intervention in occupational therapy is enhanced through the use of conceptual models. Models of practice guide holistic critical thinking in occupational therapy and theory and provide a foundation and rationale for practice (Scaffa, 1992). Recent scholars agree that occupation should be the central construct in our practices (Christiansen, Baum, & Haugen, 2004; Kielhofner, 2004; Wood, 1998; Yerxa, 1992). Occupation-centered interventions focus beyond impairment reduction toward meaningful participation in life (Lee, Taylor, Kielhofner, & Fisher, 2008). Play and leisure pursuits can be highly meaningful, adding much to the health, well-being, and social participation of human beings. In occupational practice, this important area of occupation is sometimes overlooked, perhaps because present society seems to favor work and self-care. This chapter focuses on interventions specific to play and leisure across the lifespan. It is based on goal-directed preparatory activities, purposeful activities, and occupational performance.

Play is the primary activity, and playfulness is the primary process by which occupational therapy practitioners address young children and infants (Bundy, 1997). Playfulness, according to Bundy, has three elements: intrinsic motivation, internal control, and the freedom to suspend reality. Suspending reality, or pretend or symbolic play, incorporates an imaginative element that can facilitate a child to develop the skills needed for real life (Bundy, 1993). Therefore, occupational therapy practitioners working with young children should try to create a safe environment, make activities fun, make routines part of a game or song, and engage the family or friends in the playful process. Creating contexts that enhance development is also an important aspect of the occupational therapy process because the child and the environment are interdependent in a transactional relationship (Humphry & Wakeford, 2006). Play facilitates dynamic development within and across domains in physical, cognitive, social, and emotional skills and is the underlying mechanism of learning during the developmental years. During play, a child should feel comfortable, safe, and engaged. The process needs to be enjoyable for both the client and the therapist.

Case-Smith (2010) promotes the use of intervention to enhance occupational performance that optimizes active engagement, provides a "just right challenge," provides a therapeutic relationship, and adequate intensity and reinforcement (p. 5). In Western culture, play is often considered to be the occupational role of children (Parham, 2008; Rodger & Ziviani, 1999). However, play and leisure are often interconnected to cultural and the economics of a society. In some cultures, both play and leisure are often embedded in work and self-care activities (Bazyk, Stalnaker, Llerena, Ekelman, & Bazyk, 2003; Hammell, 2009; Primeau, 1995). For this reason, it is important for occupational therapy practitioners to understand the role of play or leisure in the culture of the client and family (Parham, 2008).

Play activities throughout infancy and childhood can lead to decisions about which leisure activities to participate in later in life. Leisure activities are those that fill our free time as we take on adult roles and are important to leading a balanced life. Leisure activities have individual meaning to the persons participating in them. The complex and interconnected process of play and leisure leads contemporary adults to engage in coordinated and complementary leisure. Coordinated leisure activities are those that are work-related, such as playing on the company softball team or attending holiday parties at work. Complementary leisure is role-related, such as a mother who coaches soccer, a father who works on the set of his children's theater, or partners who accompany an elderly family member on a trip to his or her homeland (Glantz & Richman, 2001).

When complex intervention incorporates play or leisure activities, it is vital for the occupational therapist to consider the meaning a certain activity has to the client. Also, it is important to note that although occupational therapy practitioners promote play and leisure occupations, not all play and leisure occupations are healthy or positive. Children and adults can have negative occupations such as self-destructive behavior; addictions such as gambling; substance abuse; compulsions; or aggressive, illegal, or unsafe behaviors during their free time (Moyers, 1999). Clients may also have impoverished habits to be addressed in occupational therapy such as watching too much television and or over-eating high fat food. It is important for occupational therapy practitioners to promote healthy occupations and prevent or decrease unhealthy ones. Having strong and meaningful leisure occupations can prevent the development of an unhealthy interaction with the environment and promote healthy occupations for a lifetime.

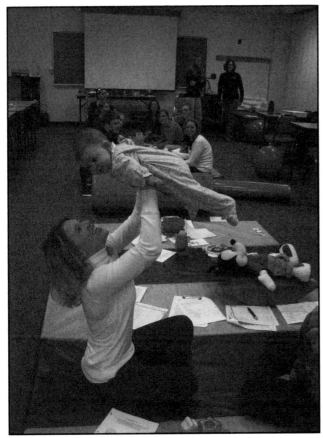

Figure 27-1. An OT student learns occupational development through play.

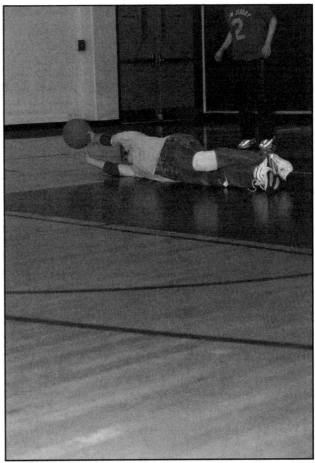

Figure 27-2. An athlete plays "Goalball," a sport designed for people who are blind or visually impaired.

Play and Leisure Across the Lifespan

Infancy and Preschool

In infancy, play focuses around exploration of surroundings and is sensorimotor based. Infants and young children discover cause-and-effect relationships to develop a purpose to their actions. Play occurs as an interaction between the infant and caregiver and later evolves to include siblings or other children (Knox, 1998). During the preschool years, play becomes more constructive and symbolic play is refined. Children start to use play to explore social roles. Play often incorporates fine motor activity, refining this skill as well. Play at this stage often occurs at home with parents or siblings (Figure 27-1).

School Age

School-aged play frequently revolves around rule-governed games, with emphasis on turn taking (Knox, 1998). Play is part of life for school-aged children on the playground at recess, in after-school activities, and during free time. School-aged children also have free leisure time that they need to find positive ways of fulfilling. Middle childhood is a time of engagement with peers in real and important ways. It is a time to make decisions about what occupations are fulfilling and meaningful to them, which can lead to decisions about what leisure activities to pursue in coming years.

Adolescence

As children approach adolescence, they begin to engage in more organized or "structured" play and leisure activities such as arts, sports, and other specific individual interests. The main focus of most play and leisure activities in adolescence is socialization. For this age group, it has been found that participation in structured activities can lead to decreased antisocial behavior (Mahoney & Stattin, 2000) and even higher academic grades (Fletcher, Nickerson, & Wright, 2003) (Figure 27-2).

Adulthood

Time spent pursuing leisure activities varies widely depending on contexts during adulthood. A single man or woman's leisure activities differ greatly from those of new parents, which differ from those of parents of adolescents or a business man or woman, which are again different from those of a retired couple. For parents, leisure activities might center around their children's activities. As adults age and children leave the house, more free time emerges for leisure activities such as reading, sewing, ballroom dancing, kayaking, or hiking. Social clubs or religious organizations might become important. Older adults and elders may engage in card groups, restaurant nights, and gardening as an empty nest, retirement, or disability allow more leisure time.

Evaluation

In-depth evaluation before intervention planning is critical when addressing play and leisure skills in order to help the practitioner gain a deeper understanding of the complex nature of this area of occupation. See Chapter 13 for more information on assessment of play and leisure skills.

INTERVENTION PLAN

The safety, health, and well-being of the client should always be the primary focus of the occupational therapy practitioner when addressing play or leisure areas of occupation. Knowing and following precautions may enable a client to feel safe and engaged in a therapeutic play or leisure setting. The intervention planning process should encompass the following domains according to the Occupational Therapy Practice Framework (AOTA, 2008):

- **Client factors.** All individual client factors, but especially the areas of values and beliefs, are critical to developing interventions of play and leisure. It is important not to project the therapist's own preconceived personal values onto the client, while maintaining a focus on health-promoting outcomes. Play and leisure skills vary widely across contexts and may have an impact on what activities are considered meaningful. For instance, a family who believes that an infant or child is too fragile for play but would benefit from motor activities could be educated to follow precautions while given specific ideas for interactive play with a medically fragile child.

- **Performance skills.** Posture, mobility, coordination, strength and effort, energy level, cognitive, emotional, sensory, social, and communication performance skills are used in the process of play and leisure. Intervention often targets specific areas of performance through interventions that are play or leisure based, creating a fun and engaging therapeutic activity.

- **Performance patterns.** Play and leisure are part of everyday occupations. Play or leisure time routines can be restorative in the balanced lives of human beings. Play, leisure habits, and routines are embedded in roles of individuals, families, and social groups.

- **Context.** The dynamic and complex nature of context, environment, and circumstances should be considered, used, and adapted for optimal therapeutic outcomes. Often play and recreational contexts are outdoors or in the community; this can have a very positive therapeutic influence on intervention outcomes. Because the natural environment is less controlled and predictable, safety considerations specific to each client, his or her age, and ability level should always be in place for any therapeutic context.

- **Activity demands.** Activity demands are inherent to many properties of play and leisure. Objects and their properties are important in consideration of use of toys, games, sports equipment, etc. Consideration of the space and social demands is an important part of decision-making process in intervention. Many sports, games, and play and leisure activities include aspects of sequencing and timing, cognitive demands, social skills, and required body functions and structures, which should be considered by the occupational therapy practitioner.

The occupational therapy intervention plan using play or leisure activities is geared toward the following common approaches (AOTA, 2008):

- **Create/promote.** Play or leisure programs that target a specific population are examples of occupational therapy intervention that promotes healthy lifestyles. An example is an after-school play and fitness program with recommendations for equipment from an occupational therapy practitioner to promote easy access for all students to promote physical activity and prevent obesity. A Tai Chi program for older adults to promote relaxation and circulation as an effort in fall prevention is another example. Occupational therapists are always finding more ways to promote health in their communities or work places. Many of these programs are play or leisure based.

- **Establish/restore.** Here the play or leisure activity is geared toward factors that are interfering with overall function. The occupational therapist creatively selects a play or leisure activity that will improve the targeted areas of function through play or leisure activities.

- **Maintain.** A maintenance approach can be used to facilitate preservation of developed skills, habits, etc.

For example, this approach might be used to develop an ongoing hiking or basketball group as part of a weight maintenance program or to educate a patient about modified cooking equipment to maintain functional independence after being discharged home from an inpatient facility.

- **Modify.** This is an approach to help clients participate in the occupations of their lives by adapting the environment, using adaptive devices, or implementing a compensatory strategy. Adapting toys or games for children with physical disabilities or enlarging text for people with visual impairment to facilitate reading are examples of this approach. Training family members to include their loved one by using adaptations is also under this area of intervention.

- **Prevent.** This area may entail helping people with disabilities engage in activities that require safe and effective movement. Examples are wearing a helmet when using the adaptive bicycle, using a reacher to pick up golf balls, or ensuring that a person with a cognitive impairment understands not to swim alone. People with chronic problems such as back injuries, chronic pain, or mental illness may need an occupational therapist to assist them with a play or leisure program that is healthy and will not exacerbate their disability.

Intervention Using Play or Leisure for Occupational Performance

Play and leisure are often used in two ways in occupational therapy practice: play and leisure as a means, or play and leisure as an end. Play and leisure as a means is described as using these activities as a tool for other goal oriented outcomes. This can be an important part of occupational therapy intervention and can be used to address many different client factors because clients are more likely to engage and cooperate in fun activities (O'Brien, 2006). Play and leisure as an end, or "outcome," is used when the occupational therapy practitioner is focused on helping the client gain skills and use daily routines in engagement in play or leisure activities (O'Brien, 2006).

Occupational therapy goals should be objective, measurable, and client centered. The following goals presented are broad in scope and are intended to facilitate ideas for intervention planning.

1. Play or leisure to improve targeted motor skills or development.
   - ◊ Johnny will improve gross and fine motor skills through play with objects and toys in his environment in a variety of developmental positions

as measured by improvement to an 18-month developmental level as measured by the Peabody Developmental Motor Scales (Folio & Fewell, 2000)
   - * Activity ideas: Creating a supportive context of developmental play incorporating the interdependent contexts of family, play, and childcare in the natural environment. Explorative play in positions such as supportive sitting, prone on elbows, or supported standing and interaction with age-appropriate sensorimotor toys should be facilitated
   - ◊ Through play-based motor activities, Christine will improve trunk control, sitting balance, and upper body control as measured by clinical observation data
     - * Activity ideas: Horseback riding, swimming, playing on a playground
   - ◊ William will engage in selected leisure activities 30 minutes per day in order to improve overall energy, bilateral arm use, and social participation as measured by self-reported journal entries
     - * Activity ideas: Involvement in an after-school program of choice such as shooting baskets, playing catch with a friend, swimming with a group, playing waffle ball, or playing volleyball

2. Goals to improve playfulness.
   - ◊ Jessie will engage in make-believe play with her sister with activity set-up as measured by sustaining pretend play activity for three interactions
     - * Activity ideas: Family training and facilitation of make-believe play such as a puppet theater, dress up, or bath-time play

3. Goals to improve psychosocial and behavioral skills.
   - ◊ Annie will improve emotional control and social interactions when engaging in peer group activities as measured by successful interactions without behavioral outburst three out of four times
     - * Activity ideas: The occupational therapist can consult with the staff to create contexts that support this goal. Other ideas include board games with one or more peers, "new games," and initiative and cooperative games (possibly done in the physical education class)
   - ◊ Mrs. Cooper will actively engage in a leisure activity daily with her husband without outburst for 30 minutes daily as measured by the husband's report
     - * Activity ideas: Consultation with the family and caregivers to create a context of support, safety, and recreation. Simple card games, walking around the block, reading a book to

their grandchild, and baking cookies together are ideas that could be incorporated into the intervention plan

4. Goals to improve social interactions and community participation.
   ◊ Dustin will interact with peers during recess to negotiate and share equipment three out of four times as measured by educational technician record keeping
     * Activity ideas: Facilitating play with a group of children along with the client, modeling and scripting communication to share the swings, helping a child wait and then try the slides, engaging a group of children in a four-square game alternating participants
   ◊ Susan will successfully join the fitness center, interacting with staff as needed as measured by therapist observation one time per month

5. Goals to add structure and leisure occupations to the daily routine.
   ◊ Isabelle will engage in three leisure activities that she will perform independently during free time as measured by group home record keeping
     * Activity ideas: Explore and engage in leisure activities to add to her list
   ◊ James will engage in three meaningful leisure-based heavy work activities to effectively transition from home to school daily as measured by sensory diet report card
     * Activity ideas: Pogo stick, medicine ball, mini trampoline, book deliveries

6. Goals with play or leisure occupations as the outcome.
   ◊ As part of the group home program, members will plan and engage in two community recreation activities per month as measured by record keeping and client report
     * Activity ideas: Choosing and going to a movie or theater event, going to the mall, walking on the high school track, going to an outdoor concert
   ◊ The Samson family will develop at least five play or leisure activities they can engage in as a family and do one family activity per week as measured by family reporting

7. Goals that use adaptation or compensation for play and leisure involvement.
   ◊ Simon will use adaptation in the community, such as his adapted bicycle, for safe and effective play participation with his siblings as measured by family report
   ◊ Given adaptations for visual deficits, including enlarging the targets, creating tactile boundaries,

and adding noise to sports equipment, Lynn will fully participate in sports at recreation camp as measured by staff reports, photos, and anecdotal data
   ◊ Given adaptations such as a card holder, Emma will effectively play with her friends on Cards Night for 30 minutes using her hemiplegic left arm as a functional assist as measured by therapist observation and record keeping

8. Goals to prevent disability.
   ◊ Amanda will learn and participate in three safe activities to engage in on the playground without injury as measured by inclusive playground therapy record keeping by the OT
   ◊ Markus will learn and use safe body mechanics while playing outdoor games such as bocce ball with his friends without pain behaviors as measured by client pain journal data

9. Goals to promote health.
   ◊ The group of people recovering from substance abuse will show increased insight about their addictions and less recidivism after the outdoor adventure program as measured by a 6-week follow-up study
   ◊ The older adults in assisted living will show improved balance after the ballroom dance session as measured by improved performance on the Berg Balance Scale

10. Goals to develop positive occupational leisure choices.
   ◊ Isabelle will learn three positive leisure activities for physical input that she will engage in instead of reverting to self-abusive behaviors (such as cutting) as measured by staff record keeping
   ◊ John will actively participate in a leisure activity of his choice three times a week and refrain from online gambling as measured by reflection journal and anecdotal records

11. Goals to improve self-esteem.
   ◊ Kayla will improve self-confidence and self-esteem through success in community programs such as Special Olympics and choir, as measured by an increase of 10% on scores of the self-esteem checklist

Summary

Occupational therapy practitioners promote and facilitate play with a purpose. Play and leisure are an important part of the triad of balance in occupational performance skills involved in life and occupational therapy practice. Using models and frames of reference as a guide, play and leisure activities in occupational therapy

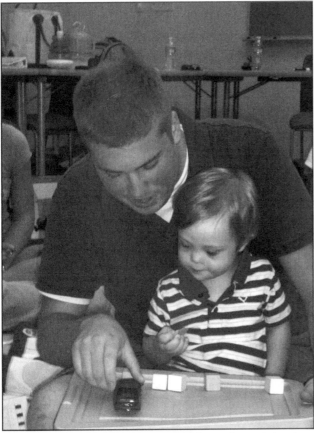

Figure 27-3. An OT practitioner playfully performs a developmental assessment.

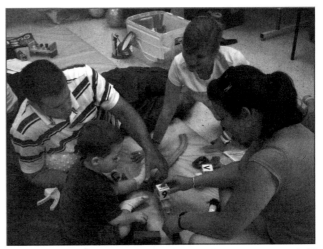

Figure 27-4. Occupational therapy students engage a child in play.

intervention should be carefully selected and performed with cultural sensitivity and individualized plans. Taking client factors into consideration—such as developmental level, physical and cognitive ability levels, psychosocial skills, and cultural considerations—a wide range of activities can be used in play and leisure interventions. The natural environment of intervention need to also be considered and modified to facilitate participation of play, leisure, and recreation in context. The outcomes of play and leisure intervention are as dynamic and broad as the occupational therapy spectrum, but they all facilitate occupational performance when they are performed with safety, fun, and enjoyment.

Student Self-Assessment

OCCUPATIONS OF CHILDREN

The instructor brings in a variety of toys and games for a wide spectrum of developmental levels and interests. Every students goes to a toy, game, or creative childhood item (Figures 27-3 and 27-4).

1. Answer the following questions:
   ◊ What thoughts or memories does this item bring back for you?
   ◊ What ages and gender would most likely use this toy or game?
   ◊ What skills are necessary to use this toy or game?
   ◊ What areas of motor development does this toy or game facilitate?
   ◊ What levels of visual, perceptual, or cognitive development does this toy or game facilitate?
   ◊ How could this toy or game develop social interaction with other people?
   ◊ How could this toy or game be modified for a person with physical special needs? For cognitive special needs?
   ◊ Is this something that an occupational therapist might use during an intervention? Describe how and with what client and client factors. Include age, diagnosis, and environment.

2. The following is a teaching, learning, and service assignment: adaptive equipment, activity, or toy fabrication.
   ◊ Description of the assignment: Students are to find a child with special needs through fieldwork or other means and design a piece of play equipment, toy, game, or sport specifically for that individual child or family. The student will then give the child or family the project. Cost limitation: $20. Lab time can be provided for this project.
   ◊ Criteria
     * Level of sophistication: complexity of project
     * Degree of individualization, client centered
     * Safety
     * Functionality: How well does it work?
     * Fun factor
     * Family friendly
     * Presentation in class

* Aesthetics
* Level of learning for the student
* Creativity

3. Leisure and recreation

    ◊ The instructor should bring in a variety of arts and crafts, games, and sports equipment such as croquet, bocce ball, checkers, Connect Four (Hasbro), Twister (Hasbro), deck of cards, Kings in the Corner, playground ball, table tennis, arts activities such as scrapbooking, etc.

    ◊ Students are divided into groups. Each group has 5 to 10 minutes to plan and 5 minutes to present or demonstrate one activity. Groups choose a scenario below and an activity to adapt for a successful occupational leisure activity.

      * The occupational therapy practitioner is working with a middle school child who is significantly visually impaired. They child is participating in a recreational after-school program with typical peers.

      * The occupational therapy practitioner needs to plan an activity evening for young adult clients with mental retardation and mild obesity who generally like to sit and watch TV and are resistant to physical activity.

      * The occupational therapy practitioner is working with a client with chronic low back pain and overmedication who is sedentary and depressed. OT goals are to promote pain-free movement.

      * The occupational therapy practitioner is working with a 60-year-old man with significant tremors and balance deficits from Parkinson's disease who wants to participate in activities with his wife.

* The occupational therapy practitioner is working with a young man with schizophrenia in a mental health group of four people who have significant difficulties with social interaction.

Activity	Goal(s)	Adaptations	Expected Outcomes

4. Experiential learning: Students who have been involved with work or volunteer work with people in adapted play, leisure, or recreational programming gain valuable insight into the importance and skills involved in adaptive activities. Consider the following experiential activities for students through volunteer experiences, work or Level 1 fieldwork:

    ◊ Therapeutic horseback riding
    ◊ Adaptive aquatics
    ◊ Transdisciplinary playgroups (Loukas, Whiting, Ricci, & Cohen-Konrad, 2012)
    ◊ Camps for children with special needs (e.g., Easter Seals)
    ◊ Martial arts for people with physical challenges
    ◊ Special Olympics
    ◊ Ski programs for people with physical challenges
    ◊ School-based summer recreational programs with inclusion
    ◊ Sensory integrative camps
    ◊ Developmental preschools

EVIDENCE-BASED RESEARCH CHART

Goal	Intervention Description	Evidence
Playfulness	Intervention targeted at improving playfulness in 4- to 6-year-old children with autism spectrum disorder	O'Brien et al., 2000
	Play behaviors of random preschool children found a positive correlation between playfulness and coping skills	Saunders, Sayer, & Goodale, 1998
	Playfulness correlated with stress coping skills on 195 university students	Qian & Yarnell, 2011
Play as goal occupation	Purposeful "play" activity more effective than rote exercise in a case study of two children with burn injuries	Melchert-McKearnan, Deitz, Engle, & White, 2000
	The parasympathetic and sympathetic nervous systems are influenced during the important developmental play activities of children	Way, 1999
	Nonplay-specific materials found to increase playfulness on a school playground with 5- to 7-year-old school children	Bundy et al., 2008
	Mastery of play was one area targeted through sensory integrative intervention for preschool children with autism	Case-Smith & Bryan, 1999
	Positioning equipment for children with physical disabilities has a positive impact on play skills as measured by parent survey	O'Brien et al., 1998
Play as a means to improve performance skills	Participation in the "Learn to Play" program over 6 months was associated with increased social interaction, connection, and language skills in 19 children with intellectual disabilities	Stagnitti, O'Connor, & Sheppard, 2012
	Occupational therapy-directed play can improve fine motor and visual motor performance in intervention in preschool-aged children with fine motor delays	Case-Smith, 2000
	Initiation and response in free-play dyads of children with delayed play skills when engaged with higher level peers	Tanta, Deitz, White, & Billingsley, 2005
Leisure as an occupational performance goal	Program implementation of the Healthy Occupations for Positive Emotions (HOPE) initiative with 70 African American students ranging in age from 7 to 12 years	Bazyk & Bazyk, 2009
Leisure as a means to improve performance skills	Reading, playing board games, playing music, and dancing are associated with a reduced risk of dementia	Verghese, Lipton, Katz, & Hall, 2003
	Sixty pet owners with serious mental illness living in the community demonstrate higher social community integration	Zimolag & Krupa, 2009
	Leisure benefits for persons with congenital disabilities by involvement in leisure activities	Specht, King, Brown, & Foris, 2002
	Structured leisure activities (clubs, sports, classes) are linked to lower levels of antisocial behavior in adolescents	Fletcher, Nickerson, & Wright, 2003; Mahoney & Stattin, 2000
	Improvement of occupational identity of older retired persons involved in creative occupations such as woodworking, painting, knitting, etc.	Howie, Coulter, & Feldman, 2004
	Evidence-based review of interventions used to improve leisure occupations of people with Alzheimer's disease shows a positive impact	Letts et al., 2011
	Interventions designed to modify activity demands of leisure were found to be effective for people with Alzheimer's disease	Padilla, 2011
	Occupation-based life review activity improved symptoms of depression in older adults	Chippendale & Bear-Lehman, 2012
Long-term benefits of leisure participation	Longitudinal study of 457 Swedish individuals indicates that late-life participation in both physical and sedentary activities, especially for men, is associated with long-term survival benefits	Agahi, Silverstein, & Parker, 2011
Cultural influences	Play is incorporated into work activities with Mayan children	Bazyk et al., 2003
	Sociocultural comparison of Nigerian and American children's games indicate a diversity of styles, values, and approach to play in different cultures	Nwokah & Ikekeonwu, 1998

References

Agahi, N., Silverstein, M., & Parker, M. G. (2011). Late-life and earlier participation in leisure activities: Their importance for survival among older persons. *Activities, Adaptation & Aging, 35,* 210-222.

American Occupational Therapy Association. (2002). The occupational therapy practice framework: Domain and process. *American Journal of Occupational Therapy, 56,* 609-639.

American Occupational Therapy Association. (2008). The occupational therapy practice framework: Domain and process, (2nd ed). *American Journal of Occupational Therapy, 62*(6), 625-683.

Bazyk, S., & Bazyk, J. (2009). The meaning of occupation-based groups for low-income urban youths attending after-school care. *American Journal of Occupational Therapy, 63,* 69-80.

Bazyk, S., Stalnaker, D., Llerena, M., Ekelman, B., & Bazyk, J. (2003). Play in Mayan children. *American Journal of Occupational Therapy, 57*(3), 273-283.

Bundy, A. C. (1993). Assessment of play and leisure: Delineation of the problem. *American Journal of Occupational Therapy, 47*(3), 217-222.

Bundy, A. C. (1997). Play and playfulness: What to look for. In L. D. Parham & L. S. Fazio (Eds.), *Play in occupational therapy for children* (pp. 52-66). St. Louis, MO: Mosby.

Bundy, A. C., Luckett, T., Naughton, G. A., Tranter, P. J., Wyver, S. R., Ragen, J., Singleton, E., & Spies, G. (2008). Playful interaction: Occupational therapy for all children on the school playground. *American Journal of Occupational Therapy, 62,* 522-527.

Case-Smith, J. (2000). Effects of occupational therapy services on fine motor and functional performance in preschool children. *American Journal of Occupational Therapy, 54*(4), 371-380.

Case-Smith, J. (2010). An overview of occupational therapy for children. In J. Case-Smith & J. C. O'Brien (Eds.), *Occupational therapy for children* (pp. 1-21). Maryland Heights, MD: Mosby Elsevier.

Case-Smith, J., & Arbesman, M. (2008). Evidence-based review of interventions for autism used in or of relevance to occupational therapy. *American Journal of Occupational Therapy, 62,* 416-429.

Case-Smith, J., & Bryan, T. (1999). The effects of occupational therapy with sensory integration emphasis on preschool-age children with autism. *American Journal of Occupational Therapy, 53*(5), 498-497.

Chippendale, T., & Bear-Lehman, J. (2012). Effect of life review writing on depressive symptoms in older adults: A randomized controlled trail. *American Journal of Occupational Therapy, 66*(4), 438-446.

Christianson, C. (1991). Occupational therapy: Intervention for life performance. In C. Christianson & C. Baum (Eds.), *Occupational therapy: Overcoming human performance deficits.* Thorofare, NJ: SLACK Incorporated.

Christiansen, C. H., Baum, C. M., & Haugen, J. B. (Eds.). (2004). *Occupational therapy: Performance, participation, and well-being* (3rd ed.). Thorofare, NJ: SLACK Incorporated.

Doig, E., Fleming, J., Cornwell, P. L., & Kuipers, P. (2009). Qualitative exploration of a client-centered, goal-directed approach to community-based occupational therapy for adults with traumatic brain injury. *American Journal of Occupational Therapy, 64,* 559-568.

Fletcher, A. C., Nickerson, P., & Wright, K. L. (2003). Structured leisure activities in middle childhood: Links to well-being. *Journal of Community Psychology, 31*(6) 641-659.

Folio, M. R. & Fewell, R. R. (2000). *Peabody Developmental Motor Scales* (2nd ed). San Antonio, TX: PsychCorp Pearson.

Glantz, C. H., & Richman N. (2001). Leisure activities. In L. W. Pedretti & M. B. Early (Eds.), *Occupational therapy practice skills for physical dysfunction* (5th ed., pp. 249-256). St. Louis, MO: Mosby.

Hammell (2009). K. @W., (2004). Dimensions of meaning in the occupations of daily life. *Canadian Journal of Occupational Therapy, 71*(5), 296-305.

Hoppes, S., & Segal, R. (2010). Reconstructing meaning through occupation after the death of a family member: Accommodation, assimilation, and continuing bonds. *American Journal of Occupational Therapy, 64,* 133-141.

Howie, L., Coulter, M., & Feldman, S. (2004). Crafting the self: Older persons' narratives of occupational identity. *American Journal of Occupational Therapy, 58,* 446-454.

Humphry R., & Wakeford, L., (2006). An occupation-centered discussion of development and implications for practice. *American Journal of Occupational Therapy, 60,* 258-267.

Kielhofner, G. (2004). *Conceptual foundations of occupational therapy* (3rd ed.). Philadelphia: F. A. Davis Company.

Kielhofner, G. (Ed.), (2008). *A model of human occupation* (4th ed.). Baltimore, MD: Williams and Wilkins.

Knox, S. H. (1998). Treatment through play and leisure. In M. E. Neistadt & E. B. Crepeau (Eds.), *Willard and Spackman's occupational therapy* (9th ed., pp 382-390). New York, NY: Lippincott Williams and Wilkins.

Lee, S. W., Taylor, R., Kielhofner, G., & Fisher, G. (2008). Theory use in practice: A national survey of therapists who use the Model of Human Occupation. *American Journal of Occupational Therapy, 62,* 106-117.

Letts, L., Edwards, M., Berenii, J., Moros, K., O'Neill, C., O'Toole, C., & McGrath., C. (2011). Using occupations to improve quality of life, health and wellness, and client and caregiver satisfaction for people with Alzheimer's disease and related dementias. *American Journal of Occupational Therapy, 64,* 497-504.

Loukas, K. M., Whiting, A., Ricci, E., & Cohen Konrad, S. (2012). Transdisciplinary playgroup: Interprofessional opportunities in early intervention practice education. *OT Practice, 17*(3), 8-13.

Mahoney, J. L., & Stattin, H. (2000). Leisure activities and adolescent antisocial behavior: The role of structure and social context. *Journal of Adolescence, 23,* 113-127.

Melchert-McKearnan, K., Deitz, J., Engel, J. M., & White, O. (2000). Children with burn injuries: Purposeful activity versus rote exercise. *American Journal of Occupational Therapy, 54*(4), 381-390.

Moyers, P. (1999). The guide to occupational therapy practice. *American Journal of Occupational Therapy, 53,* 246-322.

Nwokah, E. E., & Ikekeonwu, C. (1998). A sociocultural comparison of Nigerian and American children's games. In *Play and culture studies* (vol. 1). London, England: Ablex Publishing.

O'Brien, J. C. (2006). Play and playfulness. In J. W. Solomon & J. C. O'Brien (Eds.), *Pediatric skills for occupational therapy assistants* (pp. 321-342). St. Louis, MO: Mosby.

O'Brien, J., Boatwright, T., Chaplin, J., Geckler, C., Gosnell, D., Holcombe, J., & Parrish, K. (1998). *The impact of positioning equipment on play skills of physically impaired children. In Play and Culture Studies* (vol. 1). London, England: Ablex Publishing.

O'Brien, J., Coker, P., Lynn, R., Suppinger, R., Pearigen, T., Rabon, S.,...Ward., A. T. (2000). The impact of occupational therapy on a child's playfulness. *Occupational Therapy in Health Care, 12*(2/3), 39-51.

Padilla, R. (2011). Effectiveness of interventions designed to modify the activity demands of the occupations of self-care and leisure for people with Alzheimer's disease and related dementias. *American Journal of Occupational Therapy, 65*, 523-531.

Parham, L. D. (2008). Play and occupational therapy. In L. D. Parham & L. S. Fazio (Eds.), *Play in occupational therapy for children* (pp. 3-39). Maryland Heights, MD: Mosby Elsevier.

Parham, L. D., & Fazio, L. S. (1997). *Play in occupational therapy for children.* St. Louis, MO: Mosby.

Primeau, L. A. (1996). Work and leisure: Transcending the dichotomy. *American Journal of Occupational Therapy, 50*(7), 569-577.

Qian, X. L., & Yarnal, C. (2011). The role of playfulness in the leisure stress-coping process among emerging adults: An SEM analysis. *Leisure, 35*(2), 191-209.

Rodger, S., & Ziviani, J. (1999). Play-based occupational therapy. *International Journal of Disability, Development, and Education, 40*(3), 337-365.

Saunders, I., Sayer, M., & Goodale, A. (1999). The relationship between playfulness and coping in preschool children: A pilot study. *American Journal of Occupational Therapy, 53*(2), 221-225.

Scaffa, M. (2001). *Occupational therapy in community-based practice settings.* Philadelphia, PA: F.A. Davis Company.

Shimoni, M., Engel-Yeger, B., & Tirosh, E. (2010). Participation in leisure activities among boys with attention deficit hyperactivity disorder. *Research in Developmental Disabilities, 31,* 1234-1239.

Specht, J., King, G., Brown, E., & Foris, C. (2002). The importance of leisure in the lives of persons with congenital physical disabilities. *American Journal of Occupational Therapy, 56*(4), 436-445.

Stagnitti, K., O'Connor, C., & Sheppard, L. (2012). Impact of the Learn to Play program on play, social competence, and language for children aged 5-8 years who attend a specialist school. *Australian Occupational Therapy Journal, 59,* 302-311.

Tanta, K. J., Deitz, J. C., White, O. and Billingsley, F. (2005). The effects of peer-play level on initiations and responses of preschool children with delayed play skills. *American Journal of Occupational Therapy, 59*(4) 437-445.

Verghese, J., Lipton, R. B., Katz, M. J., & Hall, C. B. (2003). Leisure activities and the risk of dementia in the elderly. *New England Journal of Medicine, 348*(25) 2508-2517.

Way, M. (1999). Parasympathetic and sympathetic influences in neuro-occupation pertaining to play. *Occupational Therapy in Health Care, 12*(1), 71-86.

Wood, W. (1998). It is jump time for occupational therapy. *American Journal of Occupational Therapy, 52,* 403-411.

Yerxa, E. J. (1992). Some implications of occupational therapy's history for its epistemology, values, and relation to medicine. *American Journal of Occupational Therapy, 46,* 79-83.

Yuen, H. K., Huang, P., Burik, J. K., & Smith, T. G. (2008). Impact of participating in volunteer activities for residents living in long-term-care facilities. *American Journal of Occupational Therapy, 62,* 71-76.

Zimolag, U., & Krupa, T. (2009). Pet ownership as a meaningful community occupation for people with serious mental illness. *American Journal of Occupational Therapy, 63,* 126-137.

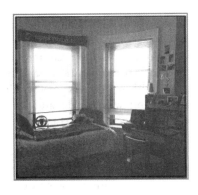

28

INTERVENTIONS TO ENHANCE OCCUPATIONAL PERFORMANCE IN REST AND SLEEP

Michelle Goulet, MS, OTR/L; Courtney S. Shufelt, MS, OTR/L; and Briana Youland, MS, OTR/L

ACOTE STANDARDS EXPLORED IN THIS CHAPTER

B.5.1-5.4, 5.8

KEY VOCABULARY

- **Cognitive behavioral therapy:** A therapy approach that is used when a practitioner is aiming to change the way a client thinks about something; this is done using the assumption that the way in which we think about a situation controls how we feel and in turn controls our actions and the consequences to those actions.

- **Compensation/adaptation:** Changing the task itself such as its necessities, the objects it uses, or how the task is accomplished in order to elicit a more desired outcome.

- **Health promotion:** Focuses on lifestyle redesign and the balance between one's body, self, and environment in order to engage in purposeful and meaningful occupations.

- **Primary disability prevention:** Addresses society as a whole, including those who do not have limitations or impairments.

- **Remediation/restoration:** Focuses on reversing/ceasing the unwanted components and repairing the desired components of one's performance including physiological, psychological, neurological, and biological aspects.

- **Secondary disability prevention:** Focuses on a group or population that is considered at risk for a disease or disability.

- **Sleep deprivation:** The result that occurs when an individual does not receive the amount of sleep his or her body requires for optimal functioning.

- **Tertiary disability prevention:** Meant to increase function and decrease the effects of an illness or injury in those who already have or currently are experiencing its effects.

Jacobs, K., MacRae, N., & Sladyk, K. (Eds.).
*Occupational Therapy Essentials for
Clinical Competence, Second Edition* (pp. 379-384).
© 2014 SLACK Incorporated.

Introduction

Continuing with the occupations of rest and sleep, this chapter discusses how occupational therapy practitioners may help to enhance these occupations. General and specific intervention guidelines and ideas are provided. The effects of sleep deprivation on our clients' activities of daily living (ADL) and instrumental activities of daily living (IADL) performance are discussed for a general knowledge of what to expect.

Interventions

Before an intervention can begin, an occupational therapy practitioner must create a comprehensive intervention plan for the client. This is developed in conjunction with not only the client and other health care professionals but also, whenever possible, the family and caregivers. The five major parts of an intervention plan are (1) long-term goals; (2) short-term goals; (3) the possible intervention procedures; (4) the amount, frequency, duration, and type of therapy sessions; and (5) any further recommendations and referrals to other health care professionals (Moyers, 1999). An intervention plan is just that, a plan. There is no guarantee that everything mentioned in the intervention plan will be achieved or even addressed during treatment. It is good practice to try to include everything listed (unless unforeseen circumstances arise such as the client succeeding much quicker than anticipated or requiring increased time to reach short-term goals) because the items were included for particular reasons.

When attending to the topic of sleep disturbances, clients are more often than not referred to occupational therapy for other reasons, and sleep disturbances are discovered during evaluation. It may come to a practitioner's attention that a client's sleep disturbances may require a referral to a physician who specializes in sleep. Physicians who specialize in sleep should be contacted when a person has not been diagnosed with a sleep disorder; if the occupational therapy practitioner suspects sleep apnea, a nocturnal seizure disorder, or periodic limb movement disorder; if a formal sleep study is needed; or if there is suspicion that medication may need to be reviewed or altered (Westley, 2004)

The intervention process can be classified, according to Moyers (1999), by four common approaches, which are used in an integrated fashion.

1. **Remediation/restoration.** Remediation/restoration focuses on the components of one's performance including physiological, psychological, neurologic, and biologic processes. It may require the occupational therapy practitioner to provide education on techniques and the review of techniques to enable the client to institute new skills, habits, and behaviors within those components that are required for successful performance. An intervention pertaining to sleep that falls within this category would be providing education on what to do and what not to do to increase the success of adequate sleep or to provide behavioral treatment interventions. When addressing rest with a client who enjoys reading books but has difficulty reading the print, an intervention that falls into this category would be introducing the use of either large-print books or an electronic reader with which font size can be changed accordingly.

2. **Compensation/adaptation.** Compensation/adaptation attends to the possibility of changing the task itself, such as its necessities, the objects it uses, or how the task is accomplished. An occupational therapy practitioner may also decide to change the task environment under this approach. A client who loves to watch his or her favorite television show as relaxation but has difficulty seeing the remote may benefit from a remote control for vision-impaired individuals or a voice-activated home system, including the television. A client who experiences sleep difficulties may benefit from a home visit with an occupational therapy practitioner to change his or her sleeping environment to make it more conducive for a restful night's sleep or providing a sleeping wedge for a client who has gastroesophageal reflux disease to decrease the likelihood of increased acid reflux while lying flat.

3. **Disability prevention.** Disability prevention is split up into three different types: primary, secondary, and tertiary. Primary prevention of disability is meant to address society as a whole, including those who do not have limitations or impairments. Providing education throughout the lifespan to all clients about the importance of maintaining good sleep habits is a great example of this. When prevention is focused on a group or population that is considered at risk, it is called secondary prevention. Providing information about how specific conditions may affect sleep is a good example of protecting those with a higher chance of sleep disturbances. The goal of tertiary prevention is to increase function and decrease the effects of an illness or injury in those who already have or currently are experiencing its effects. Providing a group for elders who experience sleeping difficulty on how to improve their sleep, and thus their everyday functioning, displays this type of prevention.

4. **Health promotion.** Health promotion focuses on lifestyle redesign and the balance between one's body, self, and environment in order to engage in purposeful and meaningful occupations. Current research has even found evidence of decreased amounts of sleep positively affecting weight gain in all age groups, but particularly in those younger than 18 years (Patel & Hu, 2008; Vorona et al., 2005). When discussing the possibilities of sleep disruptions with clients, it is important to educate them on being able to regulate a healthy daily routine juggling rest, work, play, and leisure and how it can affect our mood, relationships, and performance.

Two specific types of intervention have been shown to be very helpful when working with clients who experience sleeping difficulties. Both types of interventions have been used separately and in conjunction with one another, resulting in success within groups and on an individual basis, also yielding positive results. Studies have shown that using cognitive and behavioral treatment approaches are safe and effective alternatives to some medication (Davidson, Waisberg, Brundage, & Maclean, 2001). These two intervention approaches are different; however, they share many of the same qualities and beliefs, making them easy to use in combination with one another.

Cognitive behavioral therapy (CBT) is a therapy approach that is used quite often when a practitioner is aiming to change the way a client thinks about something. The main assumption of CBT is that the way we think about a situation controls how we feel and, in turn, controls our actions and the consequences of those actions. The goal of using CBT with clients who have sleep difficulties is to change the way they think and act in relation to their sleep. Logging the client's sleep is usually the first step, as well as receiving general education about sleep and clients' personal sleep hygiene. Next, practitioners work with clients to cognitively restructure their dysfunctional beliefs about sleep, highlighting unrealistic thoughts and irrational fears (Vitiello, 2000; Vitiello, Rybarczyk, Korff, & Stepanski, 2009). Eliminating behaviors in the bed or bedroom that are not conducive to sleep is a CBT guideline for sleep intervention. This is done to foster the thinking that the bed and bedroom are meant only for sleep, sex, and activities that help one sleep. Sticking to a sleep–wake schedule and avoiding naps during the day will train a client that there are only certain times when he or she should be sleeping. If a person does not sleep during that time, then he or she should wait until the next sleep-appropriate time frame (Vitiello, 2000).

Behavioral treatment focuses on the behaviors that one performs surrounding sleep and how changing them

---

General Sleep Interventions: The Dos and Don'ts

Do

- Eat a healthy, small snack before bed if you prefer.
- Go to bed and wake up at the same time each day.
- Use a consistent bedtime routine.
- Use relaxation techniques to reduce anxiety before bedtime.
- Take a nap for 20 minutes or less if you must take one.
- Contact your doctor if you suspect a sleep disorder.
- Decrease noise and light in your bedroom.
- Maintain a consistent exercise program.
- Get natural sunlight during the day, especially toward the end of the day.

Don't

- Drink alcohol or caffeine near bedtime.
- Take naps during the day, especially after 2 pm.
- Use your bed for anything other than sleep, activities that encourage sleep, or sex.
- Watch television close to bedtime.
- Exercise 2 hours before going to bed.
- Eat a big meal before going to bed or go to bed on a full stomach.
- Drink liquids close to bedtime if you have urinary urgency.
- Keep your bedroom too hot or cold; neutral temperatures are better.
- Go to bed unless you feel sleepy.
- Stay in bed if you cannot fall asleep.

Adapted from Rajki, 2011; Subramanian & Surani, 2007; Vitiello, 2000; and Westley, 2004.

---

can improve the quality of sleep. The aim is to positively impact the emotional connection one has between sleeping and his or her bedroom, rather than the association to the bedroom with his or her insomnia.

There are three main treatment areas used: relaxation techniques, temporal control therapy, and sleep restriction therapy. Different from CBT, behavioral treatments focus on relaxation techniques, allowing the client to let go of the emotional stressors attached to his or her sleeping difficulties by integrating biofeedback, meditation, and guided imagery as part of his or her sleep routine (Rajki, 2011; Subramanian & Surani, 2007). These strategies, in turn, reduce cognitive and physiologic arousal at bedtime (Vitiello, 2009). Similar to a CBT approach are temporal control therapy and sleep restriction therapy of behavioral intervention. Maintaining a consistent sleep/wake cycle and avoiding daytime napping are included with the temporal control aspect; this is accomplished by getting in and out of bed at the same time each day regardless of how the client's sleep went the previous night. Sleep restriction allows a sleep debt to accumulate based on the theory that it will enhance the tendency to sleep at the appropriate time (Subramanian & Surani, 2007).

Affect of Sleep on Performance in Activities of Daily Living and Instrumental Activities of Daily Living

Sleep is important for restoring energy, repairing the physical body, regulating temperature, revitalizing emotions, and recharging cognitive function (Luyster, Strollo, Zee, & Walsh, 2012; Ohlmann & O'Sullivan, 2009). Sleep allows the brain to form new neural pathways and synapses (Church, 2012). Healthy sleep habits and routines that promote optimal sleep duration and quality of sleep have a positive impact on ADL and IADL. An individual wakes feeling energized and prepared to accomplish mental and physical tasks. On the other hand, when an individual does not receive the amount of sleep his or her body requires, sleep deprivation can occur, and this can affect ADL and IADL. Sleep deprivation can affect an individual's functional capabilities by increasing his or her likelihood of accidents, decreasing productivity, increasing fatigue, and increasing health problems (Ohlmann & O'Sullivan, 2009).

Sleep deprivation can be acute or chronic. In acute sleep deprivation, individuals are awake for 24- to 72-hour periods. In chronic sleep deprivation, individuals experience a cumulative sleep loss over several consecutive nights (Kravitz, 2012). Multiple factors can contribute to sleep deprivation, including sleep disorders such as insomnia, sleep apnea, and restless leg syndrome; anxiety; depression; certain medications; and other health problems (Wells & Vaughn, 2012). Environmental factors and an individual's lifestyle or routine may also contribute to his or her sleep deprivation.

Use the following to discover if a client may be sleep deprived (Ohlmann & O'Sullivan, 2009):

- Client complains of feeling sleepy while driving.
- Client states he or she is addicted to caffeine.
- Client makes frequent mistakes.
- Client forgets information he or she should know.
- Client states that he or she feels depressed, uptight, or anxious.
- Client reports often getting sick.

Although research is still being conducted, links between sleep and physical health, psychological and neurological dysfunction, and mood have been reported (Valenza, Rodenstein, & Ferández-de-las-Peñas, 2011).

Sleep and Physical Health

Researchers have found that sleep deprivation and sleep apnea are linked to cardiovascular disease. During sleep, the body repairs cardiovascular tissues. If deep sleep is interrupted, the body does not have adequate time to repair these tissues, and damage to vital organs can occur (Ohlmann & O'Sullivan, 2009). Sleep deprivation has also been shown to increase heart rate and blood pressure and has been linked to an increase in the incidence of cardiac-related death (Valenza et al., 2011). Although damage to vital cardiovascular organs may not be directly apparent to the client or practitioner, it is important for clients and practitioners to remain mindful that sleep is imperative for cardiovascular health, and a client's cardiovascular health affects his or her ability to perform daily activities and tasks.

In addition to cardiovascular health, sleep is also important for maintaining insulin levels within the body. Research has found that after three consecutive nights of sleep loss, an individual's insulin sensitivity decreases by 25%. According to Ohlmann and O'Sullivan (2009), sleep deprivation has the potential to decrease glucose tolerance and compromise insulin sensitivity because sympathetic nervous system activity increases, which raises evening cortisol levels and decreases the use of glucose. Cardiovascular health and diabetes type II are two of the most common physical health problems associated with sleep in current research. Other health problems that have the potential to arise from or are made worse by sleep deprivation include obesity (Kravitz, 2012), certain types of cancers (Church, 2012; Luyster et al., 2012; Ohlmann & O'Sullivan, 2009), and digestive problems (Ohlmann & O'Sullivan, 2009).

Although it is hard to see the direct impacts of sleep deprivation on an individual's physical health, sleep does play an important role in restoring the health of the body's organs and physiological systems. Chronic sleep deprivation has the potential to significantly impact an individual's physical health, which could greatly impact an individual's ability to perform daily activities. Regardless of whether a client already has physical health impairments, a practitioner must encourage healthy sleep habits and routines in order to maintain optimal physical health. Even though sleep deprivation does not necessarily have immediate physical effects on the body, it does have the potential to cause life-threatening damage over the course of time. Therefore, a practitioner should think about the end goals of interventions and treatments, the client's sleep habits and routines, and how they will impact the client's goals and future.

Sleep and Cognitive Functioning

Sleep deprivation also impacts an individual's cognitive functioning. Along with restoring physical properties within the body, sleeping also restores an individual's cognitive processes. If cognitive processes are not restored during sleep, an individual's ability to engage in tasks that require cognitive functioning will be greatly impacted. Many aspects of cognitive functioning have the potential to be influenced by a lack of sleep such as memory, perception, reaction time, attention, and processing.

Sleep is essential for adequate memory processing. Sleep transforms the information we learn while we are awake into a more concrete memory within different parts of the brain. Researchers believe that during sleep, memories are allocated to other parts of the brain to be stored. This is the brain's way of sorting through important information. Research also suggests that engaging in rapid eye movement (REM) and non-REM sleep after engaging in a learning activity increases one's ability to retain the information he or she learned during the activity and results in improved performance with the activity the next day (Church, 2012; Dang-Vu et al., 2010). Therefore, sleep is important for the rehabilitation process, specifically the carryover of learned information from one day to another.

One IADL that is influenced by sleep deprivation is driving. Driving requires many cognitive skills such as reaction time, memory, attention, sequencing, and processing. When a person is tired and the brain has not received an adequate amount or quality of sleep, these cognitive functions will be impaired. The National Highway Traffic Safety Administration estimates that there are approximately 100,000 police-reported accidents, 1,550 deaths, and 71,000 injuries each year caused by sleep-deprived drivers (Wells & Vaughn, 2012).

Almost all ADL and IADL require some form of cognitive functioning. Because sleep plays an important role in cognitive functioning, not only for optimal cognitive functioning but also for gains to be made during occupational therapy interventions, the practitioner and client need to make sure the client is receiving adequate sleep

---

Case Example: Intervention Plan for an Individual Experiencing Sleep Difficulties

David is a 43-year-old single father of two adolescent boys who is having difficulties falling asleep and staying asleep at night. David is an electrician, and a typical workday is from 7:00 AM to 6:00 PM with minimal breaks. David has weekends free from work, during which he enjoys spending time with his children, often engaging in outdoor activities such as hiking, fishing, golfing, and biking. David's difficulty sleeping started approximately 1 month ago after the divorce with his wife was finalized. David gets about 3 hours of sleep per night and often feels tired when he wakes. He thinks it is starting to affect his work and the time he spends with his children. David is unable to identify why he is not able to fall asleep at night, and he states that he usually thinks about what happened with his marriage while he is trying to sleep. David is seeing outpatient mental health occupational therapy services for a diagnosis of depression.

Consider the following questions:

- What sleep disorder might David have?
- What model of practice and which assessments would you use in David's intervention plan?
- Should the performance area of rest be addressed with David? Why or why not?
- How are David's ADL and IADL being affected by his lack of sleep?
- What intervention strategies would you use to help David?

---

in order for the client to retain new information during therapy.

Sleep and Emotional Processing

Sleep affects emotional memories. How we interpret our personal experiences affects our relationships and ability to survive. It is crucial for individuals to be able to interpret experiences as either rewarding or dangerous. If one's emotional judgment is being affected by sleep deprivation, this can cause dysfunctional emotional processing. An individual who is experiencing dysfunctional emotional processing may engage in risky or dangerous behaviors. Also, sleep deprivation has been linked to mood disorders. People who are sleep deprived also find

EVIDENCE-BASED RESEARCH CHART

Topic	Evidence
Occupational therapy process	Moyers, 1999
Cognitive behavioral therapy used with sleep	Vitiello, 2000; Vitiello, Rybarczyk, Korff, & Stepanski, 2009
Behavioral treatment techniques used with sleep	Rajki, 2011; Subramanian & Surani, 2007; Vitiello, 2009
Acute and chronic sleep deprivation and its effects on the body	Kravitz, 2012; Wells & Vaughn, 2012
Sleep deprivation and how it affects an individual's physical health	Ohlmann & O'Sullivan, 2009
Sleep deprivation and how it affects an individual's cognitive functioning	Church, 2012; Dang-Vu et al., 2010
Sleep deprivation and how it affects an individual's emotional processing	Church, 2012

it more difficult to deal with criticism and painful experiences (Church, 2012).

Sleep deprivation has a grave impact on decision making and the emotions associated with this task (Church, 2010). Decision making is a large part of the occupational therapy process, and intervention often includes a great amount of emotional involvement from the client, caregivers, family, and practitioner. Therefore, if any individual involved in the intervention process is sleep deprived, emotions can be affected and may influence the therapy process, resulting in an impact on the client's ability to perform his or her ADL or IADL. Similarly, outside of therapy, an individual going about his or her daily routine who is experiencing emotional dysfunction because of sleep deprivation may have difficulties with ADL and IADL that require decision making and involve relationships.

References

Church, E. J. (2012). Imaging sleep and sleep disorders. *Radiologic Technology, 83*(6), 585-605.

Dang-Vu, T. T., Schabus, M., Desseilles, M., Sterpenich, V., Bonjean, M., & Maquet, P. (2010). Functional neuroimaging insights into the physiology of human sleep. *Sleep, 33*(12), 1589-1603.

Davidson, J. R., Waisberg, J. L., Brundage, M. D., & Maclean, A. W. (2001). Nonpharmacologic group treatment of insomnia: A preliminary study with cancer survivors. *Psycho-Oncology, 10*, 389-397.

Kravitz, L. (2012). Sleep deprivation: Cognitive function and health consequences. *IDEA Fitness Journal*, 18-21.

Luyster, F. S., Strollo, P. J., Zee, P. C., & Walsh, J. K. (2012). Sleep: A health imperative. *SLEEP, 35*(6), 727-734.

Moyers, P. A. (1999). The guide to occupational therapy practice. *American Journal of Occupational Therapy, 53*(3), 247-322.

Ohlman, K. K., & O'Sullivan, M. I. (2009). The costs of short sleep. *AAOHN Journal, 57*(9), 381-385.

Patel, S. R., & Hu, F. B. (2008). Short sleep duration and weight gain: A systematic review. *Obesity, 16*(3), 643-653.

Rajki, M. (2011). Sleep problems in older adults. *ADVANCE for NP & PAs, 2*(12), 16-22.

Subramanian, S., & Surani, S. (2007). Sleep disorders in the elderly. *Geriatrics, 62*(12), 10-32.

Valenza, M. C., Rodenstein, D. O., & Ferández-de-las-Peñas, C. (2011). Consideration of sleep dysfunction in rehabilitation. *Journal of Bodywork and Movement Therapies, 15*, 262-267.

Vitiello, M. V. (2000). Effective treatment of sleep disturbances in older adults. *Clinical Cornerstone, 2*(5), 16-24.

Vitiello, M. V., Rybarczyk, B., Von Korff, M., & Stepanski, E. J. (2009). Cognitive behavioral therapy for insomnia improves sleep and decreases pain in older adults with co-morbid insomnia and osteoarthritis. *Journal of Clinical Sleep Medicine, 5*(4), 355-362.

Vorona, R. D., Winn, M. P., Babineau, T. W., Eng, B. P., Feldman, H. R., & Ware, J. C. (2005). Overweight and obese patients in a primary care population report less sleep than patients with a normal body mass index. *Archives of Internal Medicine, 165*, 25-30.

Wells, M. E., & Vaughn, B. V. (2012). Poor sleep challenging the health if a nation. *Neurodiagnostic Journal, 52*(3), 233-249.

Westley, C. (2004). Sleep: Geriatric self-learning module. *MEDSURGE Nursing, 13*(5), 291-295.

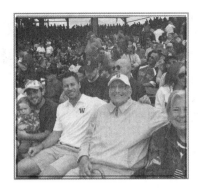

29

INTERVENTIONS TO ENHANCE OCCUPATIONAL PERFORMANCE IN SOCIAL PARTICIPATION

Jane O'Brien, PhD, OTR/L

ACOTE STANDARDS EXPLORED IN THIS CHAPTER
B.5.1–B.5.6

KEY VOCABULARY

- **Compensation:** Refers to making changes to the activity or way in which the client performs.
- **Occupation-based activity:** Involves doing the actual occupation, which provides meaning and is part of one's identity (Fisher, 1998).

- **Preparatory activity:** Help clients get ready for the intervention and may include relaxation techniques, sensory-based activities, role-playing, or discussion.
- **Remediation:** The act or process of correcting a fault or deficiency (Editors of the American Heritage Dictionaries, 2009).

Introduction

This chapter introduces readers to therapeutic use of occupations and activities for helping clients increase social participation, and self-management, and community and work integration. Techniques to provide development, remediation, and compensation for social behaviors are introduced. Examples of how to grade and adapt the environment, tools, materials, occupations, and interventions to reflect the client's social participation needs are provided. Finally, a description of compensatory strategies that may be helpful in terms of social participation is included. The roles of occupational therapists and occupational therapy assistants in intervention of social participation are differentiated throughout the chapter.

Social Participation

Social participation is an area of occupation targeted in intervention by occupational therapy practitioners. Social participation includes activities associated with

Jacobs, K., MacRae, N., & Sladyk, K. (Eds.).
Occupational Therapy Essentials for
Clinical Competence, Second Edition (pp. 385-395).

Table 29-1.	
COMMUNICATION AND INTERACTION SKILLS	
Physicality: Pertains to using the physical body when communicating within an occupation	Contacts: Makes physical contact with others Gazes: Uses eyes to communicate and interact with others Gestures: Uses movements of the body to indicate, demonstrate, or add emphasis Maneuvers: Moves one's own body in relation to others Orients: Directs one's body in relation to others or occupational forms Postures: Assumes physical positions
Information exchange: Refers to giving and receiving information within an occupation	Articulates: Produces clear, understandable speech Asserts: Directly expresses desires, refusals, and requests Asks: Requests factual or personal information Engages: Initiates interactions Expresses: Displays affect or attitude Modulates: Uses volume and inflection in speech Shares: Gives out factual or personal information Speaks: Makes oneself understood through the use of words, phrases, and sentences Sustains: Keeps up speech for appropriate duration
Relations: Relates to maintaining appropriate relationships within an occupation	Collaborates: Coordinates action with others toward a common goal Conforms: Follows implicit and explicit social norms Focuses: Directs conversation and behavior to ongoing social action Relates: Assumes a manner of acting that tries to establish a rapport with others Respects: Accommodates others' reactions and requests

Reprinted with permission from American Occupational Therapy Association. (2002). Occupational therapy practice framework: Domain & process. *American Journal of Occupational Therapy, 56,* 622.

organized patterns of behavior that are characteristic and expected of an individual or an individual interacting with others within a given social system (American Occupational Therapy Association [AOTA], 2008, adapted from Mosey, 1996, p. 340). As such, social participation includes activities that occur with community members, family, peers, or friends.

The first step in planning intervention to improve engagement in social participation is to understand the client's needs. This involves collaboration with clients, family members, and significant others. Therefore, the occupational therapist designs intervention based on "the client's goals, values, and beliefs as well as the health and well-being of the client" (AOTA, 2008, p. 655). Although the occupational therapist is ultimately responsible for the intervention plan, the occupational therapy assistant may provide input and data to the process and may be responsible for designing the activities based on the established plan (AOTA, 1990, 1994).

In addition to collaborating with clients, the occupational therapy practitioner analyzes the performance skills required for successful social participation. Performance skills are observable elements of action (AOTA, 2008; Fisher & Kielhofner, 1995) and include motor, processing, communication, and interactions skills (Table 29-1).

The occupational therapist evaluates performance skills required for social interactions by observing, interviewing, and conducting evaluations. This process is outlined in the following case example.

MOTOR SKILLS

Prior to discharge, the occupational therapist further evaluates the motor skills required to interact at the recreational center and in the support group. Using the Case Example: Mabel's Story, it is clear that Mabel needs to develop adequate sitting and standing posture, walk to and from the center entrance, and sit for extended periods of time at the center. She must get up out of the car seat and chair, use fine motor skills for activities, and eat a light meal.

PROCESSING SKILLS

The processing skills required in Mabel's case include choosing and using words, inquiring, and sequencing conversation. Mabel speaks slowly but is able to make conversation. She has difficulty with word finding and articulation, but she will have assistance at the recreational center and in the support group.

Case Example: Mabel's Story

Mabel is a 75-year-old woman who had a stroke resulting in right-sided weakness. She lives alone and has limited social contact. The occupational therapist observes Mabel interacting with other older adults as they wait for rehabilitation services. Mabel seems to "light up" and become more verbal around other people her age. She enjoys talking about television programs and listens well to others. Mabel is liked by her peers in the rehabilitation program. The occupational therapy practitioner is concerned that Mabel will have limited social contact upon discharge.

During the interview, the occupational therapist learns that Mabel has no transportation or opportunities for social activities. She speaks slowly and has trouble expressing herself since the stroke. Mabel's strengths include the ability to listen and make appropriate eye contact and that she is viewed as personable and approachable. Mabel works slowly but is capable of completing tasks.

The occupational therapy practitioner works with the social worker to arrange for weekly transportation to the local recreational center upon discharge and to a weekly support group for those with stroke. Mabel is pleased with this arrangement.

COMMUNICATION AND INTERACTION SKILLS

Communication and interaction skills are a large component of engagement in social participation (see Table 29-1). The framework (AOTA, 2008) provides guidelines to direct observation. Using these guidelines, the practitioner observes that Mabel is good at making physical contact and eye contact; she is neither too forward nor too shy and easily "connects" with others. She shows some difficulty maneuvering around others (because of motor difficulties associated with having a stroke). In terms of information exchange, Mabel asks, engages in interactions, and shares easily. However, she has articulation difficulties and speaks slowly. Although Mabel has facial weakness, she is able to convey affect and attitude through her eyes and body posture. Mabel shows strength in the area of relations. She works with others toward common goals. In the rehabilitation setting, Mabel establishes a rapport easily with others.

This case illustrates the many factors associated with social participation.

Performance Pattern

Although performance skills are important, the pattern of engagement in social activities also provides

direction for occupational therapy intervention. The practitioner determines whether the social activity is part of the client's established routine or role. Activities performed on a regular basis may become routine and part of the client's identity. Generally, clients wish to return to engaging in routines as they are conducted as part of one's role. Roles are "a set of behaviors that have some socially agreed upon function for which there is an accepted code of norms" (e.g., mother, father, student, and worker; Christiansen & Baum, 1997, p. 603).

To distinguish between roles and routines, consider Gordon, a 78-year-old grandfather who enjoys walking. As part of his routine, he walks to the store for the paper each morning, converses with others, and returns home to report. This routine has become part of his social role within the community. Gordon would be distressed if he could not partake in this routine. Furthermore, as part of his grandfather role, Gordon frequently brings back "treats" for his grandchildren. Clients may possess performance patterns that foster engagement in social participation (useful habits) or patterns of performance considered limitations (impoverished habits). Self-stimulating behaviors (e.g., head banging, hand biting) are considered dominating habits that interfere with social participation.

Habits and patterns may interfere with social participation as observed with Kenny, a 58-year-old client with traumatic brain injury, who hopes to return to "hanging out" with a group of work friends but has trouble remembering to bathe or groom himself. His habits around hygiene are impoverished because he has no routine or pattern of performance. Although Kenny has many useful habits (e.g., he takes public transportation), his impoverished pattern interferes with successful participation.

Contexts

After the practitioner has an understanding of the client's performance skills and patterns, further evaluation of the context in which the social interaction takes place is considered. The framework lists cultural, physical, social, personal, virtual, and temporal contexts as important to consider when developing occupation-based intervention. A description of how each context may be considered in terms of social participation is presented.

CULTURAL

Cultures hold different expectations for social participation. The occupational therapy practitioner evaluates expectations for such things as proximity, eye contact, and physical contact (e.g., touch). Because the expectations of participation in social events vary among cultures and influence the goals for occupational therapy, it is the occupational therapy practitioner's responsibility to be aware of cultural complexities.

Occupational therapy practitioners must be aware that cultural differences are also observed within families. For example, Tonya expressed concern that her 3-year-old son with autism could not play with his cousin at family gatherings every Sunday. The occupational therapy practitioner realized the cultural value of this to the family and worked on play skills with the child, encouraging the mom to bring in his cousin on occasion. Being sensitive to the family's values enabled the practitioner to design client-centered intervention that made a difference to the child and family.

PHYSICAL

The physical space in which the social interaction occurs becomes important when examining the activity demands on the client. Physical space includes the building, location, surroundings, objects, and setup of the event. Small intimate gatherings require different social skills than large public events. Activities that occur outside on uneven or hilly terrain may not be accessible to some clients. Background noise or even certain smells may be bothersome to some clients, especially older adults or children with olfactory sensitivity.

SOCIAL

Everyone makes social mistakes varying from wearing the wrong clothes to saying the wrong thing. Social situations require different behaviors and may become the source of occupational therapy intervention. Social manners may need to be addressed to help clients engage in social events. Helping clients address others properly, make conversation, and participate in events with others are all part of occupational therapy intervention. Other peoples' expectations affect the skills necessary to participate in social events. For example, the training and standards for success differ between formal and informal events and between familiar persons and strangers. Clients are expected to behave differently with peers or loved ones than in public settings. Social activities differ in the type and amount of personal disclosure required. Therefore, occupational therapy practitioners analyze the social requirements to prepare clients for social outings, as in the case of Max, a 20-year-old man with muscular dystrophy who freely (and inappropriately) discusses personal issues. Before the actual outing, the occupational therapy practitioner reviewed social expectations for attending the art museum and led clients in a role play activity to illustrate social behaviors appropriate for the art museum. Max and the occupational therapy practitioner developed a system to remind him when his behavior was not appropriate. After the outing, they discussed Max's performance to reinforce what he did well and to discuss what he did not.

PERSONAL

Social participation requirements may vary depending on one's age, gender, educational level, or socioeconomic status. Although the occupational therapy practitioner is not able to change personal context, this must be considered when designing intervention. Examples along the developmental continuum are offered to illuminate this aspect of social participation. As commonly understood, adults interact and express themselves differently than children. For example, occupational therapy practitioners working with clients with intellectual disabilities may need to design "age-appropriate" activities. Thus, the occupational therapy practitioner would not give a rattle to a 12-year-old girl who still mouths objects; this is not considered socially appropriate. Developing social activities commensurate with educational level requires the practitioner consider such things as the client's reading level. Socioeconomic status may include considering cost as a factor to certain social activities.

VIRTUAL

Communication via computers may provide a social outlet for some clients, but they may require help navigating Internet sources. Occupational therapy practitioners may help clients understand the social expectations and guidelines to protect themselves while using Internet sources or communicating with unknown people.

TEMPORAL

The demands for social participation vary over the lifespan. Early social experiences with children involve their parents. As children gain experience and develop social and cognitive skills, parallel play develops followed by cooperative play and games with rules. Children learn to negotiate and read others' cues early in their development (Bundy, 1997). Expectations for social behavior increase as school-aged children are expected to behave in socially appropriate manners.

Children and Youth

Frequently, young children receiving occupational therapy services have difficulty playing with others. They may experience difficulty reading nonverbal cues or "framing" play situations (Bundy, 1997). Occupational therapy intervention may be designed to increase the child's ability through role playing, practice, and verbalization. Children may exhibit other problems with social participation. For example, children may hug strangers and exhibit self-stimulating behaviors. Occupational therapy intervention may include techniques to eliminate these behaviors.

Adolescents

Social groups are important to adolescents, who are beginning to develop their personal identity. Adolescent peer groups pressure adolescents to conform to certain rules and expectations. For example, adolescents dress alike, use certain slang phrases, and collectively take up similar mannerisms. Adolescents may be working and thus have to show social skills for work. Adolescents need to learn to get along in groups, be heard, negotiate, stand up for themselves, and resist negative peer influences. Occupational therapy practitioners work with adolescents who have experienced disease, trauma, or an event that has changed or interrupted their development (Llorens, 1976). In terms of social participation, adolescents may exhibit a host of difficulties including inappropriate affect; difficulty initiating or sustaining conversation; and difficulty with boundaries, articulation, or poor judgment. The occupational therapist's role is to close the gap (Llorens) and work on foundational social skills such as making eye contact, greeting people, and social manners. Activities may be structured to help the adolescent understand social rules before spending time in social settings. The occupational therapy practitioner may decide to include peers in activities.

Adults

Social participation related to work and relationships becomes important to adolescents and adults. Work relationships require different skills than intimate relationships. Adults are expected to take the lead and participate in community and family activities, each requiring social skills. Raising a family introduces situations that require the adult to model behaviors for children.

Older Adults

Finally, older adults may experience loss as they retire and lose work relationships. As the social activities provided through work decline, they may need to establish new social avenues. Some older adults may experience a loss of a spouse or loved one, changing the social support to which they are accustomed.

After the occupational therapist evaluates and develops the goals with clients and family members, the occupational therapist and occupational therapy assistant together design an intervention plan in collaboration with the client and family. The occupational therapist is responsible for the intervention plan, but the occupational therapy assistant may design the actual activities used and communicates with the occupational therapist as needed (AOTA, 1990, 1994). Both the occupational therapist and occupational therapy assistant are skilled at adapting and grading activities so that intervention involves the "just-right" challenge. The "just-right" challenge refers to activities that are not so difficult as to cause frustration nor so easy as to cause boredom, and

consequently are not therapeutic (Ayres, 1979). The occupational therapy practitioner regularly monitors the level of difficulty of the activity in relationship to the client's skills and abilities and makes adjustments as needed.

Family, Community, Peers, or Friends

Social participation occurs with family, community, or peers and friends (Figures 29-1 to 29-3). The relationships of those involved in the social interactions change the activity demands. For example, clients are expected to behave differently in community settings (e.g., a public fair) than with family (e.g., at home). Clients exhibit closer displays of affection with significant others than with coworkers. Many social rules exist to describe the relationship boundaries and associated interactions. Thus, social training differs for community versus family activities. For example, family activities generally evoke deeper emotional responses and closer physical contact.

Socialization is an aspect of work settings; thus, helping clients return to work may require remediation of social participation skills. Role playing, practice, and cognitive awareness of social behaviors appropriate for work may help a client return to work successfully.

Development of Social Participation

PREPARATORY

Clients may experience stress or discomfort before engaging in social activities. Preparatory activities help clients get ready for the interaction and may include relaxation techniques, sensory-based activities, role playing, or discussion. Breathing techniques, mental rehearsal, or reviewing the schedule of events have been found to be helpful preparatory activities. For example, some children or adults may experience tactile defensiveness and dislike crowds, being touched, or even noises. The occupational therapy practitioner may work with the client on preparatory activities aimed at preparing the nervous system for the interaction. These preparatory activities may be used by the client on a regular basis after therapy to "calm" the system so that the client is not fearful.

Some clients may be fearful of social participation after injury and may need the practitioner to complete the activity with them. Price, Stephenson, Krantz and Ward (2011) found that clients with spinal cord injury appreciated it when the practitioners engaged in the social activity with them (as a partner) and when they conducted home visits to involve family and friends.

Figure 29-1. The O'Brien and Cohn families celebrate the holiday together.

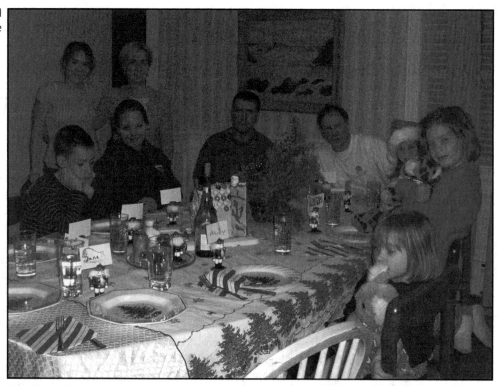

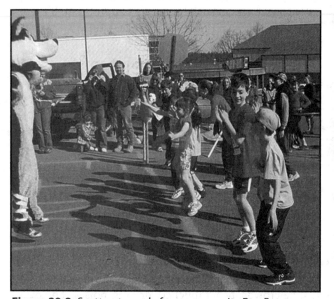

Figure 29-2. Scott gets ready for a community Fun Run.

Figure 29-3. Molly, Alison, and Shelby enjoy a day trip to StoryLand.

PURPOSEFUL ACTIVITY

When working on social participation, occupational therapy practitioners may help clients learn specific skills through engagement in purposeful activity. Purposeful activity is a goal-directed activity with an end product (Fisher, 1998). Typically, purposeful activity is used in intervention to target given client factors. See Table 29-1 for a description of client factors that may interfere with interactions. For example, the client may show poor interaction skills by sharing inappropriate personal information with strangers. Using purposeful activity, the occupational therapy practitioner may address this skill level through education, role playing, or discussion before actually having the client perform the social activity. Another example may be sharing craft supplies as one way to increase the ability to ask and communicate with others. Working on group projects may be purposeful and work on selected areas of social participation. Cooperating with others and playing a sport together are examples of how an occupational therapy practitioner may help clients improve their social participation skills. Clients may work in small groups on expressing frustration appropriately with the hope that this will transfer to the actual occupation in which the person engages. The client may work on eye contact, appropriate conversations, body language, and relating to others during many different group events. Frequently, the occupational therapy practitioner sets up scenarios for clients to role play so they may practice the skills before the actual event.

Occupation-Based Activity

Performing social activities in their actual context is the goal of occupational therapy. For example, helping children get along with others on the playground at the school or day care they attend is the preferred activity. Working with siblings so they may play and socialize together at home is an occupation-based activity. In this scenario, the occupational therapy practitioner may encourage children to play games and facilitate socialization when the client is showing signs of stress or decreased ability. Taking clients to a public event such as the swimming pool and encouraging them to use socially appropriate behaviors is an occupation-based activity. The occupational therapy practitioner may deal with difficulties the client exhibits during the occupation through many techniques depending on the client and the frame of reference (refer to Chapter 15). For example, practitioners may use a behavioral frame of reference to reward clients for positive social behaviors (e.g., verbal cue, token, or smile). Clinicians using a cognitive behavioral approach may help the client identify the behaviors that were positive during the occupation so that the client helps determine the solution.

Consultation

Consulting requires clear communication and negotiation skills. Consulting is most frequently conducted by an occupational therapist. The occupational therapist may decide to serve as a consultant to improve social participation. In this case, the role of the occupational therapist is to help the client identify the problem, try some solutions, and alter them as necessary (AOTA, 2008). The occupational therapist does not do the activity with the client but instead recommends activities to enhance the client's functioning. For example, the occupational therapist may suggest that an adolescent join the Special Olympics. The child may require consultation from the occupational therapist to be successful in the desired sport. This consultation may require the occupational therapist to visit the site and make suggestions to the coach, client, or family member.

Consultation for social participation may include identifying social groups that the client would enjoy and making specific recommendations to the client or family. The occupational therapist may serve as a consultant on an as-needed basis to help the client problem solve situations as they arise. When consulting, the occupational therapist is not directly responsible for the outcome (AOTA, 2008). Consultation may occur to increase social behaviors of clients in group homes, schools, etc. The occupational therapist provides information on the client's abilities and disabilities along with suggestions to help the client be successful. Implementation is overseen by others and responsibilities for outcomes lie with the client.

Education

Occupational therapy practitioners frequently educate others about occupations and the impact a disorder, disease, or trauma may have on a client's functioning. Imparting knowledge or educating others about the occupation is part of the intervention process (AOTA, 2008). The occupational therapy practitioner may educate family members or caregivers on social expectations consistent with a client's diagnosis. Family members may need education on how to best approach and communicate with clients who do not use traditional methods (e.g., computer systems, communication boards). Family members, caregivers, or significant others may need education on the prognosis of the client to help develop realistic expectations (which is not to be confused with giving up hope). Frequently, occupational therapy practitioners teach others what to expect developmentally from the client, how to grade and adapt activities so the client is successful, how to make social situations successful for clients with all abilities and disabilities, the legal rights that will help the clients be more successful in their occupations (e.g., access, billing), and the possibilities for engagement in occupations.

Occupational therapy practitioners are resources to those with disabilities since they frequently know which programs adapt to clients with special needs. Other resources available to clients allow them to engage in social activities such as transportation systems, adapted sailing programs, hippotherapy programs, or aquatic programs.

Designing Intervention Using Frames of Reference

Understanding the theory and rationale for a specific frame of reference helps practitioners design intervention. Occupational therapy practitioners evaluate clients based on the frame of reference and design goals that the frame of reference can address. For example, when providing intervention to improve the play skills of a child

Table 29-2.

STUDIES ON OCCUPATIONAL THERAPY INTERVENTION AND SOCIAL PARTICIPATION

Author/Year	Population	Measurement	Intervention	Results
Carter et al., 2004	Children with Asperger syndrome ages 8 to 15 ($n=12$)	Lifestyle Performance Profile Interview	An afterschool program for children	Positive results per report from children and parents
Dumont, Gervais, Fougeyrollas, & Bertrand, 2005	53 adults with traumatic brain injury	Self-Efficacy and Social Participation questionnaire		Perceived self-efficacy explained 40% variance of social participation
Gol & Jarus, 2005	Children with ADHD ($n=27$) and without ADHD ($n=24$)	Assessment of Motor Processing (AMPS)	Social skills training through meaningful occupations (e.g., art, games, cooking) in groups	AMPS for children with ADHD improved from first to second evaluation ($P = .008$)
Paul-Ward, Kielhofner, Braveman, & Levin, 2005	Staff members ($n=21$) and clients with AIDS ($n=16$)	Focus groups		Staff identified systematic and personal barriers; clients identified only systemic barriers as impacting participation
Steultjens et al., 2005	14 systematic reviews (4 reviewed stroke)	Systematic search for evidence	Comprehensive occupational therapy	Occupational therapy intervention improved social participation in clients with stroke
Thibodaux, 2005	2 years post spinal cord injury ($n=976$)	Craig Handicap Assessment		83.6% reported involvement in recreation

with developmental delays, occupational therapy practitioners frequently use the developmental frame of reference (Llorens, 1976). This frame of reference postulates that practice will improve the child's ability by improving neural synapses. Thus, the practitioner determines the level of play in which the child currently functions and addresses therapy at that level with the intent to grade the challenge slightly so the child can succeed and move to the next level. Using the intervention approaches as outlined in the framework (AOTA, 2008) provides practitioners with strategies to address.

Occupational Therapy Intervention Approaches

Overall occupational therapy intervention aimed to increase social participation has been reported to have positive results (Carter et al., 2004; Gibson, Amico, & Arbesman, 2011; Gol & Jarus, 2005; Peterson, Lovett, Cooks, & Bell, 2010; Price et al., 2011; Steultjens, Dekker, Bouter, Leemrijse, & van den Ende, 2005). However, more research is required to substantiate this claim using randomized controlled trials with larger samples and

specific populations. See Table 29-2 for a review of studies examining social participation in occupational therapy. According to the framework, occupational therapy intervention consists of five approaches: create, establish, maintain, modify, and prevent (AOTA, 2008). The following describes each approach and how occupational therapy practitioners apply the approach to enhance social participation:

- **Create, promote (health promotion).** This approach develops experiences for everyone, not just those with disabilities. Occupational therapy practitioners use this approach to create social experiences for all persons and promote healthy social activities. Examples are as varied as clients but include developing afterschool programs for children or creating social opportunities, such as a tea party or dance, appropriate to clients. An occupational therapy practitioner using this type of approach sets up the scenario under the premise that the clients have the abilities but need the opportunity.

- **Establish, restore (remediation, restoration).** This intervention approach works on establishing abilities that have not developed or restoring those that may have been lost (AOTA, 2008). Developing a client's social skills through role playing and coaching techniques is one way to establish abilities. This approach requires restoring the underlying factors interfering with the occupation. Helping a client who has had a stroke interact with loved ones is an example of attempting to restore social skills. Many of the behavioral frames of reference work on establishing appropriate social skills through reinforcement methods. Clients are rewarded when their behavior meets the appropriate social standards. Motor control or biomechanical approaches work to increase physical skills that may be interfering with social participation. The developmental frame of reference postulates that practice helps clients establish abilities.

- **Maintain.** Occupational therapy practitioners may help clients keep the skills and abilities they currently possess so they do not decline in function. This type of approach may be readily used with deteriorating conditions in which maintaining function is difficult. In this case, the client is expected to keep the appropriate skills she has without losing function. Thus, the practitioner helps the client keep the social skills she currently has and develops strategies so the client may participate in social activities. For example, the occupational therapist may work with the client to continue attending a weekly yoga class. The occupational therapist may work to help the client communicate with others despite decreased functioning. Maintaining social networks may require educating others involved or helping the client overcome fears.

- **Modify (compensation, adaptation).** This intervention approach requires the occupational therapy practitioner to make changes to the activity or the way in which the client performs the activity. In this case, the expectation is not that the client makes improvements in his or her abilities but rather learns to perform the activity differently. Compensation is used to help clients engage in occupations without trying to change the degree of disability. Clients may need to compensate in social activities for poor verbal skills by using assistive technology. More subtle but equally important compensations may be required when a client experiences psychological difficulties interfering with social participation. For example, clients anxious in new social systems may be encouraged to seek out a familiar person with whom to attend social activities. The compensation strategy may be that the client only attends those functions for short periods of time, or the client is encouraged to participate in activities with a few familiar peers.

- **Prevent (disability prevention).** Some occupational therapy practitioners develop programs to help those who may be at risk for disability such as programs targeting backpack awareness, healthy computing, childhood obesity, well elderly, work simplification, or fall prevention. The goal of this type of intervention is to prevent future impairments. Social participation programs such as Big Brother Big Sister, peer mentoring groups, day intervention, and adult recreational leagues are designed to increase socialization, friendships, and a sense of belonging. Structured groups provide resources to individuals. These groups may prevent antisocial behaviors or psychosocial disorders (e.g., depression and loneliness) caused by a lack of social interactions. The occupational therapy practitioner may develop a specific group around preventing disability or help a client participate in an existing group. Clients may be involved in book clubs, dance classes, school programs, craft classes, parenting classes, and exercise groups. Clients may form support groups with persons with similar diagnoses. These support groups provide resources and are a source of social participation. Therefore, they help the client meet his or her social needs and identify with others.

Grading and Adapting Social Participation

Grading and adapting social participation first involves a thorough analysis of the social behaviors and expectations required of the activity. Table 29-3 provides some questions to ask when grading or adapting social participation activities. These areas can be modified to make the activity more or less challenging for the client. For example, the rules and expectations of the social activity may be formal or informal, flexible or inflexible, and explicit or implicit. The social activity may be new versus old or active versus passive. Occupational therapy practitioners also consider the number of people involved in the activity and the relationships of group members. The diversity of group members and the content of the activity change the degree of difficulty. The difficulty level may be changed by altering the group structures. For example, the task group requires members to complete a given activity. Clients work on individual goals toward the end product. This group requires interactions, but the occupational therapy practitioner is able to grade interactions as needed. In a task group, the degree of sharing and negotiation required is more difficult when supplies are limited. Cooperative groups require clients to interact closely and work toward a collective end goal. Therefore, cooperative groups require a great deal of interaction,

Table 29-3.		
FACTORS TO CONSIDER WHEN GRADING AND ADAPTING SOCIAL PARTICIPATION ACTIVITIES		
Client's goal for activity		
Purpose of interactions	Project Goals of group	
Size of group		
Location	Familiar versus unfamiliar Transportation	
Physical space	Outdoors versus indoors Small versus large Quiet versus noisy Public versus private Formal versus informal	
Structure	Expectations Expectations of others Roles Degree of investment required Time commitment Degree of supervision	
Experience	Novelty Frequency of social interaction Risk	
Behavioral expectations	Rules Complexity of interactions Interaction of members	
Cultural expectations	Past experiences with activity Meaning ascribed to activity	
Performance expectations	Degree of difficulty Mobility requirements Social requirements	
Conclusion	Degree of follow-up available	
Other	Cost	
Suitability for client		
Modifications needed		

communication, and negotiation. Adapting and grading activities require that the practitioner consider the client's strengths and weaknesses when deciding on the type of social activity and how to change the activity so the client will be successful. Generally, small task-oriented groups are the least stressful socially. Pairing clients with others who have similar issues may be helpful. Working one-on-one with the client to establish a rapport before a social event may prove useful. Discussing the social rules, boundaries, and consequences before the activity promotes success. Setting firm limits and helping clients work through and socially adapt to different situations is necessary before performing the actual occupation.

Summary

Humans are social beings and, as such, social participation is an important occupation for clients of all ages and abilities. Occupational therapy practitioners evaluate the social skills required, considering the contexts of the activity, including the setting in which the activity occurs.

Occupational therapy practitioners help prepare clients for the social interactions by providing them with many opportunities to practice the prerequisite skills, consulting with them and team members, and educating clients on appropriate social behaviors. In this way, the goal of improved social participation can be reached.

Student Self-Assessment

1. Describe the social behaviors required to participate in one social activity. Describe the context in which this activity takes place.
    ◊ Change the context of the aforementioned activity.
    ◊ Compare and contrast the differences.
2. Describe the social aspects of an activity using Table 29-3.
3. Make a list of social activities in which you participate.
    ◊ Describe the motor, processing, and communication and interaction factors involved in three of them.
4. Develop a notebook of social activities and resources for children, adolescents, adults, and elderly persons.
5. Summarize three research articles describing social participation in a given population.

References

American Occupational Therapy Association. (1990). Entry-level role delineation for registered occupational therapists (OTRs) and certified occupational therapy assistants (COTAs). *American Journal of Occupational Therapy, 44*(12), 1091-1102.

American Occupational Therapy Association. (1994). Guide for supervision of occupational therapy personnel. *American Journal of Occupation Therapy, 48,* 1045-1046.

American Occupational Therapy Association. (2008). Occupational therapy practice framework: Domain and process (2nd ed.). *American Journal of Occupational Therapy, 62,* 625-683.

Ayres, A. J. (1979). *Sensory integration and the child.* Los Angeles, CA: Western Psychological Services.

Bundy, A. C. (1997). Play and playfulness: What to look for. In L. S. Parham & L. S. Fazio (Eds.), *Play in occupational therapy for children.* St. Louis, MO: Mosby.

Carter, C., Meckes, L., Pritchard, L., Swensen, S., Wittman, P. P., & Velde, B. (2004). The Friendship Club: An after-school program for children with Asperger syndrome. *Family and Community Health, 27*(2), 143-150.

Christiansen C., & Baum, C. (1997). Person-environment occupational performance: A conceptual model for practice. In C. Christiansen & C. Baum (Eds.), *Occupational therapy: Enabling function and well-being* (2nd ed.). Thorofare, NJ: SLACK Incorporated.

Dumont, C., Gervais, M., Fougeyrollas, P., & Bertrand, R. (2005). Perceived self-efficacy is associated with social participation in adults with traumatic brain injury. *Canadian Journal of Occupational Therapy, 72*(4), 222-233.

Editors of the American Heritage Dictionaries (Ed.). (2009). *The American Heritage Dictionary of the English Language* (4th ed.). Boston, MA: Houghton Mifflin Company.

Fisher, A. G. (1998). Uniting practice and theory in an occupational framework. 1998 Eleanor Clarke Slagle lecture. *American Journal of Occupational Therapy, 52*(7), 509-521.

Fisher, A. G., & Kielhofner, G. (1995). Skill in occupational performance. In G. Kielhofner (Ed.), *A model of human occupation: Theory and application* (2nd ed., pp. 113-128). Philadelphia, PA: Lippincott Williams & Wilkins.

Gibson, R., D'Amico, M., & Jaffe, L. (2011). Occupational therapy interventions for recovery in the areas of community integration and normative life roles for adults with serious mental illness: a systematic review. *American Journal of Occupational Therapy, 65*(3), 247-256.

Gol, D., & Jarus, T. (2005). Effect of a social skills training group on everyday activities of children with attention-deficit-hyperactivity disorder. *Developmental Medicine & Child Neurology, 47*(8), 539-545.

Llorens, L. A. (1976). *Application of a developmental theory for health and rehabilitation.* Rockville, MD: AOTA Press.

Mosey, A. C. (1996). *Psychosocial components of occupational therapy.* Philadelphia, PA: Lippincott Williams & Wilkins.

Paul-Ward, A., Kielhofner, G., Braveman, B., & Levin, M. (2005). Resident and staff perceptions of barriers to independence and employment in supportive living settings for persons with AIDS. *American Journal of Occupational Therapy, 59*(5), 540-545.

Peterson, B. D., Lovett, A., Cooks, K., & Bell, J. (2010). Promoting social participation for adults through arthritis self-management: A pilot study. *Physical & Occupational Therapy in Geriatrics, 28*(3), 297-306.

Price, P., Stephenson, S., Krantz, L., & Ward, K. (2011). Beyond my front door: the occupational and social participation of adults with spinal cord injury. *OTJR: Occupation, Participation & Health, 31*(2), 81-88.

Steultjens, E. M., Dekker, J., Bouter, L. M., Leemrijse, C. J., & van den Ende, C. H. (2005). Evidence of the efficacy of occupational therapy in different conditions: An overview of systematic reviews. *Clinical Rehabilitation, 19*(3), 247-254.

Thibodaux, L. R. (2005). Habitus and the embodiment of disability through lifestyle. *American Journal of Occupational Therapy, 59*(5), 507-515.

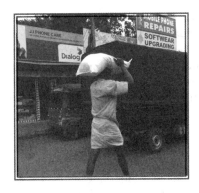

30

ENVIRONMENTAL ADAPTATION AND ERGONOMICS

Betsy DeBrakeleer, COTA/L, ROH; William R. Croninger, MA, OTR/L; and John E. Lane, Jr., OTR/L

ACOTE STANDARDS EXPLORED IN THIS CHAPTER

B.5.9

KEY VOCABULARY

- **AbleData:** An information resource funded and maintained by the National Institute on Disability and Research. It provides information, not products, relative to assistive technology and rehabilitative products as well as information about conferences, information centers, and international resources. It can be accessed via the Web page.

- **Americans with Disabilities Act (ADA):** Signed into law by Congress in 1990 this act seeks to prevent discrimination in employment, public buildings and transportation, public accommodations, and telecommunications based solely on disability.

- **Ergonomics:** A scientific discipline concerned with the understanding of interactions among humans and other elements of a system and the profession that applies theory, principles, data, and other methods to design to optimize human well-being and overall system performance.

- **Human factors engineering:** *See* ergonomics.

- **Universal design:** An idea that all environments and products, to the greatest extent possible, should be easily accessed and used by everyone regardless of age, ability, or circumstance. It includes design of environments and products that are useful across the human lifespan.

Jacobs, K., MacRae, N., & Sladyk, K. (Eds.).
*Occupational Therapy Essentials for
Clinical Competence, Second Edition* (pp. 397-406).
© 2014 SLACK Incorporated.

Introduction

The role of the occupational therapy practitioner is to consider the client's occupational performance in the environment in which is it performed. Environmental adaptation has as its goal the modification of the client's environment to maximize participation in his or her occupational roles. It is an attempt, then, to modify the environment to match the abilities of the client rather than expecting an individual to meet the demands of the environment. In assessing an environment, regardless of whether it is home, work, school, or the community, it is desirable to organize around the following tasks:

- Movement to a site (e.g., public or private transportation)
- Access to the structures or areas (e.g., parking, entering and exiting a building)
- Movement within common areas (e.g., foyers, halls, cafeteria or kitchen, bathroom)
- Tasks specific to each activity area (e.g., dressing, bathing, word processing, fabrication, note taking, shopping)

An additional point to remember is that the environment may be appropriate, but the activities, processes, or procedures within task areas may lead to injury secondary to repetition or strain.

Transportation

PUBLIC TRANSPORTATION

The Americans with Disabilities Act (ADA) of 1990, updated in 2010 with revisions implemented in 2012, prohibits discrimination against individuals with disabilities. Relative to transportation, the ultimate goal is the provision of access to "basic mobility" for all individuals with disabilities.

PRIVATE TRANSPORTATION

Private transportation is access to and the operation, either by self or a driver, of motor vehicles. Public transportation assumes an individual with a disability needs only to access a conveyance. Private transportation can place greater demands on a client if he or she is expected to also be the vehicle operator. The client must then be able to enter and exit the vehicle unassisted, store and access necessary mobility devices, and safely operate the vehicle. A standard-sized automobile may well be sufficient when the client can transfer to and from the vehicle unassisted. Vehicles with sufficient room behind the front seat can be appropriate when a client has the strength and balance to stow a wheelchair or other devices there independently.

When the weight of the mobility aid becomes prohibitive or an individual does not have the strength to load a wheelchair, car top–mounted power lifts are available. When independent transfers are impossible or not inappropriate, a van can become the best solution.

Vans may be modified to allow entrance and exit via a power lift or ramp. Some are factory made for accessibility. Independent operation of the vehicle requires the ability to access controls such as the ignition and accelerator, to control the direction of travel, and to be able to stop. Modifications may entail mechanical assists to lessen the force needed to use traditional controls such as a steering wheel, accelerator, or brake. However, adaptations using nontraditional controls, such as hand accelerators, also exist.

SITE ACCESSIBILITY

When the client arrives at a destination, access to the structure or area becomes the next potential challenge. If arriving in a personal vehicle, the initial challenge will be parking and egress followed by movement through common areas and finally passage through doorways or openings.

- *Parking places:* The ADA specifies the number of parking places that must be accessible. Additionally, regulations specify the number of these spaces that must be larger to accommodate van access.
- *Walkways:* The ADA requires at least one "accessible route" be provided that allows individuals access to and between all accessible areas.
- *Entry doors:* The following section provides guidance on the ADA regulations as they apply to the width, handle type, and force required in constructing doors in accessible structures. Doors must be 32 inches in width and require no greater than 5 lb of force to open. The handles should be lever style, such that it can be operated with the push of a closed fist.

Ramps

One common means of providing access to a private or public structure is via ramps. A ramp for a public structure must meet state and local codes. Ramps for a private residence may or may not be covered by a local code. Quite often, family, friends, or a civic organization may want to assist the client with construction.

The most common specification encountered for determining how long to make a ramp is the ratio 1:12, which translates to 12 inches in length for every 1 inch the ramp must rise. Note that this ratio is the maximum angle allowed. When possible, it is desirable to make the ramp longer to place less stress on the person propelling the chair, whether it is a client or a caregiver.

Wheelchair ramps are commonly built over concrete posts, which must be constructed so they extend lower

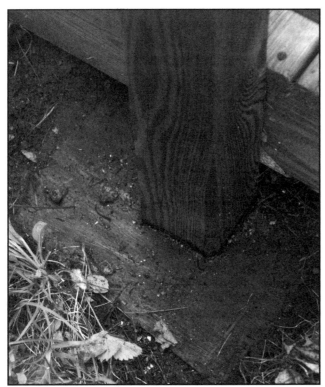

Figure 30-1. Detail of a "floating base." (Reprinted with permission from William R. Croninger.)

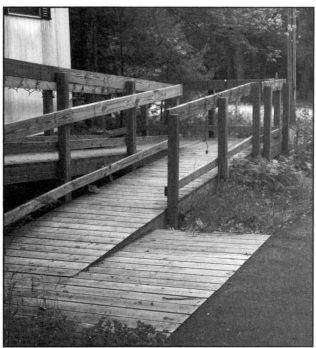

Figure 30-2. A 42-foot ramp constructed by an occupational therapist for his neighbor who is a wheelchair user. (Reprinted with permission from William R. Croninger.)

than the normal frost line found in the area. This procedure, although necessary when using concrete posts to support the ramp's uprights, greatly increases the cost and difficulty of construction.

Information on a clever alternative method of supporting uprights can be found at the Minnesota Center for Independent Living (MCIL).

The Handyman's Club of America published the original article (available at www.klownwerkz.com/ramp/rampman/articles/handyman/handyman.htm) on the ramp in Figure 30-1. In this method, the uprights sit on 12" x 12" plates. The plates are standard treated 3/4" thick plywood. The entire deck "floats" with the thawing and freezing of the underlying ground. The method used in the ramp in Figure 30-2 has the added advantage of being modular—it can be fabricated off site and later assembled at the residence. It can also be taken apart and reused in the future. Information about ramps, loan programs, and grant programs can be found at state independent living centers.

COMMON AREA ACCESS

Common areas can be thought of as areas within a structure that a client will need to navigate or use. This might include hallways, a cafeteria, and bathrooms, as well as utilization of devices such as drinking fountains. Guidance for the acceptable dimensions and location can be found under Electronic Resources.

Task Areas

Task areas may be thought of as the sites where primary occupations take place. Examples include the following:

- Home: Kitchen and bathroom
- School: Classroom and gym
- Work: Storeroom and office
- Community: Stores, restaurants, and theaters

Task areas offer occupational therapists the opportunity to use the unique training received in activity analysis.

The Case Example: Grace's Story, provides an overview for assessing any environment in which a client will function (home, school, work, community).

The Process

Using context and activity portions of the American Occupational Therapy Association (AOTA) Occupational Therapy Practice Framework (OTPF; 2008), define the demands of the environment and activities within the following:

- **Educational setting.** Watson and Wilson (2003) stressed the importance of "participation and engagement" by modifying the classroom and its demands to allow all students to participate more fully. Participation in learning activities is argued to be more effective than simply providing a piece of assistive technology, which makes it possible to

Case Example: Grace's Story

Shortly after the death of her husband, Grace's family began to notice changes in her behavior. She began calling her adult children numerous times on the same day, each time asking the same question. It became apparent that she was opening cards and letters repeatedly before mailing them to see whom she had written them to or if she had included the letter. Most alarming was that her friends began calling to report she was becoming increasingly forgetful. An assessment by a neuropsychologist returned a diagnosis of mild dementia. An occupational therapist assisted the family by using the OTPF (AOTA, 2008) to define Grace's goals and the requirements of her environment and to determine her ability to meet those requirements. With the assistance of the therapist, the family helped their mother identify her goals related to living independently, her continued operation of a motor vehicle, and her desire to continue to participate in social activities. In the areas of independent living and motor vehicle operation, Grace and her children were able to define "threshold events" that would require her to give up her driver's license or move to residential living facility. Using the Context and Activity Demands portions of the OTPF, the therapist identified the performance skills and client factors needed to be successful in the context and activity demands of Grace's environment. The therapist then requested the family use a common ADL checklist to identify both performance skills and performance patterns they had observed in their mother. The therapist stressed that it was important to look at change over time, always considering her performance in these areas at her "best" rather than focusing only on current issues.

Finally, using the assessment reports provided by the neuropsychologist, Grace, her children, and the therapist were able to develop a plan that included environmental adaptations and weekly visits by a caregiver.

participate. Thus, it is imperative for the school-based therapist to work with the classroom teacher and caregivers to fully understand the contexts of the classroom as well as performance skills and activity demands before suggesting alterations in the space or activities.

- **Adaptations.**
  ◊ Decrease clutter throughout the house
  ◊ Create "workstations" where Grace could place bills and other important mail for later pickup by a friend who paid her bills

  ◊ Place a whiteboard over the phone and have Grace write answers to her questions on the "first" call.

Grace was able to live successfully in her home for 2 additional years, relinquishing her driver's license during this period when the threshold event occurred.

- **Work setting.** Before performing an ergonomic or job task analysis at the workplace, the therapist should contact the employer to determine what safety equipment is required, such as steel-toed shoes, safety glasses, or hearing protection.

- **Computer workstation setting.** Most individuals use a computer as a regular part of their occupation. When looking at a computer workstation, the Occupational Safety and Health Administration's (OSHA's) Web site can be used as a reference. When making recommendations for equipment or a change in the work process, review these recommendations with the employer before committing them to the report or discussing with the employee. You should not make demands on the employer that cannot be immediately honored because of costs or production restraints. However, instruction to the employee regarding tool positioning, body mechanics, and other basic safety practices can be recommended at the time of the evaluation (Figure 30-3).

- **Community setting.** Interview the client to determine goals and preexisting performance patterns. Performance skills and client factors can be assessed using standardized or nonstandardized means to understand observed or potential issues related to the client's ability to successfully and safely function in the environment.

Overview of Ergonomics and Human Factors Engineering

In the preceding pages of this chapter, a process for assessing an environment before determining what modifications might be desirable has been detailed. Ergonomics provides a very useful body of knowledge that will assist practitioners in understanding the activity demands of task areas (AOTA, 2008), particularly those found in work settings, although the application of ergonomic principles are being applied to other contexts such as learning environments (e.g., schools, libraries).

Jacobs (1999) traced the understanding of the importance of ergonomics back to the earliest tools created by humanoids as they shaped stone implements to fit their own hands and abilities. An Internet search for the term yields a wide range of definitions. However, the recurring theme is that the practice of ergonomics seeks to match the demands of work with the abilities of the worker. In

Operator's Name:
Location:
Age: Dom: Vision: Phone:
Years VDT use: (total) Supervisor:
Operator's estimate of average VDT use per day:

Evaluator:
Date:
Flagged items:

Criteria	Problematic	Not Problematic	Measurements	Comments
Pain: Repetitive Strain Injury				
The operator complains of numbness or tingling in the hands while using VDT at work.				
The operator complains of numbness or tingling in the hands out of work.				
There is a positive Tinel's sign.*				
There is a positive Phalen's sign.†				
There is a positive Finkelstein's sign.‡				
The operator complains of other hand or arm pain.				
The operator complains of headaches or ophthalmologic symptoms while using the VDT.			Daily __X Week __X Month	
The operator complains of neck pain while at the VDT.			Daily __X Week __X Month	
The operator complains of back pain while at the VDT.			Daily __X Week __X Month	
The operator takes a 15-minute break during each hour of continuous typing.				
Workstation				
The operator's elbows are between 80 and 100 degrees of flexion when hands are on the keyboard.				
When positioned at the keyboard, the operator's wrists are within 5 degrees of neutral. • Keyboard height is adjustable. • Keystroke pressure is comfortable.				
Operator's chair has arm rests.				
Chair height is adjustable.				
Chair back supports lumbar curve.				

Figure 30-3. Video Display Terminal Worksheet Assessment. *(continued)*

Backrest is adjustable. • In height • In angle relative to seat surface • To alter seat depth				
Chair height or seat depth puts pressure on user's legs.				Chair height needed –
Operator's thighs are horizontal when seated.				
Operator's feet touch ground or foot rest when seated.				
Chair moves easily around workstation.				
Operator feels chair is comfortable.				
Work or writing table is at a comfortable height for writing and other work.				Counter or desk height –
There is adequate workspace.				
A document holder is available at an appropriate position.				
Needed items are within easy reach.				
A telephone cradle or head set is present.				
Monitor				
Top of monitor screen is at eye level or no less than 2 inches below.				
Screen distance is 18 to 20 inches.				
Operator is able to reach and operate the mouse without extended reach, long duration, or repetitive reaching.				
Work Environment				
Operator complains of glare on VDT screen.				
Operator thinks there is adequate light for work.				
Operator thinks noise levels are tolerable.				
The operator thinks the room temperature is appropriate.				
The operator complains of other stressors (personal or job related).				
Air circulation is adequate.				

What are the main problems you found with this study area, and how would you fix them?
Main Problem   *Recommended Solutions*

BdeB'97
*Tinel's test Tap over carpal tunnel. +for carpal tunnel if paraesthesia distal to wrist.
†Phalen's test: Wrists max flexed by holding together for 1 minute + for carpal tunnel if paraesthesia in thumb, index, middle, and lateral half of the ring finger.
‡Finkelstein's test: Make a fist with thumb inside then bend wrist ulnarly. + for DeQuervain's tenosynovitis if pain is felt.

Figure 30-3 (continued). Video Display Terminal Worksheet Assessment.

this way, worker safety, comfort, and productivity are maximized.

A term closely related to ergonomics and often used interchangeably is *human factors engineering* (HFE). Both involve knowledge of human physiology and psychology and the ability to process information (United States Army Human Engineering Laboratory, 1984).

The pilots of some World War II-era aircrafts frequently displayed puzzling behavior after landing. While taxing back to parking areas, the pilots would retract their landing gear, dropping the aircraft to the ground and causing considerable damage to the aircraft. The surprised and embarrassed pilot would later relate that he thought he was retracting the flaps, a necessary practice after landing. Investigators discovered this error was not common across all types of aircraft. Rather, it was most frequently seen in specific models of fighters and bombers. In looking deeper, it was noted that the "problem" models had flap and gear levers or switches side by side. In fact, on many aircrafts, the controls were of identical

Table 30-1.

FIELDS CONTRIBUTING TO KNOWLEDGE OF ERGONOMICS

Subject	Operational Definition	Example
Physiology	Sensory information: visual, auditory, olfactory, touch, taste	What color would make a shut-off switch most visible in an emergency situation?
Skills	What is the skill set required to operate a piece of equipment?	What is the longest password that the average person can remember?
Performance	What are the factors that influence an operator's ability to perform an operation?	How long can a long-distance truck driver safely operate his or her vehicle on the highway?
Anthropometrics	Study of human body dimensions; examines both averages and extremes	How far can the average person reach into a refrigerator?
Biomedical factors	Effects of environment on workers: sound levels, temperature, vibration, altitude, humidity, odor, etc.	What effect does temperature have on a worker's ability to perform fine adjustments on a piece of equipment?
Safety factors	What could go wrong? What are the consequences of making a wrong choice?	What are the consequences of a distracted vehicle operator shifting the transmission into "park" while moving?
Training	How long should a training program be?	What is the minimal amount of time a driver education program needs to significantly reduce the accident rate among new drivers?
Manning implications	What is the minimum number of workers we need?	How many craftspeople should be on a team that manufacturers custom-made stairways onsite?

Adapted from Headquarters Department of the Army. (1983). *Man-material systems: Human factors engineering program.* AR 602-1, Washington, DC: Author.

shape. Pilots of aircrafts that had the levers separated or those that used a different sequence for each action did not commonly embarrass themselves by retracting their plane's landing gear while on the ground. It was wartime, so one could not simply recall all of the aircrafts and move the controls. However, when HFE was applied to the problem, a quick and easily applied solution was readily found. The fix? Small rubber tires were added to the ends of the landing gear levers, while the flap lever was modified so it ended in a same wedge shape as the actual flaps. Pilots of World War II aircrafts were too busy to look away from the runway, landing at high speed, with limited control, and with the likelihood of battle damage. However, having levers that resembled the action intended could easily be interpreted through their flying gloves, and incidences of "wheels up" after landing decreased significantly (Roscoe, 1997).

Environmental Adaptation and Ergonomics

Ergonomics requires knowledge in a wide range of topics. Table 30-1 provides an overview.

The field of ergonomics then holds considerable promise for the occupational therapy practitioner. It allows for a thorough understanding of the contexts and performance skills required by a task and its environment. Furthermore, it can help the practitioner understand the interrelationship of these skills and better plan for an environment that will promote client independence. It can also assist a practitioner in analyzing an environment or process to better understand the sources of injury and in devising the means to prevent it.

Universal Design

Closely aligned with ergonomics is the concept of universal design. This term is attributed to architect Ronald Mace and means tools and spaces should be designed to be at the same time aesthetically pleasing as well as usable by all individuals, regardless of their abilities (About the Center: Ronald L. Mace, 2008). Universal design, at its core, has seven principles. They are as follows (The Center for Universal Design, 1997):

1. Equitable use
2. Flexibility in use
3. Simple and intuitive use
4. Perceptible information
5. Tolerance for error
6. Low physical effort
7. Size and space for approach and use

Case Example

A contract-manufacturing firm was required to modify its standard operating procedure to accommodate the demands of a customer. Specifically, the firm was required to retool from bottling a single flavor to bottling three flavors. Initially, the pails of product would be palletized by each flavor, then re-palletized, so three flavors were on each pallet, increasing the handling of each pail threefold and exposing workers to an increased risk of injury.

The onsite occupational therapist performed a job task analysis and recommended the pails be stacked by flavor, one flavor per row as they came off the production line, reducing the pail handling to once per pail.

To decrease the potential for shoulder injuries, an adaptive piece of equipment was designed by the occupational therapist and fabricated by the employer's maintenance department. Now, instead of reaching at arm's length with a pail weighing 40 lb, the employee places the pail on top of the first row and slides it into place (Figures 30-4 and 30-5).

By John E. Lane, Jr., OTR/L

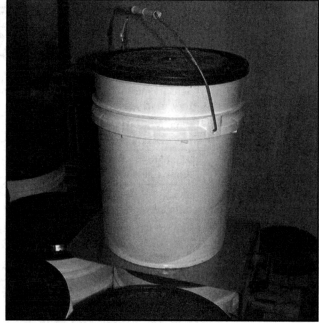

Figure 30-4. Palletizing of 40-lb buckets by hand requires frequent lifting and unsupported forward reaching at or above shoulder height. (Reprinted with permission from John E. Lane, Jr.)

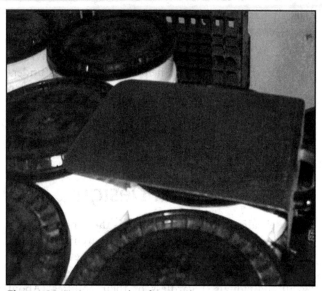

Figure 30-5. An example of a simple engineering control to reduce shoulder strain. A stainless steel "slide board" was made by an employer's in-house maintenance department per recommendation of the on-site occupational therapist. (Reprinted with permission from John E. Lane, Jr.)

Universal design could be thought of as an attempt to "get it right from the start." Rather than adapting the environment as a user's abilities change, universal design seeks to anticipate these changes by building "tolerance" for different abilities and processes.

In the case example, note how the practitioner analyzed the activity demands of the task. Using HFE principles, he recognized potential sources of hazards for the workers. His suggested fix demonstrates a low-tech, cost-effective strategy for greatly reducing worker risk.

Overview of Ergonomics and Process Modification

Job modifications to decrease risk of injury are in three categories and include the following (Cohen, Gjessing, Fine, Bernard, & McGlothing, 1997):

1. Engineering controls: Design of the job, the workstation, the tools, and work process are created from the beginning to accommodate the capability and capacities of the workers. It is independent of the worker's capabilities or techniques.

2. Administrative controls: The policies or work practices used to prevent or control exposure to ergonomic risks (e.g., frequent rest breaks to offset fatigue, limiting overtime or rotating between tasks, broadening job responsibilities to decrease repetition or awkward postures, slowing of production rates).

3. Personal protective equipment: Provides a barrier between the worker and the hazard source. This is the least preferred intervention and should only be implemented when engineering and administrative controls have not been effective.

The practitioner chose to address the task by altering the work process and workstation, found under

EVIDENCE-BASED RESEARCH CHART

Intervention	Keywords	Evidence
Americans with Disabilities Act (ADA)	Mixed results in the workplace; limited to negative results in employment; per student expenditures; preliminary findings suggested improvements in transportation and accessibility of public buildings	Bell & Heitmueller, 2005; Frieden, 2005; Gius, 2005; Wells, 2001
Ergonomics, human factors engineering (HFE)	Return to work; cost effectiveness of ergonomics improvements; parents rank repetitive stress injury low on concerns for children using computers at home, interventions; aircraft cockpit design and HFE	Anema et al., 2004; Helander & Burri, 1995; Kimmerly & Odell, 2009; Schmelzer, n.d.
Universal design	Designing instructional materials for all learners; designing computer interface (email) for seniors; potential role for physiological anthropologists in improving independence of elders; downloadable booklet: principles, history, case studies in universal design	Crews & Zovotka, 2006; Hawthorn, 2003; Pisha & Coyne, 2001; Story, Mueller, & Mace, 1998
Environmental adaptation	Positive and negative aspects of adapting homes for children with disabilities; poor housing related to poor health; justifying occupational therapy at home; effectiveness of home adaptation decreases as client limitations increase in elderly adults	Donald, 2009; Mathieson, Kronenfeld, & Keith, 2002; Richards, 2003; Roy, Rousseau, Allard, Feldman, & Majnemer, 2008

engineering controls. It was also necessary for him to convince the administration that work practices needed to be modified (administrative controls).

Occupational Therapist and Occupational Therapy Assistant Teams in Environmental Adaptation

The occupational therapy assistant may work with an occupational therapist in the provision of services in environmental adaptation. The standard, however, makes it clear that the occupational therapy assistant may also work independently to modify, adapt, and teach after service competency has been demonstrated. Service competency is a method by which both the occupational therapy assistant and the occupational therapist determine that the clinical skills of each are appropriate and by which the occupational therapist verifies that the occupational therapy assistant is functioning to the ethical, safety, and practice standards of the profession. This is most often achieved by regularly coassessing and cotreating clients and comparing results and treatment methodologies.

Summary

Environmental adaptation and ergonomics present occupational therapists with an important professional challenge. To be effective, the practitioner must be familiar with the client, environment, and tasks involved. In this chapter, a process for addressing each of these has been presented.

Student Self-Assessment

1. Specify a ramp for the residence you live in or one nearby. Your work should be specific enough that a contractor could fabricate it without additional questions. You should include the length of ramp, width, height of handrails, and wheelchair rails. If you need "switchback," you should also state the dimensions for the platform that ties the sections together. Use any of the Web sites listed to assist you.

2. Assess your computer workstation or that of a friend or member of your faculty. Create a detailed report that specifies how the workstation should be altered to meet OSHA guidelines.

3. Using a diagnosis provided by your facility, perform a home evaluation on your residence, your parents' home, or a relative's home. How should the site be modified to allow the "client" to remain in the home at a maximal level of independence?

4. Write a job description for one of your faculty members. How would the environment need to be changed to allow that person to continue to teach were he or she to lose his or her sight, hearing, or mobility?

5. Conduct an informal assessment of a supermarket aisle. How might this aisle be confusing for a client

after a head injury? How would you suggest modifying the environment to make it less problematic for this client?

Electronic Resources

- AbleData: http://www.abledata.com
- ADA standards: http://www.ada.gov/2010ADA standards_index.htm
- Adapting Vehicles for People with Disabilities: http://www.nhtsa.dot.gov/cars/rules/adaptive/brochure/brochure.html.
- Center for an Accessible Society: http://www.accessiblesociety.org/topics/universaldesign
- National Council of Independent Living: http://www.ncil.org/
- National Council on Disability (Pprovides recommendations to the Administration, Congress, and executive branch" on issues impacting individuals with disabilities.): http://www.ncd.gov/newsroom/publications
- Seven Principles of Universal Design and their guidelines: http://www.design.ncsu.edu/cud/pubs_p/docs/poster.pdf.
- U.S. Architectural and Transportation Barriers Compliance Board Americans with Disabilities Act (transportation in general): http://www.access-board.gov/publications/ADAFactSheet/a13.html.
- U.S. government site for ADA: http://www.ada.gov.

References

About the Center: Ronald L. *Mace.* Retrieved from http://www.design.ncsu.edu/cud/about_us/usronmace.htm

American Occupational Therapy Association. (2008). Occupational therapy practice framework: Domain and process (2nd ed.). *American Journal of Occupational Therapy, 62,* 625-683.

Anema, J., Cuelenaere, B., van der Beek, A., Knol, D., de Vet, H., & van Mechelen, W. (2004). The effectiveness of ergonomic interventions on return-to-work after low back pain; a prospective two year cohort study in six countries on low back pain patients sicklisted for 3-4 months. *Occupational and Environmental Medicine, 61,* 289-294.

Bell, D., & Heitmueller, A. (2008). *The Disability Discrimination Act in the UK: Helping or hindering employment among the disabled?* Retrieved from http://www.ncbi.nlm.nih.gov/pubmed/19091434?ordinalpos=9&itool=EntrezSystem2.PEntrez

The Center for Universal Design. (1997). *The principles of universal design, version 2.0.* Raleigh, NC: North Carolina State University.

Cohen, A., Gjessing, C., Fine, L., Bernard, B., & McGlothing, D. (1997). Elements of ergonomic programs. *NIOSH Pub.,* 97-117, 31-37.

Crews, D., & Zavotka, S. (2006). Aging, disability, and frailty: Implications for universal design. *Journal of Physiological Anthropology, 25,* 113-118.

Donald, I. (2009). Housing and health care for older people. *Age and Ageing, 38*(4), 364-367.

Frieden, L. (2005). *NCD and the Americans with Disabilities Act: 15 years of progress.* Retrieved from http://www.ncd.gov/newsroom/publications/2005/15yearprogress.htm

Gius, M. (2005). The effect of the American with Disabilities Act on public education expenditures, *Journal of Social Sciences, 1*(3), 162-165.

Hawthorn, D. (2003). *How universal is good design for older users?* Presented to the Proceedings of the 2003 Conference on Universal Usability.

Headquarters Department of the Army. (1983). *Man-material systems: Human factors engineering program.* AR 602-1, Washington, DC: Author.

Helander, M., & Burri, G. (1995). Cost effectiveness of ergonomics and quality improvements in electronics manufacturing. *Journal of Industrial Ergonomics, 15*(2), 137-151.

Jacobs, K. (Ed.). (1999). *Ergonomics for therapists* (2nd ed.). Newton, MA: Butterworth Heinemann.

Kimmerly, L., & Odell, D. (2009). Children and computer use in the home: Workstations, behaviors and parental attitudes. *WORK, 32*(3), 299-310.

Mathieson, K., Kronenfeld, J., & Keith, V. (2002). Maintaining functional independence in elderly adults: The roles of health status and financial resources in predicting home modifications and use of mobility equipment. *The Gerontoligist, 42*(1), 24-31.

Pisha, B. & Coyne, P. (2001). Smart from the start: The promise of universal design for learning. *Remedial and Special Education, 22*(4), 197-203.

Richards, S. (2003). *People leave hospital stable, but not necessarily able: We must help them.* Retrieved from http://0-proquest.umi.com.lilac.une.edu:80/pqdweb?did=351348661&sid=14&Fmt=3&clientId=8421&RQT=309&VName=PQD

Roscoe, S. (1997). *The adolescence of engineering psychology.* Retrieved from http://www.hfes.org/Publication Maintenance/FeaturedDocuments/27/adolescencehtml.html

Roy, L., Rousseau, J., Allard, H., Feldman, D., & Majnemer, A. (2008). Parental experience of home adaptation for children with motor disabilities. *Physical & Occupational Therapy in Pediatrics, 28*(4), 353-368.

Schmelzer, R. (n.d.). *Human interaction with aircraft cockpit displays.* Retrieved from http://www.eas.asu.edu/~humanfac/ringo.html

Story, M., Mueller, J. & Mace, R. (1998). *The universal design file: Designing for people of all ages and abilities.* Retrieved from http://eric.ed.gov:80/ERICDocs/data/ericdocs2sql/content_storage_01/0000019b/80/19/ac/11.pdf

U.S. Army Human Engineering Laboratory. (1984). *Human factors engineering: Supplement for HEO 101-108.* Aberdeen Proving Ground, MD: The Army Institute for Professional Development, Army Correspondence Course Program.

Watson, D., & Wilson, S. (2003). *Task analysis: An individual and population approach.* Baltimore, MD: AOTA Press.

Wells, S. (2001). *Is the ADA working—Americans with Disabilities Act.* Retrieved from http://findarticles.com/p/articles/mi_m3495/is_4_46/ai_73848278

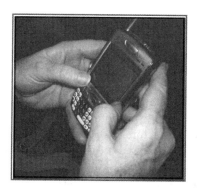

31

ASSISTIVE TECHNOLOGY

Betsy DeBrakeleer, COTA/L, ROH and William R. Croninger, MA, OTR/L

ACOTE STANDARDS EXPLORED IN THIS CHAPTER
B.5.11

KEY VOCABULARY

- **Assistive technology (AT):** Defined by Public Law 100-407, any item, piece of equipment, or product system whether acquired commercially off the shelf, modified, or customized, that is used to increase, maintain, or improve functional capabilities of individuals with disabilities.

- **High-tech AT:** Items or devices that are expensive, difficult to make or difficult to find and purchase.
- **Low-tech AT:** Inexpensive items or devices that are simple to make or easy to find and purchase.

Introduction

It is altogether too easy to think of assistive technology (AT) as being appropriate only for individuals with a deficit of some type. We may believe our clients "need" AT because they are unable to do something. In fact, the definition of assistive technologies seems to promote the disability label: "Assistive technology can be defined as any item, piece of equipment, or product system, whether acquired commercially off the shelf, modified, or customized, that is used to increase, maintain, or improve the functional capabilities of individuals with disabilities" (Office of the Federal Register, 2000).

Mann and Lane (1991) offered a different paradigm when they stated, "Tools augment existing human functions or add new functions" (p. 6). If we look at AT as a collection of tools that augment or add to the functions possible for our clients, we deemphasize the disability label. Using AT can benefit learning, safety, function, mobility, self-esteem, productivity, and so on. All humans and many animals use tools. A length of pipe added to a wrench is often used to increase the force generated when trying to free a stubborn bolt. Chimpanzees have been

Jacobs, K., MacRae, N., & Sladyk, K. (Eds.).
Occupational Therapy Essentials for
Clinical Competence, Second Edition (pp. 407-417).
© 2014 SLACK Incorporated.

observed in the wild using sticks to gather food, and otters are regularly observed to use rocks to open sea urchins. In this chapter, ATs are explored as tools that extend and augment our client's ability to function in a variety of settings and roles.

Assistive technologies have traditionally been divided into two types:

1. Low-tech devices: Characterized as being "inexpensive and easy to obtain" (Cook & Hussey, 1995, p. 7). Examples include built-up handles on utensils, adapted doorknobs, dressing sticks, and sock aids.

2. High-tech devices: Thought of as more expensive, more difficult to obtain, and often requiring training to operate. They are usually electrical or electronic. Falling into this classification are robotic assistants, augmented speaking devices, and prosthetic limbs.

Although common, there are difficulties with this classification system. Technologies continue to move from "high" to "low" in terms of their cost and availability. In 1995, computers were considered high-tech devices (Cook & Hussey, 1995). Today, they would hardly be thought of as such under this classification system. Another example is the cellular phone. The first call was placed on one in 1973 (Bellis, n.d.), and until recently, they would have been considered high-tech devices. Now they are nearly ubiquitous and affordable for many of the world's population. Possibly the best method of conceptualizing ATs is that they exist in a continuum with technologies that were once considered high tech, gradually moving to low tech as new tools come into existence.

Evaluation

Assessment should start with a thorough analysis of the demands of the task, which under the Occupational Therapy Association (AOTA) Occupational Therapy Practice Framework (OTPF) (2008) fall under the category of activity demands and performance skills. Common tasks such as those found in activities of daily living (ADL) will likely be familiar to the practitioner. Tasks that are unfamiliar, such as those found in school, work, or leisure, require additional consultation. In work settings, a job description is helpful, and team members, coworkers, and supervisors may also be able to deepen the practitioner's understanding of the demands and skills necessary. Coworkers or peers who might be affected by the device also need to be considered. To be successful, the practitioner needs a firm grasp of all of the task components.

Simultaneously, the practitioner should interview the client relative to his or her impressions of the roles, demands, and skills required. At this time, it is also appropriate to work with the client to understand performance patterns. What are the habits and routines historically used by the client? Were they successful in the past? What parts of the routine or habit does the client value and seek to maintain? Finally, what limitations does the client place on the nature of any intervention or tool?

The final set of assessments fall into the areas of performance skills and client factors (AOTA, 2008). At this point, the practitioner has assessed the skills required by the task. How do the performance skills and contextual factors of the task match with the performance skills and client factors? When mismatches are noted that cannot be addressed solely by environmental or process changes, AT devices may be appropriate.

Assistive Devices

There are a variety of methods for classifying assistive technologies. Angelo (1997) looked at mobility, methods of access, switch types, and the level of technology. Mann and Lane (1991) presented a system that sorts devices by disability: physical, sensory, speech, and cognition. Cook and Hussey (1995) arranged their work by activity area: communication, mobility, sensation, manipulation, and control. All of these ordering systems would seem to be appropriate. A look at AT using a combination of the preceding classification systems follows.

Occupational Therapy's Role in Assistive Technology Provision

Mann and Lane (1991) noted that the occupational therapist may work independently in some situations, as when training a client to use a "sock aid" after a total hip arthroplasty. When the complexity of the task(s) requires a team approach, they argued that the occupational therapist is the individual best prepared to act as its leader.

Angelo (1997) stated that the occupational therapist frequently serves as the "interface specialist" (p. 8). In this role, the responsibility of the occupational therapist is to assess the client's performance skills and client factors to determine the body part or motion over which the client demonstrates the greatest and most consistent control. Working with other team members, the specific method of access, the switch, and its mounting location can then be selected.

All authors are in agreement that one primary role for the occupational therapist and other team members is in positioning and seating. Effective, consistent control will not be possible until the client is positioned correctly.

We met Maryanne when she was in her mid-seventies. Despite severe arthritis, she had continued to live independently in her own home after the death of her husband. Maryanne had been referred for occupational therapy after replacement of the metacarpophalangeal joints of her left hand. During therapy, she related that she was experiencing significant issues centered on ADL and home management. Permission for a home evaluation was obtained from her attending physician.

Maryanne escorted us through her home, pointing out problem areas and detailing strategies she had used with various degrees of success. In coming up with a set of possible interventions, we paid attention to her impressions of the task demands, the contexts in which the tasks took place, and her habits and routines. We tried each task to get a feel of the performance skills required. Our understanding of her "space" was then compared with the formal assessments we had on her range of motion, strength, endurance, and information from the physician relative to the expected progress of both her therapy and the disease.

We then met again with Maryanne to present our list of solutions and to get her feedback on her willingness to accept changes to habit and routine. Financial considerations related to the final choice of assistive devices were also discussed. One major issue was that her limited range of motion made opening doors with traditional knobs almost impossible. We selected a commercially available device that clamps over the doorknob and featured a lever she could easily use. A second issue related to controlling the faucets in her kitchen. Replacing the controls was not a financial option. However, she was able to use the controls when we attached wooden clothespins to them. These adaptations allowed her to use her closed fist to turn the water on and off. The pins initially slid off the controls quickly, but this was rectified by a small bolt with a nut running through the open portion of the pin.

A final problem of great aggravation to her was her inability to open the windows in her living area on hot days. She was able to close windows with her fists but could not grasp the window hardware to open it. Maryanne had shown us, with great pride, how she used a back scratcher to remove her winter coat. Because she always left her windows open a small amount, we devised a plan where we attached small blocks to each of the windowsills. We then fabricated a slightly stronger "scratcher" that allowed her to use the block as a fulcrum to lever the windows up on warm days. She now had a combination scratcher–lever. A few weeks later, she demonstrated, with great pride, how she could also use the device to open her refrigerator by inserting it into the door handle and pushing against it with her chest.

All tools were decidedly "low-tech" interventions, and only the door handles entailed any cost for Maryanne. She took a considerable amount of pride in helping "her" therapists. One unintended consequence was that she also became one of the strongest advocates in our community for occupational therapy.

Augmenting or Adding Mobility

Problems with mobility have a wide variety of potential causes, which may include problems with balance, muscle strength, joint range, control, or sensation. Finally, a limb may not be present in whole or part.

- *Low-tech examples:* Canes, walkers, crutches, lower extremity orthosis, manual wheelchairs. Low-tech mobility devices such as canes, walkers, and crutches are commonly prescribed by the physical therapist, who performs the initial selection, set-up, and training. Thereafter, all team members frequently work to improve a client's functional mobility as during ADL.
  - ◊ *Lower extremity orthoses:* Lower extremity orthoses can take many forms and can impact the body at the ankle, knee, hip, or any combination of these. They are frequently used to stabilize the lower extremity, correct deformity, or slow the progression of deformity. In addition to stability functions, they are used to assist in mobility by correcting problems in gait. They are generally fabricated and fitted by an orthotist.
  - ◊ *Manual wheelchairs:* These are generally coprescribed by attending physical and occupational therapists.
- *High-tech examples:* Power wheelchairs, personal mobility devices, lower extremity prosthesis, and robotic walkers
  - ◊ *Powered wheelchairs:* These items change dramatically every year. The therapist should know the products and have a good working relationships with equipment vendors to ensure that the client receives the most appropriate equipment.
  - ◊ *Personal mobility devices:* A wide range of devices fall into this category (Figures 31-1 and 31-2), from three-wheeled scooters to electric carts to high-tech two-wheeled devices such as the Segway personal transportation device.

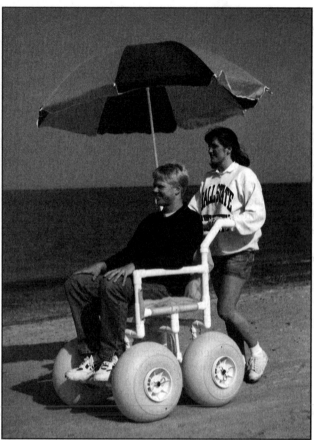

Figure 31-1. All-terrain chair. (Reprinted with permission from Assistive Technology, Inc.)

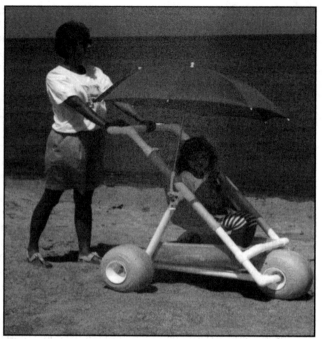

Figure 31-2. Beach baby stroller. (Reprinted with permission from Assistive Technology, Inc.)

◊ *Lower extremity prosthesis:* Although a lower extremity orthosis is used to augment an existing body part, the prosthesis functions to replace a missing body part (Bodeau, 2002). Assessment and prescription require the team to look at a diverse set of criteria that includes the cognitive status, function, environment in which the device will be used, client goals, client financial situation, and the level of amputation.

◊ *Robotic walker:* The robotic walker is a hybrid system under development that adds global positioning, obstacle avoidance, and speech recognition to a rolling walker. Researchers envision this device as a means to allow individuals with cognitive and balance deficits to ambulate more safely.

◊ *Exoskeleton walker:* Although still in the realm of science fiction, considerable research is being conducted in this area. Unlike the robot walker, the exoskeleton attaches to or is donned by the user. Current devices are aimed at augmenting or enhancing an individual's ability to walk or carry heavy loads over a variety of terrain types.

Assistive Technology for Upper Extremity Augmentation

The upper extremities are frequently impacted by a number of conditions, both congenital and acquired. This classification looks at AT for situations requiring the augmentation or extension of gross motor upper extremity functions including range of motion, strength, sensation, and control.

- *Low-tech devices:* Dressing sticks, reachers, long-handled shoe horns, long-handled bath sponges, sock aids, button hooks, nosey cups, lipped plates, plate guards, built-up utensils, card holders, mouth sticks, pointing devices, and static splints (Figures 31-3 to 31-6)

- *High-tech devices:* Environmental controls, upper extremity prosthetic, robotics, and dynamic splints

Assistive Technology for Fine Motor Augmentation

Most of the devices discussed in this chapter allow a user to approach or participate in a task. The fine motor AT is commonly some type of switch. It is critically important because it is the point of interface between user and device. AbleData is again an excellent resource

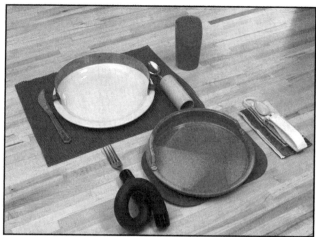

Figure 31-3. Low-tech assists for eating. (Reprinted with permission from William R. Croninger.)

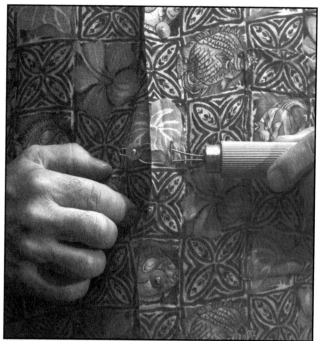

Figure 31-4. Low-tech assist for buttoning. (Reprinted with permission from William R. Croninger.)

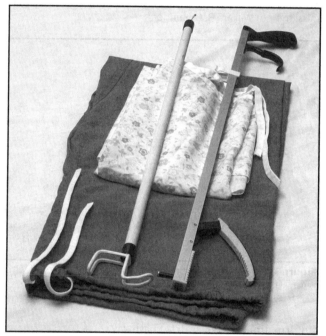

Figure 31-5. Low-tech dressing assists. (Reprinted with permission from William R. Croninger.)

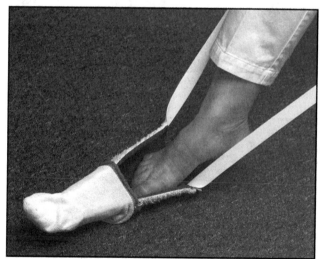

Figure 31-6. Low-tech assist for sock donning. (Reprinted with permission from William R. Croninger.)

to begin to understand the large variety and types of switches available.

Most critical is that the switch be accessible and appropriate for the client. Because it is the most heavily used portion of the intervention, it is also the most common point of failure. Therapists should always consider the impact of switch failure, both on the client's ability to access the device and on the impact to client safety if a switch fails while the device is being used. The following are two types of switches:

- *Latched:* Latched switches turn a device on or off. After being activated, the device stays in that mode until the switch is reactivated. Examples include light switches, on/off knobs on appliances, and tools that require two-handed operation (Figures 31-7 and 31-8).

- *Momentary:* Momentary switches require constant input or attention to operate. Examples include automobile accelerators and the "triggers" on tools that require fine adjustments while operating (Figures 31-9 and 31-10).

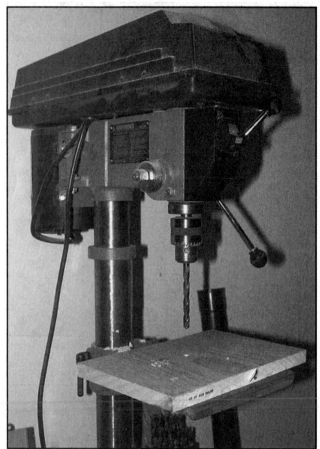

Figure 31-7. Example of tool with a latched switch. (Reprinted with permission from William R. Croninger.)

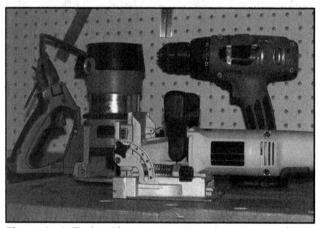

Figure 31-9. Tools with momentary switches. (Reprinted with permission from William R. Croninger.)

Assistive Technology for Sensory Augmentation

This AT area is generally thought of as including deficits in vision and hearing. To this, however, should be added technology for individuals who experience altered sensation, whether it is the epicritic or protopathic

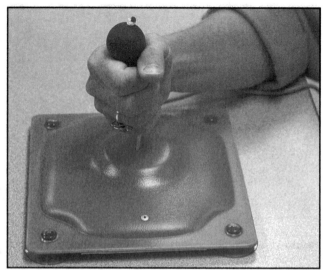

Figure 31-8. Example of a latched switch. (Reprinted with permission from William R. Croninger.)

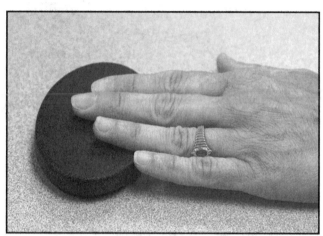

Figure 31-10. Example of a momentary switch. (Reprinted with permission from William R. Croninger.)

(informational versus safety) pathway.

Hearing

- **Environmental adaptations.** Include modifications to environment to reduce background noise and "auditory clutter."
  - *Low-tech examples:* These include sound-deadening materials, amplification, or choice or positioning of furniture. These also include modifications speakers make, such as not standing in front of bright light sources and trimming of mustaches or beards to allow a listener who lip reads a clear view of the speaker's lips.
  - *High-tech examples:* In some situations, selective amplification, as in assisted listening devices, is more appropriate. The assisted listening devices involve a microphone (speaker), transmitter, receiver, and earphone (listener) system that

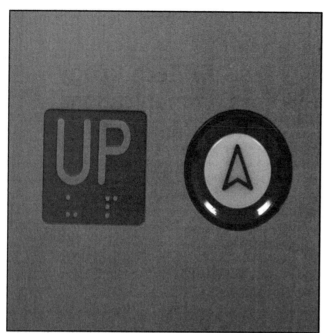

Figure 31-11. Low-tech vision assists. (Reprinted with permission from William R. Croninger.)

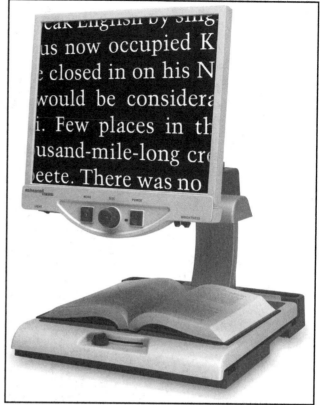

Figure 31-12. Merlin: LCD. (Reprinted with permission from Enhanced Vision.)

allows an individual with diminished hearing to adjust the sound levels produced at the earphones. In this way, an audience can be made up of those who do and do not need amplification.

- **Hearing aids (generally all high tech).** Falling into this category are devices that alert or augment hearing. Buzzers, strobes, flashing lights, and vibratory devices can signal an individual that he or she needs to attend to some event or situation. Hearing aids are classified by the National Institute of Health (National Institute on Deafness and Other Communications Disorders, 2002) using a number of categories:
  ◊ *By style:* In the ear hearing aids fit into the outer ear; behind the ear is located behind the ear with the earpiece located within the canal; canal aids fit completely within the ear canal; body aids are large devices carried external to the ear and located on the wearer's clothing.
  ◊ *By circuitry:* The analog adjustable type is built for a specific client to augment a specific level of hearing loss. The analog programmable type is fabricated to an individual's specific needs—the users can often select a variety of settings depending on the environment he or she is in. The digital programmable type contains a microchip which increases the ability of the device to adjust to the acoustics of varying environments.
- **Cochlear implants.** This AT involves implantation of a device implanted behind the ear. The device

bypasses damaged or nonfunctioning parts of the user's ear, sending information directly to the brain.

VISION

- **Low-tech examples.** Glasses, a magnifying glass, large print, large fonts, alterations to light levels, contrast enhancement, reduction of glare, books and signage in Braille, walking cane (Figure 31-11).
- **High-tech examples.** Scanning or large display device, character enhancement via computer, Braille talkers or typers, digital e-books, tablet computers (Figure 31-12).
  ◊ *Scanning or large display devices:* A large number of devices allow a user to scan print on a page and display it on a screen in real time.
  ◊ *Character enhancement:* Adds a computer that can enlarge fonts or "speak" words on a page
  ◊ *Braille talkers or typers:* Braille typers use a scanner that is moved over a printed page. The device converts the text input to Braille and raises the correct pins under the reader's fingers. Another strategy again uses a scanner to convert text to Braille, but the output is in Braille via a specialized printer.

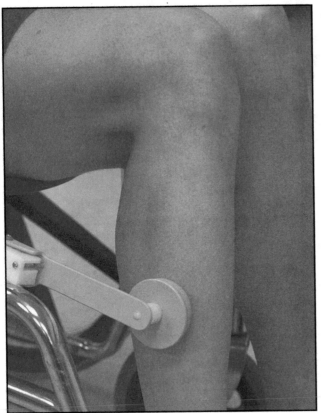

Figure 31-13. Locate the switch where the user has the greatest amount of control. (Reprinted with permission from William R. Croninger.)

Touch

Altered sensation, particularly tactile and pain, has the potential to impose a significant impact on a client's life and well-being. Because the hands are the most common means by which we interact with our environment, loss of tactile sensation makes it more difficult to choose effective AT for other existing conditions. Therapists should remember that switches need not always be activated by hand. The key is that the switch be positioned where motor ability allows consistent and accurate access (Figure 31-13).

Loss of sensation in the protopathic pathways (sharp–dull and hot–cold) brings a safety issue into the equation. Clients may not recognize they have come into contact with an object that is sharp or sufficiently cold or hot enough to cause tissue damage. Individuals with decreased peripheral sensation, such as is found after trauma or with diabetes, may not recognize that their fingers, toes, or a complete limb is too cold or hot.

The first strategy could be deemed to be "no tech," in that clients should be trained to attend visually to affected body parts. When the body part cannot be readily visualized, it can often be viewed using a hand mirror or mirror fitted with a universal cuff. Clients should always use thermometers when extremes of temperature may be encountered.

Assistive Technology for Communications Augmentation

A wide variety of conditions can lead to a decreased ability to communicate. Problems may be congenital, as in a child with dysarthria acquired after a cerebrovascular accident, or progressive, as seen in amyotrophic lateral sclerosis. Strategies involve a wide range of low- and high-tech interventions.

- **No-tech examples:** Gestures, grimaces, "mouthing," eye gaze.
- **Low-tech examples:** Paper and pencil, picture boards, symbol boards, touch talkers, and speech recognition software. Speech recognition and touch talkers were originally considered high-tech interventions. However, both have now become much more commonly available to the general public.
- **High-tech examples:** Tablet computers now have downloadable applications or "APPS" that are used as AT. Some examples, such as the Smarty Ears APP, assist in teaching pronunciation skills, articulation, stuttering, articulation, and language skills. There are also APPS that provide icons, phrases, and videos to assist or supplement speech (Lingraphica). Dedicated software and computer systems use variable strategies for word selection or prediction. Mann and Lane (1991) grouped electronic communication devices into three types by method of access, each with its own advantages and drawbacks.

1. *Direct:* Here, the user touches or uses a form of fine motor augmentation to select the response from among a group. The fine motor augmentation could be a mouth stick or one of the many head-mounted electronic pointers that use lasers, infrared, or radio waves.
2. *Scanning:* In this strategy, the device moves through the available choices in a prearranged pattern at a preset pace. When the desired choice is available, often signaled by a light-emitting diode (LED) near the choice, the user responds. This method requires less user action but is slower than direct selection.
3. *Encoding:* Symbols, numbers, colors, or letters are used for the desired words or phrases. This requires the least action on the part of the client in exchange for the client learning a new system of symbolizing.

Occupational Therapy Assistant in Assistive Technology

The occupational therapy assistant may work with an occupational therapist in the provision of services in AT provision. The Accreditation Council for Occupational Therapy Education (ACOTE) standard, however, makes it clear that the occupational therapy assistant may also work independently to modify, adapt, and teach

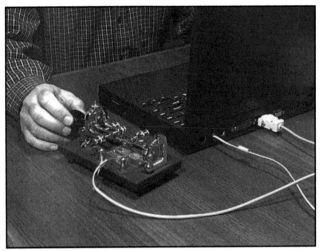

Figure 31-14. Example of a Morse code keyer (N7RZ). (Reprinted with permission from Les Kerr.)

after service competency has been demonstrated. Service competency is a method by which both the occupational therapy assistant and the occupational therapist determine that the clinical skills of each are appropriate and by which the occupational therapist verifies the occupational therapy assistant is functioning to the ethical, safety, and practice standards of the profession. This is most often achieved by regularly coassessing and cotreating clients and comparing results and treatment methodologies.

Morse Code

Morse code is an example of an encoding strategy. In this system, combinations of short and long tones stand for letters, numbers, and abbreviations. With modern equipment, very small hand movements are needed to generate the tonal sequences, which could then be displayed on a computer screen as letters. The computer would add the ability to have a short letter combination, such as "az," stand for an entire phrase just as in when a word processor is used to create a "macro" (Figure 31-14).

Summary

Assistive technology, whether it is a low-tech reacher or high-tech communication device, has the potential to greatly enhance the ability of occupational therapy clients to engage in occupations. Careful use of the practice framework (AOTA, 2008) greatly enhances the potential interventions that use these technologies will be successful. The practitioner, however, should pay particular attention to the sources cited in the following chart on evidence-based practice, which documents why and when AT interventions have failed. It is not enough to provide ATs for our clients. Practitioners must be certain that what is provided is the proper tool, that the client is

EVIDENCE-BASED RESEARCH CHART

Intervention	Keywords	Evidence
Pediatric	Improve writing, verbal communication	Lancioni et al., 2007; Lau & O'Leary, 1993; Mihailidis, Tam, McLean, & Lee, 2005
	Caregiver reasons for use versus non-use (mobility, augmentative communications)	Benedict, Lee, Marrujo, & Farel, 1999
Cognitive	Memory loss, conversation skills	Bourgeois & Mason, 1996; Van Hulle & Hux, 2006
Functional mobility, communication, ADL	Improved independence	Dahlin Ivanoff & Sonn, 2005; Eriksrud & Bohannon, 2005; Hoenig, Taylor, & Sloan, 2003; Nordenskiöld, 1997; Uustal & Minkel, 2004
	Reasons for use versus non-use	Agree & Freedman, 2003; Sonn, 1996

adequately trained, and that ongoing support after discontinuation of services is provided.

Student Self-Assessment

1. Write a definition of AT you could use to explain an AT intervention to the partner of a client.

2. Review Maryanne's story. What other ATs could have been used to assist her in her dressing, cooking, and home management activities?

3. Pick one of your instructors and imagine he or she has lost the use of his or her right upper extremity. Analyze the tasks required by his or her environment and roles. What AT interventions might assist him or her in maintaining his or her occupations? How would you assist him or her with AT if the problem were decreased memory? Decreased mobility?

Electronic Resources

- AbleData, sponsored by the U.S. Department of Education: http://www.abledata.com
- American Foundation for the Blind: http://www.afb.org/Section.asp?SectionID=3&TopicID=135&DocumentID=2424
- American Speech-Language-Hearing Association: http://www.asha.org/members/divs/div_12.htm
- Assistive technology: http://www.asha.org/public/hearing/treatment/assist_tech.htm and assistivetech.net
- Communication Disorders (NIDCD)—Cochlear implants: http://www.nidcd.nih.gov/health/hearing/coch.asp
- Gallaudet University: http://www.gallaudet.edu
- Hearing Loss Association of America: http://www.shhh.org
- International Society for Augmentative and Alternate Communication: https://www.isaac-online.org/english/home/
- Job Accommodation Network: http://www.jan.wvu.edu
- National Institute on Deafness and Other Communication Disorders (NIDCD)—Hearing aids: http://www.nidcd.nih.gov/health/hearing/hearingaid.asp
- Rehabilitation Engineering & Assistive Technology Society of North America: http://www.resna.org

References

Agree, E., & Freedman, V. (2003). A comparison of assistive technology and personal care in alleviating disability and unmet need. *The Gerontologist, 43*(3), 142-151.

American Occupational Therapy Association. (2008). Occupational therapy practice framework: Domain and process (2nd ed.). *American Journal of Occupational Therapy, 62*, 625-683.

Angelo, J. (1997). *Assistive technology for rehabilitation therapies.* Philadelphia, PA: F. A. Davis Company.

Bellis, M. (n.d.). *Martin Cooper—History of cell phone: Martin Cooper talks about the first cell phone call.* Retrieved from http://inventors.about.com/cs/inventorsalphabet/a/martin_cooper.htm

Benedict, R. E., Lee, J. P., Marrujo, S. K., & Farel, A. M. (1999). Assistive devices as an early childhood intervention: Evaluating outcomes. *Technology and Disability, 11*(1/2), 79-90.

Bodeau, V. (2002). *Lower limb prosthetics. In EMedicine from WebMD.* Retrieved from http://www.emedicine.com/pmr/topic175.htm

Bourgeois, M., & Mason, L. A. (1996). Memory wallet intervention in an adult day-care setting. *Behavioral Interventions: Theory and Practice in Residential and Community-Based Clinical Programs, 11*(1), 3-18.

Cook, A. M., & Hussey, S. (1995). *Assistive technologies: Principles and practice.* St. Louis, MO: Mosby.

Dahlin Ivanoff, S., & Sonn, U. (2005). Assistive devices in activities of daily living used by persons with age-related macular degeneration: A population study of 85-year-olds living at home. *Scandinavian Journal of Occupational Therapy, 12*(1), 10-17.

Eriksrud, O., & Bohannon, R. (2005). Effectiveness of the easy-up handle in acute rehabilitation. *Clinical Rehabilitation, 19*(4), 381-386.

Hoenig, H., Taylor, D. H., Jr., & Sloan, F. A. (2003). Does assistive technology substitute for personal assistance among the disabled elderly? *American Journal of Public Health, 93*(2), 330-337.

Lancioni, G. E., Singh, N. N., O'Reilly, M. F., Sigafoos, J., Olivia, D., & Baccani, S. (2007). Enabling students with multiple disabilities to request and choose among environmental stimuli through microswitch and computer technology. *Research in Developmental Disabilities: A Multidisciplinary Journal, 28*(1), 50-58.

Lau, C., & O'Leary, S. (1993). Comparison of computer interface devices for persons with severe physical disabilities. *American Journal of Occupational Therapy, 47*(11), 1022-1030.

Mann, W. C., & Lane, J. P. (1991). *Assistive technology for persons with disabilities: The role of occupational therapy.* Bethesda, MD: AOTA Press.

Mihailidis, A., Tam, T., McLean, M. & Lee, T. (2005). An intelligent health monitoring and emergency response system. In S. Giroux & H. Pigot (Eds.), *From smart homes to smart care* (pp. 272-281). Amsterdam, The Netherlands: IOSPress.

National Institute on Deafness and Other Communications Disorders. (2002). *Hearing aids.* Retrieved from http://www.nidcd.nih.gov/health/hearing/hearingaid.asp

Nordenskiöld, U. (1997). Daily activities in women with rheumatoid arthritis. Aspects of patient education, assistive devices and methods for disability and impairment assessment. *Scandinavian Journal of Rehabilitation Medicine Supplement, 37,* 1-72.

Office of the Federal Register, National Archives and Records Service, General Services Administration. (2000). Electronic and information technology accessibility standards. *The Federal Register, 65*(246), 80499-80528.

Sonn, U. (1996). Longitudinal studies of dependence in daily life activities among elderly persons. *Scandinavian Journal of Rehabilitation Medicine Supplement, 34,* 1-35.

Uustal, H., & Minkel, J. (2004). Study of the Independence IBOT 3000 Mobility System: An innovative power mobility device, during use in community environments. *Archives of Physical Medicine and Rehabilitation, 85*(12), 2002-2010.

Van Hulle, A., & Hux, K. (2006). Improvement patterns among survivors of brain injury: Three case examples documenting the effectiveness of memory compensation strategies. *Brain Injury, 20*(1), 101-109.

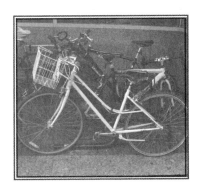

32

OCCUPATION-CENTERED FUNCTIONAL AND COMMUNITY MOBILITY

Kathryn M. Loukas, OTD, MS, OTR/L, FAOTA and Scott McNeil, OTD, MS, OTR/L

ACOTE STANDARDS EXPLORED IN THIS CHAPTER

B.5.12, B.5.13

KEY VOCABULARY

- **Body mechanics:** The utilization of appropriate muscles and positions to complete heavy work safely and efficiently (Brookside Associates, 2007).
- **Bed mobility:** Safely and effectively moving in bed for comfort, skin integrity, and function.
- **Community mobility:** Engaging in mobility resulting in successful participation in the community (American Occupational Therapy Association [AOTA], 2008).
- **Driver recommendations:** The process of making suggestions regarding the safe and efficient ability to engage in the occupation of driving.

- **Driver rehabilitation:** A specialized form of therapy that focuses on evaluation and intervention in the occupation of driving a vehicle.
- **Functional mobility:** "Moving from one position to another during performance of every day activities" (AOTA, 2008, p. 631).
- **Mobility device care:** The use and care of ambulatory devices to participate in everyday occupations.
- **Positioning and seating systems:** Selection and utilization of a comfortable, supportive wheelchair or chair seat that encourages symmetry, skin integrity, and occupational performance.

(continued)

Jacobs, K., MacRae, N., & Sladyk, K. (Eds.).
Occupational Therapy Essentials for
Clinical Competence, Second Edition (pp. 419-437).
© 2014 SLACK Incorporated.

KEY VOCABULARY (CONTINUED)

- **Transfers:** A specific process of moving effectively from one surface to another to participate in life activities.
- **Wheelchair management:** Selection, utilization, and functional mobility of a wheelchair.

- **Wheelchair selection and accessories:** A client-centered process that generates a product to maximize health and functional independence in wheeled mobility.

Introduction

Occupational engagement and participation in activities of life require people to move about their environment. Social participation is greatly enhanced when people can freely travel with purpose in their homes, communities, and gathering places. *Functional mobility intervention* is the term occupational therapy practitioners most often use to describe the therapeutic tenets of bringing a client from bed mobility through transfers and finally to community mobility and driving. Safe and effective participation in occupational performance is the goal of such intervention. Functional mobility is defined in the AOTA's Occupational Therapy Practice Framework (OTPF) (2008) as "moving from one position or place to another during performance of everyday activities...including ambulation and transporting objects" (p. 631). It is usually an interprofessional intervention because the occupational therapy practitioner must work closely with the physical therapist, who addresses gait training and functional ambulation, as well as physicians and durable medical equipment vendors involved in wheeled mobility. The occupational therapy practitioner must be fully informed of important factors involved in functional mobility through evaluation of overall important client factors including strength, range of motion, balance, coordination, cognitive processing, perceptual understanding, and visual skills (Bolding, Adler, Tipton-Burton, & Verran, 2013; Creel, Adler, Tipton-Burton, & Lillie, 2001).

Pierce (2002) proposed a basic hierarchy of mobility to address the order in which these skills should be addressed. This adapted pyramid forms the stability, positioning, and mobility necessary to participate in meaningful occupations. The pyramid of skills goes from the foundation or base and moves to the top (Figure 32-1).

The occupational therapy practitioner must keep in mind that every client is unique in his or her abilities and approach to mobility in occupation. Prerequisites to functional mobility training include critical thinking of the occupational therapy practitioner regarding client factors and performance patterns, including primary and secondary medical conditions, age, medications, family unit, and lifestyle, and how these factors might affect the client's functioning now and in the future (AOTA, 2008). Context and environmental opportunities and obstacles are also important to incorporate and adapt if necessary. It is imperative that occupational therapy practitioners learn and use proper body mechanics to safely move, position, and transfer clients.

BASIC PRINCIPLES OF BODY MECHANICS

Use of proper body mechanics is essential for the safety of both the occupational therapy practitioner and the client. Alnaser (2007) found in a literature review that patient handling was the most common occupational factor involved in work-based injuries. In addition, occupational therapy practitioners may teach caretakers or instruct clients to facilitate the proper body mechanics of handling and lifting in the home or community.

Principles and techniques to use during handling or lifting include the following (Bolding et al., 2013; Brookside Associates, 2007; Creel et al., 2001):

- Assess the context to ensure that you are capable of handling the situation; if not, seek assistance.
- Communicate with the person you are handling or lifting and facilitate involvement or independence as much as possible.
- Maintain a wide base of support and a stable center of gravity.
- Maintain proper body alignment, keeping a square orientation to the client.
- Bend at the hips and knees using the larger, stronger muscles, such as the legs, for lifting.
- Lift in one smooth motion, keeping your heels down.
- Stay as close as possible to the person you are lifting or handling.
- Avoid twisting or overstretching by moving your feet in the direction of movement.

Bed Positioning and Mobility

Movement in the bed is usually the first physical task involved in the recovery of occupational performance. The occupational therapy practitioner is often involved with the interdisciplinary team in assisting the client to position or move in the bed. It is important that the team collaborate and communicate the best positioning movement techniques for each individual client. All team members should facilitate the positioning and movement of the client in the same manner to help the client move in an independent or interdependent manner.

GOALS OF BED POSITIONING

The goals of bed positioning are as follows (Wilson, Lange, & Mandac, 2006):

- Provision of support, comfort, and pain relief
- Normalization of muscle tone
- Promotion of symmetrical positioning
- Improved awareness of affected side and safety of limbs
- Prevention of positions of deformity and pressure sores
- Facilitation of occupational mobility and meaningful activities
- Optimization of occupational performance

PRECAUTIONS

The occupational therapy practitioner should be aware of her or his own physical capabilities as well as the medical and psychosocial needs and attributes of the client when preparing for occupational mobility. Common client precautions include the following (Bolding, Adler, Tipton-Burton, & Lillie, 2006; Bolding et al., 2013):

- Absent or impaired sensation
- Pressure points and length of positioning
- Awareness of skin integrity as friction during movement may cause shearing, particularly over bony prominences
- Deep vein thrombosis (DVT) from lack of circulation in the legs
- Abnormal muscle tone (hypertonia or hypotonia) with impaired sensation
- Proper positioning of client in bed to prevent foot entrapment
- Orthostatic hypotension caused by a sudden drop in blood pressure when moving from supine to upright positions following long periods of bed rest, resulting in dizziness, nausea, or possible loss of consciousness
- Cognitive challenges

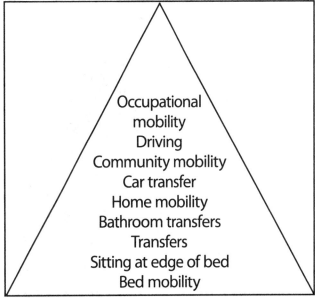

Figure 32-1. The occupation-based mobility pyramid. (Adapted from Pierce, S. [2002]. Restoring competence in mobility. In C. A. Trombly & M. V. Radomski [Eds.], *Occupational therapy for physical dysfunction* [5th ed., p. 667]. Philadelphia, PA: Lippincott Williams & Wilkins.)

General Bed Mobility Skills

The occupational therapist can facilitate the basic movements needed in the occupational performance task of bed mobility. Breaking these tasks into manageable steps can be an effective way to facilitate bed mobility. The occupational therapy practitioner should work with the interprofessional team to develop an individualized approach to bed mobility based on the evaluation of individual client factors, performance patterns, and contexts. Practicing can help the client gain skills and confidence to begin to combine movements for occupational performance. The occupational therapy practitioner needs to then facilitate the use of these skills in independent or interdependent performance patterns and daily routines. Skills needed for effective bed mobility include the following:

- Rolling (to either side)
- Bridging (pulling the hips up in supine while supporting the pelvis from the legs)
- Scooting up in bed (necessary to reposition one's self in bed)
- Supine, to side lying, to sit
- Moving to either side of the bed

ADAPTIVE DEVICES FOR BED MOBILITY

Adaptive equipment may assist a client to move effectively in bed. The occupational therapy practitioner works with the interprofessional team to facilitate

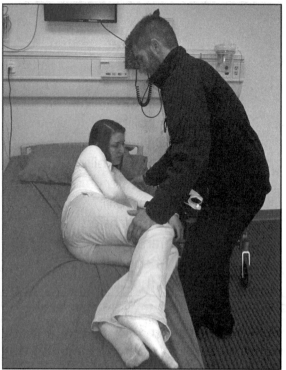

Figure 32-2. The occupational therapy practitioner assists the client to safely roll to the side of the bed.

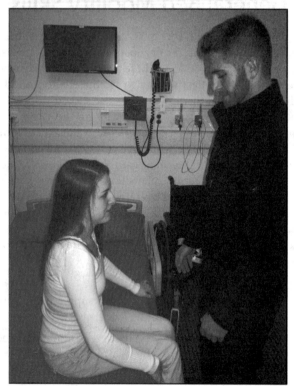

Figure 32-4. The client has transferred to the edge of the bed.

independent or interdependent bed mobility individualized to each client. Devices that can facilitate bed mobility in the medical setting or home include the following:

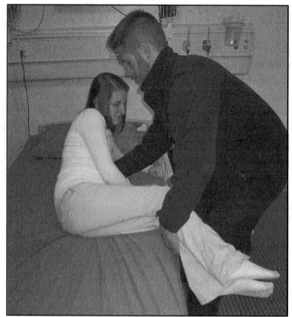

Figure 32-3. The occupational therapy practitioner facilitates the transition from side-lying to sit.

- Bed ladder pull-up
- Leg lifter
- Overhead trapeze bar
- Bed rail assist
- Transfer pole
- A draw sheet or positioning sheet can be placed perpendicular to the client under the trunk and hips for dependent bed mobility with two people on either side of the bed (Pierce, 2002)

THERAPEUTIC BED MOBILITY

Bed mobility can be used as the occupational product of therapy, such as when a client is given adaptations for independence or as an occupational process (Royeen, 2002), such as when the therapist is facilitating movement, cognitive processing, or perceptual awareness through the occupation of bed mobility. Some examples of performance skills that can be incorporated into bed mobility include the following:

- Awareness of affected side (hemiparesis) or affected extremities (spinal cord injury [SCI])
- Upper extremity movement, including scapular mobility
- Weight shift and weight bearing
- Trunk stability and postural control
- Management of affected extremities
- Safe movement and cognitive awareness

Figures 32-2 to 32-4 demonstrate steps of bed mobility.

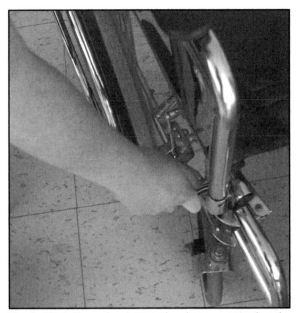

Figure 32-5. Properly position the chair assuring that the wheelchair brakes are locked.

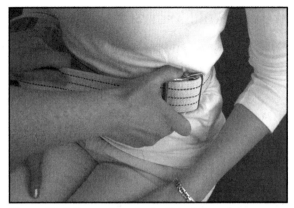

Figure 32-6. Secure transfer (gait) belt for safety.

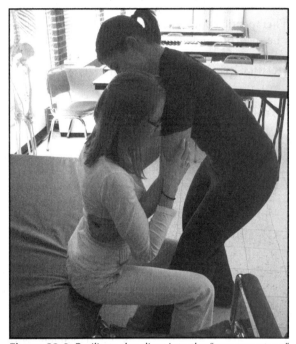

Figure 32-8. Facilitate the client into the "nose over toes" position; block the knee or knees if there is weakness.

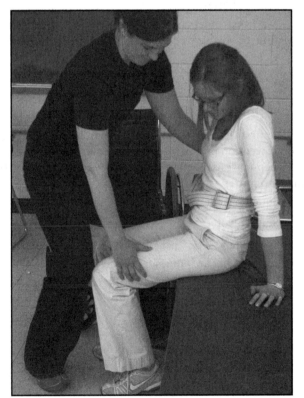

Figure 32-7. Facilitate the client to safely scoot forward.

Transfers

The next step in the occupation-based mobility pyramid is teaching your client with mobility limitations to move from one surface to another. This is called *transferring*. Some facilities and occupational therapy departments require use of a transfer belt for safety when transferring clients. Occupational therapy practitioners need to be aware of the protocol of their facility or department regarding use of a transfer belt or any protocol (Figures 32-5 to 32-8).

GENERAL SAFETY CONSIDERATIONS

- Be aware of the client factors and context.
- Set up the physical environment.
- Recognize the dynamic nature of your own physical abilities and limitations.
- Use optimal body mechanics.
- The client should be wearing shoes with a nonslip sole.
- Transfers are most efficient when the surfaces are the same height.
- A client with hemiparesis or other one-sided impairment will most easily transfer toward his or her stronger side.

Wheelchair Safety Considerations

- The wheelchair brakes should be locked during all transfers.
- The wheelchair footrests are not for the client to stand on and should be moved or removed before a transfer.
- All persons involved in the transfer need to have non-skid soles for stability during the transfer (Bolding et al., 2013).

Therapeutic Principles Incorporated in the Transfer

Therapeutic approaches and client factor remediation can be incorporated into the occupation of transferring. The following can be related to the occupational therapy intervention plan, model, or frame of reference:

- Pelvic tilt and position
- Trunk alignment
- Weight bearing and weight shifting
- Use of manual cues (neurodevelopmental treatment) (Runyan, 2006)
- Lower extremity positioning
- Upper extremity positioning and functional use
- Cognitive, perceptual, and visual awareness
- Facilitating independence by encouraging the client to do as much of the process him- or herself as possible. The occupational therapy practitioner should provide the minimal amount of physical assistance for safe transfer

In the case of a client who is interdependent with a caregiver, teach the client how to teach others including his or her family, caregivers, and paid attendants.

Preparation for the Transfer

1. Communicate with the client about the procedure and provide rapport and meaning to this mobility occupation.
2. Position the (wheel) chair at a 0- to 30-degree angle to the surface to which you are transferring.
3. Be certain that the surface is stable and the wheelchair brakes are locked. Facilitate the client's awareness and participation in the safety process.
4. The client should wear a transfer belt as facility policy indicates.
5. Remove the armrest closest to the transfer site (if necessary).
6. The client should scoot forward.
7. The client should lean forward (nose over toes).
8. Stabilize the lower extremities or the hemiplegic leg (if necessary).

9. Support any upper extremity limbs with abnormal tone.

Levels of Assistance in Transfer

The following are the levels of assistance required for transfers (Matthews & Jabri, 2001; Smith, 2013):

- One or two people assist with device, if needed
- Two or more assistants (maximum assist x 2)
- Verbal cues needed (tactile, visual cues)
- Dependent: 75% to 100% assistance
- Maximum assist: 50% to 74% assistance
- Moderate assist: 25% to 49% assistance
- Minimum assist: up to 24% assistance
- Contact guard (CG): Practitioner has her or his hand on the client at all times
- Supervised: Requires supervision for safe completion. No hands-on assistance, although a verbal cue may be required.
- Modified independence: Client requires additional time or adaptive equipment for completion of task.
- Independent: The client is independent in the task (no assistance or cueing is needed).

Transfer Techniques

The first three types of transfers can be performed as an intervention progression and are often used for clients with hemiparesis or other central nervous system impairments (Figures 32-9 to 32-11):

- Squat or bent pivot
- Stand pivot
- Stand step

The following are equipment used for transfers:

- *Sliding board:* Commonly used for people who have a SCI, overall weakness, or an above-knee or double amputation
- *Dependent transfers:* Use of mechanical device such as a Hoyer lift (Figure 32-12)
- *Cueing systems:* Clients with cognitive impairments may be physically able but may need verbal, tactile, or visual cues to break down the steps of the task for safety

Bent (Squat) Pivot

1. Remove armrest.
2. Scoot forward and lean forward (nose over toes).
3. Position affected arm.
4. Support affected leg.
5. Transfer, keeping the client in a bent forward position.

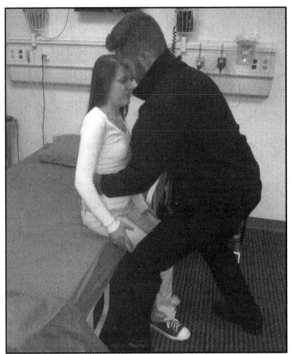

Figure 32-9. The client is seated at the edge of the bed ready to stand. Note the body mechanics of the occupational therapy practitioner, including a bent knees, straight back, and a wide base or support (stance).

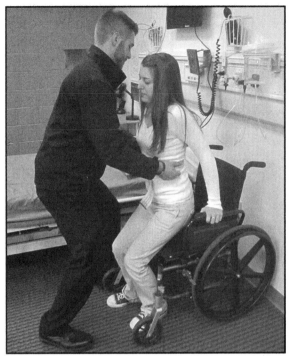

Figure 32-10. After the client was standing, the occupational therapy practitioner facilitated the client to pivot to align with the wheelchair. The client is encouraged to reach for and use the wheelchair arms to assist in the transfer.

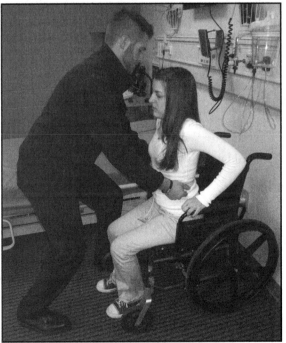

Figure 32-11. The client is safely transferred into the wheelchair while the occupational therapy practitioner maintains sound body mechanics.

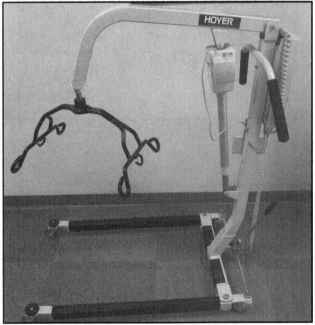

Figure 32-12. Dependent lift system.

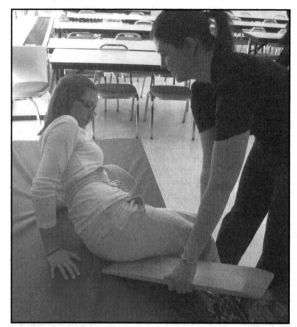

Figure 32-13. Sliding board transfer. The client supports herself in a tripod arm position while unweighting the hip closest to the wheelchair.

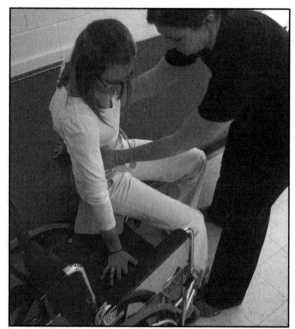

Figure 32-14. The occupational therapy practitioner facilitates the client to slide across the board from the mat to the wheelchair. Comparing this sliding process to entering booth seat at a restaurant may be helpful to the client.

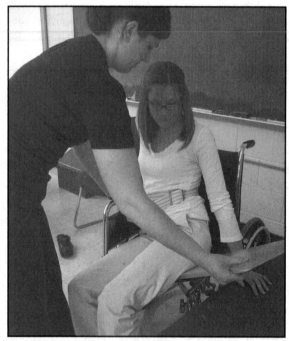

Figure 32-15. After the client has transferred to the chair, she continues to lean in the direction of the transfer to unweight the slideboard for removal. It is important to ensure that the client is properly positioned in the wheelchair at the conclusion of the transfer, which includes a neutral pelvic position and being seated deeply enough in the chair.

Stand Pivot

1. Same as Bent (Squat) Pivot, although you do not need to remove armrests.

2. Bring client to a standing position, gain equilibrium, do not rush.
3. Client pivots on unaffected leg, or both.
4. Reach back for the chair.
5. Lean the client forward as you descend as well.

Stand Step

1. Same as stand pivot, with weight shift of the lower extremities.
2. Should need less physical assistance.

Sliding Board Transfer

See Figures 32-13 to 32-15.
1. Set up wheelchair as described previously.
2. Shift weight to the opposite side of the transfer and maneuver the sliding board under the leg and buttock closest to the wheelchair (when there are sensation losses, male clients need to be careful of the positioning of their genitalia).
3. Block the client's knees with your own knees (the practitioner may be seated during the transfer).
4. The client should make sure the board is in a good position to travel into the chair.
5. Instruct the client to lean forward and put his or her hands on the board (clients with a SCI who are preserving the tenodesis grasp should keep their hands fisted so as to not overstretch the wrist and hand extensors).

6. The client slowly and carefully scoots or moves toward the wheelchair with the practitioner directly in front of him or her (the transfer should become more independent as the client's skill progresses).

DEPENDENT TRANSFERS

Many clients with significant client factors will be dependent in their transfers. It is important for occupational therapy practitioners to know their own limitations and protect their own bodies when attempting dependent transfers for clients. Dependent transfers can be accomplished by use of a team approach. However, if a client needs to transfer dependently long term, the best solution is a client lift system. If a client is very heavy, there are bariatric lift systems available to lift up to 1000 lbs. The role of the occupational therapy practitioner then becomes selection and training of the family or caregiver to use the device. The occupational therapy practitioner can work with more involved clients to ensure that they have the skills to do their own transfer training over the lifespan as caregivers may come and go. An example of this is a client with quadriplegic cerebral palsy making a digital recording of a caregiver performing a model transfer in order to train others.

Occupation-Based Mobility Considerations

BATHROOM MOBILITY

To maintain independence at home, clients must be able to safely move and complete various transfers in the bathroom. Although the transfer process may be similar, environmental factors that affect safety such as throw rugs, steam, temperature changes, and water on surfaces can increase the risk of falls. Changes in client factors can magnify this risk and result in the necessity of using a mobility device to access the bathroom or various pieces of adaptive equipment to assist with bathing and toileting tasks. Home modifications may facilitate safety and occupational performance in the bathroom (AOTA, 2011). Elevated toilet seats, shower chairs or benches, and grab bars are common client-centered adaptations or may be part of universal design to enhance independence with bathroom mobility. If architectural barriers or movement precautions prevent access to the bathroom, a bedside commode may be necessary for toileting purposes. It is essential that the occupational therapy practitioner review bathroom mobility and address the necessary contextual elements to maximize occupational performance in these areas (Bolding et al., 2013).

HOME MOBILITY

Various instrumental activities of daily living (IADL), including home management tasks, require dynamic balance and occupation-based mobility skills. In addition to the general safety considerations mentioned previously in the chapter, the home layout, furnishings, clutter, varied floor surfaces, poor lighting, and the presence of pets should be considered. During the intervention process, the occupational therapy practitioner may explore adaptations such as the use of a rolling cart during meal preparation, a long-handled duster to safely clean bookshelves, an automated pet feeder, or a walker basket to transport objects around the house (Bolding et al., 2013; Santucci, 2008).

CAR TRANSFERS

One of the more complex transfers to consider during occupational therapy intervention is car transfers (Bolding et al., 2013). Contextual considerations for car transfers include the skill level of the client or caregiver, the vehicle being used, the use of a mobility device, and if the client will be a passenger or driver. A variety of transfer techniques may be used for this process and typically, the client will enter the car using a backward approach, swinging his or her legs into the car after being seated (Meriano & Latella, 2008). Some clients find that riding in the back seat, if available, is an easier option than negotiating the front seat. When the client will be driving, it is important to consider the steering wheel during the transfer process as well as management of any mobility devices. There are various adaptations available to promote independent driving that will be discussed later in this chapter.

Occupation-Based Mobility for Persons of Size

Occupational therapy practitioners are often called upon to meet the needs of a large, heavy, or obese client. In the areas of beds, mats, transfer aids, adaptive equipment, and lift systems, specialized equipment is often needed to meet the needs of large, difficult-to-mobilize clients. It is important to use equipment that can handle the individual's weight for maximal safety and comfort of our larger clients. Occupational therapy practitioners should work with their interprofessional team, including durable equipment vendors and manufacturing representatives, to keep current with the evolving adaptive equipment and assistive technology available to meet client needs.

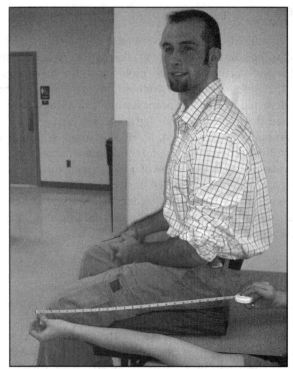

Figure 32-16. Measurements for a wheelchair should be made while the client is in the optimal sitting position.

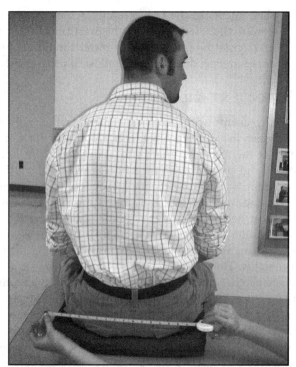

Figure 32-17. Hip measurements for wheelchair width.

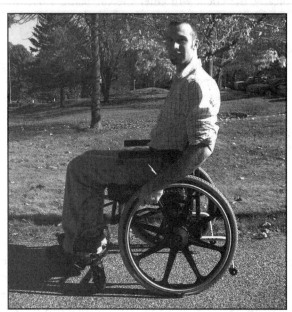

Figure 32-18. The proper type and fit of a wheelchair is necessary for optimal occupation-based community mobility and participation.

Wheelchair Management

The occupational therapy practitioner respects the physical and psychosocial difficulties a client may have with use of the wheelchair. The wheelchair is a wonderful tool to facilitate occupational mobility. However, it also carries with it stigma regarding disability and loss of ambulation, whether it is temporary or permanent. The occupational therapy practitioner who is skilled in both physical and psychosocial aspects of human life should be attuned to the client as he or she begins to be mobilized by a wheelchair. Language is essential to acceptance of mobility using a wheelchair. The occupational therapy practitioner should refer to the client as "using" or being "mobilized" by a wheelchair. Care should be taken that clients are not referred to as "confined" to a wheelchair because this statement is limiting and stigmatizing. The occupational therapy practitioner should speak to clients at wheelchair height when possible and not stand over the client to talk (Loukas, 2008).

WHEELCHAIR SELECTION

The occupational therapy practitioner works with the interprofessional team to collaboratively select the appropriate wheelchair with the client. The most common types of wheelchairs are manual and electric or power chairs. Considerations in the wheelchair selection process include specific condition and disability needs, client lifestyle, context of use, necessary accessories and modifications, payment, size and growth needs, and client factors (especially strength and functional use of the upper extremities). The occupational therapy practitioner often works with the client, physical therapist, and assistive technology professional (ATP) or durable medical equipment (DME) supplier in this process (Bolding et al., 2013). The occupational therapy practitioner uses critical thinking to ensure that the mobility device facilitates the client's occupational performance, enabling the client to participate as fully as possible in occupations in the home, worksite, and community (Figures 32-16 to 32-19).

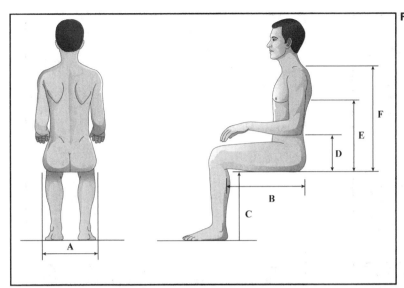

Figure 32-19. Wheelchair measurements.

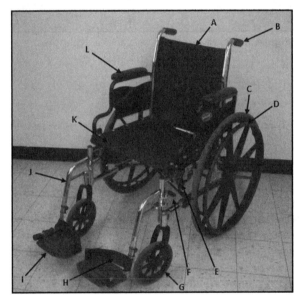

Figure 32-20. Standard wheelchair components. (A) Backrest. (B) Push handle. (C) Drive wheel. (D) Handrim. (E) Brake. (F) Front rigging release. (G) Caster wheel. (H) Heel loop. (I) Flip-up foot rest. (J) Front rigging. (K) Seat. (L) Armrest.

Manual wheelchairs are commonly used in medical facilities especially for short-term use. These chairs come in a variety of frame styles that range from a standard wheelchair (Figure 32-20) to more customized chairs with reclining backs or lightweight frames to enhance agility. Power wheelchairs provide a wide range of customization that can enhance independence for individuals who are unable to self-propel a manual wheelchair. The client must have adequate strength and control to mobilize the wheelchair. For clients who will propel their wheelchairs manually, techniques include giving clients protective gloves or lacing the wheelchair with rubber tubing to improve grip. Other techniques, such as using wheeled mobility or electric devices, can conserve energy

and improve occupational functioning and community participation for many clients. For clients with high-level paralysis, a breath-controlled or head-controlled electronic system can be used to operate the wheelchair, thus providing important independence and mobility. For children with mobility impairments, there are a myriad of pediatric mobility devices. These include push chairs, positioning chairs, and adaptable level chairs for school-based occupations.

Wheelchair Seating and Accessories

After a manual or power wheelchair has been selected, additional considerations include seating and accessories. The appropriate selection of a seating system that promotes a safe and functional body position is essential. Goals for proper wheelchair seating and positioning include the following:

- To facilitate postural control and head stability.
- To provide symmetry and prevent deformity.
- To normalize muscle tone and facilitate postural control.
- To maintain skin integrity and pressure management.
- To promote occupational performance and function to maximize sitting endurance and stamina for activity.
- To optimize respiratory function (Bolding et al., 2013).

A variety of specialized cushions are available to clients who use a manual or power wheelchair for mobility. Sling seats in a wheelchair are for very short-term, occasional use. Common cushion types include foam, gel, or air-based systems, which are recommended based on various client factors and physical assessment that may

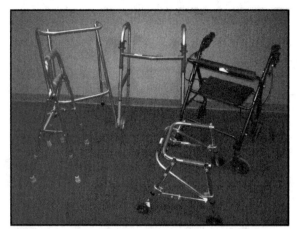

Figure 32-21. An assortment of walkers.

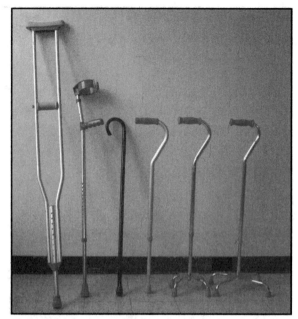

Figure 32-22. An assortment of canes and crutches.

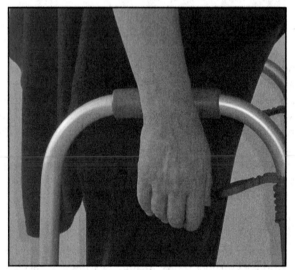

Figure 32-23. A properly fit walker or cane should place the handle of the device at the client's wrist crease.

communication system (Bolding et al., 2013; Pierson & Fairchild, 2008; Wilson, 2006).

MOBILITY DEVICES

During occupation-based mobility, clients may use a variety of mobility devices. The type of device is typically recommended by the physical therapy practitioner based on the diagnosis, prognosis, and ambulation assessment. Occupational therapy practitioners work closely with physical therapists during the intervention process and must be familiar with not only the device but also its proper fit and use. The recommended mobility device will vary in the amount of support provided to the client. Walkers provide more support than canes and include standard and various wheeled varieties (Figure 32-21). A variety of crutches and canes are available with a quad cane providing greater support than a single-point cane (Figure 32-22) (Bolding et al., 2013; Pierson & Fairchild, 2008).

Mobility devices can enhance occupational performance if the device is fitted and used properly. It is not uncommon for clients to attempt using mobility devices recommended for friends and family members, but these often do not fit the client properly. One simple way to ensure that a walker or cane is properly fit to the client is the wrist test. When the client is standing with the walker or cane at the side, the handle should be level with the patient's wrist crease (Figure 32-23) (Pierson & Fairchild, 2008). Physical therapy practitioners address ambulation patterns with the client during his or her treatment session, so it is important to collaborate with the team to ensure consistency. Generally speaking, the client will hold a cane in the hand opposite the affected

include pressure mapping. If a client requires additional postural support, various positioning devices may be added to the wheelchair frame to maintain body alignment and promote body functions and occupational performance.

Wheelchairs can be customized to meet the specific needs of each individual client. A wide variety of leg rests, armrests, and wheel styles and configurations are available. Various components of the wheelchair, especially on power chairs, can be mechanized to promote skin integrity, respiratory status, blood pressure, and circulatory issues. An interprofessional team can include the client, his or her family or caregiver, a physician, a physical therapist, an ATP or DME supplier, respiratory therapist, and an occupational therapist. Other specialists such as a speech and language pathologist may be involved when the client uses an electronic communication device. In this circumstance, the positioning and attachment of the device becomes essential to functional use of the

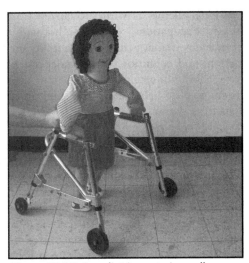

Figure 32-24. A pediatric posterior walker.

lower extremity. The cane and the affected leg should hit the ground simultaneously. When negotiating a step or stairs, the client should typically step up with the unaffected leg and "down" with the affected leg. Mobility devices for children include posterior walkers, dynamic prone standers, and other specialized equipment (Figure 32-24).

COMMUNITY MOBILITY

Community mobility is defined in the framework (AOTA, 2008) as "moving around in the community and using public or private transportation, such as driving, walking, bicycling, or accessing and riding in buses, taxi cabs, or other transportation systems" (p. 631). Client-centered community participation is a very important aspect to a full life and occupational functioning. The Americans with Disabilities Act (ADA) of 1990 has provided important accessibility rights for people with mobility challenges, and this continues to improve (U.S. Department of Justice, n.d.). For children and youth, the Individuals with Disabilities Education Act of 1990 and 1997 and the Individuals with Disabilities Improvement Act of 2004 support both physical and attitudinal accessibility changes in our communities and create more opportunities for people with disabilities (AOTA, 2006). Occupational therapy practitioners are at the forefront of these advocacy efforts. Facilitation of clients to return or emerge into the community is an important aspect of a full life and full participation (Baum, 2006).

For persons with functional mobility impairment, the first important step is for clients to have insight regarding their own abilities, opportunities, and obstacles. A client who can realistically judge his or her own strength and mobility challenges will have more success in planning for community mobility. For clients with cognitive challenges or lack of insight into their own abilities, the occupational therapy practitioner must help them understand and judge their own needs and abilities. The next step is planning. The occupational therapy practitioner can assist his or her client to plan an outing into the community, such as grocery shopping, visiting a friend, going out to eat, or attending church. Planning includes thinking about transportation, devices, safety and equipment needs, medication management, and many other client-specific factors. Finally, going out into the community in graded steps is achieved. The client should be encouraged to reflect on the experiences and to plan and adjust as he or she progresses in community participation. The occupational therapy practitioner may accompany the client on several community outings to foster mobility independence and community participation.

For infants, children, and youth, community participation includes day care centers, preschools, schools, work sites, and social events. Mobility and positioning devices can enhance the opportunities for inclusive participation of children in the community. Adaptive play equipment can facilitate community mobility on the playground or in the gym.

TRANSPORTATION

Many wheelchair-accessible vans, entry systems, and driving controls are available to clients with mobility challenges. There is also increasingly more public transportation that provides accessibility to people who use wheelchairs and other mobility devices such as independent transportation networks. Children traveling in school buses should have accessible and safe systems in place for transport. Parents with young children who have mobility impairment often transfer their children into a car seat and have portable wheelchairs or push chairs (strollers) for community mobility. It is important for the occupational therapy practitioner to assist the family to explore their adaptive equipment options as the child grows and needs a more accessible system that allows him or her to continue using a wheelchair.

Driver Rehabilitation

Driving is an integral part of independent living and is essential to a person's success in employment, education, socialization, community participation, and aging in place (American Medical Association [AMA], 2003; Bolding et al., 2006). Occupational therapy practitioners are influencing the practice of driver rehabilitation for persons with physical disabilities in greater numbers. An entry-level occupational therapy curriculum includes an understanding of driver assessment and vehicle adaptations. Advanced training and certification is available

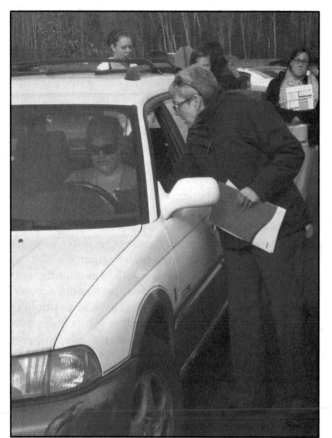

Figure 32-25. An occupational therapy practitioner works with older adults to ensure safe and efficient driving using the CarFit program.

for occupational therapy practitioners to become Driver Rehabilitation Specialists (DRS). A DRS is "one who plans, develops, coordinates, and implements driving services for individuals with disabilities" (AMA, 2003, p. 53). Further certification in driving to become a Certified Driver Rehabilitation Specialist (CDRS) is available but not required to practice (AMA, 2003). Issues that are red flags for medically impaired driving include the following:

- Acute events: A stroke or brain injury, seizure, surgery, or delirium of any type
- Patient or family member concern
- Medical history that includes chronic conditions, particularly those that affect vision, cardiovascular disease, neurologic disease, psychiatric disease, metabolic disease, musculoskeletal disabilities, chronic renal failure, and respiratory disease
- Medical conditions with unpredictable, episodic events
- Medications that can impair performance (AMA, 2003)
- A pattern of motor vehicle accidents

Occupational therapists with specialized training in driving-based occupations conduct a thorough evaluation that includes vision, perception, mobility, hand and foot function, and cognition. Many independent living centers or rehabilitation centers offer driving assessment and training services. They assist the client in choosing options such as car or vehicle considerations and the adaptive equipment needed to safely operate a motor vehicle. From there, occupational therapy practitioners develop a full plan of care to help the client return to driving, begin to drive, or recommend that driving is not a safe option (AMA, 2003; Bolding et al., 2006).

Vehicle features are also an important part of driving for older drivers and those with specific disabilities. Recommendations regarding entering and exiting the vehicle, opening and closing doors, and seat belt use are areas that occupational therapy practitioners can address specific to client needs. Programs that address person-to-vehicle fit, such as the AARP/AAA CarFit program (Thate, Gulden, Lefebvre, & Springer, 2011), can address the needs of aging drivers in vision, location of devices and controls, and emerging technology (Shaw, Polgar, Vrkljan, & Jacobson, 2010; Figure 32-25).

Issues Related to Driver Rehabilitation and Recommendations

The Aging Driver

Motor vehicle injuries are the leading cause of injury-related deaths for the 65- to 74-year-old age bracket and the second leading cause (after falls) for the 75- to 84-year-old age bracket (AMA, 2003). Many older drivers begin to change their own habits by limiting driving to familiar places, driving only during the daylight hours, and avoiding busy or congested areas of traffic. Client factors, particularly regarding vision, are important to assess and address as adults age into their elder years. The loss of the ability to drive has been correlated with risk of entering a long-term care facility in the elder population (Freeman, Gange, Munoz, & West, 2006).

Adolescents and Young Adults With Disabilities

Learning to drive is a rite of passage and important means to community participation as children and youth with disabilities transition to young adult roles and responsibilities. Students with autism spectrum disorders, physical disabilities, or other impairments are often capable of driving. It is important that occupational therapy practitioners encourage safety in all areas of transportation for the students with whom they work. Independence in transportation improves opportunities for employment, housing, social events, and educational and recreational involvement (AOTA, 2012).

ADAPTIVE DEVICE CONTROLS

Clients with paralysis or right-sided impairment may switch to hand controls. These are manufactured and can be used to help a client with paralysis return to the safe occupation of driving. Behind-the-wheel driving instruction is essential for those individuals who are reestablishing their safe driving skills using adaptive devices.

A number of devices are now being used to assist drivers who are visually impaired. Most states require a visual acuity of 20/40 to 20/70 or better and visual fields of about 140 degrees, although different states vary in their requirements (AMA, 2003). Bioptic telescopes are legal in many states for those with visual impairment, but the scopes must bring the vision to a level of 20/70 or better (AMA, 2003).

ADAPTED VEHICLES AND LIFTS

Many companies have a line for adapted vehicles and lifts. These can be very expensive for clients, so it is important to make good decisions for the best overall occupational outcomes. There has been an expansion in vehicle adaptations to such a degree that it is imperative occupational therapy practitioners collaborate with DME vendors regarding up-to-date equipment options. Behind-the-wheel assessments are vital in order to assess the actual adaptive equipment needs so that money is not needlessly spent. Nationwide, there are alternative financing programs available for low-interest loans so that individuals can borrow the money needed to buy adapted vehicles.

Summary

Occupational therapy practitioners address occupation-based functional mobility in the contexts in which clients engage in social participation. The occupational therapy practitioner and the physical therapist collaborate in the areas of functional mobility to maximize client potential. As indicated in the occupation-based mobility pyramid, skills progress developmentally from bed mobility to transfers to transportation and finally to community mobility. Many client factors are involved in occupation-based mobility across the lifespan and should be evaluated and addressed in occupational therapy interventions. Safety is a priority in the mobility-based

intervention progression. Intervention planning should include a holistic model and frames of reference. Client-centered, occupation-based mobility can be addressed within those therapeutic and often interprofessional approaches as occupational therapy practitioners facilitate participation in life.

Acknowledgments

The authors acknowledge student involvement of Ethan Drouin, Lindsey Holmes, Sarah Hume, Erin O'Brien, and Justin West. Gratitude is extended to Barb Allen, PT, for her consultative advice.

Student Self-Assessment

1. **Body mechanics.** The students should put a necklace on with string and a bolt around the string. The necklace should be long enough to hang at the navel of the student. Instruct students to bend and lift items such as books. They should bend with their legs, and the necklace should not go further than 1 or 2 inches forward as they bend. You can also practice keeping the body stable and not allowing any rotation and pulling versus pushing for bed mobility.

2. **Wheelchair experience.** Each student should spend 1 day using a wheelchair. Students should go to class, go out in the community, and perform other typical activities. They should then write a journal entry regarding the challenges and changes they experienced and their psychosocial responses to the wheelchair experience. It is very important for students to take this experience seriously and to not get out of the wheelchair in public; this could be disrespectful to people who are mobilized by a wheelchair.

3. **Bed mobility practice.** Students should practice bed mobility for various clients. Practice the basic skills and then apply these bed mobility skills for clients with the following diagnoses: hemiplegia, SCI paraplegia, and hip fracture or replacement. They should practice different teaching models in this process.

4. **Transfer practice.** Students practice all of the transfer methods reviewed in this chapter. They progress from bed or mat to wheelchair, from wheelchair to toilet or tub chair, and finally from wheelchair to car.

EVIDENCE-BASED RESEARCH CHART

Functional Mobility		
Issue	**Description**	**Evidence**
Elders	Elders who fell within 6 months after a hip fracture demonstrate poorer balance, slower gait, and decline in ADL	Restoring elders to full health after a hip fracture is indicated, including addressing mobility and balance deficits (Shumway-Cook, Ciol, Grubon, & Robinson, 2005)
Mobility device use	Qualitative, longitudinal study to assess how frequently older women use their mobility devices

Pilot study to explore falls and the fear of falling among elders using rolling walkers | Assumptions of mobility device use in the home, if recommended, are not always followed. Practitioners should consider the contextual considerations of device use in home during treatment (Porter, Matsuda, & Benson, 2011)

Fear of falling is greater among those who have fallen in the past. Inappropriate walker fit and use was identified and may be associated with falls (Liu, Grando, Zabel, & Nolen, 2009) |
| Individuals with spinal cord injury (SCI) | Functional mobility was found to be one of the top three problems identified by clients with SCI | Client-centered approaches have the best results (Donnelly et al., 2004) |
| Seating and mobility | Model for persons with SCI that considers the person, wheelchair, and environments of home, work, and community

Researchers examined segmented foam and skin protection wheelchair cushion efficacy to prevent pressure ulcers among nursing home residents | Seating and multiple considerations should be used for persons mobilized with a wheelchair (Minkel, 2006)

The combination of a properly fit wheelchair and skin protection wheelchair cushion reduce the risk of pressure ulcers (Brienza et al., 2010) |
Self-perceived physical independence	Activity limitations correlate with perceptions of independence	Community mobility and coping efficacy improve self-perception of independence (Wang, Badley, & Gignac, 2004)
Wheelchair design	Wheelchair performance was tested on a community obstacle course	Differences in wheelchair design affect performance, and wheelchair choice is important to community mobility (Rogers, Berman, Fails, & Jaser, 2003)
Wheelchair users at home	Researchers found that of 525 respondents, 37.9% of wheelchair users fell in the past 12 months; 17.7% suffered a fall-related injury	Structural modifications and functional mobility–based therapy services for safety are needed (Berg, Hines, & Allen, 2002)
Wheelchair mobility

Wheeled mobility and independence | Users' opinions on mobility devices and satisfaction with the devices

People with SCI were studied regarding types of wheeled mobility | Positive effect on activity, transportation, security, and participation in social activities (Wressle & Samuelsson, 2004)

Independent use of manual wheelchairs and the ability to travel efficiently have been correlated with community participation (Cooper, Ferretti, Oyster, Kelleher, & Cooper, 2011) |
| Severely disabled people and powered wheelchairs | Quantitative study on perceived quality of life after use of a powered wheelchair | Improvements in mobility and reduction in pain and discomfort were reported (Davies, Souza, & Frank, 2003) |
| Children | Children with cerebral palsy were compared across environmental settings in their gross motor performance | Results show differences across settings, indicating that use of the natural context is important in therapy (Tieman, Palisano, Gracely, & Rosenbaum, 2004) |

(continued)

EVIDENCE-BASED RESEARCH CHART (CONTINUED)

Functional Mobility

Issue	Description	Evidence
Spirituality and occupation-based mobility	Attendance at church by people with functional disabilities correlated with improved functioning Using prayer as a modality for healing is more common among people with mobility limitations	Church-related community mobility is important (Idler & Kasl, 1997) Practitioners should facilitate a client's own spiritual expression and connection to a higher power, or "religious pluralism" (Hendershot, 2003)

Community Mobility

Issue	Description	Evidence
Mobility devices	Pilot study indicates skills course improves mobility	Device use in the community should be addressed individually in practice (Walker et al., 2010)
Car transfers	Study of wheelchair athletes	Evidence that car transfers are most essential (Fliess-Douer, Vanlandewijck, & Van Derwoude, 2012)
Driving with a disability	Focus groups find arthritis may affect safe driving	Toolkit created to address safety concerns of this population (Vrkljan et al., 2010)
Nonstandard controls for disabled drivers	Large study of people with acquired disability; 79% had returned to driving; a significantly higher proportion had accidents	Problems associated with nonfamiliar controls (Prasad, Hunter, & Hanley, 2005)
Safety and mobility of people with disabilities in adapted cars	Safety and perceptions of safety, as well as confidence in an adapted car were reported	One of 10 had accidents, a small number attributed to special equipment in the car (Henriksson & Peters, 2004)
Effects of fatigue on driving for people with multiple sclerosis (MS)	People with MS report fatigue, leg problems, numbness, and eye problems	MS population reports driving short distances and shorter driving times because of fatigue (Chipchase, Lincoln, & Radford, 2003)
Older non-drivers (never drivers and former drivers) Drivers with dementia	Correlated as an independent risk factor for entering long-term care facilities Exploratory study examining drivers with dementia in the media	(Freeman, Gange, Munoz, & West, 2006) Significant safety issues are found in drivers with dementia who become lost (Hunt, Brown, & Gilman, 2010)
Senior driving	Safety risks occur as a result of incongruence between vehicle and driver	Intervention is needed to promote vehicle to driver fit (Shaw, Polgar, Vrkljan, & Jacobson, 2010)
People with Parkinson's disease Combat veterans with traumatic brain injury and posttraumatic stress disorder	Effects of cognitive abilities Veterans found to have more critical driving errors	Cognitive abilities were found not to be associated with fitness to drive (Radford, Lincoln, & Lennox, 2004) Intervention to address safe driving needed for veterans (Classen et al., 2011)

References

Alnaser, M. Z. (2007). Occupational musculoskeletal injuries in the health care environment and its impact on occupational therapy practitioners: A systematic review. *WORK, 29*(20), 89-100.

American Medical Association. (2003). *Physicians guide to: Assessing and counseling older drivers.* Chicago, IL: Author.

American Occupational Therapy Association. (2006). *The New IDEA: Summary of the Individuals with Disabilities Education Improvement Act of 2004 (P.L. 108-446).* Retrieved from http://www.aota.org

American Occupational Therapy Association. (2008). Occupational therapy practice framework: Domain and process (2nd ed.). *American Journal of Occupational Therapy, 62*(6), 609-639.

American Occupational Therapy Association. (2011). *Fact sheet: Home modifications and occupational therapy.* Bethesda, MD: AOTA Press.

American Occupational Therapy Association. (2012). *Fact sheet: The occupational therapy role in driving and community mobility across the lifespan.* Bethesda, MD: AOTA Press.

Baum, M. C. (2006). Centennial challenges, millennium opportunities: Presidential address, 2006. *American Journal of Occupational Therapy, 60,* 609-616.

Berg, K., Hines, M., & Allen, S. (2002). Wheelchair users at home: Few home modifications and many injurious falls. *American Journal of Public Health, 92*(1), 48.

Bolding, D., Adler, C., Tipton-Burton, M., & Lillie, S. M. (2006). Mobility. In H. M. Pendleton & W. Schultz-Krohn (Eds.), *Pedretti's occupational therapy practice skills for physical dysfunction* (6th ed., pp. 195-247). St. Louis, MO: Mosby Elsevier.

Bolding, D., Adler, C., Tipton-Burton, M., & Verran, A. (2013). Mobility. In H. M. Pendleton & W. Schultz-Krohn (Eds.), *Pedretti's occupational therapy* (7th ed., pp. 233-294). St. Louis, MO: Elsevier Mosby.

Brienza, D., Kelsey, S., Karg, P., Allegretti, A., Olson, M., Schmeler, M., & Holm, M. (2010). A randomized clinical trial on preventing pressure ulcers with wheelchair seat cushions. *Journal of the American Geriatric Society, 58,* 2308-2304.

Brookside Associates Multi-Media Edition. (2007). Nursing Fundamentals I. Retrieved from http://www.brooksidepress.org/Products/Nursing_Fundamentals_1/Index.htm

Chipchase, S. Y., Lincoln, N. B., & Radford, K. A. (2003). Measuring fatigue in people with multiple sclerosis. *Disability and Rehabilitation, 25*(14), 778-784.

Classen, S., Levy, C., Meyer, D. L., Bewernitz, M., Lanford, D. N., & Mann, W. C. (2011). Simulated driving performance of combat veterans with mild traumatic brain injury and post-traumatic stress disorder: A pilot study. *American Journal of Occupational Therapy, 65,* 419-427.

Cooper, R. A., Ferretti, E., Oyster, M., Kelleher, A., & Cooper, R. (2011). The relationship between wheelchair mobility patterns and community participation among individuals with spinal cord injury. *Assistive Technology, 23,* 177-183.

Creel, T. A., Adler, C., Tipton-Burton, M., & Lillie (2001). Mobility. In L. W. Pedretti & M. B. Early (Eds.), *Occupational therapy practice skills for physical dysfunction* (5th ed., pp. 172-178). St. Louis, MO: Mosby.

Davies, A., Souza, L. H., & Frank, A. O. (2003). Changes in the quality of life in severely disabled people following provision of powered indoor/outdoor chairs. *Disability and Rehabilitation, 25*(6), 286.

Donnelly, C., Eng, J. J., Hall, J., Alford, L., Gianchino, R., Norton, K., et al. (2004). Client centered assessment and the identification of meaningful treatment goals for individuals with a spinal cord injury. *Spinal Cord, 42,* 302-307.

Fliess-Douer, O., Vanlandewijck, Y. C., & VanDer Woude, L. H. (2012). Most essential wheeled mobility skills for daily life: an international survey among Paralympic wheelchair athletes with spinal cord injury. *Archives of Physical Medicine and Rehabilitation, 93,* 629-635.

Freeman, E. E., Gange, S. J., Munoz, B., & West, S. K. (2006). Driving status and risk of entry into long-term care in older adults. *American Journal of Public Health, 96*(7), 1254-1259.

Hendershot, G. E. (2003). Mobility limitations and complementary and alternative medicine: Are people with disabilities more likely to pray? *American Journal of Public Health, 93*(7), 1079-1080.

Henriksson, P., & Peters, B. (2004). Safety and mobility of people with disabilities driving adapted cars. *Scandinavian Journal of Occupational Therapy, 11,* 54-61.

Hunt, L., Brown, A. E., & Gilman, I. P. (2010). Drivers with dementia and outcomes of becoming lost while driving. *American Journal of Occupational Therapy, 64,* 225-232.

Idler, E. L., & Kasl, S. V. (1997). Religion among disabled and non-disabled persons, II: Attendance at religion services as a predictor of the course of disability. *Journal of Gerontology, 52B,* S306-S316.

Liu, H., Grando, V., Zabel, R., & Nolen, J. (2009). Pilot study evaluating fear of falling and falls among older rolling walker users. *International Journal of Therapy and Rehabilitation, 16*(12), 670-675.

Loukas, K. M. (2008). The evolution of language and perception of disability in occupational therapy. *The Education Special Interest Section Newsletter, 18*(2), 1-4. Bethesda, MD: AOTA Press.

Mathews, M. M., & Jabri, J. L. (2001). Documentation of occupational therapy services. In L. W. Pedretti & M. B. Early (Eds.), *Occupational therapy practice skills for physical dysfunction* (5th ed., pp. 91-100). St. Louis, MO: Mosby.

Meriano, C., & Latella, D. (2008). Activities of daily living. In C. Meriano & D. Latella (Eds.), *Occupational therapy interventions: Function and occupations* (pp. 129-236). Thorofare, NJ: SLACK Incorporated.

Minkel, J. L. (2000). Seating and mobility considerations for people with spinal cord injury. *Physical Therapy, 80*(7), 701-709.

Pierce, S. (2002). Restoring competence in mobility. In C. A. Trombly & M. V. Radomski (Eds.), *Occupational therapy for physical dysfunction* (5th ed., pp. 665-693). Philadelphia, PA: Lippincott Williams & Wilkins.

Pierson, F. M., & Fairchild, S. L. (2008). *Principles & techniques of patient care* (4th ed.). St. Louis, MO: Saunders Elsevier.

Porter, E. J., Matsuda, S., & Benson, J. J. (2011). Intentions of older homebound women about maintaining proximity to a cane or walker and using it at home. *Journal of Applied Gerontology, 30*(4), 485-504.

Prasad, R. S., Hunter, J., & Hanley, J. (2006). Driving experiences of disabled drivers. *Clinical Rehabilitation, 20*(5), 445-450.

Radford, K. A., Lincoln, N. B., & Lennox, G. (2004). The effects of cognitive abilities on driving in people with Parkinson's disease. *Disability and Rehabilitation, 26*(2), 65-70.

Rogers, H., Berman, S., Fails, D., & Jaser, J. (2003). A comparison of functional mobility in standard versus ultralight wheelchairs as measured by performance on a community obstacle course. *Disability and Rehabilitation, 25*(19), 1083-1088.

Royeen, C. B. (2002). Occupation reconsidered. *Occupational Therapy International, 9*(2), 111-120.

Runyan, C. (2006). Neuro-developmental treatment of adult hemiplegia. In H. M. Pendleton & W. Schultz-Krohn (Eds.), *Pedretti's occupational therapy practice skills for physical dysfunction* (6th ed., pp. 769-790). St. Louis, MO: Mosby Elsevier.

Santucci, M. E. (2008). Instrumental activities of daily living. In C. Meriano, & D. Latella (Eds.), *Occupational therapy interventions: Function and occupations* (pp. 238-283). Thorofare, NJ: SLACK Incorporated.

Shaw, L., Polgar, J. M., Vrkljan, B., & Jacobson, J. (2010). Seniors' perceptions of vehicle safety risks and needs. *American Journal of Occupational Therapy, 64*, 215-224.

Shumway-Cook, A., Ciol, M. A., Grubon, W., & Robinson, C. (2005). Incidence of risk factors for falls following hip fracture in community dwelling older adults. *Physical Therapy, 85*, 648-655.

Smith, J. (2013). Documentation of occupational therapy services. In H. M. Pendleton & W. Schultz-Krohn (Eds.), *Pedretti's occupational therapy* (7th ed., pp. 117-139). St. Louis, MO: Elsevier Mosby.

Thate, M., Gulden, B., Lefebvre, J., & Springer, E. (2011). CarFit: finding the right fit for the older driver. *Gerontology Special Interest Section Quarterly, 34*(4), 1-4. Bethesda, MD: AOTA Press.

Tieman, B. L., Palisano, R. J., Gracely, E. J., & Rosenbaum, P. L. (2004). Gross motor capability and performance of mobility in children with cerebral palsy: A comparison across home, school and outdoors/community settings. *Physical Therapy, 84*(5), 419-427.

U.S. Department of Justice. (n.d.). *Americans with Disabilities Act.* Retrieved from http://www.ada.gov

Vrkljan, B., Cranney, A., Worswick, J., O'Donnal, S., Li, L. C., Gelinas, I., ... Marshall, S. (2010). Supporting safe driving with arthritis: Developing a driving toolkit for clinical practice and consumer use. *American Journal of Occupational Therapy, 64*, 259-267.

Walker, K. A., Morgan, K. A., Morris, C. L., DeGroot, K. K., Hollingsworth, H. H., & Gray, D. B. (2010). Development of a community mobility skills course for people who use mobility devices. *American Journal of Occupational Therapy, 65*, 547-554.

Wang, P. P., Badley, E. M., & Gignac, M. (2004). Activity limitation, coping efficacy and self-perceived physical independence in people with disability. *Disability and Rehabilitation, 26*(13), 785-793.

Wheelchair Net. (2006). *Wheelchair and seating evaluations.* Retrieved from http://www.wheelchairnet.org/wcn_ProdServ/Consumers/evaluations.html

Wresstle, E., & Samuelsson, K. (2004). User satisfaction with mobility assistive devices. *Scandinavian Journal of Occupational Therapy, 11*(3), 143-150.

Wilson, P. E., Lange, M. L., & Mandac, B. R. (2006). *Seating evaluation and wheelchair prescription.* Retrieved from http://emedicine.medscape.com/article/318092-overview

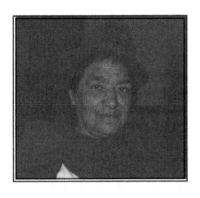

33

PHYSICAL AGENT MODALITIES

Alfred G. Bracciano, EdD, OTR/L, FAOTA

ACOTE STANDARDS EXPLORED IN THIS CHAPTER
B.5.13, B.5.14

KEY VOCABULARY

- **Deep thermal agents:** Are those modalities which penetrate to a depth of 5 cm and cause a change in tissue temperature and biophysiology. Deep thermal agents include but are not limited to ultrasound, phonophoresis, diathermy, and other commercially available technologies.

- **Electrotherapeutic agents:** Use electricity and the electromagnetic spectrum to facilitate tissue healing, improve muscle strength and endurance, decrease edema, modulate pain, decrease the inflammatory process and modify the healing process. Electrotherapeutic agents include but are not limited to neuromuscular electrical stimulation (NMES), functional electrical stimulation (FES), transcutaneous electrical nerve stimulation (TENS), high-voltage galvanic stimulation for tissue and would repair (ESTR), high-voltage pulsed current (HVPC), direct current (DC) iontophoresis, and other commercially available technologies (Bracciano, 2008).

(continued)

Jacobs, K., MacRae, N., & Sladyk, K. (Eds.).
Occupational Therapy Essentials for
Clinical Competence, Second Edition (pp. 439-456).
© 2014 SLACK Incorporated.

KEY VOCABULARY (CONTINUED)

- **Physical agent modalities:** Are those procedures and interventions that are systematically applied to modify specific client factors when neurological, musculoskeletal, or skin conditions are present that may be limiting occupational performance. PAMs use various forms of energy to modulate pain, modify tissue healing, increase tissue extensibility, modify skin and scar tissue, and decrease edema or inflammation. OAMs are used in preparation for or concurrently with purposeful and occupation-based activities (AOTA, 2012; Bracciano, 2008).

- **Superficial thermal agents:** Are those modalities that penetrate to a depth of 1 to 2 cm and cause a change in tissue temperature and biophysiology. Superficial thermal agents include but are not limited to hydrotherapy/whirlpool, cryotherapy (cold packs, ice), fluidotherapy, hot packs, paraffin, water, infrared, and other commercially available superficial heating and cooling technologies (AOTA, 2012).

Introduction

The profession of occupational therapy has long debated the role and use of physical agent modalities. There has often been heated dialogue over whether physical agent modalities were "occupational" in nature or were the purview of other disciplines and had no role in intervention. There have been controversies regarding training, preparation, and competency, with wide variability in academic and clinical preparation and training (Cornish-Painter, Peterson, & Lindstrom-Hazel, 1997; Glauner, Ekes, James, & Holm, 1997). To some extent, the debate continues between academics, theoreticians, and clinicians. The American Occupational Therapy Association (AOTA) clarified and strengthened the definition of physical agent modalities and their role and use as preparatory agents in the AOTA 2012 position statement. Partially driven by the need to strengthen regulatory oversight of physical agent modalities, the AOTA revised its position statement to assist regulatory bodies and clinicians to outline and define physical agent modality use. The 2011 Accreditation Council for Occupational Therapy Education (ACOTE) standards (B.5.15–5.16) reinforced the need and responsibility of academic institutions and occupational therapists to provide basic education and theory behind physical agent modality use. This chapter will provide a broad overview of the different categories of physical agent modalities and their clinical use. Students and clinicians are encouraged to explore additional material and educational opportunities, which can provide the physiological basis and depth of knowledge necessary to safely integrate physical agents into clinical practice and to meet specific state regulatory and licensing requirements. The reader is encouraged to review specific regulatory requirements for the state in which he or she will be practicing as well as any institutional requirements. The terms *physical agent modality, physical agent,* and *physical modality* can be used interchangeably.

Physical agent modalities are one component of the intervention process and should always be used preparatory to engagement in occupational activities and tasks. The AOTA 2012 Physical Agent Modalities position paper defines *physical agent modalities* as those procedures and interventions that are systematically applied to modify specific client factors when neurological, musculoskeletal, or skin conditions are present that may be limiting occupational performance. Physical agent modalities use various forms of energy to modulate pain, modify tissue healing, increase tissue extensibility, modify skin and scar tissue, and decrease edema or inflammation. Physical agent modalities are used in preparation for or concurrently with purposeful and occupation-based activities (Bracciano, 2008). It is important for the occupational therapist to understand the classification system of physical agents and their mechanism of action in order to select the appropriate intervention based on the clinical condition and needs of the client. Physical agent modalities are used as part of clinical intervention in order to enhance engagement in occupation and to facilitate healing and performance. Many clinicians view the application of physical agents as an external, ancillary intervention with a "generalized" reaction that may decrease pain or improve client comfort. There is little recognition by these clinicians that by using physical agents, we manipulate the healing tissue at a cellular level, or at the level of the "client factor." Clinical consideration of the appropriate timing and application may facilitate the healing process and ultimately improve occupational performance. Physical agents can be a powerful adjunct to intervention and will facilitate outcomes and speed recovery when used appropriately and judiciously. Physical agents should never be used singularly or in and of themselves. To do so is not considered occupational therapy.

Physical agents are often used in the intervention of musculoskeletal injuries, or by therapists whose primary practice is hands. This concept is both limiting to the profession and to the client. The fundamental physiological principles related to healing and the influence of physical agents on that process are consistent whether the tissue is located in the hand, shoulder, knee, or back. An appreciation of the impact physical agents have on physiological and systemic processes (the client factors) will facilitate clinical reasoning and generalization of the interventions to other conditions and injuries. Occupational therapists bring the unique perspective of occupation and performance to the use of these agents as part of the intervention process, and research has demonstrated the effectiveness of pairing movement, valued tasks, and activities with physical agents such as electrotherapy and improved outcomes. There have been dramatic advances in technology, equipment, and research related to physical agents, and to neglect their use as a part of occupational therapy intervention or to overlook their impact to facilitate healing and performance is both limiting to the profession and to the client.

Regulatory Issues and the Role of the Occupational Therapy Assistant

As physical agent modalities have taken on greater significance as an adjunct to occupational therapy intervention, so too have regulatory restrictions. Many states such as Georgia, Florida, Minnesota, Kentucky, Tennessee, Nebraska, Montana, South Dakota, Maryland, and California have specific requirements and separate licensing regulations that must be met before physical agents can be used by occupational therapists. Most of these states require a specific number of continuing education hours or experience that must be met before physical agents can be used. It is the responsibility of clinicians to know what their respective state requires

before utilizing physical agents in their clinical practice. Occupational therapy assistants must also meet these regulatory requirements. To date, Nebraska is the only state that restricts occupational therapy assistants to only superficial thermal agents. In all other states with licensing regulations, occupational therapy assistants can apply physical agents under the direction and supervision of the occupational therapist. Some hospitals or clinical settings may also have restrictions or require additional institutional credentialing before using physical agents. It is the ethical and legal responsibility of the occupational therapist to be aware of all regulatory issues prior to incorporating physical agents as a component of clinical practice.

The AOTA position paper on physical agent modalities (AOTA, 2012) outlines the role responsibilities of the occupational therapist and occupational therapy assistant. The occupational therapist is responsible for determining physical agent modality use for the specific clinical condition being treated. The occupational therapy assistant can administer physical agent modalities as a part of the intervention plan under the direction and supervision of the occupational therapist. Both the occupational therapist and assistant must meet and comply with all institutional and state regulatory requirements for supervision, licensure, and competency in order to use physical agents as an adjunct to occupational therapy intervention (AOTA, 2012).

Physical Agent Modality Classifications

There are four primary classifications of physical agents commonly used by occupational therapists: superficial thermal agents, deep thermal agents, electrotherapeutic agents, and mechanical devices. The classifications describe the depth of penetration or mechanism of action and provide a convenient method for initial selection of an agent for the clinician. Superficial thermal agents are the therapeutic application of any modality that elevates or lowers the temperature of the skin and superficial subcutaneous tissue to a depth of 1 to 2 cm. Common superficial thermal agents include hydrotherapy/whirlpool, cryotherapy, hot packs, paraffin, water, and infrared heating. Many of these modalities are historically the most commonly used agents by occupational therapists and are often considered as relatively "safe" in application and effect. However, many of these agents can cause serious burns or damage to tissues; care should be used with these applications and will be discussed further.

Deep thermal agents include therapeutic ultrasound, phonophoresis, and diathermy and are categorized according to their depth of penetration. Deep thermal agents will affect tissue to a depth of approximately 5 cm and may exert a thermal or mechanical effect. Ultrasound and diathermy are unique in that both modalities can have either a superficial or deep effect depending on the parameters used by the practitioner.

Electrotherapeutic agents are those electrical agents that possess electromagnetic properties and include biofeedback, electrical muscle stimulation (EMS), neuromuscular electrical stimulation (NMES), functional electrical stimulation (FES), transcutaneous electrical nerve stimulation (TENS), electrical stimulation for tissue repair (ESTR), high-voltage galvanic stimulation (HVGS), and iontophoresis. Electrotherapeutic agents use electricity and the electromagnetic spectrum to facilitate tissue healing, improve muscle strength and endurance, decrease edema, modulate pain, decrease the inflammatory process, and modify the healing process (AOTA, 2012; Bracciano, 2008). Mechanical devices may include vasopneumatic devices and continuous passive motion (CPM) devices that exert a mechanical force on the underlying tissue (AOTA, 2012).

This chapter will review the mechanism of action and clinical applications of the most commonly used physical agent modalities. The reader is encouraged to continue learning about physical agents through academic preparation, continuing education, reading, and research. Clinicians who will be using physical agents should be able to demonstrate competency and ensure that they have a thorough grounding in the assessment, application and precautions, indications, and contraindications of the physical agents administered. Failure to integrate the theory and application of physical agents as part of the clinical reasoning process will make clinicians mere technicians in using physical agent modalities.

Biophysiology of Wound Healing— An Occupational Perspective

Occupational therapists are adept at assessing the client holistically and providing interventions and adaptations to facilitate independence and performance. The interventions and activities we use are very often "visual" to therapists in that we can physically "see" or visualize what we or the client are doing. We can visually "see" how the client is responding in a very concrete, global fashion. In effect, we have immediate feedback on our selection of therapeutic intervention or adaptation in an almost linear fashion. As occupational therapists, we assess and address the performance skills, patterns, context, and demands of the client that have been impacted by the disease or disorder.

Because of our holistic view of the client's function, we often overlook the ability to influence the unique client factors, body functions, or physiological processes that underlie all performance and function (World Health Organization [WHO], 2001, p. 10). Because of our educational training and our theoretical and philosophical approach to illness, injury, or disability, we often fail to take into consideration the primary component of performance—cellular and physiological function. We often fail to recognize how our selection of appropriate physical agents, preparatory to occupation, can facilitate and influence the healing process in the client. We have become adept at providing holistic adaptations to performance deficits but have failed to appreciate or consider that we may actually be able to "heal" and manipulate at a cellular and physiological level those tissues and structures that have been affected. This may be due, in part, to our profession's historical evolution and movement away from the "medical model," which was viewed as limiting and reductionistic to the profession.

This view has become anachronistic with the dramatic advances in technology, neuroscience, and medicine that allow us to appreciate the basic components and details of cellular and physiological functioning and the interrelationship with health, function, and occupational performance. To overlook or neglect our ability to influence these physiological processes and healing, which ultimately facilitate occupational performance and independence, is both ethically incongruent and inconsistent with our professional development. Failure to actively embrace and engage these emerging technologies and interventions as a component of the occupational process will lead to the void being filled by other disciplines willing and able to incorporate these techniques and advancements into an integrated program of intervention leading to improved outcomes.

Physical agent modalities are those clinical interventions that are used to produce a specific response in soft tissue through the application of energy. These interventions include the use of light, water, temperature, sound, electricity, or mechanical devices to influence the healing process. This chapter will focus on superficial thermal, deep thermal, and electrotherapeutic agents. The AOTA, in their 2012 position statement, identified the specific physical agents that correspond to the categories.

Because of the impact that physical agents have at the cellular and physiological level, it is crucial for occupational therapists to have a foundational understanding of the healing process. Any injury to vascularized tissue causes a series of systemic responses that are distinct but overlapping, including inflammation, proliferation, and remodeling. This physiological "healing" response occurs in order to rid the area of any microorganisms, foreign materials, or dead tissues so that the repair process where new tissue will be formed can occur. Wound healing is an overlapping process of repair that involves a series of events that encompass chemotaxis, cell division, neovascularization, synthesis of new extracellular matrix (ECM) components, and the formation and remodeling of scar tissue (Enoch & Harding, 2003). Wounds or injuries can be caused by disease; by vascular insufficiency due to compromised venous or arterial flow leading to ischemia or insufficient blood flow; or by trauma such as abrasions, lacerations, avulsions, punctures, burns, or even surgery. These wounds and injuries are often accompanied by pain, limited motion, and decreased motor function and occupational performance. Chronic inflammation, infection, and scarring may also cause complications, preventing a full return to function and performance.

The phases of healing are overlapping and vary in length. A healing wound or injury may demonstrate all three phases at the same time. The three phases of healing include the inflammatory phase, proliferation, and remodeling or maturation (Andreadis, 2006; Bolton & van Rijswijk, 1991). Injury to soft tissues below the skin depends on the nature of the causative factor, the location (either superficial or deep), and the material properties of the tissue. Therapists should understand the phases and timing of healing, because the appropriate physical agent will facilitate or modify the response of the tissue, ultimately impacting outcomes. Improper application of physical agents may negatively influence the healing process and lead to further complications and potential tissue damage (Figure 33-1).

Wound Healing

INFLAMMATORY PHASE

The inflammatory phase is the initial response of the body to injury and lasts approximately 72 hours. Inflammation is primarily a vascular response to the injury. The initial response to an injury is vasoconstriction, which decreases blood flow to the area, followed by vasodilation and the release of chemicals, nutrients, oxygen, and specialized cells to the site. There are a number of histochemical changes that occur and promote capillary permeability and chemotaxis, which is cell movement along a chemical concentration gradient, positively or negatively. A number of histochemical mediators are released into the tissue at this time, which facilitate formation of the fibrin clot and include histamine, prostaglandins, growth factors, and others that stimulate the inflammatory process and facilitate migration of fibroblasts, macrophages, and other specialized cells that form the "granulation tissue." A combination of blood exudate and serous transudate creates a reddened, hot, swollen, painful environment in the vicinity of the damaged tissue and wound. The inflammatory edema fills all spaces within the wound, surrounding all damaged or repaired structures, thereby binding them together as a one-wound structure. Some swelling in a wound is necessary to trigger the inflammatory process. However, if too little inflammation occurs, the healing response is

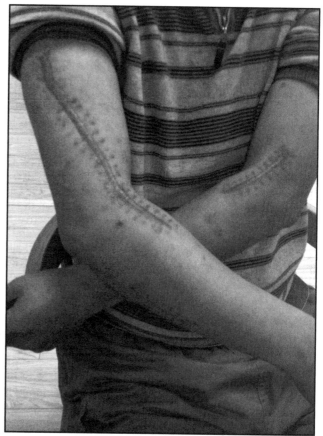

Figure 33-1. Example of remodeling phase of healing with imbalance of synthesis lysis process in a 32-year-old man post open reduction and internal fixation (ORIF) secondary to crush injury occurring at work. Note the raised hypertropic scars within the scar margins.

slow; if too much inflammation occurs, an excessive scar is produced (Hardy, 1989).

PROLIFERATIVE PHASE

During the proliferative phase of healing, granulation tissue matures to form scar tissue. This phase of healing lasts approximately 3 weeks. Two primary processes occur during this phase: fibroplasia and angiogenesis. *Angiogenesis* is the process of cell growth or cell budding to form new capillary blood vessels within injured tissue. In the body, angiogenesis is controlled through a balance of growth and inhibitory factors. Cancer is an example of the normal balance of inhibition and growth out of syncrony. Fibroblasts migrate to the area in order to repair the connective tissue of the skin and are mediated by chemicals released from the macrophages. At the same time, new capillary growth in the damaged tissue is growing in an effort to establish blood flow through the region and to remove the metabolic and repair wastes. Fibroblasts lay down collagen fibers that modify and change as the repair matures. Myofibroblasts are responsible for wound contraction and strength of the

Suzanne was a very active and dynamic 85-year-old woman. Her medical history was unremarkable, although she complained of having trouble hearing at times. Suzanne lived independently in a one-floor senior citizens' condominium complex. She no longer drove; however, she did use public transportation extensively to shop, visit her friends for lunch, and attend church services. She was very active in her church and enjoyed socializing with her friends. One wintry day while shoveling snow off the walkway to her door, she slipped and fell. In an attempt to "catch" herself, she put out her arm, extending it fully. When she landed on the ground, she fractured her distal radius, a classic "FOOSH" (fall on outstretched hand). She was taken to the emergency room, where she was placed in a soft splint to accommodate for the swelling; 2 days later, she underwent closed reduction of the fracture and was placed in a cast. X-rays indicated good apposition (alignment of the two fragments) of the fractured ends. She healed quickly, and the cast was removed at 7 weeks.

Following removal of the cast, her skin was flaky, dry, and macerated. Although her physician reassured her that the break was "solid" and she should move her wrist and use her hand as much as possible, Suzanne was apprehensive and protective of the extremity. She kept the fingers of her hand closed, and when she moved, she had a tendency to hold her hand at the wrist in a protective, guarded pattern. She was referred for occupational therapy "evaluation and intervention." On the initial visit, the occupational therapist reviewed the x-rays and report to ensure the fracture was solidly healed and in good alignment and confirmed that there were no biomechanical causes for her hesitancy and protection of the wrist and hand. When asked to move her hand and wrist, Suzanne politely, but firmly, replied she "couldn't" and was "afraid it was going to hurt." Suzanne's hesitancy to use the hand was limiting her ability to take care of her daily routines and self-care activities. She was struggling to dress herself and manipulate fastenings and was having difficulty cooking and cleaning because she would use the extremity as a "wedge" to hold objects against her body and forearm rather than using her wrist and fingers actively. Passive range of motion appeared to be within functional limits, but Suzanne would not actively use the hand to grasp objects. The occupational therapist was aware that immobilization of the forearm due to the cast could cause disuse atrophy and generalized weakness in the arm and hand and was anxious to get Suzanne moving to prevent fibrosis or adhesions in her shoulder due to lack of movement caused by the guarded position of the arm and hand. The therapist also realized that the prolonged immobilization may have contributed to distorted sensory perception in kinesthesia and proprioception, which could make Suzanne "feel" that her arm and hand were not "moving the same" as before the fall.

It was determined by the occupational therapist to prepare the tissue and area before engaging Suzanne in a variety of activities that would ensure her use of the hand and extremity. Suzanne's skin was dry and flaky, and the skin that was under the cast was "smelly." She was motivated to "clean up [her] arm and get rid of the dead skin." The occupational therapist decided to use a warm, hand whirlpool, with the water at a temperature between 102°F and 104°F with a gentle agitation. Suzanne was given a washcloth with which to "scrub" the dry skin off and was assisted by the occupational therapist in this task. Suzanne diligently "cleaned" the dead slough off her forearm and allowed the occupational therapist to assist. During this time, Suzanne was extending and flexing her fingers and actively moving her wrist in flexion and extension, as well as in supination and pronation of the forearm. After 20 minutes, the therapist removed Suzanne from the water, dried the skin, and applied lotion to the forearm and digits, gently mobilizing and manipulating the wrist and fingers in the process. Suzanne mentioned how the warm water "relaxed" her arm and hand, and she was instructed to "soak" her hand in warm water at home, rubbing the extremity with a washcloth to further clean off the dried skin and to provide sensory input into the extremity. Suzanne quickly began to use her healed arm and hand more functionally following a few short interventions, which incorporated the use of the superficial warmth in preparing the tissue to engage in a variety of activities and exercises to strengthen her arm and hand and to improve fine motor control and object manipulation. Because of the superficial heating of the tissue, Suzanne was soon riding public transportation again, visiting her friends for lunch, and engaging in her active preinjury activities and tasks.

repair by drawing the outer edges of the wound together. Importantly, the collagen fibers are oriented in response to local stress (force) that is applied to them and provide the tensile strength in the appropriate or required direction. This stress can occur internally or externally and is one of the reasons why occupational therapists use dynamic or static splinting, use physical agent modalities, and grade activities and occupational tasks. The intent of our intervention is to manipulate these healing structures through application of forces and energy that can facilitate and enhance the healing process and strength and speed of the repair (Kloth & McCulloch, 1995).

REMODELING PHASE

The remodeling or maturation phase of the healing process can continue for 1 to 2 years. Epithelialization is an important component of the remodeling phase of healing so that the wound has sufficient skin coverage. During this phase, there is continued fibroblastic activity and deposition of the collagen fibers. In addition, there is a balance between the synthesis of the collagen fibers and the subsequent lysis, or breakdown of the collagen. The collagen fibers, healing scar, and tissue continue to realign themselves and differentiate in function based on the tension and forces applied to the healing area. Remodeling overlaps the proliferative phase of healing and can continue for up to 1 year or more. The process of scar remodeling is responsible for the final orientation and arrangement of collagen fibers. Remodeling is influenced by both synthesis–lysis balance and fiber orientation. When the balance between synthesis and lysis is out of sync, the probability of keloid or hypertrophic scarring increases and may be problematic (Cuzzell, 2002; Gogia, 1995; see Figure 33-1).

During this period of maturation, the remodeling of the collagen results in the early, randomly deposited scar tissue arranged in both a linear and lateral orientation approximating the tissues that surround it. During the remodeling phase, the original wound, which resulted in a single scar, now has to differentiate itself to provide a function, such as tendon, muscle, or skin. As occupational therapists, we attempt to modify this process through our interventions including physical agents, splinting, and engagement in occupational tasks and activities. Induction theory states that the tissue will attempt to mimic the characteristics of the tissue that is surrounding it, whereas tension theory states that a low-load, long-duration stress (force) on the healing tissue—through the application of pressure, dynamic splinting, mobilization, soft tissue loading, and unloading, and other techniques—accounts for the differentiation in the healing tissue. It is through the correct and timely selection and application of the physical agent and "force" to the tissue that is crucial in effecting positive clinical outcomes (Ankrom et al., 2005).

Superficial Thermal Agents

Superficial thermal agents are those interventions that cause a temperature change in the underlying tissue. Tissue temperature can be modified through the application of heat to increase tissue temperature, or it can be cooled through the application of cold agents. The use of heat or cold to decrease pain and improve function has a long history. It is important to understand the physiological response to these modalities in order to determine how they can be used as part of the intervention process. Heat or cold is transmitted to the underlying tissue through the following five primary principles:

1. *Conduction* refers to heat transfer through direct contact with the underlying tissue. The heat loss or gain occurs when there is contact between materials that possess different temperatures. For example, heat will be absorbed by the body when a hot pack is applied, whereas a cold pack will conduct heat away from the underlying tissue. Both methods of heat transfer through the process of conduction.

2. *Convection* refers to the transfer of heat or cold to the body through the movement of air, matter, liquids, or particles over and around the extremity or body part. An example of a form of convection is fluidotherapy, where the air temperature can be adjusted and the cellulose particles are circulated by the force of the air around the treated extremity.

3. *Radiation* occurs when the radiant energy transfers heat through the air from a warm source, such as an infrared lamp, to a cooler source. The infrared lamps that are often seen in restaurants are an example of this process. Infrared lamps are rarely used in rehabilitation anymore.

4. *Conversion* occurs when there is a temperature change resulting from the transformation of energy from one form to another. Clinically, this can be seen when thermal ultrasound is used to heat tissue—the sound energy is transformed to thermal or heat energy as the cells respond to the sound waves by vibrating, changing the sound energy into kinetic energy.

5. *Evaporation* is the transformation of a liquid into a gaseous state. During this change, there is an exchange of energy with the by-product of heat being released when the liquid is transformed into a gas. The most common clinical form of evaporation occurs with the use of vapocoolant sprays, which cause a decrease in skin temperature due to the evaporative effects of the spray.

Heat Agents

There are a variety of therapeutic heat agents used by occupational therapists and these are categorized according to their depth of penetration. These thermal agents are considered either deep or superficial. Superficial heating agents include hot packs, over-the-counter "thermal wraps," fluidotherapy, paraffin, and warm whirlpool. All of these agents increase the superficial temperatures of the skin and subcutaneous tissues to a depth of approximately 1 to 2 cm. Ultrasound, in its superficial settings (3-MHz frequency), has a depth of penetration of approximately 1 to 2 cm. Short wave diathermy is another physical agent that can increase tissue temperature at deeper levels, but it is rarely used by occupational therapists.

The extent of temperature change on the underlying tissue depends on four primary factors: the temperature difference between the physical agent being applied and the underlying tissue, the duration of the exposure of the tissue to the agent, the intensity of the heat agent, and the volume or area of the tissue being treated. The thermal conductivity of the tissue is also a factor that must be taken into consideration because adipose or fat tissue will act as an insulator, whereas blood and muscle, due to their blood flow and water content, absorb and conduct heat more efficiently.

Tissue Temperature Effect

The degree of tissue temperature elevation depends on the following:

- Volume or area being treated
- Duration of the application
- Temperature variation between the tissue and the physical agent
- Thermal conductivity of the tissue

Physiological Response to Heat

The primary purpose for applying a thermal agent is to increase the temperature of soft tissue to a specific therapeutic range so a physiological response will occur. When the temperature of soft tissue is increased between the range of 104°F and 113°F, it can have a positive therapeutic effect on the client. If the soft tissue is heated to a temperature of less than 104°F, cell metabolism will not be stimulated adequately enough to elicit a therapeutic response. Conversely, if the same tissue is heated to greater than 113°F, catabolism and cell death may occur. The physiological response to heat will vary according to the duration of the application, the volume of tissue being treated, and how long the modality is applied. Heating doses are considered either mild or vigorous, with the higher temperatures producing more noticeable redness or hyperemia to the underlying tissue. The application of heat causes a number of physiological responses, including increased blood flow to the area due to vasodilation of the blood vessels and increased rate of cell metabolism, oxygen consumption, capillary permeability, inflammation, and muscle contraction velocity. Conversely, the application of heat will decrease fluid viscosity of the tissue, pain, and muscle spasm (Loten et al., 2006). It is important to take into account not only the factors related previously but also the age of the client. Older clients may have an impaired ability to dissipate the heat effectively, and care must be taken to prevent burns or systemic overheating (Petrofsky et al., 2006).

Clinical Application and Goals

The application of heat as an adjunct to intervention has many therapeutic goals. The application of heat to an extremity can aid in pain relief and decrease the muscle spasms that a client may be experiencing. Because blood flow increases as a result of heat, the outcome will be the removal of the local muscle metabolites and the reduction in sensitivity of the muscle spindles, which tend to stretch and cause pain (Michlovitz, Hun, Erasala, Hengehold, & Weingand, 2004). Heat application can also decrease

muscle guarding and muscle spasm, which often lead to the pain-spasm-pain cycle and decrease the client's functional abilities and occupational performance. Heat applications placed on soft tissue also assist in increasing the tissue extensibility (Nadler, Steiner, et al., 2003).

Superficial heating agents used in most clinics are typically capable of providing moderate and vigorous thermal dosages. A moderate dose involves elevating the tissue temperature between 102°F and 106°F and will result in only a slight increase of blood flow. This dosage level is effective when heat is indicated, but edema may occur. A vigorous dose results in a marked increase in blood flow. The temperature will increase rapidly, duration will be relatively long, and temperature elevation at the site of pathology will be high (between 107°F and 113°F). This dosage level is beneficial for ischemic conditions and for when heat is indicated and edema is not a concern. Heat will also increase viscosity and elasticity of the soft tissue–muscle tendon and joint capsule when combined with positional or dynamic stretch over a period of time. The average length of time for heat application is between 10 and 20 minutes for physiological effects to occur in the intervention tissue. The length of time depends on the factors identified earlier, the area of tissue being covered, the intensity of the heat, and the duration of application. Although there are different methods used to apply heat, the biophysiological response will always be the same. In addition, it is important to remember that there is a 10-minute window of opportunity following the application of heat within which the load or stretch must be applied, although positional stretch during the heat application can be utilized and is also effective (Kottke, Pauley, & Ptak, 1966; Laban, 1962).

Indications for using superficial thermal agents include the following:

- Stiff joints
- Subcutaneous adhesions
- Soft tissue contractures
- Chronic arthritis
- Subacute and chronic inflammation
- Cumulative trauma
- Wounds
- Neuromas
- Sympathetic nervous system disorders

Precautions and Contraindications

The choice of heat selection depends on the area of tissue being treated and the goals established for the client. If the area is large and requires the medium to contour to the area (e.g., a shoulder), then a hot pack would be an appropriate choice. Hands and wrists can be easily accommodated in either a Fluidotherapy unit or through the application of paraffin. The client's skin should be closely monitored during any heat application because the potential for thermal burns can be high if improperly applied. Heat applications should never be used over open lesions, cuts, lacerations, or sutures of the skin. The area being treated should be inspected prior to application of the thermal agent and the sensation of the area confirmed. The client's cognition, level of awareness, and ability to inform the therapist of any discomfort or pain should also be assessed and reviewed. The skin and treated area should be checked after the first 5 minutes of application, if possible, to ensure that there are no adverse reactions. Close monitoring of the client is crucial because heat applications are the most common method of burning a client.

Precautions and contraindications for superficial thermal agents include the following:

- Peripheral vascular disease
- Acute inflammation
- Cancer or malignancies
- Acute hemorrhage
- Infection
- Primary repair of tendon or ligaments
- Advanced cardiac disease
- Compromised or limited cognitive status
- External pins/plates/hardware
- Sensory deficits
- Pregnancy

Cryotherapy

Cryotherapy is the application of a cold agent to selected tissue. The physiological response to cold application is essentially the reverse of heat applications. As with heat application, the physiological response to cold application depends on the duration of application, area or volume of the tissue being treated, and the rate at which the agent is being applied. With application of cold, the initial response in the underlying tissue is one of vasoconstriction. Superficial cooling agents are recommended for the inflammatory phase of healing and most acute conditions, producing a decrease in tissue temperature resulting in an analgesic effect. Cryotherapy can be used clinically to decrease edema, spasticity, muscle spasm, and pain. As the duration of application is increased, the physiological response is one of decreased nerve conduction velocity, decreased delivery of leukocytes and phagocytes, decreased lymphatic and venous drainage, and decreased muscle excitability and muscle spindle depolarization (Barber, 2000; Gracies, 2001; Sanya &

Bello, 1999; Welch et al., 2000). With short-duration applications, most clinical applications of cryotherapy will penetrate to a depth of approximately 1 cm, although longer durations may penetrate to a depth of 4 cm (Olson & Stravino, 1972). Commonly used cryoagents include commercially available ice packs, ice ups and ice packs made up of crushed ice, and cryopressure units that are effective following surgery to decrease pain and edema (Singh, Osbahr, Holovacs, Cawley, & Speer, 2001). It is important to recognize that physiological changes will occur when the temperature of the tissue drops below 80.6°F. Care must be taken when cryomodalities are applied for extended periods of time to prevent frostbite and tissue damage.

PRECAUTIONS AND CONTRAINDICATIONS

Cryotherapy can be an effective and safe modality when used within the appropriate clinical parameters. However, patients with difficulty in thermoregulation, sensory deficits, or hypersensitivity to cold would be contraindicated or require close monitoring of the application. Cryotherapy is contraindicated in those patients with cryoglobulinemia, Raynaud's disease, or cold urticaria. Systemic responses in patients with cold sensitivity include syncope, increased heart rate, flushing, and a drop in blood pressure. Close monitoring of the client's blood pressure and systemic response should be routinely performed with any thermal application, either heat or cold (Nadler, Prybicien, Malanga, & Sicher, 2003).

Precautions and contraindications include the following:

- Impaired circulation
- Peripheral vascular disease
- Hypersensitivity to cold
- Skin anesthesia
- Open wounds or skin conditions
- Infections

Deep Thermal Agents: Therapeutic Ultrasound

Ultrasound has been used in medicine for diagnosis, in imaging structures for tissue destruction and surgery, and in rehabilitation for its thermal and nonthermal effects. Therapeutic ultrasound uses acoustic energy, which is above the frequency that humans can hear. There are two primary uses for ultrasound in rehabilitation: to heat deeper structures and tissue or to facilitate healing of soft tissues. The historical use of ultrasound was to raise the temperature of deep structures, such as tendon, ligament, and joint capsules. Ultrasound parameters can be configured to provide either a "superficial" effect, penetrating to a depth of 1 to 2 cm, or a "deep" effect, penetrating to up to 5 cm.

Ultrasound units consist of an ultrasound generator that uses alternating electrical current and creates an acoustic wave at a specific frequency. The ultrasound unit also consists of a power supply, oscillator circuit, transformer, coaxial cable, and transducer and/or sound head (the part that is actually placed on the client to administer the sound energy). The biophysical principle, which is the basis for ultrasound, is known as the *piezoelectric effect*. Essentially, when an alternating electrical current is passed through the piezoelectric crystal located in the sound head of the ultrasound transducer, the crystal responds by oscillating, expanding, and contracting. As the crystal expands and contracts in response to the electric current, it "vibrates," creating sound waves that are then transmitted through the use of a coupling agent (electrode gel) to the underlying tissue.

As the crystal expands and contracts in response to the electrical current, it produces sound waves that, when the transducer is placed on a body part, compress the underlying molecules lying in the path of the sound energy. This movement of the molecules in the underlying tissue, essentially oscillating back and forth against each other, is known as *longitudinal wave propagation*. This sound wave and molecular movement will continue to expand until the energy is absorbed. When the sound wave reaches bone, it is generated along the periosteum and reflected back toward the surface, creating a shear wave. The sound wave traveling through the body will become attenuated as the energy is either absorbed or dispersed through reflection or refraction (Ter Haar, 1978).

Body tissue is not homogeneous, and each layer of the body will transmit or absorb the ultrasound energy according to its own unique properties. Fluid elements of the body have the lowest impedance, or resistance, to the sound energy and lowest acoustic absorption values. Bone has the highest impedance value and the highest acoustic absorption coefficient. This means that bone will stop the flow of the energy and absorb the energy from the ultrasound wave, causing physiologic changes. With higher energy levels produced by the ultrasound machine, there will be a concurrent effect of heating the tissue. As the ultrasound is transmitted to the lower tissues coming in contact with the bone, most of the energy will be reflected back, where it will meet the energy that is being transmitted down into the tissue and can produce a "standing wave" or "hot spot," which can be painful and damage the tissue. To prevent the development of standing waves or hot spots, the sound head should be moved in small circular motions (Dyson, 1987).

To control the amount of energy and the biophysiological effect on the tissue, there are a number of factors that are considered and adjusted when using ultrasound equipment including the frequency, duty cycle, time, and intensity. The frequency of ultrasound determines the number of complete wave cycles that are generated each second and determines the depth of penetration. In the United States, there are two frequencies that can be selected on most ultrasound machines: 1 or 3 MHz. As the number of cycles per second increases, the duration of each cycle and wavelength decreases, which accounts for the difference in the depth of penetration. The frequency of the ultrasound will influence the amount of energy that is absorbed with higher frequencies (3 MHz), delivering more energy but superficial in depth. Intervention using a frequency of 3 MHz leads to a superficial effect (1 to 2 cm deep) compared to an intervention using a frequency of 1 MHz (2 to 5 cm deep) (Fyfe & Bullock, 1985). Areas of the body such as the dorsal aspect of the hand, lateral and medial epicondyles, fingers, and other superficial structures would be more effectively treated using a frequency of 3 MHz. Deeper soft tissue structures such as the shoulder joint should be treated with a frequency of 1 MHz (Bracciano, 2008).

The biophysical effects of ultrasound depend on a number of factors, with the primary one being the intensity of the ultrasound. If the intensity is high enough, it will cause heating of the tissues, whereas low-intensity and pulsed-mode delivery will result in nonthermal changes due to the "mechanical" effect of the ultrasound energy. Tissues are heated through the transfer of the sound energy into kinetic energy due to the oscillation of the molecules in the tissue responding to the sound waves. To increase the total amount of heat delivered to the targeted tissue, the duration of the ultrasound application and/or the intensity must be increased. Thermal effects of tissue heating will do the following (Enwemeka, 1989; Hong, Liu, & Yu, 1988; Rimington, Draper, Durrant, & Fellingham, 1994):

- Decrease pain perception
- Decrease nerve conduction velocity
- Increase the metabolic rate
- Increase blood flow
- Stimulate the immune system
- Decrease the fluid viscosity in the tissue
- Increase tissue extensibility

Factors influencing the physiological effects of ultrasound include the following:

- Frequency (1 or 3 MHz)
- Duty cycle
- Time
- Intensity

The thermal effects of ultrasound can be decreased through either decreasing the intensity of the ultrasound or by "pulsing" the ultrasound. Pulsing the ultrasound refers to the duty cycle, or that period of time when the sound energy is being delivered to the tissue divided by the pulse period, which is the on time and off time. Most of the ultrasound equipment will have a 50%, 20%, or 10% duty cycle setting. The nonthermal or "mechanical" effects of ultrasound result in second-order physiological effects, which are effective for wound healing. These mechanical effects occur through the process of acoustic streaming and micro-massage at the cell membrane. Benefits have been shown for inflammation, proliferation, and maturation processes, with the primary site of ultrasound interaction and activity occurring at the cell membrane. From a clinical standpoint, nonthermal ultrasound (pulsed, low intensity) will facilitate tissue repair (Chan et al., 2006; Ebenbichler & Resch, 1994; Fyfe & Bullock, 1985; Giannini, Giombini, Moneta, Massazza, & Pigozzi, 2004; Turner, Powell, & Ng, 1989). *Phonophoresis* is the therapeutic application of ultrasound using a topical medication. The intent of phonophoresis is to direct the drug delivery directly to the site where the desired effect is sought. Phonophoresis is noninvasive and essentially painless. There is a discrepancy over whether the mechanism of action is thermal or due to the mechanical effects of the ultrasound. In addition, there are some inconsistencies regarding the effectiveness of ultrasound due to the wide variability of intervention parameters (Casarotto, Adamowski, Fallopa, & Bacanelli, 2004; Klucinec, 1996; Klucinec, Scheidler, Denegar, Domholdt, & Burgess, 2000; Oziomek, Perrin, Herold, & Denegar, 1991; Reshetov, Tverdokhleb, & Bezmenov, 2000).

PRECAUTIONS AND CONTRAINDICATIONS

Prior to the application of ultrasound, it is important that the therapist determine which frequency he or she is using as well as whether the intention of the intervention is to "heat" tissue or to "heal" tissue. Many of the contraindications and precautions of therapeutic ultrasound are with thermal, high-intensity applications. As with any physical agent, care must be used when the client has areas of decreased sensation, mentation, or cognitive abilities. Caution should also be used in patients with pacemakers. Ultrasound is contraindicated in patients with malignant tumors, during pregnancy, over epiphyseal plates of children, with joint cement, and with thrombophlebitis. Ultrasound should never be applied over the eyes, reproductive organs, or central nervous system tissue.

Precautions and contraindications for ultrasound include the following:

- Malignant tumors
- Joint cement
- Pacemakers
- Thrombophlebitis
- Reproductive organs
- Eyes
- Central nervous system tissue
- Pregnancy

Electrotherapy Principles and Applications

There are a variety of therapeutic applications of electrotherapy available to the occupational therapist. Because of the wide variability in applications and language used in the research and by the manufacturers, there is also a great deal of confusion that exists. The American Physical Therapy Association (APTA) attempted to standardize the terminology related to electrotherapeutic agents by classifying the agents according to their therapeutic goals. The following applications are the ones most frequently used by occupational therapists in clinical practice:

- *EMS:* Used for denervated muscles
- *NMES:* Used with innervated muscles
- *FES:* Used for electrical stimulation as an orthotic substitute
- *ESTR:* Electrical stimulation for tissue repair
- *TENS:* Used for decreasing pain

The most commonly used applications by occupational therapists include NMES, FES, TENS, HVGS (used for tissue repair and healing), and iontophoresis (used to administer medications to targeted tissue).

Electricity is a form of energy that exhibits magnetic, chemical, mechanical, and thermal effects. Electrical current involves the flow or movement of ions or electrons from one area to another and from a high concentration to a low concentration. The human body is electrically conductive, and tissue is either excitable and responsive to the electrical current or is nonexcitable and will be modified by the electrical fields but nonresponsive to the electrical current flow. When electricity is applied to excitable tissue, there is physiological and physiochemical changes that occur due in part to the water in the tissues. If the electrical current is of sufficient intensity, duration, and frequency, a muscle contraction will occur. A primary difference between electrically stimulated movement and voluntary contractions is the sequence of movements. In a voluntary contraction, small motor nerves are recruited first, then larger motor nerves, and finally muscles in an asynchronous sequence as gradually greater strength is required. In electrically stimulated movement, however, the reverse occurs with the larger fibers and muscles being recruited first in a synchronous, linear fashion. This accounts for the often "robot-like" movements of electrically stimulated muscles.

NEUROMUSCULAR ELECTRICAL STIMULATION

The choice of an appropriate electrical device depends on the goals set by the occupational therapist during the evaluation and intervention. NMES uses a pulsed alternating current to stimulate intact peripheral motor nerves to produce a motor response or muscle contraction. This form of stimulation is used to decrease muscle spasms, increase muscle strength, and decrease edema through the pumping action of alternating muscle contractions. NMES is indicated to improve muscle strength without increasing cardiovascular output; it can increase range of motion, decrease or inhibit spasticity, and improve strength and endurance; it is also used for muscle re-education or facilitation (Baker, Parker, & Sanderson, 1983; Billian & Gorman, 1992; Carmick, 1995, 1997; Chae & Hart, 1998; Scheker & Ozer, 2003). Electrodes are placed on the bulk of the muscle belly over the motor nerve with a second electrode placed distal to the first, usually near the muscle attachment. Correct electrode placement is crucial for effective response, and it is recommended to practice electrode placement on yourself or a colleague to ensure appropriate location. The amplitude or strength of the electrical current is increased until the nerve becomes depolarized and the muscle reaches tetany, causing a muscle contraction.

NMES can also be used for orthopedic injuries, particularly those conditions that have been immobilized, causing muscle weakness or hesitancy in moving the affected extremity through the available range of motion. Combining NMES with occupational activities and movements facilitates outcomes, strengthens the response, and increases strength more than just by conventional exercise alone (Hesse, Werner, Bardeleben, & Brandl-Hesse, 2002; Weingarden, Kizony, Nathan, Ohry, & Levy, 1997). NMES has also been used to decrease or modulate spasticity in neurologically impaired or orthopedic patients. Success with neurologically involved patients may vary due to the underlying cause. There are two primary methods for improving range of motion and decreasing spasticity: stimulating the spastic muscle to fatigue or stimulating the antagonist muscle to attempt to strengthen it and overpower the spastic muscle. Combining these NMES techniques with static and dynamic splinting, positional stretch, and other "conventional" methods of intervention may facilitate better outcomes (Daly et al., 1996; Detrembleur, Lejeune, Renders, & Van Den Bergh, 2002; Hesse et al., 2002; Scheker, Chesher, & Ramirez, 1999; Scheker & Ozer, 2003).

FES is a form of NMES, but the application is that the targeted stimulation and application is used as a substitute for an orthotic device or to produce a specific motor movement and activity. NMES and FES are frequently used with patients who have suffered from a stroke and hemiplegia. FES has been used as a substitute for the conventional "slings" that patients with shoulder subluxation frequently have following a stroke. Other applications of FES may be for reaching activities of the upper extremity or to strengthen or enhance grasp-and-release activities in order to allow the client to pick up and manipulate objects. There is a great deal of research and interest in the use of NMES with patients who have suffered a cerebrovascular accident (CVA) and in the ability to facilitate return and decrease shoulder subluxation and pain in patients at the early stage of recovery (Aoyagi & Tsubahara, 2004; Chae et al., 2005; Liu, You, & Sun, 2005; Yu, 2004). As the technology and research continues to expand and progress, occupational therapists should stay current with these therapeutic applications in order to facilitate occupational performance in patients with hemiplegia. Electrode placements for shoulder subluxation include over the supraspinatus and the upper trapezius, with a second electrode over the posterior deltoid. FES can also be configured to target two or more muscles in order to facilitate active movements such as mass extensor patterns or grasp-and-release activities. A creative approach to the intended movement and activity is required to determine the appropriate placement of electrodes.

Electrical Stimulation for Wound Healing

It is beyond the scope of this chapter to outline the various parameters of ESTR. It is recommended that the reader interested in this electrotherapeutic application review other materials and information available. There are some factors salient to many of the clinical conditions discussed earlier. Following an injury or surgery, there is a disruption of the body's normally occurring electrical field, with a change in polarity of the adjacent area. The application of electrical stimulation through the use of direct current and high-voltage pulsed current facilitates the transfer of the energy from the electrical current to the wound due to the change in polarity caused by the injury. The electrical current and stimulation affects not only the circulation, but also the histochemical effects and functions as well as the orientation of the cell structures and facilitation of the healing process. ESTR is indicated for pressure ulcers (stages I through IV), diabetic ulcers, venous ulcers, traumatic and surgical wounds, ischemic ulcers, wound flaps, and burn wounds. Precautions and contraindications are essentially the same as those discussed for electrotherapy in general (Baker, Chambers, DeMuth, & Villar, 1997; Bayat et al., 2006; Bogie, Reger,

Levine, & Sahgal, 2000; Gardner, Frantz, & Schmidt, 1999; Houghton et al., 2003; Langevin et al., 2006).

Transcutaneous Electrical Nerve Stimulation

Pain is a complex, multifaceted experience that can have unique social and cultural components. Electrical stimulation in the form of TENS can be an effective adjunct to conventional intervention. Pain is modulated through the use of TENS by affecting the perception and sensation of pain rather than correcting any underlying clinical condition. There are two primary theories related to the efficacy of TENS to modulate pain: the gate control theory and the endorphin- or opiate-mediated control theory. The reader is encouraged to explore these theories further to familiarize him- or herself with the intricacies of each. TENS is most often used in the intervention of musculoskeletal disorders, back pain, arthritis, and inflammatory disorders of soft tissue or for postoperative pain. There are a variety of intervention parameters available, and many TENS units are preprogrammed with the regimens that are the most effective.

TENS uses pulsed or alternating current, and the manufacturers have programmed different combinations of stimulation patterns directly into the equipment. There are four common forms of TENS used clinically: subsensory-level, sensory-level, motor-level, and noxious-level stimulation; a combination of all four levels may be used as well:

1. Subsensory-level stimulation is also known as microcurrent electrical neuromuscular stimulation (MENS), microcurrent electrical stimulation (MES), subliminal stimulation, or low-intensity stimulation (LIS). The characteristic of subsensory-level stimulation is that the intensity of the equipment is so low (less than 1 milliamp) that it does not stimulate a muscle contraction and is considered "subthreshold." Much of the research generated by this form of TENS has been in fractures and skin wounds and is based on the movement of the ions in the tissues at such low magnitude that there is no cutaneous sensation (Currier & Mann, 1983; Denegar, 1993).

2. Sensory-level stimulation is also known as conventional or high-rate TENS and is primarily used during the acute phase of injury. This form of stimulation is based on the gate control mechanism or opiate-mediated pain control and uses amplitudes and durations between 50 and 100 pulses per second (Melzack, 1993). Sensory-level TENS activates the cutaneous tactile sensory fibers and causes cutaneous paresthesia or a tingling sensation. The intensity of this form of stimulation does not elicit a motor response, although the client can "feel" the sensation. This form of TENS has a relatively quick response in decreasing pain, but the long-term effects are not usually longer than 1 hour. Extended periods of pain relief may be due to the stimulation interrupting the pain-spasm-pain cycle.

3. Motor-level stimulation is also known as strong low-rate (SLR) or acupuncture-like TENS and uses a high-amplitude and low-frequency pulse duration. This form of stimulation is also based on the gate control or opiate-mediated theories of pain control. Motor-level stimulation uses an amplitude high enough to produce a motor response in the underlying tissue. As the amplitude is increased, greater numbers of muscle fibers and motor axons are recruited and can reach a titanic contraction. Electrode placement for motor-level stimulation is directly over the motor point, which correlates with the location of the client's pain or on the segmental nerve roots. Motor-level stimulation is often used to treat chronic pain or pain that is caused by damage to deeper tissues, muscle spasms, and myofascial pain (Al-Smadi et al., 2003; Bjordal, Johnson, & Ljunggreen, 2003; Breit & Van der Wall, 2004; Chang, Lin, & Hsieh, 2002).

4. Noxious-level stimulation is also known as electro-acupuncture, hyperstimulation, or noxious-level TENS. This form of TENS is of motor-level intensity and uses longer pulse durations and frequencies. As the name suggests, noxious-level stimulation is reached when the stimulation amplitude is increased and perceived by the client to be "painful." This intense stimulation activates the ascending neural mechanisms and is based in part on the endogenous opiate theory. Noxious-level stimulation produces relatively high levels of analgesia. However, the effects are short lived and transitory. Most often, this form of stimulation is used prior to surgical procedures or debridement of tissue (Chandran & Sluka, 2003; Chang et al., 2002; Likar et al., 2001).

Most TENS units have two channels with four electrodes. When used with patients reporting pain, electrodes are positioned over or around the painful site. Other sites that may be used include motor points, which correspond with the area of pain; trigger points; or acupuncture points. All of these locations are considered electrically active and will facilitate the current flow into the selected tissue. Other potential stimulation sites include areas along the peripheral nerves, the tissue overlying the painful areas, specific dermatomes, or over the spinal segmental myotomes, which correspond to the patient's reported pain. Clinically, the therapist needs to determine whether the desired outcome will involve a motor response, sensory analgesia, or a noxious level of stimulation for analgesia. If the client does not report any improvement in the pain level or is unable to tolerate the stimulation, the clinician should change the electrode placement or adjust the stimulation parameters. Intervention is continued if the client is able to tolerate the sensation, reports a decrease in pain, and indicates an improvement in occupational performance or movement (Bracciano, 2008).

Precautions and Contraindications

As with any physical agent modality, a thorough examination and assessment of the client is necessary to identify the source of the client's pain and symptoms. Reviewing the past medical history of the patient and subjective history of the current condition assists in clarifying and identifying contraindications or precautions that might be required. Precautions and contraindications are essentially the same as those for any form of electrical stimulation. Precautions include those patients with known cardiac disease or cardiac arrhythmias. These patients should be monitored for any sign of distress or adverse effects. Care should be used if TENS is being placed over the lumbar paraspinals or abdominal region during pregnancy, except when used during labor and delivery in uncomplicated pregnancies. If a client has been diagnosed with cancer or malignancies, TENS may be used to assist with pain control. Informed consent of the client and attending physician should be obtained when using electrical stimulation or TENS with both the client with cancer and during pregnancy.

TENS and electrical stimulation are contraindicated in patients with demand-type cardiac pacemakers. Electrical stimulation should never be used over the carotid sinus because stimulation over this region of the neck may cause a hypotensive incident and cardiac irregularities. TENS and electrical stimulation should never be applied over the eye or over areas of decreased or abnormal sensation or used in patients with undiagnosed pain, epilepsy, metastasis, or peripheral vascular disease.

TENS contraindications include the following:

- Peripheral vascular disease
- Infection
- Impaired cognition or mentation
- Demand-type pacemakers
- Over the carotid sinus
- Over the eye
- Patients with epilepsy
- Cancer malignancies
- Decreased or absent sensation

Summary

The rehabilitation field has seen a dramatic increase in the use of technology and physical agent modalities. Physical agents can be used as part of the therapeutic intervention for a variety of clinical conditions that impact occupational function and independence. Because of reimbursement, efficacy, and demand for evidence-based practice, research related to physical agent modalities continues to grow, with research and intervention parameters more standardized and objective. Large, random controlled trials remain limited, however. The occupational therapist who is considering the use of physical agents as an adjunct to engagement in occupation needs to consider the context and unique client factors relevant to the disease or impairment to facilitate determination of therapeutic parameters. Rather than using a "technician-like" approach to physical agents, the skilled clinician needs to determine which client factors and which physiological functions are impacted by the impairment or disorder and determine how best to facilitate the desired healing response that will improve occupational performance and function. The ability to discern the underlying physiological components and cause of the impairment or condition, and the clinical experience and knowledge to determine how best to impact that component, requires additional training and experiential learning to ensure that we use physical agents in a timely, systematic, and effective fashion. Failure to consider physical agents and their potential for benefiting our patients through improved occupational functioning not only limits our effectiveness as occupational therapists and the profession, but also limits our ability to fully help patients achieve their highest level of independence.

Student Self-Assessment

THERAPEUTIC APPLICATION OF COLD: DETERMINING CLINICAL RESPONSE

Objective

The student will determine the effectiveness of different cold applications in decreasing skin temperature, achieving an analgesic response, and in determining its effect on grip/pinch strength. Students will monitor the form of application, duration, and the client's subjective comments during the application of cold. The student will take a pre- and post-grip and/or pinch test in the same upper extremity to which the cold modality will be applied.

EVIDENCE-BASED RESEARCH CHART

Intervention	Keywords	Evidence
Superficial thermal agents—cryotherapy, heat agents	Cryotherapy/instrumentation, pain, analgesics, superficial heat agent, heat agent, thermal agent, superficial thermal agent, paraffin bath, Fluidotherapy, hot pack, contrast bath, whirlpool, thermotherapy, physical agent modality, hydrotherapy, bath, paraffin embedding, hyperthermia	Ayling & Marks, 2000; Brosseau et al., 2002; Conroy & Hayes, 1998; Eversden, Maggs, Nightingale, & Jobanputra, 2007; Hirvonen, 2007; Hochberg, 2001
Superficial thermal agents—heat	Pain, pain measurement, heat/therapeutic use, intervention outcome	Michlovitz et al., 2004
Therapeutic ultrasound	Ultrasonic therapy, ultrasonic therapy/methods	Citak-Karakaya, Akbayrak, Demirturk, Ekici, & Bakar, 2006; Lazar et al., 2001; Sarrafzadeh, Ahmadi, & Yassin, 2012; Trudel et al., 2004; Uhlemann, 1993
Electrotherapy—NMES, TENS	Neuromuscular electrical stimulation, electrical stimulation, functional electrical stimulation, task practice, functional activity, practice, repetition, tasks, exercise	Alon, Levitt, & McCarthy, 2008; Breit & Van der Wall, 2004; Hara, Ogawa, Tsujiuchi, & Muraoka, 2008; Kesar & Binder-Macleod, 2006; Knutson, Hisel, Harley, & Chae, 2009; Lourençao, Battistella, de Brito, Tsukimoto, & Miyazaki, 2008; Mangold, Schuster, Keller, Zimmermann-Schlatter, & Ettlin, 2009; Paci, Nannetti, & Rinaldi, 2005; Shields, Dudley-Javoroski, & Cole, 2006; Sullivan & Hedman, 2004; Thrasher, Zivanovic, McIlroy, & Popovic, 2008

Equipment

Select from the various methods of administering cryotherapy, including the following:

- Crushed ice bag
- Ice immersion bucket
- Ice massage cup
- Reusable cold pack
- Stopwatch or watch with second/minute hand
- Dynamometer and/or pinch gauge

Procedure

1. Select a method of applying cryotherapy. Identify which upper extremity will be targeted for the application. The modality should be applied to the forearm of the selected upper extremity. Before applying the cold modality, take a baseline grip strength using the dynamometer. Apply the cold modality to the body part for a maximum total of 10 minutes, or less if using the ice massage method (approximately 4 minutes).

2. Using the Numerical Rating Scale (NRS) (0 = no pain; 10 = unimaginable pain), have the client "rate" his or her pain level at each temperature measurement (each minute).

3. Note the client's response (verbal and behavioral) as well as the skin appearance during each measurement period.

4. Immediately after discontinuing the application, use the dynamometer/pinch gauge and remeasure grip and/or pinch strength in the upper extremity.

5. Using a different area or body part, apply a different application technique and repeat steps 1 through 4.

6. Following completion of the lab and measurements, note any differences in grip/pinch strength. What did you find? Was one type of application more effective than another? What were the client's subjective comments? Did you notice any patterns?

Electronic Resources

- AliMed: www.alimed.com
- Amrex Electrotherapy Equipment: www.amrexusa.com
- Biodex Medical Systems Inc.: www.biodex.com

- Chattanooga Group: www.chattgroup.com
- Empi: www.empi.com
- GNR Health Systems, Inc.: www.gnrcatalog.com
- Medical Science Products Inc.: www.medsciencepro.com
- Mettler Electronics Corp.: www.mettlerelectronics.com
- North Coast Medical: www.ncmedical.com
- Omni Medical Supply: www.omnimedicalsupply.com
- Vonco Medical: www.voncomed.com
- Whitehall Manufacturing: www.whitehallmfg.com

References

Alon, G., Levitt, A. F., & McCarthy, P. A. (2008). Functional electrical stimulation (FES) may modify the poor prognosis of stroke survivors with severe motor loss of the upper extremity: A preliminary study. *American Journal of Physical Medicine and Rehabilitation, 87*(8), 627-636.

Al-Smadi, J., Warke, K., Wilson, I., Cramp, A. F., Noble, G., Walsh, D. M., et al. (2003). A pilot investigation of the hypoalgesic effects of transcutaneous electrical nerve stimulation upon low back pain in people with multiple sclerosis. *Clinical Rehabilitation, 17,* 742-749.

American Occupational Therapy Association. (2012). Physical agent modalities: A position paper. *American Journal of Occupational Therapy, 66,* S78-S89. Retrieved from http://dx.doi.org/10.5014/ajot.2012.66S78

American Occupational Therapy Association. (2008). Physical agent modalities: A position paper. *American Journal of Occupational Therapy, 62,* 691-693.

Andreadis, S. T. (2006). Experimental models and high-throughput diagnostics for tissue regeneration. *Expert Opinion on Biological Therapy, 6,* 1071-1086.

Ankrom, M. A., Bennett, R. G., Sprigle, S., Langemo, D., Black, J. M., Berlowitz, D. R., et al. (2005). Pressure-related deep tissue injury under intact skin and the current pressure ulcer staging systems. *Advances in Skin & Wound Care, 18,* 35-42.

Aoyagi, Y., & Tsubahara, A. (2004). Therapeutic orthosis and electrical stimulation for upper extremity hemiplegia after stroke: A review of effectiveness based on evidence. *Topics in Stroke Rehabilitation, 11,* 9-15.

Ayling, J., & Marks, R. (2000). Efficacy of paraffin wax baths for rheumatoid arthritic hands. *Physiotherapy, 86*(4), 190-201.

Baker, L. L., Chambers, R., DeMuth, S. K., & Villar, F. (1997). Effects of electrical stimulation on wound healing in patients with diabetic ulcers. *Diabetes Care, 20,* 405-412.

Baker, L. L., Parker, K., & Sanderson, D. (1983). Neuromuscular electrical stimulation for the head-injured patient. *Physical Therapy, 63,* 1967-1974.

Barber, F. A. (2000). A comparison of crushed ice and continuous flow cold therapy. *American Journal of Knee Surgery, 13,* 97-101; discussion 102.

Bayat, M., Asgari-Moghadam, Z., Maroufi, M., Rezaie, F. S., Bayat, M., & Rakhshan, M. (2006). Experimental wound healing using microamperage electrical stimulation in rabbits. *Journal of Rehabilitation Research and Development, 43,* 219-226.

Billian, C., & Gorman, P. H. (1992). Upper extremity applications of functional neuromuscular stimulation. *Assistive Technology, 4,* 31-39.

Bjordal, J. M., Johnson, M. I., & Ljunggreen, A. E. (2003). Transcutaneous electrical nerve stimulation (TENS) can reduce postoperative analgesic consumption. A meta-analysis with assessment of optimal treatment parameters for postoperative pain. *European Journal of Pain, 7,* 181-188.

Bogie, K. M., Reger, S. I., Levine, S. P., & Sahgal, V. (2000). Electrical stimulation for pressure sore prevention and wound healing. *Assistive Technology, 12,* 50-66.

Bogie, K. M., & Triolo, R. J. (2003). Effects of regular use of neuromuscular electrical stimulation on tissue health. *Journal of Rehabilitation Research and Development, 40,* 469-475.

Bolton, L., & van Rijswijk, L. (1991). Wound dressings: Meeting clinical and biological needs. *Dermatology Nursing/Dermatology Nurses' Association, 3,* 146-161.

Bracciano, A. G. (2008) *Physical agent modalities: Theory and application for the occupational therapist* (2nd ed.). Thorofare, NJ: SLACK Incorporated.

Breit, R., & Van der Wall, H. (2004). Transcutaneous electrical nerve stimulation for postoperative pain relief after total knee arthroplasty. *Journal of Arthroplasty, 19,* 45-48.

Brosseau, L., Robinson, V., Pelland, L., Casimiro, L., Milne, S., Judd, M., & Shea, B. (2002). Efficacy of thermotherapy for rheumatoid arthritis: A meta-analysis. *Physical Therapy Reviews, 7*(1), 5-15.

Carmick, J. (1995). Managing equinus in children with cerebral palsy: Electrical stimulation to strengthen the triceps surae muscle. *Developmental Medicine and Child Neurology, 37,* 965-975.

Carmick, J. (1997). Use of neuromuscular electrical stimulation and [corrected] dorsal wrist splint to improve the hand function of a child with spastic hemiparesis. *Physical Therapy, 77,* 661-671.

Casarotto, R. A., Adamowski, J. C., Fallopa, F., & Bacanelli, F. (2004). Coupling agents in therapeutic ultrasound: Acoustic and thermal behavior. *Archives of Physical Medicine and Rehabilitation, 85,* 162-165

Chae, J., & Hart, R. (1998). Comparison of discomfort associated with surface and percutaneous intramuscular electrical stimulation for persons with chronic hemiplegia. *American Journal of Physical Medicine and Rehabilitation, 77,* 516-522.

Chae, J., Yu, D. T., Walker, M. E., Kirsteins, A., Elovic, E. P., Flanagan, S. R., et al. (2005). Intramuscular electrical stimulation for hemiplegic shoulder pain: A 12-month follow-up of a multiple-center, randomized clinical trial. *American Journal of Physical Medicine and Rehabilitation, 84,* 832-842.

Chan, C. W., Qin, L., Lee, K. M., Zhang, M., Cheng, J. C., & Leung, K. S. (2006). Low intensity pulsed ultrasound accelerated bone remodeling during consolidation stage of distraction osteogenesis. *Journal of Orthopaedic Research, 24,* 263-270.

Chandran, P., & Sluka, K. A. (2003). Development of opioid tolerance with repeated transcutaneous electrical nerve stimulation administration. *Pain, 102,* 195-201.

Chang, Q. Y., Lin, J. G., & Hsieh, C. L. (2002). Effect of electroacupuncture and transcutaneous electrical nerve stimulation at hegu (LI.4) acupuncture point on the cutaneous reflex. *Acupuncture and Electro-Therapeutics Research, 27,* 191-202.

Citak-Karakaya, I., Akbayrak, T., Demirturk, F., Ekici, G., & Bakar, Y. (2006). Short and long-term results of connective tissue manipulation and combined ultrasound therapy in patients with fibromyalgia. *Journal of Manipulative and Physiological Therapeutics, 29,* 524-528.

Conroy, D. E., & Hayes, K. W. (1998). The effect of joint mobilization as a component of comprehensive treatment for primary shoulder impingement syndrome. *Journal of Orthopaedic and Sports Physical Therapy, 28*(1), 3-14.

Cornish-Painter, C., Peterson, C. Q., & Lindstrom-Hazel, D. K. (1997). Skill acquisition and competency testing for physical agent modality use. *American Journal of Occupational Therapy, 51,* 681-685.

Currier, D. P., & Mann, R. (1983). Muscular strength development by electrical stimulation in healthy individuals. *Physical Therapy, 63,* 915-921.

Cuzzell, J. (2002). Wound healing: Translating theory into clinical practice. *Dermatology Nursing, 14,* 257-261.

Daly, J. J., Marsolais, E. B., Mendell, L. M., Rymer, W. Z., Stefanovska, A., Wolpaw, J. R., et al. (1996). Therapeutic neural effects of electrical stimulation. *IEEE Transactions on Rehabilitation Engineering, 4,* 218-230.

Denegar, C. (1993). The effects of low-volt microamperage stimulation on delayed onset muscle soreness. Journal of Sports Rehabilitation, 1, 95-102.

Detrembleur, C., Lejeune, T. M., Renders, A., & Van Den Bergh, P. Y. (2002). Botulinum toxin and short-term electrical stimulation in the treatment of equinus in cerebral palsy. *Movement Disorders, 17,* 162-169.

Dyson, M. (1987). Mechanisms involved in therapeutic ultrasound. *Physiotherapy, 73,* 116-120.

Ebenbichler, G., & Resch, K. L. (1994). Critical evaluation of ultrasound therapy. *Wiener Medizinische Wochenschrift (1946), 144,* 51-53.

Enoch, S., & Harding, K. (2003). Wound bed preparation: The science behind the removal of barriers to healing. *Wounds, 15,* 213-229.

Enwemeka, C. S. (1989). The effects of therapeutic ultrasound on tendon healing: A biomechanical study. *American Journal of Physical Medicine and Rehabilitation, 68,* 283-287.

Eversden, L., Maggs, F., Nightingale, P., & Jobanputra, P. (2007). A pragmatic randomised controlled trial of hydrotherapy and land exercises on overall well being and quality of life in rheumatoid arthritis. *BMC Musculoskeletal Disorders, 8,* 23.

Fyfe, M. C., & Bullock, M. (1985). Therapeutic ultrasound: Some historical background and development in knowledge of its effects on healing. *Australian Journal of Physiotherapy, 31,* 220-224.

Gardner, S. E., Frantz, R. A., & Schmidt, F. L. (1999). Effect of electrical stimulation on chronic wound healing: A meta-analysis. *Wound Repair and Regeneration, 7,* 495-503.

Giannini, S., Giombini, A., Moneta, M. R., Massazza, G., & Pigozzi, F. (2004). Low-intensity pulsed ultrasound in the treatment of traumatic hand fracture in an elite athlete. *American Journal of Physical Medicine and Rehabilitation, 83,* 921-925.

Glauner, J. H., Ekes, A. M., James, A. E., & Holm, M. B. (1997). A pilot study of the theoretical and technical competence and appropriate education for the use of nine physical agent modalities in occupational therapy practice. *American Journal of Occupational Therapy, 51,* 767-774.

Gogia, P. (1995). *Clinical wound management.* Thorofare, NJ: SLACK Incorporated.

Gracies, J. M. (2001). Physical modalities other than stretch in spastic hypertonia. *Physical Medicine and Rehabilitation Clinics of North America, 12,* 769-92, vi.

Hardy, M. A. (1989). The biology of scar formation. *Physical Therapy, 69,* 1014-1032.

Hara, y., Ogawa, S., Tsujiuchi, K., Muraoka, Y. (2008). A home-based rehabilitation program for the hemiplegic upper extremity by power-assisted functional electrical stimulation. *Disability and Rehabilitation, 30*(4), 296-304.

Hesse, S., Werner, C., Bardeleben, A., & Brandl-Hesse, B. (2002). Management of upper and lower limb spasticity in neurorehabilitation. *Acta Neurochirurgica, 79* (Suppl.), 117-122.

Hirovnen, J., Kajander, J., Hagelberg, N., Mansikka, H., Någren, K., Hietala, J., & Pertovaara, A. (2007). Correlation of human cold pressor pain responses with 5-HT(1A) receptor binding in the brain. *Brain Research,* (10)1172: 21-31

Hochberg, J. (2001). A randomized prospective study to assess the efficacy of two cold-therapy treatments following carpal tunnel release. *Journal of Hand Therapy, 14,* 208-215.

Hong, C. Z., Liu, H. H., & Yu, J. (1988). Ultrasound thermotherapy effect on the recovery of nerve conduction in experimental compression neuropathy. *Archives of Physical Medicine and Rehabilitation, 69,* 410-414.

Houghton, P. E., Kincaid, C. B., Lovell, M., Campbell, K. E., Keast, D. H., Woodbury, M. G., et al. (2003). Effect of electrical stimulation on chronic leg ulcer size and appearance. *Physical Therapy, 83,* 17-28.

Kesar, T., & Binder-Macleod, S. A. (2006). Effect of frequency and pulse duration on human muscle fatigue during repetitive electrical stimulation. *Experimental Physiology, 91*(6), 967-976.

Kloth, L. C., & McCulloch, J. M. (1995). The inflammatory response to wounding. In J. M. MuCulloch, L. C. Kloth, & J. A. Feedar (Eds.), *Wound healing: Alternatives in management* (2nd ed., p. 3). Philadelphia, PA: F. A. Davis Company.

Klucinec, B. (1996). The effectiveness of the aquaflex gel pad in the transmission of acoustic energy. *Journal of Athletic Training, 31,* 313-317.

Klucinec, B., Scheidler, M., Denegar, C., Domholdt, E., & Burgess, S. (2000). Transmissivity of coupling agents used to deliver ultrasound through indirect methods. *Journal of Orthopaedic and Sports Physical Therapy, 30,* 263-269.

Knutson, J. S., Hisel, T. Z., Harley, M. Y., Chae, J. (2009). A novel functional electrical stimulation treatment for recovery of hand function in hemiplegia: 12 week pilot study. *Neurorehabilitation and Neural Repair, 23*(1), 17-25.

Kottke, F. J., Pauley, D. L., & Ptak, R. A. (1966). The rationale for prolonged stretching for correction of shortening of connective tissue. *Archives of Physical Medicine and Rehabilitation, 47,* 345-352.

Laban, M. M. (1962). Collagen tissue: Implications of its response to stress in vitro. *Archives of Physical Medicine and Rehabilitation, 43,* 461-466.

Langevin, H. M., Storch, K. N., Cipolla, M. J., White, S. L., Buttolph, T. R., & Taatjes, D. J. (2006). Fibroblast spreading induced by connective tissue stretch involves intracellular redistribution of alpha- and beta-actin. *Histochemistry and Cell Biology, 125,* 487-495.

Lazar, D. A., Curra, F. P., Mohr, B., McNutt, L. D., Kliot, M., & Mourad, P. D. (2001). Acceleration of recovery after injury to the peripheral nervous system using ultrasound and other therapeutic modalities. *Neurosurgery Clinics of North America, 12,* 353-357.

Likar, R., Molnar, M., Pipam, W., Koppert, W., Quantschnigg, B., Disselhoff, B., et al. (2001). Postoperative transcutaneous electrical nerve stimulation (TENS) in shoulder surgery (randomized, double blind, placebo controlled pilot trial). *Schmerz, 15,* 158-163.

Liu, J., You, W. X., & Sun, D. (2005). Effects of functional electric stimulation on shoulder subluxation and upper limb motor function recovery of patients with hemiplegia resulting from stroke. *Di Yi Jun Yi Da Xue Xue Bao, 25,* 1054-1055.

Loten, C., Stokes, B., Worsley, D., Seymour, J. E., Jiang, S., & Isbistergk, G. K. (2006). A randomized controlled trial of hot water (45 degrees C) immersion versus ice packs for pain relief in bluebottle stings. *Medical Journal of Australia, 184,* 329-333.

Lourençao M. I. P., Battistella, L. R., de Brito, C. M., Tsukimoto G. R., & Miyazaki, M. H. (2008). Effect of biofeedback accompanying occupational therapy and functional electrical stimulation in hemiplegic patients. *International Journal of Rehabilitation Research, 31*(1), 33-41.

Mangold, S., Schuster, C., Keller, T., Zimmermann-Schlatter, A., & Ettlin, T. (2009). Motor training of upper extremity with functional electrical stimulation in early stroke rehabilitation. *Neurorehabilitation and Neural Repair, 23*(2), 184-190.

McPhee, S. D., Bracciano, A. G., Rose, B. W., Brayman, S. J., & Commission on Practice. (2003). Physical agent modalities: A position paper. *American Journal of Occupational Therapy, 57,* 650-651.

Melzack, R. (1993). Pain: Past, present and future. *Canadian Journal of Experimental Psychology, 47,* 615-629.

Michlovitz, S., Hun, L., Erasala, G. N., Hengehold, D. A., & Weingand, K. W. (2004). Continuous low-level heat wrap therapy is effective for treating wrist pain. *Archives of Physical Medicine and Rehabilitation, 85,* 1409-1416.

Nadler, S. F., Prybicien, M., Malanga, G. A., & Sicher, D. (2003). Complications from therapeutic modalities: Results of a national survey of athletic trainers. *Archives of Physical Medicine and Rehabilitation, 84,* 849-853.

Nadler, S. F., Steiner, D. J., Erasala, G. N., Hengehold, D. A., Abeln, S. B., & Weingand, K. W. (2003). Continuous low-level heatwrap therapy for treating acute nonspecific low back pain. *Archives of Physical Medicine and Rehabilitation, 84,* 329-334.

Olson, J. E., & Stravino, V. D. (1972). A review of cryotherapy. *Physical Therapy, 52,* 840-853.

Oziomek, R. S., Perrin, D. H., Herold, D. A., & Denegar, C. R. (1991). Effect of phonophoresis on serum salicylate levels. *Medicine and Science in Sports and Exercise, 23,* 397-401.

Paci, M., Nannetti, L., & Rinaldi, L. A. (2005). Glenohumeral subluxation in hemiplegia: An overview. *Journal of Rehabilitation Research and Development, 42,* 557-568.

Petrofsky, J. S., Lohman III, E., Suh, H. J., Garcia, J., Anders, A., Sutterfield, C., et al. (2006). The effect of aging on conductive heat exchange in the skin at two environmental temperatures. *Medical Science Monitor, 12,* CR400-CR408.

Reshetov, P. P., Tverdokhleb, I., & Bezmenov, V. A. (2000). The use of hydrocortisone combined with ultrasound with gonarthrosis patients. *Voprosy Kurortologii, Fizioterapii, i Lechebnoi Fizicheskoi Kultury, 4,* 47-48.

Rimington, S. J., Draper, D. O., Durrant, E., & Fellingham, G. (1994). Temperature changes during therapeutic ultrasound in the precooled human gastrocnemius muscle. *Journal of Athletic Training, 29,* 325-327.

Sanya, A. O., & Bello, A. O. (1999). Effects of cold application on isometric strength and endurance of quadriceps femoris muscle. *African Journal of Medicine and Medical Sciences, 28*(3-4), 195-198.

Sarrafzadeh J., Ahmadi A., & Yassin M. (2012) The effects of pressure release, phonophoresis of hydrocortisone, and ultrasound on upper trapezius latent myofascial trigger point. *Archives of Physical Medicine and Rehabilitation, 93*(1), 72-77.

Scheker, L. R., Chesher, S. P., & Ramirez, S. (1999). Neuromuscular electrical stimulation and dynamic bracing as a treatment for upper-extremity spasticity in children with cerebral palsy. *Journal of Hand Surgery (Edinburgh, Lothian), 24,* 226-232.

Scheker, L. R., & Ozer, K. (2003). Electrical stimulation in the management of spastic deformity. *Hand Clinics, 19*(4), 601-606, vi.

Shields, R. K., Dudley-Javoroski, S., & Cole, K. R. (2006). Feedback-controlled stimulation enhances human paralyzed muscle performance. *Journal of Applied Physiology: Respiratory, Environmental and Exercise Physiology, 101*(5), 1312-1319.

Singh, H., Osbahr, D. C., Holovacs, T. F., Cawley, P. W., & Speer, K. P. (2001). The efficacy of continuous cryotherapy on the postoperative shoulder: A prospective, randomized investigation. *Journal of Shoulder and Elbow Surgery, 10,* 522-525.

Sullivan, J. E., & Hedman, L. D. (2004). A home program of sensory and neuromuscular electrical stimulation with upper-limb task practice in a patient 5 years after a stroke. *Physical Therapy, 84,* 1045-1054.

Ter Haar, G. (1978). Basic physics of therapeutic ultrasound. *Physiotherapy, 64,* 100-103.

Thrasher, T. A., Zivanovic, V., McIlroy, W., & Popovic, M. R. (2008). Rehabilitation of reaching and grasping function in severe hemiplegic patients using functional electrical stimulation therapy. *Neurorehabilitation and Neural Repair, 22*(6), 706-714.

Trudel, D., Duley, J., Zastrow, I., Kerr, E. W., Davidson, R., & MacDermid, J. C. (2004). Rehabilitation for patients with lateral epicondylitis: A systematic review. *Journal of Hand Therapy, 17*(2), 243-266.

Turner, S. M., Powell, E. S., & Ng, C. S. (1989). The effect of ultrasound on the healing of repaired cockerel tendon: Is collagen cross-linkage a factor? *Journal of Hand Surgery, 14,* 428-433.

Uhlemann, C. (1993). Pain modification in rheumatic diseases using different frequency applications of ultrasound. *Zeitschrift Fur Rheumatologie, 52,* 236-240.

Van Til, J. A., Renzenbrink, G. J., Groothuis, K., & Ijzerman, M. J. (2006). A preliminary economic evaluation of percutaneous neuromuscular electrical stimulation in the treatment of hemiplegic shoulder pain. *Disability and Rehabilitation, 28,* 645-651.

Weingarden, H. P., Kizony, R., Nathan, R., Ohry, A., & Levy, H. (1997). Upper limb functional electrical stimulation for walker ambulation in hemiplegia: A case report. *American Journal of Physical Medicine and Rehabilitation, 76,* 63-67.

Welch, V., Brosseau, L., Shea, B., McGowan, J., Wells, G., & Tugwell, P. (2000). Thermotherapy for treating rheumatoid arthritis. *Cochrane Database of Systematic Reviews, 4,* CD002826.

World Health Organization. (2001). *International classification of functioning, disability and health (ICF).* Geneva, Switzerland: Author.

Yu, D. (2004). Shoulder pain in hemiplegia. *Physical Medicine and Rehabilitation Clinics of North America, 15,* vi-vii, 683-697.

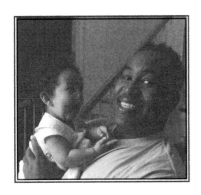

34

INTERVENTIONS TO ENHANCE FEEDING, EATING, AND SWALLOWING

Kristin Winston, PhD, OTR/L and Kathryn M. Loukas, OTD, MS, OTR/L, FAOTA

ACOTE STANDARDS EXPLORED IN THIS CHAPTER
B.5.14

KEY VOCABULARY

- **Aspiration:** Entrance of food or secretions into the larynx below the level of the vocal cords (Avery-Smith, 2002, p. 1092).
- **Bolus:** Food or liquid in the mouth (Avery-Smith, 2002, p. 1092).
- **Deglutition:** The act of swallowing (Avery-Smith, 2002, p. 1092).
- **Dysphagia:** Difficulty with any stage of swallowing (Avery-Smith, 2002, p. 1092).
- **Eating:** The ability to keep and manipulate food/fluid in the mouth and swallow it (O'Sullivan, 1995, p. 191).
- **Enteral tube feedings:** Tubes that deliver nutrition directly to the gastrointestinal system (Morris & Klein, 2000).
- **Feeding:** The process of bringing food from plate or cup to the mouth (O'Sullivan, 1995, p. 191).

- **Gastroesophageal reflux disease (GERD):** Described as the chronic return of gastric contents into the esophagus.
- **Gastroesophageal scintigraphy:** Sometimes referred to as a "milk scan," this medical test looks at stomach emptying as well as extent and severity of reflux (Morris & Klein, 2000).
- **Gastrostomy tube (G-tube):** Bypasses the mouth and is inserted directly into the stomach surgically.
- **Jejunostomy tube:** Is placed directly into the jejunum, bypassing the stomach.
- **Nasogastric tube:** A feeding tube inserted through the oral pharyngeal area, supplying liquid nutrition by passing the mouth.

(continued)

Jacobs, K., MacRae, N., & Sladyk, K. (Eds.).
*Occupational Therapy Essentials for
Clinical Competence, Second Edition* (pp. 457-471).
© 2014 SLACK Incorporated.

ACOTE STANDARDS EXPLORED IN THIS CHAPTER
B.5.14

KEY VOCABULARY (CONTINUED)

- **NPO (nil per os):** Latin for "nothing by mouth," no food, liquid, or medication is to be given orally (Avery-Smith, 2002).
- **Parenteral tube feedings:** Tubes that deliver nutrition via bypassing the gastrointestinal system to deliver nutrition into the bloodstream (Morris & Klein, 2000).
- **pH probe:** Medical test used to help identify amount and severity of gastroesophageal reflux.

- **Positioning:** The most important first step in the eating and feeding process.
- **Suck, swallow, breathe synchrony:** The smooth coordination of sucking, swallowing, and breathing to allow for efficient and effective eating.
- **Video fluoroscopy or modified barium swallow:** "Recording on video of moving radiographic images of structure and physiology; in this case of swallowing (Avery-Smith, 2002).

Introduction

Feeding, eating, and swallowing are important occupational performance skills across the lifespan that can be interrupted through a number of neurological, developmental, or orthopedic conditions.

Kedesdy and Budd (1998) stated, "No human activity has greater biological and social significance than feeding" (p. 1). As such, the occupations of feeding and eating have great significance for the practice of occupational therapy. Across the lifespan, feeding, eating, and swallowing are necessary to support nutritional intake and hydration that in turn support growth and overall health (Baer, 2005). For infants and young children, success in the occupations of feeding, eating, and swallowing satisfies their sense of hunger, provides pleasure related to taste and textures of foods, and creates opportunities for parent–child bonding (Kedesdy & Budd, 1998). For the parents of young children, success in the occupations of feeding, eating, and swallowing signifies competence in the role of caregiver and in turn facilitates the bonding experience between parent and young child (Kedesdy & Budd, 1998). From early childhood through adulthood, the occupations related to feeding, eating, and swallowing continue to fulfill a nutritional need, but these occupations also begin to take on strong social and cultural significance (Baer, 2005; Jenks, 2002). The sharing of food and the occupations of mealtimes are frequently a part of celebrations large and small; cultural events; and other social activities at home, at school, in the workplace, and within the community (Figure 34-1).

Secondary to the complex nature of concerns within the occupations of feeding, eating, and swallowing, occupational therapy practice in this area has different levels at which therapists are able to intervene due to varying degrees of competency (American Occupational Therapy Association [AOTA], 2003, 2007). Intervention depends on a thorough assessment and evaluation of factors relating to the person, the context, and occupation. AOTA (2007) states the following: "Occupational therapists and occupational therapy assistants have the knowledge and skills necessary to take a lead role in the evaluation and intervention of feeding, eating, and swallowing problems. Further, occupational therapists have the entry-level knowledge and skills to evaluate oral and pharyngeal swallowing function" (p. 2). As such, occupational therapy practitioners should understand not only the sensory and motor concerns that might be influencing the feeding, eating, and swallowing process but also complex cognitive, perceptual, contextual, and psychosocial factors that influence occupational performance in the areas of feeding, eating, and swallowing. The progression from entry-level practitioner to advanced practitioner in this area of practice is unique for each individual therapist and his or her practice setting. Competence in feeding, eating, and swallowing intervention may involve continuing education, on-the-job training, mentoring, independent study, and practice for the occupational therapy practitioner.

As entry-level practitioners, occupational therapists and occupational therapy assistants are educated to address many concerns related to this area of clinical practice as guided by the theoretical principles that are the foundation for practice. Occupational therapy practitioners provide intervention in this area that relates to occupational performance, performance skills, performance patterns, context, activity demands, and client factors facilitating a holistic approach to intervention (AOTA, 2008). Entry-level practitioners can refer to AOTA's paper entitled *Specialized Knowledge and Skills in Feeding, Eating, and Swallowing for Occupational Therapy Practice* (2007) for guidelines related to specific roles for each practitioner.

Occupational therapy practitioners are especially skilled to address the performance of feeding, eating, and swallowing from multiple perspectives secondary to the emphasis on client factors, occupational analysis, and contextual factors as outlined by the Occupational Therapy Practice Framework (AOTA, 2008). These factors include but are not limited to motor skills, sensory processing skills, cognitive skills, perceptual skills, contextual factors (such as cultural and social), and performance patterns including habits and routines around meals.

The occupational therapist assumes the primary responsibility for the delivery of assessment and intervention in this practice area. Occupational therapy assistants provide services related to feeding, eating, and swallowing under the supervision of and/or collaboration with the occupational therapist as per the AOTA as well as individual state rules and regulations regarding the practice of occupational therapy (AOTA, 2004). "During intervention, both occupational therapists and occupational therapy assistants select, administer, and adapt activities that support the intervention plan developed by the occupational therapist. Practitioners must always adhere to state and agency regulatory laws when providing services across these continua of care" (AOTA, 2007, p. 3). The amount of supervision that is provided to an occupational therapy practitioner in the area of feeding, eating, and swallowing depends on the individual's training, experience, and competency as well as guidelines within state licensure laws and practice guidelines. "Occupational therapy assistants and entry-level occupational therapists should seek supervision and mentoring from a more experienced occupational therapist or an occupational therapist with advanced knowledge and skills in feeding, eating, and swallowing" (AOTA, 2007, pp. 3-4). As stated previously, AOTA's specialized knowledge and skills paper on feeding, eating, and swallowing contains detailed information regarding the roles of the occupational therapist and occupational therapy assistant in this practice area (AOTA, 2007).

Occupational therapy practitioners work with individuals who receive their nutritional intake through oral or non-oral means. The following information seeks to clarify issues related to intervention for individuals receiving oral nutrition, non-oral nutrition, or a combination of

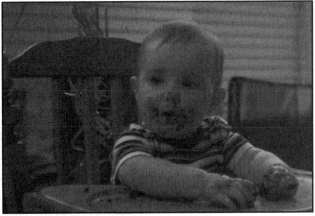

Figure 34-1. Enjoying a first birthday cupcake as part of a family celebration.

methods. Non-oral nutrition may be via enteral systems that feed directly into the gastrointestinal tract or via parenteral feeding where nutrition is supplied intravenously.

Oral Feeding

Oral feeding encompasses the process of gaining nutrition through the intake of fluids and solids by mouth. In the young child, the parent or caregiver facilitates feeding because the young child is dependent in many feeding/eating skills until the motor, sensory, cognitive, and perceptual skills necessary for independence in the area of feeding and eating develop (Case-Smith & Humphry, 2005). Once young children develop the necessary skills, independence in these occupations continues through adulthood, unless illness or disability affects the skills necessary to maintain independence.

Whenever possible, occupational therapy practitioners work with the client to develop the skills needed to feed him- or herself to facilitate occupational performance and promote independence. The occupational therapy practitioner should be aware of the possible stigma of being fed for adults, elders, and older children and move toward self-feeding as soon as possible if this is a meaningful goal.

Examples of adaptive equipment that can facilitate self-feeding include but are not limited to the following (these items can be found in adaptive equipment catalogues) (Figure 34-2):

- Dycem to stabilize the plate or bowl
- Plate guards to assist getting food onto a utensil
- Weighted, bendable, strapped, or built-up utensils or self-feeding systems such as the Neater Eater (Sammons Preston) or Stable Slide (Sammons Preston) self-feeding system
- Rocker knives, which can be helpful to cut food when bilateral coordination is compromised

Figure 34-2. Assorted adapted equipment commonly used for eating and feeding. Clockwise from left to right: Dycem, chewy stick, built-up utensil, weighted utensil, spoon with universal cuff, nosey cup, weighted plate with plate guard, bolus spoon, rocker knife, and wrap-around utensil.

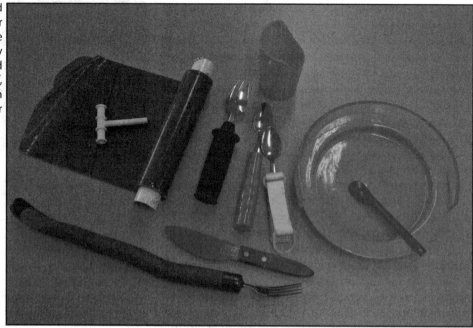

- Universal cuffs, which can be helpful for those with limited hand control
- A cup with a cut-out (nosey cup) to assist those who experience difficulty with head control

Independence and occupational performance may also be promoted in feeding, eating, and swallowing for those who depend on a caregiver for nutritional intake. This is accomplished by assisting the individual with difficulty in these areas to become an active participant in the relationship that forms between the individual and the caregiver.

Expanding the individual's options for making choices about types of foods/liquids eaten, times of meals, and other contextual or environmental factors related to feeding and eating fosters independence, engagement, and participation in these occupations. This, in turn, facilitates independence as individuals are encouraged to make decisions regarding their own lives (Crittenden, 1990).

Four Phases of Oral Eating

The Anticipatory/Preparatory Phase

This phase is described as a process in which the food or drink is brought to the mouth either by the person engaged in the eating or by the feeder (AOTA, 2003). The phase incorporates a combination of motor and sensory skills that include how the food looks and smells as well as the person's ability to reach for the food and bring it to his or her mouth. This phase also includes the sensory processing skills necessary to assist in determining the taste, texture, and temperature of foods and the initial motor skills needed to prepare and position the food for swallowing.

Intervention in this phase may be directed at assisting with sensory, motor, cognitive, or perceptual skills that inhibit an individual's occupational performance in the areas of feeding and eating.

Examples of intervention techniques in this phase include the following:

- Cheek and jaw support and facilitation of movement can improve feeding effectiveness in preterm infants (Hwang, Lin, Coster, Bigsby, & Vergara, 2010), as well as other clients of all ages who may have weak facial musculature.

- To address weakness of lips or cheeks and concerns regarding range of motion, the use of tapping, vibration, quick stretch or slow stretch, resistive sucking and blowing exercises (Avery, 2008; Jenks, 2002; Jenks & Smith, 2006) may help with strength and range of motion.

- For the presence of atypical oral reflexes, training caregivers to avoid stimulation of the reflex through positioning and adaptive techniques, as well as positioning with stability, may help reduce the impact of atypical reflexes (Avery, 2008).

- To support postural control for muscle efficiency, position with stability in the trunk and pelvis (Avery-Smith, 2002; Smith & Jenks, 2013).

- For concerns related to oral hypersensitivity, try deep pressure or proprioceptive input in and around the mouth, work with food textures that are comfortable for the individual (some clients with sensory processing concerns prefer smooth textures, whereas others prefer crunchy), and develop sensory diet activities that calm and organize the oral area before and during a meal or snack (Logemann, 1998).

- For concerns related to oral hyposensitivity, therapists may try using warmer/colder and more flavorful tastes to stimulate sensation, as well as developing sensory diet techniques that are alerting to increase input to the oral area before and during a meal or snack (Arvedson, Brodsky, & Reigstad, 2002; Logemann, 1998).

- For children experiencing difficulties with the sensory properties of food, food chaining is a technique that is emerging to help children who are restrictive or "picky" eaters (Fraker, Fishbein, Cox, & Walbert, 2007). This technique includes expanding the repertoire of foods by matching color, texture, or context to increase types of food intake in a systematic fashion. Behavioral techniques can enhance this method, which is often used with children who are on the autism spectrum.

THE ORAL PHASE

This phase is described as the phase in which the bolus of food or liquid is propelled by the tongue; masticated by the teeth and gums; and manipulated by the lips, cheeks, and tongue (AOTA, 2003; Avery, 2008; Jenks, 2002; Smith & Jenks, 2013). In this phase, the action is to move the food to the back of the mouth in preparation for initiating the swallow. This phase of the swallow is voluntary and typically takes about 1 second to complete (Jenks, 2002; Smith & Jenks, 2013).

Intervention in this phase for individuals who are considered safe for oral feeding is typically directed at assisting with sensory and motor skills that inhibit an individual's occupational performance in the areas of feeding and eating.

Examples of intervention techniques in this phase include the following:

- For concerns with slow oral transit time, interventions might include the use of cold or sour boluses, or infusing a sour into foods (such as lemon).

- The occupational therapy practitioner may try thermal stimulation because cold temperatures may facilitate the initiation of the swallow (Avery, 2008; Logemann, Kahrilas, Kobara, & Vakil, 1989).

- For concerns related to positioning of the head and neck for a safe swallow, encourage a chin tuck, which moves the base of the tongue back and protects the airway when the larynx is low and the swallow

is weak (Case-Smith & Humphry, 2005; Ohmae, Logemann, Kaiser, Hanson, & Kahrilas, 1996).

- The occupational therapy practitioner may also try encouraging the individual to use an effortful swallow that helps to elevate the base of the tongue and then encouraging the individual to squeeze hard with throat muscles while swallowing (Avery-Smith, 2002; Pouderoux & Kahrilas, 1995).

- Encourage the use of the Mendelsohn maneuver following training and supervision in the use of this technique, where the individual pushes the tongue to the roof of the mouth and tries to keep the Adam's apple up while swallowing (Avery, 2008; Logemann et al., 1989).

- For clients with hemiparesis, suggest using neck rotation to turn the head toward the weaker side, which can help to close the weaker side of the pharynx, utilizing the stronger side (Avery, 2008; Logemann et al., 1989).

- Therapists may also try intervention strategies aimed at improving oral motor control and coordination as suggested previously in the oral preparatory phase.

- Additional references for assessment and intervention in the oral phase include Arvedson and Brodsky, 2002; Case-Smith and Humphry, 2005; and Wolf and Glass, 1992.

THE PHARYNGEAL PHASE

This phase is described as the phase in which the swallowing response is initiated and breathing is briefly interrupted (Avery, 2008; Avery-Smith, 2002; Jenks, 2002; Smith & Jenks, 2013). Intervention in the pharyngeal phase is often directed toward working with the individual's team to determine the ability to safely swallow.

This intervention is typically accomplished through facilitated head and neck positioning, including a chin tuck for safe swallowing. Diagnostic testing is frequently recommended to examine the individual's ability to safely swallow a variety of food and liquid consistencies without risk of aspiration (i.e., videofluoroscopy). Intervention may involve working with the team to train an individual and his or her caregivers as to what types of foods/liquids are recommended and safe. For example, it may be recommended that the individual have no thin liquids. Strategies would then be discussed to avoid thin liquids and meltables (e.g., ice cream, popsicles, or ice), or to thicken liquids to an appropriate consistency as determined by the individual's intervention team (Smith & Jenks, 2013).

Individuals with concerns in the pharyngeal phase of swallowing frequently are diagnosed with dysphagia. If the client has swallowing problems or an inability to

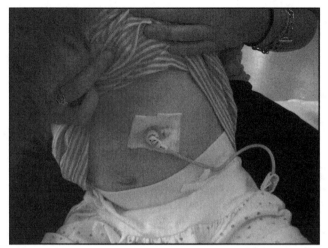

Figure 34-3. Placement of a gastrostomy tube for non-oral feeding.

swallow, the occupational therapy practitioner should be aware that continuing education and specialized training is necessary for competent interventions in this area. Specialized medical intervention in addition to individualized precautions are often indicated when a client is experiencing dysphagia. Speech pathologists and occupational therapy practitioners frequently work collaboratively with the client with dysphagia after diagnostic testing is performed. Additional team members may include the physician, a radiologist, a nurse, and nutrition or dietary services (AOTA, 2003, 2007).

Esophogeal Phase

This phase is described as the phase in which the bolus enters the esophagus and travels through the esophagus and into the stomach (Avery, 2008; Smith & Jenks, 2013). Occupational therapy practitioners do not provide direct intervention for concerns identified in this area. However, as a team member working on concerns related to feeding, eating, and swallowing, occupational therapy practitioners need to be aware of concerns that could arise in this phase of eating.

Occupational therapy practitioners may assist in developing interventions focusing on positioning or other factors to improve safety and comfort. In addition, occupational therapy practitioners may assist in team decisions regarding further diagnostic assessment to determine concerns in this phase of eating (AOTA, 2007).

Non-Oral Feeding

Non-oral feedings are utilized to support nutritional intake when risk of aspiration is a concern and it does not appear to be safe for the individual to eat by mouth. Non-oral feeding may also be utilized to support nutritional intake when the individual is not able to effectively and efficiently take in enough calories by mouth to support growth and overall health (Morris & Klein, 2000). Feeding tubes or enteral nutrition may be a temporary or a permanent solution to nutritional intake concerns. Occupational therapy practitioners work with individuals and teams to facilitate the transition from non-oral to oral feedings as appropriate. In addition, occupational therapy practitioners work closely with individuals and their families/caregivers to integrate tube feedings into the habits and routines that exist around mealtimes (Jenks & Smith, 2006; Morris & Klein, 2000).

Non-oral feedings are delivered through various tube placements. A few types (defined in the glossary) include nasogastric tubes, gastrostomy tubes, and jejunostomy tubes. A nasogastric tube is inserted through the nasal cavity into the stomach, a gastrostomy tube bypasses the mouth and is inserted surgically directly into the stomach (Figure 34-3), and a jejunostomy tube is surgically inserted into the jejunum (a branch of the small intestine). For some individuals, non-oral feedings will continue secondary to structural issues or neurological issues that prevent safe oral feedings. For others, the goal is to transition from non-oral feedings to oral feedings. The process of weaning from non-oral to oral feedings is complex. Schauster and Dwyer (1996) suggest that promoting a positive relationship between the individual and caregiver is an important first step in facilitating the transition to oral feedings. In addition, the transition is facilitated by intervention aimed at normalizing feeding and eating through safe and structured exploration of oral experiences (Figure 34-4).

General Factors to Consider

Developmental Progression

The infant is born with a small oral cavity. The fatty cheek pads and tongue are in close proximity to each other and nearly fill the oral cavity such that a typically developing infant can easily achieve suction and compress a nipple because of the tight fit when placed in the mouth (Case-Smith & Humphrey, 2005; Morris & Klein, 2000; Wolf & Glass, 1992). The structures of the throat in the infant are also in close proximity to one another. This arrangement of structures allows for the flow of liquid to pass safely from the base of the tongue to the esophagus. Protection of the trachea from liquid occurs as the larynx elevates the epiglottis and falls over the trachea. The structure of the oral cavity allows for a safe swallow when held in a reclined position for early breast- and bottle-feeding. Aspiration is unlikely in the first 4 months due to these structural arrangements, allowing the safe feeding of infants in a reclined position (Case-Smith

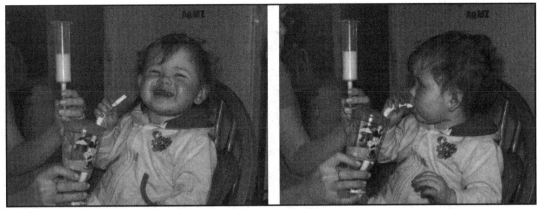

Figure 34-4. Providing oral opportunities during non-oral feedings.

& Humphrey, 2005; Morris & Klein, 2000). This factor becomes important when working with young children with feeding concerns as structural changes begin to occur between 4 and 6 months and continue through the first year of development (Morris & Klein). This is important in terms of intervention because therapists need to assist parents in developing options for upright feeding and eating when developmentally appropriate to support safe swallowing without aspiration.

POSITIONING

The position of the trunk, head, and neck directly affects the ability to swallow safely in children and adults; therefore, the first and most important aspect of feeding and eating intervention is ensuring that the client is in the proper position for eating (Smith & Jenks, 2013). When positioning a client, the occupational therapist should typically begin at the pelvis. As an anonymous saying goes, "What happens at the lips begins at the hips." The client should be positioned symmetrically from the head through the neck, trunk, and to the hips. A firm surface is best with the knees and ankles at 90 degrees. The pelvis can be in a slight anterior pelvic tilt with the hips at about 100 degrees (Smith & Jenks, 2013). The trunk should be flexed slightly forward with the back straight. The head should be slightly forward with the chin slightly tucked. Arms can be positioned on the table if necessary for support. It should be noted that in some cases, due to structural or neurological impairments, it might be difficult to achieve symmetry. However, this should be the overall goal to encourage safe swallowing, facilitate postural alignment, and prevent structural deformity (Figure 34-5).

SUCK, SWALLOW, BREATHE SYNCHRONY

An infant as well as a client recovering from neurological insult must begin with a suck, swallow, breathe synchrony. The smooth coordination between sucking, swallowing, and breathing is what allows the individual to eat effectively and efficiently (Wolf & Glass, 1992). This is evident, as seen with infants suckling from the breast or bottle. It should be noted that clients with breathing difficulties might experience feeding and eating difficulties because of the necessary breathing component in the rhythm of this synchrony of eating.

DIET SELECTION

Diet selection is an important component of the feeding and eating program. Precautions for clients with suspected swallowing difficulties may include avoiding foods with multiple textures; fibrous or stringy vegetables, meats, or fruits; crumbly or flakey foods; foods that liquefy; and foods with skins or seeds (Smith & Jenks, 2013). Diet selection is a team decision that includes the client. It is a decision that must be determined following comprehensive evaluation of the individual's feeding and eating skills (Smith & Jenks).

DIET PROGRESSION

After making a diet selection, developmental and rehabilitative approaches suggest that the diet should move in the following order from the easiest to manage to the most difficult (Avery, 2008; Smith & Jenks, 2013):

- Solids
  ◊ Level 1—Puréed (the lowest level of consistency for solids)
  ◊ Level 2—Minced ground
  ◊ Level 3—Mechanical soft
  ◊ Level 4—Regular soft
  ◊ Level 5—Regular diet

- Liquids
  ◊ In general, thickened liquids may be the easiest to manage based on thorough assessment of swallowing. Liquid consistency may progress to thinner liquids as tolerated by the client.

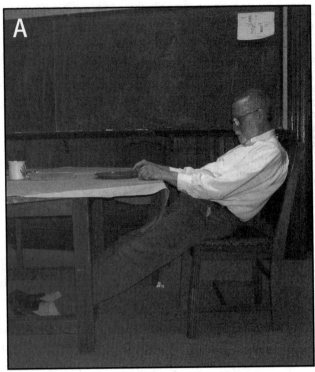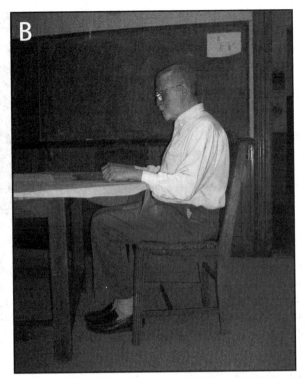

Figure 34-5. (A) Improper eating position versus (B) proper eating position.

Most dysphagia diet progressions include four liquid consistencies. For further information regarding dysphagia diet details, please refer to http://www.anfponline.org/Publications/articles/2004_03_008Dysphagia.pdf.

Ongoing assessment is indicated when considering changing or progressing a client's diet. The decision to move an individual to a modified consistency should be a team decision based on diagnostic assessment and clinical reasoning. It should be noted that thin liquids are typically the most difficult consistency to swallow and the easiest to aspirate. Thin liquids should only be given if you are certain the client has an intact swallow. A safe swallow can be determined through videofluoroscopy or a modified barium swallow. Signs and symptoms of possible aspiration include but are not limited to the following (Avery, 2008):

- Prolonged or inefficient cough
- A wet, gurgly quality to the individual's voice before, during, or after eating
- Any color change in the individual during or after eating
- Breathiness or loss of voice when eating

If the occupational therapy practitioner has any concerns regarding the individual's ability to swallow safely, he or she should discuss concerns with the client and his or her team to determine the need for further assessment prior to intervention.

Additional Issues for Feeding and Eating

Nil Per Os

Nil per os is the Latin term for "nothing by mouth" is a very important and strict precaution. All occupational therapy practitioners should check a client's chart and strictly adhere to this precaution.

No Thin Liquids

Difficulty with thin liquids is common with people after a neurological insult such as a cerebrovascular accident (CVA) or brain injury. The individual with aspiration precautions should be watched carefully. Liquids can be thickened with products such as applesauce or Thick-It (Precision Foods, Inc.). Thickening of liquids should only occur following thorough assessment including appropriate medical testing and team discussion. The client should be closely monitored while eating.

Special Diets

Clients with diabetes, food allergies, or special precautions will be on special diets. The occupational therapy practitioner should be vigilant about knowing precautions and making sure that the client and caregivers fully understand the precautions as well.

SENSORY IMPAIRMENT/ SENSORY PROCESSING

An assessment of the client's sensory processing is an important component of feeding, eating, and swallowing evaluation and intervention. Clients with hyposensitivity or decreased sensation will often be unaware of foods in the cheeks or under the tongue. It is important to work with these clients on sensory re-education or sensory processing strategies to increase awareness and tolerance when eating and drinking. Clients with hypersensitivity or increased sensitivity are often defensive or hyperaware of temperature, taste, and other sensory properties of foods, such as smell, and the visual aspects of foods. A sensory-based intervention program can be helpful to overcome these difficulties (Case-Smith & Humphry, 2005; Chatoor, 2009).

GENERAL INTERVENTION TECHNIQUES

A variety of techniques might be recommended for the client or for caregiver carryover of feeding, eating, and swallowing strategies. Caregiver programs are individualized and need to be developed based on the individual's current areas of need. As occupational therapy practitioners, we must be responsive to creating education materials that are "understandable, accessible and usable by the full spectrum of consumers" (AOTA, 2011, p. 1).

Positioning

- Ensure proper positioning while feeding, eating, and swallowing by providing the client, caregiver, and/or interprofessional team with a picture or diagram of best positioning for eating. Provide necessary external supports to help facilitate or maintain proper positioning with hips and knees flexed at 90 degrees, feet supported, and trunk symmetrical and erect. The seated position for the eating process is best if the person is leaning forward from the hips 20 to 30 degrees. Head and neck position should be neutral with a slight chin tuck. Positioning to facilitate optimal feeding, eating, and swallowing might include lateral supports, pillows, cushions, or other supports as determined by the intervention team.

- Encourage the client to tuck the chin to better align the head and neck for a safe swallow.

Presentation of Foods and Liquids

- Assist client and caregivers to follow specifics related to dietary consistency and food choices for each individual's nutrition, independence, and safety.

- Consider the pace of the presentation of foods/liquids—some individuals will need more time between bites of foods or sips of liquid to process, whereas others will need less time.

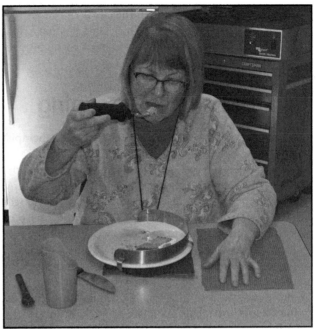

Figure 34-6. An adult uses adaptive equipment for independent feeding.

- Be aware of the amount of food or liquid being presented—too much or too little food or liquid may impact the individual's ability to safely participate in the mealtime and may impact independence as well.

Sensory Information

- The occupational therapy practitioner may recommend providing sensory input prior to and during feeding to improve sensory awareness in and around the mouth as long as the input is not aversive to the client.

- Provide tactile cues to encourage the use of the correct movement patterns to facilitate the processes of feeding, eating, and swallowing.

Adaptive Equipment and Adaptive Techniques

- Use adapted equipment as needed to facilitate safety, efficiency, and independence in the occupations of feeding, eating, and swallowing (Figure 34-6).

- Teach the client to clear the throat of food and liquid by coughing, and/or teach the clients' caregivers/team to cue the client to clear the throat.

Contextual Considerations

- Be aware of how cultural considerations may affect your intervention choices. Are there certain foods that are important to the client and/or family? Are there certain routines around mealtimes that need to be addressed?

- You may need to work with the client and caregivers to create an environment that facilitates participation, such as a quieter mealtime, more social interaction, or fewer distractions.

Professional Reasoning

What are the questions the occupational therapist should ask that begin to guide his or her choice of intervention strategies? The framework (AOTA, 2008) outlines the domain of practice of occupational therapy. "A profession's domain of concern consists of those areas of human experience in which practitioners of the profession offer assistance to others" (Mosey, 1981, p. 51). "The domain of occupational therapy frames the arena in which occupational therapy evaluations and interventions occur" (AOTA, 2008, p. 626).

Professional reasoning and evidence-based practice guide the occupational therapist in planning and implementing intervention in the area of feeding and eating using the framework (AOTA, 2008). This process is not intended to be prescriptive; each individual occupational therapy practitioner and client will bring unique areas of strength and areas of concern to be considered. It is also not exhaustive in nature and, as stated previously, is intended to provide a guide for assisting occupational therapy practitioners and the individuals with whom they work in planning intervention.

Occupational Performance

PERFORMANCE SKILLS

What motor skills and body functions (Thomas, 2012) are influencing the individual's ability to feed him- or herself or participate in the process of being fed?

EXAMPLE: There is difficulty with stability and postural control of the trunk, neck, head, and upper or lower extremities while eating.

- Intervention strategies
  - ◊ Remediation/restoration
    - * Therapeutic positioning
    - * Neurodevelopmental treatment techniques or other facilitation/inhibition techniques to address muscle tone
    - * Graded participation in functional activities to increase occupational performance
  - ◊ Compensation/adaptation
    - * Addition of lateral supports, head/neck supports, or other positioning aids
    - * Mobile arm supports or foot supports

EXAMPLE: There is decreased strength, coordination, and/or range of motion (ROM) necessary to bring a cup or a spoon to the mouth.

- Intervention strategies
  - ◊ Remediation/restoration
    - * Therapeutic activities to promote active ROM as indicated
    - * Therapeutic activities to facilitate muscle strength
    - * Neuromuscular facilitation or inhibition techniques to facilitate active use of the upper extremities in feeding and eating
  - ◊ Compensation/adaptation
    - * Adaptive equipment such as a universal cuff, built-up spoon, or adaptive cup
    - * Self-feeding devices

EXAMPLE: The individual is demonstrating concerns regarding the ability to swallow safely. This area requires advanced skills and knowledge to intervene. The entry-level practitioner should refer this individual to a more experienced team member or seek consult with a feeding and eating specialist.

What process skills, including level of arousal, attention to task, perceptual awareness, impulse control, and cognitive functioning, are influencing the individual's ability to feed him- or herself or to be fed?

EXAMPLE: The individual does not have the necessary energy, endurance, and/or breath support to facilitate occupational performance in the areas of eating and feeding.

- Intervention strategies
  - ◊ Remediation/restoration
    - * Postural control activities
    - * Activities designed to improve breath support
    - * Activities designed to build endurance
  - ◊ Compensation/adaptation
    - * Positioning
    - * Adaptation of the context to facilitate reduced activity, promote relaxation when eating
    - * Teach the use of energy conservation techniques and pacing techniques

EXAMPLE: The individual lacks the necessary skills to motor plan and sequence the actions needed for occupational performance in the areas of feeding, eating, and swallowing.

- Intervention strategies
  - ◊ Remediation/restoration
    - * Provide consistent instruction during feeding, eating, and swallowing
    - * Establish routines for the individual and his or her caregivers around feeding and eating

◊ Compensation/adaptation
  * Provide checklists for visual cues
  * Design verbal, written, and/or visual cues to facilitate feeding, eating, and swallowing

EXAMPLE: For a client who depends on a caregiver for physical assistance or cueing during feeding, eating, and swallowing, there is a concern related to the relationship between the individual and the caregiver that does not support occupational performance.

- Intervention strategies
  ◊ Remediation/restoration
    * Role model the appropriate level of assistance for the caregiver using a coaching model
    * Assist the client to be assertive in the feeding, eating, and swallowing process
  ◊ Compensation/adaptation
    * Give the caregiver a checklist of appropriate steps
    * Put verbal cues on a tape recorder
    * Provide adaptive equipment such as a self-feeder to eliminate the need for assistance

Please note that client factors should be individually evaluated and addressed in the occupational therapy process. Many client factors vary and require advanced practice skills for intervention.

Performance Patterns

As the occupational therapy practitioner, use or develop the individual's habits to assist in facilitating his or her occupational performance in the areas of feeding, eating, and swallowing. Establish or facilitate routines that positively influence occupational performance in the areas of feeding, eating, and swallowing. Establish or facilitate roles to positively impact the individual's occupations related to feeding and eating. Integrate cultural or religious rituals or functions that are important to this individual's occupational performance in the area of feeding and eating into intervention.

Context

The practitioner should assess the environment for optimal function for each individual client concerning noise and distractions, visual stimuli, room temperature, and olfactory input. Some clients benefit from the company of others, whereas others eat more efficiently alone, especially if eating is challenging for them. A typical, natural setting is usually best for clients of all ages.

Context includes the following considerations for intervention:

- Cultural context: What are the beliefs, values, or attitudes related to feeding and eating? Examples include consideration of religious holidays and family roles for the occupations of feeding and eating.
- Physical context: What are the qualities of the environment or objects within the environment as they relate to feeding and eating? Examples include the use of utensils and the ability to eat in noisy or distracting environments.
- Social context: What are the relationships that are important in terms of feeding and eating? Examples include the individuals who are present at the family table at meals and how relationships change when eating at home versus eating out.
- Personal context: Who is the individual receiving intervention for concerns related to feeding and eating? Examples include how intervention differs for a parent versus a child.
- Spiritual factors: What might inspire or motivate the individual receiving intervention? Examples include the natural environment of the individual and special meals/foods.
- Temporal context: What factors related to time might influence performance in the areas of feeding and eating? Examples include considering when the client is used to eating meals—is a large meal preferred at noon or at 5 p.m.?

Activity Demands

Consideration of activity demands is an important part of intervention planning for feeding and eating. The occupational therapy practitioner should carefully consider the demands of each activity chosen to ensure that a "just-right challenge" is achieved during the therapeutic process.

Client Factors

Client factors include body functions and body structures (AOTA, 2008). Body functions include but are not limited to motor, sensory, cognitive, and perceptual functions. Body structures include but are not limited to the structures of the nervous system; structures related to sensory receptors; structures related to movement; and structures related to digestive, cardiovascular, and respiratory systems.

	Table 34-1. ACTIVITY ANALYSIS OF THE SENSORY/MOTOR PATTERNS FORM		
Food Type	**Motor Patterns Needed** (Discuss and document motor patterns for the lips, tongue, jaw, cheeks)	**Sensory Considerations of Each Food** (Taste, texture, visual, olfactory, proprioceptive)
Cracker		
Applesauce		
Carrot stick		
Milkshake		
Rice		
Gummy bear		

These factors should be considered individually to determine how the factors might affect occupational performance in feeding, eating, and swallowing. Intervention would then be directed at restoration or remediation of areas of concern or at developing compensatory or adaptive strategies to improve performance.

For example, restoration or remediation would be actually improving the ability to bring hand to mouth, whereas compensation would be implementing the use of an assistive device to bring hand to mouth.

Summary

Feeding and eating are necessary and pleasurable occupations of daily life. Because of the potential risk of aspiration, the occupational therapist should carefully evaluate and plan intervention for each client in relationship to the model of intervention chosen. The occupational therapy practitioner can carry out that plan with interdisciplinary input for effective eating and feeding interventions. Independence or effective interdependence in safe feeding and eating are important components of occupational therapy intervention planning.

Student Self-Assessment

1. Break up into small groups and discuss how context is important to you, your friends, and your family in terms of eating and feeding. Now consider how you would include contextual factors in your intervention planning for individuals across the lifespan who are experiencing concerns in the area of eating and feeding. Refer to the framework (AOTA, 2008).

2. Working in pairs or small groups as an experiential learning exercise, complete an activity analysis of the sensory/motor patterns that are necessary for eating different textures. Fill out the chart in

Table 34-1 with your findings. (This chart can be expanded for classroom purposes.)

3. Using Thick-It, thicken water and juice to each of the following thicknesses: honey, nectar, and pudding. Try the same activity but use applesauce or another fruit purée. What are the differences between Thick-It and fruit purée? Are there other foods you might be able to use to thicken thin liquids or purées for a modified diet? Discuss the team members and assessment procedures that will determine what modifications need to be made to an individual's diet.

4. The instructor will need tables and chairs with armrests, applesauce, graham crackers, lollipops, vibration devices, adaptive equipment of all types, spoons, and paper or nosey cups. Students need to wash their hands and use protective gloves. Hand washing and gloving should be emphasized. Be sure to ask if any students have latex or food allergies. Students will work in pairs, each taking a turn at being a "client" and a "therapist." Students actually do hands-on positioning, feeding, and facilitation of eating.

5. For each of the two case studies that follow, fill out Table 34-2 and actually perform the tasks to help your client eat.

   ◊ Client A: Your client, Bob Brown, is a 65-year-old man who had a CVA about 1 month ago. He is a friendly, kind man who served as a police officer until his recent retirement. Bob has right-sided flaccid hemiparesis with overall low tone and a low level of alertness. He is right dominant, has some language-based expressive aphasia, and enjoys being with his wife but is overwhelmed with too much stimulation. Bob sometimes seems embarrassed when he dribbles food in front of his wife. He has impaired sensation on the right side of his face and is having difficulty

Table 34-2.

FEEDING, EATING, AND SWALLOWING INTERVENTIONS

	Client A	Client B
Environment or context		
Positioning: hips, trunk, head, neck, and jaw		
Adjunctive methods		
Hand-to-mouth technique		
Diet progression/types of food		
Cues or assistance needed		
Adaptive equipment or devices that may be helpful		
Handling ideas		
Observations needed		

EVIDENCE-BASED RESEARCH CHART

Topic	Evidence
Behavioral approaches to feeding and eating intervention	Babbitt et al., 1994; Linscheid, 2006; Roche et al., 2011; Twachtman-Reilly, Amaral, & Zebrowski, 2008
Refusal to eat	Bazyk, 2000; Fraker & Walbert, 2011
General feeding intervention	Bober, Humphry, Carswell, & Core, 2001; Case-Smith & Humphrey, 2005; Edwards & Martin, 2011
Management of drooling	Brei, 2003; Domaracki & Sisson, 1990; Fairhurst & Cockerill, 2011; Iammatteo, Trombly, & Luecke, 1990; Squires, Wills, & Rowson, 2012
Sensory motor concerns related to feeding and eating	Case-Smith, 1989; Overland, 2011; Palmer & Heyman, 1993; Toomey & Sundeth-Ross, 2011
Feeding tube dependency	Schauster & Dwyer, 1996; Tarbell & Allaire, 2002

with lip closure on the right side of the mouth. He has hypotonia and poor postural control of the trunk. His head control is weak but responds well to facilitation techniques. You are beginning an eating and feeding program and know that there are no swallowing problems. Mr. Brown hopes to return home in 2 weeks.

◊ Client B: Susan Smith is a 28-year-old woman who sustained a brain injury 3 months ago. Susan was a blackjack dealer in Las Vegas until her car accident. Susan has overall high muscle tone, has ataxia, and is hyper-alert. She is easily over-stimulated, becoming irritated with noise or too many verbal instructions. She has a very short attention span and is impulsive. Susan is able to use her arms but has difficulty with coordinated hand function. She tends to eat all the time and to stuff her mouth too full, causing her to choke or spit out food. She is restless and moves around as she eats, sometimes even getting up out of the chair. Susan may be discharged to a group home in the near future.

6. Have your students watch a DVD of a videofluoroscopy. These are often available through medical centers with swallowing programs. Watch a typical swallow and have students discuss what they are seeing in the progression. Watch an atypical swallow and see if students can see the areas of difficulty. Discuss the case and why swallowing deficits are dangerous and need to have special attention and a team approach. Occupational therapy practitioners should note the signs and symptoms of an abnormal swallow and make appropriate referrals. Occupational therapy practitioners require further education to perform dysphagia intervention.

References

American Occupational Therapy Association. (2003). Specialized knowledge and skills in eating and feeding for occupational therapy practice. *American Journal of Occupational Therapy, 57,* 670-678.

American Occupational Therapy Association. (2004). Guidelines for supervision, roles, and responsibilities during the delivery of occupational therapy services. *American Journal of Occupational Therapy, 58,* 663-667.

American Occupational Therapy Association. (2007). Specialized knowledge and skills in eating and feeding for occupational therapy practice. *American Journal of Occupational Therapy, 61,* 686-700.

American Occupational Therapy Association. (2008). Occupational therapy practice framework: Domain and process (2nd ed.). *American Journal of Occupational Therapy, 62,* 625-683.

American Occupational Therapy Association. (2011). AOTA's societal statement on health literacy. *American Journal of Occupational Therapy, 65*(Suppl.), S78-S79. doi: 10.5014/ajot.2011.65S78

Arvedson, J. C., & Brodsky, L. (2002). *Pediatric swallowing and feeding assessment and management.* Albany, NY: Singular Publishing Group.

Arvedson, J. C., Brodsky, L., & Reigstad, D. (2002). Clinical feeding and swallowing assessment. In J. C. Arvedson & L. Brodsky (Eds.), *Pediatric swallowing and feeding assessment and management* (2nd ed., pp. 283-340). Albany, NY: Singular Publishing Group.

Avery, W. (2008). Dysphagia. In M. V. Radomski & C. A. Trombly (Eds.), *Occupational therapy for physical dysfunction* (6th ed., pp. 1321-1344) Philadelphia, PA: Lippincott Williams & Wilkins.

Avery-Smith, W. (2002). Dysphagia. In C. A. Trombly & M. V. Radomski (Eds.), *Occupational therapy for physical dysfunction* (pp. 1091-1109). Philadelphia, PA: Lippincott Williams & Wilkins.

Babbitt, R. L., Hoch, T. A., Coe, D. A., Cataldo, M. F., Kelly, K. J., Stackhouse, C., et al. (1994). Behavioral assessment and treatment of pediatric feeding disorders. *Developmental and Behavioral Pediatrics, 15*(4), 278-291.

Baer, C. T. (2005). Addressing feeding with adults with developmental disabilities: A team approach part 1. *Developmental Disabilities Special Interest Section Quarterly, 28,* 1-3.

Bazyk, S. (2000). Addressing the complex needs of young children who refuse to eat. *Occupational Therapy Practice, 17,* 10-15.

Bober, S. J., Humphry, R., Carswell, H. W., & Core, A. J. (2001). Toddler's persistence in the emerging occupations of functional play and self-feeding. *American Journal of Occupational Therapy, 55*(4), 369-376.

Brei, T. (2003). Management of drooling. *Seminars in Pediatric Neurology, 10*(4), 265-270.

Case-Smith, J. (1989). Intervention strategies for promoting feeding skills in infants with sensory deficits. *Developmental disabilities: A handbook for occupational therapists.* Philadelphia, PA: Haworth Press.

Case-Smith, J., & Humphry, R. (2005). Feeding intervention. In J. Case-Smith (Ed.), *Occupational therapy for children* (5th ed., pp. 481-520). St. Louis, MO: Elsevier Mosby.

Chatoor, I. (2009). *Diagnosis and treatment of feeding disorders in infants and young children.* Washington, DC: Zero to Three.

Crittenden, P. M. (1990). Toward a concept of autonomy in adolescents with a disability. *Child Health Care, 19,* 162-168.

Domaracki, L. S., & Sisson, L. A. (1990). Decreasing drooling with oral motor stimulation in children with multiple disabilities. *American Journal of Occupational Therapy, 44*(8), 680-684.

Edwards, D. K., & Martin, S. M. (2011). Protecting children as feeding skills develop. *Perspectives on Swallowing and Swallowing Disorders, 29*(3), 88-93. doi: 10.1044/sasd20.3.88

Fairhurst, C. B. R., & Cockerill, H. (2011). Management of drooling in children. *Archives of Disease in Childhood: Education and Practice Edition, 96,* 26-30. doi: 10.1136/adc.2007.129478

Fraker, C., Fishbein, M., Cox, S., & Walbert, L. (2007). *Food chaining.* Philadelphia, PA: DaCapo Press.

Fraker, C., & Walbert, L (2011). Treatment of selective eating and dysphagia using Pre-chaining and Food Chaining© therapy programs. *Perspectives on Swallowing and Swallowing Disorders, 29*(3), 75-81. doi: 10.1044/sasd20.3.75

Hwang, Y.-S., Lin, C.-H., Coster, W. J., Bigsby, R., & Vergara, E. (2010). Effectiveness of cheek and jaw support to improve feeding performance of pre-term infants. *American Journal of Occupational Therapy, 64,* 886-894. doi: 10.5014/ajot.2010.09031

Iammatteo, P. A., Trombly, C., & Luecke, L. (1990). The effect of mouth closure on drooling and speech. *American Journal of Occupational Therapy, 44*(8), 686-691.

Jenks, K. (2002). Dysphagia. In L. W. Pedretti & M. B. Early (Eds.), *Occupational therapy skills for physical dysfunction* (5th ed., pp. 730-766). St. Louis, MO: Mosby.

Jenks, K. N., & Smith, G. (2006). Eating and swallowing. In H. M. Pendleton & W. Schultz-Krohn (Eds.), *Pedretti's occupational therapy practice skills for physical dysfunction* (6th ed., pp. 609-645). St. Louis, MO: Mosby.

Kedesdy, J. H., & Budd, K. S. (1998). *Childhood feeding disorders biobehavioral assessment and intervention.* Baltimore, MD: Paul H. Brookes Publishing Co.

Linscheid, T. (2006). Behavioral treatments for pediatric feeding disorders. *Behavior Modification, 30*(1), 6-23.

Logemann, J. A. (1998). *Evaluation and treatment of swallowing disorders.* Austin, TX: Pro-Ed.

Logemann, J. A., Kahrilas, P. J., Kobara, M., & Vakil, N. B. (1989). The benefit of head rotation on pharyngoesophogeal dysphagia. *Archives of Physical Medicine and Rehabilitation, 70,* 767-771.

Morris, S. E., & Klein, M. D. (2000). *Pre-feeding skills: A comprehensive resource for mealtime development* (2nd ed.). Austin, TX: Therapy Skills Builders.

Mosey, A. C. (1981). *Occupational therapy: Configuration of a profession.* New York, NY: Raven.

Ohmae, Y., Logemann, J. A., Kaiser, P., Hanson, D. G., & Kahrilas, P. J. (1996). Effects of two breath-holding maneuvers on oropharyngeal swallow. *Annals of Otology, Rhinology, and Laryngology, 105,* 123-131.

Overland, L. (2011). A sensory motor approach to feeding. *Perspectives on Swallowing and Swallowing Disorders, 29*(3), 60-64. doi: 10.1044/sasd20.3.60

O'Sullivan, N. (1995). Dysphagia care: Team approach with acute and long-term patients (2nd ed.) New York, NY: Cottage Square Press.

Palmer, M. M., & Heyman, M. B. (1993). Assessment and treatment of sensory- versus motor-based feeding problems in very young children. *Infants and Young Children, 6*(2), 67-73.

Pouderoux, P., & Kahrilas, P. J. (1995). Deglutitive tongue force modulation by volition, volume, and viscosity in humans. *Gastroenterology, 108,* 1418-1426.

Roche, W. J., Eicher, P. S., Martorana, P., Berkowitz, M., Petronchak, J., Dzioba, J, & Vitello, L. (2011). An oral motor, medical, and behavioral approach to pediatric feeding and swallowing disorders: An interdisciplinary model. *Perspectives on Swallowing and Swallowing Disorders, 29*(3), 65-74. doi: 10.1044/sasd20.3.65

Schauster, H., & Dwyer, J. (1996). Transition from tube feedings to feedings by mouth in children: Preventing eating dysfunction. *Journal of the American Dietetic Association, 96,* 277-281.

Smith, J., & Jenks, K. J. (2013). Eating and swallowing. In H. M. Pendelton & W. Schulz-Krohn (Eds.), *Pedretti's occupational therapy practice skills for physical dysfunction* (7th ed., pp. 678-717. St. Louis, MO: Elsevier Mosby.

Squires, N., Wills, A., & Rowson, J. (2012). The management of drooling in adults with neurological conditions. *Current Opinion in Otolaryngology & Head and Neck Surgery, 20*(3), 171-176.

Tarbell, M. C., & Allaire, J. H. (2002). Children with feeding tube dependency: Treating the whole child. *Infants and Young Children, 15*(1), 29-41.

Thomas, H. (2012). *Occupation-based activity analysis.* Thorofare, NJ: SLACK Incorporated.

Toomey, K., & Sundeth-Ross, E. (2011). SOS approach to feeding. *Perspectives on Swallowing and Swallowing Disorders, 29*(3), 82-87. doi: 10.1044/sasd20.3.82

Twachtman-Reilly, J., Amaral, S. C., & Zebrowski, P. P. (2008). Addressing feeding disorders in children on the autism spectrum in school based settings: Physiological and behavioral issues. *Language, Speech and Hearing Services in Schools, 39,* 261-272.

Wolf, L. S., & Glass, R. G. (1992). *Feeding and swallowing disorders in infancy: Assessment and management.* San Antonio, TX: Therapy Skill Builders.

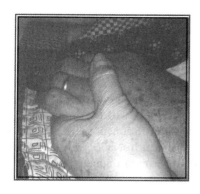

35

CASE MANAGEMENT AND COORDINATION

Diane P. Bergey, MOT, OTR/L and Erica A. Flagg, OT

ACOTE STANDARDS EXPLORED IN THIS CHAPTER
B.5.26–B.5.29

KEY VOCABULARY

- **Care coordination:** A process that facilitates the linkage of individuals and their families with appropriate services and resources in a coordinated effort to achieve good health.
- **Case management:** A collaborative process that assesses, plans, implements, coordinates, monitors, and evaluates the options and services required to meet the client's health and human services needs.
- **Clinical pathway:** A method used in health care settings as a way of organizing, evaluating, and limiting variations in expected client care secondary to diagnosis and other client-specific factors.

- **Managed care:** A variety of methods of financing and organizing the delivery of health care in which costs are contained by controlling the provision of services.
- **Transition services:** A results-oriented process that facilitates movement between settings and providers based on changing client needs. This term is most often used in the school setting but is an essential part of care coordination across the continuum.

Jacobs, K., MacRae, N., & Sladyk, K. (Eds.).
*Occupational Therapy Essentials for
Clinical Competence, Second Edition* (pp. 473-480).
© 2014 SLACK Incorporated.

Introduction

The role of the occupational therapy practitioner in care coordination, case management, and transition services is not only an area of emerging practice but is already a role that occupational therapists are filling in traditional practice environments. With our education, we are prepared to fill case management roles, utilizing our skills well and meeting the demands of society and our clients effectively. In order to be marketable in an environment highly influenced by managed care, it is important to realize case management as a career option.

What Is Case Management?

The Case Management Society of America (CMSA) defines case management as:

> A collaborative process that assesses, plans, implements, coordinates, monitors, and evaluates the options and services required to meet the client's health and human services needs. It is characterized by advocacy, communication, and resource management, and promotes quality and cost-effective interventions and outcomes. (Blass & Reed, 2003, p. 81)

Case management is a practice area and not a profession; therefore, it allows practitioners from a variety of disciplines and work settings to enter the field. For decades, health care organizations have used case managers to manage resources and reduce costs. This trend in managed care has only increased in recent years, becoming even more relevant. Van Deusen (1995) stated that managed care is here to stay; as such, the issue is how occupational therapists can function effectively within this system. Case managers are utilized in numerous settings including traditional health care settings as well as educational programming and community health services. Lohman (1999) proposed that occupational therapy be "proactive" in the current health care environment and take on nontraditional roles, such as case manager.

The term *case manager* is a title; *care coordination* is the function. Care coordination entails looking at the big picture, assessing needs and goals, identifying resources, and efficiently coordinating services to best meet the client's needs. The case manager's support and coordination facilitates and sustains movement through the health care system toward optimal health. An individual's health care needs often change based on a variety of factors, including nature of condition, age, availability of services, environmental factors, and individual choices. As the single point of entry, the case manager will coordinate care and facilitate transitions. Transition services are an integral part of case management. For instance, per the Individuals with Disabilities Education Act (IDEA) 2004, a student with an identified disability will receive services through the school system until graduation. This individual will then require transition services that are vocational, residential, and life-skill based. Additionally, a person with a hip replacement will first require acute services in a hospital for stabilization, possible transfer to a skilled facility, and home health services. Each example benefits from the skills of a case manager to ensure a smooth transition.

How Is Managed Care Affecting Case Management?

"The purpose of managed care is to provide affordable, quality health care with functional outcomes in a reasonable time frame. Access, quality, cost, and satisfaction are the usual goals that exist in health care" (Pope, 1995, p. 110). Case management and managed care are not synonymous. Trends in health care reflect the need for continued and creative resource management, which is driven by managed care. Case managers provide a vehicle to reach these goals. The demand for case management services is likely to increase given limited financial and human resources. We are living in a society that is aging, clients are returning home after shorter acute inpatient stays, people are living longer with chronic conditions (Markle, 2004), and more children are being identified with persistent medical conditions. With these demands on our system, limited resources are available, necessitating cost efficiency and streamlining of services. Even though insurers use case management to obtain timely and cost-effective outcomes, we need to stress the importance of doing this in a positive way to meet the client's needs (Fricke, 2006). Most importantly, we are there to improve quality of life for the client and family by continued assessment and evaluation. To summarize, managed care is creating a need for case managers, but there is a shortage of nurses and social workers who often fill this role. This should encourage more allied health professionals to enter the practice area of case management (Baldwin, 2005).

Why Is Case Management an Appropriate Role for Occupational Therapists?

Occupational therapy is the only discipline with the sole focus of understanding function. We evaluate occupational performance, routines, and volition as these factors interact with the client's environment. Our training provides us with strong human interaction skills, knowledge of occupational performance, and the ability

Table 35-1. COMPARISON OF CASE MANAGER FUNCTIONS AND STANDARDS OF PRACTICE	
Case Manager Functions (Case Management Society of America, 2010)	**Standards of Practice for Occupational Therapy (AOTA, 2010)**
Standard B—Client Assessment: Client assessment includes but is not limited to physical/functional, mental health, cognitive, spiritual, environmental and residential, caregiver(s) capability and availability, and self-care capability.	Standard II—Screening, Evaluation, Re-evaluation: The occupational therapist assesses a client's ability to participate in daily occupations in their context through collaboration with the client and support providers.
Standards C and D—Problem/Opportunity Identification and Planning: Identifies short- and long-term needs, as well as development of appropriate strategies to address needs.	Standard III—Intervention: Develops intervention based on evaluation goals, evidence, and clinical reasoning.
Standard E—Monitoring: Employs ongoing assessment and documentation to determine client's response to the plan of care.	Standard IV—Outcomes: Measures, documents, interprets, and monitors expected or achieved outcomes in client-centered plan through achievement of occupational performance.
Standard F—Outcomes: Utilizes evidence-based guidelines to demonstrate efficacy of interventions in achieving goals.	Standard IV—Outcomes: Determines and documents changes in performance and capacities; discontinues services when client has achieved goals and reached maximum benefit or client lacks desire to continue services.
Standard G—Termination of Case Management Services: Appropriately terminates case management services based on achievement of targeted outcomes.	Standard IV—Outcomes: Prepares and implements a transition or discontinuation plan based on client needs and achievement of goals.
Standard H—Facilitation, Coordination, and Collaboration: Develops and maintains proactive, client-centered relationships with the client and other associated professionals.	Standard III—Intervention: Networks with appropriate others to establish progress toward goals including safety, benefits, and risks.

to see the "big picture." Occupational therapists are a "tremendous untapped talent in terms of case management" (Hettinger, 1996).

There are clear parallels between the criteria for case management and the Standards of Practice for Occupational Therapy (American Occupational Therapy Association [AOTA], 2010). Thurkettle and Noji (2003) described case management as a process consisting of assessing, planning, implementing, coordinating, monitoring, and evaluating. These six functions depend on effective communication skills. The case manager must communicate with a number of people including the client, family members, service providers, vendors, insurance companies, and employers.

As illustrated in Table 35-1, educational standards prepare entry-level occupational therapists to take on case management roles. Delineated later are some of the standards of practice for each profession. Standards such as confidentiality, cultural competency, advocacy, and ethics, although not discussed, are standard components of an occupational therapist's education as well.

The specific qualities that have supported excellence in occupational therapy will also foster competency as a case manager. The occupational therapy perspective considers meaning in context of the client's condition and environment. The client's medical, spiritual, and psychosocial needs are holistically considered. Consideration of all contexts and participants is essential, both in occupational therapy and case management. All factors, including family interaction, environment, and response to illness and intervention measures, are critical when determining a person's ability to engage in meaningful occupations.

Occupational therapists often consider factors missed by other disciplines. "In the case management role, occupational therapists can help to facilitate a continuum of care from the acute setting to the community by developing clinical pathways that include the whole episode of care that emphasize functional status" (Lohman, 1999, p. 112). Additionally, other professionals may focus more on symptomatic relief and less on functional outcomes. For example, a particular individual with a lower limb amputation may be more functional utilizing a wheelchair rather than being fitted for a prosthetic. In the school system, the push to focus on proper grip and handwriting is not appropriate for all. Some students are better served by technology, meeting needs with the use of a keyboard, saving energy, and achieving success in the academic environment.

Clinical pathways are an essential function of care coordination. Occupational therapists acting as case managers can incorporate their knowledge about work, play, daily activities, disability, and environment into realistic clinical pathways. Accurate assessment is critical in the application of reasonable clinical pathways. Our assessment tools are geared toward understanding occupational impact and will possibly lead to better intervention planning.

Any case manager coordinating the care of a client is concerned with the functional level of the person's ability to complete activities of daily living (ADL). The skills that case managers need are an understanding of the injury or illness, ability to act as a lifespan coordinator (i.e., being able to project future care and responsibilities of the person who is ill or injured), knowledge of costs for specific health care procedures and intervention, and understanding of clinical pathways (Fisher, 1996). Consequently, better quality of care emerges.

The basic tenets of occupational therapy have long focused on client-centered planning and care. It is the occupational therapist's intention to ensure that each individual is able to meet personally chosen goals. "The client/patient is an active partner in care, sharing risk for the impact of choices on quality of life, functional ability, and subsequent income generation" (Thurkettle & Noji, 2003, p. 90). At times, goals are set without input of the individual and are based on assumptions of need. Occupational therapy embraces education as a vital step in including the client in the decision-making process. Clients are provided with information that allows decisions reflective of possible consequences and risks. In order to remain person centered, it is important to empower clients, educating them about their disease process and giving them a larger voice in their care delivery and more personalized attention to their needs (Mullahy, 1998).

Occupational therapy's holistic nature allows us to get a broader picture and supports client-centered planning. Our view of the environment does not focus solely on the physical environment. It also considers the sensory environment, recognizing the fact that we all must function within larger systems. There are a number of factors that must be considered in care coordination. Awareness of cultural differences; medical, spiritual, and psychosocial needs; unique gender and role beliefs; and generational norms are essential to client-centered planning. Our holistic view recognizes that we affect change by addressing individual factors as well as the broader system. For instance, when working within the school system, it may

be necessary to educate direct care staff, educational technicians, special staff, teachers, and administrators in order to achieve good outcomes. In order to support the student, all team members must be working toward a common goal. The holistic focus of occupational therapy allows for case management to occur in the most supportive environment. Although specific clinical pathways are prescribed, it is always necessary to take into consideration the unique characteristics of the individual case that may influence the norm and the success of the plan. Fricke (2006) asserted that the client still remains the priority in an environment of resource management. Within the current system, which demands cost-effectiveness, the client's needs must be considered foremost.

Barriers to Case Management

The realm of case management is an exciting area of potential growth for occupational therapists. However, breaking into a new niche can have its challenges. To be best prepared to meet challenges, it is important for occupational therapists to be aware of the potential barriers that may be encountered.

Occupational therapy programs are currently providing a good base of education to prepare new therapists for the specialty practice area of case management. However, therapists are likely to find that there will be skills that need to be developed in order for therapists to be proficient as case managers. As an occupational therapist enters the realm of case management, weaker skills will become more apparent. Once need areas are determined, further education, networking, or exploration can occur. The need areas will highly depend on the setting, client base, community resources, and so forth. Lohman (1999) noted that in her experience as a "participant observer of case management" in an acute care setting, she found that she did not have all of the medical background necessary to be an effective case manager in that particular context. However, through networking with other professionals and reading current journals and textbooks, she was able to gain a better understanding of pertinent issues. She noted that it was important to understand the medical chart by using a functional perspective. This observation is likely to be consistent across many settings. She also noted that advanced training or continuing education addressing the specifics of case management, such as the development of multidisciplinary clinical pathways and economic aspects of interventions, would be beneficial (Lohman).

Also significant is the current shortage of resources for case managers. For example, there are more nonprofessionals involved in the carry-through of care for our consumers (i.e., personal care assistants, nursing technicians, and other paraprofessionals) (Boling & Hoffman, 2001). Paraprofessionals and family members are commonly used at this time in order to control costs. However, with this trend, more oversight is necessary to ensure good care for our clients. "[C]ase managers must become an even stronger link along the care continuum to oversee the efficient implementation of intervention plans and, at the same time, become instrumental in developing innovative solutions to fill those care gaps already emerging" (Boling & Hoffman, 2001, p. 54). Family support and community programming are essential to good outcomes.

Case management positions have traditionally been held by social workers and nurses. At the time of this writing, there is a shortage of nurses, which will inevitably affect the provision of case management services. If occupational therapists choose to fill these roles effectively, they are likely to have to prove themselves. As outsiders, the challenge is to demonstrate the ability to fill these roles well. Tensions regarding boundaries can be overcome with good interdisciplinary communication. Communication can be enhanced with an understanding of each profession's educational background, values, roles, norms, and thinking differences (Lohman, 1999). An effective interdisciplinary team requires solid communication skills, the ability to resolve conflict, and respect for each team member's role. Occupational therapists as case managers must be willing to collaborate with those better equipped to address their client's particular needs. Seeking the assistance of other professionals will lead to better care, as well as increased respect from one's peers. Through effective case management, turf barriers should eventually dissolve. "Effective case managers understand the organization's informal political system. They have good communication skills, show a willingness to do a fair workload, respect differences, and have good conflict resolution and negotiating skills" (Lohman, 1999, p. 112).

Barriers to effective care coordination include the following (American Academy of Pediatrics, 2005; Boling & Hoffman, 2001):

- Lack of knowledge with regard to chronic conditions, resources, or the coordination process
- Lack of effective communication
- Poor team building
- Lack of clearly defined roles
- Insufficient acknowledgment for amount of time/work spent
- Inadequate reimbursement
- Lack of an organized system
- Language/cultural barriers
- Decreased client education
- Increased percentage of clinical complications
- Increased nursing/medical error rates

- Decreased client satisfaction
- Decreased clinical outcomes
- Documentation too heavy
- High-volume caseload/burnout

How to Become a Certified Case Manager

Since its inception, case management has evolved as a multidisciplinary specialty practice, with the case manager position filled by those trained in a variety of health care disciplines including nursing, social work, and rehabilitation counseling. Several years ago, case management was not a profession but rather a practice area. Presently, there are accredited degree programs specifically for case management. However, it continues to be more common for case managers to receive on-the-job training through employee training, supervision, and team meetings. "The Case Management Society of America (CMSA), through the development of its core curriculum for case managers, established the first national, standardized, basic knowledge and skill set for case managers" (Boling & Hoffman, 2001, p. 54). The CMSA now has standards of practice as noted in Table 35-1. Both methods still allow qualified health care professionals from a variety of disciplines to enter the field.

In addition to completing a degree program in case management, an occupational therapy practitioner can also become a certified case manager (CCM). The CCM designation is offered through the Commission for Case Manager Certification (1996). Certification is a voluntary process, as it is possible to fulfill the role of case manager without this credential. The credentialing process is described next. One must do the following:

- At a minimum, the professional license for certification shall be based on an educational requirement of a post-secondary program in a field that promotes the physical, psychosocial, or vocational well-being of the persons being served. Applicants must hold a current, active, unrestricted license or certification in another health or human services discipline.

- The license must allow the individual to practice independently without the supervision of another licensed professional.

- The individual must show documented employment experience as a case manager or as a supervisor of case management services. The following are three categories of acceptable employment based on time frames for employment and the amount of supervision provided by either a CCM or non-CCM:
  ◊ Category 1: Twelve months of full-time employment under the supervision of a CCM

◊ Category 2: Twenty-four months of employment as a case manager, with no requirements for supervision

◊ Category 3: A minimum of 12 months directing case management services

- Use the eight essential case management activities of assessment, planning, implementation, coordination, monitoring, evaluation, outcomes, and "general" to perform six core practice components, as documented in one's job description.

- Pass a certification examination that covers the six core practice components of psychosocial aspects, health care reimbursement, rehabilitation, health care management and delivery, principles of practice, and case management concepts.

- Display good moral character and reputation.

As it would be in any practice area, it is important to remain current no matter how the credentials of case manager are acquired. The CMSA hosts professional conferences that provide case managers with the opportunity to maintain professional licensure and credentials through continuing education. Training that pertains to a case manager's specific client population is also available to remain current.

Applications

Case manager skills parallel those used by therapists in all settings. Occupational therapists use the skills of case management for best practice in daily decision making, therapeutic intervention, collaboration, and transition planning. Currently, occupational therapists fill essential roles as team members, providing direct service as needed. They provide information on baseline functioning, work collaboratively with the team, and support the care plan with the ultimate goal of discharge from service. Insurance companies, including workers' compensation and return-to-work programs, depend on occupational therapy to provide the information for planning and coverage.

Occupational therapy practitioners understand productive living. They understand job analysis, job accommodations, and many of the issues facing injured workers. Because of this knowledge and their background in the psychosocial sciences, occupational therapists are a natural possibility as case managers for the worker's compensation population . . . understanding a variety of occupations and skills necessary to do certain jobs is an advantage to case management in this area as is understanding specific task modifications and job accommodations. (Fisher, 1996, p. 453)

An occupational therapist provides input regarding job descriptions, considering physical and cognitive requirements rather than simply a job posting. The concept of meaningful work is understood by occupational therapists as the difference between meaningful engagement and busy work and is clearly valued by the profession (Mattaliano, 2008).

Less traditionally, occupational therapists as compared to other health care professionals can act as case managers, making valuable contributions in high-risk communities, community-based health centers located in schools, churches, day care centers, or other population centers (Thurkettle & Noji, 2003). Occupational therapists are also qualified to work directly with these companies as case managers.

Occupational therapists have a unique perspective on functioning, viewing the whole system and the person within their context. They are a valuable asset to case management because of their understanding of function. Occupational therapists are unique because their education includes the intensive study of all vital components of human functioning, recognizing how the interrelationships of the components affect well-being and quality of life (Hafez & Brockman, 1998). Occupational therapy programming may be helpful in developing services for health promotion. This may include self-care management, cognitive assessments, activities-based programming, and home safety screening for modifications (Chapleau & Meyers, 2011).

Occupational therapists' education addresses physical and lifestyle factors and their application in the complex task of helping a client continue to live a meaningful and purposeful life. Occupational therapists are likely to be the only professionals analyzing all factors influencing a client to determine how to build supports that are truly compatible. For instance, a vocational rehabilitation counselor might select a job coach based on availability and not compatibility. If the client required motor-based modeling and demonstration to learn tasks but was paired with a coach who used an extensive verbal cueing system, success would be diminished. It is the ability of an occupational therapist to analyze each component of support that increases the potential for success. The cornerstone of a healthy team process must be consumer driven, and all parts must be well matched. Good case management is achieved through a team process. This is well supported by occupational therapy philosophy, making occupational therapists a natural match for the role.

Occupational therapists might coordinate care through consultation services. Although not labeled case management, the services provided directly impact the intervention plan, thus driving care coordination. Functional occupational therapy assessment provides recommendations for the client based on the client's occupational capabilities and areas of needs. Clear identification of strengths and weaknesses in the areas of sensory processing, visual perceptual abilities, cognition/ learning style, psychosocial engagement, and contextual factors allows the team to use the dynamic process in a truly client-centered approach. Recommendations target areas of need identified by the functional assessment and consider contextual factors and the need for skill building. The format of a typical occupational therapy evaluation reflects an all-inclusive view of a person's functioning. The following sidebar illustrates how this process might unfold.

Another example of an occupational therapist's effectiveness in case management can be seen in coordinating transition services for a young person "aging out" of high school or foster care. This is an appropriate role for an occupational therapist whose expertise in human development facilitates the client's transition from childhood/ adolescence occupational roles to those of a young adult.

Case management can also take the form of clinical consultation. For example, on a regular basis, an occupational therapist can review intervention plans for individuals with mental illness and/or mental retardation who attend a community-based day program. A care plan, created from information supplied by direct support providers, can be used to guide intervention between scheduled consultation, at which time adjustments are made to the plan to address new or different needs. The plan would provide specific guidelines that drive the direct support for provider interventions as well as a means for documentation and a crisis intervention plan. Team collaboration may reveal the need to bring in additional professionals to address goals and support function.

The goal of case management is to manage limited resources. A means of reaching this goal is to provide comprehensive training to address functional needs. If we provide functionally based training with the intent of teaching direct care providers how to better support their clients, we will be supporting more efficient use of resources. For example, a referral for a behaviorally dysregulated client would require functional assessment. Assessment may determine that, in order to support the least restrictive living environment, additional one-on-one staffing is needed. By providing a structured routine full of motor-based activities, the client would be able to remain calm and organized. For this routine and the interventions to truly be supportive, proper training would need to be offered to direct service providers. This training would identify the needs of persons with sensory defensiveness, detail his or her learning style, and describe sensory interventions and how to structure the environment. Given effective services, the individual's needs would be met safely and efficiently, enabling significant changes to day-to-day function.

Occupational therapists are able to look at the big picture by using a systems approach to drive services in an effective manner. The examples presented previously detail how case management can be applied in

Occupational Therapy Evaluation Example

An occupational therapist would be called in when an individual is not functioning effectively in his or her environment. For instance, a resident with unhealthy eating habits, aggression, and poor hygiene is at risk of losing housing placement. The first step in working with this individual would be to complete a functional assessment. Next, feedback involving the individual and the team would be provided. Through this feedback and the process of collaboration, an intervention plan is developed. This intervention plan needs to address how the system will assist this person, what skill building needs to occur, and how the environment can be set up to facilitate individual growth and functioning. After the completion of a thorough functional evaluation, a number of strategies to address the resident's clinical needs can be determined. For instance, the individual may require more joint compression to calm the nervous system and minimize aggression. It would be important to work with the direct care providers to find appropriate activities to increase deep pressure, weight bearing, and heavy muscle work. The case manager may want to make a referral to vocational rehabilitation services to match this person with an appropriate job with physical components. This would be in addition to helping the individual develop and use strategies to reduce arousal level and minimize aggressive outbursts. In this example, the occupational therapist is not officially assuming the role of case manager but is acting as a consultant to help direct the provision of services.

both traditional settings and in emerging practice areas. Although these are only a few examples, many opportunities exist in our discipline. Three important differences between a traditional case manager and an occupational therapist as a case manager are as follows:

- Our understanding of functional abilities that are needed to match the person to the task.
- Our occupational analysis skills, which allow us to adapt and be creative with support systems and solutions.
- Our ability to guide support providers to facilitate effective interventions.

Summary

Understanding the clear connections between the skills of a case manager and the skills of an occupational therapist magnifies the many opportunities that exist. Occupational therapists can use these skills in roles specifically designated as "case manager." There are also alternative applications that may not carry the title but

EVIDENCE-BASED RESEARCH CHART

Issue	Evidence
Impact of managed care on case management	Baldwin, 2005; Fricke, 2006; Markle, 2004; Pope, 1995
Occupational therapy attributes that are a match for case management	Fisher, 1996; Hettinger, 1996; Lohman, 1999; Mullahy, 1998; Thurkettle & Noji, 2003
Understanding barriers to case management	Boling & Hoffman, 2001; Chapleau & Meyers, 2011; Lohman, 1999
Case management outcomes	Allison, 2004; Blass & Reed, 2003; Lohman, 1999; Van Deusen, 1995

have the same end result. Occupational therapists can be part of care coordination, transition services, management of resources, and good outcomes in any role that they fill. Good case management demands excellent communication with the client and the interdisciplinary team. It requires comprehensive knowledge of available human, financial, and community-based resources and an ability to use these in the most cost-effective manner. Flexibility as well as ability to adjust the plan based on the client's functional level and changing goals are vital. Occupational therapists only add to these general principles, bringing a truly holistic view of the client and their context.

Electronic Resource

- Case Management Society of America: www.cmsa. org
- Commission for Case Manager Certification: www. ccmcertification.org

References

Allison, L. (2004). Evidence-based practice as tool for case management. *Case Manager, 15*(5), 62-65.

American Academy of Pediatrics. (2005). Policy statement: Care coordination in the medical home: Integrating health and related systems of care for children with special health care needs. *Pediatrics, 116*(5), 1238-1244.

American Occupational Therapy Association. (2010). Standards of practice for occupational therapy. *American Journal of Occupational Therapy, 64*, S106-S111.

Baldwin, T. M. (2005). Case management: Entry-level practice for occupational therapists? *Case Manager, 16*(4), 47-51.

Blass, T. C., & Reed, T. L. (2003). Consider case management. *Nursing Management, 34*(10), 81-83.

Boling, J., & Hoffman, L. (2001). The nursing shortage and its implications for case management. *Case Manager, 12*(6), 53-57.

Chapleau, A., & Meyers, S. (2011). Occupational therapy consultation for case managers in community mental health: Exploring strategies to improve job satisfaction and self efficacy. *Professional Case Management, 16*(2), 71-79.

Commission for Case Manager Certification. (1996). *CMM certification guide.* Rolling Meadow, IL: Author.

Fisher, T. (1996). Roles and functions of a case manager. *American Journal of Occupational Therapy, 50*(6), 452-454.

Fricke, K. (2006). Client centered case management in today's health care. *Lippincott's Case Management, 11*(12), 112-114.

Hafez, A., & Brockman, S. (1998). Occupational therapists: Essential team members as service providers and case managers. *Journal of Care Management, 4*(2), 10-20.

Hettinger, J. (1996). Case management: Do OTs have what it takes? Yes! *OT Week, 10*, 12-14.

Lohman, H. (1999). What will it take for more occupational therapists to become case manager? Implications for education, practice and policy. *American Journal of Occupational Therapy, 53*(1), 111-113.

Markle, A. (2004). The economic impact of case management. *Case Manager, 15*(4), 54-58.

Mattaliano, R. (2008). Beyond the adhoc approach: Putting a return-to-work program "on the books." *Professional Case Management, 13*(5), 290-292.

Mullahy, C. (1998). *The case manager's handbook* (2nd ed.). Gaithersburg, MD: Aspen.

Pope, T. (1995). Case managers help define managed care. *Case Manager, 6*(4), 109-114.

Thurkettle, M., & Noji, A. (2003). Case management: A source of support and stability for the client and the health care system. *Lippincott's Case Management, 8*(2), 88-94.

Van Deusen, J. (1995). What is the role of the occupational therapist in managed care? *American Journal of Occupational Therapy, 49*(8), 833-834.

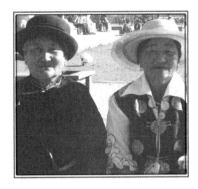

36

CONSULTATION, REFERRAL, MONITORING, AND DISCHARGE PLANNING

Julie Savoyski, MS, OTR/L, MPA

ACOTE STANDARDS EXPLORED IN THIS CHAPTER
B.5.21, B.5.22, B.5.25, B.5.26, B.5.28

KEY VOCABULARY

- **Consultation:** The exchange of ideas with an expert who is called on for professional advice (American Occupational Therapy Association, 2010).
- **Discharge planning:** The process of determining what happens after therapy services are discontinued.

- **Monitoring:** The act of observing a client's response to intervention.
- **Referral:** Making a professional judgment to have another occupational therapy specialist, discipline, or facility evaluate the client.

Introduction

The client has been evaluated and an intervention plan has been established. At this point, it is not just day-to-day intervention that occupies the mind of a competent occupational therapy practitioner. Continual monitoring and reassessment of goals in the intervention plan will ensure that the client is working toward the achievement of a desired level of function at discharge. As changes occur in the client's functional status, an alteration of the intervention plan may become necessary. Such a change may require consultation with another professional from within the occupational therapy field or an expert from a different discipline. As intervention nears an end, the role of the occupational therapy practitioner is to coordinate services that relate to the client's occupational performance needs. At times, referrals to other professionals or community agencies that are suited to meet the unique needs of the client are necessary. The end of the therapeutic relationship between the client and occupational therapy practitioner occurs at discharge; however, discharge planning should begin far earlier—as soon as the initial evaluation in some cases. At this point, the course of intervention is documented in a

Jacobs, K., MacRae, N., & Sladyk, K. (Eds.).
Occupational Therapy Essentials for
Clinical Competence, Second Edition (pp. 481-487).
© 2014 SLACK Incorporated.

discharge summary to pass on to other professionals the client may work with in the future.

Monitoring and Reassessment

Throughout the course of intervention, the client should be consistently monitored and reassessed in order to gauge the effectiveness of intervention. These actions will ensure that the client's areas of need are being addressed appropriately. After the initial evaluation has been completed and the intervention plan is in place, progress continues to be documented. This documentation ensures that goals and objectives concerning appropriate performance areas, performance components, and performance contexts are in place. Refer to Chapter 22 for more information about progress notes.

Periodic reassessment is also an important part of tracking a client's progress. Reassessment can occur on a formal or informal basis. Under the supervision of an occupational therapist, occupational therapy assistants should participate in the process of reassessment (American Occupational Therapy Association [AOTA], 2010). As the client transforms throughout the course of intervention, hopefully gaining skills, the occupational therapist makes changes to the intervention plan as necessary. Occupational therapy assistants should be a part of such alterations, under the supervision of an occupational therapist (AOTA, 2010). The supervising occupational therapist maintains the discretion to determine the extent to which the occupational therapy assistant participates in various processes. The occupational therapist's responsibility is to establish that the occupational therapy assistant has the skills and knowledge necessary to complete such tasks (known as determining service competency). In some situations, the occupational therapy assistant may have more experience than the occupational therapist and would certainly be incorporated in the process as much as possible. In other situations, the occupational therapy assistant may make suggestions while the occupational therapist does a majority of the task. Each occupational therapist/occupational therapy assistant relationship is different; however, it is important that a sense of mutual respect be maintained at all times (Dillon, 2001).

The Consultative Process

Although occupational therapy education is broad in scope, occupational therapy practitioners may not have all of the knowledge necessary to address every facet of a client's needs. It is the responsibility of the occupational therapy practitioner to acknowledge this and seek the expertise of other specialists when necessary (AOTA, 2010) (Table 36-1). This may result in consultation or referral. Consultation is the exchange of ideas with an expert who is called on for professional advice (AOTA, 2010). There are many niches within the field of occupational therapy in which an individual may specialize (Table 36-2). As a result, there may be times when the occupational therapy practitioner is called on as a consultant for his or her expertise. Consultation, beyond the scope of direct intervention, is a growing area of practice in occupational therapy (Dudgeon & Greenberg, 1998).

The first step in the consultative process is to identify the need for consultation (West, 1973). For example, Kamari is a 12-year-old boy of Haitian descent. He currently resides in a residential treatment facility for children with emotional and behavioral disturbances. He works with an occupational therapy assistant who is the activity director, under the supervision of an occupational therapist. The occupational therapy assistant is exploring self-regulation strategies with Kamari that will prevent him from becoming assaultive when he is upset. The occupational therapy assistant has recognized that Kamari becomes frustrated when he is unable to communicate what he wants and needs to others as a result of a significant speech impairment. There is no speech and language pathologist on staff at the residential facility.

Once the client's needs have been identified, the next step is to locate a group, program, organization, or community that can provide the service (West, 1973). In the example of Kamari, the occupational therapy assistant locates a company that provides speech and language pathologists as consultants to residential treatment programs. The consultants should be experts in their field and comfortable with giving advice while having limited exposure to the client or environment (West, 1973).

When a suitable organization has been determined, the availability of both parties is then established. A consultation referral or contract should be drawn up, including the services that will be provided by the consultant as well as when and where the services will be provided. Referral is making a professional judgment to have another occupational therapy specialist, discipline, or facility evaluate the client. According to the AOTA's Statement of Occupational Therapy Referral (AOTA, 1994), "Certified occupational therapy assistants, under the supervision of and in collaboration with registered occupational therapists and in compliance with AOTA'S Standards of Practice for Occupational Therapy and Occupational Therapy Code of Ethics, acknowledge requests for services, whatever their source... and identify and screen individuals for potential referral (p. S109)." The consultative referral is a contract that provides a picture of the necessary case information to be sure that the details of the consultative relationship are understood. The expectations of both parties should be clearly outlined to eliminate confusion. Specific sponsorship issues should be clarified, including exactly who is seeking the

Table 36-1.

SPECIALISTS OUTSIDE OF OCCUPATIONAL THERAPY

Professional	Roles and Responsibilities
Speech and language pathologist (SLP)	Specializes in intervention of physical and/or cognitive disorders resulting in difficulty with verbal communication, speech, language, and feeding/swallowing disorders
Physical therapist (PT)	Concerned with the assessment and intervention of disabilities through physical means including strength, endurance, coordination, balance, and mobility
Physician (MD, DO)	Medical doctor or doctor of osteopathy
Pediatrician	Physician who specializes in treating children
Neurologist	Physician who specializes in treating disorders of the nervous system
Orthopedist	Physician who specializes in treating disorders of the musculoskeletal system
Psychiatrist (MD, DO)	Medical specialist whose primary goal is the intervention of mental illness through medication, psychotherapy, and psychosocial interventions
Social worker (LCSW, LICSW)	Involved in coordinating clients with agencies that will meet their psychosocial needs through psychotherapy and human services management; social welfare policy analysis, community organizing, advocacy, teaching, and social science research are also areas of interest in social work
Nurse (LPN, RN)	Responsible for the care and safety of well and ill individuals in institutional and community settings
Physician assistant (PA); advanced practice registered nurse (APRN)	Medical professional with advanced training who, under the supervision of an MD or DO, can assess, implement, and coordinate medical intervention
Teacher	Responsible for developing and implementing curriculum in a school setting to educate students
Therapeutic recreation	Professional who promotes health through engagement in recreational activity
Architect	Involved in the planning, designing, and oversight of a building's construction; familiar with Americans With Disabilities Act (ADA) codes and universal design specifications for private and public structures
Administrator	Individual or group who ensures implementation of policies and procedures in a health care organization
Dietician (RD, DTR)	Expert in food and nutrition who promotes good health through proper eating

consultation (an organization, group, or individual?), the purpose of the consultation (is the consultation client specific, staff specific, or program specific?), and the authority of the consultee to implement suggestions made by the consultant (Dutton, 1986). At this point, an agreement can been made for the arrangement of services (Jaffe & Epstein, 1992). Kamari's occupational therapy assistant shares his developmental history and the concerns of his grandmother, who is his primary caretaker outside of the program, with the speech and language pathologist who is assigned the case. Services are arranged to be delivered every other week at the facility with Kamari, his occupational therapy assistant, and the consulting speech and language pathologist. Through this early process of

information, an exchange rapport is established, fostering a sense of trust and respect that can be helpful in the course of the partnership. Consultative relationships can take on a number of different dynamics. A partnership is the preferred and most cooperative type; however, there are times when the interaction may either be led by the consultant or consultee (Jaffe & Epstein, 1992).

Once the details of consultation have been identified in the referral, both parties can discuss expectations and a plan can be made for achieving the desired outcomes. Kamari's occupational therapy assistant and speech and language pathologist develop goals to assist him in slowing down his speech so that others are able to understand him more easily. Throughout the course of the

Table 36-2.
SPECIALTIES WITHIN THE FIELD OF OCCUPATIONAL THERAPY*
• Administration and management (including private practice subsection) • Developmental disabilities • Education (including faculty and fieldwork) • Gerontology • Hand therapist (not a special interest section) • Home and community health (including home modification network) • Mental health • Physical disabilities (including hand subsection and driving/driver rehabilitation network) • School systems • Sensory integration • Technology • Work programs
*Based on AOTA special interest sections.

partnership, reassessment should take place to ensure that progress is being made toward the predetermined goals. Kamari's speech and language pathologist monitors his progress every time they meet and also does formal reassessment on a regular basis. The occupational therapy assistant also monitors and reassesses Kamari's ability to access the sensory strategies that he uses to help him stay regulated. Additionally, the occupational therapy assistant informally consults with Kamari's schoolteacher to pass along both the communication and self-regulation strategies that have worked best for him and may improve his ability to access the educational curriculum.

When goals have been achieved or the client has made as much progress as he or she is able, the case may be closed. In our example, Kamari's discharge from the residential program at 13 years of age is the natural end point for his speech services. The consultative relationship between the occupational therapy assistant and speech and language pathologist does not end there, however. A few months later, a resident is admitted who needs communication services that the occupational therapy assistant is unable to provide.

Throughout the consultative relationship, adequate communication is necessary to ensure that both parties are in agreement about the course of action. Consultation can take place in person or via telephone, email, faxed documentation, and/or meetings. The consultant may be called in regard to a specific case for direct services, as with Kamari's case, but may also provide education to other team members or lend program development ideas (Dudgeon & Greenburg, 1998; Jaffe & Epstein, 1992; West, 1973).

It is helpful to be familiar with resources in the community that may be potential sites for referral or consultation. Maintaining positive relationships with various organizations can be helpful when setting up services for clients (AOTA, 2010). Examples of such organizations include but are not limited to vocational rehabilitation programs, assisted living communities, psychiatric day programs, medical equipment vendors, recreational organizations, and services for the visually or hearing impaired.

At times, the services that may be best for a client are not feasible due to socioeconomic, cultural, or psychosocial barriers. Once such a barrier has been identified, there may be community organizations that provide assistance in that specific area of need. For example, a client being discharged home from a rehabilitation hospital may not have the means to purchase a necessary piece of adaptive equipment. With the work of a diligent occupational therapy practitioner, the equipment could be provided by a community organization that offers outreach to low-income individuals in need (AOTA, 2010).

Consultation is a popular way to provide occupational therapy services, although it is not always easy. At times, there are barriers that can get in the way of services being delivered (Dutton, 1986). This is especially true when working with larger programs, organizations, and communities rather than individuals. Often, the occupational therapy practitioner experiences a lack of power when working with these larger entities. Many people still do not know what occupational therapy is or the role that occupational therapy practitioners may have in a specific setting. Although this is an excellent opportunity to enlighten the public, it can also stand in the way of efficiency. Poor carryover can also have an impact as well as issues when recommendations may conflict with the operating policies and procedures of the facility being consulted. At times, there may be a lack of resources in the program that may make it difficult to fulfill the recommendations made by the occupational therapy practitioner. Lastly, how the facility wants things done may conflict with the advice given by the occupational therapist. Ultimately, it is the program's decision as to whether and how to apply the knowledge that they gain from this consultation. This application may not always be exactly how the occupational therapy practitioner envisioned it (Dutton, 1986; see Table 36-2).

Discharge Planning

Discharge planning often begins at the time of initial evaluation and continues throughout the intervention process in order to set realistic goals and allow adequate time for all necessary services to be arranged (AOTA, 2010). As with the entire intervention process, the client, his or her family members, caregivers, and significant others should participate in the discussion to determine the most feasible options for discharge. This process includes but is not limited to identification of the client's current status within the continuum of care, and the identification of community, human, and fiscal resources; recommendations for environmental adaptations; and home programming to facilitate the client's progression along the continuum toward outcome goals.

For example, the discharge plan for a client in a rehabilitation setting may involve being discharged home in the care of a significant other. A referral for occupational therapy home care service will be sent to the client's insurance company. A planned home visit may reveal that a raised toilet seat will better support the client's ability to be independent. The seat is ordered from a vendor, paid for out-of-pocket by the client, and will be installed prior to the date of discharge. A home exercise program will be developed and taught to the client and other caregivers. On the day that the client leaves the rehabilitation facility, all services will be in place to ensure a smooth transition.

The life roles of the client must also be taken into account during transition planning. The occupational therapy practitioner, the client, and relevant caregivers must examine the client's level of independence and if he or she is capable of community living. It should be determined if the client is capable of self-care. Additionally, the occupational therapy practitioner, in collaboration with the client, must establish that he or she is able to perform the tasks necessary to engage in work, play, and leisure activities (AOTA, 2010).

As part of the intervention team, the occupational therapy practitioner facilitates the transition process in cooperation with the client. The wishes of his or her family members and loved ones are also considered. At this time, it may be appropriate to refer to the services of other professionals within the field and outside of occupational therapy (see Tables 36-1 and 36-2). Referrals can be arranged to appropriate community agencies for

psychosocial, cultural, and socioeconomic barriers and limitations that may need modification (AOTA, 2010).

There are multiple factors that can determine where a client will go when he or she leaves the care of an occupational therapy practitioner. For example, did the client live alone prior to intervention? Does the client have a person who can serve as a caretaker or was he or she providing care to another person prior to the event that brought the person to this level of care? What is the next functional level? Depending on the setting, there are many paths to choose from when determining the next step for a client. In mental health arenas, clients may move from an inpatient setting to a day program or to their home with wraparound services. Wraparound services are supports that are implemented to allow a client to live at home with as much independence as possible. Wraparound services may include a phone number to call for peer or professional support. This line may be designated for crisis or non-crisis situations. Other wraparound services include safe houses, case management, home visits, peer advocacy, and other programs designed to support an individual as needed. Following knee replacement surgery, a client may move from an acute inpatient hospital to a rehabilitation hospital to learn how to perform his or her occupations safely with a new joint. From the rehabilitation hospital, the client may go on to an assisted living facility, return to the home with regularly scheduled home care occupational therapy services, or return home with a relative.

A number of events may precipitate the transition process and termination of services. Ideally, discharge occurs when the client has achieved all intervention goals and is no longer in need of occupational therapy services. However, sometimes this is not the case when the therapeutic relationship comes to an end. If a client is unable to achieve his or her goals after a predetermined period of time, a third-party payer may require that the services cease (AOTA, 2010). In addition, the client may be discharged from one facility to be admitted to another. For example, a client may be discharged from an acute care setting after a certain time period, only to be admitted to a rehabilitation facility or a skilled nursing facility. Lastly, a change in environment may necessitate the transition process. For example, an elementary school student receiving occupational therapy services eventually must move on to middle school (AOTA, 2010).

Summary

In addition to developing and conducting each occupational therapy intervention session, the occupational therapy practitioner must simultaneously consider numerous other processes. Depending on the setting, the discharge plan is often developed from the very first time the client interacts with the occupational therapy

EVIDENCE-BASED RESEARCH CHART

Chapter Focus	Evidence
Consultation	Bazyk et al., 2009; Davies & Gavin, 1994; Dreiling & Bundy, 2003; Kemmis & Dunn, 1996; McDermott et al., 2002; Reid, Chiu, Sinclair, Wehrmann, & Naseer, 2006; Wehrmann, Chiu, Reid, & Sinclair, 2005
Monitoring	Chen, Heinemann, Bode, Granger, & Mallison, 2004; Golos, Sarid, Weill, & Weintraub, 2011; Murphy & Tickle-Degnen, 2001; Tickle-Degnen, 2000
Referral	Crabtree, 1991; Deitch, Gutman, & Factor, 1994; Hammerschmidt & Sudsawad, 2004; Kelly & Steinhauer, 1991; Mitchell, Rourk, & Schwarz, 1989
Discharge planning	Atwal & Caldell, 2002; McAnanama, Rogosin-Rose, Scott, Jaffe, & Kelner, 1999; Spencer & Davidson, 1998
OT-OTA relations	Dillon, 2001

practitioner. Throughout the course of intervention, the occupational therapy practitioner engages in a conversation about discharge options with the client and his or her family members and significant others to determine the most appropriate course of action. During intervention sessions, the occupational therapy practitioner engages in monitoring and reassessment to determine that goals in the treatment plan are accurate and achievable. At some point, a consultation or referral may be necessary to meet all of the clients needs. Additionally, the occupational therapy practitioner may be called on to provide consultation in an area of expertise to another professional.

Student Self-Assessment

1. Read and summarize two of the articles about occupational therapy and consultation, referral, monitoring, or discharge in the Evidence-Based Research Chart.

2. Think about an individual you have observed or worked with during fieldwork. How would your approach be different in the consultant role than if you were providing direct intervention?

3. List the many possible practice settings for an occupational therapy practitioner. Now, list the individuals who may be part of the interdisciplinary team in each setting. What are the unique roles and responsibilities of each professional?

4. In the course of discharge planning, there are times when occupational therapy practitioners must have difficult, and at times emotionally charged, conversations with clients and family members. In pairs, role-play a scenario where an occupational therapy practitioner in a skilled nursing facility must recommend that the client should not return home alone, where he or she lived prior to admission, due to safety concerns. What resources may be available to the client?

References

American Occupational Therapy Association. (1994). Statement of occupational therapy referral. *American Journal of Occupational Therapy, 48*(11), 1034. doi:10.5014/ajot.48.11.1034

American Occupational Therapy Association. (2010). Standards of practice for occupational therapy. *American Journal of Occupational Therapy, 64*(6), S106-S111. doi:10.5014/ajot.2010.64S106

Atwal, A., & Caldwell, K. (2002). Do multidisciplinary integrated care pathways improve interprofessional collaboration? *Scandinavian Journal of Caring Sciences, 16*(4), 360-367. doi: 10.1046/j.1471-6712.2002.00101.x

Bazyk, S., Michaud, P., Goodman, G., Papp, P., Hawkins, E., & Welch, M. A. (2009). Integrating occupational therapy services in a kindergarten curriculum: A look at the outcomes. *American Journal of Occupational Therapy, 63,* 160-171. doi: 10.5014/ajot.63.2.160

Chen, C. C., Heinemann, A. W., Bode, R. K., Granger, C. V., & Mallison, T. (2004). Impact of pediatric rehabilitation services on children's functional outcomes. *American Journal of Occupational Therapy, 58*(1), 44-53. doi: 10.5014/ajot.58.1.44

Crabtree, J. L. (1991). The effect of referral for profit on therapists' and clients' autonomy and fair competition. *American Journal of Occupational Therapy, 45,* 464-466. doi: 10.5014/ajot.45.5.464

Davies, P., & Gavin, W. (1994). Comparison of individual and group consultation treatment methods for preschool children with developmental delays. *American Journal of Occupational Therapy, 48*(2), 155-161. doi: 10.5014/ajot.48.2.155

Deitch, C. J., Gutman, S. A., & Factor, S. (1994). Medical residents' education about occupational therapy: Implications for referral. *American Journal of Occupational Therapy, 48,* 1014-1021. doi: 10.5014/ajot.48.11.1014

Dillon, T. H. (2001). Practitioner perspectives: Effective intraprofessional relationships in occupational therapy. *Occupational Therapy in Health Care, 14*(3/4), 1-15. doi: 10.1080/J003v14n03_01

Dreiling, D., & Bundy, A. (2003). A comparison of consultative model and direct-indirect intervention with preschoolers. *American Journal of Occupation Therapy, 57*(5), 566-569. doi: 10.5014/ajot.57.5.566

Dudgeon, B. J., & Greenberg, S. L. (1998). Preparing students for consultation, roles, and systems. *American Journal of Occupational Therapy, 52*(10), 801-809. doi: 10.5014/ajot.52.10.801

Dutton, R. (1986). Procedures for designing an occupational therapy consultation contract. *American Journal of Occupational Therapy, 40*(3), 160-166. doi: 10.5014/ajot.40.3.160

Golos, A., Sarid, M., Weill, M., & Weintraub, N. (2011). Efficacy of an early intervention program for at-risk preschool boys: A two-group control study. *American Journal of Occupational Therapy, 65,* 400-408. doi: 10.5014/ajot.2011.000455

Hammerschmidt, S. L., & Sudsawad, P. (2004). Teachers' survey on problems with handwriting: Referral, evaluation, and outcomes. *American Journal of Occupational Therapy, 58,* 185-192. doi: 10.5014/ajot.58.2.185

Jaffe, E. G., & Epstein, C. F. (Eds.). (1992). *Occupational therapy consultation: Theory, principles and practice.* St. Louis, MO: Mosby.

Kelly, P. A., & Steinhauer, M. J. (1991). Strategies for increasing referrals for occupational therapy in home health care. *American Journal of Occupational Therapy, 45,* 656-658. doi: 10.5014/ajot.45.7.656

Kemmis, B., & Dunn, W. (1996). Collaborative consultation: The efficacy of remedial and compensatory interventions in school. *American Journal of Occupational Therapy, 50*(9), 709-717. doi: 10.5014/ajot.50.9.709

McAnanama, E. P., Rogosin-Rose, M. L., Scott, E. A., Jaffe, R. T., & Kelner, M. (1999). Discharge planning in mental health: The relevance of cognition to community living. *American Journal of Occupational Therapy, 53,* 129-135. doi: 10.5014/ajot.53.2.129

McDermott, S., Nagle, R. J., Wright, H., Swann, S. S., Leonhardt, T., & Wuori, D. (2002). Consultation in pediatric rehabilitation for behavior problems in young children with cerebral palsy and/or developmental delay. *Pediatric Rehabilitation, 5*(2), 99-106. doi: 10.1080/1363849021000013531

Mitchell, M., Rourk, J. D., & Schwarz, J. (1989). A team approach to vocational services. *American Journal of Occupational Therapy, 43*(6), 378-383. doi: 10.5014/ajot.43.6.378

Murphy, S., & Tickle-Degnen, L. (2001). The effectiveness of occupational therapy-related treatments for persons with Parkinson's disease: A meta-analytic review. *American Journal of Occupational Therapy, 55*(4), 385-392. doi: 10.5014/ajot.55.4.385

Reid, D., Chiu, T., Sinclair, G., Wehrmann, S., & Naseer, Z. (2006). Outcomes of an occupational therapy school-based consultation service for students with fine motor difficulties. *Canadian Journal of Occupational Therapy, 73*(4), 215-224. Retrieved from www.caot.ca/CJOT_pdfs/CJOT73/reid2.pdf

Spencer, J. C., & Davidson, H. A. (1998). The community adaptive planning assessment: A clinical tool for documenting future planning with clients. *American Journal of Occupational Therapy, 52,* 19-30. doi: 10.5014/ajot.52.1.19

Tickle-Degnen, L. (2000). Monitoring and documenting evidence during assessment and intervention. *American Journal of Occupational Therapy, 54,* 434-436. doi: 10.5014/ajot.54.4.434

Wehrmann, S., Chiu, T., Reid, D., & Sinclair, G. (2006). Evaluation of occupational therapy school based consultation service for students with fine motor difficulties. *Canadian Journal of Occupational Therapy, 73*(4), 225-235. doi: 10.2182/cjot.05.0016

West, W. (1973). Principles and process of consultation. In L. Llorens (Ed.), *Consultation in the community: Occupational therapy in child health* (pp. 51-58). Dubuque, IA: Kendall/Hunt Publishing Company.

VI

CONTEXT OF SERVICE DELIVERY

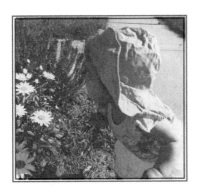

37

EMERGING AREAS OF PRACTICE

Jeffrey L. Crabtree, OTD, MS, FAOTA

ACOTE STANDARDS EXPLORED IN THIS CHAPTER
B.2.1, B.3.4, B.6.1–B.6.3, B.6.5, B.6.6, B.8.1

KEY VOCABULARY

- **Client-centered practice:** "[A]n approach to service which embraces a philosophy of respect for, and partnership with, people receiving services" (Law, Baptiste, & Mills, 1995, p. 253).
- **Evidence-based occupational therapy:** "Client-centred enablement of occupation based on client information and a critical review of relevant research, expert consensus, and past experience" (Canadian Association of Occupational Therapists, 2009, p. 1).

- **Moral treatment:** "[A] period in American psychiatry in the first half of the nineteenth century when retreats and asylums, following the example of the York Retreat in England, began to offer humane care to the mentally ill" (Dunkel, 1983).
- **Neuroscience-based treatment:** An approach to treatment that incorporates neuroscientific evidence, technology such as functional magnetic resonance imaging (fMRI), and techniques such as constraint-induced movement treatment (CIMT).
- **Technology:** A general term that refers to tools and technologies developed to solve human-related problems.

Jacobs, K., MacRae, N., & Sladyk, K. (Eds.).
*Occupational Therapy Essentials for
Clinical Competence, Second Edition* (pp. 491-508).
© 2014 SLACK Incorporated.

Introduction

The purpose of this chapter is to discuss some of the significant changes or trends within the profession and the impact of demographic changes and technology. Many would agree that the world, society, and the occupational therapy profession—virtually everything—changes. On the other hand, not all agree whether a particular change was good or would agree on the meaning of that change. The concept of a trend is no more objective. Statistically, we know that it takes several data points to establish a trend. For example, in the case of consumer spending, when one has data on a dozen holiday seasons of consumer spending, one can estimate a trend. But it is quite another thing to understand why the trend line went in one direction or another, whether the trend will continue, or whether any causal relationship between the trend and background forces can be established. The field of occupational therapy is no different. We see changes and have glimpses of what are likely trends, but it is still quite difficult to understand the forces behind those trends, what the trends predict, or whether the trends will continue. Consequently, the changes and trends discussed here are a combination of the author's personal perspective and literature supporting that perspective.

A Professional Perspective

In this section, select changes and trends occurring in occupational therapy within the United States, within other Western English-speaking countries, and—to a lesser extent—within other countries are reviewed. To do this, the author focused on selected American Occupational Therapy Association (AOTA) documents and English-speaking journals. In most cases, the journals are instruments of national occupational therapy or related professional associations. Consequently, these journals contain not only scholarly works but also information about the professional association and its members. It is important to keep in mind that as the world shrinks because of technology such as the Internet, traditional distinctions between national and international ideas become blurred. So in the strict sense of the word, and from an American perspective, the Canadian, British, and Australian journals of occupational therapy could be considered foreign or international journals, yet a search of English-speaking literature on a particular topic would likely yield pertinent articles in at least one if not all occupational therapy journals from Canada to Australia. These journals publish authors from a variety of countries, and the studies and evolving ideas published in these journals have become an integral part of Americans' notions of occupational therapy.

Three significant examples show the international quality of our current domestic notions about effective occupational therapy. One is the concept of client-centered practice (Canadian Association of Occupational Therapists [CAOT], 1997; Law, Baptiste, & Mills, 1995). In addition to many articles published in the *Canadian Journal of Occupational Therapy* (the developers of this concept are Canadian), client-centered practice has been discussed in the *Indian Journal of Occupational Therapy* (Morgan, Kelkar, & Vyas, 2002), the *British Journal of Occupational Therapy* (Unsworth, 2004), the *Scandinavian Journal of Occupational Therapy* (Hammell, 1995), *Occupational Therapy International* (Rigby, Ryan, From, Walczak, & Jutai, 1996), and the *American Journal of Occupational Therapy* (Snodgrass, 2011), just to cite one example from each of these journals.

The other example is the Canadian Occupational Performance Measure (COPM) (Law et al., 1998). This measure, too, was originated by Canadian occupational therapists, but the measure has been used and statistically verified in a variety of countries and on a variety of conditions. The results of the research have been published in the *British Journal of Occupational Therapy* (Warren, 2002), the *Scandinavian Journal of Occupational Therapy* (Wressle, Samuelsson, & Henriksson, 1999), *Occupational Therapy International* (Chen, 2002), *Occupational Therapy in Mental Health* (Boyer, Hachey, & Mercier, 2000), the *Australian Occupational Therapy Journal* (Farnworth, 2003), *World Federation of Occupational Therapists Bulletin* (Jansa, Sicherl, Angleitner, & Law, 2004), and *American Journal of Occupational Therapy* (Simmons, Crepeau, & White, 2000), to name a few.

In addition, the COPM exemplifies how a measure can break national and diagnosis boundaries. It has been translated into over 20 languages, and its reliability and validity has been studied for a number of different conditions. To cite a few examples, Spadaro and colleagues (2010) examined the internal consistency, external validity, and reliability of an Italian version of the COPM. They found the Italian version to be a valid and reliable outcome measure for people with ankylosing spondylitis. Dielacher and Höss (2011) used the COPM in a pre–post design to show the effectiveness of vocational reintegration for Austrian people with mental illness. Finally, Oestergaard and colleagues, used the COPM to understand its usefulness with Danish patients with lumbar spinal fusion.

Change and Trends Within Occupational Therapy in the United States

To put into perspective the changes and trends that have led to what we understand as occupational therapy today, it is useful to briefly describe the social and medical context of the turn of the 20th century when occupational therapy was a fledgling profession (see Chapter 4). By the late 1800s, the Civil War and reconstruction periods were over. "Moral treatment of the mentally ill" was a specific approach to treating people in the mental hospitals of the day (Bockoven, 1971).

Medicine and health care during the decades before and after 1900 were changing at a fast rate. On July 9, 1893, Dr. Daniel Hale Williams performed the world's first open heart surgery (Buckler, 1968; Cobb, 1953); the Curies shared the Nobel Prize in physics with Henri Becquerel for their work on radioactivity; vitamins were discovered; Robert Kotch discovered the tubercle bacillus; Wilhelm Conrad Röntgen discovered x-rays (Sutcliffe & Duin, 1992); and only a few "resurrectionists," or grave robbers, were still supplying some medical schools with cadavers. Hospital care changed rapidly during this time. These discoveries, activities, and new approaches to health care only begin to characterize the changes that took place in medicine and health care around the turn of the 20th century.

The early years of the 20th century were a time when the founders of occupational therapy in the United States and their supporters were nurturing the infant profession that essentially came from what has been called the *moral treatment era* (Bockoven, 1971; Lilleleht, 2002; Luchins, 1992; Peloquin, 1989, 1994; Tuke, 1813). Moral treatment of the mentally ill started in the 19th century at about the same time in England, France, and Italy (Lilleleht, 2002). It was then brought to the United States.

Furthermore, Licht (1949) noted that around the turn of the 20th century, occupational therapy was being provided by teachers and craftspeople. The educational programs were composed of a few weeks post–high school training until the early 1920s when the education grew to 1 year post high school (West, 1979). In March 1917, a group of supporters met in Clifton Springs, New York, to form the National Society for the Promotion of Occupational Therapy (Quiroga, 1995). By 1921, the name was changed to the AOTA, and the association started publishing the *Archives of Occupational Therapy* in that year. Furthermore, the types of clients seen by occupational therapy practitioners were becoming more diversified, and by the early 1900s, practitioners were providing services to clients with physical problems such as arthritis and tuberculosis as well as those with mental illness (Bing, 1981; Quiroga, 1995).

In the fall of 1978, the AOTA's Representative Assembly invited a number of the leaders of the profession to develop a framework that addressed issues affecting the profession (AOTA, 1979a). The presenters' topics included the following:

- A historical perspective of the profession
- A discussion of practice, education, and research issues
- A discussion of the occupational therapy professional identity
- A review of the external influences impacting the profession
- An exploration of traditional and nontraditional practice arenas

All of the critical concerns of that era fit into three areas: education, research, and practice. Some of the presenters were concerned about the quality of professional education and the influence of formal education on practitioners (Gillette, 1979; Johnson, 1979; Wiemer, 1979). Others expressed the need for developing client assessments that were unique to occupational therapy (West, 1979), and for developing research upon which to base our interventions (Yerxa, 1979). It is important to note that education, research, and practice compose dynamic parts of a whole. To be a practitioner, one must be educated in the theories and skills of the profession. Sound theories and skills are founded on evidence from research and on the clinical expertise that comes from practice. Therefore, the following sections are arbitrarily divided into education, research, and practice only to be able to highlight some of the changes that have occurred in those areas during the last few decades.

Education

One of the overarching concerns noted in *Occupational Therapy: 2001 AD: Papers presented at the special session of the Representative Assembly, November 1978,* which touched upon research, education, and practice, was our professional status. During the 1970s and 1980s, there were many discussions about what constituted being a profession as opposed to a semiprofession or a technical field (AOTA, 1979a; Fleming, Johnson, Marina, Spergel, & Townsend, 1987). Fidler (1979) identified and compared the various characteristics of these levels of professionalism (technical, semiprofession, and profession) and suggested that for several reasons, occupational therapy was a semiprofession. The reasons included that because of our level of education, we did not have adequately evolved specialized knowledge abstracted and codified into a specific body of theories and principles, and we lacked full control over our practice. Fidler cited our educational training of the time as being "less vigorous or substantive than, for example, the art therapist, the special education teacher, the dance therapist, the nurse, social worker, or therapeutic re-creator (sic)" (p. 35).

The first education for occupational therapists in the second decade of the 20th century was composed of a few weeks post high school; then it grew to 1 year post high school by 1923; and then to 34 months with a diploma by 1938 (West, 1979). According to the Council on Medical Education and Hospitals of the American Medical Association, which was the occupational therapy accrediting body in 1947, there were 18 approved schools that offered either a diploma, certificate, or bachelor of science degree in occupational therapy (Council on Medical Education and Hospitals of the American Medical Association, 1947, p. cover 3).

In the 1970s, of those graduating from professional programs, 90% received a bachelor of science degree, whereas others received certificates in occupational therapy (Jantzen, 1979). According to the AOTA (1974), by 1974 there were 51 accredited professional programs in the United States and Puerto Rico. Of those, 10 programs offered a master's degree to those who had a bachelor's degree in other fields, and 17 programs offered a Master of Science degree for occupational therapists. It is interesting to note that New York University (NYU) was the only school that offered a doctoral degree at that time. Occupational therapists wishing to get a degree beyond the master's level either went to NYU or received degrees in education, psychology, or other areas outside of occupational therapy.

According to the AOTA Academic Programs Annual Data Report, Academic Year 2011–2012 (AOTA, 2012), there were four accredited occupational therapy doctoral programs, 145 occupational therapy master of science programs, and 159 occupational therapy assistant programs. In addition, 39 universities offer post-professional occupational therapy master's degrees; 15 offer other post-professional master's degrees in such areas as health science, 15 offer post-professional professional doctorates (OTD), 28 offer other post-professional doctorates such as doctor of health sciences, 5 offer post-professional PhD degrees, and one offers the post-professional doctor of science degree (ScD). This increase in the level of education offered by education programs represents a significant change in occupational therapy education that was mandated by the AOTA (1999), requiring by 2007 that all entry-level occupational therapy professional programs in the United States be at the post-baccalaureate level.

Elsewhere, the University of Western Ontario, Canada, the University of Sydney in 1998, and a preregistration master's degree program in Scotland in 1999 were the first to establish entry-level master of science programs prior to the 21st century (Allen, Strong, & Polatajko, 2001). More recently, the CAOT mandated entry-level master of science degree programs by 2010 (CAOT, 2002). According to a report by the Council of Occupational Therapists for the European Countries (COTEC), 276 of the 368 occupational therapy schools throughout are approved by the World Federation of Occupational Therapists (WFOT), and 11 COTEC member countries offer master's degree programs specific to occupational therapy (COTEC, 2012).

According to Hilton's (2005) analysis of the current transition to post-baccalaureate entry, there were five documented expectations of that transition (p. 67):

1. Elevate the status of the profession.
2. Increase research competency, contributions to professional literature, and accountability to the public.
3. Expand to incorporate the growth of knowledge and practice.
4. Increase doctorally prepared occupational therapists.
5. Increase enrollment of the professional-level therapist.

It is interesting to note that these expectations, in various forms, are also often put forth as justification for the occupational therapy profession moving to the entry-level doctorate. As stated earlier, as of June 2008 there were 5 occupational therapy doctoral programs in the United States (AOTA, n.d.a). Some are entry-level professional doctoral programs and others are post-professional doctorates (OTD). Some are offered as a distance education program. As of the 2012 report, there were 5 candidate and 5 applicant occupational therapy doctoral programs. In addition to doctoral degrees in OT, there are schools that offer the doctor of philosophy (PhD) and doctor of science (ScD) degrees. The number of doctoral programs is increasing. This suggests that there will be more changes ahead for occupational therapy education.

Of the occupational therapy doctoral programs, the OTD is most controversial. The results of a recent study of academic occupational therapy programs (Griffiths & Padilla, 2006) suggest that there are several reasons for this controversy. However, there seems to be as many different opinions about the degree as there are people with opinions. The reasons for controversy identified in the study ranged from some respondents thinking that there is little support within the profession for the degree, to there being little evidence of the need for the degree in the health care system, to there being too little research, and therefore, an insufficient knowledge base in the profession to justify the degree.

Research

The need for research within occupational therapy has existed from the early years of the profession. For example, Licht (1947), when addressing some of the challenges facing occupational therapy in the mid-1940s, said that "little or no statistical data which are suitable for scientific scrutiny and evaluation have been published" (p. 455), and there was only one answer to that challenge—research. The state of research in our profession in the 1970s was characterized by Ethridge and McSweeney's (1970) assessment that "experimental research has thus far been quite rare in occupational therapy literature" (p. 491). Johnson (1979) suggested that the profession relied more on theory based on "a system of beliefs or a philosophy . . . than upon research that provides confidence in the knowledge we acquire" (p. 60). To the extent that professional journals reflect the profession's academic structure and professional maturity, Madhill, Brintnell, and Stewin's (1989) review of the number and content of occupational therapy journals may exemplify the growth of research in our profession over the past several decades. Although the *American Journal of Occupational Therapy* existed from the beginning of the profession, these researchers found an increase in the number of professional journals internationally as well as in the number of research articles reflecting professional maturity.

The *Occupational Therapy Journal of Research* was one of the professional journals initiated in the 1980s. The journal represented one of several initiatives by the American Occupational Therapy Foundation (AOTF) to stimulate research in the United States. In addition to launching the *Occupational Therapy Journal of Research*, the AOTF funded an ambitious and enlightening study—the Clinical Reasoning Study (Mattingly & Fleming, 1994). In her editorial in the 10th anniversary issues of *Occupational Therapy Journal of Research*, Gillette (1990) reported that the AOTF had been successful in meeting those mandates. Bonder and Christiansen (2001), at the *Occupational Therapy Journal of Research*'s 20th anniversary, reported that based on the number of manuscripts submitted to the *Occupational Therapy Journal of Research*, "occupational therapy has more active researchers now than ever in its history" (p. 5).

Although Bonder and Christiansen saw great progress in the profession's research endeavors, they noted that there were at least two goals yet to be reached. The first was to create an occupational therapy culture rich in research traditions. The second was to place research emphasis on "activity and participation rather than body structure and function" (p. 10). An important part of the research is its application to practice. By the 21st century, occupational therapy was becoming committed to evidence-based occupational therapy—further proof of the profession's growth and maturity.

As mentioned previously in this chapter, education, research, and practice compose dynamic parts of a whole. To be a practitioner, one must be educated in the theories and skills of the profession. Sound theories and skills are founded on evidence from research and on clinical expertise that comes from practice. The academic preparation of clinicians, researchers, and scholars is one of many examples of the need for dynamic interaction between education, research, and practice. To accomplish

this dynamic interrelationship and ultimate AOTA's Centennial Vision, Bear-Lehman (2012, p. 252) recommends educational curricula that meet the following standards:

- Understand and be conversant about the similarities and differences between basic and applied scientific inquiry and their interrelationships

- Be comfortable with and confident in being an occupational therapy practitioner and knowledgeable regarding the profession's focus, goals, and means

- Understand the knowledge deficits and research needs of the occupational therapy profession and the ways that these can be ameliorated through the work of multidiscipline, cross-profession, multi-skilled research teams

- Describe the nature of occupational therapy in language that is understood by the biosocial disciplines, other health-related professions, and community members (e.g., using, where appropriate, language of the International Classification of Functioning, Disability and Health [ICF])

- Hear, understand, and appreciate the various agendas (stated and unstated) of multidiscipline, cross-profession, multiskilled research teams

- Participate in the necessary give, take, and compromise of multidiscipline, cross-professional, multi-skilled research teams

Practice

As suggested previously, education, research, and practice are all facets of the same concept. Evidence-based occupational therapy is an approach that blends research and practice. Evidence-based occupational therapy evolved from the awareness that best practice requires practitioners to use the best available evidence to support their intervention, and that education, research, and practice compose dynamic parts of a whole. However, occupational therapy practice also has a strong tradition in what has been referred to as *the era of humane intervention* for the mentally ill and has always rested on a strong humanistic foundation. Entry into the 21st century and the rigors of evidence-based practice in the latter part of the 20th century has brought occupational therapy face-to-face with positivistic science in which measurement and objectivity are valued over intuition and subjectivity.

Johnson (1979) analyzed why education in her era seemed to not bridge the education-practice gap or bring about the changes she felt would help the profession meet its potential. She speculated that "the emotional impact upon young students in the clinical setting is so great that they turn almost immediately to the models of practice they see being demonstrated rather than to the theoretical models they studied but have seldom seen incorporated in practice" (p. 60). This education-practice gap is likely common to other practice professions and not just occupational therapy. Efforts to both maintain high educational standards and to strengthen the relationship between professional education in occupational therapy and practice have traditionally been the role of each national professional association and of transnational organizations such as the WFOT, the European Network of Occupational Therapy in Higher Education (ENOTHE), and the COTEC.

"The aim of the Council [COTEC] is to enable National Associations of Occupational Therapists of the European Countries to develop, harmonize, and promote standards of professional practice and education of Occupational Therapists and to advance the science of occupational therapy throughout Europe" (COTEC, n.d.). The ENOTHE aims to unite European occupational therapy educational programs and proposed programs to advance the education changes and trends in education research and practice and the body of knowledge of occupational therapy and to work with COTEC to promote occupational therapy education in Europe (ENOTHE, n.d.). The mission of the WFOT is to promote occupational therapy as an art and science internationally. The Federation supports the development, use, and practice of occupational therapy worldwide, demonstrating its relevance and contribution to society (WFOT, n.d.).

In the United States, the role of maintaining high educational standards has been taken by AOTA's Accreditation Council for Occupational Therapy Education (ACOTE). The AOTA Commission on Practice has the role of establishing high standards of practice and over the years has produced official documents meant to help practitioners maintain best practice. Of these documents, AOTA's *Uniform Terminology for Occupational Therapy* exemplifies the national association's efforts to establish best practice standards. The first edition of the uniform terminology document was published in 1979 (AOTA, 1979b). It has been revised two times (AOTA, 1989, 1994). The third edition was modified, and the product is called the *Occupational Therapy Practice Framework: Domain and Process* (AOTA, 2008a). To ensure that these documents would help other health professions understand the scope of occupational therapy, the framework uses the terminology and language of the ICF (AOTA, 2008a). All of the documents are meant to provide practitioners with a description of the domain of occupational therapy, which "grounds the profession's focus and actions" (p. 609), and to outline the process of evaluation and intervention or interventions.

Over the years, the AOTA has developed and published other significant documents affecting practice, including the Occupational Therapy Code of Ethics (2005),

Guidelines for Supervision, Roles, and Responsibilities During the Delivery of Occupational Therapy Services (2004), Standards for Continuing Competence (2005), and the Standards of Practice for Occupational Therapy (2005), to name a few. The AOTA Web site (www.aota.org) has a complete listing of its official documents. In terms of specific practice approaches, the early 21st century could jokingly be referred to as the dash-based era of health care; that is, current occupational therapy practice is influenced by the concept of occupation-based therapy, and virtually all health care professions—including occupational therapy—espouse client-centered practice, evidence-based occupational therapy, and neurology-based practice. Furthermore, we treat in hospital-, school-, or community-based settings. The following section briefly describes several of these current approaches to practice.

Client-Centered Practice

The client-centered practice approach in occupational therapy was developed in Canada over the past two decades (CAOT, 1997). As Law et al. (1995) stated, this approach "is a philosophy of practice built on concepts that reflect changes in the attitudes and beliefs of clients and occupational therapists" (p. 253). These attitudes and beliefs include the notion that clients need to express their needs and make choices regarding their occupations, that clients share responsibility for the therapeutic process, that the client-centered approach represents a shift from seeing the person as disabled to seeing the person as enabled, and that clients' "roles, interests, environments, and culture are central to the occupational therapy process" (Law et al., p. 252; Table 37-1).

Occupation-Based Practice

It is important to note that the concept of occupation as a special form of doing has been part of the occupational therapy ethos since the profession's infancy. Just to cite examples from one of the early proponents of occupational therapy, Dr. Adolf Meyer maintained that "occupation is, with good right, called the most essential side of hygienic treatment of most insane patients" (Meyer & Winters, 1951, p. 46). When speaking of his efforts to organize medical work in large state hospitals, Meyer stated that "since most mental disorders are, to a large extent, disorders of conduct, a regulated existence with occupation is, on the whole, the. . . most efficient form of treatment" (p. 95). Meyer believed that the intervention of people with gastrointestinal disturbances, which he felt also caused mental disorders, should include:

> [O]ccupation treatment [over] mere talking . . . due to the fact that, after all, we have not yet as excellent control over the things that form the fancy and the thought life of the individual; whereas we look upon performance and

Table 37-1.

CONTRIBUTIONS OF THE CLIENT AND THERAPIST IN EVIDENCE-BASED OCCUPATIONAL THERAPY

Client's Contributions	Therapist's Contributions
Knowledge, beliefs, hopes, and so forth, necessary for determining meaningful occupational intervention priorities	Knowledge of client's environment and other information relevant to enabling occupational performance
Beliefs about what medical, developmental, or social problems prohibit meaningful occupational performance	Using evidence-based occupational therapy principles and professional expertise, assists client to identify and prioritize occupational performance goals
Subjective evaluation of present occupational performance	Offers suggestions and encourages client to explore new ways of viewing occupational performance deficits
Knowledge and perceptions of personal and environmental resources and limitations	Offers suggestions and encourages client to consider new uses of personal and environmental resources
Hopes for outcomes and agreement with possible therapy plans and measures of success	
With the therapist, identifies intervention outcomes and commits to the proposed intervention and measures of desired outcomes	

Adapted from Canadian Association of Occupational Therapists. (1999). *Joint position statement on evidence-based occupational therapy.* Toronto, ON: CAOT Publications. Retrieved from http://www.caot.ca/default.asp?ChangeID =166 & pageID =156

activity as the actual functioning and the test of the working of the individual's drives and life. (p. 629)

Although the notion of the power of occupation is a part of our early history, it fell into disfavor between World War I to about the 1980s, when occupational therapy was dominated by the traditional, reductionistic medical model, which was the health care system of the day. Mattingly and Fleming (1994), in their study of occupational therapist clinical reasoning, capture the essence of this period of our history when describing what it means to be a "good therapist" in the eyes of non-occupational therapists. They found that "to ensure that services were billable, therapists were driven to narrow the scope of treatment goals and activities along more biomedical lines—to treat the physical body" (Mattingly & Fleming, p. 296) without concern for the phenomenological side of their practice. Yet these researchers saw that their subjects seemed naturally drawn to understanding the clients' disabling experience and the broader meanings of disrupted or lost occupations but could not formally incorporate interventions that would help "patients to formulate, either through words or actions, deeper understandings of themselves and their experiences" (p. 296).

A number of current models exist that espouse the notion that occupation should form the basis of occupational therapy intervention, and that in addressing

occupations, therapists address not only functional deficits but broader issues of meaning, purpose, and spirituality—issues that must be addressed if we are going to assist in a client's construction or reconstruction of the self (Baum & Christiansen, 1997; Christiansen, 1999; Crabtree, 2003; Howard & Howard, 1997; Mattingly & Fleming, 1994). These include the Canadian Occupational Performance Measure (CAOT, 1997) and the Occupational Performance Model (Australia) (Chapparo & Ranka, 1997). In addition, the concept of occupational performance forms the core of the framework (AOTA, 2008a). Suffice it to say, these models place occupation, or purposive doing, at the center of occupational therapy intervention and assume that humans are occupational beings who express their meaning and purpose through their occupations. Many of these models are discussed in more depth in other chapters.

EVIDENCE-BASED OCCUPATIONAL THERAPY

As discussed earlier, evidence-based occupational therapy has received lots of attention from health care professionals. This approach started with the advent of evidence-based medicine, which was defined as "the conscientious, explicit, and judicious use of current best evidence in making decisions about the care of individual patients" (Sackett, Rosenberg, Muir Gray, Haynes, & Richardson, 1996, p. 71). The Joint Position Statement on

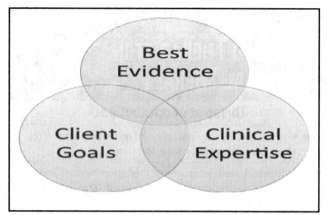

Figure 37-1. The elements of evidence-based practice.

Evidence-Based Occupational Therapy was endorsed by the 2004 AOTA Online Representative Assembly (AOTA, n.d.b) and applies the best concepts from evidence-based medicine to the needs of occupational therapy. Recognition of the need for evidence-based occupational therapy has now reached an international level (Ilott, Taylor, & Bolanos, 2006). Essentially, evidence-based occupational therapy is a collaborative effort between the client and the therapist in which the client (or patient) contributes what is uniquely his or hers to offer, and the therapist contributes his or her expertise (see Table 37-1).

As one might imagine, the application of evidence-based practice across all health care disciplines, many of which have limited research-based knowledge, can be challenging at best and discouraging at worst. Consequently, each profession needs to identify an appropriate blend of the best evidence, clinical expertise, and the client's goals to its practice (Figure 37-1). The concept of best evidence in some ways may pose the greatest challenge to evidence-based occupational therapy. Best evidence is generally based on the idea that certain research designs provide a stronger level of evidence, or greater control of bias, than other research designs. However, there is disagreement among researchers, whether they are part of qualitative or quantitative traditions, as to the precise definitions of evidence, let alone which types of research designs provide the best evidence (Bannigan & Moores, 2009; Cicerone, 2005; Hammell, 2002; Law & MacDermid, 2007; MacDermid, 2004; Sackett et al., 1996).

No particular hierarchy of evidence exists within the qualitative research traditions; rather, there are criteria of credibility, transferability, dependability, and confirmability that must be met to support best evidence in qualitative research (Finlay, 2006). A hierarchy of evidence does exist within quantitative research traditions (Table 37-2). These hierarchies have evolved from traditional lists of specific types of research designs, such

as case studies, cohort studies, randomly controlled trials, and meta-analyses, to what Haynes (2001) called "the most 'evolved' information services for the topic areas of concern" (p. 37). These more "evolved" evidence-based resources include *systems* such as computerized decision support systems (CDSS) (Kawamoto, Houlihan, Balas, & Lobach, (2005); *synopses* such as evidence-based journal abstracts (Teasell, Foley, Bhogal & Speechley, 2002); *syntheses* such as Cochrane reviews (www.cochrane.org); and original *studies* published in journals.

Neuroscience-Based Treatment and Related Evolving Technologies

The 1990s were designated as the Decade of the Brain "to enhance public awareness of the benefits to be derived from brain research" (Library of Congress, n.d.a, n.d.b). During that decade, the Library of Congress and the National Institute of Mental Health of the National Institutes of Health sponsored a number of initiatives to advance the goals set forth by the President. This proclamation stimulated scientific research across the globe (Tandon, 2000).

During and since the Decade of the Brain, in addition to breakthroughs in specific diseases such as stroke, Parkinson's, and Alzheimer's, and in the development of imaging technologies such as the positron emission tomography (PET) scanning, magnetic resonance imaging (MRI), and functional magnetic resonance imaging (fMRI), scientists have come to understand the plasticity of the nervous system—an important characteristic of the nervous system for occupational therapists to appreciate, study, and apply to their practice. Simply put, neuronal plasticity conceives the nervous system to be dynamic and capable of cortical reorganization (Curt, Schwab, & Dietz, 2004; Hamzei, Liepert, Dettmers, Weiller, & Rijntjes, 2006; Liepert, 2006; Taub, 2004) and regeneration of nerve tissues. Animal model researchers, in particular, have discovered a number of examples of plasticity from dendritic arborization (generation of new dendrites) (McAllister, 2000) to axonal regeneration (Curt et al.).

As more basic neuroscience research results are translated to health care practice, occupational therapy practitioners will need to become "neuroscience literate" in order to communicate with physicians and others involved in health care about the science supporting health care services and interventions. Recent advances in upper extremity prosthetics provide a good example. Near the end of 2012, the *Baltimore Sun* reported a young woman had received a "high-tech, thought-controlled prosthetic capable of nearly matching the dexterity of flesh and bone" (Dance, 2012). When talking with family members, physicians, physical therapists, and others

Table 37-2.

EXAMPLE OF A HIERARCHY OF LEVELS OF EVIDENCE IN QUANTITATIVE RESEARCH

Level	Description
I	Systematic review of the literature; meta-analyses; multiple randomized controlled trials
II	Case-control design; non-randomized control/cohort design
III	Cross-sectional design; non-randomized before-after/pretest-posttest design
IV	Single-subject design
V	Expert opinion

about how this sort of high-tech prosthesis works, occupational therapists' explanation will need to be far more sophisticated and accurate than explaining that *thinking* controls the prosthesis. At the minimum, with this example, practitioners who do not work with prosthetics will need to recognize the ever-evolving biotechnical complexity of upper extremity prosthesis. It is also important to remember that neuroscience and technology are progressing swiftly and all current explanations of the science and technology soon become yesterday's news.

Those working in the field of upper extremity prosthetics, or any other area impacted by the growth in the neurosciences, will need a more nuanced and practical understanding of the neuroscience that supports those fields. Again, to use an upper extremity prosthesis as an example, if occupational therapy practitioners intend to continue training in the use of prostheses, they will need to understand targeted nerve reinnervation (TR) surgery and how the resulting nerve connections are able to generate sufficient electromyogram signals to operate high-tech prostheses (Kim, Colgate, Santos-Munne, Makhlin, & Peshkin, 2010; Kuiken et al., 2009).

Clinical application of neuroscientific findings and evolving technologies holds great promise for occupational therapy practice. These applications range from constraint-induced movement therapy (CIMT) to new and evolving technologies such as high-tech prostheses mentioned earlier, to neuromuscular electrical stimulation, to virtual reality. CIMT is one example of neuroscience-based therapy. In this approach, the nonaffected limb is constrained, and for a period of time, the client must practice using the affected limb to perform various tasks, often to perform activities of daily living (ADL) (Roberts, Vegher, Gilewski, Bender, & Riggs, 2005; Taub & Uswatte, 2006). Although the timing, frequency, and duration of the intervention and the means of constraining the nonaffected limb vary depending on the severity of the disability, the intervention setting (e.g., outpatient clinic, home, hospital), and other factors, the outcomes appear to be good (Wolf et al., 2010).

Various forms of electrical stimulation technology, such as functional electrical stimulation (FES), inferential current (IFC), neuromuscular electrical stimulation (NMES), and transcutaneous electrical nerve stimulation (TENS), can be traced to ancient times and have had medical uses for several decades (Knight & Draper, 2007; Tyler, Caldwell, & Ghia, 1982). TENS and IFC are used to provide relief from pain (Sluka & Walsh, 2003), whereas FES and NMES are used to improve blood flow, to strengthen and reduce muscle atrophy, among other therapeutic purposes (Sheffler & Chae, 2007). Although these technologies currently have mixed scientific backing, as scientists' understanding of the nervous system improves, they are likely to become increasingly more effective.

Newer evolving technologies, such as rhythmic auditory stimulation (RAS), computer-enhanced visual feedback associated in conjunction with other technologies such as high-tech prosthetics and orthotics, and computer games such as the Wii (Nintendo), suggest a trend toward technology that is becoming increasingly available in practice. To cite a few examples, for gait training, RAS incorporates auditory rhythmic cues matched to the patient's gait cadence. As treatment sessions progress, the cue frequencies are increased and physical challenges such as walking on a ramp or stairs are added (Thaut et al., 2007). There appears to be compelling evidence that because of likely audiomotor projections to the spinal cord and cerebellum, among other neurological findings, RAS can "produce functional change in motor therapy for stroke, Parkinson's disease, traumatic brain injury, and other conditions" (Thaut & Abiru, 2010, p. 263).

It appears that there is much interest in using the Wii and similar games in therapy. One can follow this trend in blogs such as the Wiihabtherapy blog (wiihabtherapy.blogspot.com) and the popular press. However, the enthusiasm expressed in these venues should be tempered with the recognition that using such games may be appealing to only certain generations (Laver et al., 2011). The effectiveness of the games may also be limited to certain populations. For example, Wuang, Chiang, Su, and Wang (2011) demonstrated improved sensorimotor function among people with Down syndrome, and others have found that using the Wii may have positive results with children with cerebral palsy (Deutsch, Borbely, Filler, Huhn, & Guarrera-Bowlby, 2008) and adults with stroke (Saposnik et al., 2010).

As one can surmise from reading this section, boundaries between neuroscience and technology are disappearing. The two fields, combined in various ways and in different degrees, generate incredible therapeutic advances in health care. An interesting example of the combination of neuroscience, different technologies, and occupation-based interventions comes from the work of Hermann et al. (2010), who are exploring the feasibility and efficacy of client-centered, occupation-based, telerehabilitation and functional electrical stimulation, thus combining standard occupational therapy approaches with telecommunication and electrical stimulation technologies.

Interfield theory (Darden & Maull, 1977) helps to explain the usefulness of amalgamating, in this case, neuroscience and other disciplines. Simply put, the result of combining two separate fields of study that share an interest in explaining the same problem or phenomenon yields an understanding of a problem that neither field can offer alone. To cite examples in the fields of life and human sciences, *neuroanthropology* brings together neuroscience and anthropology to study dimensions of human neural activity and culture, and *neuroengineering* combines engineering and neuroscience to better understand, repair, replace, or enhance neural systems. In the fields of business, *neuromarketing* combines neuroscience and marketing to examine buyer response to marketing stimuli; *neurotheology* unites neuroscience and theology to study the relationship of the spiritual experiences to neuroscience; and *neuroesthetics* employs neuroscience and esthetics to explore, among many things, the relationship of art appreciation and levels of brain function (Crabtree, 2011).

Specific to occupational therapy, Padilla and Peyton (1997) coined the term *neuro-occupation* and introduced the notion of the reciprocal relationship between the central nervous system and occupational performance. Since then, a number of occupational theorists and practitioners have explored how combining neuroscientific knowledge related to human performance with occupational science helps us better understand how occupational performance can affect the nervous system, and how the nervous system effects occupational performance. To cite a few examples, Lohman and Royeen (2002) explored how a neuro-occupational perspective in therapy helps practitioners better understand the neurological correlates of posttraumatic stress disorder (PTSD) and in turn better understand how engaging in purposive occupation can help reduce PTSD symptoms. Others have explored neuro-occupation as the

"interaction between occupational therapists and their clients, and between clients and other human systems, in order to understand the complexity of the dynamic human system and the interplay of the environment" (Haltiwanger, Lazzarini, & Nazeran, 2007, p. 355). Still others have explored intention as a critical partner in the marriage of occupation and neuroscience, or neuro-occupation (Crabtree, 2010; Lazzarini, 2004).

Emerging Practice Areas

According to the 1973 AOTA member data survey, most occupational therapists (about 55%) practiced in traditional settings such as acute hospitals, rehabilitation hospitals, and school systems (Jantzen, 1979), but there have likely always been occupational therapists who have provided services for which they treat nontraditional clients. For example, in 1973, about 8% of registered occupational therapists worked in community programs, such as community mental health centers and day care centers. In this era, a little more than 1% of the members stated that they were in private practice. More than 30 years later, hospitals and rehabilitation units, skilled nursing and other long-term care facilities, and school systems including early intervention make up more than 80% of the settings in which occupational therapists work (AOTA, 2006). Throughout the years, a small percentage of occupational therapists have always worked in what might be referred to as nontraditional or emerging practice areas.

The AOTA has identified a number of what they call emerging niches that fit well within the occupational therapy scope of practice in the United States (AOTA, n.d.c). This section identifies only a few of these areas of practice. The reader is encouraged to go to the AOTA members' area on the AOTA Web site (www.aota.org) for detailed information about these emerging practice areas. With each area, the Web site includes hot links to more detailed information useful to the practitioner.

The following briefly explores three of these emerging niches: bullying, chronic disease management, and veterans and wounded warrior care. According to the American Psychological Association (APA),

> Bullying is a form of aggressive behavior in which someone intentionally and repeatedly causes another person injury or discomfort. Bullying can take the form of physical contact, words or more subtle actions. The bullied individual typically has trouble defending him or herself and does nothing to "cause" the bullying. (APA, n.d.)

The AOTA (2008b) has articulated the importance of occupational therapy practitioners addressing bullying and has provided a number of resources for practitioners on the AOTA Web site. It is important to note there is a plethora of Internet information and program resources ranging from the Pacer Center (www.pacer.org), which focuses on children with disabilities, to MedlinePlus (www.nlm.nih.gov/medlineplus/bullying.html), a National Institutes of Health Web resource for patients and families.

According to the Centers for Disease Control and Prevention (2012), more than half of the deaths among Americans each year result from chronic diseases such as heart disease, cancer, and stroke. Of those with chronic conditions, 25% are limited in one or more ADL. Until recently, management of chronic diseases has been the role of health care providers. However, with the increase in chronic disease has come a significant increase in the cost of caring for people with chronic diseases. Chronic disease management is an emerging approach to address both the health-related problems and to help reduce the cost of health care for those with chronic conditions. The AOTA (2013) offers a number of resources and information about how occupational therapy practitioners can become involved in helping those with chronic disease both manage the symptoms and engage in meaningful ADL.

The United States Department of Defense reported that nearly 34,000 American troops will be coming home from Afghanistan during 2013 (http://www.defense.gov/News/NewsArticle.aspx?ID=119278). That is a relatively small portion of the approximately 1.9 million troops who have deployed in Afghanistan and Iraq in 3 million tours since 2001 (Committee on the Initial Assessment of Readjustment Needs of Military Personnel, Veterans, and Their Families, 2010). Men and women returning from service bring home complex medical and mental health problems from amputations of both upper and lower extremities, to mental disorders and mental health problems, to cancer and high risks of suicide. As with all of the emerging practice areas, the AOTA offers a number of resources for those interested in working in any emerging area of practice. As identified in the "Veterans' and Wounded Warriors' Mental Health" Web page (www.aota.org), occupational therapy practitioners have the skills needed to address the stress and health problems that military personnel experience when attempting to reintegrate into civilian life.

Demographics and Technology

The practice of occupational therapy does not exist in a vacuum. Practitioners and what they practice are situated in political, cultural, social, geographical, religious, and many other contexts. Of the many possible contexts to consider, this chapter focuses on demographics and technology. These appear to likely have significant implications for occupational therapy practitioners in this century.

DEMOGRAPHICS OF THE UNITED STATES

Hiemstra (2003), a futurist, has identified five demographic trends that will have a significant impact on the United States and, by extension, will have important implications for occupational therapy practitioners:

1. Americans are getting older.
2. Americans are becoming more ethnically diverse.
3. The Baby Boomers are retiring, and generation Y is reaching adulthood.
4. Americans will move back to urban inner cities.
5. The United States population will likely peak in the mid- to late 21st century.

The Pew Research Center predicts that the nation's population will rise to 438 million in 2050 compared to 269 million in 2005. In 2050, nearly 20% of Americans will be foreign born. Those 65 years and older will increase from 37 million in 2005 to 81 million in 2050, representing nearly 20% of the total population (Passel & Cohn, 2008). There is no way of knowing today whether these trends will come to pass exactly as predicted, but regardless of the precision of these trends, demographic changes in the United States are likely to have a significant impact on occupational therapy in varying degrees and ways. The aging and increased ethnic diversity of Americans, in particular, will have an impact on occupational therapy in that the increase in the number of older adults will create an increased demand for occupational services, and the increase in the ethnic diversity of our clients will require increased skill on the part of practitioners to be culturally proficient (Royeen & Crabtree, 2006). When you add the increasing numbers of United States citizens with disabling conditions to this equation, the demand for occupational therapy services increases even more.

For example, according to the National Health Interview Survey, 2010, "15% of adults had great difficulty with at least one of nine physical activities performed without help and without the use of special equipment" (Schiller, Lucas, Ward, & Peregoy, 2012, p. 9). About 4.9 million adults (2%) required the help of another person with ADL such as eating, dressing, or bathing, and 9.1 million (4%) required help with instrumental activities of daily living (IADL) such as household chores or shopping. Among adults 75 years and older, about 11% required the help of another person with ADL and 19% required help with IADL (Adams, Martinez, Vickerie, & Kirzinger, 2011).

The National Center for Health Statistics (2005) reported that more than a third of those community-dwelling people 65 years and older reported activity limitations.

The chronic conditions most common to this age group are heart or other circulatory conditions and arthritis and other musculoskeletal conditions. The other conditions that caused activity limitations included "senility," diabetes, vision, and hearing disorders. Although these data were not related directly to the need for occupational therapy services, it is fair to say that the demand for occupational therapy will increase as more Americans enter this age group.

As our nation becomes increasingly ethnically diverse, so will our clinics, hospitals, schools, and other occupational therapy service settings. With this diversity comes differences between therapists and clients or clients' basic values, attitudes, and beliefs about what it means to be an individual; the importance (or lack of importance) of independence or the ability to make decisions; and many other aspects of culture. Disagreement concerning such values and beliefs need not confound the occupational therapy practitioner's efforts to provide effective services. However, to minimize the chances of such conflicts undermining therapy, occupational therapy practitioners need to be culturally proficient, as discussed in Chapter 2.

TECHNOLOGY

In this section, there is a focus on technology in general, not on the technology that is available for use in therapy. For specific information on assistive technology, please see Chapter 31; for information on telehealth, please see Chapter 38. There is a need to focus on the possible problems related to technology because, as occupational therapy practitioners, we are most likely to treat people who may be negatively affected by technology as well as those who benefit from technology.

As consumers of technology, we may seldom give a critical thought to the worth of technology, let alone its possible problems. After all, because of technology, we can see and speak in real time to someone on the other side of the globe, we can prepare a tasty meal in only minutes, we can listen to our favorite music, we can communicate with our friends from virtually anywhere and at any time, and our automobiles can tell us where we are and how to get to our destination. Furthermore, if we need a vital organ, because of modern technology, we can receive either a synthetic organ or an organ transplant.

There is no question that technology has made doing some things easier (Smith, 2000), but has it contributed to the good of humanity, and how is a person's occupational performance affected by technology? These are both philosophical and practical questions—the sort of critical questions occupational therapy practitioners need to ask themselves if they are to make sound clinical judgments about the effect of technology on their clients and society. To make these clinical judgments, it is important to be able to distinguish between the concepts of positive

and negative benefits of technology. A negative benefit is the removal or decrease of something considered bad or negative (Rescher, 1980). For example, using a gas-powered automobile to drive to work might be a negative benefit compared to walking, because walking to work takes 2 hours compared to 15 minutes to drive and walking requires much more human energy. Another example of a negative benefit, again saving time and energy, could be using a microwave oven to prepare a frozen meal compared to preparing a meal from scratch and using a conventional stove or oven. In both examples, the negative benefit is found in reducing the amount of time and energy required to perform the activity.

A positive benefit is one that involves an intrinsic good or a positive condition like happiness, joy, pleasure, and the like (Mejias, 2006; Rescher, 1980). No number of negative benefits, on their own, add up to a positive benefit. In other words, one can have the latest automotive technology that keeps you safe from injuries, as well as technology that cooks a delicious meal and washes, dries, and stacks the dishes without effort, and still be unhappy or still feel unfulfilled. By the same token, people can be very happy and lead a meaningful life and have these magnificent labor- and time-saving devices. In other words, peoples' happiness is not directly related to technology. From the occupational therapy practitioner's perspective, peoples' happiness is related to being able to perform in ways that meet their goals and help them live meaningful, productive, and satisfying lives.

There are two classes of implications of technology for occupational therapy practitioners. One is the obvious, physical effect of using technology, which includes a variety of repetitive stress injuries, many of which are discussed elsewhere in this textbook (Amini, 2006). The second is the not-so-obvious implication in which people, as a result of a poor match of technology to the individual's needs, may develop "Internet addiction" (Beard & Wolf, 2001; Hansen, 2002; Michaels, 1988), leading to a sense of alienation, of being disenfranchised, or of having no meaningful goals or purpose in life. It is important to note that technology can be very useful and rewarding for some. However, for others, having the latest and best technology may mask their need to be connected to others and to be engaged in meaningful occupations (Bakhtin, Liapunov, & Holquist, 1993; Gergen, 1991; Hall, 1981; Jonas, 1982, 1984; Rivers, 1993, 2005).

When we consider that doing, or occupational performance, is critical to peoples' health and ability to make meaning and quality in their life, occupational therapy practitioners need to be able to critically evaluate their client's knowledge and use of technology. As Rogers (1983) stated, "Therapeutic action must be the right action for ... [the] ... individual. This implies that it must be as congruent as possible with the patient's concept of

EVIDENCE-BASED RESEARCH CHART

Topic	Evidence
Client-centered practice	Law, Baptiste, & Mills, 1995
Constraint-induced movement therapy	Taub & Uswatte, 2006
Bullying	Bundy et al., 2008
Wounded Warrior mental health	Sayer et al., 2009

the 'good life'" (p. 602). For many, the use of technology can make the difference between isolation and participation and between independence and dependence. However, what might be a liberating technology helping one live the good life for one person, might be a form of subtle enslavement for another. Take the simple case of a woman who loves to bake desserts from scratch and who has pleased her multigenerational family for years with her cooking skills. After a stroke that leaves her paralyzed on one side, her occupational therapist might be tempted to include preparing frozen desserts as part of the intervention because such an approach would be easy and take less therapy time. The older woman might not criticize the therapist or complain about using microwave technology, but she might be very disheartened to think that she may never return to cooking in the manner to which she is accustomed. In this case, technology has perhaps offered a negative benefit by reducing a burden (clumsy, frustrating, and unsafe cooking techniques) but inadvertently has taken from the woman one of her reasons for living. A more appropriate approach to therapy might be to take the time necessary to help the woman relearn how to bake "the old-fashioned way" using an oven.

Summary

This chapter discusses some of the significant changes, or trends, within the profession and situated occupational therapy in the broad context of the 21st century. The author addresses changes in education, research, and practice. Although there have been some significant changes in the number of occupational therapy practitioners in the United States, the level of education and the amount of research undertaken, the scientific basis of our intervention and intervention, and other factors, many elements of our practice remain essentially the same. At the very least, we continue to provide services to those who have been seriously disabled due to illness, accidents, disease, and other factors. These people, as Jennings (1993) suggested, still need "the restoration of wholeness and integrity ... and the preservation of a meaningful life" (p. S25)—the essence of occupational therapy. Regardless of the era, people want to be happy, well, and satisfied with their life; to participate in the daily course of social and economic events; and to be able to construct worthy goals and meet those goals. As the occupational therapy profession has grown and matured, it has become more able than ever to meet the needs of those people.

Student Self-Assessment

1. Search the literature on an occupational therapy assessment or intervention and then identify how many professional journals from other countries have published articles on that topic. Were there significant differences in the ways the topic was addressed? If so, how were they different or similar?

2. Compare and contrast two journal articles on a given occupational therapy topic—one from an article published prior to 1970 and one from an article published after 1990.

3. Using U.S. Census data, examine the demographics of your state or county. Explain the implications of your findings related to the need for occupational therapy services in your area. Find examples of people's need for assistive technology in your local newspaper. What were the needs, and who provided the services or applied the technology? Did an occupational therapy practitioner provide the service? If not, speculate why.

4. Considering the current trends in practice, education, and research, explain how you think the trend will continue in each of those areas and explain why.

Electronic Resources

- Evidence-based occupational therapy resources, AOTA official documents, and emerging practice areas: www.aota.org

- Information about the American Occupational Therapy Foundation and the Wilma West Library: www.aotf.org

- Client-centered practice resources: www.caot.ca
- Information about international resources and international occupational therapy programs: www.wfot.org.au

References

Adams, P. F., Martinez, M. E., Vickerie, J. L., & Kirzinger, W. K. (2011). Summary health statistics for the U.S. population: National Health Interview Survey, 2010. *Vital and Health Statistics,10*(251), 1-117.

Allen, S., Strong, J., & Polatajko, H. J. (2001). Graduate-entry masters' degrees: Launch pad for occupational therapy in this millennium? *British Journal of Occupational Therapy, 64*(11), 572-576.

American Occupational Therapy Association. (1974). *The 1974-1975 yearbook.* Rockville, MD: AOTA Press.

American Occupational Therapy Association. (1979a). *Occupational therapy: 2001 AD: Papers presented at the special session of the Representative Assembly, November 1978.* Rockville, MD: AOTA Press.

American Occupational Therapy Association. (1979b). Uniform terminology for occupational therapy (1st ed.). *Occupational Therapy News, 35,* 1-8.

American Occupational Therapy Association. (1989). Uniform terminology for occupational therapy (2nd ed.). *American Journal of Occupational Therapy, 43,* 808-815.

American Occupational Therapy Association. (1994). Uniform terminology for occupational therapy (3rd ed.). *American Journal of Occupational Therapy, 48,* 1047-1054.

American Occupational Therapy Association. (1999). ACOTE sets timeline for post-baccalaureate degree programs. *OT Week, 13*(33), i, iii.

American Occupational Therapy Association. (2006). *AOTA 2006 occupational therapy workforce and compensation report.* Bethesda, MD: AOTA Press.

American Occupational Therapy Association. (2008a). Occupational therapy practice framework: Domain and process (2nd ed.). *American Journal of Occupational Therapy, 62,* 625-683

American Occupational Therapy Association. (2008b). AOTA's societal statement on youth violence. *American Journal of Occupational Therapy, 62,* 709-710.

American Occupational Therapy Association. (2012). *Academic Programs Annual Data Report, Academic Year 2011-2012.* Retrieved from http://www.aota.org/~/media/Corporate/Files/EducationCareers/Accredit/47682/2011-2012-Annual-Data-Report.ashx.

American Occupational Therapy Association. (2013). Chronic disease management. Retrieved from http://www.aota.org/Practice/Health-Wellness/Emerging-Niche/Chronic-Disease-Management.aspx.

American Occupational Therapy Association. (n.d.a). *Schools, June 2008.* Retrieved from http://www.aota.org/media/Corporate/Files/EducationCareers/Accredit/47683/2007-2008%20Annual%20Data%20Report.ashx.

American Occupational Therapy Association. (n.d.b). *Top 10 emerging practice areas to watch in the new millennium.* Retrieved from http://www.aota.org/nonmembers/area1/links/link61.asp

American Occupational Therapy Association. (n.d.c). Emergiing niches in practice. http://www/aota.org/Search/SearchResults.aspx?q=emerging.

American Psychological Association. (n.d.). *Bullying.* Retrieved from http://www.apa.org/topics/bullying/index.aspx

Amini, D. (2006). Repetitive stress injuries and the age of communication. *OT Practice, 11*(9), 10-15.

Bakhtin, M. M., Liapunov, V. (Trans. & Ed.), & Holquist, M. (Ed.). (1993). *Toward a philosophy of the act.* Austin, TX: University of Texas Press.

Bannigan, K., & Moores, A. (2009). A model of professional thinking: Integrating reflective practice and evidence based practice. *Canadian Journal of Occupational Therapy, 76*(5), 342-350.

Baum, C., & Christiansen, C. (1997). The occupational therapy context: Philosophy-principles-practice. In C. Christiansen & C. Baum (Eds.), *Occupational therapy: Enabling function and well-being* (2nd ed., pp. 27-45). Thorofare, NJ: SLACK Incorporated.

Bear-Lehman, J. (2012). Comparison of the occupational therapy research agenda with the National Institutes of Health Roadmap for Medical Research. *The American Journal of Occupational Therapy, 66*(2), 250-253.

Beard, K. W., & Wolf, E. M. (2001). Modification in the proposed diagnostic criteria for Internet addiction. *Cyberpsychological Behavior, 4*(3), 377-383.

Bing, R. K. (1981). Occupational therapy revisited: A paraphrastic journey. *American Journal of Occupational Therapy, 35*(8), 499-518.

Bockoven, J. S. (1971). Legacy of moral treatment—1800s to 1910. *American Journal of Occupational Therapy, 25*(5), 223-225.

Bonder, B., & Christiansen, C. (2001). Editorial: Coming of age in challenging times. *Occupational Therapy Journal of Research, 21*(1), 3-11.

Boyer, G., Hachey, R., & Mercier, C. (2000). Perceptions of occupational performance and subjective quality of life in persons with severe mental illness. *Occupational Therapy in Mental Health, 15*(2), 1-15.

Buckler, H. (1968). *Daniel Hale Williams. Negro surgeon.* New York, NY: Pitman Publishing Corporation.

Bundy, A. C., Luckett, T., Naughton, G. A., Tranter, P. J., Wyver, S. R., Ragen, J., Singleton, E., & Spies, G. (2008). Playful interaction: Occupational therapy for all children on the school playground. *American Journal of Occupational Therapy, 62*(5), 522-527.

Canadian Association of Occupational Therapists. (1997). *Enabling occupation: An occupational therapy perspective.* Toronto, Ontario, Canada: CAOT Publications.

Canadian Association of Occupational Therapists. (2002). *CAOT announces professional master's degree as entry requirement starting 2010.* Retrieved from http://www.caot.ca/pdfs/mastersentryfacts.pdf

Canadian Association of Occupational Therapists. (2009). *Joint position statement on evidence-based occupational therapy.* Retrieved from http://www.caot.ca/default.asp?ChangeID=166&pageID=156

Centers for Disease Prevention and Health Promotion. (2012). Retrieved from: http://www.cdc.gov/chronicdisease/overview/index.htm.

Chapparo, C., & Ranka, J. (1997). *Occupational performance model (Australia), Monograph 1.* Sydney, Australia: Total Print Control.

Chen, Y-H. (2002). Experiences with the COPM and client-centered practice in adult neurorehabilitation in Taiwan. *Occupational Therapy International, 9*(3), 167-184.

Christiansen, C. H. (1999). Eleanor Clarke Slagle Lectureship—1999. Defining lives: Occupation as identity: An essay on competence, coherence, and the creation of meaning. *American Journal of Occupational Therapy, 53*(6), 547-558.

Cicerone, K. D. (2005). Evidence-based practice and the limits of rational rehabilitation. *Archives of Physical Medicine and Rehabilitation, 86,* 1073-1074.

Cobb, W. M. (1953). Medical history. *Journal of the National Medical Association, 45*(5), 379-385.

Committee on the Initial Assessment of Readjustment Needs of Military Personnel, Veterans, and Their Families. (2010). *Returning home from Iraq and Afghanistan: Preliminary assessment of readjustment needs of veterans, service members, and their families.* Atlanta, GA: National Academies Press.

Council on Medical Education and Hospitals of the American Medical Association. (1947). Approved schools for occupational therapy technicians. *Occupational Therapy and Rehabilitation, 26*(3), cover 3.

Council of Occupational Therapists for the European Countries (COTEC). (n.d.). *History of COTEC: Introduction.* Retrieved from http://www.cotec-europe.org

Council of Occupational Therapists for the European Countries (COTEC). (2012). *Summary of the occupational therapy profession in Europe, 2012.* Retrieved from http://www.cotec-europe.org/

Crabtree, J. L. (2003). On occupational performance. *Occupational Therapy in Health Care, 17*(2), 1-18.

Crabtree, J. L. (2010). No one dresses accidentally: A research synthesis on intentional occupational performance. *OTJR: Occupation, Participation, and Health, 30*(3), 100-110.

Crabtree, J. L. (2011). Neuro-occupation: The confluence of neuroscience and occupational therapy. *Japanese Journal of Occupational Therapy, 45*(7), 879-886.

Curt, A., Schwab, M. E., & Dietz, V. (2004). Providing the clinical basis for new interventional therapies: Refined diagnosis and assessment of recovery after spinal cord injury. *Spinal Cord, 42,* 1-6.

Dance, S. (2012, December 23). Amputee eager for arm moved by thought. *Indianapolis Star,* A9.

Darden, L., & Maull, N. (1977). Interfield theory. *Philosophy of Science, 44*(1), 43-64.

Deutsch, J. E., Borbely, M., Filler, J., Huhn, K., & Guarrera-Bowlby, P. (2008). Use of a low-cost, commercially available gaming console (Wii) for rehabilitation of an adolescent with cerebral palsy. *Physical Therapy, 88*(10), 1196-1207.

Dielacher, S., & V., Höss. (2011). Occupational therapy in vocational rehabilitation of adults with mental illness. *Die Rehabilitation, 50*(05), 308-315.

Dunkel, L. M. (1983). Moral and humane: Patients' libraries in early nineteenth-century American mental hospitals. *Bulletin of the Medical Library Association, 73*(3), 274-281.

Ethridge, D. A., & McSweeney, M. (1970). Research in occupational therapy part 1. *American Journal of Occupational Therapy, 24*(7), 490-494.

European Network of Occupational Therapy in Higher Education (ENOTHE). (n.d.). *Organization: Introduction.* Retrieved from http://www.enothe.hva.nl

Farnworth, L. (2003). Sylvia Docker lecture. Time use, tempo and temporality: Occupational therapy's core business or someone else's business? *Australian Occupational Therapy Journal, 50*(3), 116-126.

Fidler, G. (1979). Professional or nonprofessional. In *Occupational therapy: 2001 AD: Papers presented at the special session of the Representative Assembly, November 1978* (pp. 31-36). Rockville, MD: AOTA Press.

Finlay, L. (2006). "Rigour", "ethical integrity" or "artistry"? Reflexively reviewing criteria for evaluating qualitative research. *British Journal of Occupational Therapy, 69*(7), 319-326.

Fleming, M. H., Johnson, J. A., Marina, M-H., Spergel, E. L., & Townsend, B. (1987). *Occupational therapy directions for the future.* Report of the Entry-Level Study Committee of the American Occupational Therapy Association. Rockville, MD: AOTA Press.

Gergen, K. J. (1991). *The saturated self: Dilemmas of identity in contemporary life.* New York, NY: Basic Books.

Gillette, N. (1979). Practice, education and research. In *Occupational therapy: 2001 AD: Papers presented at the special session of the Representative Assembly, November 1978* (pp. 18-25). Rockville, MD: AOTA Press.

Gillette, N. (1990). Guest editorial: 10th anniversary volume of OTJR: An update of research programs. *Occupational Therapy Journal of Research, 10*(6), 67-73.

Griffiths, Y., & Padilla, R. (2006). National status of the entry-level doctorate in occupational therapy (OTD). *American Journal of Occupational Therapy, 60*(5), 540-550.

Hall, E. T. (1981). *Beyond culture.* New York, NY: Anchor Press.

Haltiwanger, E., Lazzarini, I., & Nazeran, H. (2007). Application of nonlinear dynamics theory to neuro-occupation: A case study of alcoholism. *British Journal of Occupational Therapy, 70*(8), 349-357.

Hammell, K. W. (1995). Application of learning theory in spinal cord injury rehabilitation: Client-centered occupational therapy. *Scandinavian Journal of Occupational Therapy, 2*(1), 34-39.

Hammell, K. W. (2002). Informing client-centred practice through qualitative inquiry: Evaluating the quality of qualitative research. *British Journal of Occupational Therapy, 65*(4), 175-184.

Hamzei, F., Liepert, J., Dettmers, C., Weiller, C., & Rijntjes, M. (2006). Two different reorganization patterns after rehabilitative therapy: An exploratory study with fMRI and TMS. *Neuroimage, 31*(2), 710-120.

Hansen, S. (2002). Excessive Internet usage or 'Internet Addiction'? The implications of diagnostic categories for student users. *Journal of Computer Assisted Learning, 18*(2), 235-236.

Haynes, R. B. (2001). Of studies, summaries, synopses, and systems: The "4S" evolution of services for finding current best evidence. *Evidence Based Mental Health, 4*(2), 37-38. doi: 10.1136/ebmh.4.2.37

Hermann V. H., Herzog, M., Jordan, R., Hofherr, M., Levine, P., & Page, S. J. (2010). Telerehabilitation and electrical stimulation: An occupation-based, client-centered stroke intervention. *American Journal of Occupational Therapy, 64*(1), 73-81. doi: 10.5014/ajot.64.1.73

Hiemstra, G. (2003). Population myths, trends and transportation planning. *FuturistNews.* Retrieved from http://www.futurist.com

Hilton, C. L. (2005). The evolving postbaccalaureate entry: Analysis of occupational therapy entry-level master's degree in the United States. *Occupational Therapy in Health Care, 19*(3), 51-71.

Howard, B. S., & Howard, J. R. (1997). Occupation as spiritual activity. *American Journal of Occupational Therapy, 51*(3), 181-185.

Ilott, I., Taylor, M. C., & Bolanos, C. (2006). Evidence-based occupational therapy: It's time to take a global approach. *British Journal of Occupational Therapy, 69*(1), 38-41.

Jansa, J., Sicherl, Z., Angleitner, K., & Law, M. (2004). The use of Canadian Occupational Performance Measure (COPM) in clients with an acute stroke. *World Federation of Occupational Therapists Bulletin, 50,* 18-23.

Jantzen, A. (1979). The current profile of occupational therapy and the future—professional or vocational? In *Occupational therapy: 2001 AD: Papers presented at the special session of the Representative Assembly, November 1978* (pp. 71-75). Rockville, MD: AOTA Press.

Jennings, B. (1993). Healing the self: The moral meaning of relationships in rehabilitation. *American Journal of Physical Medicine and Rehabilitation, 72,* 401-404.

Johnson, J. (1979). Reorganization in relation to the issues. In *Occupational therapy: 2001 AD: Papers presented at the special session of the Representative Assembly, November 1978* (pp. 60-68). Rockville, MD: AOTA Press.

Jonas, H. (1982). *The phenomenon of life.* Chicago, IL: University of Chicago Press.

Jonas, H. (1984). *The imperative of responsibility.* (H. Jonas & D. Herr, Trans.) Chicago, IL: University of Chicago Press.

Kawamoto, K., Houlihan, C. A., Balas, E. A., & Lobach, D. F. (2005). Improving clinical practice using clinical decision support systems: A systematic review of trials to identify features critical to success. *BMJ, 330*(7494), 765. doi: 10.1136/bmj.38398.500764.8F

Kim, K., Colgate, J. E., Santos-Munne, J. J., Makhlin, A., & Peshkin, M. A. (2010). On the design of miniature haptic devices for upper extremity prosthetics. *IEEE/ASME Transactions on Mechatronics, 15*(1), 27-39. doi: 10.1109/TMECH.2009.2013944

Knight, K. L., & Draper, D. O. (2007). *Therapeutic modalities: The art and science with clinical activities manual.* Baltimore, MD: Lippincott Williams & Wilkins.

Kuiken, T., Li, G., Lock, B. A., Lipschutz, R. D., Miller, L. A., Stubblefield, K. A., & Englehart, K. (2009). Targeted muscle reinnervation for real-time myoelectric control of multifunction artificial arms. *Journal of the American Medical Association, 301*(6), 619-628. doi: 10.1001/jama.2009.116

Laver, K., Ratcliffe, J., George, S., Burgess, L., & Crotty, M. (2011). Is the Nintendo Wii Fit really acceptable to older people?: A discrete choice experiment. *BMC geriatrics, 11*(1), 64.

Law, M., Baptiste, S., Carswell, A., McColl, M. A., Polatajko, H., & Pollock, N. (1998). *The Canadian occupational performance measure* (3rd ed.). Toronto, Ontario, Canada: CAOT Publications.

Law, M., Baptiste, S., & Mills, J. (1995). Client-centered practice: What does it mean and does it make a difference? *Canadian Journal of Occupational Therapy, 62*(5), 250-257.

Law, M. C., & MacDermid, J. (2007). *Evidence-based rehabilitation: A guide to practice.* Thorofare, NJ: SLACK Incorporated.

Lazzarini, I. (2004). Neuro-Occupation: the nonlinear dynamics of intention, meaning and perception. *The British Journal of Occupational Therapy, 67,* 342-352.

Library of Congress. (n.d.a). *The decade of the brain 1999-2000.* Retrieved from http://www.loc.gov/loc/brain

Library of Congress. (n.d.b). *Presidential proclamation 6158.* Retrieved from http://www.loc.gov/loc/brain/proclaim.html

Licht, S. (1947). Modern trends in occupational therapy. *Occupational Therapy and Rehabilitation, 26*(6), 455-460.

Licht, S. (1949). The changing role of the occupational therapist. *Occupational Therapy and Rehabilitation, 28*(3), 260-264.

Liepert, J. (2006). Motor cortex excitability in stroke before and after constraint-induced movement therapy. *Cognitive and Behavioral Neurology, 19*(1), 41-47.

Lilleleht, E. (2002). Progress and power: Exploring the disciplinary connections between moral treatment and psychiatric rehabilitation. *Philosophy, Psychiatry, and Psychology, 9*(2), 167-182.

Lohman, H., & Royeen, C. (2002). Posttraumatic stress disorder and traumatic hand injuries: a neuro-occupational view. *The American Journal of Occupational Therapy , 56*(5), 527.

Luchins, A. S. (1992). The cult of curability and the doctrine of perfectibility: Social context of the nineteenth century American asylum movement. *History of Psychiatry, 3,* 203-220.

MacDermid, J. C. (2004). *An introduction to evidence-based practice for hand therapists. Journal of Hand Therapy, 17*(2), 105-117. doi: 10.1197/j.jht.2004.02.001

Madhill, H., Brintnell, S., & Stewin, L. (1989). Professional literature: One view of a national perspective. *Australian Occupational Therapy Journal, 36,* 110-119.

Mattingly, C., & Fleming, M. H. (1994). *Clinical reasoning: Forms of inquiry in a therapeutic practice.* Philadelphia, PA: F. A. Davis Company.

McAllister, A. K. (2000). Cellular and molecular mechanisms of dendrite growth. *Cerebral Cortex, 10*(10), 963-973.

Mckinnon, A. L. (2000). Client values and satisfaction with occupational therapy. *Scandinavian Journal of Occupational Therapy, 7*(3), 99-106.

Medical Surveillance Monthly Report. (2012). Medical surveillance monthly report. In F. L. O'Donnell (Ed.), *The medical surveillance monthly report* (Vol. 19). Silver Spring, MD: Armed Forces Health Surveillance Center.

Mejias, U. A. (2006). *Technology without ends: A critique of technocracy as a threat to being.* Retrieved from http://blog.ulisesmejias.com/2006/06/03/technology-without-ends-a-critique-of-technocracy-as-a-threat-to-being

Meyer, A., & Winters, E. E. (Eds.). (1951). *The collected papers of Adolf Meyer* (Vol. 2). Baltimore, MD: Johns Hopkins Press.

Michaels, R. J. (1988). Addiction, compulsion, and the technology of consumption. *Economic Inquiry, 26*(1), 75-88.

Morgan, S. B., Kelkar, R. S., & Vyas, O. A. (2002). Client-centered occupational therapy for acute stroke patients. *Indian Journal of Occupational Therapy, 34*(1), 7-12.

National Center for Health Statistics. (2005). *Health, United States, 2005 with chart book on trends in the health of Americans.* Hyattsville, MD: Author.

Oestergaard, L., G., Maribo, T., Bünger, C. E.,& Christensen, F. B. (2012). The Canadian Occupational Performance Measure's semi-structured interview: its applicability to lumbar spinal fusion patients. A prospective randomized clinical study. *European Spin Journal 21*(1), 115-121.

Padilla, R., & Peyton, C. B. (1997). Neuro-occupation: Historical review and examples. In C. B. Royeen (Ed.), *Neuroscience & occupation: Links to practice.* Bethesda, MD: AOTA Press.

Passel, J. S., & Cohn, D. (2008). *U.S. population projections: 2005-2050.* Washington, DC: Pew Research Center:

Peloquin, S. M. (1989). Moral treatment: Contexts considered. *American Journal of Occupational Therapy, 43,* 537-544.

Peloquin, S. M. (1994). Moral treatment: How a caring practice lost its rationale. *American Journal of Occupational Therapy, 48,* 167-173.

Quiroga, V. A. M. (1995). *Occupational therapy: The first 30 years: 1900 to 1930.* Bethesda, MD: AOTA Press.

Rescher, N. (1980). *Unpopular essays on technological progress.* Pittsburgh, PA: University of Pittsburgh Press.

Rigby, R., Ryan, S., From, W., Walczak, E., & Jutai, J. (1996). A client-centered approach to developing assistive technology with children. *Occupational Therapy International, 3*(1), 67-79.

Rivers, J. R. (1993). *Contra technologiam: The crisis of value in a technological age.* Lanham, MD: University Press of America.

Rivers, J. R. (2005). An introduction to the metaphysics of technology. *Technology in Society, 27,* 551-574.

Roberts, P. S., Vegher, J. A., Gilewski, M., Bender, A., & Riggs, R. V. (2005). Client-centered occupational therapy using constraint-induced therapy. *Journal of Stroke and Cerebrovascular Diseases, 14*(3), 115-121.

Rogers, J. C. (1983). Eleanor Clarke Slagle Lectureship—1983; clinical reasoning: The ethics, science, and art. *American Journal of Occupational Therapy, 37*(9), 601-616.

Royeen, M., & Crabtree, J. L. (2006). *Culture in rehabilitation: From competency to proficiency.* Upper Saddle River, NJ: Prentice Hall.

Sackett, D. L., Rosenberg, W. M. C., Muir Gray, J. A., Haynes, R. B., & Richardson, W. S. (1996). Evidence-based medicine: What it is and what it isn't. *British Medical Journal, 312,* 71-72.

Saposnik, G., Mamdani, M., Bayley, M., Thorpe, K., Hall, J., Cohen, L., & Teasell, R. (2010). Effectiveness of Virtual Reality Exercises in STroke Rehabilitation (EVREST): Rationale, design, and protocol of a pilot randomized clinical trial assessing the Wii gaming system. *International Journal of Stroke, 5*(1), 47-51.

Sayer, N. A., Cifu, D. X., McNamee, S., Chiros, C. E., Sigford, B. J., Scott, S., & Lew, H. L. (2009). Rehabilitation needs of combat-injured service members admitted to the VA Polytrauma Rehabilitation Centers: The role of PM&R in the care of wounded warriors. *PM & R: The Journal of Injury, Function, and Rehabilitation, 1*(1), 23-28.

Schiller, J. S., Lucas, J. W., Ward, B. W., & Peregoy, J. A. (2012). Summary health statistics for U.S. adults: National Health Interview Survey, 2010. *Vital and Health Statistics, 10*(252), 1-207.

Sheffler, L. R., & Chae, J. (2007). Neuromuscular electrical stimulation in neurorehabilitation. *Muscle and Nerve, 35*(5), 562-590. doi: 10.1002/mus.20758

Simmons, D. C., Crepeau, E. B., & White, B. P. (2000). The predictive power of narrative data in occupational therapy evaluation. *American Journal of Occupational Therapy, 54*(5), 471-476.

Sluka, K. A., & Walsh, D. (2003). Transcutaneous electrical nerve stimulation: Basic science mechanisms and clinical effectiveness. *Journal of Pain, 4,* 109-121.

Smith, R. O. (2000). The role of occupational therapy in a developmental technology model. *American Journal of Occupational Therapy, 54*(3), 339-340.

Snodgrass, J. (2011). Effective occupational therapy interventions in the rehabilitation of individuals with work-related low back injuries and illnesses: A systematic review. *American Journal of Occupational Therapy, 65*(1), 37-43.

Spadaro, A., Lubrano, E., Massimiani, M., P., Gaia, P., Perrotta, F. M., Parsons, W. J.,...Valesini, G. (2010). Validity, responsiveness and feasibility of an Italian version of the Canadian Occupational Performance Measure for patients with ankylosing spondylitis. *Clinical and experimental rheumatology, 28*(2), 215-222.

Sutcliffe, J., & Duin, N. (1992). *A history of medicine.* New York, NY: Barnes & Noble Books.

Tandon, P. N. (2000). The decade of the brain: A brief review. *Neurology India, 48*(3), 199-207.

Taub, E. (2004). Harnessing brain plasticity through behavioral techniques to produce new treatments in neurorehabilitation. *American Psychologist, 59*(8), 692-704.

Taub, E., & Uswatte, G. (2006). Constraint-induced movement therapy. *NeuroRehabilitation, 21*(2), 93-176.

Teasell, R. W., Foley, N. C., Bhogal, S. K., & Speechley, M. R. (2002). An evidence-based review of stroke rehabilitation. *Topics in Stroke Rehabilitation, 10*(1), 29-58.

Thaut, M., Leins, A., Rice, R. R., Argstatter, H., Kenyon, G. P., McIntosh, G. G., Bolay, H. V., & Fetter, M. (2007). Rhythmic auditory stimulation improves gait more than NDT/Bobath training in near-ambulatory patients early poststroke: A single-blind, randomized trial. *Neurorehabilitation and Neural Repair, 21*(5), 455-459.

Thaut, M. H., & Abiru, M. (2010). Rhythmic auditory stimulation in rehabilitation of movement disorders: A review of current research. *Music Perception, 27*(4), 263-269.

Tuke, S. (1813). *Description of the retreat, an institution near York, for insane persons.* London, England: Oxford University. [Digitized May 3, 2007].

Tyler, E., Caldwell, C., & Ghia, J. N. (1982) Transcutaneous electrical nerve stimulation: An alternative approach to the management of postoperative pain. *Anesthesia & Analgesia 61*(5), 449-456.

Unsworth, C. A. (2004). Clinical reasoning: How do pragmatic reasoning, worldview and client-centredness fit? *British Journal of Occupational Therapy, 67*(1), 10-19.

Warren, A. (2002). An evaluation of the Canadian Model of Occupational Performance and the Canadian Occupational Therapy Measure in mental health practice. *British Journal of Occupational Therapy, 65*(11), 515-522.

West, W. (1979). Historical perspectives. In *Occupational therapy: 2001 AD: Papers presented at the special session of the Representative Assembly, November 1978* (pp. 9-17). Rockville, MD: AOTA Press.

Wiemer, R. (1979). Traditional and nontraditional practice arenas. In *Occupational therapy: 2001 AD: Papers presented at the special session of the Representative Assembly, November 1978* (pp. 42-53). Rockville, MD: AOTA Press.

Wolf, S. L., Thompson, P. A., Winstein, C. J., Miller, J. P., Blanton, S. R., Nichols-Larsen, D. S., Morris, D. M., Uswatte, G., Taub, E., Light, K. E., & Sawaki, L. (2010). The EXCITE stroke trial comparing early and delayed constraint-induced movement therapy. *Stroke, 41*(10), 2309-2315.

World Federation of Occupational Therapists. (n. d.). *History.* Retrieved from http://www.wfot.org.au

Wressle, E., Samuelsson, K., & Henriksson, C. (1999). Responsiveness of the Swedish version of the Canadian Occupational Performance Measure. *Scandinavian Journal of Occupational Therapy, 6*(2), 84-89.

Wuang, Y. P., Chiang, C. S., Su, C. Y., & Wang, C. C. (2011). Effectiveness of virtual reality using Wii gaming technology in children with Down syndrome. *Research in Developmental Disabilities, 32*(1), 312-321.

Yerxa, E. (1979). The philosophical base of occupation. In *Occupational therapy: 2001 AD: Papers presented at the special session of the Representative Assembly, November 1978* (pp. 26-30). Rockville, MD: AOTA Press.

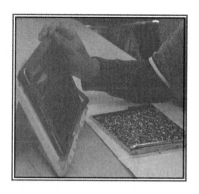

38

TELEHEALTH

Nancy Doyle, OTD, OTR/L

ACOTE STANDARDS EXPLORED IN THIS CHAPTER
B.1.8, B.2.1, B.3.4, B.6.1–B.6.3, B.6.5, B.6.6, B.8.1

KEY VOCABULARY

- **Encrypted communication technologies:** Communication technologies that are encoded in order to protect client privacy and confidentiality across the lines of communication between service provider and client.
- **In-person:** Where the service provider and client are in the same location and work together face-to-face.
- **Service delivery model:** A method for providing services to clients.

- **Telehealth:** The delivery of health services using telecommunication technology by providers who are at a distance from clients.
- **Telerehabilitation:** Area of telehealth that is focused on rehabilitation with clients who have had an illness or injury.

Introduction

Telehealth is a service delivery model utilized across various health professions, including occupational therapy. It is a "mode of delivering health care services and public health utilizing information and communication technologies to enable the diagnosis, consultation, treatment, education, care management, and self-management of patients at a distance from health care providers" (Telehealth Advancement Act of 2011, p. 3).

Within occupational therapy, telehealth is an emerging niche (American Occupational Therapy Association [AOTA], 2013a) that can be used in any practice area (Cason, 2012b), including children and youth, health and wellness, mental health, productive aging, rehabilitation, disability, participation, and work and industry (AOTA, 2013b). It has been used, for example, to provide early intervention services to children in rural areas (Cason, 2009) or to provide energy conservation educational courses to individuals with multiple sclerosis (Holberg &

Jacobs, K., MacRae, N., & Sladyk, K. (Eds.).
*Occupational Therapy Essentials for
Clinical Competence, Second Edition* (pp. 509-515).
© 2014 SLACK Incorporated.

Finlayson, 2007). Typically, it is utilized to provide occupational therapy services to clients who would otherwise have difficulty accessing services in person. Such difficulties may include remote location, mobility or transportation, and long travel distances to specialists.

Research has shown telehealth to be at least as therapeutically effective as in-person services in many settings (Jacobs, Blanchard, & Baker, 2012) with high client satisfaction ratings (Steel, Cox, & Garry, 2011). It has also been shown to be cost-effective and efficient for practitioners and clients alike (Cason, 2009; Dreyer, Dreyer, Shaw, & Wittman, 2001; Hermann et al., 2010). When guided by clinical reasoning, evidence, and appropriate technical training (AOTA, 2010c), it can be a positive and efficacious model for delivering occupational therapy services. Certainly, it provides an additional method for providing services across the country and around the globe to promote "the health and participation of people, organizations, and populations through engagement in occupation" (AOTA, 2008, p. 625).

This chapter will define *telehealth*; present how it is currently being used in occupational therapy; and discuss practical, legal, ethical, and reimbursement issues related to telehealth. These topics are intended to demonstrate how telehealth can be used to support the "performance, participation, health and well-being" (Accreditation Council for Occupational Therapy Education [ACOTE], 2012, p. S34) of occupational therapy clients. Additionally, this chapter will analyze the telehealth service delivery model and its "potential effect on the practice of occupational therapy" (p. S52).

Terminology

Traditionally, health services have been provided when the provider and client are face-to-face in the same physical location, termed *in-person services*. In contrast, telehealth allows health services to be provided when the practitioner and client are in different physical locations. *Telehealth* is a broad term that encompasses many different aspects of promoting and providing health and public health services using telecommunication technology. *Telecommunication technology* is technology that allows communication at a distance. Today, interactive technologies such as synchronous videoconferencing and streaming of video and audio media through the Internet and wireless devices can provide access to face-to-face telehealth for many practitioners and clients (Health Resources and Services Administration [HRSA], 2012).

Telemedicine and *telerehabilition* are related terms that fit under the umbrella of telehealth. Telemedicine focuses specifically on providing medical care and services using telecommunication technology. Telerehabilition is the provision of rehabilitation services by allied health professionals using telecommunication technology. Cason

(2012a) advocates that occupational therapy use the term *telehealth* to fully represent what we can and do provide to clients via telecommunication technology. Our services are more than just rehabilitative for clients with disabilities; they may also include education, habilitation, prevention, health promotion, and wellness services.

History of Telehealth

Telemedicine was first introduced in the 20th century. Early instances include a published illustration of a physician remotely viewing his patient on a "radio-screen" in a 1924 issue of *Radio News*, a cross-state demonstration of telemedicine at the 1951 New York World's Fair, and teleradiology in 1957 by Albert Jutras in Montreal, Canada (Dreyer et al., 2001). The National Aeronautics and Space Administration (NASA) began using telemedicine to monitor the health of astronauts in space as early as the 1960s (Dreyer et al., 2001). Hospitals in the United States began utilizing telemedicine in the late 1960s and in Australia in the early 1980s (Dreyer et al., 2001).

AOTA president Mary Foto began introducing the concept of telerehabilitation to occupational therapists in the United States in the late 1990s (Foto, 1996, 1997). Utilization and research of telecommunication technology began in the 21st century (Dreyer et al., 2001) and is growing as an emerging service delivery model in occupational therapy (AOTA, 2013a).

The AOTA has published position papers on telerehabilitation and occupational therapy's role in and contributions to this model of service provision (AOTA, 2005, 2010c). As telehealth evolves, the position papers will continue to be revised and published every 5 years to keep current with evidence-based provision of occupational therapy through telecommunication technologies. The American Telemedicine Association (ATA) has also worked across disciplines to develop a blueprint, or guidelines, for "providing effective and safe services that are based on client needs, current empirical evidence, and available technologies" (Brennan et al., 2010, p. 263). The guidelines from AOTA (2010c) and the ATA (Brennan et al., 2010) should be reviewed when implementing a telehealth service provision model; they provide strong guidance for developing the appropriate administrative, clinical, technical, and ethical aspects of telehealth services.

Telehealth and Occupational Therapy

Telehealth has the potential to be used in all areas of occupational therapy practice (Cason, 2012b). Just as with in-person occupational therapy services, telehealth provided by occupational therapy practitioners focuses on occupational performance. The overall goal of occupational therapy provided through telehealth is to support a client's "health and participation in life through engagement in occupation" (AOTA, 2008, p. 626). Telehealth may be used for occupational therapy services that include prevention, health promotion, evaluation, intervention, consultation, and long-term monitoring of health (AOTA, 2010c).

Research has shown that a variety of assessments are valid and reliable when utilizing telehealth technologies (AOTA, 2010c; Cason, 2012a). These include the Kohlman Evaluation of Living Skills, Canadian Occupational Performance Measure, Functional Reach Test, European Stroke Scale, Functional Independence Measure, Jamar Dynamometer, Preston Pinch Gauge, Nine-Hole Peg Test, Unified Parkinson's Disease Rating Scale, and Functioning Everyday With a Wheelchair.

Telehealth has been used across the occupational therapy domain. This service delivery model has been used to provide early intervention, school-based, stroke rehabilitation, and ergonomic services; long-term monitoring of chronic conditions; and virtual reality interventions for individuals with cognitive impairments (AOTA, 2010c; Cason, 2012b). Practitioners have used telehealth to provide services to clients with a variety of concerns including traumatic brain injuries, multiple traumas, prostheses, autism spectrum disorders, cerebral palsy, and stroke (Cason, 2012a, 2012b; Jacobs et al., 2012).

Cason (2009) points out the potential for telehealth to be used in areas of practice that "have a strong consultative and/or educational component" (p. 44). Additionally, she has recently written on the opportunities for telehealth occupational therapy services as supported by the Patient Protection and Affordable Care Act of 2010. This law works to "improve access, quality, efficiency, and transparency of health care services" (Cason, 2012b, p. 131). As noted in her study of telehealth occupational therapy services for children receiving early intervention in rural Kentucky, telehealth can provide quality services at a lower cost to families, practitioners, and companies in terms of travel time and cost (Cason, 2009), thereby improving access, quality, efficiency, and transparency.

Efficacy of Telehealth

Occupational therapy interventions have also been shown to be effective in a variety of practice settings and geographical locations around the world (Heimerl & Rasch, 2009). These include early intervention to children in rural Kentucky (Cason, 2009) and post-stroke rehabilitation (Hermann et al., 2010). Heimerl and Rasch (2009) report on additional telehealth occupational therapy services as diverse as for school children in Hawaii, individuals with mental illness in rural Japan, and clients with neurological issues in rural Minnesota and American Samoa.

Researchers and practitioners must continue to develop and study occupational therapy telehealth services in order to build our evidence base. In addition to our own profession, we are able to pull from telehealth studies across disciplines that look at mental and physical health. For example, a recent systematic review examines telehealth studies published since 2000 by occupational therapy, psychiatry, counseling, and physical therapy researchers (Steel et al., 2011). Studies comparing the efficacy of in-person and telehealth service provision have found no significant difference in clinical outcomes (Jacobs et al., 2012; Steel et al., 2011). In addition to clinical efficacy, telehealth may reduce costs for some clients and interventions, particularly if in-person services require significant therapist time and travel (Cason, 2009). Costs may also be reduced in long-term monitoring of chronic health conditions (Jacobs et al., 2012).

Overall, clients are satisfied with telehealth services (Jacobs et al., 2012). It can improve access to services, reduce costs, and improve communication with professionals (Jacobs et al., 2012). Clinicians are also generally satisfied by service delivery by telehealth, although they may be more affected by challenges managing the telecommunication technology than their clients (Jacobs et al., 2012).

Selecting Telehealth

The decision to use telehealth with occupational therapy clients must be based on sound clinical reasoning and must utilize the best available evidence for effective service provision. It enables occupational therapy services for clients who otherwise might experience significant access barriers, and who will, in the best judgment of the occupational therapist, positively benefit from services provided through telecommunication technologies.

Cason (2012a) presents three main reasons to select telehealth occupational therapy services for a client. This service delivery model may (1) enable clients to receive services when there are significant barriers to in-person services, (2) allow consultation with "expert practitioners with specialized knowledge and skills" (Cason, 2012a, p. CE2), and (3) provide occupational therapy services in the natural contexts and environments of the client. First, barriers to receiving in-person services may include a shortage of occupational therapy professionals in a given location, distance to services, difficulty with transportation to services, and a client's preference for discreet evaluation or services (Cason, 2012a). Second, telehealth allows clients and generalist occupational therapy professionals to consult with expert practitioners in order to provide more specialized care (Cason, 2012a). An added benefit to this specialized consultation process is the potential for increasing the knowledge and ability of generalist occupational therapy professionals; this may be particularly helpful when generalists are working in areas where specialized clinicians are not readily available. Third, telehealth also affords the opportunity to work with clients in their natural contexts and environments. This can enhance occupational therapy services by helping a client apply new strategies and adaptations to their daily occupations and natural settings. For example, telehealth may be used for in-home consultation regarding falls prevention and other modifications for older adults who wish to age in place.

It is important to keep in mind that telehealth may present particular barriers to certain clients and practitioners, and therefore is not a panacea for clients who are long distances from in-person services. Individuals who have difficulty utilizing telecommunication technology, maintaining such technology, or sustaining participation when utilizing such technology may not be ideal candidates for telehealth services (AOTA, 2010c).

Technology

The ability to deliver telehealth occupational therapy services is undergirded by the telecommunications technology selected. Technology can range from telephone use, to asynchronous communication through voice or written memos, to face-to-face live interaction utilizing cameras by both therapists and clients. The latter is the most akin to in-person occupational therapy service delivery and therefore may be most satisfactory to many clients and therapists. Today, the cameras utilized are often Web based and rely on wireless or Internet access, computer and camera hardware, and some type of Web camera communication software. Clients may have the ability to use their own home computers and Web cameras; others may benefit from another service provider's access to these resources; still others may travel short distances to telehealth centers set up by their state's public health department (Cason, 2009).

As with any technology, telecommunication technologies can present opportunities for, but also sometimes challenges to, communication. For example, the speed of an Internet connection can determine whether the video and audio communication between therapist and client are seamless and efficient or halting and time-consuming. Additionally, difficulty with hardware or software can present challenges on either side of the telehealth communication partnership. It is helpful to have technical support available to both parties before and during the scheduled sessions. It is important to note that this technical support should be involved only to problem solve any technical issues. In order to maintain client confidentiality and privacy, occupational therapy services such as assessment and intervention should be provided when only the therapist and client are present.

Occupational therapy practitioners can benefit from understanding the technology requirements of the telecommunication technologies they will use in providing telehealth services (AOTA, 2010c). They may engage in formal or informal training with more experienced telehealth providers or with technical support staff (AOTA, 2005). Finally, occupational therapy professionals who wish to become experts in providing telehealth services can seek out mentorship from other professionals who are advanced in their use of telecommunication technologies and knowledge of best practice and evidence in telehealth (AOTA, 2010b).

Legal Considerations

It is important to be aware of legal considerations before engaging in telehealth. Such considerations include appropriate state licensure, state laws, and insurance for providing occupational therapy through telecommunication technologies. Current consensus indicates that occupational therapy professionals must be licensed in the state where they are physically located as well as in the states where their clients are located (AOTA, 2010c; Brennan et al., 2010). For example, if a therapist in Virginia is working with a client in West Virginia, the therapist must be licensed in West Virginia as well as Virginia in order to provide such services legally.

In addition to licensure, occupational therapy professionals should check with the state laws in any states where they are providing telehealth services. It is critical to know any rules and regulations guiding the provision of services, and whether it is legal to provide occupational therapy services through telecommunication technologies.

Finally, occupational therapy professionals should work with their employers and insurers to determine the extent of coverage for professional liability, malpractice, and other applicable forms of insurance. It is important to be clear with insurers about how telehealth services are provided and whether they will be provided to clients in the same or different state as the location of the occupational therapy professional.

Ethical Considerations

Using telehealth as a service delivery model for occupational therapy necessitates consideration of two main categories of ethics: those pertaining to the profession generally and those related to telehealth specifically. As in all areas of practice, occupational therapy professionals must adhere to the code of ethics related to their professional organization; certification and/or licensure; and national, state, and/or local regulations. For example, in the United States, occupational therapy professionals are guided by AOTA's Code of Ethics and Ethic Standards (AOTA, 2010a). The main elements of this code and set of standards are beneficence, nonmaleficence, autonomy and confidentiality, social justice, procedural justice, veracity, and fidelity.

There are aspects of the AOTA Code of Ethics and Ethical Standards (AOTA, 2010a) that have particular resonance when utilizing a telehealth service delivery model. In terms of caring for others (beneficence), occupational therapy professionals are obligated to practice telehealth only if it is within their range of competence (Principle 1.E), if it utilizes best available evidence (Principle 1.F), and if they have current knowledge of this service delivery model and are able to "weigh potential for client harm when generally recognized standards do not exist in emerging technology or areas of practice" (Principle 1.G; AOTA, 2010a, p. S19). In terms of not causing harm to clients (i.e., nonmaleficence), telehealth may be a way to "ensure continuity of services or options for transition to appropriate services to avoid abandoning the service recipient if the current provider is unavailable due to medical or other absence or loss of employment" (Principle 2.B; AOTA, 2010a, p. S20).

In terms of autonomy and confidentiality, an occupational therapy professional should be sure to provide clients receiving services through telehealth delivery with "disclosure of the benefits, risks, and potential outcomes of any intervention" (Principle 3.A; AOTA, 2010a, p. S21), including those delivered via telehealth. Particularly critical when using telecommunication technologies in telehealth is to ensure the privacy and confidentiality of clients (Principles 3.G and 3.H). Encrypted telecommunication across interfaces such as the Internet are important to ensure the security, privacy, and confidentiality of clients (Chiu & Henderson, 2005) and compliance with Health Insurance Portability and Accountability Act (HIPAA) regulations (Cason & Brannon, 2011). It is also essential that only individuals given permission by the client to participate in the session, such as therapist, client, and family members, are able to participate. Therefore, for example, although there may be technical support staff available to troubleshoot telecommunication technology issues in real time with the therapist and client, they are not included in the actual session's therapeutic interaction and conversation between therapist and client.

The use of telehealth to deliver occupational therapy services and its ability to reach underserved populations resonates particularly strongly with the ethical principle of social justice. One particular aspect of this social justice is making "efforts to advocate for recipients of occupational therapy services to obtain needed services through available means" (Principle 4.E; AOTA, 2010a, p. S22); one such mean may be through telehealth. In delivering such services, it is critical that not only ethical standards but also procedural justice principles are addressed, including meeting any legal obligations (e.g., institutional policies, state licensure, national certification) and reimbursement regulations.

Reimbursement

Reimbursement for services rendered through telehealth may vary for type of service provider, clients, and clients' health insurers. For example, although some states' Medicaid programs reimburse for occupational therapy delivered through telehealth, Medicare does not provide reimbursement for telehealth occupational therapy services at this time (Cason & Brannon, 2011). The Department of Defense and the Veterans Administration do currently provide funding for some occupational therapy telehealth services to active military and veterans, respectively (Cason, 2012a). Some third-party insurance companies will reimburse for telehealth services; however, it is critical to determine whether occupational therapy practitioners can deliver telehealth services, and if there are only certain services delivered by telehealth that will be reimbursed. Finally, it is important to be sure that when services are delivered through telecommunication technologies, that they are billed accordingly under telehealth codes (AOTA, 2010c; Brennan et al., 2010).

Summary

Telehealth is a viable, efficacious, cost-effective service delivery model for occupational therapy. It is particularly useful for clients who might not otherwise be able to access occupational therapy services in person. This chapter defined telehealth, described current research and practice areas utilizing telehealth, and discussed legal, ethical, and reimbursement implications for using a telehealth service delivery model in occupational therapy practice. Of particular note is the ability of this emerging niche in occupational therapy practice to provide new ways for clients to access services. This service delivery model may therefore promote social justice (AOTA, 2010a) by adding to in-person services and facilitating the occupational engagement of at-a-distance individuals, organizations, and populations.

Suggested Web Sites

- American Occupational Therapy Association: www.aota.org
- American Telemedicine Association: www.americantelemed.org
- International Journal of Telerehabilitation: http://telerehab.pitt.edu
- Office for Advancement of Telehealth: www.hrsa.gov/telehealth/

EVIDENCE-BASED RESEARCH CHART

Topic	Evidence
AOTA's position on telehealth	AOTA, 2010c
AOTA statement on specialized knowledge and skills in technology	AOTA, 2010b
Developing telehealth services	Chiu & Henderson, 2005; Dreyer et al., 2001; Heimerl & Rasch, 2009
Efficacy of telehealth	Cason, 2009; Dreyer et al., 2001; Hermann et al., 2010; Jacobs et al., 2012; Steel et al., 2011

Student Self-Assessment

1. Consider a recent fieldwork experience. How could you translate this area of practice to a telehealth service delivery model? What would be the benefits of or barriers to such implementation?

2. List at least two areas of practice that are of interest to you. How could using telehealth increase the range of clients you would be able to serve in each area?

3. Imagine that in your first job, you advocate for the inclusion of telehealth as a service delivery model for your practice. Your manager asks you to create a presentation on this topic. How would you define telehealth? What evidence would you cite to argue for the implementation of telehealth?

4. Considering the scenario in #3, what state licensure, legal, ethical, and reimbursement considerations for utilizing telecommunication technologies would you include in your presentation?

References

Accreditation Council for Occupational Therapy Education. (2012). 2011 Accreditation Council for Occupational Therapy Education (ACOTE) standards. *American Journal of Occupational Therapy, 66,* S6-S74. doi: 10.5014/ajot.2012.66S6

American Occupational Therapy Association. (2005). Telerehabilitation position paper. *American Journal of Occupational Therapy, 59,* 656-660. doi: 10.5014/ajot.59.6.656

American Occupational Therapy Association. (2008). Occupational therapy practice framework: Domain and process (2nd ed.). *American Journal of Occupational Therapy, 62,* 625-683. doi: 10.5014/ajot.62.6.625

American Occupational Therapy Association. (2010a). Occupational therapy code of ethics and ethics standards. *American Journal of Occupational Therapy, 64,* S17-S26. doi: 10.5014/ajot.2010.64S17

American Occupational Therapy Association. (2010b). Specialized knowledge and skills in technology and environmental interventions for occupational therapy practice. *American Journal of Occupational Therapy, 64,* S44-S56. doi: 10.5014/ajot.2010.64S44

American Occupational Therapy Association. (2010c). Telerehabilitation. *American Journal of Occupational Therapy, 64,* S92-S102. doi: 10.5014/ajot.2010.64S92

American Occupational Therapy Association. (2013a). *Emerging niche: Telehealth.* Retrieved from http://www.aota.org/Practice/Rehabilitation-Disability/Emerging-Niche/Telehealth.aspx

American Occupational Therapy Association. (2013b). *Practice areas.* Retrieved from http://www.aota.org/Practice.aspx

Brennan, D. M., Tindall, L., Theodoros, D., Brown, J., Campbell, M., Christiana, D., ... Lee, A. (2010). A blueprint for telerehabilitation guidelines—October 2010. *Telemedicine and e-Health, 17,* 662-665. doi: 10.1089/tmj.2011.0036

Cason, J. (2009). A pilot telerehabilitation program: Delivering early intervention services to rural families. *International Journal of Telerehabilitation, 1*(1), 29-37. doi: 10.5195/ijt.2009.6007

Cason, J. (2012a). An introduction to telehealth as a service delivery model within occupational therapy. *OT Practice, 17*(7), CE1-CE7.

Cason, J. (2012b). Telehealth opportunities in occupational therapy through the Affordable Care Act. *American Journal of Occupational Therapy, 66,* 131-136. doi: 10.5014/ajot.2012.662001

Cason, J., & Brannon, J. A. (2011). Telehealth regulatory and legal considerations: Frequently asked questions. *International Journal of Telerehabilitation, 3*(2), 15-18. doi: 10.5195/ijt.2011.6077

Chiu, T., & Henderson, J. (2005). Developing Internet-based occupational therapy services. *American Journal of Occupational Therapy, 59,* 626-630. doi: 10.5014/ajot.59.6.626

Dreyer, N. C., Dreyer, K. A., Shaw, D. K., & Wittman, P. P. (2001). Efficacy of telemedicine in occupational therapy: A pilot study. *Journal of Allied Health, 30*(1), 39-42.

Foto, M. (1996). Presidential address—trends, tools, and technology. *American Journal of Occupational Therapy, 50,* 619-625. doi: 10.5014/ajot.50.8.619

Foto, M. (1997). Preparing occupational therapists for the year 2000: The impact of managed care on education and training. *American Journal of Occupational Therapy, 51,* 88-90. doi: 10.5014/ajot.51.2.88

Health Resources and Services Administration. (2012). *Telehealth*. Retrieved from http://www.hrsa.gov/telehealth/

Heimerl, S., & Rasch, N. C. (2009, September). Delivery developmental occupational therapy consultation services through telehealth. *Developmental Disabilities Special Interest Section Quarterly, 32*(3), 1-4.

Hermann, V. H., Herzog, M., Jordan, R., Hofherr, M., Levine, P., & Page, S. J. (2010). Telerehabilitation and electrical stimulation: An occupation-based, client-centered stroke intervention. *American Journal of Occupational Therapy, 64,* 73-81. doi: 10.5014/ajot.64.1.73

Holberg, C., & Finlayson, M. (2007). Factors influencing the use of energy conservation strategies by persons with multiple sclerosis. *American Journal of Occupational Therapy, 61,* 96-107. doi: 10.5014/ajot.61.1.96

Jacobs, K., Blanchard, B., & Baker, N. (2012). Telehealth and ergonomics: A pilot study. *Technology and Health Care, 20,* 445-458. doi: 10.3233/THC-2012-0692

Steel, K., Cox, D., & Garry, H. (2011). Therapeutic videoconferencing interventions for the treatment of long-term conditions. *Journal of Telemedicine and Telecare, 17,* 109-117. doi: 10.1258/jtt.2010.100318

Teleheath Advancement Act of 2011. (2011). *Assembly Bill No. 415.* Retrieved from http://www.leginfo.ca.gov/pub/11-12/bill/asm/ab_0401-0450/ab_415_bill_20111007_chaptered.pdf

VII

MANAGEMENT OF
OCCUPATIONAL THERAPY SERVICES

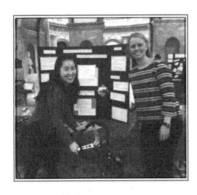

39

LAWS, CREDENTIALS, AND REIMBURSEMENT

Dory E. Holmes, MPH, OTR/L and Lisa L. Clark, MS, OTR/L, CLT

ACOTE STANDARDS EXPLORED IN THIS CHAPTER
B.6.2, B.7.1, B.7.2, B.7.4

KEY VOCABULARY

- **Affordable Care Act:** Known as Patient Protection and Affordable Care Act, P/L/ 111-148 is referred to as "federal health reform." The provision is to expand access to insurance, increase consumer protection, emphasize wellness and prevention, and improve system performance.
- **Case mix groups:** A patient classification system to group patients with similar characteristics and in terms of resources used during care.
- **Durable medical equipment:** Reusable medical equipment such as walkers, wheelchairs, and hospital beds. It must be medically necessary and is prescribed by a physician, nurse practitioner, physician assistant, or clinical nurse specialist.

- **Prospective payment system:** Method of reimbursement in which payment is made on predetermined, fixed amounts. It was established in 1983 to address increasing inpatient hospital costs and now extends to acute rehabilitation, home health, and skilled. It is based on codes coded to a client's bill.
- **Resource utilization group (RUG):** A patient classification system that categorizes skilled nursing home patients by functional status and anticipated use of services and resources. The RUG score is used to determine a per diem rate of reimbursement.
- **Utilization review:** A process that reviews requests for medical treatment. It is a safeguard against unnecessary and inappropriate medical care.

Jacobs, K., MacRae, N., & Sladyk, K. (Eds.).
Occupational Therapy Essentials for Clinical Competence, Second Edition (pp. 519-532).
© 2014 SLACK Incorporated.

Introduction

Twenty-five years ago, it was considered somewhat unethical for an occupational therapist or occupational therapy assistant to ask about a client's reimbursement mechanism. In the last few years, it has become increasingly common to ask and to be aware of how occupational therapy services will be compensated. Indeed, it is almost unethical now not to have information about payment. Many hospitals, outpatient settings, and private practices hire people whose sole purpose in the organization is to access reimbursement information. The practitioner is expected to maximize this reimbursement for the client's benefit. This information is now added to the already existent complexities in providing care to consumers in this evidence-based health system. This chapter introduces the basics of reimbursement systems. It is important to understand that for every rule, there is an exception, and for every payment system, there is a large amount of additional information that cannot be included in an introductory chapter.

For new practitioners, the world of payment can be overwhelming. However, the following is a simple formula to consider:

- Reimbursement = Location of Service + Coding + Documentation + Payer

Each section of the formula will be discussed in this chapter.

Reimbursement

Reimbursement is the fee received for a service rendered. That fee may be paid in several ways: a fee schedule, fee-for-service, discounts, per diem rate, or per episode of care rate. Fees are based on a formula and may be paid in many different ways. These formulas consist of a relative value unit (RVU) and a monetary conversion factor. Components of the RVU are the following: time used by the provider, expenses of running a practice, and professional liability expenses. The conversion factors are determined by geographic cost differences. Set by agreement between the contractor/facility (provider) of service and the payer, the reimbursement payment is typically determined in advance.

Location of Service

It is occupational therapy's good fortune that services are reimbursed today in so many settings. From hospitals, skilled nursing facilities, outpatient settings, home health and community settings, schools, and private practice, the occupational therapist is viewed as a skilled professional health care provider. These various locations have separate and distinct regulatory rules that govern the facilities' operation, billing, and reimbursement practices. The sites of service are examined in depth in this chapter.

Coding

Coding is fundamental to reimbursement (Practice Management Information Corporation [PMIC], 2005). It can involve three parts: the diagnosis code (International Classification of Diseases, Ninth Revision, Clinical Modification, ICD-9-CM), procedural code (current procedural terminology [CPT]), and procedure code (Healthcare Common Procedure Coding System [HCPCS]). The primary diagnosis determination is the responsibility of the physician. Occupational therapy practitioners do not typically set the diagnosis code. These diagnosis codes are found in the ICD-9-CM manual (PMIC, 2005). The ICD-9 manual categorizes a client's medical condition by anatomical systems. Coding must match the diagnosis written on the physician's referral/prescription. You or your facility/agency will be ensuring that this is on the bill.

Occupational therapy practitioners should become very familiar with the CPT. CPT codes are the primary set of codes practitioners use and should understand (Centers for Medicare & Medicaid Services [CMS], 2006a). They help allocate charges to the occupational therapy intervention program. The CPT manual provides a uniform language for reliable national communication and makes reporting easier (American Medical Association [AMA], 2005). It facilitates claims processing, guides medical review, and contributes to education and research (Fearon, 2004).

Within the CPT manual is a chapter titled "Physical Medicine and Rehabilitation." The Physical Medicine and Rehabilitation codes describe the majority of interventions provided by occupational therapy personnel. Occupational therapy personnel may also use the HCPCS-II codes. These codes describe supplies, procedures, and services not listed in the CPT manual. An example would be the "L" codes, which are used for orthotics and splinting services billing.

Documentation

As noted in the chapter on documentation (Chapter 22), written documentation is the true and legal record of the occupational therapy evaluation, plan of care, interventions, and outcomes. It is a tool to support and manage reimbursement. The occupational therapy practitioner's documentation will be examined by auditors or reviewers for the following (Fearon, 2004):

- Medical necessity
- Appropriateness of interventions for the diagnosis

- Appropriate frequency and duration for a client's rehabilitation potential
- Expectation of functional improvement
- The client's response to the service
- The level of staff rendering the service

The documentation, whether narrative or computerized, must support the codes billed to receive the payment expected (AMA, 2006). It must be concise, clear, and should minimize abbreviations. Different plans may have specific documentation criteria such as requiring specific forms or mandating a schedule for progress updates. They may also require preapproval for the stay and limit the length of stay according to setting. On a rare occasion, a client's insurance plan may not pay for occupational therapy services. Therefore, it is important to ascertain the coverage that is (and is not) provided with each policy. Under most circumstances, it is the provider who is responsible for knowing whether the service is covered. Payers' expectations are that documentation justifies the purpose of occupational therapy and reports the benefits of the intervention specific to the client's goals. Therefore, learning the documentation for each setting is essential.

Payer

Occupational therapy is a commonly covered benefit. The common payment sources are Medicare, Medicaid, private health insurance, Workers' Compensation, and federally funded programs such as for veterans, railroad workers, and other federal employees. These payers will reimburse for "skilled" therapy. Skilled means that the intervention requires the unique professional abilities of occupational therapy personnel. Simply stated, only an occupational therapist or occupational therapy assistant under the supervision of an occupational therapist can safely and effectively provide the complexity of service. The occupational therapy practitioner should never assume coverage and should always inquire about a client's benefit. It is sometimes helpful for practitioners to think about their educational backgrounds. At times, some interventions may seem to be "common sense"; however, when reflecting on the requirements of occupational therapy educational programs, it becomes clear that a significant background of information and study is what led the practitioner to the conclusion about an intervention or recommendation.

One example of the importance of understanding reimbursement is Medicare, which is divided into Part A and Part B. Part A covers inpatient hospitals, home health agencies (HHAs), and skilled nursing facilities. Part B, a voluntary and supplemental benefit, covers physician services, outpatient services, and durable medical equipment (American Occupational Therapy Association [AOTA],2005). It is possible that a client could have coverage for occupational therapy in settings covered by Part A but not Part B. Often, individuals make insurance coverage choices and decisions based on the ability to pay without realizing what might be forfeited in the long term. In addition, Medicare is managed regionally via "intermediaries"—insurance companies contracted to review and manage Medicare expenditures. Facility billing may go to the regional intermediary, so there is a possible range of interpretation of reimbursement rules for Medicare based on each intermediary.

Another example of the need for the practitioner to be informed about benefits is illustrated in Medicaid programs, which are administered by individual states. Because Medicaid is funded jointly by the state and federal governments, the federal government mandates that states provide a minimum set of specific services. Regrettably, occupational therapy is an "optional" service in these mandates and may not be covered in the state where you work.

A third example of practice limitations is Tricare, the federal insurance program for active military. Occupational therapy is defined in the Tricare Policy Manual (Tricare, 2008). Practitioners must be aware of how services are defined so as to practice and document in a way that follows payer guidelines. Tricare has selected CPT codes they approve for reimbursement. Notably, they exclude vocational assessment and training, sensory integration training, and cognitive retraining, despite the fact that these are within occupational therapy's scope of practice.

In an effort to control national health expenditures, the majority of the payers today are managed. Health care expenditures spiraled upward as a result of an increasing population, expansion of health care personnel, the explosion of medical technology, pharmaceutical advances, and the growth in financing of health care (Bernstein et al., 2003). Therefore, managed care was created to decrease the growing cost of national health care expenditures and to keep the Medicare Trust Fund solvent. Regardless of the payer group, all managed care systems possess some or all of the following characteristics: precertification, preauthorization, concurrent review, utilization review, and pre-discharge planning. These concepts are reviewed as we examine the various settings in the continuum of care.

Occupational therapy practitioners should possess a grounded understanding of the basics of reimbursement. They should also understand that it is important to access information directly from original sources to the extent possible. At times, even employers and billing supervisors cannot follow the intricacies of every system. If a practitioner has a question, he or she should take the time to get to the source and find someone who will explain the issue in understandable language. Although intimidating, asking for information to be clear and understandable is not an unreasonable request. Regardless of payer, the occupational therapy practitioner's focus is on skilled intervention. The practitioner is ethically bound to provide services that are reasonable and necessary.

Now that some basics of reimbursement concepts have been introduced, this chapter continues with discussion about payment options typically available in each setting within the continuum of care. Introductory reimbursement information is highlighted for each practice setting. This organizes the information in a way that mirrors how practitioners must understand it in the context of practice settings.

Acute Hospital Care

Hospitals are the cornerstone of the American health care system. They differ in size, ownership, mission, financing, and population served. All hospitals are designed to serve communities on a bed-to-population ratio. Some types of hospitals include community hospitals, teaching hospitals, specialty hospitals, public hospitals, and multihospital systems. Hospitals consume 31% of national health care expenditures (Cowan, Catlin, Smith, & Sensenig, 2004). They focus on client care as well as cost-containment, decreasing length of stay, managing utilization of resources, and staff performance. Regardless of type, the mission of any hospital is curing and caring. Hospitals are licensed by the individual states and may voluntarily participate in regulatory accreditations as Joint Commission on Accreditation of Healthcare Organizations (JCAHO) and Commission on Accreditation of Rehabilitation Facilities (CARF). Individual state licensing may require that occupational therapy is provided as a service.

Medicare

With the increasing number of elderly in all our communities, the predominant payer for hospital care is Medicare. As mentioned previously, inpatient hospital stays are paid by Part A. Medicare is a federally funded program that is available to people ages M65 and older, individuals with disabilities and their dependents, and those with chronic kidney disease.

Occupational therapy services are "bundled" into an inclusive rate that Medicare pays the hospital. This daily rate is based on the person's diagnosis. Medicare has designed "diagnosis related groups" (DRGs), which take into consideration how much medical care a person usually needs given each particular diagnosis. The payment is to cover the usual and customary hospital stay. If the person needs to stay longer than usual, the hospital may lose money. If the person is able to leave the hospital and return home, or move to another level of care earlier than usual, the hospital may make money on the stay. Occupational therapy is part of what the hospital provides, for which they receive a payment related to the diagnostic group under which the client falls.

Medicaid

Medicaid is the state and federally funded program for health care. Each state has its own program. There are federal guidelines that mandate a minimum set of services that states must provide with their Medicaid programs (CMS, 2005a). As noted previously, occupational therapy falls under "optional" services, meaning individual states may decide whether their Medicaid programs will cover occupational therapy services. Not all states have opted for occupational therapy coverage. Practitioners must learn about their own states' coverage in order to practice knowledgeably. They can do this via their state occupational therapy membership organizations, or they can get on their states' Web sites and search for occupational therapy- and rehabilitation-covered services.

Private Health Insurance

Hospitals have contractual agreements with the various private health insurance companies. Contracts typically denote a percent discount on the cost of care, a fee schedule, and/or a predetermined payment amount for an episode of care. Inpatient acute care that is managed may require precertification for someone to be admitted from the emergency room to the hospital or to have a surgical procedure performed. While an inpatient, the individual's case is monitored by an external case manager who is reviewing the medical record for daily progress. Utilization review often occurs internally and examines the efficiency of the facility or how services are being utilized. Pre-discharge planning will coordinate the transfer of the client to the next level of care. These subsequent locations usually also have contracts with the payer.

Inpatient Rehabilitation Facilities

Inpatient rehabilitation facilities (IRFs) are either free-standing hospitals or rehabilitation units in acute care hospitals. Their role is to provide intensive rehabilitation services for an inpatient population. IRFs differ from acute care hospitals because of their focus on function and rehabilitation. Clients who are admitted must be able to tolerate 3 hours of intense therapy per day. Occupational therapy is identified as one of those essential services for a client's recovery.

MEDICARE

Just like the acute care hospital, which is paid by Part A, an IRF is reimbursed on a predetermined rate system that classifies client discharges into categories called the case mix groups (CMGs; CMS, 2006b). These are based on the top most common diagnostic groups admitted to IRFs. The CMG is based on "rehabilitation impairment categories, functional state (both motor and cognitive), age, and other comorbidities. The CMG determines the payment the facility receives for an episode of care.

On admission, data are collected on the client using the Minimum Data Set for Post-Acute Care (MDS-PAC) client assessment instrument. The assessment instrument emphasizes client care needs. With reimbursing of the facility based on the resources used, the CMG is designed just like the DRG that is used in acute hospital care. The focus is on efficiency and coordinating the care within a timeframe. IRFs also operate under the "75% Rule." This means a certain percentage of the facilities' admissions must require intensive multidisciplinary rehabilitation services. This compliance percentage was designed to ensure that IRFs are distinct from other levels of care (i.e., acute care or skilled care).

MEDICAID

Medicaid is seldom the primary payer on a rehabilitation unit. There are instances where it is used as a secondary payer.

PRIVATE HEALTH INSURANCE

This payer responds similarly in the IRF setting as it does in the skilled nursing facility (SNF).

Skilled Nursing Facilities

Occupational therapy services are very often provided in SNF settings. The SNFs are typically designed to take clients who are medically stable but require additional ancillary and/or nursing care. They are designed to transition the client to a community setting, home, or to a lower level of care such as a long-term care setting. In the mid- to late 1980s, SNFs were the fastest growing settings for the employment of occupational therapy practitioners (Kane, Chen, Blewett, & Sangl, 1996; Figure 39-1). In 1985, 55.7% of the nursing homes in the United States offered occupational therapy services, rising to 87.2% in 1995, and then to 94% in 1999 (Bernstein et al., 2003). This growth was attributed to payment policies reducing acute hospital stays (Torrens, 1993), improvement in technological and pharmaceutical advances, and the passage of the Balanced Budget Act (BBA) of 1997.

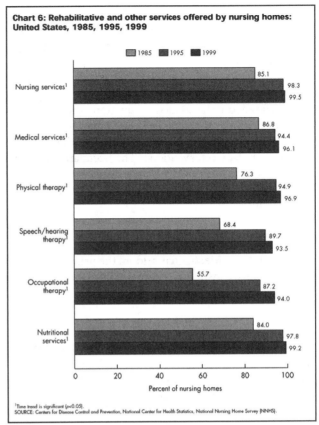

Figure 39-1. Rehabilitative and other services offered by nursing homes: United States, 1985, 1995, 1999. (Reproduced with permission from the National Center for Health Statistics.)

MEDICARE

Partly as a result of this growth, Medicare (which is the primary payer for rehabilitation in this setting) decided that costs needed to be controlled. The BBA of 1997 was passed and significantly changed how payment was made to these facilities. Medicare enacted a Prospective Payment System (PPS) in 1999 as a result of the BBA. Prior to 1999, sites were reimbursed retrospectively via a formula including how much it cost them to provide rehabilitation services. With the onset of PPS, payments were made based on a daily rate (per diem).

This rate is figured by performing an assessment (minimum data set [MDS]) for the client that helps determine the resources needed to serve him or her. The client is then placed in a resource utilization group (RUG) category. This must be based on how much service he or she appears to need (CMS, 2005b). Occupational therapists sometimes assist in the determination of which RUG the client will fall under. The RUG is important, as it determines the per diem payment rate the skilled nursing facility will receive for the client's stay. The RUG is directly related to the total number of minutes of therapy the consumer receives for the week. This is a total of the weekly minutes occupational, physical, and speech therapists have spent with the person. Therefore, it behooves the facility from a financial standpoint to offer therapies seven days per week (CMS, 2009a).

It is important for therapists to consider the ethical dimensions of deciding the amount of therapy a patient needs, based on the skilled evaluation, the therapist's scope of practice, and state licensure laws about practice responsibilities. These factors should be the primary driver of therapy interventions. The occupational therapist should also be ethically knowledgeable as to how the practice considerations will mesh with the business needs of the facility.

Medicaid

As with IRFs, Medicaid is seldom the primary payer in SNFs. There are instances where it is used as a secondary payer.

Private Health Insurance

As noted in the acute hospital section, a client may have been transferred to a specific SNF because of contractual agreements. The therapy plan of care will need to be reviewed by a case manager to determine if it is reasonable and necessary. Often the length of stay is determined by the diagnosis and limits of the plan. Progress notes will be reviewed concurrently by the external reviewers and internal utilization review team. Occupational therapy practitioners may find that durable medical equipment (DME) purchases may be made only through vendors who are approved by the insurance company and who may not be local.

Home Health Care

Home is the setting of choice for recuperation for many individuals, and it has become an integral part in the continuum of comprehensive health care. It integrates health, social, and supportive services that nurture the health and well-being of an individual. The passage of the BBA of 1997 had the opposite effect on HHAs as it did with SNFs. During the time when the utilization of SNFs was growing, HHAs experienced a reduction in the length of time clients remained in home health care and the average number of visits.

Medicare

Eligibility for home care is clearly defined in the Medicare Part A regulations. The client must meet four qualifying criteria. The individual must be the following (CMS, 2005c):
1. Homebound

2. Require intermittent skilled services
3. Have a physician-established plan of care
4. The HHA must be Medicare certified

The definition of homebound is critical. It has the following five components (CMS, 2005c):
1. A defined place of residence
2. Normal inability to leave home
3. Leaving takes considerable and taxing effort
4. Absences are infrequent and of short duration
5. The client may attend a certified/licensed day care program

Absences from the home should be of short duration and include, for example, attending a religious service; occasional trip to physician or barber; or a unique event such as a family reunion, funeral, or graduation.

Place of residence is defined as a house/apartment, an assisted living facility, group home, or a relative's home. Services cannot take place in a hospital, SNF, or long-term care facility. "Inability to leave home" means that leaving is medically contradicted, and it requires a supportive device or support from another. By definition, taxing effort to leave the home results in shortness of breath, dyspnea on exertion, or weakness.

Homebound status is evaluated on admission and throughout the episode of care. An HHA uses the Outcome and Assessment Information Set (OASIS), which sets the payment rate for each 60 days of service. Rates are based on skilled need. After a period of time, the client may switch from Medicare Part A coverage to his or her Part B benefits. Skilled need must include intermittent skilled nursing, physical therapy, speech pathology, or a continued need for occupational therapy. Only nursing, physical therapy, or speech pathology can initially qualify a client for home care services. Qualifying means that the client must have at least one of these three needs prior to receiving occupational therapy. Once the case is established, occupational therapy can continue as a sole service. The plan of care must be certified by the physician, and the course of care must have a finite and predictable ending period.

Medicaid

Medicaid is most often a secondary payer for home health services, if accessed at all, and not a primary payer. Some states have created certain provisions for Medicaid reimbursement for certain populations, such as children.

Private Health Insurance

Each private health insurance policy or managed care policy will allow for different amounts (duration/payment rates) of home health care or may not provide for care in the home setting at all. The occupational therapy practitioner must know what each policy will cover.

Outpatient Services

The delivery of outpatient services can be confusing for the new practitioner because of rules pertaining to licensing, site of service, and ownership. Originally envisioned to be delivered in private practice, outpatient services have expanded into multiservice agencies such as Medicare Part B nursing facilities, home health agencies, outpatient rehabilitation facilities, comprehensive outpatient rehab facilities (CORFs), or hospital outpatient departments (HOPDs). Many third party insurers use the Medicare guidelines; however, there are exceptions. Because the majority do, personnel authorized to provide outpatient therapy services under Medicare are defined as physical therapists, occupational therapists, speech-language pathologists, physicians, nonphysician practitioners ([NPPs]; e.g., physician assistants, nurse practitioners, clinical nurse specialists), and qualified physical and occupational therapy assistants who are supervised. Personnel not authorized to provide occupational therapy outpatient therapy services are aides, athletic trainers, massage therapists, exercise physiologists, recreational therapists, kinesiotherapists, low vision specialists, lymphedema specialists, Pilates instructors, rehab technicians, and life skills trainers. Students can participate in the provision of care but services are not reimbursable under Medicare.

MEDICARE

Regardless of setting, occupational therapy is paid for by procedure on the Medicare fee schedule. Medicare will pay 80% of the fee after the client has paid the annual deductible. Medicare administration has developed local coverage determination (LCD) policies to interpret the provisions as they apply to different geographic jurisdictions. The LCD includes consideration for local and regional practice norms. Occupational therapy services are payable under the following conditions (CMS, 2013):

- Medically necessary.
- A plan for furnishing services has been established by a physician/NPP. An NPP is a physician assistant, clinical nurse specialist, or nurse practitioner. The physician must be a doctor of medicine, osteopathy, podiatric medicine, or optometry. Doctors of dental surgery, dental medicine, or chiropractors cannot refer or establish a plan of care under Medicare Part B.

- The individual is under the care of a physician.
- Care is provided on an outpatient basis.

Reimbursement of a therapy claim is provided when an outpatient plan of care for therapy is certified by a physician/NPP every 90 days (CMS, 2008). CMS requires regular updates about progress that have been reviewed by the physician/NPP for the initial certification and ongoing certification process, respectively. These must be completed by an occupational therapist and not an occupational therapy assistant. The therapist must be able to produce required approved documentation intervention information for the Medicare intermediary upon request.

As noted earlier in this chapter, BBA of 1997 attempted to level reimbursement methods across the various sites of service (i.e., inpatient hospital/DRG, inpatient rehabilitation hospitals/CMG, skilled facilities/RUGS, and home health agencies/OASIS). However, a standardized method for outpatient began in October 2012 (Center for Medicare & Medicaid Services, 2012). This standardization came in three phases. The first phase was that all entities began on the medical provider fee schedule (MPFS). The second phase was the therapy cap (CAP): The annual financial limitation placed on a Medicare beneficiary for a calendar year. Initially, the therapy caps applied only to private practice; however, the BBA of 1997 eventually extended CAP to nursing homes, HHAs, outpatient rehab facilities, and CORFs. HOPDs remained the exception. Currently, in 2013, the therapy cap for occupational therapy is $1,900.00. A combined cap of $1,900.00 exists for physical and speech therapy. The third phase of standardization was the exception process, which was enacted in the Deficit Reduction Act of 2005. The exception process is a mechanism for a patient to continue to receive needed outpatient services above the CAP. Providers place a –KX modifier on a CPT code to request an exception. The –KX modifier indicates that the therapy is reasonable and necessary and that there is documentation in the patient's chart to support the need. Again, all outpatient providers had been using this coding system except HOPDs.

Finally, the Middle Class Tax Relief and Job Creation Act (MCTRJCA) of 2012 finalized standardization and brought HOPDs under the same rules. Starting in October, 2012, hospitals from all over the country were phased into the system. This act also established a manual review process for claims over $3,700.00. Therapists need to submit a preapproval request for up to 20 visits. The act also implemented a new claims-based data collection system on function. The data are a prerequisite to building a bundles payment system on an episode of care. Ultimately, all sites of service will be on some sort of case-mix payment.

Comprehensive Outpatient Rehabilitation Facilities

"A CORF [comprehensive outpatient rehabilitation facility] is a facility that engages in diagnostic, therapeutic, and restorative services to outpatients for the rehabilitation of the injured and disabled or to clients recovering from illness" (CMS, 2004). It is located in an outpatient setting and the program must be comprehensive, coordinated, and skilled. Minimum services required by regulation are physicians' services, physical therapy, and social or psychological services. Occupational therapy is considered a skilled service, but it is optional. Most CORFs employ occupational therapy practitioners.

MEDICARE

CORF services are paid under Medicare Part B. Payment is made under the Medicare Physician Fee Schedule (MPFS) for all services except biologicals (i.e., specialized wound dressings) and drugs. It is mandated by Medicare that adequate space and equipment are provided for any service offered. Generally, all services must be delivered onsite. Exceptions are home evaluations, physical therapy, occupational therapy, and speech-language pathology. Home assessments occur in the client's residence. Coverage is limited to the services of only one professional who is selected by the CORF.

MEDICAID AND PRIVATE HEALTH INSURANCE

For information regarding Medicaid and private insurances, refer to the following section. The mechanisms are similar for both settings.

Outpatient—Hospital-Based

As cost containment and prospective payment have reduced hospital stays, more hospital services are delivered in outpatient settings, often called "ambulatory care." Subsequently, outpatient therapy departments have experienced enormous growth over the last decade. These therapy departments can offer a single service or provide multidisciplinary interventions. For an occupational therapy practitioner, these settings offer opportunities for those who are generalists or specialists.

MEDICARE

Outpatient occupational therapy services are reimbursed by Medicare Part B. However, depending on the service site, reimbursement can pay for two distinct sets of services. Occupational therapy personnel can work in either behavioral health partial hospitalization programs (PHPs) or in physical rehabilitation outpatient therapy departments.

Clients eligible for Medicare Part B coverage of PHPs are those who were discharged from an inpatient psychiatric intervention program or those who, in absence of available partial hospitalization, would require inpatient hospitalization. The PHP can also be provided at a community mental health center. The reimbursement system that pays for partial hospitalization is called outpatient prospective payment system (OPPS). OPPS was designed for ambulatory care procedures and pays a per diem rate for the total resources used for a single outpatient visit. Occupational therapy can be one of those resources in a PHP, but it is not mandated. Although prevocational and vocational assessments are within the occupational therapy scope of practice, services related primarily to employment opportunities, work skills, or work settings are not covered.

Hospital outpatient occupational therapy departments are key to providing that continuum of care to recently hospitalized patients. Hospitals often have specialty outpatient clinics that complement physician practices and enable the patient to be monitored closely by their physician. Hospitals provide about 24% of all outpatient therapy services. Medicare has been its largest payer over the years. Now being included under the CAP and the start of the new G-code system, a more comprehensive reporting system of all outpatient providers can begin. This system fits into the goals and implementation of health care reform.

MEDICAID

Medicaid payments for outpatient occupational therapy services vary by state if the service is a covered service for that state. It is the practitioner's responsibility to acquire information about Medicaid payment in his or her state. If occupational therapy services are reimbursed, it is often at a reduced fee schedule or for a limited number of visits.

PRIVATE HEALTH INSURANCE

In the outpatient setting, the primary care physician is the gatekeeper to referrals and services. In most situations, the physician must make a request to the insurer for services. Once this is confirmed, the occupational therapy provider will evaluate the client and submit the plan of care to the insurer. The insurer will review for medical necessity and certify a specific number of visits within a timeframe. It is the provider's responsibility to track the number of visits and timeframe. Should the plan of care exceed the limits without prior authorization, the practitioner will not be reimbursed and it may become the client's responsibility to pay. The practitioner may use a variety of methods to track the number of visits or time frames, such as specialized scheduling systems, customized flow sheets for documentation, and appointment logs.

Outpatient—Private Practice

Clinics or practices owned by private individuals are considered to be private practices. To qualify as a private practice, an individual must be enrolled as a private practitioner and be employed in an unincorporated solo, partnership, or group practice; physician/NPP group that is not a professional corporation; or an occupational therapist employed by a physician/NPP group practice if state or local law permits. In addition, private practices could include therapists who are practicing therapy as employees of a supplier or a professional corporation. Occupational therapists in private practice provide only 1% of outpatient services.

Services are offered in the therapist's or group's office or a patient's home. The definition of "office" is the location(s) where the practice operates during the time that the therapist is treating at that location. If occupational therapy services are provided in a private office space, that space must be owned, leased, or rented by the practice and used for exclusive purpose of operating the practice (CMS, 2013).

These businesses often specialize in a particular area of rehabilitation, such as low vision, or even one or two particular areas of the occupational therapy scope of practice. Settings can vary widely in the services they offer—from wellness or alternative therapy sites to more traditional orthopedic or ergonomic interventions. Some practitioners act as private practices and contract their services out to schools or nursing homes, for example.

MEDICARE

All documentation, certification, and utilization guidelines pertain to private practice. In addition, private occupational therapy practitioners can participate in Medicare's Physician Quality Reporting system (PQRS). PQRS is a reporting system of selected Medicare quality measures. Medicare physicians; practitioners, such as physician assistants, nurse practitioners, social workers, and audiologists; and therapists, such as occupational therapists, can report on select measures or groups voluntary. If a provider reports, there is a financial incentive or bonus payment.

Practitioners who have private practices with Medicare reimbursement must apply for a National Provider Identifier (NPI) number through Medicare. An NPI is a 10-digit number that is intelligence free. Intelligence free means that the number contains no identifying information about the provider. No payment for services will be made without an assigned provider number. Medicare requires proof of a practitioner's credentials before they will issue a provider number.

MEDICAID

Providing occupational therapy services in a private practice and receiving Medicaid payment also requires that a provider number be procured from the state. Practitioners will need to ensure that occupational therapy is a reimbursed service in their state and research what services are paid for and at what rate. As a Medicaid provider, therapists should be aware that Medicaid has the right to perform an audit of the practice's financial records at any time.

PRIVATE HEALTH INSURANCE

Often these payers will negotiate contracts with private practices or clinics for a predetermined reimbursement amount. This amount can be based on the number of visits, amount paid per visit, or types of intervention that are approved.

Community Settings

Some community settings offer services that may be paid for on a "fee-for-service" basis. In this instance, the site decides the cost for each service and charges consumers accordingly. In these cases, consumers are funding their own health and wellness care.

School services are often covered by federal Department of Education funds. Legislation over the last 30 years has guaranteed the funding and dramatically changed the provision of services to young children. In 1975, The Education For All Handicapped Children Act (Cengage Learning, n.d.) guaranteed a free and appropriate public education for all handicapped children. Within the law, occupational therapy was defined as a "related " service because it enabled a child to access his or her education. Services needed to be educationally relevant for the school setting. In 1986, the law was amended to include special education and related services to handicapped preschoolers. This amendment focused on family training and education. The significance for our profession was that occupational therapy was clearly identified as a primary early intervention service.

The Individuals with Disabilities Education Act (IDEA) of 1990 was the new name for the 1975 act and was a reauthorization of the earlier commitment to public education for children with disabilities. It defined the minimum amount of services that a state must provide to various student groups (i.e., infants, toddlers, children, and older youth with disabilities). In 1997, IDEA was amended to include rights and protection for children with disabilities. It also stressed learning results for children (U.S. Department of Education, n.d.).

As the price of public education has increased with the expansions and federal education funds have been reduced, some states are also choosing to access Medicaid funds for eligible children in the schools. This can be complex, and practitioners will need to explore the regulations in each state.

Military Health Services

Our military health system is unique. The system is divided into two groups: active military and retired/disabled. The active military system provides health care wherever enlisted personnel are assigned. This can be anywhere around the world. It has a focus on wellness and is highly organized and integrated. The most unique feature of the military system is the master client record, which travels with the enlistee. The military has developed the most comprehensive medical record in the United States health system. Should a health issue become long-term and the enlistee cannot return to active duty, the individual receives a medical discharge and is referred to Veterans Affairs (VA). VA hospitals have seen a huge increase in clients as aging veterans have developed medical issues. Originally designed as hospitals, the VA facilities have experienced growth in their outpatient programs that parallels civilian health care.

Dependents and family members of active military have a separate health system that combines the active military system with the general health care system. Previously known as CHAMPUS (Civilian Health and Medical Program of the Uniformed Services), it is today called the U.S. Family Health Care Program. Dependents of military personnel receive routine services at military clinics and are referred to local community providers for specialty services. This system is managed and adheres to the Tricare provision of care.

Occupational therapy is an essential service in both military hospitals and VA hospitals. Therapists and assistants are serving around the globe. Although reimbursement is not the focus, our military health system was the first national movement toward managed care.

Affordable Care Act

U.S. health care spending has grown so much that it is outpacing the annual economic growth rate of the United States. With the coming of age of the Baby Boomers, Medicare has seen an increase in enrollment rates that will increase its spending. Individual states have seen a growth of their Medicaid budgets because of these sluggish economic conditions. The growth in personal out-of-pocket expenses has resulted from employers shifting more cost of health insurance onto their employees. Hospital costs have been spiraling with an increase in free care. Given the combination of all these factors with the growth of prescription drug spending, our health care system was not sustainable.

Reform of the payment and delivery system was identified as necessary. These reforms needed to include the expansion of access to care to 32 million Americans; evidence-based medicine and practice with a focus on quality and outcomes; and cost management. Ultimately, the federal Patient Protection and Affordable Care Act (P.L. 111-148) was signed March 23, 2010 and amended by the Health Care and Education Reconciliation Act signed March 31, 2010. This piece of legislation is commonly known as the Affordable Care Act (ACA), the "federal health reform," or Obamacare. "The Congressional Budget Office (CBO) has determined that the ACA will be fully paid; provide coverage for the limit that President Obama established; bend the health care cost curve, and reduce the deficit over the next ten years" (National Conference of State Legislatures [NCLS], 2011)

The ACA contains nine key elements and they are to be effective January 1, 2014. The highlights with examples are the following:

1. Quality, affordable health care for all Americans—market reform to eliminate discriminatory practices to preexisting condition exclusions

2. The role of public programs—expand eligibility to Medicaid

3. Improving the quality and efficiency of health care—creation of new patient care models

4. Prevention of chronic disease and improving public health—initiatives to develop healthy communities

5. Health care workforce—enhancing health care workforce education and training

6. Transparency and program integrity—combating fraud and abuse in private and public programs

7. Improving access to innovative medical therapies—biologic price competition

8. Community living assistance services and supports—establish a new, voluntary, self-funded long-term care insurance

9. Revenue provisions—new excise tax of 40% on insurance companies for insurance plans with an annual premium that is above the threshold of $8,500 for single coverage and $23,000 for family coverage

How will occupational therapy benefit under ACA and all its reform? First, there is opportunity for occupational therapy in the new patient models of care. Accountable Care Organizations (ACOs) are a new delivery model tool. ACOs are local health care organizations with a related set of providers who are primary care physicians, specialists, and hospitals. The goal is coordinated and efficient and it must be provided across the continuum of care. ACOs that achieve cost and quality targets will receive a financial bonus and those who fail will be levied a financial penalty. Occupational therapy personnel across the continuum of these ACOs should collaborate and use best practice to achieve the highest functional outcomes for their patients.

Another opportunity exists in the development of new patient-centered medical home models. These models have an emphasis on primary care, working in teams, and coordinating and tracking care over time. Its focus is to strengthen relationships among patients, physicians, and families. Care is facilitated through registries, information technology, health information exchange, and other means to ensure that patients get the indicated care when and where they need and want it in a culturally and linguistically appropriate manner (NCCA.org). Medical homes are working on keeping populations/communities healthy and focusing its care and treatment on chronic conditions.

Today is the opportunity to advocate for the value and contributions of occupational therapy. Today's practitioner should look to our own growing professional body of evidence and outcome reporting to be part of these new provisions. Many of you are future occupational therapists and assistants preparing for your role in "therapy." However, it is critical for all of us to commit to the tenets of occupational science and develop a deeper understanding of the linkage of occupation to health/wellness. Being able to articulate this linkage will enable occupational therapy to be a vital member of the new evolving health care team. As one of our esteemed founders, Mary Reilly, once stated during the 1961 AOTA Eleanor Clark Slagle address: "Man, through the use of his hands, as they are energized by mind and will, can influence the state of his own health" (Reilly, 1962).

Social Justice Issues and Advocacy

As may have become obvious, there are considerable ways for ethical, moral, and social policy issues to arise in the world of reimbursement. Chapters 2, 40, and 47 provide more information on these topics.

Occupational therapy practitioners are bound by the Code of Ethics developed by AOTA (Purtillo & Doherty, 2011) and by the code from their places of employment, but how do these play out when there is no funding for someone to receive needed services? Conversely, if organizations consistently provide services for no or minimal payment, how do they stay viable in order to help the most number of people in need of health care? In our

culture, we have struggled with the terms we use for people who need health care (patients, clients, consumers, etc.). Kronenberg and Pollard (2006) pointed out that these terms that we strive to use to adequately reflect who our consumers are have a common denominator: they all imply that the person is someone who can pay for our services. How is this consistent with our professional beliefs about social justice and who "deserves" intervention? Occupational therapy practitioners must continue to engage in the struggle of how, where, and why people receive services.

In instances where consumers have no health care coverage, there are some options. Facilities may opt to set up payment plans for clients. In some cases, organizations decide to write off payment for care rendered.

Occupational therapy practitioners should possess strong knowledge about their communities and supports that are available. Help might come from community religious or fraternal organizations who offer financial support to people with significant health care needs. Contact with local agencies such as The United Way can inform the practitioner of myriad community offerings.

Occupational therapy practitioners act as advocates for clients. This includes having awareness of overarching public health issues and working to be part of the solution. As a member of the larger health care team, it is occupational therapy's responsibility to participate in public health education campaigns to urge consumers to follow recommendations (e.g., weight control, exercise, smoking cessation, backpack safety) and intervention regimens (e.g., medication schedules).

Meaning for the Practice of Occupational Therapy

In present times, all care is managed in some form. There have been benefits to managed care. The expansion of outpatient and community services has opened up new employment opportunities for practitioners. Because of cost-saving tenets of managed care, occupational therapy assistants are in greater demand. The early emphasis on quality assurance has fueled the profession's efforts for evidence-based practice and the publication of new professional journals. It has promoted specialty certification and the development of new practice parameters. Cost savings have come from limiting unneeded care and keeping people healthy through prevention.

For every benefit there is a drawback. Care today has benefit limitations, whether in cost, time frame, or choice. These limitations have created role conflicts within some settings. They have affected access and availability. They have also created increased concerns about confidentiality and "indirect" intervention time. In response to these concerns, the Health Insurance Portability and

Accountability Act (HIPAA) of 1996 was passed to establish national standards for electronic health care transactions and to ensure privacy and security for health data (CMS, 2005d).

From a historical and public health perspective, reimbursement issues have fueled many changes in practice over the years. The push to move care from acute hospital settings to other (less expensive) levels of care has significantly shortened the length of stay (LOS) in acute settings. This shift has also increased the medical acuity of clients moving on to skilled or rehabilitative care, home health care, and even nursing home care. Occupational therapy practitioners have had to learn new skills, reflect on practice, and adapt to new documentation as these changes have infiltrated their work places.

Shrinking reimbursement has forced occupational therapy practitioners, and others, to offer 7-days-a-week coverage in settings, whereas "Monday through Friday" used to be a more typical routine. It has also asked practitioners to ensure that interventions are effective. Evaluation skills are crucial in skillfully administering comprehensive assessments needed for establishing baselines, setting appropriate interventions that meet clients' needs for service, and attending to the parameters of the payment system. Productivity standards have shifted over the years to meet the financial needs of provider institutions. This can be stressful in many settings and requires the occupational therapy practitioner to be flexible and creative with scheduling. In the midst of this complex context, practitioners must decide where their ethical and professional boundaries lie, and how to hold fast to them.

Practitioners must understand the big picture of health care reimbursement. It is easy to forget the other part of the reimbursement equation as occupational therapy practitioners work in the "helping" professions. Money for payment has to come from somewhere. Insurance companies, Medicare, or the state Medicaid reimbursement systems are not always adversarial in the sometimes limited services they cover. At times, these organizations are working with limited funds themselves. For example, consider that state Medicaid funds come from people's tax dollars. Someone, somewhere, makes hard decisions about how and where those funds are spent. At times, occupational therapy practitioners need to advocate about insurance coverage. Self-advocacy and consideration for people's best interest from a social justice standpoint is core to the profession's espoused ethics and philosophy. Principle 1 of the Occupational Therapy Code of Ethics requires practitioners show concern for the well-being of the people they serve (see Appendix F).

In 2005, Slater was already warning about ethical conflicts around reimbursement. She offers examples of scenarios where legal and ethical and regulatory lines may be crossed, such as clinicians not being allowed to discharge patients when they had ascertained that therapy was completed. She cited incidences of therapists being told to count patient rest periods in their therapy billing, or having facility administrators or directors in other disciplines mandate the amount of therapy an individual will receive. These concerns continue today and are warnings for therapy practitioners to stay informed and on top of their code of ethics and state and federal regulations around practice and reimbursement (Slater, 2005).

Summary

The occupational therapy consumer ultimately pays all health care costs. Over a lifetime, the consumer pays premiums for health care insurance through an employer, payroll taxes under Social Security for Medicare in later years, insurance premiums for private secondary coverage, general out-of-pocket expenses, and state taxes and federal taxes that are paid to support the Medicaid system. Consumers of occupational therapy services include clients, insurance companies, vendors, and employers, and they are all demanding quality. It is tantamount that each professional is committed to the standards of practice set by AOTA and is knowledgeable about and using evidence-based interventions.

Occupational therapists derive benefits from engaging with their state and national membership associations (see Chapter 41). These groups advocate for the profession and provide education regarding reimbursement considerations. Encouraging clients to be active participants, valuing life-long learning in the profession, refining teaching skills, and thoughtfully promoting wellness are key characteristics of practitioners who are able to effectively meet the payment challenges of today's health care continuum. The important issue for the practitioner is to be responsibly informed, provide services thoughtfully and responsibly, and have the confidence to ask questions about reimbursement.

Student Self-Assessment

1. Explore your own and a family member's insurance policies. Can you understand them? Do they provide for occupational therapy service reimbursement?

2. Review the case in Chapter 31 (p. 409). In pairs, work on coding the diagnostic information in the case using the CPT codes for rehabilitation.

3. Access the AOTA Web site and discuss at least three of the questions listed under the Reimbursement

EVIDENCE-BASED RESEARCH CHART

Topic	Evidence
History of health care	Torrens, 1993
Health care economics	Harrington & Estes, 2004
Health care utilization	Bernstein et al., 2003
Affordable Care Act	www.dpc.senate.gov.healthreformbill/healthbill04.pdf

section's Frequently Asked Questions. What are the current issues/trends in reimbursement?

4. Break into groups of four or five. Discuss the following:

   ◊ Why occupational therapy is not a primary or covered service in some insurance plans or settings.

   ◊ What steps can be taken by the profession to remedy this?

Electronic Resources

- Centers for Disease Control and Prevention, National Center for Health Statistics: www.cdc.gov/nchs

- Centers for Medicare & Medicaid Services, Department of Health and Human Services—Valuable resource for manuals, transmittals, and education: www.cms.hhs.gov

- Health Net Federal Services provides provider manuals for military beneficiaries: www.hnfs.net

- Oasis Training provides CMS-sponsored training for home health care providers and surveyors: www.oasistraining.org

- PT Manager—Resource on management for private practitioners: www.ptmanager.com

- American Occupational Therapy Association: www.aota.org

- National Committee on Quality Assurance: www.NCQA.org

- National Technical Information Services—Largest resource for government funded scientific, technical, engineering, and business information: www.ntis.gov

- Blue Cross Blue Shield Association—Resources for health plans: www.bluecares.com

- U.S. Department of Veteran Affairs—Resource for health benefits and services: www.va.gov

References

Akamigbo, A., & Wintter, A. (2012) *Mandated Report: Improving Medicare's payment system for Outpatient Therapy Services.* Retrieved from http://www.MEdpAC.gov/transcripts/outpatient%20Therapy_september2012.pdf

American Medical Association. (2005). *CPT standard edition—2006: Current procedural terminology.* Clifton Park, NY: Thomson Delmar Learning.

American Occupational Therapy Association. (2005). *Fact sheet: Medicare basics.* Retrieved from http://aota.org/Practitioners/Reimb/Pay/Medicare/FactSheets/37788.aspx

American Occupational Therapy Association. (2012). *Essential health benefits.* Retrieved from http://www.aota.org/Practitioners/Advocacy/Health-Care-Reform/Essential-Benefits.aspx

Bernstein, A. B., Hing, E., Moss, A. J., Allen, K. F., Siller, A. B., & Tiggle, R. B. (2003). *Health care in America: Trends in utilization.* Hyattsville, MD: National Center for Health Statistics. Retrieved from http://www.cdc.gov/nchs/data/misc/healthcare.pdf

Cengage Learning. (n.d.). *The Education For All Handicapped Children Act (PL 94-142) 1975.* Retrieved from http://college.cengage.com/education/resources/res_prof/students/spec_ed/legislation/pl_94-142.html

Centers for Medicare & Medicaid Services. (2004). Comprehensive outpatient rehabilitation facility (CORF) coverage, section 20.1: Required services. In *Medicare benefit policy manual.* Retrieved from http: //www.cms.hhs.gov/manuals/Downloads/bp102c12.pdf

Centers for Medicare & Medicaid Services. (2005a). *Medicaid-at-a-glance 2005.* Retrieved http://www.cms. hhs.gov/medicaiddatasourcesgeninfo/02_maag2005.asp

Centers for Medicare & Medicaid Services. (2005b). Medicare program; prospective payment system and consolidated billing for skilled nursing facilities for FY 2006. Final rule. *Federal Register, 70* (149), 45025-45127.

Centers for Medicare & Medicaid Services. (2005c). *Home health services, section 30.1: Confined to the home.* In *Medicare benefit policy manual.* Retrieved from http://www.cms.hhs.gov/manuals/Downloads/bp102c07.pdf

Centers for Medicare & Medicaid Services. (2005d). *HIPAA Overview.* Retrieved from http://www.cms.hhs.gov/hipaa-GenInfo

Centers for Medicare & Medicaid Services. (2006a). *CMS manual system: Pub 100-04 Medicare claims processing, transmittal 805.* Retrieved from http://www.cms.hhs.gov/Transmittals/Downloads/R805CP.PDF

Centers for Medicare & Medicaid Services. (2006b). *Certification and compliance: Inpatient rehabilitation facilities.* Retrieved from http://www.cms.hhs.gov/CertificationandCompliance/16_InpatientRehab.asp#TopOfPage

Centers for Medicare & Medicaid Services. (2008). *Therapy personnel qualifications and policies effective January 1, 2008. MLN Matters, MM5921.* Retrieved from http://www.cms.hhs.gov/MLNMattersArticles/downloads/MM5921.pdf

Centers for Medicare & Medicaid Services. (2009a). Hospital services covered under part B, section 70.3: Partial hospitalization services. In *Medicare benefit policy manual.* Retrieved from http://www.cms.hhs.gov/manuals/downloads/bp102c06.pdf

Centers for Medicare & Medicaid Services. (2009b). Covered medical and other health services, section 220.1: Conditions of coverage and payment for outpatient physical therapy, occupational therapy, or speech-language pathology services. In *Medicare benefit policy manual.* Retrieved from http://www.cms.hhs.gov/Manuals/downloads/bp102c15.pdf

Centers for Medicare & Medicaid Services. (2012). *Transmittal 2457: Revisions of the financial limitation for outpatient therapy services -Section 3005 of the Middle Class Tax Relief and Job Creation Act of 2012.* Retrieved from http://www.nhic.org

Centers for Medicare & Medicaid Services. (2013). *Local Coverage Determination (LCDs) for NHIC, Corp. (14101, MAC-Part A. Local Coverage Determination (LCD) for Outpatient Physical and Occupational Therapy Services (L29833).* Retrieved from http://www.nhic.org

Cowan, C., Catlin, A., Smith, C., & Sensenig, A. (2004). National health expenditures, 2002. *Health Care Financing Review, 25* (4), 143-166.

Fearon, H. (2004). *Tools for managing reimbursement in the outpatient physical therapy setting.* APTA Conference, Maine Chapter, September 24, 2004.

Harrington, C., & Estes, C. L. (2004). *Health policy: Crisis and reform in the U.S. health care delivery system* (4th ed.). Boston, MA: Jones & Bartlett Publishers.

Kane, R. L., Chen, Q., Blewett, L. A., & Sangl, J. (1996). Do rehabilitative nursing homes improve the outcomes of care? *Journal of the American Geriatrics Society, 44* (5), 545-554.

Kronenberg, F., & Pollard, N. (2006). Political dimensions of occupation and the roles of occupational therapy. *American Journal of Occupational Therapy, 60* (6), 617-625.

National Conference of State Legislatures. (March, 2011) *States Implement Health Reform. The Affordable Care Act: A Brief Summary.* Retrieved from http://www.ncsl.org/healthreform

Practice Management Information Corporation. (2005). *ICD-9-CM International Classification of Diseases, clinical modification* (9th rev., 6th ed.). Los Angeles, CA: Author.

Purtillo, R., & Doherty, R. F. (2011). *Ethical dimensions in the health professions* (5th ed.). Philadelphia, PA: Elsevier Saunders.

Reilly, M. (1962) Occupational Therapy can be one of the great ideas of 20th century medicine. *American Journal of Occupational Therapy, 16,* 300-308.

Slater, D. Y. (2005). Ethics in practice: whose responsibility? *OT Practice, 10*(19):13-15.

Tricare. (2008). Chapter 7–Medicine: Section 18.3, occupational therapy. In *Tricare policy manual 6010.57-M, February 2008.* Retrieved from http://manuals.tricare.osd.mil

Torrens, P. R. (1993). Historical evolution and overview of health services in the United States. In S. Williams & P. R. Torrens (Eds.), *Introduction to health services* (5th ed., pp. 3-35). Clifton Park, NY: Delmar Cengage Learning.

U.S. Department of Education. (n.d.). *Building the legacy: IDEA 2004.* Retrieved from http://idea.ed.gov

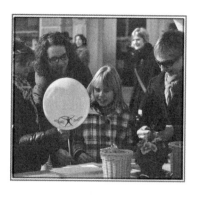

40

Marketing and Management of Occupational Therapy Services

Karen Jacobs, EdD, OTR/L, CPE, FAOTA

ACOTE STANDARDS EXPLORED IN THIS CHAPTER

B.7.7

KEY TERMS

- **Marketing:** "Marketing is the analysis, planning, implementation, and control of carefully formulated programs designed to bring about voluntary exchanges of values with target markets for the purpose of achieving organizational objectives. It relies heavily on designing the organization's offering in terms of the target markets' needs and desires, and on using effective pricing, communication, and distribution to inform, motivate, and service the markets" (Kotler & Clarke, 1987).

- **Promotion strategies:** These can be used to influence the demand for a product or service.

Introduction

We are on the verge of an era when the needs for our services are so great as to push us to the brink of glory, if *we can only deliver; or we may stumble, because we shall, I fear, cling tenaciously to what we have done without looking at what we might do if we were to take bold new directions. (Cromwell, 1984)*

Jacobs, K., MacRae, N., & Sladyk, K. (Eds.).
*Occupational Therapy Essentials for
Clinical Competence, Second Edition* (pp. 533-541).

If the concept of marketing had been applied to the profession of occupational therapy over 40 years ago, just imagine how much more of a significant role we may have been playing in the health care marketplace today!

The need for occupational therapy practitioners and students to fully understand and apply the concepts of marketing has become even more critical today.

> *We live in a world of limited resources that is technologically complex, economically competitive, and growing more politically accountable with consumer power on the rise. The good news is that this is a world of limitless opportunities for occupational therapy. However, we must work diligently—individually and collectively—to ensure that occupation is recognized as our central construct and to communicate how it shapes and informs our methods and outcomes through infusion in education, research, and practice. We must be aggressive in our support of, and advocacy for, scientific inquiry and pragmatic investigation that build the profession's evidence-based body of knowledge. We must participate in strategic partnerships and interprofessional teams (see Chapter 3) to construct communities where human occupation is recognized as fundamental to quality of life and social participation, as well as central to social, educational, and health care policies in the United States and the global community. We can and will reach this envisioned future...* (Jacobs, 2012, p. 652)

We will reach this by understanding and incorporating marketing into our daily activities. Indeed, it will help us reach the American Occupational Therapy Association's (AOTA) Centennial Vision for the profession: "We envision that occupational therapy is a powerful, widely recognized, science-driven, and evidence-based profession with a globally connected and diverse workforce meeting society's occupational needs" (AOTA, n.d.).

What Is Marketing?

Marketing has been a misunderstood term, most often used synonymously with public relations, selling, fundraising, or development. However, according to marketer Peter Drucker, "The aim of marketing is make selling superfluous" (Kotler & Murray, 1975).

Marketing consists of meeting people's needs in the most efficient and, therefore, profitable manner (Cromwell, 1984). Kotler and Clarke (1987) defined marketing in the following manner:

> *Marketing is the analysis, planning, implementation, and control of carefully formulated programs designed to bring about voluntary exchanges of values with target markets for the purpose of achieving organizational objectives. It relies heavily on designing the organization's offering in terms of the target markets' needs and desires, and on using effective pricing, communication, and distribution to inform, motivate, and service the markets.*

Successful marketing planning begins with an idea that serves as the framework for all marketing efforts. It is an orientation that makes satisfying the customer's needs the integrating organizational principle. Although the first impulse of the marketing novice is to design a program, such as a school-based, work-related occupational therapy program, and then look for customers (e.g., adolescents with developmental disabilities), effective marketing dictates that the process be reversed. One first looks at the market and listens carefully to potential customers, and then designs the program to match the needs and desires of these potential customers.

Marketing Planning

The main benefits of marketing planning can be summarized as follows (Branch, 1962):

- Encourages systematic thinking ahead
- Leads to better coordination of organizational efforts
- Leads to the development of performance standards for control
- Causes the individual/organization to sharpen its guiding objectives and policies
- Results in better preparedness for sudden developments

Marketing planning can be viewed as a three-step process. Figure 40-1 delineates this process with planning as the first step. It encompasses identifying attractive markets, and developing marketing strategies and programs. Execution is the second step. It includes carrying out the action programs. The third and final step involves marketing control. This final step requires measuring results, analyzing the causes of poor results, and taking corrective action. Adjustments in the plan, its execution, or both would include corrective actions that could be implemented.

Identifying Attractive Target Markets

Identifying the demands of the market is the first step in marketing. The market is defined as all actual or potential buyers of a product, service, or idea and can be considered in its entirety, such as all referral sources to an

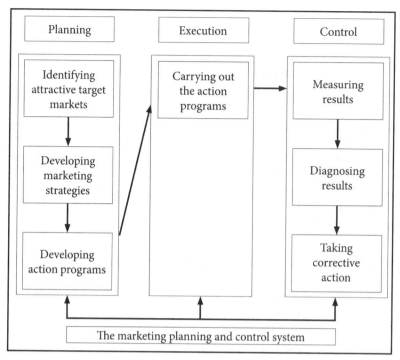

Figure 40-1. Example of marketing planning as a three-step process.

early intervention program, or divided into relevant segments according to variables, such as types of professionals (e.g., physicians, special education teachers, or nurses). Identifying attractive target markets includes the analysis of marketing opportunities. This analysis consists of the following:

- A self-audit
- Consumer analysis
- An analysis of other providers of similar services
- An environmental assessment

Self-Audit

A self-audit assesses the strengths, weaknesses, opportunities, and threats (SWOT analysis) of your department and/or specific program. Factors to be assessed may include the following:

- The reputation of your facility in the community
- The staff and their qualifications, such as certification as a hand therapist, or board-certified professional ergonomist (BCPE), or any of the specialty certification available through AOTA
- Physical size of the program
- Location of the program (e.g., hospital/rehabilitation setting, community-based)
- Convenience of your location to mass transit, highways, and parking
- Type and quality of equipment

- Available budget
- Support from administration. This self-audit assists in understanding how well or poorly prepared you are to meet the marketplace demands. Ascertaining what you do well and maintaining that product (service) at an optimal level is part of marketing.

Consumer Analysis

It is important to assess the potential consumers of your occupational therapy department's services within your catchment area. An analysis of some of the consumers who might use your products may include the following:

- Physicians
- Rehabilitation managers and consultants
- Other health and rehabilitation professionals
- Nurses
- Vocational counselors
- Special education teachers
- Attorneys
- Business and industry
- Administrators
- Workers with injuries
- Social workers
- Business and industry
- Third-party payers

- Colleagues, such as physical therapists and athletic trainers

ANALYSIS OF OTHER PROVIDERS OF SIMILAR SERVICES

How adequately the needs of the marketplace are being met, what areas are not being served, where duplication and overlap are occurring, and where opportunities for collaboration or joint venture exist can be ascertained through an analysis of other providers of similar services. One simple way to obtain information is to place your name on the mailing list of facilities/companies providing a similar product line. Reading through newsletters and brochures from the competition can be insightful. You want to learn as much as possible about the providers of similar services so you can be 10% better or 10% different from them.

Environmental Assessment

The changes and trends that may have an impact on occupational therapy services and perhaps the future of the profession comprise an environmental assessment. These include the following:

- Demographic variables
- Political and regulatory systems
- Cultural environment
- Economic/financial environment
- Psychographics
- Technological developments

Demographic Variables

Demographics is the study of human populations according to variables such as age, sex, family size, family life cycle, income, occupation, education, religion, race, and nationality. For example, the increasing number of aging "baby boomers" is a demographic trend that is having an impact on occupational therapy services.

Political and Regulatory Systems

Both political and regulatory systems may have an impact on occupational therapy services. The Patient Protection and Affordable Care Act of 2010 (PPACA) (P.L. 111–148), Physician Fee Schedule Final Rule for CY 2013, Multiple Procedure Payment Reduction (MPPR), and the Americans with Disability Act (ADA) Amendments Act of 2008 (P.L. 110-325, ADAAA) are some examples that impact occupational therapy. The reasonable accommodations are in place so that the individual with a disability can perform the essential functions of the job (United States Department of Justice, 2007).

Cultural Environment

Culture is a force that affects behaviors, values, perceptions, and preferences of individuals within a society. The United States is becoming a more multicultural society, and it is imperative that occupational therapy practitioners and students develop an understanding of and sensitivity to the culture profiles of clients within their catchment area. Having practitioners and students who are bilingual can be most beneficial and may be the variable that assists in making our services even more successful.

Economic/Financial Environment

An analysis of the economic/financial environment is important because it allows occupational therapy practitioners and students to target occupational therapy services to trends. Some interesting health care trends include the following:

- Compliance with the Affordable Care Act
  ◊ For example, State and Federal Health Insurance Exchanges will be available in 2013.
- Increased number of retail health clinics

The number of United States retail clinics is expected to climb to 2,500 in 2013, an increase of about 38% over 2012. Companies like Stayhealthy and Healthspot are accelerating this trend by providing health kiosks that offer services that would otherwise be provided in a doctor's office. Health kiosks can be used to take basic readings, perform primary care, and even deliver minor urgent care. Schools, work sites, prisons, health clubs, and pharmacies are all potential locations for these kiosks (Retrieved from http://medcitynews.com/2012/12/181872/).

Psychographics

Psychographics is the technique of measuring consumers' social class, lifestyle, and personality characteristics and can provide information on activities, interests, and opinions of these individuals. Understanding the psychographic profile of your clients helps provide information to assist in strategizing products and services to them.

Technological Developments

The technology arena is greatly advancing and has an almost daily effect on the type of assessment and intervention used by occupational therapy practitioners.

Specifically, information technology allows for information to be exchanged in a more efficient manner.

Selecting Target Markets and Market Segments

Once analysis is completed, there are three steps in target marketing. Market segmentation refers to the act of dividing a market into distinct groups of buyers who might require separate products and marketing mixes. For example, physicians can be segmented into pediatricians or neurologists and health and rehabilitation professionals can be segmented into speech pathologists, physical therapists, and athletic trainers. Market targeting is the act of evaluating and selecting one or more of the markets to enter. An example of this is targeting orthopedic surgeons as the main referral source for a hand therapy program. Product positioning is the act of formulating a competitive position for the product and a detailed marketing mix.

Developing Marketing Strategies

Developing marketing strategies includes the development of objectives for each identified target market and their implementation. The 4 P's—product, place, price, and promotion—are the strategies that can be used to influence the demand for a product (Kotler, 1983a; McCarthy, 1999). Here is how each of these "P's" is used in the marketing mix.

PRODUCT

Simply stated, what we do as occupational therapy practitioners is our product. That is, we help people, organizations, and populations through engagement in occupation. Ideally, the goal is to offer a product line—a variety of products associated with one another by an overall theme. For example, an occupational therapy department may have an industrial rehabilitation or occupational health program product line that includes post-offer screening, functional capacity evaluation, and ergonomics consultation. A school-based occupational therapy program may offer product line identifying assessment accommodations for the No Child Left Behind mandate and violence prevention programs.

How a product is packaged may influence its success. It is important to make sure all paperwork (e.g., brochures, business cards, stationary, and reports) have a professional appearance. The ability to access information quickly and be able to present it in a professional manner to the target markets is an asset.

Many new product ideas are generated by understanding our clients' needs and wants through direct surveys, projective tests, focus group discussions, and letters and complaints received. It is important to note that for every unhappy customer, you lose 50 others, and that 80% of your business is coming from 20% of your customers (Baum & Luebben, 1986).

Place

Occupational therapy services can be provided in a variety of places. Some of these include the following:

- Free-standing facilities located in professional buildings, industrial parks, and shopping centers
- Free-standing facilities affiliated with outpatient service departments, rehabilitation centers, or hospitals
- As part of a comprehensive rehabilitation or acute-care facility/program/hospital
- At work-site programs provided by a company to serve the needs of a specific business or industry
- Schools
- Skilled nursing facilities (SNFs)
- Sub-acute/transitional care unit

When analyzing the place aspect of marketing planning, other variables that should be considered are the hours the program is offered for business. For example, is your program open during hours convenient to your markets or your staff?

PRICE

The price or fee schedule for occupational therapy services (products) should be based on cost, competitive factors, geographic area, and what the consumer is willing to pay. It is important for the price to be commensurate with perceived value (Miller & Jacobs, 2007).

PROMOTION

Promotion is the vehicle of communicating information to your markets about the product's merits, place, and price. Instruments of promotion are advertising, sales promotion, publicity, and personal selling.

Advertising

Advertising involves the use of a paid message presented in a recognized medium and by an identified sponsor, with the purpose of informing, persuading, and reminding. Some advertising vehicles include the following:

- Print ads found in newspapers, journals, and magazines

Biographical Sketch of Karen Jacobs

Karen Jacobs, EdD, OTR/L, CPE, FAOTA* is a past president and vice president of the American Occupational Therapy Association (AOTA). She is a 2005 recipient of a Fulbright Scholarship to the University of Akureyri in Akuryeri, Iceland; the 2009 recipient of the Award of Merit from the Canadian Association of Occupational Therapists (CAOT); received the Award of Merit from the American Occupational Therapy Association in 2003; and the 2011 Eleanor Clarke Slagle Lectureship Award. The title of her Slagle Lecture was: *PromOTing Occupational Therapy: Words, Images and Action.*

Dr. Jacobs is a clinical professor of occupational therapy and the program director of the distance education post-professional occupational therapy programs at Boston University. She has worked at Boston University for 30 years and has expertise in the development and instruction of online graduate courses.

Dr. Jacobs earned a doctoral degree at the University of Massachusetts, a Master of Science at Boston University, and a Bachelor of Arts at Washington University in St. Louis, Missouri.

Dr. Jacobs' research examines the interface between the environment and human capabilities. In particular, she examines the individual factors and environmental demands associated with increased risk of functional limitations among populations of university and middle school aged students, particularly in notebook computing, use of tablets such as iPads, backpack use, and the use of games such as WiiFit.

In addition to being an occupational therapist, Dr. Jacobs is also a certified professional ergonomist (CPE) and the founding editor-in-chief of the international, interprofessional journal *WORK: A Journal of Prevention, Assessment and Rehabilitation* (IOS Press, The Netherlands) and is a consultant in ergonomics, marketing, and entrepreneurship.

*EdD: Doctorate in Education; OTR/L: registered and licensed occupational therapist; CPE: Certified Professional Ergonomist; FAOTA: Fellow of the American Occupational Therapy Association

Figure 40-2. Example of a biosketch.

- Brochures
- Direct mail
- Broadcasts
- Transits
- Billboards
- Quarterly newsletters
- Business cards

Sales Promotion

Sales promotion is the use of a wide variety of short-term incentives to encourage the purchase of the product. This approach is most effective when used in conjunction with advertising. For example, at an open house for an occupational therapist in a solo ergonomics practice, a successful sales promotion was giving out mouse pads with tips for setting up a computer workstation. Of course, the occupational therapist's contact information was printed on the mouse pad, too.

Publicity

Publicity is often a relatively underused aspect of promotion in relation to the real contribution it can make (Kotler, 1983b). The most positive aspect of publicity is

that it is free. However, one has little control over the placement of it and thus it becomes difficult to focus publicity on specific target markets. An example of publicity might be to contact the local media through a press release about an upcoming event at your facility (e.g., activities to celebrate AOTA's National Backpack Awareness Day). If the media finds the event newsworthy and they are not understaffed, they will often send a reporter to cover the event. Whether the reporter writes a story can be dependent on variables out of your control, such as available time and space in the newspaper, television, or radio. However, a successful strategy in utilizing publicity more effectively has been to develop a rapport with the media personnel. Personally contact your local newspaper, radio, and television stations and introduce yourself. Let them know about occupational therapy and what you do as an occupational therapy practitioner or student and offer to be available to them if they need a resource. Follow-up your email/telephone call with your résumé and biosketch for their files (Figure 40-2).

Personal Selling

Face-to-face communication between you and your audience is the most effective form of promotion, the most expensive, and also the method most used by occupational therapy practitioners (Jacobs, 1987). Word-of-mouth recommendation by staff and consumers of occupational therapy products and services is a powerful sales pitch. Other successful personal selling methods include the following:

- Exhibiting at various conferences
- Developing a free speakers' bureau
- Presenting in-service training to physicians and health and rehabilitation professionals
- Presenting continuing education workshops
- Lecturing
- Attending professional meetings for various organizations
- Holding an open house
- Holding continuing education seminars for referral sources

Social Marketing

Social marketing takes the techniques of marketing and deploys them to create a positive social change… the AOTA National School Backpack Awareness Day campaign is a good example of social marketing. Rebuilding Together (a nonprofit providing rebuilding services to low-income homeowners) and CarFit (an educational program for older drivers) are other examples. (Jacobs, 2012, pp. 663-664)

Social Media

Social media, which include social networking sites such as Facebook and LinkedIn, microblogs such as Twitter, and content communities such as YouTube may be used for effective marketing. Social media are considered a hybrid of promotion and a highly magnified form of word of mouth. Consumers are turning more frequently to social medical outlets to conduct information searches that aid in health care or purchasing decisions (Lempert, 2006; Vollmer & Precourt, 2008). That is not to say that all sources had equal impact. Sillence, Briggs, Harris and Fishwick (2007) found that individuals preferred sites that were run by reputable organizations or had a medical or expert "feel." They especially trusted the information when the credentials of the site and its authors were made explicit. They also appreciated inclusion of "familiar" (plain) rather than "technical"

language, and personalized content (i.e., stories from clients like themselves)" (Jacobs, 2012, p. 664).

Focus Groups

Focus groups have been found to be an effective marketing technique. These techniques can be used with primary referral sources, such as physicians and employers, or with reimbursement agencies or the direct recipient of our services to provide feedback on current programming efforts and recommendations for future program modifications. The use of focus groups allows you to quickly incorporate this feedback into the delivery of your product and services or the product itself. This in turn should generate an increased commitment on the part of the referral sources to the program.

Focus group interviewing is one of the major marketing research tools for gaining insight into consumer thoughts and feelings (Kotler, 1983a). Focus group interviewing consists of inviting 6 to 10 participants to spend a few hours with a skilled interviewer to discuss any designated subject matter, such as the feasibility of developing a school-based occupational therapy work program. Focus group practitioners are usually paid a small sum for attending the meeting. These are typically held in pleasant surroundings, with refreshments served. The interview begins with broad questions such as, "What do you think about occupational therapy services for elementary school-aged students?" leading to focusing in on more specific questions on the subject matter such as, "What do you think about the feasibility of an occupational therapy ergonomics program addressing the use of information and communication technical being established at Butler Elementary School?" The interviewer encourages free and easy discussion among participants, hoping that the group dynamics will bring out deep feelings and thoughts (Kotler & Clarke, 1984). Although the results cannot generalize the market as a whole due to its small sample size, the information gathered can provide insight into participants' perceptions, attitudes, and satisfaction. Information obtained can help define what issues need to be researched more formally or may provide the foundation for being able to develop a product that will meet the consumer's needs (Kotler & Clarke, 1984).

Execution of the Marketing Plan

Once you have selected your target market, develop a specific marketing mix (product, price, place, and

EVIDENCE-BASED RESEARCH CHART

Topic	Evidence
Social media	Feick & Price, 1987; Kietzmann, Hermkens, McCarthy & Silvestre, 2011; Sillence, Briggs, Harris & Fishwick, 2007; Vollmer & Precourt, 2008
Social marketing	Chou, Hunt, Beckjord, Moser & Jesse, 2009; Kotler & Zaltman, 1971

promotion) for your market that stresses the benefits of your product(s). When executing action programs, a timeline should be delineated, such as a 12-month period, to measure whether objectives and goals are being met. The action plan should be dynamic and able to be changed throughout the year as new opportunities and problems arise. Ideally, actions should be assigned to specific individuals who are given exact completion dates. For example, an action that might be assigned to an occupational therapy practitioner can include developing a single paragraph description of the violence prevention programs provided by the occupational therapy department. The practitioner is given a 1-week timeline to complete this action. Once the description is completed, the supervisor has 2 weeks to incorporate this information into a brochure being developed to promote the expanded product line of occupational therapy to potential referral sources. In this case, as in all aspects of promotion, it is important to communicate in a language that is familiar to your market. Avoid professional jargon!

Marketing Control

Marketing is an area where rapid obsolescence of objectives, policies, strategies, and programs is a constant possibility (Kotler & Clarke, 1984). Marketing control attempts to circumvent this dilemma and assists in maximizing the probability that a product will achieve its short- and long-term objectives. It is important to measure program results, diagnose these results, and take corrective action, if necessary. There are three types of marketing control (Kotler & Clarke, 1984):

1. Annual plan control consists of the steps used during the year to monitor and correct deviations from the marketing plan to ensure that annual sales and profit goals are being achieved.

2. Profitability control refers to the efforts used to determine the actual profit or loss of different marketing entities such as the products (services) or market segments.

3. Strategic control is a systematic evaluation of the organization's market performance in relation to the current and forecasted marketing environment.

Summary

A bright future can be a certainty for occupational therapy practitioners and students who are prepared to accept the reality of today's and tomorrow's health care environment. It will be increasingly competitive with various professions vying for control of limited resources that are increasingly complex and increasingly controlled by third-party payers and the government.

Occupational therapy practitioners and students' abilities to market their skills and knowledge to those that control the dollars will be an ever-present requirement for success. It will likely make the difference between encroachment by other professions, a resulting second-class specialty, and a proud and effective profession placed squarely in a leadership position within the health care industry (Pickelle & Ramos, 1991).

Having access to an expert in marketing to assist in the development of a marketing plan would be the ideal situation, but this is not always the case. On the other hand, the worst possible scenario would be one where even an informal market analysis does not precede product or service development. If this is the case for you, a word of caution: remember that designing a program and then looking for customers typically leads to facing an uphill battle to success. At the very least, before investing a great deal of useless time, effort, and money, attempt to perform a market analysis on your own following the guidelines presented in this chapter and in other available literature.

Student Self-Assessment

1. Describe, design, and discuss content for a Web page promoting occupational therapy to high school students.

2. Write a biosketch about yourself using Figure 40-2 as an example.

3. Create a brochure about the occupational therapy's contribution to any of the six broad areas of practice: mental health; productive aging; children and youth; health and wellness; work and industry; or rehabilitation, disability, and participation.

References

American Occupational Therapy Association. (n.d.). *The road to the Centennial Vision.* Retrieved from http://www.aota.org/News/Centennial.aspx

Baum, C. M., & Luebben, A. J. (1986). *Prospective payment systems: A handbook for health care clinicians.* Thorofare, NJ: SLACK Incorporated.

Borger, C., Smith, S., Truffer, C., Keehan, S., Sisko, A., Poisal, J., et al. (2006). *Health spending projections through 2015: Changes on the horizon. Health Affairs, 25*(2), w61-w73.

Branch, M. (1962). *The corporate planning process.* New York, NY: American Management Association.

Catlin, A., Cowan, C., Heffler, S., Washington, B., & National Health Expenditure Accounts Team. (2006). National health spending in 2005: The slowdown continues. *Health Affairs, 26*(1), 142-153.

Chou, W., Hunt, Y., Beckjord, E., Moser, R., & Hesse, B. (2009) Social media use in the United States: Implications for health communication. *Journal of Medical Internet Research, 11*(4), e48.

Cromwell, F. (1984). The changing roles of occupational therapists in the 1980s. *Occupational Therapy in Health Care, 1*(1), 8.

Feick, L., & Price, L. (1987). The market maven: A diffuser of marketplace information. *Journal of Marketing, 51*, 83097. Retrieved from http//dx.doi.org/10.2397/1251146.

Jacobs, K. (1987). Marketing occupational therapy. *American Journal of Occupational Therapy, 41*(5), 315-320.

Jacobs, K. (2012). PromOTing occupational therapy: Words, images, and actions (Eleanor Clarke Slagle lecture). *American Journal of Occupational Therapy, 66*, 652-671.

Kietzmann, J., Hermkens, K., McCarthy, I., & Silvestre, B. (2011). Social media? Get serious! Understanding the functional building blocks of social media. *Business Horizons, 54*, 241-251. Retrieved from http://dx.doi.org/10.1016/j.bushor.2011.01.005.

Kotler, P. (1983a). *Principles of marketing* (2nd ed.). Englewood Cliffs, NJ: Prentice Hall.

Kotler, P. (1983b). *Principles of marketing—Instructor's manual with cases.* Englewood Cliffs, NJ: Prentice Hall.

Kotler, P., & Clarke, R. (1984). *Marketing management* (5th ed.). Englewood Cliffs, NJ: Prentice Hall.

Kotler, P., & Clarke, R. (1987). *Marketing for health care organizations.* Englewood Cliffs, NJ: Prentice Hall.

Kotler, P., & Murray, M. (1975). Third sector management: The role of marketing. *Public Administration Review, 35*(5), 469.

Kotler, P., & Zaltman, G. (1971). Social marketing: An approach to planned social change. *Journal of Marketing, 35*, 3-12. Retrieved from http://dx.doi.org/10.2307/1249783.

Lempert, P. (2006, Sept. 1). Caught in the Web. *Progressive Grocer, 85*, 18.

McCarthy, E. J. (1999). *Basic marketing: A managerial approach* (13th ed.). Homewood, IL: Irwin.

Miller, D., & Jacobs, K. (2007). Economics and marketing of ergonomic services. In K. Jacobs (Ed.), *Ergonomics for therapists.* St. Louis, MO: Elsevier.

National Center for Education Statistics. (n.d.). *National Center for Education Statistics Web site.* Retrieved from http://nces.ed.gov

Pickelle, C., & Ramos, T. (1991). Publishers' message. *Rehab Management, 9.*

Sillence, E., Briggs, P., Harris, P. R. & Fishwick, L. (2007). How do patients evaluate and make use of online health information? *Social Science and Medicine, 64*, 1853-1862. Retrieved from http://dx.doi.org/10.1016/j.socscimed.2007.01.012.

United States Department of Justice. (2007). *U.S. Department of Justice Web site.* Retrieved from http://www.usdoj.gov

Vollmer, C., & Precourt, G. (2008). Always on: Advertising, marketing and media in an era of consumer control. New York: McGraw-Hill.

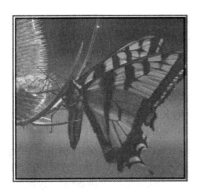

41

QUALITY IMPROVEMENT

Nancy MacRae, MS, OTR/L, FAOTA and Karen Jacobs, EdD, OTR/L, CPE, FAOTA

ACOTE STANDARDS EXPLORED IN THIS CHAPTER
B.7.6

KEY VOCABULARY

- **Benchmark:** Quantifiable measures of the outcomes of a process used as comparison to current performances or targets for an improved outcome (Braveman, 2006, p. 289).
- **Quality:** "The degree to which health care services for individuals and populations increase the probability of desired health outcomes and is consistent with current professional knowledge of best practice" (IOM, 2001, p. 232).

- **Quality assessment:** Measure of quality against a standard.
- **Quality improvement:** Management philosophy and method for structuring problem solving.

Introduction

Quality is an extremely complex construct and can be defined in many ways. It is dependent on the individual and the context, not only for definition but also for how to measure.

Quality has a value component, which is typically the relationship between cost and quality.

Health care players (clients, providers, and payers) define quality differently, usually from their unique perspectives. Some of the possible defining concepts of quality include safety, timeliness, courtesy, availability, technical support, accessibility, reliability, economic impact, accuracy, waste, durability, flexibility, and follow-up. In 2001, the Institute of Medicine (IOM) defined quality as "the degree to which health care services for individuals

Jacobs, K., MacRae, N., & Sladyk, K. (Eds.).
*Occupational Therapy Essentials for
Clinical Competence, Second Edition* (pp. 543-551).
© 2014 SLACK Incorporated.

and populations increase the probability of desired health outcomes and is consistent with current professional knowledge of best practice" (IOM, p. 232).

Service is also a likely consideration, with the following five dimensions often cited as important (Parasuraman, Berry, & Zeithaml, 1991):

1. Reliability of service

2. Tangible product or service

3. Responsiveness of service to client/customer

4. Assurance of quality to consumer

5. Empathy exercised toward consumer

There are also levels of quality for a product or service. There is the *expected* quality, the *perceived* quality, and the *actual* quality. Expected quality is influenced by opinion, whereas perceived quality is subjective; both are difficult to measure. Actual quality can consider multiple factors and be based on statistical data, so it is easier to measure (Snoby, 2004, p. 69)

Quality improvement is also a management philosophy and method for structuring problem solving. Its goal is to meet/exceed customer/client requirements for quality services through a process of improvement. The process is a continuous, nonlinear process and always involves change. However, all change is not improvement, so the process needs to be carefully and intentionally implemented. Bataldan and Davidoff (2013) propose the following five elements by which improvement can be produced: generalizable scientific evidence, particular context awareness, performance measurement, plans for change, and execution of planned changes. The data that are gathered are used to make decisions, just as for evidence-based practice. A frequently used model, developed by Donabedian (1980), lists three portions of a quality improvement program:

1. Structure: The resources available within the specific environment are used to do this

2. Process: The actual delivery of services

3. Outcomes: The final result(s) of the program

All aspects of this model and the one proposed by Bataldan and Davidoff are complementary. In addition, quality for practitioners can be understood from a micro as well as a macro view. The micro view deals with clinical aspects of care and the technical quality with which they are delivered. Geographic differences may influence this view. Interpersonal aspects of care have significance for clients—the provider's interest in and concern for the client makes an indelible impression. Quality-of-life definitions usually involve the client's sense of overall well-being and ability to participate in those activities/occupations found to be meaningful (Shi & Singh, 2012).

The macro view of quality includes a broader view of the system-wide efficiencies and outcomes, such as cost, access, and population health status (Shi & Singh, 2012, pp. 515-517). National initiatives, as well as state and community actions, are required to address these concerns.

For a quality improvement process to be successful, the following components need to be in place:

- Administrative support of this philosophy

- Training of all staff on the concepts, strategies, tools, and techniques of quality improvement

- Adoption of the norm of customer preferences being the primary determinant of quality (Table 41-1)

- Support for a team approach that encourages all to work together to improve quality; motivation must be apparent for this approach to process analysis and change to be effective

Successful quality improvement efforts work because consumers discern a greater value from the service/product than from that of the competition and a number of the following components. Five "C" components of valid customer requirements are as follows (Braveman, 2006):

1. Product is *current*

2. Outcome is *calculable*

3. Plan can be *completed*

4. Plan is *consumer* based

5. Plan is *consistent* with organizational goals

Quality improvement plans are often dictated by improving client safety and outcomes in health care, whereas in organizations they are associated with less waste and improved services, resulting in lower costs and leading to a higher profit margin, asset utilization, and competitive position. All of this improves the "bottom line," thereby satisfying shareholders and key supporters as well as consumers.

Stages and Principles

The outcome assessment process is a critical part of evaluating and improving quality. The process consists of the following:

- Identifying goals for organization, program, client, or self

- Developing a plan to achieve goals

- Implementing the plan

- Measuring and reporting outcomes

Another way to understand this process is to explain the one Deming (2000) created. It is a quality chain reaction consisting of a four part cycle:

1. Plan: Determine what will be measured

2. Do: Collect data on chosen indicators

3. Check: Analyze data and identify areas for improvement

4. Act: Implement improvements, first in pilot program; provide rewards and recognition for the team

Deming insisted that these domains were integrated and needed to be used together. In addition, users of

Table 41-1.

CLIENT-DRIVEN ACTIONS

Becoming a Client-Driven Entity Means Moving

From	To
Motivation through fear and loyalty	Motivation through shared vision
An attitude of "It's their problem."	Ownership of every problem that affects the client
"That's the way we've always done it."	Continued improvement
Making decisions based on assumptions	Making decisions based on client data
Everything begins and ends with management	Everything begins and ends with the client
Organizational foxholes	Cross-functional cooperation
Being good at crisis management and recovery	Doing it right the first time

Adapted from Whiteley, R. C. (1993). *The customer-driven company: Moving from talk to action.* New York, NY: Basic Books.

this system needed to have an appreciation for a systems approach, the likelihood of variation of performance, the theory of the scientific method of knowledge generation, and an understanding of both intrinsic and extrinsic factors affecting motivation and participation in change within an organization (Braveman, 2006).

In addition to following Deming's organized cycle, the rationale for such a plan needs to address queries such as the following:

- Who are the stakeholders?
- How do you improve responsiveness of the program?
- How do you ensure high quality standard?

Application to Clinical Settings

In an environment of constant change, cost containment, mergers, and managed health care, professionals must strive to provide quality care. Examining efficiency, effectiveness, and adherence to standards of quality management in health care is a systematic process for evaluating health care services (Joint Commission on Accreditation of Healthcare Organizations [JCAHO], 2013). Efficiency refers to services that are both cost effective and timely in their delivery. Clinical services must be effective in achieving set objectives or outcomes for care.

Quality improvement or management programs are designed to measure and assess performance to ensure adherence to pre-established standards. These standards are established by state, federal, and accreditation organizations, such as the JCAHO and the Commission on Accreditation of Rehabilitation Facilities (CARF). Hospitals and other health care facilities refer to this process with many terms: continuous quality improvement, total quality management, quality assurance, and

performance improvement. The processes of quality assurance, quality improvement/assessment, and performance are all methods of assessment. Motivations (external versus internal), focus (problem-based versus quality processes), delegation (departmentally versus interdepartmentally), and outcomes (hiding problems versus improvement) may vary (Jacobs & Logigian, 1999).

Table 41-2 provides the differences among quality assurance, similar to quality improvement but a step beyond quality assessment; quality assessment, a measure of quality against standards; and performance improvement, a combination of both.

There are many methods for evaluating quality, such as the following:

- *Clinical audits* refer to a group of peers working collectively to review case records for adherence to established standards pre-established by the peer group.
- *Peer review* is a type of record review based on criteria established by the individual department, for what is determined to be quality care (JCAHO, 1995; Rakich, Logest, & Darr, 1992). Maslin (1991, p. 177) stated: "Common to both peer review and clinical audit procedures is the term process criteria, referring to the activities or procedures undertaken as part of good patient care."
- Accreditation is sought by many hospitals and health care organizations as proof of providing services that meet established minimum standards for Medicare reimbursement (Jacobs & Logigian, 1999; JCAHO, 1995). When performance fails to meet these standards, the organization must assess the performance and attempt to improve the areas of deficit. Changes can occur organizationally, departmentally, or individually. When discussing quality improvement, we must not only look to the organization, but to each

Table 41-2.

DIFFERENCES AMONG QUALITY ASSURANCE, QUALITY ASSESSMENT, AND QUALITY IMPROVEMENT

Quality Assurance	Quality Assessment	Quality Improvement
Externally driven	Internally motivated	Internally and externally motivated
Self-oriented	Customer driven	Customer/data and assessment driven
Vertical	Horizontal	Organization wide
Delegated to a few	Embraced by all	Embraced by all
Focused on people	Focused on processes	Focused on outcomes, intervention, and systems
Hiding problems	Seeking problems	Seeking opportunities for improvement; utilizes benchmarking or comparative data
Seeks endpoints	Has no endpoints	Has no endpoints

Adapted from Rakich, J. S., Logest, B. B., & Darr, K. (1992). *Managing health services organizations* (3rd ed.). Baltimore, MD: Health Professions Press.

individual occupational therapy practitioner, whether a registered occupational therapist or a certified occupational therapy assistant, who is providing the services.

Data Collection Methods

Data collection methods include qualitative or quantitative methodology, or a combination of both, as well as the use of benchmarks. *Benchmarks* are the quantifiable measures of the outcomes of a process used as comparisons to current performances or targets for an improved outcome (Braveman, 2006, p. 289). Many methods can be used to collect data. They include observation, interviews, surveys/questionnaires, and focus groups.

Data analysis drives change. It closes the loop of quality improvement. A determination about whether the data support the focus on the goals of an organization or its view of success must be determined with an adjustment plan conceived based on the data. Data can also be utilized to indicate the effectiveness of a practitioner's performance (Table 41-3).

The ultimate goal of quality improvement programs is to have a continuous focus on quality to become the way of doing business. Success occurs when there is a constant focus on clients and their satisfaction, a constant readiness for change and process improvement, the daily use of quality improvement tools, an abiding belief that use of data to make decisions is the right way to proceed, and a commitment to balance these tasks with those of the needs of people as standard operating procedures (Braveman, 2006).

FOCUS-PDCA Model

A method used by many organizations to implement a quality improvement process is the one developed by the Hospital Corporation of America in 1980. It is known as FOCUS-PDCA. It is a "stepwise approach to teach how to design, implement, and evaluate a quality improvement initiative" (Skledar & McKaveney, 2009, p. 80). The acronym FOCUS is described below:

- Find way(s) to improve by identifying what needs improvement
- Organize a team of individuals who understand both the process and the targeted area
- Clarify issues of specified area, addressing who, what, when, and where information
- Understand causes of targeted area, addressing why question
- Select most appropriate method for improvement

The PDCA portion is based on Deming's process, already described.

Departmental communication is essential in facilitating a process, such as the preceding, fostering team development and motivating staff members to maximize efficiency and effectiveness of intervention.

Occupational therapy practitioners who are involved in the quality improvement process will have increased understanding of the indicators and their potential effects on the client, the department, and the organization.

Table 41-4 provides a more detailed outline of such a process for monitoring and evaluating assessment and improvement programs.

Table 41-3.

INDICATORS AND THRESHOLDS

Indicator	Threshold	Data Collection Method	Possible Causes for Thresholds Not Being Met
Falls prevention education was completed and thoroughly documented as evidence by	95%	Quarterly chart review of 30 records by the occupational therapist Reports to occupational therapist director and QM committee	
Clients received	95%	Falls assessment	Short length of stay Illness Family Client refusal
Documentation	95%	Documentation of education and client/family understanding	
Treatment	98%	Testing/procedures 3 hours of therapy daily to include occupational therapy and physical therapy and at times, Speech-Language Pathology (SLP) as documented in client's chart	

Table 41-4.

THE MONITORING AND EVALUATION PROCESS FOR ASSESSMENT AND IMPROVEMENT

Assign responsibility	The organization leaders oversee the design and foster and approach to continuously improve quality including the use of intradepartmental and extradepartmental activities
Delineate the scope	The organization, as a whole or as a department, delineates its scope of care and service
Identify importance	The organization, as a whole or as a department, identifies high-priority key functions, processes, activities, etc., to be monitored
Identify indicators	Teams of experts, inter- or intradepartmental, identify indicators for the important aspects of care and service; indicators pertaining to structures of care are no longer emphasized
Establish evaluation	Teams of experts establish the level, pattern, or trend triggers in data for each indicator that will trigger intensive evaluation. Statistical methods are emphasized, as is the fact that thresholds are not the only way evaluation is triggered
Collect and organize	The data collection methodology often includes a data means by which feedback from sources other than ongoing monitoring is used to indicate areas for evaluation and improvement
Initiate evaluation	When thresholds are reached and when other feedback (e.g., client reports) identifies other opportunities for improvement, leaders set priorities for evaluation and establish teams, which evaluate the client care or service function in question
Take action	Greater emphasis is placed on focusing actions on processes, especially the "hands off" between departments and services
Assess effectiveness	A greater emphasis is placed on ensuring that improvement is sustained over time
Communicate results	Findings of those performing monitoring and evaluation of the findings are forwarded to the leaders and affected individuals and groups
Other feedback	Receive surveys, comments, suggestions, and complaints

Adapted from Logigian, M. K. (1999). In K. Jacobs & M. K. Logigian (Eds.), *Functions of a manager in occupational therapy* (3rd ed., p. 124). Thorofare, NJ: SLACK Incorporated.

With a strong quality improvement program, departments and organizations will show improved efficiency with decreased cost and waste and improved productivity and effectiveness, with positive outcomes and client satisfaction. Quality care should always be thought of as an ongoing process for the organization as a whole and for each individual working within the organization.

Impact on the Profession

Quality improvement processes are important to the profession of occupational therapy. The principles mirror those of evidence-based practice and support a strengthening and growth of our profession and its foundation of occupation. Our profession maintains a unique definition of quality outcomes: occupational therapy outcomes need to be based on engagement in occupation (O'Sullivan, 2004). Measures can include the following (Case-Smith, 2005, pp. 8-9):

- Occupational performance
- Client satisfaction
- Role competence
- Adaptation
- Health and wellness
- Prevention
- Quality of life

Clinical assessment tools need to be critically analyzed with a determination made as to what they assess, how they will be used, and their limitations. Tools also need to be reliable, valid, and sensitive. Some examples of currently used tools are as follows:

- **Functional Independence Measure (FIM).** A national tool used in rehabilitation settings
- **Minimum Data Information Set (MDIS).** Used to determine level of intervention needed in nursing homes
- **Outcomes Assessment Information Set (OASIS).** Home health standardized assessment
- **SF-36.** National quality of life assessment
- **Canadian Occupational Performance Measure (COPM).** Can be used with multiple populations

Outcome Measures

Quality outcome measures also need to be applied at the individual practitioner level to ensure quality care for the clients and the continuing competence of practitioners. Looking at quality care, occupational therapy practitioners must look at the overall outcomes of client intervention and their individual professional competence as

occupational therapy practitioners. Hinojosa et al. (1998) defined continuing competence as "a dynamic multidimensional process in which the professional develops and maintains the knowledge, performance skills, interpersonal abilities, critical reasoning skills, and ethical reasoning skills necessary to continue in his or her evolving roles throughout a professional career" (p. 4). This process requires the occupational therapy practitioner to understand that this is a continuous process of improvement.

The American Occupational Therapy Association (AOTA), the national organization for occupational therapy practitioners, is committed to assisting its members in keeping abreast of advancements in the profession and establishing standards that define quality services.

AOTA has established a council, the Committee on Continuing Competence and Professional Development (CCCPD), as a committee of the Representative Assembly to develop and maintain Standards for Continuing Competence (AOTA, 2010b) and offer guidelines and tools to support professional development. With financial and time constraints commonly experienced by many occupational therapy practitioners, AOTA has developed continuing education (CE) articles, self-paced clinical courses, workshops on DVD/CD, etc., and online courses to assist its members in meeting continuing education (CE) requirements and obtaining CE units (CEUs) to keep current in a growing profession.

Occupational therapy practitioners must maintain and demonstrate the appropriate knowledge and skill level for client intervention in varied roles. Many state licensure boards require documentation of CE (refer to your state licensure laws) in order to maintain current licensure. These CE credits should be related to the occupational therapy practitioner's individual roles within their position.

As of 2002, the National Board for Certification in Occupational Therapy (NBCOT) requires practitioners to accrue 36 hours of professional development units (PDUs) over a 3-year period to maintain certification and to use the credentials of certified occupational therapy assistant or registered occupational therapy. The requirement is intended to complement state licensure terms. Of the 36 units, two-thirds (24 PDUs) must be directly related to the delivery of occupational therapy services (NBCOT, 2013).

CEUs are converted to PDUs according to a formula established by NBCOT. In addition, NBCOT offers a listing of a wide variety of professional activities that may be applied to PDUs (NBCOT). Practitioners must keep records, usually in the form of a portfolio of their professional development activities. At recertification time, NBCOT will randomly audit recertification applicants for the required PDUs (NBCOT, 2013).

Skills Needed by Practitioners

Occupational therapy practitioners must be able to demonstrate appropriate communication (Joint Commission White Paper on Patient-Centered Communication), interpersonal abilities, and problem solving in order to maintain professional relationships with clients, family members, peers, and other health care professionals. Being able to adapt in order to meet the needs of the client, family, or health care professional will foster greater understanding and may improve overall intervention outcomes. Lastly, occupational therapy practitioners must always adhere to the Code of Ethics established by the AOTA (2010a). This code guides our practice and allows occupational therapy practitioners to make appropriate decisions and actions. Each occupational therapy practitioner is responsible for his or her own ethical practice.

Given the demand for accountability within the health care field and the rapid changes within the profession of occupational therapy and areas of technology, it becomes essential for occupational therapy practitioners to continuously update individual skills and knowledge level. As a new graduate or an advanced practitioner, it is important to have a professional development plan in order to compete in an ever-changing health care environment. AOTA has a Professional Development Tool online that enables the occupational therapy practitioner to assess his or her own strengths and weaknesses, develop goals and objectives to improve skills or knowledge, implement the plan, create a space to document credentials and continuing competency, identify possible resources to meet the goals, and engage in cyclical self-reflection. NBCOT also has a self-assessment tool available to practitioners.

Skills that you will apply to the quality improvement process include the following:

- Effective communication is necessary in organizing, implementing, and reporting quality improvement activities. Practitioners need to share information with colleagues who are also involved in the study, with the head of the quality improvement study team and possibly with facility administration.

- The tasks of management are frequently part of a quality improvement study. Therefore, knowledge of their procedures and purpose will be of benefit to the practitioner who participates in quality improvement activities.

- Leadership can be displayed in a number of ways. Occupational therapy practitioners may lead the entire study or a portion of it. Certified occupational therapy assistants are encouraged to assume a leadership role by noting areas in practice that could benefit from quality monitoring.

Case Example

The occupational therapy department in a 16-bed inpatient rehabilitation unit has developed a quality management program to review the following:

- Splinting schedules and adherence to the schedules by the staff.

- Falls prevention education and carry-over of the information for the clients.

- Intervention minutes.

The department, including the occupational therapy director, registered occupational therapists, and certified occupational therapist assistants, collected data and completed a chart review. Splinting schedules were to be placed in the chart and documented in the nursing daily sheets for adherence to the schedule. Falls prevention education was to be documented in the occupational therapy daily notes, including client understanding and carry-over. Intervention documentation was to be documented in the daily notes and billing records for a minimum of 45 minutes twice a day (BID).

Goals were established as follows:

- Splinting schedules and adherence to the schedule were documented 95% of the time.

- Falls prevention education was completed and thoroughly documented with client understanding 95% of the time.

- Clients received occupational therapy intervention in 45-minute sessions BID 95% of the time; if therapy was missed, thorough documentation was included for missed session 100% of the time.

Thresholds for splinting and falls prevention were met at 95%, whereas thresholds for intervention minutes were not met and achieved 85% compliance. The occupational therapy department held a meeting to discuss the results. The occupational therapy department has two full-time registered occupational therapists, two full-time occupational therapy assistants, and an occupational therapy aide. Department hours are from 8 AM to 5 PM, Monday through Saturday, and Sunday from 8 AM to 12 PM.

Quality improvement activities are frequently a requirement of accrediting bodies and state regulatory boards. Assessing and improving the quality of care to the clients we serve is an ethical responsibility, as is continually improving and upgrading our own skills. Results of quality improvement activities provide a sound basis for change, improvement, and growth. Practitioners' participation in quality improvement activities will hopefully make the resultant changes easier to implement.

EVIDENCE-BASED RESEARCH CHART

Topic	Evidence
Evidence-based quality improvement	Chassin, Loeb, Schmaltz, & Wachter, 2010; Schmaltz & Wachter, 2010
Effectiveness of quality improvement strategies and programs	Grimshaw et al., 2003; Mittman, 2004; Shojania & Grimshaw, 2005; Skledar & McKaveney, 2009; Snoby, 2004

Summary

Keys to success in a quality improvement endeavor are to consider it as a continuous circular process, not a onetime deal or solely as a cost-cutting maneuver. Such a process requires a culture change and a full buy-in from all concerned. Devising the end results (outcomes) can lead to increased satisfaction for the stakeholders and makes the task even more worthwhile.

Quality improvement is an ongoing, circular process that includes administration, professionals, and consumers. The process is completed to ensure the highest quality care possible. To sustain quality, administration and professionals must communicate and actively participate in the quality improvement process. The FOCUS-PDCA process demonstrates how the development of a comprehensive quality improvement program can be used to monitor and evaluate quality standards. Assessment of quality does not stop at the clinic or organization; occupational therapy practitioners must strive to provide quality and ethical services and take the responsibility for their own professional development.

Albrecht (1993, p. 116) underscores, in the following, the critical importance of the occupational therapy profession investing in continually improving the quality of their services: "the moment of truth is an episode in which the customer (client) comes into contact with the organization and gets an impression of its service."

Student Self-Assessment

1. Identify the FOCUS-PDCA process for monitoring and evaluating quality standards.

2. Further discuss possible solutions to remedy the intervention minutes problem within the department.

References

Albrecht, K. (1993). *The only thing that matters: Bringing the power of the customer into the center of your business* (p. 54). New York, NY: Harper Paperbacks.

American Occupational Therapy Association. (2010a). Occupational therapy code of ethics and ethics standards, *American Journal of Occupational Therapy, 64*(Suppl. 6).

American Occupational Therapy Association. (2010b). Standards for Continuing Competence. *American Journal of Occupational Therapy, 64*(Suppl. 6).

American Occupational Therapy Association. (2013). *Professional development tool.* Retrieved from http://www1.aota.org/pdt/p2_4.htm#

Bataldan, P. B., & Davidoff, F. (2013). *What is "quality improvement" and how can it transform healthcare?* Retrieved from http://qualitysafety.bmj.com/content/16/1/2.full?sid=60556d89-bb15-4c47-8e54-edc85fe71af4

Braveman, B. (2006). *Leading & managing occupational therapy services: An evidence-based approach.* Philadelphia, PA: F.A. Davis Company.

Case-Smith, J. (2005). Using client outcome data to guide your professional development. *OT Practice, 10*(4), 8-9.

Chassin, M. R., Loeb, J. M., Schmaltz, S. P., & Wachter, R. M. (2010). Accountability measures: Using measurement to promote quality improvement. *New England Journal of Medicine, 363,* 638-688.

Deming, D. E. (2000). *Out of crisis.* Cambridge, MA: The MIT Press.

Donabedian, A. (1980). *Explorations in quality assessment and monitoring: The definition of quality and approaches to its assessment* (Vol. 1.). Ann Arbor, MI: Health Administration Press.

Griffin, R. W. (1993). *Management* (4th ed.). Boston, MA: Houghton Mifflin.

Grimshaw, J., McAuley, L. M., Bero, L. A., Grilli, R., Oxman, A. D., Ramsay, C., et al. (2003). Systematic reviews of the effectiveness of quality improvement strategies and programmes. *Quality and Safety in Health Care, 12,* 298-303.

Hinojosa, J., Bowen, R., Epstein, C., Scwope, C., Davis Rourk, J., Berg Rice, V., et al. (1998). *Continuing competency task force report to the executive board.* Bethesda, MD: AOTA Press.

Institute of Medicine (2001). Crossing the quality chasm: A new health system for the twenty-first century. Washington, DC: National Academy Press.

Jacobs, J. S., & Logigian, M. K. (Eds.). (1999). *Functions of a manager in occupational therapy* (3rd ed.). Thorofare, NJ: SLACK Incorporated.

Jencks, S., Huff, T., & Cuerdon, T. (2003). Change in the quality of care delivered to Medicare beneficiaries, 1998-1999 to 2000-2001. *Journal of the American Medical Association, 289,* 305-312. Retrieved from http://domrg.stanford.edu/compliance/focus.html

Joint Commission on the Accreditation of Healthcare Organizations. (1995). *Using performance improvement tools in home care and hospice organizations.* Oakbrook Terrace, IL: Author.

Joint Commission on the Accreditation of Healthcare Organizations. (2013). Facts about patient-centered communications. Retrieved from http://www.jointcommission.org/assets/1/18/Patient_Centered_Communications_7_3_12.pdf

Lindenauer, P., Remus, D., Roman, S., Rothberg, M., Benjamin, E., Ma, A., et al. (2007). Public reporting and pay for performance in hospital quality improvement. *New England Journal of Medicine, 356*(5), 486-496.

Maslin, Z. B. (1991). *Management in occupational therapy.* San Diego, CA: Singular Publishing Group.

Mittman, B. (2004). Creating the evidence base for quality improvement collaboratives. *Annals of Internal Medicine, 140*(11), 897-901.

National Board for Certification in Occupational Therapy. (20). *Certification renewal handbook.* Retrieved from http://www.nbcot.org/webarticles/anmviewer.asp?a=66&z=13

National Board for Certification in Occupational Therapy. (2013). *Self-assessment tool:* Retrieved from http://www.nbcot.org/index.php?option=com_content*view=article&id=218&Itemid=136

O'Sullivan, G. (2004). Leisure activity programming: Promoting life satisfaction and quality of life for residents in long-term care. *New Zealand Journal of Occupational Therapy, 51*(2), 33-38.

Parasuraman, A., Berry, L. L., & Zeithaml, V. A. (1991). Understanding customer expectations of service. *Sloan Management Review, 32*(3), 39-48.

Punwar, A. J. (1998). *Occupational therapy: Principles & practice.* Baltimore, MD: Williams & Wilkins.

Rakich, J. S., Logest, B. B., & Darr, K. (1992). *Managing health services organizations* (3rd ed.). Baltimore, MD: Health Professions Press.

Rosenthal, M., Fernandopulle, R., Song, H., & Landon, B. (2004). Paying for quality: Providers' incentives for quality improvement. *Health Affairs, 23*(2), 127-141.

Shi, L., & Singh, D. (2012). *Delivering health care in America: A systems approach* (5th ed.). Burlington, MA: Jones & Bartlett Publishers.

Shojania, K., & Grimshaw, J. (2005). Evidence-based quality improvement: The state of the science. *Health Affairs, 24*(1), 138-150.

Skledar, S. J., & McKaveney, T. P. (2009). A method for teaching continuous quality improvement to student pharmacists through a practical application project. *Currents in Pharmacy, Teaching, and Learning, 1,* 79-86.

Snoby, P. (2004). Performance improvement boot camp. *Radiology Nursing, 23*(3), 68-77.

Whiteley, R. C. (1993). *The customer-driven company: Moving from talk to action.* New York, NY: Basic Books.

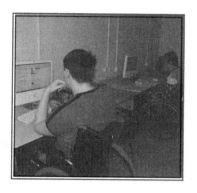

42

SUPERVISION OF
OCCUPATIONAL THERAPY PERSONNEL

Amy Jo Lamb, OTD, OTR/L, FAOTA

ACOTE STANDARDS EXPLORED IN THIS CHAPTER
B.7.7

KEY VOCABULARY

- **Occupational therapy practitioners:** Term used to encompass occupational therapists and occupational therapy assistants.
- **Service competency:** The ability of an occupational therapy assistant to obtain the same information in an evaluation tasks or perform treatment procedures in a manner that outcomes and documentation are equivalent to that of the supervising occupational therapist.

- **Site:** Setting in which practice occurs.
- **Supervisee:** One who receives direction and undergoes evaluation by a qualified practitioner.
- **Supervision:** Direct and evaluate performance.

Introduction

The advancement of the occupational therapy profession is multifaceted. At the heart of this advancement is the necessary inter-collaborations of occupational therapy professionals of all levels. This chapter identifies the participants in the supervisory relationship; examines the professional guidelines for supervision in occupational therapy; and provides an overview of strategies for effective, competency-based, legal, and ethical supervision of occupational therapy and non-occupational therapy personnel.

Jacobs, K., MacRae, N., & Sladyk, K. (Eds.).
Occupational Therapy Essentials for
Clinical Competence, Second Edition (pp. 553-558).
© 2014 SLACK Incorporated.

Participants in the Supervisory Relationship

The term *occupational therapy professional* includes occupational therapists, occupational therapy assistants, and students of occupational therapy. In some practice settings, occupational therapy or rehabilitation aides are also a part of the supervisory relationship. The functions of a supervisor are in three areas: educational, administrative, and supportive.

The official documents of American Occupational Therapy Association (AOTA) define supervision as a:

> *Cooperative process in which two or more people participate in a joint effort to establish, maintain, and or elevate a level of competence and performance.* (AOTA, 2009, p. 173)

GENERAL SUPERVISION ISSUES

Supervision is a continuing and dynamic process that encourages professional development in both the supervisee and supervisor. Supervision is considered a professional responsibility and, therefore, an important aspect of good clinical practice. Both the occupational therapy assistant and occupational therapist should seek supervision according to the Code of Ethics and good clinical judgment (Sladyk, 2005).

Being a supervisor for another practitioner is a process that is sure to spark development and growth in both the supervisor and the supervisee. Communication is a key factor in the supervisory process. It is often the supervisor who takes the lead in initiating this process. It is best accomplished by scheduling time to sit together and discuss how each of you communicates. For example, if the supervisor is very direct in his or her communication, a supervisee who is more timid may read that as a lack of openness and may refrain from engaging in dialogue or asking questions out of fear. Opening the lines of communication allows for each party to share how they communicate up front before any issues emerge and grow. These open lines also provide a good avenue to offer feedback. Frequent feedback is essential to learning. How does your supervisee prefer feedback? Perhaps he or she prefers it immediately or perhaps all lumped together at the end of the day or week in a summary session. Does the supervisee prefer the nuts and bolts of what needs to be worked on, or does he or she prefer a cushioned approach to feedback, such as stating areas of development in between comments about strengths they have in their practice? This information can all be discovered by keeping open communication lines.

As a supervisee, putting your best foot forward first is a great way to build a strong relationship with your direct supervisor. Prior to the starting the position, examine what it is you need and expect from the supervisor. Share this information with your supervisor on the first day to help define what you look for from the supervisory relationship. Know what to expect, review the materials the facility has regarding clients and department organization as well as your job description. Write down questions and ask for clarification; do not assume. Use the documents reviewed for your own reflection as to what kind of supervision you are expecting and in what manner you would prefer to receive supervision. A positive attitude by both parties is fundamental to success. When supervisors and supervisees approach the relationship with a positive attitude, are open to feedback, and participate with open communication, good things happen for the clients, departments, and facilities. Supervision is fundamental to skill development and learning, and being open to the process is the first step toward a successful relationship.

SUPERVISION OF THE OCCUPATIONAL THERAPIST

Although no supervision is required, supervision by an occupational therapist with advanced skills is recommended and will enhance clinical practice. Novice practitioners can benefit from supervision from mid-career and advanced practitioners. Mid-career practitioners can often benefit from occasional supervision by advanced practitioners as they continue to grow in their practice and skill set. The regular interaction of practitioners at all experience levels enhances the practice of all involved and encourages the use of best practices, evidence, and innovative treatment approaches.

SUPERVISION OF THE OCCUPATIONAL THERAPY ASSISTANT

Services of occupational therapy assistants are provided under supervision from an occupational therapist. Supervision of the occupational therapy assistant by an occupational therapist is a requirement both professionally and legally.

PROFESSIONAL GUIDELINES FOR SUPERVISION

The manner in which this supervision occurs is guided by the general principles outlined by the AOTA in the *Guidelines for Supervision, Roles, and Responsibilities During the Delivery of Occupational Therapy Services.* Key principles in the occupational therapist/occupational therapy assistant supervisory relationship include the following:

- Provision of safe and effective service delivery is essential; therefore, the occupational therapist and occupational therapy assistant should collaborate to determine the manner and frequency of supervision.

- Both the occupational therapist and occupational therapy assistant should recognize when supervision is needed.

- Frequency, methods, and content of supervision is dependent on the practice setting and needs of clientele.

- Supervision that is more stringent than the facility or regulatory body requires may be necessary in settings where clients are complex.

- Methods of supervision should vary and include both direct and indirect contact.

- Occupational therapists and occupational therapy assistants must adhere to facility and state requirements for supervision.

- The occupational therapist must recognize and be responsive to the occupational therapy assistants' professional growth and support their advancing practice skill set (AOTA, 2009, p. 174).

It is important to recognize that the guidelines provided are to serve as a guide as you develop the framework for the occupational therapist/occupational therapy assistant partnership. It is essential that you look at state licensing and reimbursement agency requirements for supervision, as they supersede the preceding guidelines from AOTA.

ROLES AND RESPONSIBILITIES IN THE DELIVERY OF OCCUPATIONAL THERAPY SERVICES

There are several points that are important to emphasize in the roles and responsibilities of occupational therapists and occupational therapy assistants in the delivery of occupational therapy services as it pertains to the supervision process.

- The occupational therapist is responsible for all aspects of occupational therapy service delivery.

- The occupational therapist must be involved in the initial evaluation and regularly throughout the client's intervention.

- The occupational therapy assistant delivers occupational therapy services under supervision of an occupational therapist.

- The occupational therapist determines when to delegate responsibilities to an occupational therapy assistant when service competency has been demonstrated.

- The occupational therapists and occupational therapy assistants demonstrate and document service competency for clinical reasoning and judgment as well as treatment techniques and interventions (AOTA, 2009, p. 175).

Within this area it is important to recognize that service competency means that an occupational therapy assistant gets the same information, or performs treatment procedures in a manner that the outcome and documentation are equivalent to what would have been achieved if the supervising occupational therapist had performed the services. Service competency is often established by the occupational therapist and occupational therapy assistant working together to establish such competencies. In the establishment of service competency, open communication is important as is consistent feedback between both the supervisor and supervisee.

OCCUPATIONAL THERAPY OR REHABILITATION AIDES

Aides are individuals who provide support services to the occupational therapist, occupational therapy assistant, physical therapist, or physical therapist assistant. They are trained by the skilled rehabilitation professional and must demonstrate competency to complete delegated client and non-client tasks (AOTA, 2010, p. 177). When aides are being used in a practice setting, the occupational therapist is responsible for developing, documenting, and implementing a supervisory plan for the aide. Occupational therapy assistants can provide supervision to the aide.

Skills for Supervisory Success

Supervision is a process by which both the supervisor and supervisee are learning from the other. The supervisory relationship provides partners with a planned opportunity to talk about practice, exchange ideas, and ensure appropriate delivery of services. Supervisors should clarify expectations surrounding their responsibilities as a supervisor within their profession at large and also within their organization to develop a foundation for success.

COMMUNICATION

Communication is a must in a successful supervisory relationship. Being successful in your occupational therapy role is not limited to the technical aspects of the job or being willing to work hard. Success is intricately related to being able to transmit information and ideas to others (with clients, occupational therapy team members, and other health care practitioners alike). The ability to communicate in a clear, consistent manner is vital to the supervisory process. Supervisors also need to recognize the importance of listening, establishing rapport, and motivating others. Effective communication leads to productive relationships.

Appropriate Delegation

It is the responsibility of the supervisor to ensure that when tasks are delegated to a supervisee that they are ready for that responsibility and qualified to adequately complete the task. Delegating does not take responsibility away from the supervisor. When delegating, it is important to consider the practice context, knowledge and skill level of the supervisee, and complexity of the task. It is often helpful to use a method frequently used in documentation for communication in delegating tasks. The SMART method (specific, measurable, achievable, realistic, and time bound) can be used as a framework in which you delegate tasks to a supervisee; this method supports clear communication so both the supervisor and supervisee understand the task and its associated responsibilities.

Feedback

Clear, consistent regular feedback is useful in keeping the supervisory/supervisee relationship moving forward. Feedback encourages growth among both parties and is essential to learning and development. Feedback should not just happen once a year at an annual performance review but is most effective when it occurs regularly and is consistent. Feedback should also be mixed; things the supervisee is doing well should be emphasized along with the areas for growth. It is also recommended that you observe your supervisee in a variety of venues, such as a treatment session, documentation, communication with clients and/or families, and communication with other professionals in the setting to provide feedback in each of these areas.

Create multifaceted mechanisms for delivering feedback. Each of us processes information differently. Provide avenues to reach the supervisee in multiple ways. Written feedback can be provided in weekly progress forms and shared with the supervisee. Feedback in writing allows the supervisee to reflect back on your comments. Verbal feedback can be provided in conjunction with the written feedback and ideally reviewed in a weekly meeting. Verbal feedback can also occur immediately after an observation session, and depending on the observation setting, you can ask the supervisee to reflect on what happened, what went well, and what they would have done differently. This sparks reflective thinking and opens the door for you to offer feedback after they have shared their reflections with you. Finally, demonstrations can effectively serve as feedback as well. Establish opportunities for staff to learn from one another. It creates a strong sense of team and builds the culture within in a department.

Supporting Professional Growth

Each occupational therapy practitioner has their own desires and interests for professional growth. Working together as a team does not mean that both the supervisor and supervisee need to have similar professional growth interests. One of the benefits of working as a team is supporting one another in professional growth. As a supervisor, when an individual under your supervision expresses an interest in gaining additional skills in a particular area or seeking increased experience in an area they find intriguing, it is your responsibility to assist the supervisee in identifying and supporting appropriate professional growth opportunities.

Evaluation of Performance

Almost all facilities require a minimum yearly written review of work productivity. Feedback on this form should not come as a surprise to the supervisee, as a good supervisor has talked about the issues well before a formal written evaluation is completed. Feedback should be specific, balanced, and focused on behaviors. The supervisee should initially develop professional goals for the next review period that fit the program's mission statement. Then together the supervisor and supervisee should develop a plan to meet these goals (Sladyk, 2005). A helpful strategy for supervisors to use is to provide the supervisee with a copy of the annual performance documents to utilize as a self-evaluation tool prior to the meeting, as it opens the door to enhanced dialogue in the meeting and allows the supervisee to have done some reflection on their performance in a more organized way.

Reflective Learning in Supervision

Reflection is defined as "careful consideration of a subject matter, idea or purpose" (Merriam-Webster, 2012). Reflection is a primary vehicle for learning but it is not a process that comes easily for all. The process of supervision aims to facilitate reflection to deepen understanding (Davys & Beddoe, 2009). When reflection occurs as a part of the supervisory process, the supervisee is driven to learn from the experience and thought rather than pure knowledge of the supervisory. When a supervisor provides opportunity for the supervisee to reflect, they encourage the supervisee to take ownership of experiences while enhancing learning and development.

Generational Differences

Another important factor in the supervisory process is found in understanding the generational differences currently found in practice and in our upcoming generation of occupational therapists and occupational therapy assistants.

When examining generations, we look at the commonalities among individuals from hugely different

Table 42-1.

TRAITS ACROSS THE GENERATIONS

Generation (Born between)	Outlook	Work Ethic	View of Authority	Leadership Through	Perspective
Baby Boomers (1940 to 1960)	Optimistic	Driven	Love/hate	Consensus	Team
Generation X (1960 to 1980)	Skeptical	Balanced	Unimpressed	Competence	Self
Millennial (1980 to 2000)	Hopeful	Ambitious	Relaxed, polite	Achievement	Civic

Adapted from Raines, C., & Ewing, L. (2006). *The art of connecting: How to overcome differences, build rapport, and communicate effectively with anyone.* New York, NY: American Management Association.

backgrounds within a defined period of time (Raines, 2003). How does this information play a role in occupational therapy supervision? Consider who we are often pairing together within the supervisory relationship. Think about how practice has evolved and changed and how rapidly the system in which we practice is changing. Areas of practice have shifted, educational programs have evolved, and the entry-level practitioner today is different from that 20 years ago. For this discussion, we will focus on three generations, all of which are key players within occupational therapy clinical education: the baby boomers, generation X, and generation Y. Table 42-1 explores these generations further.

Generational differences cannot go ignored as we examine the supervisor/supervisee relationship. Let us examine the supervisor/supervisee concept further and then look at case studies that include the generational mixes found in practice today.

Ethical Dilemmas in Supervision

It is inevitable that we will encounter ethical challenges in practice. When ethical issues emerge around supervisory relationships, each person is watching the other to see how it will be handled. There are models of decision making related to ethics that can be of use in demonstrating the process of handling ethical dilemmas. Gervais (2005) identified six steps to assist practitioners in this process. These steps include gathering background knowledge of the situation; examining the case based on its facts and context; completing a self-assessment, including the personal capacity for your decision, weighing options for what is most right, acting on the option you feel is ethically correct, and evaluating via reflection to examine what you learned in your review and handling

of this situation; and what you would do the same or what you would do differently should the situation arise again.

Supervisors should model ethical reasoning to supervisees to assist them in learning how they will approach ethical situations that arise. When an ethical issue arises with a client with whom both you and your supervisee have both been working, it is helpful to engage the supervisee with you as you navigate your decision making.

Summary

Supervision is a process through which both the supervisor and supervisee can develop professionally. The process of supervision is one that when done with open communication, consistent and frequent feedback, and in a manner that promotes professional growth can enhance the professional relationship among those involved. Using reflection in the supervision process enhances the learning for the supervisee and should be utilized regularly to promote professional development. In establishing supervisory partnerships, it is important to considering the generational differences to allow those of different generations to appreciate their colleagues' approach to the supervisory process.

Student Self-Assessment

1. In pairs, practice verbalizing what you envision to be the ideal supervisor/supervisee relationship.

2. On paper, write out how you would best describe your learning style is, how you prefer feedback, and your communication style.

3. Practice communicating with a partner and focus on clear direct communication to get them to complete a task.

EVIDENCE-BASED RESEARCH CHART

Issue	Evidence
Supervision	AOTA, 2008, 2009, 2010; Davys & Beddoe, 2010; Gervais, 2005
Reflective learning	Davys & Beddoe, 2009; Thorpe, 2004
Generational differences	Raines & Ewing, 2006; Zemke, Raines, & Filipczak, 2013

References

American Occupational Therapy Association. (2008). Occupational therapy practice framework: Domain and process (2nd ed.). *American Journal of Occupational Therapy, 62*(6), 625-683.

American Occupational Therapy Association. (2009). *Guidelines for supervision, roles, and responsibilities during the delivery of occupational therapy services.* Retrieved from http://www.aota.org/Practitioners/Official/Guidelines/36202.aspx?FT=.pdf

American Occupational Therapy Association. (2010). *Standards of practice for occupational therapy.* Retrieved from http://www.aota.org/Practitioners/Official/Standards/36194.aspx?FT=.pdf

American Occupational Therapy Association. (2011). *Accreditation Council for Occupational Therapy Education Standards and Interpretative Guidelines.* Retrieved from http://www.aota.org/Educate/Accredit/Draft-Standards/50146.aspx?FT=.pdf

Davys, A., & Beddoe, L. (2009). The reflective learning model: Supervision of social work students. *Social Work Education, 28*(8), 919-933.

Gervais, K. G. (2005). A model for ethical decision making to inform the ethics education of future health care professionals. In R. B. Purtilo, G. M. Jensen, & C. B. Royeen (Eds.), *Educating for moral action: A sourcebook in health and rehabilitation ethics.* Philadelphia, PA: F.A. Davis Company.

Merriam-Webster. (2013). *Webster online dictionary.* Retrieved from http://www.merriam-webster.com/dictionary/reflection

Raines, C. (2003). Connecting generations: The sourcebook for a new workplace. Menlo Park, CA: Crisp Publications.

Raines, C., & Ewing, L. (2006). *The art of connecting: How to overcome differences, build rapport, and communicate effectively with anyone.* New York, NY: American Management Association.

Sladyk, K. (Ed.) (2005). OT study cards in a box. Thorofare, NJ: SLACK Incorporated.

Thorpe, K. (2004). Reflective learning journals: From concept to practice. *Reflective Practice, 5*(3), 327-343.

Suggested Readings

Davys, A., & Beddoe, L. (2010). *Best Practice in Professional Supervision: A guide for the helping professions.* Philadelphia, PA: Jessica Kingsley Publishers.

Zemke, R., Raines, C., & Filipczak, B. (2013). *Generations at Work: Managing the Clash of Boomers, Gen Xers, and Gen Yers in the Workplace.* New York, NY: American Management Association.

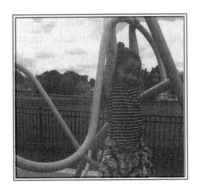

43

FIELDWORK EDUCATION

Julie Ann Nastasi, OTD, OTR/L, SCLV, FAOTA

ACOTE STANDARDS EXPLORED IN THIS CHAPTER

B.7.8

KEY VOCABULARY

- **Fieldwork coordinator:** A faculty member who is responsible for overseeing student fieldwork placements.
- **Fieldwork supervisor:** An occupational therapy practitioner who provides supervision to the student during the fieldwork placement.

- **Level I fieldwork:** Fieldwork that introduces the student to the fieldwork experience.
- **Level II fieldwork:** Fieldwork that transitions the student to the role of an entry-level practitioner.

Introduction

Fieldwork education is crucial to the field of occupational therapy. Occupational therapy relies on fieldwork supervisors, who work in collaboration with fieldwork coordinators to train and evaluate students to meet the minimal standards for entry-level practice (Accreditation Council for Occupational Therapy Education [ACOTE], 2011). Successful completion of fieldwork is required to graduate from an accredited program and to sit for the national board examinations (ACOTE, 2011; National Board for Certification in Occupational Therapy [NBCOT], 2009). Occupational

therapy practitioners have a professional responsibility to ensure the future of the profession through fieldwork education. Roles, criteria, and components of fieldwork education are explored in this chapter.

Occupational Therapy Education Programs

Occupational therapy education programs are responsible for training students in the fundamental knowledge and skills necessary to become occupational therapists and occupational therapy assistants. Each occupational

Jacobs, K., MacRae, N., & Sladyk, K. (Eds.).
Occupational Therapy Essentials for
Clinical Competence, Second Edition (pp. 559-565).

therapy education program designs its curriculum to address its mission and vision for the program. The fieldwork coordinator selects fieldwork sites for students that match the program's mission and vision.

FIELDWORK COORDINATOR

Each occupational therapy education program has a fieldwork coordinator who is responsible for the program's compliance with fieldwork education requirements. The fieldwork coordinator serves as a liaison between the program and the fieldwork sites to ensure that students are being properly trained and that the fieldwork placement aligns with the program's curriculum. The fieldwork coordinator oversees the fieldwork placements and works with the fieldwork supervisor and students in facilitating fieldwork placements.

FIELDWORK SUPERVISOR

The fieldwork supervisor is the person responsible for supervising occupational therapy students on Level I or Level II fieldwork placements. The fieldwork supervisor is responsible for the student completing the fieldwork placement. The supervisor guides, facilitates, and evaluates the student throughout the placement. At the end of the placement, the fieldwork supervisor evaluates whether the student has accomplished the requirements of the fieldwork placement. If the student achieves the requirements, the student passes the fieldwork placement. If the student does not meet the requirements, the fieldwork supervisor collaborates with the fieldwork coordinator and the student for the purpose of preparing for another placement. They discuss the areas that the student needs to improve before completing a new placement.

ELIGIBILITY REQUIREMENTS FOR FIELDWORK SUPERVISORS

The ACOTE (2011) requires that Level II fieldwork supervisors have successfully completed initial certification through the NBCOT and have a minimum of 1 year of practice before supervising students on fieldwork placements. In addition, the fieldwork supervisor must be adequately prepared to supervise the student. Training in fieldwork supervision may be provided by the academic program or the fieldwork site. The requirements for Level I fieldwork supervisors are less stringent. Occupational therapists and occupational therapy assistants may supervise students on Level I fieldwork as well as other qualified professionals, including psychologists, physician assistants, teachers, social workers, nurses, and physical therapists (ACOTE, 2011).

STUDENTS

Students on fieldwork must first complete their academic program's requirements to be eligible for a fieldwork placement. In addition, some fieldwork sites may require students to complete additional requirements. Some of these requirements may include, but are not limited to, a physical examination, cardiopulmonary resuscitation (CPR) training, a criminal background check, fingerprinting, and individual malpractice insurance. The fieldwork coordinator or the fieldwork supervisor typically notifies the students of the requirements for specific fieldwork placements. Some fieldwork sites also require students to complete orientation through their human resources department before starting fieldwork. Students should check to ensure that all requirements are met before starting fieldwork in order to avoid a delay or cancellation in the placement.

While on fieldwork, the students report directly to their assigned fieldwork supervisors. In some settings, students may have more than one supervisor. Students should collaborate and communicate with their assigned fieldwork supervisors. If students find they are having problems at their fieldwork site, they should notify their program's fieldwork coordinator. The fieldwork coordinator serves as a liaison between the students and the fieldwork site where the students are placed. It is in the students' best interest to communicate with their fieldwork coordinators about their fieldwork progress.

Fieldwork

Fieldwork should provide students "with the opportunity to carry out professional responsibilities under supervision of a qualified occupational therapy practitioner serving as a role model" (ACOTE, 2011, p. 32). Students have the opportunity to participate in Level I and Level II fieldwork experiences.

LEVEL I FIELDWORK

The goal of Level I fieldwork is to introduce students to the fieldwork experience, to apply knowledge to practice, and to develop understanding of the needs of clients. (ACOTE, 2011, p. 33)

During Level I fieldwork, students complete observations in an assigned setting. Settings are often associated with a particular practice course that the students have taken. For example, some programs have students complete Level I fieldwork in pediatrics during or after their pediatric practice course. The Level I fieldwork experience allows the students to observe and participate in clinical practice settings that relate to their coursework. Students are not required to be supervised by an occupational therapist or occupational therapy assistant during Level I fieldwork. Other qualified professionals include psychologists, physician assistants, teachers, social workers, nurses, and physical therapists (ACOTE, 2011).

It should be noted that ACOTE now requires students to complete a Level I or a Level II fieldwork experience that "focuses on psychological and social factors that influence engagement in occupation" (ACOTE, 2011, p. 33). Students should expect to be placed in a Level I or Level II fieldwork placement that addresses psychological and social factors that impact engagement in occupation.

LEVEL II FIELDWORK

The goal of Level II fieldwork is to develop competent, entry-level, generalist occupational therapists and occupational therapy assistants (ACOTE, 2011). "Level II fieldwork must be integral to the program's curriculum design and must include an in-depth experience in delivering occupational therapy services to clients, focusing on the application of purposeful and meaningful occupation and research" (ACOTE, 2011, p. 34). Occupational therapy students must complete a minimum of 24 weeks of full-time Level II fieldwork. Typically, the occupational therapy students complete two 12-week fieldwork placements in two different practice settings. Occupational therapy assistant students must complete a minimum of 16 weeks of full-time Level II fieldwork, which typically is in two different practice settings for 8 weeks each.

SPECIALTY LEVEL II FIELDWORK

Some programs allow students the option to select a third Level II fieldwork placement in a specialty area; other programs require students to complete a third Level II fieldwork placement. The third Level II fieldwork placement provides students with the opportunity to complete a fieldwork placement that is in a specialized practice area. Programs are required to prepare students as entry-level generalists (ACOTE, 2011). The third fieldwork placement goes beyond the accreditation requirements, thus providing students with the opportunity for specialization (Nastasi, 2012). For example, a student may want to complete a third Level II fieldwork placement in low vision rehabilitation or in a neonatal intensive care unit.

Steps for a Successful Fieldwork Placement

The goal for fieldwork coordinators, fieldwork supervisors, and students is to have students pass their fieldwork placements. Some steps for a successful fieldwork placement include a pre-fieldwork interview, formal orientation, student self-assessment, shared supervision by two fieldwork supervisors, and technological tools to promote independent learning.

PRE-INTERVIEW

Fieldwork supervisors should request that students complete an interview before their fieldwork placement.

The interview provides the students and the fieldwork supervisors with the opportunity to meet and gain a better understanding of the expectations of the placement, as well as to determine if there will be a good working relationship. Research has found that students benefit from a pre-fieldwork interview (Gutman, McCreedy, & Heisler, 1998; Holloway & Neufeldt, 1995). Grades are not effective indicators for fieldwork success. When students communicated with fieldwork supervisors, they are more successful on their fieldwork placements (Gutman et al., 1998). Students who are interpersonally attractive to their supervisors have been rated as being more effective by their supervisors than by their clients (Holloway & Neufeldt, 1995). The personality fit of the fieldwork supervisors and students plays a critical role in the scores that the students received from their fieldwork supervisors. Therefore, scheduling an interview before a fieldwork placement allows the fieldwork supervisors and the students to determine if there is a good fit as well as establish strong communication and a good working relationship.

FORMAL ORIENTATION

Students also benefit from formal orientation at their fieldwork sites. Formal orientation provides students with a better understanding of the expectations of the fieldwork supervisors and the fieldwork site. Kirke, Layton, and Sims (2007) used focus groups to determine the key elements of fieldwork education. The groups identified that fieldwork supervisors need to have a planned orientation during which the requirements of the placement are covered. Providing role clarity, team members' responsibilities, and a better understanding of the skills required during fieldwork facilitates the fieldwork placement (Robertson & Griffiths, 2009). In addition, structure is needed for continual development of students' skill progression during the fieldwork placement (Kleiser & Cox, 2008). Formal orientation provides a way to communicate the expectations of the fieldwork placement and provides students with key training and resources to support their participation in fieldwork education.

STUDENT SELF-ASSESSMENT

During fieldwork, students need to assess their performance and determine if they are meeting the expectations of their fieldwork supervisors and the site. Different forms of self-assessment have been incorporated into fieldwork education. Duke (2004) reported "that students who had self-awareness of their own strengths and weaknesses, and were not afraid to ask for help, were more competent than the students who were not able to reflect on their practice and to highlight areas of difficulty" (p. 207). One form of self assessment includes the use of journals (Buchanan, van Niekerk, & Moore, 2001; Maizels et al., 2008). Students complete a daily log during their fieldwork experience. Then at weekly supervision meetings, the students share portions of their journals with their fieldwork supervisors. This provides the students the opportunity to go over their thoughts and concerns during the past week. Upon completion of fieldwork, students should reread their journals and submit their journals to the program's fieldwork coordinator. The journal provides students with the opportunity to communicate with their fieldwork supervisors and to see their growth over the fieldwork placement. Other forms of self-assessment include learning contracts. Whitcombe (2001) studied the use of learning contracts in fieldwork education among 68 participants. The study found that the majority of respondents supported using learning contracts. Students reported that learning contracts allowed them to control their own learning. The fieldwork supervisors reported that the learning contracts helped them to focus on the individual learner's needs.

In conjunction with journals and a learning contract, a formal self-assessment should take place at the midterm and final evaluations. These formal self-assessments provide a reflective process, allowing the students, via collaboration with their fieldwork supervisors, to identify the progressive skill requirements and assess their performance during the placement, including what they need to do to successfully complete the placement.

STRUCTURE AND VALIDATION FOR SHARED SUPERVISION

Fieldwork coordinators and students know that it is not always easy finding fieldwork placements. A shortage of fieldwork placements and changes in occupational therapy practice have led the field of occupational therapy to examine different models of fieldwork supervision. Literature supports students having one or two fieldwork supervisors during their fieldwork placements (Bonello, 2001; Nolinske, 1995; Thomas et al., 2007). Supervision by two fieldwork supervisors provides students with opportunities to complete fieldwork in settings that do not have full-time occupational therapists. In addition, it provides students with the opportunity to complete fieldwork in emerging practice settings (Bonello, 2001). A recent study in Australia reported that 96% of participating students were supervised by one or two supervisors during fieldwork (Thomas et al., 2007). By allowing shared supervision between two fieldwork supervisors, both the shortage in fieldwork placements and the opportunity for students to engage in emerging practice areas are met.

TECHNOLOGICAL TOOLS TO PROMOTE INDEPENDENT LEARNING

Technology provides students with opportunities to learn and collaborate with their fieldwork coordinator and their fieldwork supervisors. Current research supports the use of technology in fieldwork education and for self-directed learning. "A growing body of evidence supports the conclusion that technology-enhanced teaching is equivalent in effectiveness compared with traditional methods when student-learning outcomes are the focus of the measurement" (Fullerton & Ingle, 2003, p. 426). Fullerton and Ingle reviewed 19 studies that focused on allied health professions and evaluated student grades, grade point averages, self-assessment competencies, practice guidelines, test scores, learner satisfaction, and use of technical support. They concluded that there was no difference in scores or grades for students learning on campus and students learning through asynchronous learning environments (Fullerton & Ingle, 2003). Overall, the evidence suggests that online learning allows for flexibility in studying in a virtual environment and is playing a more important role in supporting learning (Lui & Wang, 2009). Creating online materials for students during their fieldwork experience enhances their fieldwork experience. The use of Web-based instruction during fieldwork provides fieldwork coordinators with the opportunity to communicate with students during fieldwork. Such instruction may include synchronous or asynchronous discussions or meetings via Web camera. In addition, it provides students with the opportunity to network with each other, gain treatment ideas, and remain updated on the profession. In a study by Creel (2001), 89% of students involved in Web-based instruction during fieldwork indicated a strong interest in participating in it again for their next Level II fieldwork.

Training Materials for Fieldwork Education

Training and training materials are essential to fieldwork education. Training materials help fieldwork supervisors guide students through the fieldwork experience. Training materials include, but are not limited to, a manual, competency checklist, site-specific objectives, and developmental timeline.

MANUAL

Manuals provide fieldwork supervisors and students with a mechanism to store pertinent information about the fieldwork placement. The fieldwork supervisors may decide to review the materials with the students or have the students review the materials on their own time. Manuals should include a competency checklist, site-specific objectives, and a developmental timeline for the students.

Competency Checklist

A competency checklist provides fieldwork supervisors and students with information on the areas that the students need to be competent in to pass a fieldwork placement. The checklist allows the fieldwork supervisors and students to develop a plan on how to achieve the specific requirements during the fieldwork placement. The checklist should be reviewed on a weekly basis to ensure that the students are making progress on the required competencies. Fieldwork supervisors should develop and use a competency checklist that corresponds to the entry-level requirements for occupational therapists and occupational therapy assistants at their sites because the goal of Level II fieldwork is to achieve entry-level status. This assists the fieldwork supervisors at the site and the students in understanding the specific requirements of the fieldwork placement.

Site-Specific Objectives

Site-specific objectives should align with the Fieldwork Performance Evaluation (American Occupational Therapy Association [AOTA] 2002). Each fieldwork site should identify specific objectives for each of the items on the evaluation. Some sites may opt to use site-specific objectives that are provided by the educational program sending fieldwork students. Whether the site or the educational program creates the site-specific objectives, ACOTE (2011) requires that fieldwork sites have site-specific objectives. Structure and guidance are needed during fieldwork (Kleiser & Cox, 2008; Whitcombe, 2001). Having written guidelines and assessment criteria for fieldwork students assists the students (Buchanan et al., 2001; Meyers, 1995). Both occupational therapy students and fieldwork supervisors have reported that it was important to have defined objectives focusing on the fieldwork experience and the overall learning experience (Whitcombe, 2001). Site-specific objectives help define the students' fieldwork learning experiences.

Developmental Timeline

Finally, a developmental timeline provides fieldwork supervisors and students with an understanding of how students should progress through their fieldwork experience. Timelines break down the students' responsibilities in terms of case load and knowledge. By the end of the fieldwork placement, students should be carrying their supervisor's full caseload. A timeline provides students and fieldwork supervisors with a natural progression for the student's competency development. It provides structure and guidance for supervision (Kleiser & Cox, 2008).

Training Fieldwork Supervisors

Fieldwork supervisors generally receive on-the-job training to become fieldwork supervisors as well as training from the educational programs that send students to their sites. Formal training is available through the AOTA's Fieldwork Educators Certificate Workshop (AOTA, 2012). The workshop provides instruction in administration, education, supervision, and evaluation to fieldwork coordinators and fieldwork supervisors. It is important that occupational therapy practitioners are trained to become fieldwork supervisors because their participation is critical to the continued development and growth of the occupational therapy profession.

The ultimate goal for training fieldwork supervisors is to have a positive impact on practice, education, and research. This is established through collaboration with the fieldwork coordinators. Training ensures the fieldwork supervisors' competency as well as comfort with the tools developed for supervising and evaluating students. By providing ongoing support to fieldwork supervisors, occupational therapy education programs enhance their students' experiences on fieldwork.

Summary

"The purpose of fieldwork education is to propel each generation of occupational therapy practitioners from the role of student to that of practitioner" (AOTA, 2009, p. 821). If practitioners did not supervise students, the field of occupational therapy would eventually come to an end. Supervision of students brings forth the next generation of practitioners and leaders for the profession. Without future practitioners, societal needs will not be met. Supervising students on fieldwork placements not only benefits the profession but also benefits the fieldwork sites that take students, the fieldwork supervisors, and the students. For fieldwork sites, supervision of students brings new ideas to the setting as well as opportunities to recruit new employees. The fieldwork site benefits from training the students to meet the entry-level requirements specific to their site. The fieldwork site often is the first contact the student will have from an employer offering employment; this may allow the student an easy transition into his or her first position as an occupational therapist or occupational therapy assistant. For the fieldwork supervisor, NBCOT recognizes the value of supervising students (AOTA, 2009). Fieldwork supervisors are eligible to receive credit towards their continuing education requirements for renewing their certification as an OTR (occupational therapist) or COTA (certified occupation therapist assistant) through NBCOT by supervising students on Level I and Level II fieldwork placements. In addition, serving as a fieldwork supervisor is often a practitioner's first chance to serve in the role of mentor or manager. Fieldwork supervision provides practitioners with the opportunity to develop their own skills for career promotion. Finally, for students, fieldwork education provides them with the opportunity to complete the final steps to becoming a practitioner. Without fieldwork,

EVIDENCE-BASED RESEARCH CHART

Topic	Evidence
Pre-fieldwork interview	Gutman, McCreedy, & Heisler, 1998; Holloway & Neufeldt, 1995
Formal orientation	Kirke, Layton, & Sims, 2007; Kleiser & Cox, 2008; Robertson & Griffiths, 2009
Student self-assessment	Buchanan, van Niekerk, & Moore, 2001; Duke, 2004; Kramer & Stern, 1995; Lui & Wang, 2009: Maizels et al., 2008; Whitcombe, 2001
Structure and validation for shared supervision	Bonello, 2001; Kleiser & Cox, 2008; Nolinske, 1995; Thomas et al., 2007
Technology tools to promote independent learning	Creel, 2001; Fullerton & Ingle, 2003; Liu & Wang, 2009; Maizels et al., 2008; Nastasi, 2012
Fieldwork manual	Holloway & Neufeldt, 1995; Nastasi, 2012; Whitcombe, 2001
Competency checklist	Allison & Turpin, 2004; Buchanan et al., 2001; Duke, 2004; Kleiser & Cox, 2008; Maizels et al., 2008; Meyers, 1995; Nastasi, 2012; Robertson & Griffiths, 2009; Whitcombe, 2001
Site-specific objectives	Buchanan et al., 2001; Kleiser & Cox, 2008; Maizels et al., 2008; Meyers, 1995; Nastasi, 2012; Robertson & Griffiths, 2009; Thomas et al., 2007; Whitcombe, 2001
Developmental timeline	Buchanan et al., 2001; Kleiser & Cox, 2008, Maizels et al., 2008; Meyers, 1995; Nastasi, 2012; Robertson & Griffiths, 2009; Whitcombe, 2001
Training fieldwork supervisors	AOTA, 2012; ACOTE, 2011; Duke, 2004; Gutman et al., 1998; Kirke et al., 2007; Kleiser & Cox, 2008; Kramer & Stern, 1995; Meyers, 1995; Nastasi, 2012; Robertson & Griffiths, 2009

students would not be allowed to graduate or to sit for the board exams. "In summary, fieldwork education is an essential bridge between the academic education and the authentic occupational therapy practice" (AOTA, 2009, p. 822).

Electronic Resources

- AOTA fieldwork education resources: http://www.aota.org/Educate/EdRes/Fieldwork.aspx
- AOTA fieldwork-related products: http://www.aota.org/Educate/EdRes/Fieldwork/Products.aspx
- AOTA resources for new fieldwork programs: http://www.aota.org/Educate/EdRes/Fieldwork/NewPrograms.aspx
- AOTA site-specific objectives: http://www.aota.org/Educate/EdRes/Fieldwork/SiteObj.aspx
- AOTA student supervision: http://www.aota.org/Educate/EdRes/Fieldwork/StuSuprvsn.aspx

Student Self-Assessment

1. Identify five fieldwork sites where you would like to complete a fieldwork placement.

2. Visit the Web sites for each of the places that you have identified and gather information for each site. What services are provided? What is the setting? Who are the clients? What are the mission and vision of the site?

3. What do you need to do to prepare for fieldwork at the site?

4. Before your fieldwork placement, you should prepare for your interview. In pairs, discuss the kind of questions that may be asked on an interview and how you would answer the questions.

5. Journals are commonly used for self-assessment. Have you kept a journal in the past? If so, what were some of the benefits of keeping a journal? If not, how will keeping a journal help you?

References

Accreditation Council for Occupational Therapy Education. (2011). *2011 Accreditation Council for Occupational Therapy Education (ACOTE) Standards and Interpretive Guide.* Retrieved from www.aota.org/~/media/Corporate/Files/EducationCareers/Accredit/Draft-Standards/2011%20Standards%20and%20Interpretive%20Guide%20-%20December%202012%20Version.ashx

Allison, H., & Turpin, M. (2004). Development of the student placement evaluation form: A tool for assessing student fieldwork performance. *Australian Occupational Therapy Journal, 51*, 125-132.

American Occupational Therapy Association. (2002). *Fieldwork performance evaluation for occupational therapy students.* Bethesda, MD: AOTA Press.

American Occupational Therapy Association. (2009). Occupational therapy fieldwork education: Value and purpose. *American Journal of Occupational Therapy, 63*, 821-822.

American Occupational Therapy Association. (2012). *Fieldwork educators certificate workshop.* Retrieved from http://www.aota.org/Educate/EdRes/Fieldwork/Workshop.aspx

Bonello, M. (2001). Fieldwork within the context of higher education: A literature review. *British Journal of Occupational Therapy, 64*, 93-99.

Buchanan, H., van Niekerk, L., & Moore, R. (2001). Assessing fieldwork journals: Developmental portfolios. *British Journal of Occupational Therapy, 64*, 398-402.

Creel, T. (2001). Chat rooms and level II fieldwork. *Occupational Therapy in Health Care, 14*, 55-59.

Duke, L. (2004). Piecing together the jigsaw: How do practice educators define occupational therapy student competence? *British Journal of Occupational Therapy, 67*, 201-209.

Fullerton, J. T., & Ingle, H. T. (2003). Evaluation strategies for midwifery education linked to digital media and distance delivery technology. *Journal of Midwifery and Women's Health, 48*, 426-436.

Gutman, S. A., McCreedy, P., & Heisler, P. (1998). Student level II fieldwork: Strategies for intervention. *American Journal of Occupational Therapy, 52*, 143-149.

Holloway, E. L., & Neufeldt, S. A. (1995). Supervision: Its contributions to treatment efficacy. *Journal of Consulting and Clinical Psychology, 63*, 207-213.

Kirke, P., Layton, N., & Sims, J. (2007). Informing fieldwork design: Key elements to quality in fieldwork education for undergraduate occupational therapy students. *Australian Occupational Therapy Journal, 54*(Suppl.), S13-S22.

Kleiser, H., & Cox, D. L. (2008). The integration of clinical and managerial supervision: A critical literature review. *British Journal of Occupational Therapy, 71*, 2-9.

Kramer, P., & Stern, K. (1995). Approaches to improving student performance on fieldwork. *The American Journal of Occupational Therapy, 49*, 156-159.

Lui, Y., & Wang, H. (2009). A comparative study on e-learning technologies and products: From the east to the west. *Systems Research and Behavioral Science, 26*, 191-209.

Maizels, M., Yerkes, E., Macejko, A., Hagerty, J., Chaviano, A. H., Cheng, E. Y., et al. (2008). A new computer enhanced visual learning method to train urology residents in pediatric orchiopexy: A prototype for accreditation council for graduate medical education. *Journal of Urology, 180*, 1814-1818.

Meyers, S. (1995). Exploring the costs and benefits drivers of clinical education. *American Journal of Occupational Therapy, 49*, 107-111.

Nastasi, J. (2012). Specialty level II fieldwork in low vision rehabilitation. *OT Practice, 17*(11), 13-16.

National Board for Certification in Occupational Therapy. (2009). *Eligibility requirements.* Retrieved from NBCOT: http://nbcot.org/index.php?option=com_content&view=article&id=247&Itemid=154

Nolinske, T. (1995). Multiple mentoring relationships facilitate learning during fieldwork. *American Journal of Occupational Therapy, 49*, 39-43.

Robertson, L. J., & Griffiths, S. (2009). Graduate's reflections on their preparation for practice. *British Journal of Occupational Therapy, 72*, 125-132.

Thomas, Y., Dickson, D., Broadbridge, J., Hopper, L., Hawkins, R., Edwards, A., et al. (2007). Benefits and challenges of supervising occupational therapy fieldwork students: Supervisor's perspectives. *Australian Occupational Therapy Journal, 54*(Suppl.), S2-S12.

Whitcombe, S. W. (2001). Using learning contracts in fieldwork education: The views of occupational therapy students and those responsible for their supervision. *British Journal of Occupational Therapy, 64*, 552-558.

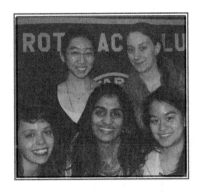

44

LEADERSHIP

Lisa L. Clark, MS, OTR/L, CLT and James Marc-Aurele, MBA, OTR/L

ACOTE STANDARDS EXPLORED IN THIS CHAPTER
B.7.1, B.7.5, B.9.2, B.9.10

KEY VOCABULARY
• **Context:** Environment and pragmatic considerations within which leadership takes place. • **Leader:** A person with authority who influences others toward a set of goals.	• **Leadership:** A process of leading and influencing others, which involves a range of theories of types of leadership. • **Manager:** A person in a position of power who directs others in their work or tasks.

The growth and development of people is the highest calling of leadership.

—Harvey S. Firestone

Introduction

When we first think of leadership, what comes to mind? Do we think about world leaders, whose position of power influences national and international public policies? Do we think about impassioned advocates who bring about sweeping social change against the odds of convention and misplaced conviction? Often, particular people come to mind: Golda Meir, Gandhi, Martin Luther King, Jr., Winston Churchill, and

so on. They embody what we think of as leaders—people who create a vision, move others to believe in it, and aspire to achieve it.

At first thought, leadership is a descriptor of the actions of those who have achieved exceptional status and influence as a result of accomplishments credited to their efforts. Although this is often the case, leadership in its truest sense is far more common. Opportunities for leadership present themselves every day. As occupational therapy practitioners, we are in a position to be leaders in our profession, our communities, and our day-to-day interactions with others.

This chapter explores the importance of leadership in the occupational therapy profession. The chapter discusses different types of leadership as a necessary background to thinking about effective leading. Personal, social, and

Jacobs, K., MacRae, N., & Sladyk, K. (Eds.).
*Occupational Therapy Essentials for
Clinical Competence, Second Edition* (pp. 567-575).
© 2014 SLACK Incorporated.

cultural contexts are important influences in leadership abilities and styles. Being a leader can be an occupation. The framework is used to examine the contexts that define leadership (American Occupational Therapy Association [AOTA], 2008). Although leadership occurs in political, community, and global settings, it is also very present in occupational therapy practitioners' daily work. This chapter illustrates several forms of leadership and makes it clear that leadership opportunities—and even obligations—exist for all occupational therapy practitioners in all settings. Finally, the chapter closes with an emphasis on how leadership in occupational therapy can play an important role in promoting social justice and social change.

Leadership as Occupation

Leadership and learning are indispensable to each other.

—*John F. Kennedy*

The AOTA Occupational Therapy Practice Framework (2008) informs internal and external audiences of the unique scope of service of occupational therapy and replaces the Uniform Terminology III document. The framework uses the following definition of occupation: "Activities . . . of everyday life, named, organized, and given value and meaning by the individuals and a culture. Occupation is everything people do to occupy themselves, including looking after themselves . . . enjoying life . . . and contributing to the social and economic fabric of their communities . . . " (Law, Polatajko, Baptiste, & Townsend, 2002). The occupation of leadership can be described using the Practice Framework as a background.

Acting as an effective leader involves performance skills, motor and process abilities, as well as communication and interaction skills. Leadership influences and is influenced by individual roles, habits, and routines. Particular activity demands are involved in leadership, and these demands differ in each situation. Context significantly influences leadership. The framework names several types of context: cultural, social, physical, temporal, virtual, and personal. Below is a brief exploration of each context and its relation to leadership.

- *Cultural context:* The culture in which leadership takes place is important. This context includes beliefs, customs, standards of behavior, and laws that are all part of an accepted culture of which an individual is a member (AOTA, 2008). These are generally factors that are external to the person. However, much of a cultural context can be internalized by the person as well. Laws that govern employee–employer relations can be part of a leader's cultural context. The internal culture of an organization also influences how leadership is performed.

- *Social context:* Social context includes expectations of other people who are important to the individual, as well as accepted norms of larger social groups (AOTA, 2008). Leaders may have particular ways of dressing or using specific words or language as part of their social context. The social context can significantly influence leading.

- *Physical context:* Physical context is the "environment" factor typically thought of when discussing context. It includes nonhuman aspects of the environment such as tools, plants, furniture, objects, animals, and natural terrain (AOTA, 2008). The physical context of where an individual engages in leading can greatly influence performance of leadership abilities. A concrete example of this is Martin Luther King, Jr.'s opportunity to use a microphone when leading and speaking to large groups. In this example, his physical context greatly enhanced his ability to lead effectively.

- *Temporal context:* This "time" context refers to the influence time can have on the performance of occupations (AOTA, 2008). A leader who holds meetings at the end of a long workday may find his or her effectiveness limited by the temporal context. Some leaders may feel influenced in their work by the time of year.

- *Virtual context:* This term refers to communication that occurs without physical contact and takes place over the airways or with a computer (AOTA, 2008). The virtual context has greatly influenced how and when communication takes place, as well as how effective it is. Leadership involves a great deal of communication (Hamm, 2006). Leaders must pay attention to the influence of the virtual context on the effectiveness of their leading.

- *Personal context:* According to the framework, personal context is made up of personal factors about the individual—age, gender, and other demographic information such as educational status and socioeconomic status. One example of this is studies where gender is examined as an influence on leadership styles (George & Jones, 2002).

The framework also describes a specific factor about the person that is important in the consideration of leadership, and that is spirituality. Spirituality takes into account what motivates or is inspirational to an individual. *Servant leadership* is a relatively new term for leadership that defines servant leaders as those who put others' needs before their own (Dillon, 2011). Servant leaders believe in self-knowledge, justice, and caring for the people they lead. Relationships are important. All leaders, in large or small ways, must be in touch with what is meaningful to them (Sadler-Smith & Shefy, 2004). Kouzes and Posner (2007) discussed exemplary leadership as having five important components. One of these is "encouraging the heart." They maintained that leaders need to "hear the heart and see the soul" (Kouzes & Posner, p. 329). Spirituality is an important factor to consider in terms of how each person participates in leadership behaviors.

Leadership as an occupation can be analyzed using the framework (AOTA, 2008), the latest written work describing what occupational therapy practitioners do and how and where they do it. It informs us about what motor, process, and communication abilities are helpful in leading, and it promotes discussion on the importance of contexts as they influence occupations.

Theories of Leadership

In developing leadership abilities, it is useful to understand how leadership theories and models have evolved over time. In some ways, the movement of leadership models to ones of more participatory, or shared, philosophies as well as transformational constructs more closely mirrors the way occupational therapy practitioners have been working to interact with people for the last century.

TRAIT THEORIES

There are many definitions and interpretations of leadership. In the past 75 years, countless theories have been espoused in an attempt to identify and explain the characteristics of leaders and effective leadership. DeYoung (2005) described how Lewin proposed that most leaders engaged in three leadership styles based on personality traits. These included authoritarian, democratic, and laissez-faire. Additional studies (George & Jones, 2002) focused on specific traits or characteristics displayed by leaders. Researchers identified several traits thought to have the strongest correlation with effective leadership. These included intelligence, task-relevant knowledge, energy, tolerance for stress, integrity, emotional maturity, and self-confidence. These traits were thought to be relatively fixed and not amenable to change. This view implies a predetermined ability to lead based on the possession of certain traits.

BEHAVIORAL THEORIES

DeYoung (2005) identified the specific behaviors engaged in by leaders to promote organizational effectiveness when he referred to the Ohio State research, which has been cited by many authors in leadership. According to these studies, leadership behavior can be classified as either consideration behaviors or as initiating structure behaviors. Consideration behavior is defined as behavior indicating that a leader trusts, respects, and values good relationships with his or her followers. Initiating structure behaviors are defined as actions a leader performs to make sure the work gets done. It is important to recognize that these leadership behaviors are not mutually exclusive. Leaders can and do engage in both initiating structure and consideration behaviors. The behavioral models provide insight into leader characteristics but do not address how and why leadership happens (George & Jones, 2002).

Leadership and Context

One of the early theorists credited with considering the context of leadership was Frederick Fiedler (1978). He attempted to explore the interrelationship between leader characteristics and the specific situation in which leadership takes place. The framework would refer to this as the influence of context. Fiedler defined the situation as having three specific dimensions: leader–follower relations, task structure, and the position power of the leader. In Fiedler's view, these three relationships, identified as contingency dimensions, significantly impacted leadership effectiveness (Fiedler, 1967). These characteristics were thought of as existing on a continuum from low to high. Together, the characteristics would determine "situational favorableness" for a particular leadership style (George & Jones, 2002). According to Fiedler, leaders engage in two specific styles of leadership: relationship oriented and task oriented (DeYoung, 2005). Relationship-oriented leaders place primary value on establishing positive working relationships with those they are leading. Leaders who are task oriented primarily emphasize task completion. Fiedler suggested that leaders are most effective in situations that most closely match their leadership styles. It is significant that he viewed leadership styles to be relatively fixed, such that leaders could not easily move from one style to the other. Thus, in his view, leadership style was a first-order variable with the situation (or context) as a determinant as to how effective a leadership style would be.

Fiedler's work began to look at situational factors and gave rise to the Situational Leadership Model. Developed by Hersey and Blanchard, the Situational Leadership Model examined the relationship among three dimensions: task behavior, relationship behavior, and the maturity of the individuals being led. The task behavior refers to the degree of structure and clarity that the leader provides (clearly defined work roles and responsibilities). The relationship dimension refers to the emotional and psychological relationship between the leader and the individual being led (Hersey & Blanchard, 1982). According to Hersey and Blanchard, these first two dimensions are greatly influenced by the maturity level of the individual being led. The maturity level is characterized by three specific criteria: level of motivation, willingness to assume responsibility, and the individual's experience and education level. Based on these criteria, the leader modifies his or her leadership approach. For example, when working with an entry-level occupational therapy practitioner, a leader will likely provide more structure for a given task to promote success, but a practitioner with considerable experience in the same situation may require less direction from the leader. Likewise, the leader must consider the level of motivation of the individual in altering his or her leadership behavior.

Leadership and Intuition

More recently, the role of intuition has gained increased attention. Some leadership abilities can be innate (Sadler-Smith & Shefy, 2004). Intuition is formed by individual feelings based on experience. Once regarded as anything but useful, intuition is now being recognized as a component to leadership. The role of intuition is supported by some researchers who postulate "much if not most of cognition occurs automatically outside of consciousness" (Sadler-Smith & Shefy, p. 78). Some studies indicate that senior leaders lead more intuitively than middle managers, highlighting the impact of experience in developing intuition.

Participatory Leadership

As the evolution of leadership continued over the decades, participatory leadership models gained increasing acceptance (McLagen & Nell, 1995). Given the multitude of societal and cultural change factors in organizations, participatory leadership models have become more popular. "With these changes, coaching and commitment cultures have replaced the command, control, and compartmentalization orientations of the past" (Kets de Vries, 2005, p. 62). Participatory leadership embraces change and readily involves others (Kouzes & Posner, 2007). Leadership in day-to-day work can move from person to person depending on the tasks involved and competencies needed. The leader facilitates and guides transitions (Ackerman & MacKenzie, 2006; McLagen & Nell). Participatory leaders readily defer to others' expertise. The parallels with occupational therapy client-centered practice are easily discerned. Engaging in participatory leadership is a powerful way to help people grow their strengths and enable future leaders. In participatory leadership, the focus is on collaboration, commitment, and context. Participatory leadership incorporates much of the multifaceted tenets of previous leadership theories. Pearce (2004) advocates that the more complex a task is, the more there is a need for shared or participatory leadership. This model is less a body of new work than a coming together of earlier approaches, melding traits, behaviors, and contextual factors.

Transformational Leadership

Transformational leaders also inspire and motivate people in their groups. They tend to be thought of as inspirational and are able to share credit and recognize the people who have contributed to shared work for an organization. Transformational leaders also stimulate people intellectually. Transformational leadership has been found to be effective in health care (Bowles & Bowles, 2000).

In this brief review of leadership theories, it is noted that early theories focused on individual traits and characteristics. This was followed by a study of specific behaviors, and more recent work has focused on the context of leadership. Although this review is limited, the theories here were chosen to provide a degree of insight into the components of leadership to help us begin to understand the what, why, and how of leadership. The effectiveness of leadership is a complex and ongoing field of study. The most effective leaders are able to use knowledge, experience, and consideration of personal and contextual factors when determining a style of interaction. The issue is not to excel at one particular type of leadership but to determine which approach is best given each particular scenario and context (Pearce, 2004; Shortell & Kaluzney, 2000).

Use the Case Example on the following page to look at the following problems.

PROBLEM #1

To comply with new insurance regulations, a directive has come down from senior management that billing documentation from each department must be on the same form. Ann's preferred leadership style is one of participatory leadership. However, this is an example of an issue that requires a directive leadership approach.

- **Virtual context.** Virtual communication may negatively influence Ann's ability to lead around this issue. Ann may find sending out a blanket email about this relatively large change in documentation does not engender effective communication with staff.

- **Temporal context.** This change needs to be implemented immediately. This temporal context constrains Ann's effectiveness as a leader in making this change.

- **Cultural context.** The organization understands the value of communicating directives when needed. They believe that the leader (Ann) can give these directives in whatever style she prefers.

- **Personal context.** Ann's years of experience may help her leadership with staff when delivering the billing form information.
- **Social context.** Ann's family values include a strong work ethic, and she realizes that some things just need to happen to keep organizations working effectively. Ann's staff members' contexts become part of her social context at work and do influence her leading abilities around this problem. She will have to consider Brad's time constraints and Jennie's penchant for questioning the system.
- **Physical context.** The fact that the staff members Ann leads are in different physical locations influences her effectiveness in leading them to work with this new form. Ann's sense of spirituality and her understanding of this in her own life can influence how she performs her leadership role. Her fundamental orientation to life is one of a belief in calm centeredness. This part of her person positively influences her leading, especially in potentially stressful times.

Problem #2

The occupational therapy staff wishes to infuse the framework into their daily documentation. The first step will be to revamp the initial assessment form for the outpatient department. Ann's preferred participatory leadership style can be put into play more in this scenario.

- **Virtual context.** The use of email can enhance Ann's leadership here, as suggestions and drafts of assessment forms may be easily shared among occupational therapy staff in different physical locations.
- **Temporal context.** This context will not significantly influence Ann's leading because there are no time constraints to the project.
- **Cultural context.** The organization values employee input for some projects. This context will help Ann lead her team to a successful conclusion in changing their assessment.
- **Personal context.** There is no change from the previous problem.
- **Social context.** Again, the staffs' contexts become part of Ann's social context at work. She will need to be cognizant of Brad's work schedule. Jennie will probably be helpful because her input is included in this project. Ann's appreciation of a strong work ethic leads her to value employees in all categories and will assist her in positive leading with the occupational therapy assistant and the occupational therapists alike. This will enhance her leadership and thus the outcome of the project. Ann values Juliette's attention to detail and this will also help the project.
- **Physical context.** Ann chooses a conference meeting that contains plush chairs, good lighting, and

---

Case Example

Ann is the manager of occupational therapy at a community medical center. Ann has 18 years of experience as an occupational therapist. Her specialty area of practice has been working with people with repetitive strain injuries. Ann possesses a very strong work ethic and believes that others should embrace this as well. She is responsible for overseeing the delivery of occupational therapy services in three different settings at two different locations. Her job responsibilities include scheduling and supply inventories. She initially found both tasks overwhelming without administrative support. She is now thankful that she enrolled in a continuing education course to learn to use software that helps to manage work schedules and inventories.

The level of experience of the staff Ann supervises is mixed. Brad is a new graduate occupational therapist. He is the father of two toddlers. He struggles occasionally to juggle his important roles of father, husband, and professional. Jennie has 25 years of experience as an occupational therapy assistant in rehabilitation with people experiencing neurologic deficits. She has a strong belief in self-advocacy and at times finds herself working in opposition to established systems. Juliette is an occupational therapist with 8 years of general experience with people who have physical disabilities. She is Franco American and works long hours to complete her work to her own high standards.

The organizational culture of the medical center is one of careful consideration of problems. The leadership values employee contributions for many, but not all, tasks. Some issues are clearly handled in a directive style. Many middle managers are allowed to lead in the manner they see fit.

---

plenty of workspace room for their first brainstorming meeting. Healthy snacks are provided. Ann knows that the physical context can greatly influence success in occupational performance.

Conclusion

The contexts of the leading, which are part of each problem, are important even though Ann must use different leadership styles in each scenario. Her effectiveness as a leader is greatly enhanced when she carefully considers the influences of the different contexts. Her abilities as a reflective leader help her consider the influence that context can have on her leading. She also recognizes when she needs to use different management strategies. By engaging her staff in a participatory fashion in the second scenario, Ann is able to capitalize on the strengths and experiences of the staff. Their participation, along with her leadership skills, combines to create an ultimately successful project.

Management Versus Leadership

Management is efficiency in climbing the ladder of success; leadership determines whether the ladder is leaning against the right wall.

—*Stephen R. Covey*

Leadership and *management* are often thought of as synonymous terms, implying that leaders manage and managers lead. Although this may be the case in some instances, it is arguably more complex than this. Effective leaders readily embrace change—they facilitate and guide transitions. Leaders involve others and are aware of their own limitations. Leaders are able to create a shared vision among people. Leaders inspire and coach others to work toward a shared vision of a group or organization.

Managers are often described in terms of the tasks to which they ably attend. They are responsible for resource allocation (staffing and budgets), generating reports, and managing programs (Borkowski, 2005; Grady, 2003).

Let us go back to our case study. Ann was in a position of leadership. In the first scenario, it could be said that she was managing. The new billing form information came in the form of a directive, which needed to be communicated. In the second scenario, she was able to lead more effectively. She valued input, understood and had thought about her own limitations, and inspired a shared vision with her coworkers around their project.

It is important to note that management and leadership are not mutually exclusive entities, nor is the comparison meant to diminish the functions of a manager. Management functions provide necessary parameters for operations to take place. Leaders may or may not be responsible for managerial components within their situations of leadership.

Leadership From Occupational Therapy Practitioners

Leadership should be, and is, undertaken by occupational therapists and occupational therapy assistants, as well as students. Some leadership skills can be similar to skills that practitioners use in their daily practice (McCormack, 2003; Strzelecki, 2007). Practitioners recognize that leadership skills and abilities can be present in everyone. Many state occupational therapy member associations, such as Maine and New York, are free to elect occupational therapists and occupational therapy assistants as president or other executive board positions. The New York State Occupational Therapy Association elected an occupational therapy assistant for a second term as president, starting in June 2005 (AOTA, 2005). There are many other examples of occupational therapists and occupational therapy assistants providing exemplary leadership within and outside of the profession.

Occupational Therapy Code of Ethics

Another key document for the profession that can shed light on leadership is the AOTA Occupational Therapy Code of Ethics. The Code is covered in greater detail in Chapter 48 but is briefly mentioned in this chapter.

The Occupational Therapy Code of Ethics (Slater, 2010) is a list of seven important principles that define how occupational therapy practitioners should conduct themselves in practice of the profession. Many of the principles seem to strictly apply to working with clients at first glance. However, the document asks that we understand that occupational therapy practice involves attention to work with others beyond clients, including the community. It is clear that occupational therapy practitioners are asked to be responsive to individuals, communities, and beyond. Leadership can be an effective occupation to help accomplish this. Occupational therapy practitioners can practice leadership in far-reaching, even political, ways and can thoughtfully recognize that every therapeutic interaction with another can be an act of leadership. Our professional Code of Ethics calls us to "virtuous practice of artistry and science . . . and to noble acts of courage" (AOTA, p. 639).

Leadership is not merely an opportunity but an obligation. By carefully increasing awareness and intentional concern for context, all practitioners can engage in leadership. Opportunities for leadership may present themselves in formal ways such as holding a position as manager or supervisor, but there are other equally important opportunities for leadership (Strzelecki, 2007). Using the information presented about the framework and how leadership can be analyzed as an occupation and having a better understanding of leadership models can engender a discussion about the influence of context on each individual's leadership abilities. Occupational therapy practitioners and students can think about their leadership abilities and desires by reflecting on their process and communication skills in addition to pondering their own individual contextual influences.

Personal context, such as age and education level, can affect how someone leads. Some of these individual factors are also influenced by the social context (society) and the cultural context (see Chapter 2). How do we tend to respond to a leader who has recently graduated from college? Or a leader who is in his or her 80s? Do we have societal or cultural expectations of how old or young a person must be to lead effectively? If so, does it behoove us to reconsider these perceived limitations? According to the framework, laws and societal changes are all part of the cultural context. Reflective and ethical leaders need to consider how laws and changes occurring in the larger community (e.g., changes in reimbursement) are affecting their leadership. How do these influences change what leaders must do, and how they do it?

On a smaller scale, individual leaders should also examine the influence of expectations and norms of their closer circles. These include beliefs, behavioral standards, or norms, and they can have an enormous effect on how people communicate and process information. Is the leader's family supportive of achievement? Do friends encourage or disparage moral standards? People who lead effectively reflect on what strategic tasks and occupations have been successful in the past. Also, has the use of virtual communication methods been a hindrance or a help in leading others? Leadership may also be influenced by the spiritual context, and this is an important area to ponder. The final context considered here in personal reflection of leaders is the physical. The physical environment (e.g., furniture, lighting, air quality, plants, objects) can stifle or encourage leading and the activities that accompany it. Each person should determine the importance of each of these contexts in his or her leadership practices.

The ways in which the framework breaks out different contextual influences can be a start in helping individuals assess their leadership abilities and experiences. Most occupational therapy practitioners will find that, upon reflection, many of the tasks they already complete can be seen in a leadership frame. Leadership theories and models can be infused into this complex weave of leading as an occupation. This weaving is a mechanism for individuals to reflect on how, where, and when leadership interfaces with their own lives. Occupational therapy practitioners understand people as occupational beings (Jarman, 2004). We can contemplate ourselves as occupational beings and become aware of how leading is an occupation that is important to the profession. Leadership in occupational therapy is an adventure in which all can participate in some way.

Spreier, Fontaine, and Malloy (2006) recognized that teams working together are more effective than individuals moving toward a goal on their own. This is part of participatory leadership. Every time an occupational therapy practitioner works with someone, he or she is leading in a participatory sense. When we embrace this realization, it is a small step to move to leading in a community or global context. Occupational therapy practitioners are especially well positioned to create and influence systems of care and wellness (social and cultural contexts)

because of our client-centered beliefs and the leadership abilities that we exemplify every day.

Leadership as an Ingredient of Social Change and Justice

Clearly, occupational therapy practitioners are uniquely situated to practice effective leadership. This can create social change. We can lead in our daily interactions with others as well as in the larger community. The framework clarifies how context and abilities are important in influencing occupations. Our code of ethics demands that we consider individuals and communities in our professional activities. Discovery about leadership philosophies and models informs our learning and reflection on different beliefs and styles.

Kronenberg and Pollard (2006) reminded us that, globally, the largest number of occupational therapy practitioners reside and work in the United States. This national group "significantly influences thinking, practice, education, and research of OT practitioners all over the world " (Kronenberg & Pollard, p. 1). Perhaps in the United States, we are especially obligated to think outside the box. We must critically assess our core professional values and how well they do or do not fit with our social and cultural contexts. Kronenberg and Pollard asserted that our profession's work is "always under construction" and "essentially never finished " (p. 1). They went on to suggest that with our expertise in occupations, perhaps we need to "problematize situations in which 'occupations' contribute to the construction of communities and societies that are exclusive" (Kronenberg & Pollard, p. 2).

Townsend and others discussed the term *occupational justice* as a way to think about social justice issues through the lens of occupation (Arnold & Rybski, 2010; Townsend & Whiteford, 2005; Townsend & Wilcock, 2004). If we understand that occupations are key in the health and wellness of human beings, then it is a short journey to realizing that occupations and people's opportunities to participate in them are very much part of social justice considerations (Sinclair, 2006). Conversely, there are occupational justice issues in communities where some occupations may be forced on people. In the wake of Hurricane Katrina in the southern United States in 2005, many people who experienced the force of the storm probably found themselves participating in the occupations of acquiring food and shelter in a very different manner than before the storm. News stories chronicled the socioeconomic issues about which strata of the population was more likely to be caught in the storm versus the socioeconomic status of the people who moved to safer ground.

Kronenberg and Pollard (2006) asked us to consider how continued study in occupational therapy and

EVIDENCE-BASED RESEARCH CHART

Topic	Evidence
Leadership theories and models	Borkowski, 2005; George & Jones, 2002; Hamm, 2006
Leadership contexts as occupational therapy practitioners think of them	AOTA, 2008
Reflective leadership	Kets de Vries, 2005; Kouzes & Posner, 2002; Sadler-Smith & Shefy, 2004
Social justice implications in leadership	Kronenberg, Algado, & Pollard, 2005; Townsend & Wilcock, 2004
Transformational leadership	Nahavandi, 2012; Kouzes & Posner, 2010

occupational science can inform "societies' responses to these complex and global realities" (p. 2). Consideration of occupational justice is a leadership issue in the occupational therapy profession.

Summary

Never doubt that a small group of thoughtful, concerned citizens can change the world. Indeed, it is the only thing that ever has.

—*Margaret Mead*

This chapter has explored leadership by discussing different leadership theories and analyzing the occupation of leading using the framework. The framework emphasis was on the role of context and the importance of reflection in developing leadership abilities. Participatory leadership and transformational leadership offer particular benefits to occupational therapy practitioners in many situations. Ultimately, leaders should possess abilities in various types of leadership and use them based on situation and context. Finally, issues of occupational justice are crucial ones to address in occupational therapy leadership. Leadership occurs every day in the profession. When we recognize and name these happenings, we are in a position to respond to our obligation to lead in community and global arenas.

Student Self-Assessment

1. Construct a personal leadership plan that addresses a particular task or goal (simple or complex), the type of leadership you plan to use in completing the task, and the strengths and weaknesses of your chosen style.

2. In groups of four to eight, choose a leadership scenario from a national or global incident that is in the news. Discuss the social justice implications of people's leadership and participation in the incident. What leadership styles and skills were used? Were they effective? Why or why not? What other leadership abilities could have been used that might have been more effective?

3. Consider one leadership experience you have witnessed or of which you have been a part. Discuss and analyze the different contexts, according to the framework, and how each of them influenced the leadership scenario.

References

Ackerman, R., & MacKenzie, S. (2006). Uncovering teacher leadership. *Educational Leadership, 63*, 66-70.

American Occupational Therapy Association. (2005). OTA exchange. *OT Practice, 10*(4), 23.

American Occupational Therapy Association. (2008). Occupational therapy practice framework: Domain and process (2nd ed.). *American Journal of Occupational Therapy, 62*, 625-683.

Arnold, M. J., & Rybski, D. (2010). Occupational justice. In M. E. Scaffa, S. M. Reitz, & M. A. Pizzi (Eds.), *Occupational therapy in the promotion of health and wellness* (pp. 135-156). Philadelphia, PA: F. A. Davis Company.

Borkowski, N. (2005). *Organizational behavior in health care.* Sudbury, MA: Jones & Bartlett Publishers.

Bowles, A., & Bowles, N. B. (2000). A comparative study of transformational leadership in nursing development units and conventional clinical settings. *Journal of Nursing Management, 8*(2), 69-76.

DeYoung, R. (2005). Behavioral theories of leadership. In N. Borkowski (Ed.), *Organizational behavior in health care* (pp. 173-185). Boston, MA: Jones and Bartlett.

Dillon, T. H. (2011). A legacy of leadership: transforming the occupational therapy profession. In K. Jacobs & G. McCormack (Eds.), *The occupational therapy manager* (5th ed.). Bethesda, MD: AOTA Press.

Fiedler, F. E. (1967). *A theory of leadership effectiveness*. New York, NY: McGraw-Hill.

Fiedler, F. E. (1978). The contingency model and the dynamics of the leadership process. In L. Berkowitz (Ed.), *Advances in experimental psychology*. New York, NY: Academic Press.

George, J., & Jones, G. (2002). *Organizational behavior* (3rd ed.). Upper Saddle River, NJ: Prentice Hall.

Grady, A. (2003). From management to leadership. In G. H. McCormack, E. Jaffe, & M. Goodman-Levy (Eds.), *The occupational therapy manager* (4th ed., pp. 331-347). Bethesda, MD: AOTA Press.

Hamm, J. (2006). The five messages leaders must manage. *Harvard Business Review, 84*, 114-123.

Hersey, P., & Blanchard, K. (1982). *Management of organizational behavior: Utilizing human resources*. Upper Saddle River, NJ: Prentice Hall.

Jarman, J. (2004) What is occupation? Interdisciplinary perspectives on defining and classifying human activity. In C. Christiansen & E. Townsend (Eds.), *Introduction to occupation: The art and science of living* (pp. 47-61). Upper Saddle River, NJ: Prentice Hall.

Kets de Vries, M. F. R. (2005). Leadership group coaching in action: The Zen of creating high performance teams. *Academy of Management Executive, 19*, 61-76.

Kouzes, J., & Posner, B. (2002). *The leadership challenge* (3rd ed.). San Francisco, CA: Jossey-Bass.

Kouzes, J., & Posner, B. (2007). *The leadership challenge* (4th ed.). San Francisco, CA: John Wiley & Sons.

Kronenberg, F., Algado, S. S., & Pollard, N. (Eds.). (2005). *Occupational therapy without borders: Learning from the spirit of survivors*. Philadelphia, PA: Elsevier.

Kronenberg, F., & Pollard, N. (2006). Political dimensions of occupation and the roles of occupational therapy. *American Journal of Occupational Therapy, 60*(6), 617-625.

Law, M., Polatajko, H., Baptiste, S., & Townsend, E. (2002). In American Occupational Therapy Association. *Occupational therapy practice framework: Domain and process*. Bethesda, MD: AOTA Press.

McCormack, G. (2003). Historical and current perspectives of management. In G. H. McCormack, E. Jaffe, & M. Goodman-Levy (Eds.), *The occupational therapy manager* (4th ed., pp. 331-347). Bethesda, MD: AOTA Press.

McLagan, P., & Nell, C. (1995). *The age of participation—New governance for the workplace and the world*. San Francisco, CA: Berrett-Koehler.

Nahavandi, A. (2012). The art and science of leadership (6th ed.), Boston, MA: Prentiss-Hall/Pearson, 193-197.

Pearce, C. (2004). The future of leadership: Combining vertical and shared leadership to transform knowledge work. *Academy of Management Executive, 18*, 47-57.

Sadler-Smith, E., & Shefy, E. (2004). The intuitive executive: Understanding and applying "gut feel" in decision making. *Academy of Management Executive, 18*(4), 76-91.

Shortell, S., & Kaluzney, A. (2000). *Health care management: Organizational design and behavior*. Florence, KY: Delmar Cengage Learning.

Sinclair, K. (2006) Occupational therapy worldwide: WFOT. *Australian Occupational Therapy Journal, 53*, 49-150.

Slater, D. Y. (2010). *Reference guide to the occupational therapy code of ethics and ethics standards*. Bethesda, MD: AOTA Press.

Spreier, S., Fontaine, M., & Malloy, R. (2006). Leadership run amok: The destructive power of overachievers. *Harvard Business Review, 84*, 72-82.

Strzelecki, M. (2007). Leaders of the pack. *OT Practice, 12*(7), 16-19.

Townsend, E., & Whiteford, G. (2005) A participatory occupational justice framework. In F. Kronenberg, S. Algado, & N. Pollard (Eds.), *Occupational therapy without borders: Learning from the spirit of survivors* (pp. 110-125). London, England: Elsevier.

Townsend, E., & Wilcock, A. (2004). Occupational justice. In C. Christiansen & E. Townsend (Eds.), *Introduction to occupation: The art and science of living* (pp. 243-273). Upper Saddle River, NJ: Prentice Hall.

VIII

SCHOLARSHIP

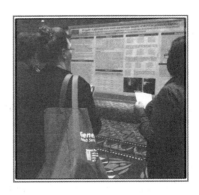

45

THE IMPORTANCE OF SCHOLARSHIP AND SCHOLARLY PRACTICE FOR OCCUPATIONAL THERAPY

Linda H. Niemeyer, OT, PhD

ACOTE STANDARDS EXPLORED IN THIS CHAPTER

B.8.0–B.8.8

KEY VOCABULARY

- **Dependent variable:** One or more clinical findings, behaviors, personal attributes, or internal experiences that are measured in research; the dependent variable might be hypothesized to change as the result of the independent variable or to differ between independent variable groupings.

- **Independent variable:** A factor in research such as an intervention that can be manipulated by the investigator; also, a stable characteristic of individuals by which they can be grouped.

- **Qualitative research:** Exploratory gathering of in-depth, detailed descriptions of problems or conditions from the point of view of the group or individual experiencing them in order to discover themes and their interrelationships or linkages.

- **Quantitative research:** Use of the scientific method to gather data that can be expressed numerically and analyzed statistically in order to describe population characteristics or determine the relationship between one or more independent and dependent variables.

- **Rigor:** Close adherence to experimental research methodology; in broader usage, embedding of sound principles and practices—agreed upon by the scientific community—into each step of the quantitative or qualitative research process in order to ensure trustworthiness of results.

- **Scholarly practice:** Evidence-based practice; using the knowledge base of the profession in occupational therapy practice and teaching.

- **Scholarship:** Research activities designed to build the knowledge base of occupational therapy so as to further advance practice and teaching.

Jacobs, K., MacRae, N., & Sladyk, K. (Eds.).
*Occupational Therapy Essentials for
Clinical Competence, Second Edition* (pp. 579-601).
© 2014 SLACK Incorporated.

Introduction

At the beginning of the new millennium, Holm (2000), in her Eleanor Clarke Slagle Lecture, reflected on the challenges that would face occupational therapy practitioners in the next century. Beginning in the mid 1970s, occupational therapy practitioners had encountered new developments in health care delivery and reimbursement, including managed care, prospective payment, capitation, and changes in staffing ratios, which greatly affected the way services were provided. Moreover, there was an increasing demand for justifying practice patterns via research-based evidence demonstrating that occupational therapy interventions resulted in improved client outcomes. The demand was not only that research evidence should demonstrate positive outcomes but also that it should provide enough information about what was done in the intervention and how it was done so that others could replicate it with comparable clients and achieve similar outcomes.

Indeed, this new emphasis on justifying occupational therapy practice patterns was reflected in an influx of published evidence. On the surface, this was encouraging news, but unfortunately, two problems were created. First, the quantity of the published evidence that practitioners would need to sift through was daunting. Dubouloz, Egan, Vallerand, and von Zweck (1999), based on semistructured in-depth interviews of eight selected participants, identified barriers related to this problem that included a therapist's perceived lack of skill and feelings of inadequacy with regard to finding, interpreting, and using evidence, as well as lack of time and administrative or organizational support. The authors further noted an attitudinal barrier in the form of therapist perception that any evidence that was located might threaten routine practice methods perceived to be effective. Second, quantity did not necessarily mean quality. For example, Holm (2000) analyzed the quality of the evidence in articles published by the *Occupational Therapy Journal of Research* between 1995 and 1999 and found that more than 50% provided the weakest evidence in the form of descriptive studies or the opinions of experts, but barely 8% represented what the author would consider the strongest evidence in the form of true experimental studies.

When occupational therapy practice is based on limited or insufficient evidence, this clearly creates an ethical dilemma. Holm (2000) cited sections of the 1994 version of the occupational therapy code of ethics to make her point. This document has been updated, and relevant sections of the 2010 current version of the *Occupational Therapy Code of Ethics and Ethics Standards* read as follows (American Occupational Therapy Association [AOTA], 2010, pp. 3-5):

- Principle 1. Occupational therapy personnel shall demonstrate a concern for the well-being and safety of the recipients of their services.
  - ◊ Avoid the inappropriate use of outdated or obsolete tests/assessments or data obtained from such tests in making intervention decisions or recommendations.
  - ◊ Use, to the extent possible, evaluation, planning, intervention techniques, and therapeutic equipment that are evidence-based and within the recognized scope of occupational therapy practice.
  - ◊ Take responsible steps (e.g., continuing education, research, supervision, training) and use careful judgment to ensure their own competence and weigh potential for client harm when generally recognized standards do not exist in emerging technology or areas of practice.
  - ◊ Take responsibility for promoting and practicing occupational therapy on the basis of current knowledge and research and for further developing the profession's body of knowledge.
- Principle 2. Occupational therapy personnel shall intentionally refrain from actions that cause harm.
  - ◊ Avoid inflicting harm or injury to recipients of occupational therapy services, students, research participants, or employees.
- Principle 3. Occupational therapy personnel shall respect the right of the individual to self-determination.
  - ◊ Establish a collaborative relationship with recipients of service including families, significant others, and caregivers in setting goals and priorities throughout the intervention process. This includes full disclosure of the benefits, risks, and potential outcomes of any intervention; the personnel who will be providing the intervention(s); and/or any reasonable alternatives to the proposed intervention.

Furthermore, Holm identified what she considered to be key obligations of occupational therapists to fulfill the ethical responsibilities of the profession, namely to "become competent in, and make a habit of, searching for the evidence, appraising its value, and presenting it to those we serve in an understandable manner" and to "improve our research competencies, to develop the habit of using those competencies in everyday practice, and to advance the evidence base of occupational therapy in the new millennium" (Holm, 2000, p. 584).

As occupational therapy academicians and practitioners tackled this challenge, a new conceptual framework for *scholarship* emerged that went beyond the traditional association with purely academic study or achievement. In a visionary paper aimed at occupational therapists, Haertlein and Coppard (2003) stated, "An expanded conception of scholarship offers a way for identifying and characterizing an array of methods by which all occupational therapy academicians and practitioners, through collaborative efforts, can succeed at their institutions while contributing to the teaching, research, and service needs of the profession" (p. 641).

Scholarly Endeavors and Their Contribution to the Occupational Therapy Body of Knowledge

Several types of scholarly endeavors are identified in the occupational therapy literature that can be perceived of as being separate yet interrelated. A new conceptual framework for scholarship was outlined in a 2009 AOTA position paper. First, the authors distinguished between scholarly practice and scholarship. Scholarly practice, otherwise known as *evidence-based practice* (EBP), was defined as "using the knowledge base of the profession or discipline in one's practice" and in teaching (AOTA, 2009, p. 790). On the other hand, *scholarship* was equated with activities designed to build the knowledge base and further advance the practice and teaching of occupational therapy; these activities also came under the heading of research. With regard to the evidence gained through scholarly practice and scholarship, the authors concluded, "All occupational therapists and occupational therapy assistants, regardless of their individual practice roles, have the professional responsibility to not only use that evidence to inform their professional decision making but also to generate new evidence through independent or collaborative research, or both" (AOTA, 2009, p. 793).

The term *evidence-based practice* had its start as evidence-based medicine in the 1980s at McMaster University Medical School in Ontario, Canada (Law & MacDermid, 2008; Taylor, 2007). *Evidence-based medicine* was defined by Sackett, Rosenberg, Gray, Haynes, and Richardson (1996) as "the conscientious, explicit, and judicious use of current best evidence in making decisions about the care of individual patients," which entailed "integrating individual clinical expertise with the best available external clinical evidence from systematic research" (p. 71). This concept quickly gained acceptance in the health care field and was soon recognized worldwide. Tickle-Degnen (1999) helped to further the understanding of the role of EBP in occupational therapy by characterizing it as a set of organizing and evaluating tools "designed to integrate research study evidence into the clinical reasoning process" in order to "help the practitioner select the best assessments and intervention procedures from an array of possibilities" (p. 537) and achieve the best possible outcomes.

According to the classic definition of EBP, the occupational therapy practitioner is asked to integrate his or her own internal clinical expertise with the best available relevant external systematic research to inform practice decisions (Kielhofner, 2006; Law & MacDermid, 2008; Taylor, 2007). The recommended procedure for conducting an EBP inquiry will be discussed later in this chapter. This process calls for a certain amount of flexibility in the practitioner's willingness to modify assessment or intervention in response to the new knowledge gained. The rewards of improved competency in both research skills and clinical practice are much valued by stakeholders, particularly those whose primary focus is consumer protection and judicious use of resources (Christiansen & Lou, 2001; Kielhofner, 2006).

Fortunately, ongoing debate and discussion has led to some evolution regarding implementation of EBP, which has enhanced its applicability to occupational therapy (Christiansen & Lou, 2001; Kielhofner, 2006; Law & MacDermid, 2008). Most notable is the acknowledgement of the importance of the values, needs, and preferences of the client and his or her family. In this adapted format, the occupational therapy practitioner bases clinical decisions on his or her own expertise and the best evidence available while also consulting with the client and family to help determine the most suitable option. The client's perspective is thus taken into account; the evidence and its meaning are translated into user-friendly terms, and choices are made based on client–practitioner collaboration (Dijkers, Murphy, & Krellman, 2012; Tickle-Degnen, 1999). In this way, EBP becomes better suited to the client-centered values and philosophy of occupational therapy.

Let us now turn our attention from scholarly practice, or EBP, to an expanded conception of scholarship. Haertlein and Coppard (2003), as well as the AOTA (2009), described four dimensions of scholarship, which are based on the seminal work of American educator Ernest L. Boyer. These four dimensions are as follows:

1. **The scholarship of discovery.** Conducting original scientific research; this type of scholarship contributes to the growing knowledge base of occupational therapy.

2. **The scholarship of integration.** Seeking new insights from existing original research, both within occupational therapy and across disciplines, by integrating, interpreting and synthesizing in a search for new patterns of connection; this type of scholarship contributes to the formation of new perspectives and theories in occupational therapy.

3. **The scholarship of application.** Forging a link between theory and practice and between academia

and service provision; this type of scholarship contributes to the use of knowledge and insights gained from the scholarship of discovery and integration to address societal problems, occupational therapy assessments or interventions, or classroom teaching of clients or occupational therapy practitioners in a practical way.

4. **The scholarship of teaching and learning.** Systematic study based on the recognition of the complementary nature of teaching and learning; this type of scholarship contributes to the knowledge base needed for high-quality teaching of occupational therapy students and also public sharing of the knowledge of the profession.

The challenge inherent in the scholarship of application dimension opened exciting new opportunities for research but also increased awareness of problems with approaches to occupational therapy research at the millennium (Hammel, Finlayson, Kielhofner, Helfrish, & Peterson, 2002; Kielhofner, 2005a, 2005b; Taylor, Fisher, & Kielhofner, 2005). Of particular concern was the observation that practice tended to lag behind research and that occupational therapy practitioners were disillusioned by theory and research that seemed to be irrelevant to methods used in their everyday work. This observation led to recognition of the need for a more inclusive participatory approach to research that would serve to better connect academicians and practitioners.

One model for enhancing the scholarship of application, termed *the community of scholars*, was designed to incorporate scholarship into the education of occupational therapy students by immersing them in a social context where they could learn "not only from their advisor or instructors but also from a community of scholars that includes student peers, other faculty, staff, clients, practitioners, and community members involved in the scholarship" (Hammel et al., 2002, p. 160). Wilding, Curtin, and Whiteford (2012) used the term *community of practice scholars* to describe an approach wherein a group of occupational therapy academicians worked collaboratively with occupational therapy practitioners. Via monthly teleconference meetings, "members of the community of practice scholars went through a cyclic process of reflection, discovery, planning, implementation, evaluation and re-evaluation" (p. 313). This model made possible an ongoing collaborative interchange that promoted critical reflection on practice and consideration of ways where practice could be improved.

The occupational therapy faculty at the University of Illinois at Chicago (UIC) developed a model based on what was termed engaged scholarship in which institutions of higher education pursued research in collaboration with community settings. In the UIC model, called *A Scholarship of Practice,* longstanding partnerships with multiple community-based organizations were

established that became "the foundation for curriculum development, research initiatives, and the development and evaluation of clinical service" (Braveman, Helfrich, & Fisher, 2002, p. 110). A Scholarship of Practice, defined as a "a dialectic in which theoretical and empirical knowledge is brought to bear on the practical problems of therapeutic work and in which the latter raise questions to be addressed through scholarship" (Kielhofner, 2005a, p. 9), represents linking of occupational therapy practitioners and academicians with the community "based on the assumption that those who ultimately will use the knowledge must be partners in its generation" and "begins with the premise that researchers and theorists in the field must work together with practitioners to not only generate the field's theory and research but also to advance practice" (Kielhofner, 2005a, p. 10). This model lays the groundwork for participatory action research (PAR). PAR is not so much a research method as an approach that uses the committed involvement of stakeholders to examine how scientific knowledge can be joined with the experiential knowledge inherent in the community, resulting in action that addresses complex social problems (Kielhofner, 2005a; Suarez-Balcazar et al., 2005).

Since the beginning of the new millennium, the breadth and depth of scholarly endeavors has grown, leading to emerging possibilities for expanding the occupational therapy body of knowledge. The types of scholarly endeavors that were discussed in this section are reviewed in Figure 45-1. Ongoing work by occupational therapy academicians and practitioners has led to the understanding that building of the occupational therapy body of knowledge via scholarly practice and scholarship entails an ongoing dialog that brings together occupational therapy theoretical concepts, empirical research to verify those concepts, and real-world application of those concepts by means of clinical practice and active collaboration with the community. Any occupational therapy practitioner, regardless of his or her role in the profession, thus has the opportunity to help fulfill the ethical responsibility to contribute to the generation of knowledge that leads to steady progression of the profession of occupational therapy.

The Nature and Quality of Evidence

The core of any scholarly endeavor, including scholarly practice (or EBP) and scholarship (or research), is the ability to judge the quality of evidence. Basically, quality of evidence might be conceived of as the degree of confidence an occupational therapy practitioner or academician can have in the trustworthiness, accuracy, relevance, and usefulness of information from a published

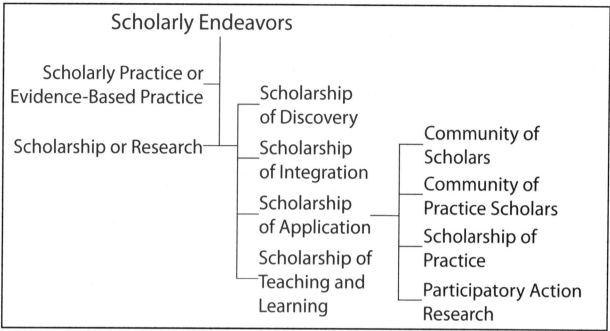

Figure 45-1. An expanded conception of scholarship as the means for building the occupational therapy body of knowledge.

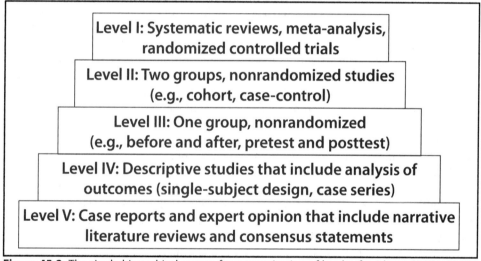

Figure 45-2. The single hierarchical system for categorization of levels of evidence (AOTA, 2012a; Tomlin & Borgetto, 2011) shown as a two-dimensional pyramid with the weakest sources of evidence at the base and the strongest sources of evidence at the apex.

research approach for making practice decisions. An understanding of the quality of evidence is also of critical importance for designing the best possible research approach to substantiate occupational therapy theory or practice methodology. The traditional guideline for judging the quality of evidence was largely established in evidence-based medicine as a single hierarchical system based on study categories and usually termed *levels of evidence* (Law & MacDermid, 2008; Sackett et al., 1996; Taylor, 2007; Tomlin & Borgetto, 2011). This hierarchical system has been widely adopted, sometimes with minor modifications, and is found in AOTA Web-based materials (AOTA, n.d., 2012a). It can be visualized as a simple

two-dimensional pyramid, as seen in Figure 45-2, with the weakest or lowest quality sources of evidence at the bottom and the strongest or highest quality sources of evidence at the apex.

However, limitations in the traditional single hierarchical system, as it pertains to occupational therapy scholarly endeavors, have been recognized (Taylor, 2007; Tomlin & Borgetto, 2011). First, this system is mainly directed to research questions about the success of interventions in promoting positive outcomes. It does not take into account the full range of research questions that an occupational therapy practitioner or academician might ask, and different types of research questions might call

Figure 45-3. The research pyramid model for depicting of levels of evidence, drawn as the top view of a three-dimensional pyramid with each of its three sides representing a distinct category of research. The weaker sources of evidence occupy lower positions on each side with the stronger sources of evidence approaching the apex. Descriptive studies are shown as a flattened pyramid forming the base or foundation of the main pyramid. (Adapted from Tomlin, G., & Borgetto, B. [2011]. Research pyramid: A new evidence-based practice model for occupational therapy. *American Journal of Occupational Therapy*, 65[2], 189-196.)

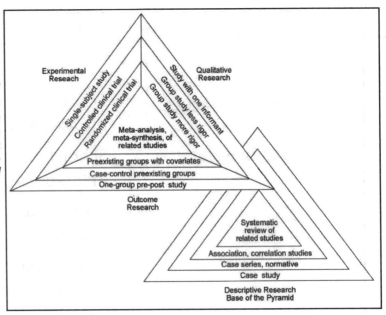

for different best research approaches. Second, it is rooted in classical experimental methodology in which randomized controlled clinical trials (RCTs) are considered to provide the best evidence. A well-designed, rigorous clinical trial is ideally suited to demonstrate the *efficacy* of an intervention, meaning the extent to which it can bring about its intended effect under ideal circumstances, such as the controlled conditions of an experiment. This research approach may not always be appropriate for establishing the *effectiveness* of an intervention, or the extent to which it can achieve its intended effect in a natural clinical, social, or community setting (Ottenbacher & Hinderer, 2001; Wholey, Hatry, & Newcomer, 2010).

Occupational therapy practitioners and academicians are often concerned with "outcomes in the real world of physical, social, and spiritual participation" (Tomlin & Borgetto, 2011, p. 189), for which the restrictions of clinical trials may not always be suitable to provide the best evidence. Rather, an occupational therapy research question about the effectiveness of an intervention in a natural setting might call for a single subject design study. Similarly, a research question about the lived experiences and perceptions of clients might call for a qualitative study, a question about the appropriateness of a screening measure for a comparison group study, or a question about the relationship between home assessment and safety training in elderly community-dwelling adults and incidence of falls over the life course for a longitudinal study (Taylor, 2007).

Tomlin and Borgetto (2011), in response to the recognized need for an alternative model for depicting levels of evidence, proposed the research pyramid. This model was designed to be a more accurate representation of the kinds of evidence needed by occupational therapy practitioners to inform professional decision making.

Instead of a single two-dimensional hierarchy, as in the traditional system illustrated in Figure 45-2, the authors' model is three dimensional. It can be seen in Figure 45-3 that the research pyramid portrays three separate hierarchies representing three distinct types of research, each located on one side of the pyramid. Descriptive studies are shown as a flattened pyramid that forms the base or foundation of the main pyramid. As in the single hierarchical model, weaker or lower quality sources of evidence for each type of research occupy lower positions on each side of the pyramid, with the stronger or higher quality sources of evidence approaching the apex.

The authors note that the research pyramid offers theoretical advantages for occupational therapy practitioners over the traditional system in the way that it separates, yet values as being equal, experimental, outcome, and qualitative research. They state, "The point of shifting from a single-hierarchy model of evidence evaluation to the pyramid model is not to claim that experimental studies are not important for occupational therapists. It is instead to assert that trustworthy evidence of different types can be discovered through disciplined inquiry, and all are important to the profession" (Tomlin & Borgetto, 2011, pp. 193-194). Thus, all forms of research have their place, and all contribute to the whole occupational therapy body of knowledge. Although RCTs may be appraised as the pinnacle of research, in truth what are considered lesser forms of research help provide the foundation that makes the more sophisticated experimental approaches possible. Outcome and qualitative research broaden occupational therapy scholarship to embrace real-world research questions as well as the lived experiences of clients. Moreover, in larger research projects (e.g., PAR), investigators have used mixed methods and gathered both quantitative and qualitative data (Mortenson & Oliffe, 2009; Westhues,

Table 45-1.

DESCRIPTIVE RESEARCH

Level I	Systematic review of related descriptive studies	Identification, selection, critical appraisal, and summary of published literature on descriptive studies that address a common research question
Level II	Associative, correlational studies	Studies that look at the degree of relationship between two or more naturally occurring phenomena or population characteristics of interest
Level III	Multiple-case studies (series)	A collection of individual case studies; a report on a series of clients with a similar characteristic of interest
	Normative studies	Research undertaken to establish usual or average values for a characteristic, trait, or performance parameter in a population of interest; related types of studies might document incidence or prevalence data on a health-related condition or patterns of growth or change in a population of interest (e.g., studies of developmental patterns in children)
	Descriptive survey	Collection of self-reported information from a population of interest using a structured questionnaire
Level IV	Individual case studies	An in-depth report of the experiences or behaviors of a single individual using interviews, observation, testing, or examination of records

Ochocka, Jacobson, Simich, Maiter, Janzen, & Fleras, 2008).

The Tomlin and Borgetto (2011) system is well suited to organize a discussion of the different categories of research approaches. The placement of descriptive research as the base of the research pyramid is fitting because this research approach is very useful for gathering evidence when little is known. Descriptive research "often takes advantage of naturally occurring events or available information in order to generate new insights through inductive processes" (Kielhofner, 2006, p. 58). Its most characteristic function is exploratory and researchers frequently use preexisting databases. Descriptive studies assemble and organize information on a single individual, population, phenomenon, or problem, typically with no investigator manipulation. The research approaches representing the different levels of evidence for descriptive research, from the highest to the lowest level, are presented in Table 45-1 (Kielhofner, 2006).

The *experimental research hierarchy* can be seen as residing on one side of the main research pyramid. A detailed explanation of the full variety of experimental designs can easily take up most or all of an entire textbook, yet they characteristically have certain aspects in common. At the core of any experimental design is the intent to establish, by means of statistical tests, the probability that an intervention—called the *independent variable*—caused change in one or more clinical findings—called the *dependent variable(s)*—in a population of interest (Kielhofner, 2006). In classical evidence-based medicine, experimental studies, or clinical trials, the independent variable is a medication, clinical procedure, or treatment, and investigators select the dependent

variable(s) based on clinical relevance. True experiments are *prospective*, meaning that data from measurement of the dependent variable(s) are gathered both before and after the intervention and are used to determine the degree to which the intervention led to change. This is in contrast to *retrospective* research, wherein data that are collected can refer to both current and past events, phenomena, or clinical findings. Individuals chosen to participate in experimental research ideally can be shown to be representative of a much larger population of individuals based on a close approximation of relevant characteristics such as age, gender, education, diagnosis, or impairment.

Experimental research extends beyond classical applications, particularly in studies conducted by occupational therapy and other allied health professionals. The independent variable can be a treatment, and it also can be a prevention or screening protocol, a form of diagnostic testing, a health care setting, or an educational program. Allied health investigators may select a relevant physical or physiological clinical finding, such as heart rate, breathing patterns, specific laboratory test results, joint range of motion, or muscle strength, as a dependent variable. They may also consider clinical findings that are behaviors or personal attributes, particularly those of importance to clients and their families, caregivers, teachers, or employers because they are related to functioning in one or more aspects of everyday life. A behavior might be chosen as a dependent variable because it is considered inappropriate, disturbing, or disruptive. A selected personal attribute might be the ability to process sensory information or to perform activities of daily living or might be a skill such as handwriting. Finally, the

Table 45-2.		
EXPERIMENTAL RESEARCH		
Level I	Meta-analysis or synthesis of related experimental studies	Synthesis: A systematic method of reviewing, critically analyzing, and integrating evidence from published studies that address a common research question. Meta-analysis: Use of statistical procedures to combine the results of multiple related studies to ascertain consistency of findings. Typically, calculation of effect size, or the magnitude of change in a dependent variable as the result of an intervention, is used as a common metric to compare individual studies.
Level II	Individual (blinded) randomized controlled clinical trials	A true prospective experimental design in which groups of participants are randomly assigned to intervention and control conditions. Blinding can be single, double, or triple. Tests the efficacy of an intervention.
Level III	Controlled clinical trials	A type of prospective experimental study in which an intervention group is compared with a control group. Both the participant and practitioner or researcher may be blinded. The system for assignment to group is not statistically randomized but is based on a quasi-random assignment system (e.g., days of the week or participant social security or medical record numbers).
Level IV	Single-subject studies	A true experimental design that uses a sample of one participant who serves as his or her own control. The experiment may be replicated with three or four participants. Serial measurements of the behavior or attribute of interest (the dependent variable) are taken before, during, and sometimes after the intervention. Tests the effectiveness of an intervention to change a relevant clinical finding, problem behavior, or attribute. Specific design approaches help to establish causality.

dependent variable of interest can be an internal experience such as perceived pain or quality of life.

The three key characteristics of true experimental studies, which are also chief considerations for establishing levels of evidence in experimental research, are control, randomization, and blinding. *Control* customarily describes the presence of a control group in which participants receive no intervention or engage in neutral activity unrelated to the intervention. Participants can also be assigned to a comparison group in which they receive an alternate intervention. The inclusion of control groups helps support the scientific conclusion that any notable differences in the dependent variable between groups can be attributed to the intervention and not to some other unidentified causal factor. One can conceive of another aspect of control, which is the assurance that all individuals within each experimental group are treated identically. Often the term *fidelity* is used to indicate that the independent variable is administered exactly as planned and is true to the underlying theory of the intervention.

Randomization means that assignment of participants to an intervention or control group is made using a statistical technique such as a random number table, so that each participant has an equal likelihood of being a member of any group. This means that the investigators, the individuals providing the intervention, or the study participants in no way directly influence assignment to group. If randomization is properly carried out, there is a high likelihood that the characteristics of participants in each group will be similar. *Blinding* refers to a process

of concealing knowledge of which participant in the experimental population is receiving what intervention or control condition; it can be extended to participants, individuals engaged in providing an intervention or recording dependent variables, or individuals analyzing data from the study. The purpose of blinding is to prevent conscious or unconscious expectations from coloring a participant's response to an intervention, an intervention provider's response to the participant, or the recording or analysis of information by members of the research team. Blinding is not always possible for a number of practical reasons. For example, it might not be feasible to conceal from a practitioner or participant the nature of the intervention that is being administered. The research approaches representing the different levels of evidence for experimental research, from the highest to the lowest level, are presented in Table 45-2 (Cooper, Hedges, & Valentine, 2009; Kazdin, 2010; Kielhofner, 2006; Wholey et al., 2010).

The *outcome research hierarchy* occupies a second side of the research pyramid. According to the Agency for Healthcare Research and Quality (AHRQ) (2000), outcome research, which is also called *outcomes research*, "seeks to understand the end results of particular health care practices and interventions" (Para. 1). As a method of monitoring program performance, outcome research can address, in addition to clinical findings and the internal experiences of recipients of care, a broad array of health care delivery factors such as regulations and reimbursement policies, benefits and risks, cost, timeliness,

Table 45-3.		OUTCOME RESEARCH
Level I	Meta-analysis or synthesis of related outcome studies	Synthesis: A systematic method of reviewing, critically analyzing, and integrating evidence from published studies that address a common research question. Meta-analysis: Use of statistical procedures to combine the results of multiple related studies to ascertain consistency of findings. Typically, calculation of effect size, or the magnitude of change in a dependent variable as the result of an intervention, is used as a common metric to compare individual studies.
Level II	Preexisting groups comparisons with covariate analysis	Also called a nonrandomized comparison group design. Assignment to an intervention or control condition is typically based on naturally occurring preexisting groups (e.g., children in two different classrooms or individuals at the top and bottom of a waiting list for the intervention). A prospective design in which pre- and postintervention measures establish differences between groups in terms of dependent variables or outcomes of interest. A variation is the cohort study, wherein assignment to group is based on differences in key participant characteristics such as certain risk factors. Individuals are followed for a period of time to establish the degree of relationship between these characteristics and subsequent outcome. Lack of random assignment increases the chance of systematic differences between groups that act as confounding variables. A confounding variable is a factor that distorts the actual relationship between the independent and dependent variables or between risk factors and outcomes. Covariate analysis is used to identify and make adjustments for these systematic differences. An alternate strategy is to select individuals that are closely matched between groups in terms of potentially confounding variables.
Level III	Case-control studies; preexisting groups comparisons	Also called a case comparison design. A retrospective study with no investigator manipulation. Preexisting groups of individuals (cases) who achieved an outcome of interest are compared with those who achieved a different outcome by means of data gathered from systematic review of relevant records or from participant interview. Often an attempt is made to match the two groups in terms of member characteristics that could be confounding variables. The goal is to determine the degree to which any variables of interest from the past discriminated between the two outcome groups.
Level IV	One-group pre–post studies	A prospective study that looks only at the group receiving the intervention. Selected dependent variables are measured before and after the intervention to establish outcome in terms of degree of change. Participants are often selected via convenience sampling, meaning that they were the most available to recruit for the study and therefore may not be representative of the larger population of interest.

efficiency, and consumer preferences (Wholey et al., 2010). "For health care managers and purchasers, outcomes research can identify potentially effective strategies they can implement to improve the quality and value of care" (AHRQ, 2000, Para. 4).

Although the RCT has been extolled as the most robust method for providing evidence linking health care to outcomes, conducting this type of experimental research is not always logically feasible for the clinical setting (Ottenbacher & Hinderer, 2001). Clinical trials are demanding of available resources. For example, they call for a large number of participants who have similar characteristics and for highly controlled experimental conditions. Moreover, ethical considerations can arise when participants who are randomly assigned to a control condition receive no intervention. The *quasi-experimental* outcome research designs depicted in Table 45-3 represent viable alternatives that, if conducted with sufficient attention to detail, can provide a quantitative estimate of the impact of an intervention or of certain

participant characteristics on outcome (Cooper et al., 2009; Kielhofner, 2006; Wholey et al., 2010).

Qualitative research, which is represented on the third side of the research pyramid, is an approach that resonates well with the holistic and client-centered worldview and the core concerns, assumptions, and values of occupational therapy (Cook, 2001; Kielhofner, 1982b, 2006; Merrill, 1985). It constitutes a naturalistic method of scientific inquiry that is fundamentally exploratory and subjective and whose primary aim is to gather in-depth, detailed descriptions of a phenomenon of interest (e.g., a problem or condition) from the point of view of the group or individual experiencing it. Inquiry does not stop at the level of describing the problem or condition but seeks to interpret each phenomenon in light of physical, social, economic, regulatory, and cultural contexts as well as personal viewpoints, meanings, and perceptions. (Kielhofner, 1982a, 2006; Merrill, 1985; Papadimitriou, Magasi, & Frank, 2012). Quantitative experimental and outcome research approaches cannot adequately capture these interwoven and sometimes elusive complexities for

Table 45-4.		
QUALITATIVE RESEARCH		
Level I	Meta-synthesis of related qualitative studies	An interpretive process of identifying, extracting and integrating the findings of related qualitative studies in order to generate new insights, leading to a "fuller understanding of the phenomenon of interest" (Thorne, Jensen, Kearney, Noblit, & Sandelowski, 2004, p. 1346)
Level II	Group qualitative studies with more rigor (a, b, c)	Gathering of in-depth and detailed information pertaining to the phenomenon of interest from multiple individuals, using recognized strategies to enhance trustworthiness including (a) prolonged engagement with participants, (b) triangulation of data from multiple sources, and (c) confirmation of data analysis and reinterpretation by means of peer and member checking
Level III	Group qualitative studies with less rigor (a, b, c)	Gathering of in-depth and detailed information pertaining to the phenomenon of interest from multiple individuals but without using recognized strategies to enhance trustworthiness
Level IV	Qualitative studies with single informant	Gathering of in-depth and detailed information from a single key individual judged to be a knowledgeable source of experiences, meanings, and events connected to the phenomenon of interest

a number of reasons (Kielhofner, 1982a; Merrill, 1985). First, when conducting quantitative research, investigators characteristically test hypotheses based on existing theories. Second, quantitative investigators use standardized methods of data collection and numerical analysis to yield findings on preestablished variables. Third, the quantitative discovery process is linear, proceeding from the definition of a research problem through a sequence of steps and concluding with reporting of findings and often generation of new research questions.

In qualitative approaches, however, the discovery process is cyclical and open ended, driven by the perspectives of the participants and not of the researchers (Cook, 2001). Methodology, concepts, and theory develop gradually as the research progresses and are derived as the accumulated data and interpretations lend structure and focus (Kielhofner 1982a, 2006; Merrill, 1985). Methods of data collection include in-depth unstructured or semi-structured interviews, focus groups, participant or field observation, and review of pertinent records and other documents (Cook, 2001; Mack, Woodsong, MacQueen, Guest, & Namey, 2005). Data are documented via written notes, photos, audio recordings, and video recordings. The goal of analysis and interpretation is to reduce data to recurring patterns of conceptual categories and themes via a painstaking process of review. As meaning and significance emerge, a model is constructed depicting interrelationships or linkages (Wholey et al., 2010).

The qualitative research hierarchy used by Tomlin and Borgetto (2011) and depicted in Table 45-4 takes into account three important strategies that enhance the quality of evidence and that are consistent with a conceptual model proposed by Guba (1981) and discussed by Krefting (1991), which is addressed in the next section. These strategies are as follows:

- *Prolonged engagement with participants:* Spending adequate time observing, speaking with or

interviewing, and developing relationships to fully understand the phenomenon of interest and to allow participants to adjust to the presence of investigators

- *Triangulation of data from multiple sources:* Verifying and cross-checking information by collecting it from several sources, using more than one research, interpretation, or analysis technique, and cross-referencing

- *Confirmation of data analysis and reinterpretation by means of peer and member checking:* In member checking, the researcher's data, interpretations, and conclusions are repeatedly tested with informants. Peer examination involves the researcher in discussing the research process, emerging assumptions, interpretations, and problems with experienced impartial colleagues.

Another concept addressed by Tomlin and Borgetto is qualitative *meta-synthesis,* which has been described as an evolving systematic approach to consolidating the findings of group of qualitative studies in order to facilitate knowledge development and contribute to an explanatory theory or model (Pearson, Wiechula, & Lockwood, 2005; Thorne, Jensen, Kearney, Noblit, & Sandelowski, 2004; Walsh & Downe, 2005).

Two types of research bear mentioning that do not fit neatly into either the single hierarchical system for assigning levels of measurement or the multidimensional Tomlin and Borgetto (2011) research pyramid. These are cross-sectional and longitudinal designs. Cross-sectional data are gathered during a single defined time period and are used to provide descriptive information on two or more preexisting groups that have certain immediately identifiable characteristics or dependent variables of interest. Typically, there is no investigator manipulation and the primary objective is to statistically identify differences or similarities between the groups (Kielhofner,

2006). Some studies explore factors that may have influenced outcome in a population of interest (Law et al., 1998a) or investigate the properties and usability of a newer measure compared with a more established or "gold standard" instrument (DeVellis, 2012). One benefit of using a cross-sectional design is that it allows researchers to address many different characteristics simultaneously.

In longitudinal research, data are collected on selected characteristics or dependent variables in a population of interest at multiple points in time, possibly over months or years. Data might also be collected on interventions or other aspects of health care received by the population, and groups who did or did not receive this care are compared. As in cross-sectional research, there is no investigator manipulation; the primary objective is to detect numerical patterns of stability and change that develop over time and that allow investigators to make statistical inferences regarding how and why change did or did not take place (Kielhofner, 2006). Some sources use the term *cohort designs* for this type of research (Law et al., 1998a).

Understanding Validity

Although determining the nature of a research design and its position on a hierarchy are important for judging the quality of evidence, that is just the beginning. Another important hallmark of quality is *research validity,* which is a core issue for all scientific inquiry, regardless of design (Kielhofner, 1982a). Research validity serves as an indication of the degree to which research methods and findings are sound in that they reflect actual phenomena in the world and are not distorted by inaccuracies in conceptual or theoretical foundations, design, measurement, or analysis. Other terms for research validity are *rigor* and *trustworthiness.* In traditional usage, rigor refers to close adherence to experimental research methodology; in broader usage, it can be described as embedding of sound principles and practices—agreed upon by the scientific community—into each step of a quantitative or qualitative research process in order to ensure trustworthiness of results (Kielhofner, 2006).

A well-developed conceptual model put forth by Guba (1981) and Krefting (1991) and summarized in Table 45-5 identifies four key criteria for evaluating research validity or trustworthiness that can be applied to both the quantitative and qualitative perspectives. The terminology used reflects the distinct philosophical, conceptual, and methodological differences of these two perspectives. Yet it should be kept in mind that one approach can be used to complement and corroborate the other and thereby extend the scope of inquiry (Mortenson & Oliffe, 2009).

Making Evidence-Based Decisions

Knowledge of research designs and an understanding of what constitutes rigorous investigation will enhance any occupational therapy scholarly endeavor. In addition to providing a framework for developing an original study, this knowledge underscores the critical appraisal of published research literature, which is essential for making EBP decisions. A number of sources offer specific detailed guidelines for scholarly practice, or EBP; these sources include Kielhofner (2006), Melnyk and Fineout-Overholt (2011), and Taylor (2007). This process begins when a clinical situation or problem is encountered in which not all the needed information is at hand. Then inquiry proceeds as a series of steps (Lin, Murphy, & Robinson, 2010).

An occupational therapy practitioner seeking specific knowledge to guide clinical decision making begins by formulating a clear, sufficiently focused, answerable *clinical question.* PICO, or PICOT (Melnyk & Fineout-Overholt, 2011), is the acronym for a practical structured approach to framing clinical questions pertinent to the care of a specific client or a category of clients seen routinely. P refers to the person, problem, or population of interest; I to the issue or intervention being considered; C to a comparison such as an alternate intervention or no intervention; O to the outcome that would be affected by the intervention; and T to a time frame. Here are two examples:

1. For adolescents with clinical depression receiving antidepressant medication (P), what is the effect of a group occupational therapy program (I) consisting of biweekly 1-hour sessions over 4 weeks (T) on participation in the community (O) compared with antidepressant medication alone (C)?

2. For elders 65 years of age and older with a history of falls who are living at home (P), does in-home fall prevention education by an occupational therapist (I) result in lower incidence of falls in the home (O) compared with outpatient clinic-based occupational therapy fall prevention education (C) at 6-month follow-up (T)?

The PICO or PICOT system prompts the occupational therapy practitioner to formulate a clinical question that supports an effective *systematic search* of the published literature for directly related research evidence, which is the second step in the EBP process. Up-to-date published peer-reviewed studies can be located via Internet sources such as Google Scholar or SpringerLink or the electronic database search system of a college or university library.

Table 45-5.

FOUR CRITERIA FOR EVALUATING THE TRUSTWORTHINESS OF RESEARCH FROM BOTH THE QUANTITATIVE AND QUALITATIVE PERSPECTIVES

Criterion	Qualitative Research Perspective	Quantitative Research Perspective
Truth value: The level of confidence in the veracity of research findings that the investigators were able to establish, given the study's design, subjects or informants, and context	Credibility: The degree of accuracy in preserving and representing the holistic situation and participants being studied, as well as in describing and interpreting the experiences of participants in way that is immediately recognizable by these individuals	Internal validity: The extent to which a causal connection can be established between an intervention, or independent variable, and one or more outcomes, or dependent variables; identification and ruling out of factors other than the independent variable that could influence or mask the research findings
Applicability: The extent to which the findings of a research study can be applied to other contexts, settings, and groups or generalized to larger populations	Transferability: The level of representativeness of the informants or participants for the particular group being studied, such that other program providers can apply the findings to their context	External validity: The extent to which research findings can be generalized or applied beyond the groups or contexts specific to the study
Consistency: The degree to which the research findings are reproducible, given that the study is duplicated with the same participants and setting or context	Dependability: The extent to which the uniqueness or repeatability of a study has been established by means of thorough and exact description of the methods of data gathering, analysis, and interpretation, as well as by use of methods to replicate and confirm the accuracy of this information	Reliability: The extent to which an experimental or outcome study would yield the same result if repeated independently; the extent to which a measurement used in a study would produce the same results with different raters or repeat administration over time
Neutrality: The level of freedom from bias, meaning that research findings are not influenced by the personal motivations or perspectives of the investigators but are the sole function of the conditions of the study.	Confirmability: The degree of understanding how and why decisions were made in a study, such that another researcher would arrive at comparable conclusions given the same data and research context, established using an external or internal auditing process to review data, findings, interpretations, and recommendations	Objectivity: The extent to which judgments made and data recorded during the research process are based solely on observed phenomena without the influence of personal agendas, emotions, prejudices, assumptions, or predispositions

Adapted from Guba, E. G. (1981). ERIC/ECTJ annual review paper: Criteria for assessing the trustworthiness of naturalistic inquiries. *Educational Communication and Technology Journal, 29*(2), 75-91; Krefting, L. (1991). Rigor in qualitative research: The assessment of trustworthiness. *American Journal of Occupational Therapy, 45*(3), 214-222; and Wholey, J. S., Hatry, H. P., & Newcomer, K. E. (2010). *Handbook of practical program evaluation* (3rd ed.). San Francisco, CA: John Wiley & Sons.

Electronic databases applicable to occupational therapy practice range from specialized (e.g., OTseeker) (Bennett et al., 2003) to broad-based compilations of thousands of journals, including EBSCOhost, CINAHL, Medline/PubMed, and PsychINFO. Collected systematic reviews and meta-analyses are published in the Cochrane Library database. The practitioner typically begins the search for relevant literature by using keywords suggested by the clinical question. However, search terms must sometimes be adapted to the standardized medical vocabulary used by some electronic databases. Fortunately, a number of excellent resources teach the often-arduous process of searching the literature and accessing pertinent research articles (Kielhofner, 2006; Melnyk & Fineout-Overholt, 2011; Taylor, 2007).

Step three is *critical appraisal of the evidence*. The occupational therapy practitioner carefully assesses the quality and trustworthiness of the research evidence in the published literature that has the most direct bearing on the clinical question. Guiding questions for critically appraising a report of quantitative and of qualitative research are presented in Tables 45-6 and 45-7. These tables are based on appraisal questions developed by the McMaster University Occupational Therapy Evidence-Based Practice Research Group.

After the available evidence has been critically appraised, in step four, the occupational therapy

Table 45-6.

GUIDING QUESTIONS FOR APPRAISING QUANTITATIVE RESEARCH

Study purpose	Was the purpose of the study or research question(s) stated clearly? How does it apply to occupational therapy and the clinical question guiding my efforts to seek evidence for clinical decision making?
Literature review	Was relevant background literature reviewed? How well did it justify the need for the study? Was the justification clear and compelling?
Design	What was the study design; was it easy or difficult to ascertain? Was it appropriate for the research question(s)? Did the design admit the possibility of the potential influence of biases (e.g., issues of randomization, control, blinding); if so, what might be the direction of their influence on the results? (These questions help to establish internal validity and objectivity.)
Study sample population	Was the population sample used in the study described in detail? If a two-group study, was the similarity between groups established? Did the investigators justify the sample size used? Was informed consent obtained? (These questions help to establish external validity and statistical conclusion validity.)
Outcomes	What outcome measures did investigators use? What clinical findings (e.g., physical or physiological, behaviors, personal attributes, internal experiences) were measured? Were the measures reliable; were they valid? What was the frequency of measurement (e.g., pretest, post-test, follow-up)? (These questions help to establish internal validity and reliability.)
Intervention	Was the intervention described in detail? Could it be replicated in occupational therapy practice? Were steps taken to maintain intervention fidelity? Was contamination bias (members of control group inadvertently exposed to the intervention) or co-intervention bias (other unaccounted for interventions received by participants during the study) avoided? (These questions help to establish internal validity and reliability.)
Data analysis	What were the methods of data analysis used? Were the analysis methods appropriate, given the study design? If there were multiple outcomes, was this taken into account in the statistical analysis? (These questions help to establish statistical conclusion validity.)
Results	Did any participants drop out from the study; if so, how many dropped out? Were reasons given and drop-outs handled appropriately? Were the research findings reported in terms of statistical significance? If results were not statistically significant, was the size of the study population large enough to show an important difference or change if in truth it did exist? Were the differences between groups clinically meaningful (e.g., effect size calculation)? Was the clinical importance or usefulness of the results reported? (These questions help to establish statistical conclusion validity.)
Overall rigor	What is the overall degree of rigor of the study, based on the four components of trustworthiness (e.g., internal validity, external validity, reliability, objectivity) plus statistical conclusion validity? How did the investigators ensure each component of trustworthiness? What meaning and relevance does the study have for my clinical question?
Conclusion and clinical implications	What did the investigators conclude? Were the conclusions appropriate given the study methods and results? What were the implications of these results for occupational therapy practice? What were the main limitations and biases in the study?

Statistical conclusion validity refers to the degree to which the investigator's statistical analysis led to a correct decision about the relationship between the intervention and outcome but not to whether a causal relationship exists between these variables (Wholey, Hatry, & Newcomer, 2010).
Adapted from Law, M., Stewart, D., Pollock, N., Letts, L., Bosch, J., & Westmorland, M. (1998a). Guidelines for critical review form: Quantitative studies. Retrieved from http://www.srs-mcmaster.ca/Portals/20/pdf/ebp/quanguidelines.pdf and Law, M., Stewart, D., Pollock, N., Letts, L., Bosch, J., & Westmorland, M. (1998b). Critical review form: Quantitative studies. Retrieved from http://www.srs-mcmaster.ca/Portals/20/pdf/ebp/quanreview.pdf

practitioner draws an unbiased conclusion, based on integration of information from the multiple studies, as to how the evidence answered the clinical question. This action, sometimes called formulating the "clinical bottom line" (Kielhofner, 2006, p. 680), is followed by step five in which the practitioner integrates the answer to the clinical question with his or her clinical expertise and considers the values, preferences, and unique situation of the client or client group to make a decision regarding the most suitable intervention (Dijkers et al., 2012). Finally,

in step six, the practitioner evaluates the outcome of the clinical decision.

QUANTITATIVE AND QUALITATIVE ANALYSIS

Knowledge of methods of data analysis for qualitative and quantitative research is essential for both scholarship and scholarly practice. In the former, it supports selection of appropriate analysis procedures or approaches

Table 45-7.	
GUIDELINES FOR APPRAISING QUALITATIVE RESEARCH	
Study purpose	Was the purpose of the study or research question(s) stated clearly? How does it apply to occupational therapy and the clinical question guiding my efforts to seek evidence for clinical decision making?
Literature	Was relevant background literature reviewed? How well did it justify the need for the study? Was the justification clear and compelling?
Study design	What was the basis of the study design (e.g., phenomenology: understanding of a lived experience, ethnography: understanding of a culture, grounded theory: theory construction, participatory action research: knowledge leading to social change); was it easy or difficult to ascertain? Was it appropriate for the research question(s)? Was a theoretical or philosophical perspective related to the phenomenon of interest identified?
Methods used	What methods of data collection were used to answer the research question(s) (e.g., in-depth unstructured or semistructured interviews, focus groups, participant or field observation, review of pertinent records and other documents)? Are the methods congruent with the philosophical underpinnings and purpose of the study?
Sampling	Was the process of purposive selection of study participants described? Did this sampling maximize the range of information uncovered? Were the sampling methods appropriate to the research purpose and question(s)? Did sampling proceed until redundancy in data was reached? (These questions help to establish credibility and transferability.) Was informed consent obtained?
Descriptive clarity	Was there a clear and complete (i.e., "thick" or "dense") description of the study context, site or setting and the participants? Was the description sufficient to impart a sense of personally experiencing the phenomenon being studied? (These questions help to establish transferability.) Was the role of the researcher and his or her relationship with participants explained? Were the assumptions and biases of the researcher identified (e.g., reflexivity via a daily introspective journal)? (These questions help to establish credibility and confirmability.) What information was missing, and how does that influence my understanding of the research?
Data collection	Did the researchers provide an adequate "dense" description of data collection procedures (e.g., gaining access to the site, field notes, training of data gatherers)? What flexibility was there in the design and data collection methods? Was there prolonged engagement at the site to allow full understanding of the phenomenon of interest? Were data gathered from multiple sources (e.g., different investigators and methods, documents, video or audio recordings)? (These questions help to establish credibility and dependability.)
Data analyses	What were the methods of data analysis used; were the methods appropriate? Did the researchers describe how the findings (e.g., codes, categories, and themes) emerged from the data? Did data analysis include verification and cross checking (i.e., triangulation) of data from multiple sources? Were the researcher's data, interpretations, and conclusions repeatedly tested with informants (i.e., member checking)? Did the investigator(s) discuss the research process, emerging assumptions, interpretations, and problems with experienced impartial colleagues (i.e., peer examination)? (These questions help to establish credibility, dependability, and confirmability.) What were the major findings of the analyses? Were findings logically consistent with and reflective of the data?
Auditability	Was the process of analyzing the data sufficiently described, such that an audit could certify that there are data to support every interpretation and that interpretations are consistent with the available data? Did the investigators provide a decision trail (e.g., for any changes in design or data collection methods or for transformation of data into codes, themes, and interrelationships)? What rationale was given for the development of themes? (These questions help to establish dependability and confirmability.)
Theoretical connections	Did a meaningful picture of the phenomenon under study emerge? How were concepts under study clarified and refined and relationships made clear? What conceptual frameworks emerged?
Overall rigor	What is the overall degree of rigor of the study, based on the four components of trustworthiness (e.g., credibility, transferability, dependability, confirmability)? How did the investigators ensure each component of trustworthiness? What meaning and relevance does the study have for my clinical question?
Conclusions and implications	What did the investigators conclude? What were the implications of findings for occupational therapy practice and research? What are the main limitations of the study? Were the conclusions appropriate given the study findings; were they meaningful to me? Did the findings contribute to theory development and future occupational therapy practice and research?

Adapted from Guba, E. G. (1981). ERIC/ECTJ annual review paper: Criteria for assessing the trustworthiness of naturalistic inquiries. *Educational Communication and Technology Journal, 29*(2), 75-91; Krefting, L. (1991). Rigor in qualitative research: The assessment of trustworthiness. *American Journal of Occupational Therapy, 45*(3), 214-222; Letts, L., Wilkins, S., Law, M., Stewart, D., Bosch, J., & Westmorland, M. (2007a). *Guidelines for critical review form: Qualitative studies*. Retrieved from http://www.srs-mcmaster.ca/Portals/20/pdf/ebp/qualguidelines_ version2.0.pdf; and Letts, L., Wilkins, S., Law, M., Stewart, D., Bosch, J., & Westmorland, M. (2007b). *Critical review form: Qualitative studies*. Retrieved from http://www.srs-mcmaster.ca/Portals/20/pdf/ebp/qualreview_version2.0.pdf

in original research; in the latter, it provides the basis to critically appraise the analyses used by investigators in a published study. This section provides a general overview of important terminology and concepts. Because of the breadth and complexity of the science of data analysis, occupational therapy practitioners embarking on any scholarly endeavor are encouraged to engage in further study.

Quantitative analysis is based on statistics, which "is a branch of applied mathematics that deals with the collection, description and interpretation of quantitative data" (Kielhofner, 2006, p. 213). For a quick reference, readers are invited to explore the Web Center for Social Research Methods at http://www.socialreserchmethods.net. A good first step in selecting the appropriate statistical methodology is to determine whether the core purpose of analysis is descriptive or inferential. Descriptive statistics summarize the basic features of study data and are used in the kinds of descriptive research presented in Table 45-1. If a single variable or group is represented in the data, descriptive statistics can be used to depict the frequency or range of individual values, the central tendency, and the spread of values around the central tendency. *Descriptive analysis* in which there is more than one group or variable consists of computation of the degree of relationship or association between two sets of values. The statistic that is generated is typically called a *contingency* or *correlation coefficient.*

Inferential statistics are used to reach conclusions that extend beyond the study data. In experimental and outcome research depicted in Tables 45-2 and 45-3, investigators use this family of analyses to infer the likelihood that what was observed in the study sample is also true for the larger population from which the sample was taken. A key aspect of inferential statistics is the determination of *significance*, which is derived from the probability that the difference between groups or the change seen as a result of an intervention occurred because of random chance. A significant research finding has a high probability of being true.

The additional piece that must be in place before the appropriate statistic can be selected is determination of the type of scale used in the measurement of variables. *Parametric* statistical operations lend themselves to interval or ratio measurement scales, which are based on real numbers. When the measurement scale is nominal, meaning categorical, or ordinal, requiring rank ordering of categories, *nonparametric* statistics must be used. There are additional requirements for use of parametric statistics based on the pattern of distribution of data points around the mean. Each parametric statistic has at least one corresponding nonparametric statistic. Table 45-8 provides a listing of some parametric and corresponding nonparametric statistical operations for basic

quantitative research designs, given the core purpose of the analysis, that readers might encounter in a published study or statistics computer program.

The inferential statistics in Table 45-8 refer to research designs that have one independent and one dependent variable. More complex designs that have two or more independent or dependent variables call for parametric statistics such as two-way analysis of variance (ANOVA), multivariate analysis of variance (MANOVA), analysis of covariance (ANCOVA), and multivariate analysis of covariance (MANCOVA).

Investigators might also use parametric predictive statistics such as linear regression. In simplest terms, linear regression is a statistical determination of the strength of the relationship between an independent, or predictor, variable and a dependent variable that is being predicted. This means that, given a value of the independent variable, a corresponding value of the dependent variable can be calculated. Regression statistics can determine whether the relationship between the independent and dependent variable is significant and the degree to which one or more predictor variables contribute to change in the dependent variable. An advantage of regression analysis for outcome research is its ease of application with naturally occurring variables, as contrasted with experimentally manipulated variables. In multiple regression there is more than one predictor variable, and in logistic regression, the dependent variable is dichotomous (e.g., example success or failure) (Kielhofner, 2006; Wholey et al., 2010).

An occupational therapy practitioner who is analyzing data from original qualitative research, depicted in Table 45-4, does not use statistical methods but rather might be characterized as playing the role of detective. With the purpose of the research in mind, disciplined examination and creative insight are applied to discover patterns that reveal meaning and significance. Qualitative data analysis and interpretation might be conceived of as separate but interrelated processes. During analysis, the researcher's goals are to bring order to the data and reduce it to manageable components by identifying recurring categories (Bernard & Ryan, 2010; Wholey et al., 2010). Categories are themes that make sense in the context of the study. A theme that emerges with high frequency in the data is often called a *core category*. Categories that surface are assigned codes, which are essentially labels. By working back and forth between the emerging coded categories and the raw data, the individual conducting the analysis refines the coding system until it appears to contain the existing data. When no new categories are appreciable, it is said that the analysis has reached *saturation.*

In the interpretive process, meaning and significance are attached to the categories, and a model is constructed depicting the interrelationships or linkages between or

Table 45-8.

OVERVIEW OF SOME APPROPRIATE PARAMETRIC AND NONPARAMETRIC STATISTICAL OPERATIONS GIVEN THE CORE PURPOSE OF THE ANALYSIS

Core Purpose	Parametric	Nonparametric
Descriptive: single group or variable	Mean, percentage, standard deviation	Mode, median, range
Descriptive: association between two groups or variables	Pearson's r correlation coefficient	Pearson's contingency coefficient Phi squared; Cramer's V Goodman & Kruskal's tau Lambda Spearman Rho Kendall coefficient of concordance Kendall's Tau; Stuart's T Gamma coefficient Somers' D
Inferential: experimental and outcomes research Single sample	t or Z test	Binomial test or chi-square
Two independent samples	t-Test for independent samples One way between groups Analysis of variance (ANOVA)	Chi-square Wald-Wolfwitz runs test Man-Whitney U test Kolmogorov-Smirnov two-sample test
Two dependent samples	t-Test for dependent samples One way repeated measures Analysis of variance (ANOVA)	McNemar chi-square Wilcoxon matched-pairs signed-ranks test
More than two independent samples	One way or two way between groups Analysis of variance (ANOVA)	Chi-square test for k independent samples Kruskal-Wallis one-way analysis of variance
More than two dependent samples	One way or two way repeated measures Analysis of variance (ANOVA) repeat measures Binomial test or chi-square	Friedman two-way analysis of variance Cochran's Q test

Adapted from Kielhofner, G. (2006). *Research in occupational therapy: Methods of inquiry for enhancing practice.* Philadelphia, PA: F.A. Davis Company and Siegel, S., & Castellan Jr., N. J. (1988) *Nonparametric statistics for the behavioral sciences.* New York, NY: McGraw-Hill.

among them (Bernard & Ryan, 2010). During data collection and data analysis, investigators may write memos consisting of thoughts about an observational theme or category and its relationship to other categories or to the research questions. These thoughts can take the form of preliminary hypotheses, questions, or inferences. Memos are often written in the margins of an interview transcript or a field journal. In published literature, the model might be depicted diagrammatically. Categories can also be described numerically in terms of frequency or proportion of occurrence. It can be seen that analysis of qualitative data requires skill and persistence, yet it allows the occupational therapy practitioner to gain understanding beyond numbers and statistical significance.

Designing a Scholarly Proposal

Well-known occasions when an occupational therapy practitioner is called upon to write a scholarly proposal are the application for a research grant and completion of the requirements for a graduate degree. However, there is good reason to prepare a detailed proposal for any scholarly project, in particular one aimed at evaluating the effectiveness or efficacy of a program or intervention. The process of writing a scholarly proposal prompts the occupational therapy practitioner to think through the project in order to explore options and anticipate any difficulties that could arise and thus avoid common pitfalls that would impede successful execution of the research or lessen the trustworthiness of the findings and conclusions (Locke, Spirduso, & Silverman, 2007; Wholey et al., 2010). "To put it bluntly, one's research is only as good as one's proposal" (Wong, 2005, p. 1).

A scholarly proposal can serve as a mode of communication, a plan of action, and a contract or bond of agreement (Locke et al., 2007). Although the audience may be a panel of experts on a grant review board or faculty members on a thesis or dissertation committee, it can also be composed of stakeholders in the community or practice setting. The primary objective is to convince the audience that the research idea is important, that it is based on a clear grasp of relevant literature and issues, that the methodology is sound and that the author of the proposal has a well-thought-out plan of action for the project—ideally, within a realistic time frame and incurring reasonable expenses—and sufficient competence to complete it. To achieve this objective, the scholarly proposal should effectively convey *why* the occupational therapy practitioner desires to embark upon the study, *what* the he or she plans to accomplish, and *how* he or she plans to proceed.

Each funding agency or university has its own set of guidelines for submissions, and there are no generally agreed upon rules that dictate the content or order of a scholarly proposal. However, the audience members will universally look for a writing style characterized by precision, simplicity, and clarity as well as the accomplishment of specific communication tasks. "In the mass of detail that goes into the planning of a research study, the writer must not forget that the proposal's most immediate function is to inform readers quickly and accurately" (Locke et al., 2007, p. 6). Fundamental communication tasks that address key elements of the research process and provide any essential information that the writer's audience needs to evaluate the proposed study are presented below (Locke et al., 2007; Wong, 2005).

- *Introduction of the study:* Meticulously prepared opening paragraphs designed to capture the interest of the readers of the document and lay the foundation for the more detailed discussion that follows. Here the writer familiarizes the readers with the problem or area of concern that prompted the investigation (e.g., the recognition of a gap, deficiency, or need in the field of inquiry), touches upon the theoretical or practical significance of the problem, and sketches the core constructs that will be represented.

- *Statement of purpose:* A declaration, made early in the proposal, of why the writer wishes to embark upon the study and what he or she intends to achieve

- *Rationale:* Justification of the importance and significance of the proposed study by explaining the potential practical and theoretical impact of

findings. In stating his or her case, the writer might bring in applicable facts, use logical reasoning, and provide a diagram of factors and relationships evident in the problem. The aim is to persuade the readers of the proposal that the investigator has sufficiently and correctly defined the problem and that the planned research is unique and worth doing, such that completion of the study will lead to a better understanding of the problem and to opening of new possibilities for a constructive course of action and further investigation.

- *Research questions or hypotheses:* Logical and concise statements that are linked to the purpose of investigation and that identify the specific direction of inquiry; they provide the foundation of the scholarly proposal and identify the independent and dependent variables or the phenomenon of interest. Research questions are most appropriate when the study tends to be exploratory in nature or uses qualitative methodology; they should be foreshadowed by prior studies or theoretical work. In study hypotheses, testable predictions are made about the relationship between two variables (e.g., an intervention and outcome) based on established knowledge and theory. A well-stated research question can lead directly into a study hypothesis. Typically, elements of a scholarly proposal appear in the published study after it is completed. Table 45-9 shows examples of the stated purpose and related research questions or hypotheses in four studies. All were published in the *American Journal of Occupational Therapy* and represent each of the four types of research discussed in this chapter.

- *Delimitations and limitations:* Statements of defined limits in the context of the scholarly proposal. Delimitations refer to factors related to use of constructs or the planned study population that would affect generalizability of findings. Factors in a study that cannot be controlled (e.g., because of feasibility or ethics) may lead to limitations that constrain the conclusions.

- *Definitions:* Clarification of any terms or language specific to the field of research addressed in the scholarly proposal

- *Background of the problem:* Review of relevant research literature and other influential papers such that "the author inserts the proposed study into a line of inquiry and a developing body of knowledge" (Locke et al., 2007, p. 17) and shows how each published source is relevant and contributes to the planned investigation. It is important to demonstrate that the conceptual and theoretical bases and research questions or hypotheses in the proposed study arise from existing knowledge and move inquiry from the answered to the unanswered

Table 45-9.

EXAMPLES OF THE STATED PURPOSE AND RELATED RESEARCH QUESTIONS OR HYPOTHESES FROM FOUR PUBLISHED STUDIES REPRESENTING EACH OF THE FOUR TYPES OF RESEARCH DISCUSSED IN THIS CHAPTER

Source	Type of Research	Purpose of the Study	Related Research Questions or Hypotheses
Duncan-Myers & Huebner, 2000	Descriptive or associative	"[T]o investigate the relationship between quality of life and personal control as measured by opportunities for choice in self-care and leisure activities among residents of long term care facilities" (p. 505), using two self-report instruments, the Quality of Life Rating and the Duncan Choice Index	Research questions: "1. What is the relationship between the residents' perceptions of the number of choices available in daily life and how they rate quality of life? 2. What level of quality of life do residents perceive? 3. In which daily tasks do residents have choices in and desire more choice?" (p. 505)
Hayner, Gibson, & Gordon, 2010	Experimental	"[T]o contribute to the understanding of constraint-induced movement therapy (CIMT) by comparing two treatments for chronic UE dysfunction in people in the post-CVA period [namely] (1) a modification of the standard CIMT protocol and (2) bilateral treatment provided with intensity equal to the CIMT condition"(p. 530)	Hypotheses: "1. All participants will demonstrate improved total Wolf Motor Function Test (WMFT) scores after [completion of both interventions]. 2. Participants in the CIMT group will demonstrate greater improvement in total WMFT scores than participants in the bilateral group after treatment of comparable intensity, frequency, duration, and activity selection" (p. 530).
Dankert, Davies, & Gavin, 2003	Outcome	"[T]o evaluate the assumption that occupational therapy provided to preschool children with developmental delays and preschool children without disabilities will significantly improve their visual-motor skills" (p. 544), as measured by the Developmental Test of Visual-Motor Integration (VMI)	Research questions: "1. Do preschool children with developmental delays demonstrate significant improvements in visual-motor skills . . . following occupational therapy for 1 school year when compared to their performance . . . prior to therapy? 2. Will preschool children with developmental delays exhibit a rate of gain consistent with typical peers . . . ?" (p. 544)
Lyons, Orozovic, Davis, & Newman, 2002	Qualitative	To study the "occupational nature of a group of persons with life-threatening illnesses, couched within the group's experiences as day hospice program participants, [framed around] a doing-being-becoming conceptualization of occupation [in order to] breathe new life into the profession's occupational gaze" (pp. 293-294).	Research question (phenomenon of interest): "Within an interpretive framework of doing-being-becoming . . . [w]hat are the occupational experiences of the men and women with life-threatening illnesses attending a day hospice program?" (p. 287)

questions. Discussion might also include critical analysis of methodologies used previously in the area of inquiry as a basis for the selection of procedures for the current study.

- *Explanation of methods:* Precise description, using concrete details, of the research design, study setting and environment, selection and recruiting of participants, and the nature of quantitative tests and measurements, as well as qualitative approaches used to collect data, intervention procedure(s), analytical techniques, and time frame. If financial information is called for, the budget might include such costs as staff and consultants, supplies and equipment, use of recording media, and travel. Information on the

planned methodology should be sufficient for the audience to determine its overall degree of rigor.

- Biographical sketch of the investigator(s): An overview of the academic, clinical, and research training and experience of the investigators relevant to the area of proposed research

It is important for the occupational therapy practitioner to think of the scholarly proposal as a work in progress. Maintaining openness to new insights and questions that may arise and readiness to modify the project to accommodate this information are often called for. "It is flexibility, not rigidity, that makes strong proposal documents" (Locke et al., 2007, p. 7).

Writing a Scholarly Report for Presentation or Publication

After a scholarly project is completed and found to generate new knowledge, the next logical step is *dissemination*, defined by the National Institutes of Health as "the targeted distribution of information and intervention materials to a specific public health or clinical practice audience. The intent is to spread knowledge and the associated evidence-based interventions" (2007, Para 5). This is in keeping with the stated priorities of the AOTA (2012), which include dissemination of occupational therapy outcomes and evidence. The traditional paths for dissemination are publishing in peer-reviewed journals and presentation at academic or professional conferences. Other dissemination activities can include briefings to stakeholders and educational sessions conducted with clients, colleagues, or policy makers. In addition, there are emerging vehicles for dissemination as promotion, including media coverage, fact sheets, flyers and brochures, Web-based text and video publications, and social media outlets (AOTA, 2012b; Jacobs, 2012; Yale Center for Clinical Investigation, 2010).

However, the gap between new knowledge generated from research findings and its implementation in practice, which was discussed earlier in this chapter, continue to be ongoing concerns in medicine, public health, and rehabilitation, as well as in occupational therapy (Burke & Gitlin, 2012; Cramm, White, & Krupa, 2013; National Center for the Dissemination of Disability Research, 2005). As an outgrowth of this concern, the model of *knowledge translation* (KT) arose as a means to reduce the gap (Backus & Jones, 2013; Bowen & Graham, 2013). Straus, Tetroe, and Graham (as cited by Cramm et al., 2013) define KT as "a dynamic and iterative process that includes the synthesis, dissemination, exchange and ethically sound application of knowledge to improve health, provide more effective health services and products and strengthen the health care system" (p. 119). This paradigm shift represents movement away from regarding knowledge generated from research as a product to instead seeing it as the result of collaboration between those who conduct the research and those who use the findings.

Dissemination is recognized to be a key element in KT but is more broadly defined as "a planned process that involves consideration of target audiences and the settings in which research findings are to be received and, where appropriate, communicating and interacting with wider policy and health service audiences in ways that will facilitate research uptake in decision-making processes and practice" (Wilson, Petticrew, Calnan, & Nazareth, 2010, p. 1). It thus behooves the occupational therapy practitioner seeking to disseminate knowledge gained from his or her scholarly project, whether via presentation or publication, to move beyond the assumption that simply informing colleagues about the new knowledge and its benefits will lead to implementation. Rather, inducing colleagues to implement the scholar's evidence-based findings requires communication based on an understanding of what constrains or expedites change in that area of practice. Factors to consider are the health system players in the area of practice (e.g., legislators, regulators, administrators, practitioners, professional organizations, clients and family members), the players' values and beliefs, the culture and climate of practice, and the ways in which new information flows through the system (Burke & Gitlin, 2012).

The most familiar means for an occupational therapy practitioner to disseminate his or her research findings is the full scholarly report, which is a complete description of the study. This format is suitable for presenting the research at an academic conference or submitting a manuscript to a peer-reviewed journal. Practitioners are generally asked to adhere to specific submission guidelines, often based on the current *Publication Manual of the American Psychological Association*. As a rule, a report of this kind begins with a descriptive title and abstract followed by introductory paragraphs and sections presenting methods, results, and discussion (Rudner & Shafer, 1999).

The ideal title of the full scholarly report piques the reader's interest and concisely communicates the essential features of the investigation, for example, by stating the nature and relationship of the targeted intervention and outcome(s). The abstract reproduces the study in about 300 words and usually covers the research question or purpose, design, methods or procedures, participants, measures, findings, and conclusions. A well-crafted scholarly proposal can provide the basis for the introduction and methods sections, with adjustments made to reflect what was actually done in the study. Typically included in the introduction are a description of the nature of problem that led to the investigation; the definition of key terms; a statement of the importance of the study; and review of relevant literature, leading to the research purpose and questions or study hypotheses. The methods section provides a detailed description of the research design, participants, measures, and procedures. Data analysis techniques and results, as well as any problems encountered during analysis, comprise the results section. In the discussion section, the scholar might highlight key results, discuss the limitations of the study, interpret the findings in light of the research questions or hypotheses, draw conclusions regarding implications of the findings, make recommendations, and suggest questions for future research.

Six other formats for reporting the results of a scholarly project, which are listed below, were described by Wholey et al. (2010). Each has applications for either presentation or publication:

- *The two-sentence summary*: A statement that effectively conveys the main message of the study. It can be a challenge for a scholar to boil down an entire research project to its essence, but it is that kernel that will attract the attention of the audience members and hold their interest. The two-sentence summary works well as a verbal introduction to the study and can also serve as the uniting theme for longer reports.

- *The compelling paragraph*: A concrete and concise overview of the major research findings and their implications for practice, with highlights of the methodology that was used. A report of this kind can be the basis of a news release, a stand-alone summary that appears on the Internet or in a professional organization's newsletter, an introductory letter or memo sent to a stakeholder with an invitation to read the longer report, or a short oral presentation at a meeting.

- *The outline*: A set of phrases or sentences that depicts the key topics for the scholarly report and their relative order and importance. The act of composing an outline helps the scholar to set priorities and refine the logical flow of ideas. In a verbal report, the outline can be converted into a slide show and handouts, which provide visual reinforcement for the audience members and help them to focus on the presentation and remember what was said. The outline functions as the backbone of a comprehensive written report and helps to eliminate potential areas of weakness or lack of focus. It can be used on its own to accompany briefings or to create a table of contents.

- *The two-page executive summary*: A document directed to decision makers or busy higher level stakeholders that highlights the most relevant information while requiring a minimal time commitment to review. Plain language makes it understandable by all readers regardless of their knowledge level or expertise. An executive summary concentrates on findings, implications for practice, and recommendations, with no more than a paragraph devoted to description of the methodology. When used as a means for persuasion, it becomes a call to action that states outcomes and benefits, substantiates benefits using the data, applies the benefits to the reader's particular context, and recommends a solution.

- *The 10-page report*: A fleshed-out version of the executive summary with added context, supporting facts, and explanation. This format is ideal for Internet publication.

- *The technical report*: A document aimed at specialists, such as academicians or policy analysts, who need or desire to know the technical details of the methodology, data collection, and data analysis used in the investigation. An important application of the technical report is for research collaboration.

Some additional guiding principles can enhance the impact of a scholarly report directed to consumers, decision makers, or stakeholders (Wholey et al., 2010). First, focus is essential to maintain the interest and attention of the audience; even in a comprehensive report, a good deal of information usually must be omitted. Second, avoid overly long sentences and paragraphs, technical jargon, and abbreviations and write in the "active voice," wherein the subject appears near the beginning of a sentence and is followed by the verb. Finally, follow the rules of effective document layout and graphic design. Keep the presentation clean and uncluttered; use font styles and sizes that look professional and that are easy to read; use clearly-labeled graphs, tables, and pictures that add relevant information; include judicious use of color where allowed; and be certain that main points are easy to discern.

Summary

Scholarship and scholarly practice are essential for the professional growth of any occupational therapy practitioner, as well as for developing the knowledge base of the discipline of occupational therapy. Understanding of the types of quantitative and qualitative research designs and their suitable applications, as well as of determinants of level of evidence for each and what constitutes rigorous investigation, is needed to support both research and EBP. Finding the evidence needed for clinical decision-making entails following a series of steps from formulating a question to integrating the results of a focused literature search into practice. When an occupational therapy practitioner embarks on a research project, writing a scholarly proposal provides the means to think through the project and make any refinements; after the study is completed, there are a number of vehicles and formats available for dissemination of findings. In any occupational therapy scholarly endeavor, collaboration is a key to narrowing the gap between the new knowledge gained from research and its implementation in everyday practice settings.

Student Self-Assessment

1. Think of a real-life practice situation that has given rise to a question. For example, it could be a recent clinical event (positive or negative) where you would like to better understand why or how this circumstance occurred. It could also be an assessment or intervention method that you use routinely in your practice for which you would like to have supporting evidence.

EVIDENCE-BASED RESEARCH CHART

Topic	Evidence
AOTA's Code of Ethics and Ethics Standards, which underscore the need for occupational therapy scholarship	AOTA, 2010
AOTA position paper on scholarship	AOTA, 2009
Models for depicting levels of evidence	AOTA, 2012a; Tomlin & Borgetto, 2011
Quantitative research	Kielhofner, 2006; Melnyk & Fineout-Overholt, 2011
Qualitative research	Bernard & Ryan, 2010; Cook, 2001; Mack, Woodsong, MacQueen, Guest, & Namey, 2005
Conducting evidence-based practice	Law & MacDermid, 2008; Taylor, 2007
Writing a scholarly proposal	Locke, Spirduso, & Silverman, 2007

2. Develop a clinical question that can be used to gather evidence about the practice situation that you have identified. Compose the question using the PICO or PICOT format. For questions that relate to an assessment or that are exploratory, the "C" or comparison aspect of the question might not be indicated.

3. Consider how you might approach searching for evidence to answer the clinical question that you have decided upon. Options to consider include electronic databases, Internet sources, "brick and mortar" libraries, and contact with colleagues. Decide on the keywords you will use in your search.

4. Locate a research article relevant to your clinical question in a peer-reviewed journal. Determine whether the type of study is quantitative or qualitative. Read the article carefully to discover the following information, as appropriate to the type of study: the purpose of investigation and research questions or hypotheses, the nature of the study participants, the research design, the independent and dependent variables, how the dependent variables were measured, the methods that were used to administer the intervention and gather the data, and the authors' findings.

5. Based on your review of the article, come to a conclusion regarding the trustworthiness of the research findings and their implications for your original clinical question.

References

American Occupational Therapy Association. (n.d.). *Levels of evidence for occupational therapy outcomes research.* Retrieved from http://www.aota.org/Educate/Research/EB/HowtoUse/35637.aspx

American Occupational Therapy Association. (2009). Scholarship in occupational therapy. *American Journal of Occupational Therapy 63*(6), 790-796.

American Occupational Therapy Association. (2010). *Occupational therapy code of ethics and ethics standards.* Retrieved from http://www.aota.org/consumers/ethics/39880.aspx

American Occupational Therapy Association. (2012a). *Guidelines for evidence tables.* Retrieved from http://www.aota.org/DocumentVault/AJOT/Guidelines-Tables.aspx

American Occupational Therapy Association. (2012b). *AOTA Board of Directors approves priorities for FY 2013.* Retrieved from http://www.aota.org/News/Announcements/Priorities-2013.aspx

Agency for Healthcare Research and Quality. (2000) *Outcomes research. Fact sheet.* Retrieved from http://www.ahrq.gov/clinic/outfact.htm

Backus, D., & Jones, M. L. (2013). Maximizing research evidence to enhance knowledge translation. *Archives of Physical Medicine and Rehabilitation, 94*(1 Suppl.), S1-S2.

Bennett, S., Hoffman, T., McCluskey, A., McKenna, K., Strong, J., & Tooth, L. (2003). Introducing Otseeker (Occupational Therapy Systematic Evaluation of Evidence): A new evidence database for occupational therapists. *American Journal of Occupational Therapy, 57*(6), 635-638.

Bernard, H. R., & Ryan, G. W. (2010). *Analyzing qualitative data: Systematic approaches.* Thousand Oaks, CA: Sage Publications.

Bowen, S. J., & Graham, I. D. (2013). From knowledge translation to engaged scholarship: Promoting research relevance and utilization. *Archives of Physical Medicine and Rehabilitation, 94*(1 Suppl.), S3-S8.

Braveman, B. H., Helfrich, C. A., & Fisher, G. S. (2002). Developing and maintaining community partnerships within "a Scholarship of Practice." *Occupational Therapy in Health Care, 15*(1-2), 109-125.

Burke, J. P., & Gitlin, L. N. (2012). How do we change practice when we have the evidence? *American Journal of Occupational Therapy, 66*(5), e85-e88.

Christiansen, C., & Lou, J. Q. (2001). Ethical considerations related to evidence-based practice. *American Journal of Occupational Therapy, 55*(3), 345-349.

Cook, J. V. (2001). *Qualitative research in occupational therapy: Strategies and experiences.* San Diego, CA: Singular Publishing.

Cooper, H., Hedges, L. V., & Valentine, J. C. (2009). *The handbook of research synthesis and meta-analysis* (2nd ed.). New York, NY: Russell Sage Foundation.

Cramm, H., White, C., & Krupa, T. (2013). From periphery to player: strategically positioning occupational therapy within the knowledge translation landscape. *American Journal of Occupational Therapy, 67*(1), 119-125.

Dankert, H. L., Davies, P. L., & Gavin, W. J. (2003). Occupational therapy effects on visual-motor skills in preschool children. *American Journal of Occupational Therapy, 57*(5), 542-449.

DeVellis, R. F. (2012). Scale development: Theory and applications (3rd ed.). Los Angeles, CA: Sage Publications.

Dijkers, M. P., Murphy, S. L., & Krellman, J. (2012). Evidence-based practice for rehabilitation professionals: Concepts and controversies. *Archives of Physical Medicine and Rehabilitation, 93*(8 Suppl.), S164-S176.

Dubouloz, C., Egan, M., Vallerand, J., & von Zweck, C. (1999). Occupational therapists' perceptions of evidence-based practice. *American Journal of Occupational Therapy, 53*(5), 445-453.

Duncan-Myers, A. M., & Huebner, R. A. (2000). Relationship between choice and quality of life among residents in long-term-care facilities. *American Journal of Occupational Therapy, 54*(5), 504-508.

Guba, E. G. (1981). ERIC/ECTJ annual review paper: Criteria for assessing the trustworthiness of naturalistic inquiries. *Educational Communication and Technology Journal, 29*(2), 75-91.

Haertlein, C., & Coppard, B. M. (2003). Scholarship and occupational therapy (2003 concept paper). *American Journal of Occupational Therapy, 57*(6), 641-643.

Hammel, J., Finlayson, M., Kielhofner, G., Helfrish, C., & Peterson, E. (2002). Educating scholars of practice: An approach to preparing tomorrow's researchers. *Occupational Therapy in Health Care, 15*(1-2), 157-176.

Hayner, K., Gibson, G., & Gordon, M. G. (2010). Comparison of constraint-induced movement therapy and bilateral treatment of equal intensity in people with chronic upper-extremity dysfunction after cerebrovascular accident. *American Journal of Occupational Therapy, 64*(4), 528-539.

Holm, M. B. (2000). The 2000 Eleanor Clarke Slagle lecture. Our mandate for the new millennium: Evidence-based practice. *American Journal of Occupational Therapy, 54*(6), 575-585.

Jacobs, K. (2012). PromOTing occupational therapy: Words, images, and actions. *American Journal of Occupational Therapy, 66*(6), 652-671.

Kazdin, A. E. (2010). *Single-case research designs: Methods for clinical and applied settings* (2nd ed.). New York, NY: Oxford University Press.

Kielhofner, G. (1982a). Qualitative research: Part one. Paradigmatic grounds and issues of reliability. *OTJR: Occupation, Participation, and Health, 2*(2), 67-79.

Kielhofner, G. (1982b). Qualitative research: Part two. Methodological approaches and relevance to occupational therapy. *OTJR: Occupation, Participation, and Health, 2*(3), 150-170.

Kielhofner, G. (2005a). A scholarship of practice: Creating discourse between theory, research and practice. *Occupational Therapy in Health Care, 19*(1-2), 7-16.

Kielhofner, G. (2005b). Scholarship and practice: Bridging the divide. *American Journal of Occupational Therapy, 59*(2), 231-239.

Kielhofner, G. (2006). *Research in occupational therapy: Methods of inquiry for enhancing practice.* Philadelphia, PA: F.A. Davis Company.

Krefting, L. (1991). Rigor in qualitative research: The assessment of trustworthiness. *American Journal of Occupational Therapy, 45*(3), 214-222.

Law, M., & MacDermid, J. (2008). Evidence-based rehabilitation: A guide to practice. Thorofare, NJ: SLACK Incorporated.

Law, M., Stewart, D., Pollock, N., Letts, L., Bosch, J., & Westmorland, M. (1998a). Guidelines for critical review form: Quantitative studies. Retrieved from http://www.srs-mcmaster.ca/Portals/20/pdf/ebp/quanguidelines.pdf

Law, M., Stewart, D., Pollock, N., Letts, L., Bosch, J., & Westmorland, M. (1998b). Critical review form: Quantitative studies. Retrieved from http://www.srs-mcmaster.ca/Portals/20/pdf/ebp/quanreview.pdf

Letts, L., Wilkins, S., Law, M., Stewart, D., Bosch, J., & Westmorland, M. (2007a). *Guidelines for critical review form: Qualitative studies.* Retrieved from http://www.srs-mcmaster.ca/Portals/20/pdf/ebp/qualguidelines_version2.0.pdf

Letts, L., Wilkins, S., Law, M., Stewart, D., Bosch, J., & Westmorland, M. (2007b). *Critical review form: Qualitative studies.* Retrieved from http://www.srs-mcmaster.ca/Portals/20/pdf/ebp/qualreview_version2.0.pdf

Lin, S. H., Murphy, S. L., & Robinson, J. C. (2010). Facilitating evidence-based practice: Process, strategies and resources. *American Journal of Occupational Therapy, 64*(1), 164-171.

Locke, L. F., Spirduso, W. W., & Silverman, S. J. (2007). *Proposals that work: A guide for planning dissertations and grant proposals.* (5th ed.). Thousand Oaks, CA: Sage Publications.

Lyons, M., Orozovic, N., Davis, J., & Newman, J. (2002). Doing-being-becoming: occupational experiences of persons with life-threatening illnesses. *American Journal of Occupational Therapy, 56*(3), 285-295.

Mack, N., Woodsong, C., MacQueen, K. M., Guest, G., & Namey, E. (2005). *Qualitative research methods: A data collector's field guide.* Research Triangle Park, NC: Family Health International. Retrieved from http://www.fhi360.org/resource/qualitative-research-methods-data-collectors-field-guide

Melnyk, B., & Fineout-Overholt, E. (2011). *Evidence-based practice in nursing & healthcare: A guide to best practice* (2nd ed.). Riverwoods, IL: Wolters Kluwer Health/Lippincott Williams & Wilkins.

Merrill, S. C. (1985). Qualitative methods in occupational therapy research: An application. *OTJR: Occupation, Participation, and Health, 5*(4), 209-222.

Mortenson, W. B., & Oliffe, J. L. (2009) Mixed methods research in occupational therapy: A survey and critique. *OTJR: Occupation, Participation, and Health, 29*(1), 14-23.

National Center for the Dissemination of Disability Research. (2005). *Focus technical brief no. 10: What is knowledge translation?* Retrieved from http://www.ncddr.org/kt/products/focus/focus10/

National Institutes of Health. (2007). *NIH conference on: Building the science of dissemination and implementation in the service of public health.* Retrieved from http://obssr.od.nih.gov/di2007/about.html

Ottenbacher, K. J., & Hinderer, S. R. (2001). Evidence-based practice: Methods to evaluate individual patient improvement. *American Journal of Physical Medicine and Rehabilitation, 80*(10), 786-796.

Papadimitriou, C., Magasi, S., & Frank, G. (2012). Current thinking in qualitative research: Evidence-based practice, moral philosophies, and political struggle. *OTJR: Occupation, Participation and Health, 32*(1 Suppl.), S2-S5.

Pearson, A., Wiechula, R., Court, A., & Lockwood, C. (2005). The Joanna Briggs Institute model of evidence-based healthcare. *International Journal of Evidence-Based Healthcare, 3*(8), 207-215.

Rudner, L. M., & Schafer, W. D. (1999). How to write a scholarly research report. *Practical Assessment, Research & Evaluation, 6*(13). Retrieved from http://www.uic.edu/depts/educ/mesalab/MESA%20Downloads/Writing%20Resources/WriteScholarlyResearch.pdf

Sackett, D. L., Rosenberg, W. M. C., Gray, J. A. M., Haynes, R. B., & Richardson, W. S. (1996). Evidence based medicine: What it is and what it isn't. *British Medical Journal, 312*(7023), 71-72.

Siegel, S., & Castellan Jr., N. J. (1988) *Nonparametric statistics for the behavioral sciences.* New York, NY: McGraw-Hill.

Suarez-Balcazar, Y., Hammel, J., Helfrich, C., Thomas, J., Wilson, T., & Head-Ball, D. (2005). A model of university-community partnerships for occupational therapy scholarship and practice. *Occupational Therapy in Health Care, 19*(1-2), 47-70.

Taylor, M. C. (2007). *Evidence-based practice for occupational therapists* (2nd ed.). Malden, MA: Blackwell Publishing.

Taylor, R. R., Fisher, G., & Kielhofher, G. (2005). Synthesizing research, education, and practice according to the scholarship of practice model: Two faculty examples. *Occupational Therapy in Health Care, 19*(1-2), 107-122.

Thorne, S., Jensen, L., Kearney, M. H., Noblit, G., & Sandelowski, M. (2004). Qualitative metasynthesis: Reflections on methodological orientation and ideological agenda. *Qualitative Health Research, 14*(10), 1342-1365.

Tickle-Degnen, L. (1999). Organizing, evaluating, and using evidence in occupational therapy practice. *American Journal of Occupational Therapy, 53*(5), 537-539.

Tomlin, G., & Borgetto, B. (2011). Research pyramid: A new evidence-based practice model for occupational therapy. *American Journal of Occupational Therapy, 65*(2), 189-196.

Walsh, D., & Downe, S. (2005). Meta-synthesis method for qualitative research: A literature review. *Journal of Advanced Nursing, 50*(2), 204-211.

Westhues, A., Ochocka, J., Jacobson, N., Simich, L., Maiter, S., Janzen, R., & Fleras, A. (2008). Developing theory from complexity: Reflections on a collaborative mixed method participatory action research study. *Qualitative Health Research, 18*(5), 701-717.

Wholey, J. S., Hatry, H. P., & Newcomer, K. E. (2010). *Handbook of practical program evaluation* (3rd ed.). San Francisco, CA: John Wiley & Sons.

Wilding, C., Curtin, M., & Whiteford, G. (2012). Enhancing occupational therapists' confidence and professional development through a community of practice scholars. *Australian Occupational Therapy Journal, 59*(4), 312-318.

Wilson, P., M., Petticrew, M., Calnan, M. W., & Nazareth, I. (2010, November 22). Disseminating research findings: What should researchers do? A systematic scoping review of conceptual frameworks. *Implementation Science, 5*(91), 1-16.

Wong, P. T. P. (2005). *How to write a research proposal.* Retrieved from http://ielcass.tripod.com/proposalwriting.pdf

Yale Center for Clinical Investigation. (2010). *Beyond scientific publication: Strategies for disseminating research findings.* Retrieved from http://www.yale.edu/bioethics/contribute_documents/CARE_Dissemination_Strategies_FINAL_eversion.pdf

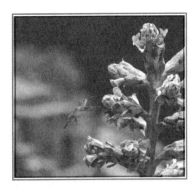

46

GRANTS

Wendy B. Stav, PhD, OTR/L, SCDCM, FAOTA

ACOTE STANDARDS EXPLORED IN THIS CHAPTER
B.8.9

KEY VOCABULARY

- **Funding agencies:** Federal, state, local, or community organizations; corporations; foundations; and trusts offering monetary support to develop programs or run research projects.
- **Grants:** Monies disbursed by a funding agency to another agency or person for the purpose of a specific program, research study, or products.

- **Proposal:** The collective materials used to apply for a grant, including an application and supporting documents.

Introduction

The majority of occupational therapy services are reimbursed through third-party payers, such as insurance companies, or are covered within the larger system in which the clients are treated, as is the case in the school system. However, there are instances in which there is no existing funding mechanism to support the work performed by occupational therapy practitioners or provide the necessary resources. These instances include research activities, new program development,

innovative programs outside of the medical model, and provision of resources to clients necessary for optimal occupational engagement but not deemed medically necessary by third-party payers. Although occupational therapy practitioners are generally altruistic and giving of their time and expertise, actual financial support is required to engage in research, develop programs, execute innovative and nontraditional programs, and provide resources to clients. Financial support is available for many of these activities through grant funding from a variety of sources. Grants are funds disbursed by

Jacobs, K., MacRae, N., & Sladyk, K. (Eds.).
*Occupational Therapy Essentials for
Clinical Competence, Second Edition* (pp. 603-612).
© 2014 SLACK Incorporated.

a funding agency to another agency or person for the purpose of a specific program, research study, or products. Grants funds are not loans and do not have to repaid; however, the expectations of the project and reporting of the activity must be completed.

There are several different sources of grant funding, including federal agencies, state agencies, corporations, foundations, trusts, and community organizations. Typically, but not exclusively, these funding agencies award grant monies to nonprofit agencies (also referred to a 501[c][3] organizations) and require an application for the funds. The application process is referred to as grant writing and requires that applicants adhere to guidelines set forth by the funding agency, including the required information to be considered for funding. This chapter reviews the types of funding sources, identification of funders, application process, and deliverables expected by the funders.

Sources of Grant Funding

A broad range of funding sources can meet a variety of research and programmatic needs. It is important that funding seekers identify the most appropriate funding source for the best chances of successfully receiving a grant. The alignment of the match between the project and funding source is critical and can be the difference between full funding and a rapid rejection letter. Larger agencies such as the federal government and state agencies tend to offer larger grant awards than smaller agencies such as local civic organizations (Doll, 2010).

The federal government is the largest grant funder in the United States. A large portion of federal grants comes from the National Institutes of Health (NIH) with more than $30.9 billion awarded annually for medical research (NIH, 2012a). The NIH distributes that investment across numerous conditions, including $490 million in mind-body research, $352 million in rehabilitation, $316 million in stroke, $103 million in macular degeneration, $334 million in intellectual and developmental disabilities, $151 million in Parkinson's disease, and $264 million in schizophrenia (NIH, 2012b). Choosing the NIH as a funding source is an appropriate selection if one is planning to conduct a research project related to health because the NIH funds only health-related projects and primarily research projects and a smaller number of program and resource grants. The NIH grant funding system includes several types of grants, each of which supports a different type of project. Table 46-1 outlines the types of NIH grants. In addition to selecting the proper type of grant, it is important to submit the grant application to the most appropriate NIH Institute because each has a unique focus and agenda. Table 46-2 lists the NIH Institutes.

Although the NIH awards a substantial portion of federal funding, other federal agencies also support research relevant to and involving occupational therapy, including the Centers for Disease Control and Prevention, Department of Transportation, and Department of Education's National Institute on Disability and Rehabilitation Research. A valuable source of available federal grants is Grants.gov (www.grants.gov). Regardless of which agencies are selected, the applicant must be cognizant of the agency's vision, identified gaps, and research agenda to create the best match between the funder's purpose and the project for which funding is sought.

Federal grants typically support projects with tens to hundreds of thousands of dollars and even as high as over $1 million. Projects that are smaller in scale, address a statewide issue, and can operate on a smaller budget can benefit from funding from state agencies. Statewide initiatives often parallel federal initiatives or are managed at a state level with federal dollars that have been sent to state agencies for distribution. For example, the campaign to reduce drunk driving–related injuries and fatalities is a national initiative with federal dollars passed to state agencies for distribution via grants to the state Departments of Transportation. The benefit of applying for state grants is the focus on programs and demonstration projects because state agencies are concerned with meeting the needs of the residents of the state through programs and services as opposed to discovering new knowledge through research. The organization and titles of state agencies vary from state to state, so applicants seeking funding should explore their own state agencies to discover the initiative of each governmental unit to create the best match. In some instances, the identification of a state agency is obvious. For example, therapists wishing to develop a child passenger safety resource center and lending library should apply to the state's department of transportation whose concern is traffic-related injury prevention. In other instances, the best agency match may not be apparent and could require additional exploration of agency vision and focus. For example, an interprofessional team trying to develop a lifestyle redesign or wellness program for retirees might apply to the state's department of elder affairs or the department of health and human services, depending on the allocation of responsibilities and focus on each agency.

Another source of grant funding is foundations. A foundations is "a non-governmental entity that is established as a nonprofit corporation or a charitable trust, with a principal purpose of making grants to unrelated organizations, institutions, or individuals for scientific, educational, cultural, religious, or other charitable purposes" (Foundation Center, 2012, Para. 1). Each foundation is created with a specific purpose and vision and as such will only fund proposals that are consistent with its agenda. For example, the mission of the Christopher and Dana Reeve Foundation states, "The Reeve Foundation

Table 46-1.

TYPES AND PURPOSE OF
SELECT NATIONAL INSTITUTE OF HEALTH GRANTS

Type	Name	Purpose
R01	NIH Research Project Grant Program	Used to support a discrete, specified, circumscribed research project
R03	NIH Small Grant Program	Provides limited funding for a short period of time to support a variety of types of projects, including pilot or feasibility studies, collection of preliminary data, secondary analysis of existing data, small, self-contained research projects, development of new research technology, and so on
R13	NIH Support for Conferences and Scientific Meetings	Support for high quality conferences and scientific meetings that are relevant to the NIH's scientific mission and to the public health
R15	NIH Academic Research Enhancement Award	Supports small research projects in the biomedical and behavioral sciences conducted by students and faculty in health professional schools and other academic components that have not been major recipients of NIH research grant funds
R21	NIH Exploratory/ Developmental Research Grant Award	Encourages new, exploratory and developmental research projects by providing support for the early stages of project development; sometimes used for pilot and feasibility studies
R41/R42	Small Business Technology Transfer	Intended to stimulate scientific and technological innovation through cooperative R/R&D carried out between SBCs and research institutions Assists the small business and research communities in commercializing innovative technologies
R43/R44	Small Business Innovative Research	Intended to stimulate technological innovation in the private sector by supporting R/R&D for for-profit institutions for ideas that have potential for commercialization
P01	Research Program Project Grant	Support for integrated, multi-project research projects involving a number of independent investigators who share knowledge and common resources
P20	Exploratory Grants	Often used to support planning activities associated with large multi-project program project grants
P30	Center Core Grants	Support shared resources and facilities for categorical research by a number of investigators from different disciplines who provide a multidisciplinary approach to a joint research effort or from the same discipline who focus on a common research problem
R24	Resource-Related Research Projects	Used in a wide variety of ways to provide resources for problems for which multiple expertise is needed to focus on a single complex problem in biomedical research or to enhance research infrastructure

NIH, National Institutes of Health; R/R&D, research/research and development; SBC, small business concern.

Adapted from National Institutes of Health. (2012c). *Grants and funding: Types of grant programs.* Retrieved from http://grants.nih.gov/grants/funding/funding_program.htm#PSeries

is dedicated to curing spinal cord injury by funding innovative research, and improving the quality of life for people living with paralysis through grants, information and advocacy" (2013, Para.1) and therefore will only approve grant proposals specific to spinal cord injury. Other foundations have broader interests such as the Robert Wood Johnson Foundation, which has program areas that include childhood obesity, public health, quality of health care, uninsured Americans, vulnerable populations, and training health care providers (Robert Wood Johnson Foundation, 2013). There are hundreds of foundations in existence with each one targeting a different population, need, or problem. Therapists seeking funding can search for individual foundations if they know of a funder with interests in a particular area or they can use a foundation search database such as Foundation Center (http://www.foundationcenter.org), Foundation Search (http://www.foundationsearch.com), or Big Online America (http://www.bigdatabase.com). If a therapist or organization is going to continuously seek foundation funding, the paid membership in these databases is worthwhile. Another option for seeking

Table 46-2.

INSTITUTES IN THE NATIONAL INSTITUTES OF HEALTH WITH RELEVANCE TO OCCUPATIONAL THERAPY

Abbreviation	Title of Institute
NEI	National Eye Institute
NIA	National Institute on Aging
NIAAA	National Institute of Alcohol Abuse and Alcoholism
NIAMS	National Institute of Arthritis and Musculoskeletal and Skin Diseases
NICHD	National Institute of Child Health and Human Development
NIDA	National Institute on Drug Abuse
NIDCD	National Institute on Deafness and Other Communication Disorders
NIMH	National Institute of Mental Health
NIMHD	National Institute on Minority Health and Health Disparities
NINDS	National Institute of Neurological Disorders and Stroke

Adapted from National Institutes of Health. (2012d). *Institutes, centers, & offices.* Retrieved from http://www.nih.gov/icd/

grant funding from a foundation is through partnerships with occupational therapists in academia because universities typically have a grant office with ongoing memberships to these or similar databases.

A final source of funding that can be useful for occupational therapy practitioners are community and civic organizations. Several organizations give back to the community in the form of grant funding and can meet the modest fiscal needs of a community program. CVS, for example, has community grants aimed at inclusive programming for children with disabilities to promote independence and support physical movement and play (CVS Caremark, 2013). Civic organizations, specifically local chapters of the Rotary Club, Lion's Club, and Kiwanis, often support small one-time grants for the local community.

Selection of a potential funding source should involve consideration of several factors, including but not limited to the following:

- Type of project (research, program or service, resource)
- Size and scope of the project
- Duration of the project
- Population involved
- Amount of money needed to support the project
- Match between project purpose and funding agency vision, mission, and agenda

Grant Proposals

Selecting the right potential funding source is an important step in the grant process, but the application process is critical to securing funding. The application document and associated requested material is referred to as a proposal. The first determination is whether the funder has sent out a call for grant applications or a request for proposals, commonly referred to as an RFP, or if the funder will accept unsolicited proposals. If the funder's materials state they do not accept unsolicited proposals, they will not award any money for proposals that have not answered a specific RFP. Applicants can increase their chances of getting funding if the proposal is thorough and accurate, includes all the information requested, and strictly adheres to the proposal guidelines.

The guidelines for proposals should be taken very literally and followed exactly. Funders make judgments about an applicant's ability to perform and spend their money wisely by how well the proposal follows the guidelines. Therefore, if proposal guidelines identify page length, font size, font style, and margin width, the proposal should follow those guidelines exactly; otherwise, the proposal will be immediately rejected before being read. Deadlines for submission are another guideline that should not be taken lightly because late submissions will not be accepted. Finally, all sections and information requested on a proposal should be completed because there are no second chances or revisions permitted. All proposals are slightly different depending on the funding source and what information they need to make a decision to award funding, but standard elements exist across most grant proposals. The common parts of a proposal, include institutional information, summary of the project with goals and objectives, biographical information of the personnel, budget with budget justification, and a plan for sustainability (Gitlin & Lyons, 2008). Throughout the entire proposal, applicants try to sell themselves and their institutions to the funder by proving the project is worthy of receiving a grant award and the applicant is qualified to see the project completed.

INSTITUTIONAL INFORMATION

Funders ask for information about the institution in which the project will take place to ensure eligibility for funding as well as to determine whether the institution has the experience, infrastructure, and resources to execute the project. Typically, applicants are asked to provide general background information about the organization, which is the same content regardless of the grant being sought. This content includes information about the type of institution; size; why type of business is conducted there; and most importantly, the tax status to prove the organization is nonprofit. The sum of this information is referred to as boilerplate content and is usually available from the organization's administration.

In addition to the boilerplate information, applicants must demonstrate how the proposed project can be successfully executed based on experience in research or program development, expertise with the described population of clients, size of the organization, proximity to clientele, and available resources. Funders consider grants to be investments in their agenda and toward their vision, so they want to be sure they are making a sound investment.

SUMMARY OF THE PROJECT

Grant proposals require a detailed description of what will be done with requested funds. For research proposals, this description should detail the population being studied, study design, proposed measurement tools, and planned data analysis. Grant proposals requested for the development of a program or services should demonstrate how the proposed program or service fills an existing gap, identifies the population to be served, and describes the program or services. In addition to a detailed description of the program, applicants identify program or research goals they plan to accomplish. Depending on the nature of the project, the goals may be related to discovering the effect of a certain intervention, identifying the relationships among variables, creating a fully operational program, or serving a specific number of clients. Practitioners who receive grant funding are held accountable for reporting the status toward goal achievement throughout the project. The information in this section of the proposal should illustrate the alignment between the proposed project and the funder initiatives and vision, and if applicable, satisfy the intent of the RFP. Any elements of the proposed project that stray from the funder's mission or initiatives will be grounds for rejection of the request.

BIOGRAPHICAL INFORMATION OF THE PERSONNEL

Funders request detailed information about the applicant and any members of the project team to determine whether the applicants have the experience and capability to carry out the proposed project. Typically, the RFP identifies exactly what the funder is looking for in terms of education, work experience, prior program development experience, previous scholarship, and often past grant funding received. As in other parts of a grant application, the applicant should provide all of the information and only the information requested by the funder. This is the applicant's opportunity to sell him- or herself and prove to be a worthy grant recipient. Often a grant funder will provide a format for the applicant's biographical information. If such a form is provided, the applicant should use only that template to provide the requested information. A form commonly completed by grant applicants is the NIH Biographical Sketch, which includes a template along with open-ended sections to complete, including a personal statement, positions and honors, selected peer-reviewed publications, and research support. Figure 46-1 is an example of an abbreviated NIH Biographical Sketch form.

BUDGET WITH BUDGET JUSTIFICATION

Development of a budget at the time of the proposal is an important step in the process because the funders will make judgments about the worthiness of the proposed project based on several factors, including the total amount of money being requested, the suggested distribution of funds across the categories in the budget, the anticipated tasks to be accomplished with the money, the proposed scope of impact of the project (i.e., local, regional, statewide, or national), adherence to budgetary guidelines in the RFP, and how realistic the request is. Applicants of all grants are required to specify exactly how much money they are suggesting will be spent across several categories within the budget. Some funders identify categories of the budget that are required; other funders allow the applicants to identify the areas of the budget.

Regardless of the structure of the grant application, several categories of the budget are common to most proposals. These categories include personnel, materials and supplies, travel, and indirect costs (Gitlin & Lyons, 2008). The more detailed and comprehensive the budget is, the

24

BIOGRAPHICAL SKETCH

Provide the following information for the Senior/key personnel and other significant contributors in the order listed on Form Page 2.
Follow this format for each person. **DO NOT EXCEED FOUR PAGES.**

NAME	POSITION TITLE
Stav, Wendy Beth	Chair and Professor of Occupational Therapy
eRA COMMONS USER NAME (credential, e.g., agency login)	

EDUCATION/TRAINING *(Begin with baccalaureate or other initial professional education, such as nursing, include postdoctoral training and residency training if applicable.)*

INSTITUTION AND LOCATION	DEGREE *(if applicable)*	MM/YY	FIELD OF STUDY
Quinnipiac University	B.S.	10/91	Occupational Therapy
Nova Southeastern University	Ph.D.	01/02	Occupational Therapy

A. Personal Statement

I have a long history of clinical and scholarly inquiry in the area of on driving and community mobility over the past 15 years related to program development, medical reporting policies, driver licensing guidelines for medically at-risk drivers, assessment predictability, and occupational therapy practice. My research and professional involvement includes activities at the state and national levels including AOTA's Older Driver Initiative, co-authorship of AOTA official documents and Occupational Therapy Practice Guidelines of Driving and Community Mobility for Older Adult, collaboration with the American Medical Association's Older Driver Project, the American Association of Motor Vehicle Administrator's Older Driver Working Group, and contribution to three separate based literature reviews on older drivers.

B. Positions and Honors

Positions

2006 – 2011 Associate Professor, Department of Occupational Therapy & Occupational Science, Towson University
2011 – 2012 Assistant Professor, Department of Occupational Therapy & Occupational Science, Towson University
2012 – Chair and Professor, Occupational Therapy Department, Nova Southeastern University

Honors

2008 Nova Southeastern University Distinguished Alumni Achievement Award
2008 Maryland Occupational Therapy Association Award of Merit
2009 American Occupational Therapy Association Roster of Fellow Award

C. Selected Peer-reviewed Publications

Stav, W., Hallenan, T., & Lane, J., & Arbesman, M. (2012). Evidence related to occupational engagement and health outcomes among older adults. *American Journal of Occupational Therapy, 66*(3), 301-310. doi: 10.5014/ajot.111.003699

Stav, W., (2012). Developing and implementing driving rehabilitation programs: A phenomenological approach. *American Journal of Occupational Therapy, 66*(1), e11-e16. doi: 10.5014/ajot.2012.000950

Stav, W., Snider Weidley, L., & Love, A. (2011). Barriers to developing and sustaining driving and community mobility programs. *American Journal of Occupational Therapy, 65*(4), e38-e45. doi: 10.5014/ajot.2011.002097

D. Research Support

American Occupational Therapy Association   Stav (PI)   2/11 – 12/11
Older Driver Evidence-Based Literature Review Update

American Association of Motor Vehicle Administrators Stav (EB Literature Review Contractor) 1/08 – 12/08
Driving Fitness Working Group

National Highway Traffic Safety Administration   Stav (PI)   1/07 – 12/09
Barriers to Developing Driving and Community Mobility Programs for Older Americans

Figure 46-1. Abbreviated National Institutes of Health Biographical Sketch form.

Table 46-3.

EXAMPLE OF A BUDGET

Category	Amount	Match	Total
Personnel	$27,560.00	$25,825.00	$53,385.00
• Principal investigator @ $67,120 + benefits x 40%	$17,500.00	$8,425.00	$25,295.00
• Project associate	$0.00	$17,400.00	$17,400.00
• Research assistant	$10,060.00	$0.00	$10,600.00
Travel	$2,700.00	$0.00	$2,700.00
• Lifesavers conference	$1,500.00	$0.00	$1,500.00
• American Occupational Therapy Association conference	$1,200.00	$0.00	$1,200.00
Contractual services	$4,600.00	$0.00	$4,600.00
• Video production @ $500/day for 2 days	$1,000.00	$0.00	$1,000.00
• Postproduction @ $40/hour for 90 hours	$3,600.00	$0.00	$3,600.00
Equipment	$0.00	$5,300.00	$5,300.00
• Computers 3 @ $1,500	$0.00	$4,500.00	$4,500.00
• Printers 3 @ $600.00	$0.00	$1,800.00	$1,800.00
• Fax machine	$0.00	$200.00	$200.00
Other direct costs	$970.00	$0.00	$970.00
• Recordable CD-ROMs (100 pack)	$25.00	$0.00	$25.00
• Three-ring binders (60)	$180.00	$0.00	$180.00
• Packing materials	$240.00	$0.00	$240.00
• WebEx account for training	$225.00	$0.00	$225.00
• Copying	$300.00	$0.00	$300.00
Indirect costs	$1,734.00	$1,156.00	$2,890.00
Total	$37,564.00	$32,281.00	$69,845.00
Percentage	53.78%	46.22%	100%

better able the funder will be to make an assessment on whether to fund the proposed project. See Table 46-3 for an example of a budget and Table 46-4 for a sample budget justification.

In an effort to provide the detail needed, the broad categories are often further broken down into individual items. For example, the personnel category, which is often the largest portion of the budget, clearly delineates each individual person involved in the project, each person's salary along with percent of time investment in the project, and the amount of their fringe benefits so all values are understood by the funder. The personnel category includes the principal investigator, who leads the entire project; other team members; subcontractors; graduate assistants; and support staff. Occupational therapy assistants applying for grants should be sure to include an occupational therapist in the project to ensure adherence to state practice guidelines in the jurisdiction of the project. If a project is planned for more than 1 year, the budget needs to reflect all of these values across each individual year of the budget. Another large portion of

the budget is the materials and supplies category. This section includes all of the items and services necessary to execute the project. The obvious items in this portion of the budget are the clinical instruments for use in the project such as assessment tools, furniture, and intervention equipment. Additional costs covered in this section include phone charges, paper and envelopes, copying, postage, food, marketing materials, consultation fees, computers, and laptops. Travel costs are also covered in a grant budget and incorporate local travel for day-to-day operation of the project as well as distance travel for dissemination of the results. Applicants should plan ahead at the time of the proposal and consider where they would like to present the study results or project outcomes. Preliminary research on the cost of travel to the location of conferences is necessary for inclusion in the budget. A final area of the budget is indirect costs, which represent the administrative and facility expenses to run a program or project. Some funders state that no indirect costs will be covered, but others identify a maximum percentage allowable. Often indirect costs are calculated

Table 46-4.	
BUDGET JUSTIFICATION	
Category and Item	**Justification**
Personnel: principal investigator	The principal investigator will coordinate the project, oversee development of materials, and supervise the tasks of the other personnel. The principal investigator has more than 20 years of experience as an occupational therapist with associated expertise in the relationship between the person and the environment as well as more than 15 years of expertise in the area of driver safety. Forty percent of the principal investigator's time will be dedicated to the project.
Personnel: research assistant	The research assistant will assist with the project coordination, information gathering, scheduling of events, and dissemination of materials developed.
Travel: Lifesavers conference	Travel to present project experiences and outcomes at a national traffic safety conference
Travel: AOTA conference	Travel to present project experiences and outcomes at a national occupational therapy conference
Contractural services: video production	The educational curriculum created from the project will be created in a video format, requiring the skilled work of video production. The project will include 2 days of video shooting at $500 per day.
Contractural services: postproduction	After video shooting, all footage will be edited for content and flow with the addition of graphics and text where necessary at a fee of $40 per hour for 90 hours.
Direct costs: recordable CD-ROMs	The video format educational program will be copied onto CD-ROMs for distribution statewide.
Direct costs: three-ring binders	Educational materials to supplement the video (handouts, tests, instructions, and so on) will be printed and placed in binders for dissemination to programs statewide
Direct costs: packing materials	Packing materials will be used to pack CD-ROMs and three-ring binders for shipping via the intra-state mail system.
Direct costs: WebEx account	A WebEx account will be used to provide synchronous training program statewide in the use of the program.
Copying	Copying services will be used to generate hard copies of the educational materials for dissemination statewide.

by a percentage of the direct costs. The monies supporting indirect costs cover expenses such as building costs, utilities, and the administrative fees associated with coordinating a grant within an institution.

Additional considerations when developing the budget for a grant are matching funds and in-kind contributions. Many funding sources require matching funds from the organization in order to receive an award. Matching funds are dollars or services contributed by the institution equal to a specified percentage of money awarded by the funding agency. In some cases, the institution has money set aside just for the purpose of matching; however, in-kind contributions can add up to a dollar amount required by the funder as long as those contributions are given a value. For example, if an institution offers to contribute a computer and printer worth $1,500 toward a project, that amount is documented. Personnel time can also be considered as an in-kind contribution as in the case of a volunteer working 10 hours per week as an estimate worth of $10 per hour or 25% of an administrative assistant's time not financially supported by the grant.

After each category and year of the budget is subtotaled and the sum of the total money requested is calculated, the applicant must write a budget justification. The justification is a rationale for each individual line in the budget to clarify exactly how the money will be spent. Budget justifications are written in a narrative format, but depending on the funder, they may also be allowable in a table format infused with budget values. As with any other portion of a grant proposal, it is incumbent upon the applicant to read the instructions and understand the expectation before writing the proposal.

PLAN FOR SUSTAINABILITY

Most proposals for programs ask the applicants to describe a plan for sustainability of the program. It is not the intention or desire of a funding agency to provide fiscal support for a program into perpetuity. Rather, funding agencies offer grants to programs as a means for start-up and development costs. Applicants must include a plan to generate revenue or another source of sustainability. Without such a plan documented in the proposal,

EVIDENCE-BASED RESEARCH CHART

Term	Evidence
Grants	Cameron & Luvisi, 2012; Cole, 2006; Doll, 2010; Jacob & Lefgren, 2007
Funding	Bear-Lehman, 2011; Lambert, 2001; Lin, 2011

funders may have concerns that their investment is not worthwhile over just a short period of time of the funding. Depending on the nature of the program, applicants should consider several options for sustainability, which may include reimbursement from a third party, out-of-pocket payments by clients, integration into another existing program, or training and delegation to other practitioners or disciplines.

Deliverables

After a grant is awarded, the grantee has an obligation to execute what was promised in the proposal. In addition to carrying out the research study or program as proposed, the grantee must provide evidence of the activities. This evidence is often referred to as deliverables. Any and all products, reports, articles, and materials generated by the project should be sent to the funder for their review. This includes marketing materials created, outcome studies, documents and forms developed, and articles published as a result of the project. In addition, many funders request reports at predetermined intervals such as annually or quarterly so they can maintain awareness of how their monies are being spent. Failure to comply with these requests or any other legally mandated or funder imposed guidelines, such as protection of health information, appropriate allocation of funds, and ethical treatment of study participants, can result in revocation of funds.

Grant Case Example

The sample budget and associated justification presented in Tables 46-3 and 46-4 represent a portion of the grant proposal written to develop a driver–vehicle fit program for teenage novice drivers. The principal investigator, having significant experience in driver safety and the CarFit program, was approached by the state highway safety office inquiring about driver–vehicle fit for teenage drivers. The request for proposals was approaching, so the principal investigator wrote a proposal for funding to meet the state's needs. The proposed program involved the development of an evidence-based educational curriculum specific to driver–vehicle fit for teenagers. The program included the development of a curriculum with

a video, worksheets, informational handouts, tests, and an instructional handbook. The plan and desire of the funder was to disseminate the curriculum to all state sanctioned driver education schools statewide. The dissemination process would include full copies of the curriculum and associated materials as well as train the trainer sessions delivered by the program staff to the driving schools via a Web-based instructional platform. Strengths of the proposal included experienced personnel, collaboration between resource-rich agencies (a state university and the regional office of a national traffic safety organization), and a plan to develop an evidence-based program. This particular grant proposal was very strong in design as well as funder interest, but it was written and submitted just before a significant downward shift in the economy, so all grant funding from the state agency was reduced, and the project was not funded.

Summary

Receiving a grant comes with a tremendous responsibility to execute the project, sustain professional and ethical standards, manage the funds and personnel properly, and complete the reports in a timely manner. It is not recommended that individuals pursue large grant funding opportunities because it requires a vast skills set and extensive time commitment beyond what an individual can dedicate. Despite the challenges associated with grants, receiving external funding to support research and projects is necessary. Grant funding allows occupational therapy practitioners to grow the profession, discover new and innovative methods to measure and enhance occupational performance, and create new forays into areas of practice that would otherwise not be reimbursed in the traditional health care system.

References

Bear-Lehman, J. (2011). The NIH roadmap: An opportunity for occupational therapy. *OTJR: Occupation, Participation and Health, 31*(3), 106-107.

Cameron, K. A. V., & Luvisi, J. (2012, March). Grants: Fulfilling dreams and needs for occupational therapy. *Administration & Management Special Interest Section Quarterly, 28*(1), 1-3.

Christopher and Dana Reeve Foundation. (2013). *About us.* Retrieved from http://www.christopherreeve.org/site/c.ddJFKRNoFiG/b.4409743/k.C825/About_Us.htm

Cole, S. S. (2006). Researcher behavior that leads to success in obtaining grant funding: A model for success. *Research Management Review, 15,* 16-32.

CVS Caremark. (2013). *Community grants.* Retrieved from http://info.cvscaremark.com/community/our-impact/community-grants

Doll, J. (2010). *Program development and grant writing in occupational therapy: Making the connection.* Sudbury, MA: Jones and Bartlett.

Foundation Center. (2012). *Knowledge base.* Retrieved from http://www.grantspace.org/Tools/Knowledge-Base/Funding-Resources/Foundations/What-is-a-foundation

Gitlin, L. N., & Lyons, K. J. (2008). *Successful grant writing: Strategies for health and human service professionals* (3rd ed.). New York, NY: Springer.

Jacob, F., & Lefgren, L. (2007). The impact of research grant funding on scientific productivity. *Journal of Public Economics, 95,* 1168-1177.

Lambert, R. (2001). The money is out there: One route to a major research funding award. *British Journal of Occupational Therapy, 64*(6), 311-313.

Lin, S. H. (2011). Increasing research capacity and advocating for research. *OT Practice, 16*(17), 33.

National Institutes of Health. (2012a). *About NIH: NIH budget.* Retrieved from http://www.nih.gov/about/budget.htm

National Institutes of Health. (2012b). *Estimates of Funding for various research, condition, and disease categories.* Retrieved from http://report.nih.gov/categorical_spending.aspx

National Institutes of Health. (2012c). *Grants and funding: Types of grant programs.* Retrieved from http://grants.nih.gov/grants/funding/funding_program.htm#PSeries

National Institutes of Health. (2012d). *Institutes, centers, & offices* Retrieved from http://www.nih.gov/icd/

Robert Wood Johnson Foundation. (2013). *Our work.* Retrieved from http://www.rwjf.org/en/our-work.html

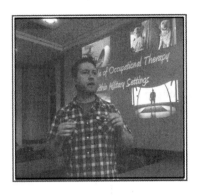

47

PROFESSIONAL PRESENTATIONS

Christine Sullivan, OTD, MS, OTR/L

ACOTE STANDARDS EXPLORED IN THIS CHAPTER

B.8.8

KEY VOCABULARY

- **American Psychological Association format:** The standard format used in health science literature for in-text citation and reference information.
- **Peer review:** A process in which a panel of experts in the field is responsible for judging the merit of a proposal for a scholarly publication or presentation.
- **Plagiarism:** The use of information that was created by another individual as though it were original.
- **Professional presentation:** An oral report of research findings or other evidence-based practice information.
- **Scholarly reports:** Documents that are written by reflective practitioners for the advancement of a profession.

Introduction

Occupational therapy practitioners have many roles to play regarding being a professional. A review of the literature reveals the multitude of activities that are the hallmark of fulfilling a professional role. Braveman (2006) discussed involvement in the professional association as being important, naming professional associations in the United States as being the "primary vehicle" that allows a profession to "promote and develop its services." This sentiment is clearly echoed

in the American Occupational Therapy Association's (AOTA) Centennial Vision (AOTA, 2007): "We envision that occupational therapy is a powerful, widely recognized, science-driven, and evidence-based profession with a globally connected and diverse work force meeting society's occupational needs."

This vision was created to be a "road map" to commemorate the AOTA's 100th anniversary in 2017. Member and nonmember feedback was sought to ensure that this was a shared vision. Demonstrating the skills to writing a scholarly report for either a presentation

Jacobs, K., MacRae, N., & Sladyk, K. (Eds.).
*Occupational Therapy Essentials for
Clinical Competence, Second Edition* (pp. 613-625).
© 2014 SLACK Incorporated.

or for publication is in direct line with the need for the profession to be visible and science based throughout the world. The *Centennial Vision's* goal of linking education, research, and practice will only be reached by ensuring that occupational therapy practitioners are able to communicate effectively both in scholarly writing and in professional presentations.

Scholarship in Occupational Therapy

In the official AOTA document titled *Scholarship in Occupational Therapy* (AOTA, 2009), scholarship is described to be important to the "growth, development, and vitality of the profession" and the necessity for it so that the profession can advance. The document describes "scholarly practice" as the use of "the knowledge base of the profession in one's practice" (p. 790). Scholarly practice is viewed by the AOTA as *evidence-based practice* that is delivered by "reflective practitioners."

In contrast, the official document describes *scholarship* akin to research, in which the emphasis is more on an investigation that is made more available to the public, subject to review and that adds to the field. Scholarship builds on what has been published before and allows the profession to advance. The belief of the AOTA is that participating in scholarship and scholarly activities is a professional responsibility, similar to the professional responsibility referred to in the introduction regarding the need to belong to our professional associations.

The *Official Document* describes the work of Boyer's definitions of the various types of scholarship (1990): the scholarship of discovery, the scholarship of integration, the scholarship of application, and the scholarship of teaching and learning. Boyer presented these categories in 1990 in *Scholarship Reconsidered: Priorities for the Professoriate.* His descriptions of the following classifications were not hierarchical.

SCHOLARSHIP OF DISCOVERY

This type of scholarship is work in an activity that leads to the development of "knowledge for its own sake" (Boyer, 1990, p. 17). The scholarship of discovery consists of primary, original research, the purpose of which is to expand the base of knowledge of a specific discipline. This is the type of scholarship that is most often completed by faculty members who are engaged in research. The AOTA recognizes the need for this type of scholarship in terms of understanding human occupation and how the participation in meaningful occupations can maintain the physical and mental health of our citizens. This is

the "science driven" phrase that is a salient feature of the *Centennial Vision.*

SCHOLARSHIP OF INTEGRATION

The AOTA official document uses Boyers' (1990) definition of this type of scholarship as "...making creative connections both within and across disciplines to integrate, synthesize, interpret and create new perspectives and theories." The difference between this and the scholarship of discovery is that this type of scholarship poses different research questions. It examines original research findings within a specific discipline and then looks to integrate them in a more interdisciplinary way. Boyer refers to finding the information that "...lies in the intersections of disciplinary boundaries," which leads to the formation of new knowledge. In the field of occupational therapy, this type of research would facilitate an improved understanding of how we can meet societal needs. This focus then brings us full circle to the goals of the *Centennial Vision.*

SCHOLARSHIP OF APPLICATION

In this type of scholarship, practitioners can *apply* the knowledge gained by the two previously discussed types: scholarship of discovery and scholarship of integration. The scholar then *applies* how the knowledge gained can be put to practical use at all levels of society. The AOTA *Official Document on Scholarship in Occupational Therapy* gives several examples of this type of scholarship. One example given is "the value of occupations as a health determinant to address health disparities of populations" (AOTA, 2009, p. 791). Some authors (as identified by the AOTA document) use the term *scholarship of practice* (Braveman, Helfrich, & Fisher, 2001). This type of scholarship focuses on occupational therapy intervention. One final type of *scholarship of application* has been identified in the AOTA document as the *scholarship of engagement* (Boyer, 1996). In this type of scholarship, multiple stakeholders (within and without the occupational therapy professional community) produce scholarly works with persons and organizations.

SCHOLARSHIP OF TEACHING AND LEARNING

This type of scholarship has more of a research frame of reference, with the systematic study of teaching and learning. Because of the nature of the subject, it is more prone to public sharing via either publications or presentations (AOTA, 2009). Because it tends to be more open to the public than the other types of scholarship, it is open to outside comment and "critical review."

Scholarly Writing and Publication

Occupational therapy practitioners must understand not only the importance of scholarly writing but also the "how to's" of successful writing and all of the component parts: from the inception of the idea to the literature review to the writing and finally to the submission for peer review and optimally, acceptance for publication! Many skilled clinicians have anxieties about writing. Some of the areas of concern of novice authors are regarding whether they chose a topic that has enough information; that they have done adequate research; and finally, whether or not they are competent in writing at such a professional level.

WHAT CONSTITUTES "SCHOLARLY WRITING?"

Aitchison and Lee (2006) posited that the purpose of scholarly writing is to "...create knowledge rather than [to write]...merely as knowledge-recording" (p. 270). Their view is echoed by others throughout the literature (Lavelle & Bushrow, 2007) in which writing skills combine with oral skills. Dallimore, Hertenstein, and Platt (2008) coined the phrase *communication competence*, which describes both the written word and the ability to present the ideas after a manuscript or article is written.

TYPES OF ARTICLES

The American Psychological Association (APA) classifies written works for the behavioral and social sciences according to the study of the subject and content of the manuscript. The *Publication Manual of the American Psychological Association* (2010) is the primary source for the health sciences style of source citation and works cited. Readers will see and hear this described as "APA format." The APA manual describes journal articles as "...reports of empirical studies, literature reviews, theoretical articles, methodological articles or case studies" (p. 10).

The following is a description of each category as per the manual.

Empirical Studies

Empirical studies are always articles that are primary resources, which means that these articles describe original research that is written by researchers. Articles regarding empirical studies follow a typical format in which there is an introduction section followed by a method section, a results section, and finally a discussion section. The methods section must be written so that any scholar or scientist would be able to reproduce the study using the same research design and sequence. The discussion section includes the author's summary of the results, any limitations of the study, and questions for further research study.

Literature Reviews

Literature reviews are considered to be a secondary source. This category of scholarly writing analyzes previously published works that have been written by researchers and scholars. Textbooks, such as this, are secondary sources that use literature reviews to draw upon the knowledge base in a discipline. The APA (2010) further defines this category of scholarly writing as being "research synthesis and meta-analyses" (p. 10). In this type of writing, the author searches for previously published writings on a particular topic, organizes the data, and uses quantitative and substantiated data to make comparisons and conclusions about current knowledge.

Theoretical Articles

Theoretical articles are those in which the author uses existing literature to propose new hypotheses to advance existing theories. In a theoretical article, the author examines both the "...internal consistency and external validity" (APA, 2010, p. 10) and forms a judgment as to whether the previous theoretical frameworks are sound. Study limitations or research design flaws are considered as the author suggests new or revised theories for study.

Methodological Articles

Methodological articles introduce new approaches to existing research designs. The focus of methodological articles is on the examination of empirical data and how current methods might be altered for a different research protocol. The intent of methodological articles is to be "user friendly" to readers within the body of the article. More complex information may be included in tables and appendices at the end of the article for more experienced readers to use as a reference.

Case Studies

Case studies are articles that describe reports of information obtained while the researcher rendered care or services to "...an individual, a group, a community or an organization" (APA, 2010, p. 11). Case studies define a problem, discuss the interventions used to ameliorate the problem, and open the door for further study of similar cases. Confidentiality is an important consideration for authors who choose to write case study articles.

Other Types of Articles

The *Publication Manual of the American Psychological Association* (2010) lists other less frequently published types of articles, including brief reports, book reviews, letters to the editor, and monographs (p. 11). Anyone considering submission of an article must be aware of the required criteria of a journal before submitting a manuscript.

The Peer Review and Editorial Process

Scholarly articles are always reviewed by a panel of experts in the same field as the submission. This is to ensure authenticity and originality of the work as well as a determination that the article presents information or research that is significant to the field. The terms *peer-reviewed, refereed,* and *juried* are generally used interchangeably to describe this process. Scholarly journal articles are expected to be original, *primary* publications (APA, 2010). Scholarly journal articles have not been published before. In addition, it is also common expectation that an author will not submit an article to more than one journal at a time (Belcher, 2009).

In the peer-review process, an editor is responsible for overseeing the quality and content of a scholarly journal. There may also be *associate, consulting,* and *advisory editors* in addition to *ad hoc reviewers,* who might be brought on to review specialty areas. The associate editor might also assist in the communications with the authors in regard to acceptance, rejection, and edits of the manuscript that might be requested of the author. The editor has the right to reject an article before it is sent for review to others on the peer-review board. Editors may also request a "masked review" in which all identifying information of the author is removed before the review (APA, 2010; Belcher, 2009).

The amount of time it takes for a review is said by the APA (2010) to be approximately 2 to 3 months. After a manuscript has been reviewed, the author should expect an answer regarding whether the article is accepted or not. There are three answers that an author might expect: acceptance, rejection, or rejection with an invitation to revise the article and resubmit it. If an author has not been informed of any decision after a period of 3 months, it would be acceptable to contact the editor. If the author is ultimately notified that the article is not accepted at all, it is then permissible to submit it to another journal for review (Belcher, 2009).

Types of Citation Formats

There are several styles, or formats, of citation styles. Style manuals give authors explicit instructions as to how to cite in-text quotations and list references and how to incorporate tables and illustrations in a manuscript, among other requirements. Some styles are designed to identify standards for authors; others are geared more toward providing standards for editors and publishers. Although several science disciplines have developed their own styles (e.g., chemistry and physics), Lipson (2006) and Belcher (2009) list that there are three *major* citation styles. These are Chicago (sometimes referred to as *Turabian,* after the name of the originator of the system), Modern Language Association (MLA), and APA.

CHICAGO STYLE

Chicago style covers a variety of topics from manuscript preparation and publication to grammar, usage, and documentation. This is generally considered the standard for preparation of books (rather than having a focus on journal articles). It covers a wide variety of book publishing issues, ranging from the writing of the book to sections regarding the actual printing and binding of books. For further information, refer to *The Chicago Manual of Style,* 16th edition (2010).

MODERN LANGUAGE ASSOCIATION STYLE

Modern Language Association style is most commonly used to set the publication standards of manuscripts within the liberal arts and humanities. This style addresses standards for writing books and articles on literature and language. It is geared toward the preparation for authors rather than for editors. For further information, please refer to the *MLA Style Manual and Guide to Scholarly Publishing,* 16th edition (2010).

AMERICAN PSYCHOLOGICAL ASSOCIATION STYLE

American Psychological Association style is most commonly used to cite sources within the social sciences. Because of the nature of the standards, APA format is designed for use by the author more than for that of the editor. This resource centers on the preparation of scholarly journal articles with standards for in-text citations, endnotes and footnotes, and the reference page. For more information, please consult the *Publication Manual of the American Psychological Association,* 6th edition, second printing (APA, 2010).

Although most writings that are done in the field of occupational therapy require APA format, it is important for scholarly writers to be cognizant of the required journal style, especially at the point of the initial submission. Having a manuscript in the required format may even improve the chances for acceptance of a submission because it allows the publisher the ability to visualize if the work would be appropriate for acceptance.

There are also some reliable and valid online resources that can be helpful for each of the various formats. One valid and frequently updated resource is a Web page designed and maintained by Purdue University. It is called the *Online Writing Lab* (OWL) and can be found at http://owl.english.purdue.edu/owl.

ACCEPTABLE TIME FRAME FOR REFERENCES

Most editors require references to be used that are no older than 5 to 7 years; however, there can be exceptions. If one of the sentinel works on a particular topic is greater than 7 years old and describes a foundational theory for a particular topic, older references may be appropriate.

Occupational Therapy and Scholarly Writing

Occupational therapy practitioners have several venues for submission of peer-reviewed publications. The *American Journal of Occupational Therapy (AJOT)* is the "...official peer-reviewed journal of the American Occupational Therapy Association" (AOTA, 2012, p. S104). This journal is published in hard copy and in an online format. The author's responsibilities, types of articles, format, and requirement for APA reference style are listed in *The Guidelines for Contributors to AJOT*, which was published as a supplement to volume 66 of the journal in 2012 (AOTA, 2012).

This guideline document is especially helpful to novice writers who have not had the experience of submitting manuscripts for review. In addition to providing the specific responsibilities required of all authors, the article lists the various types of articles that will be reviewed by the peer review board.

TYPES OF ARTICLES ACCEPTED BY THE *AMERICAN JOURNAL OF OCCUPATIONAL THERAPY*

Several types of articles will be accepted for review, including feature-length articles on original research (25 pages or a maximum of 5,000 words), critical reviews (related to works on occupational therapy), brief reports (15 pages or a maximum of 3,000 words) that addresses a pilot program or a research need, and case reports (20 pages maximum or 4,000 words) that address a short report of original work on a "case example of a clinical situation."

One interesting possibility for an *AJOT* submission is called *"The Issue Is."* These articles address current issues in the field that are being debated in the literature. These submissions have an 18-page or 3,500-word maximum.

Letters to the editor are published only in the online version of the journal. These are the only submissions to AJOT that are not peer reviewed for the journal.

MANUSCRIPT PREPARATION

There is an entire section devoted to the requirements for manuscript preparation, including a requirement that authors submit a *masked* (AOTA, 2012) version of the manuscript to ensure that there is no identifying information. This is called a *blind review*, in which the reviewers do not know the source of the submission. In addition, requirements for the title page and the inclusion of an abstract and key words are described. The author is instructed on how to list practice implications and an acknowledgement page and to use the 6th edition of the *Publication Manual of the American Psychological Association* (APA, 2010) for referencing.

Information regarding the inclusion of figures, illustrations, tables, statistics, tests and assessment tool, abbreviations, permissions is also specifically defined in the author instructions.

The process of how the manuscript is reviewed is described in detail, as well as the fact that after a manuscript is accepted, authors must give AOTA copyright ownership of the publication: "Manuscripts published in the journal are copyrighted by AOTA and may not be published elsewhere without permission" (AOTA, 2012).

Last, there is a reference for the author to complete an online registration at http://ajot.submiy2aota.org. This registration includes a checklist so the authors ensure compliance with all of the requirements of a submission.

ADDITIONAL WRITING OPPORTUNITIES FOR THE AMERICAN OCCUPATIONAL THERAPY ASSOCIATION

The AOTA has a program called *The Evidence Exchange for Critically Appraised Papers* (Arbesman, Lieberman, & Bondoc, 2012). This program is a storehouse for evidence-based practice articles that are judged for their scientific validity and value to the profession. Articles that are accepted for this program are generally submitted from articles classified as "CATS," which stands for "critically approved topics," through the AOTA. These topics are divided into practice areas that address evidence-based studies and are then posted in the Evidence-Based Practice and Research section of the AOTA's Web site. Criteria for this submission process are included on the AOTA's Web site. The criteria include the following:

- The article or study describes an intervention within the scope of occupational therapy practice.
- The article was published in a peer reviewed journal.
- The article has Level I, II, or III evidence.
- The article was published within the past 10 years of date of CAP submission
- Study was published more than 10 years from date of CAP submission but is considered "classic or seminal" (e.g., influential impact on the field, frequently cited, etc.)
- The CAP does not duplicate an article currently included in the *AOTA Evidence Exchange*.

Finally, the purpose of this program is to support the *Centennial Vision* by giving practitioners the opportunity to participate in a science and evidence-based practice.

Competency in Scholarly Writing

There have been few studies in the literature regarding the perceptions of graduate students and what they have found useful in programs that have *taught* them how to write scholarly papers (Fallahi, Wood, & Austad, 2006). The little that is documented in the literature discusses the fact that writing skills, in general, are usually taught in undergraduate level composition courses. The level of writing required for scholarly works is certainly beyond what would be acceptable for these lower level courses. Fallahi et al. (2006) discussed the "...dearth of evidence-based methods of writing instruction for undergraduate psychology students" as meeting an unmet need in most curricula.

Reasons to Write a Scholarly Paper

The task before us is to ascertain how to gain the skills necessary to write in a scholarly manner. Skills for this are not usually taught to occupational therapy practitioners in the same manner as our skills for client assessment and treatment. Tonette and Hatcher (2011) describe scholarly writing as ". . a difficult undertaking, and a challenge that produces growth and satisfaction—all at the same time." The authors discuss the fact that getting started with a piece of writing is a daunting task—one that can take hours, days, or sometimes months of work just to get started!

People choose to write for different reasons, both personal and professional. Academics (especially those in new faculty positions) write to keep their positions, earn promotions in rank, and increase their visibility or prestige within a university or discipline. Some universities and colleges offer merit raises based on a faculty member's productivity in being published. Undertaking scholarly writing with the idea of immediate profit is not supported in the literature (Tonette & Hatcher, 2011). Profit is rather a long-term effect in that a show of advanced knowledge, prominence, and prestige in a field can open the doors to better professional opportunities. In the case of academia, publications in specialty areas can lead to invitations for presentations at conferences that can pay handsomely, as well as provide the opportunity for reimbursement for all expenses and the added benefit of travel to places that one might not otherwise ever visit.

Tonette and Hatcher (2011) present an excellent example of how students can get involved in the area of scholarly writing. Two graduate students in a Master in Health Education program decided that they wanted to submit a paper for acceptance at a local conference. Their professor was very experienced in both doing professional presentations and submitting juried scholarly articles. The students worked hard at many rewrites and incorporated the revisions that were suggested by their skilled professor. They were accepted to present their paper at the conference, and then based on feedback from discussions at the conference; they revised their manuscript and submitted it to a peer-reviewed journal. Not only was the paper accepted for publication, but the article won an award for the best student paper!

Having won the award for the best article, the students had many exciting doors open to them. They were both offered positions at an institute that provided continuing education courses on weekends all throughout the United States. So in addition to gaining a lucrative side job (the salary was not quoted, but speaking engagements such as this can pay from $1,000 to $2,000 per day), they traveled the country with all expenses paid! One of them eventually successfully competed for a position as a keynote speaker and was awarded an all-expenses-paid trip to a health conference in South Africa.

Although this is an extreme example, it illustrates what can happen when someone becomes adept and competent with scholarly writing and presentations. The need to determine why a person is doing the scholarly writing can greatly help with the motivation and perseverance it takes to do it. Some scholars write to so they can secure or advance in faculty positions, but most engage in the activity of writing to "...clarify ideas, explore areas, and contribute to [their] profession" (Tonette & Hatcher, 2011, p. 4). This relates back to the section in this chapter that addressed the AOTA's official document on the various types of scholarship.

It is apparent throughout the literature that there are many reasons to write. For most authors, financial reward is the least of all motivators. Most scholars write so they are a part of the professional conversation. The motivation for others may be the sense of power, self-satisfaction, or the pure sense of happiness in seeing their name in print when the work is accepted and published.

How Does One Create Writing Opportunities?

Establishing a network of colleagues is one of the best ways to begin the journey of scholarly writing. Reading the work of good writers and reflecting on *what* makes it good can help. Attending lectures and seminars given by writers can assist in honing the craft of writing.

Networking at conferences is an excellent way to meet new colleagues and share what your skills are and what you would be interested in writing about. Some reflection is required in that you need to determine if you would feel more comfortable writing alone or in a group. Certainly, if you are involved in any group research projects, a joint effort is best for publications that are submitted for peer review. You also need to verbalize and let others know that you are interested in this endeavor. It is important to solidify connections and be sure to follow through on any opportunities that might present themselves. In the case of students, it is important to be proactive in setting up and attending meetings. Attend the meeting with an agenda and take notes, being especially careful to pay attention to the process required and the deadlines to be met (Tonette & Hatcher, 2011). Notes taken in an "action item" format with dates can help keep you on track.

Other opportunities that can arise are the *call for papers* that are published in professional and trade journals requesting writings for conferences, journals, and books.

The AOTA sends out a call for papers for the annual conference each year. Criteria for submission are listed, as well as the need for an abstract to describe the work. Careful detail must be paid to the deadlines. Most conference submissions are now done online via the use of computerized systems. These systems ensure anonymity on the part of the submitter for when the application is reviewed.

The Importance of Correct Citation in Scholarly Writing

Scholarly writing is a challenge to all who attempt it. Not only must the author present information that is based on fact, but the author must also write with the integrity necessary to cite the sources of information and then do so correctly. Sutherland-Smith discussed "...what it means to be an author—and the rights attached to authorship" (2008, p. 3). She further posited that one of the difficulties in original writing and the avoidance of plagiarism is that individuals view it differently (especially in the world of higher education). Proper citations lead to full disclosure of one's sources of information; therefore, the occurrence of plagiarism (whether intended or accidental) can be lessened.

Lipson (2006) outlines three reasons to cite materials used as (1) to give credit to the work of others, (2) to inform the reader as to the source of the material on which you have based your ideas, and (3) to direct the audience on how to find the information so they can either verify a written work or complete further investigations on a topic. Therefore, when an author uses correct citations, this accomplishes several things. It gives the author credit for his or her work, legitimizes the ideas presented by outlining what is current in the literature, and gives the cited authors credit for their original work.

Definition of Plagiarism

Many authors discuss the various intricacies of the meaning of the word *plagiarism* (Dee & Jacob, 2010; Lipson, 2006; Sutherland-Smith, 2008) all comment on the fact that plagiarism is a complex issue, the base of which is fraud. The following is the definition of plagiarism from *Webster's Online Dictionary*: "The act of using another person's words or ideas without giving credit to that person: the act of plagiarizing something" (*Merriam-Webster Online Dictionary*, 2013).

Dee and Jacob (2010) completed a study of more than 1,200 undergraduate student papers. In the experiment, half of the students completed an antiplagiarism tutorial before submitting their papers. The results of the study showed that the rate of plagiarism decreased substantially, and a follow-up study led the authors to theorize that incidents of plagiarism are a student "behavior" that can be changed by increasing knowledge of the act of plagiarism. The authors posited that the act of plagiarism is indicative not just of poor academic integrity, but in more of the cases, a lack of understanding on the part of the student regarding what constitutes plagiarism. Students were less likely to plagiarize because they had a better understanding of what plagiarism is and how it can be avoided.

Plagiarism in Today's World

In a world in which we have unlimited access to sources because of electronic databases and the Internet, novice writers may not understand the importance of avoiding noncitation of sources that are "out there" on the Internet. According to Baehr and Schaller (2010), having the information at our fingertips may be easier than when authors had to physically go to a library, look in card catalogs, and retrieve their sources. With this convenience comes the onus of "mastering many skills...even within the last decade due to shifts in technology, expectations of the [reader] and content" (p. 3). Online searching and use of key words can bring up many results. Many authors do not read entire articles because of the volume of search results. If one is not extremely conscientious about tracking this flood of information, unintended plagiarism might occur.

Tips for Avoiding Plagiarism

Antiplagiarism programs, such as Turn It In (http://turnitin.com) can be useful tools that are used primarily by institutions of higher education to evaluate whether written information is original or if it has been plagiarized. Programs such as these can be used not just by academics who are grading papers but also by students or writers who wish to employ online plagiarism and grammar checks. Turn It In also offers online tutoring. All of these services are fee based, according to which portion of the program is selected.

Free online resources that are valid, regularly updated, and reliable can be helpful to writers. Two of these are Thesaurus.com (http://thesaurus.com), which enables writers to search for synonyms, antonyms, and definitions, and OWL (http://owl.english.purdue.edu), an excellent educational Web site that offers more than 200 free resources, including information on academic writing and source citations in APA, MLA, and Chicago citation formats.

Professional Presentation of Scholarly Works

An essential part of the scholarly process is the presentation of the work at professional conferences and other venues so an author can share his or her work with others. Conference proposals may be identified as a call for papers, which is posted in both scholarly and trade journals. There may or may not be a required theme for proposals.

INITIATING THE PROCESS FOR PRESENTATION

The first thing to consider when you see a "call for papers" is to read the requirements, criteria, and deadline for submission. If possible, it is advantageous to submit it before the deadline. Late submissions may make a poor initial impression on the reviewers because it may suggest to them poor planning or time management skills. Most proposals require an abstract of between 250 to 300 words, and these are submitted online with a character limit for each section. It is imperative that the writing be concise and makes an impression on those who will be reviewing the submission. Key words should have high impact and relate directly to the topic being proposed.

IMPORTANT CONSIDERATIONS FOR PROPOSAL WRITING

The initial item to be considered is who the future audience will be. This will help determine the level of information and how detailed the proposal and eventually the presentation will be. Questions such as whether the presentation will be for all occupational therapy practitioners or for the general public must be considered.

Smith and Gutman (2011) addressed the issue of health literacy as the ability of people to understand the terms connected with health care. This factor must be taken into account if a presentation is delivered to an audience of various types of stakeholders who are not cognizant of scientific or medical terminology. Presentation proposals for large groups require the author to speak in such a way that everyone in the audience will understand and benefit from the information presented.

Quotations should be used judiciously and only to emphasize an idea. It is important that the text in the proposal conveys the meaning of the author's intent and does not overuse of quotations from others. If a writer is comparing studies or the work of others, clarity is required that connotes original ideas for the proposal.

Types of Papers

There are several types of presentations, including paper presentations, panel presentations, roundtables, and poster presentations.

PAPER PRESENTATIONS

Paper presentations are usually read aloud at a conference; most times, the presenter uses audiovisual equipment to illustrate the points. PowerPoint presentations, graphs, tables, and other pictorial images are used to demonstrate the salient points of the presentation. The depth and breadth of the presentation depend on the audience. Some audiences are well versed in research and interested in the design of a study. Other audiences may be less educated in the topic and might be attending the presentation for more useful and practical information. The speaker will be aware of the level of the audience because of the process of the proposal and from which professional body the call for papers originated.

PANEL PRESENTATIONS

Panel presentations usually consist of three to four participants. Formats vary regarding how the information is presented. Most panels are designed so that each member gives a 15- to 20-minute presentation, which may or may not use PowerPoint or other audiovisual aids. The leader of the panel will generally decide if questions should immediately follow each presentation or if there will be time incorporated into the presentation for questions and answers at the end. It is always best practice (both for the speaker and the audience) to announce at the beginning of the presentation how questions will be handled.

ROUNDTABLES

Roundtable presentations average five to six speakers. Each speaker is generally allowed 5 to 10 minutes to discuss his or her topic. This format can be slightly less formal than a panel discussion, and the topic is generally a timely issue that is shared by the participants. Written materials may be distributed before the discussion to have more targeted questions posed by the attendees.

POSTER PRESENTATIONS

Poster presentations are those in which the presenter prepares a visual display about his or her research or topic. It is a medium that lends itself well to graphs, tables, artwork, and photographic images. Generally, the author of the poster is present at a specified time and is able to converse with attendees in this most informal style of presentation. Materials used for the poster can range from inexpensive cardboard displays to professionally produced laminated posters. The laminated posters offer the most professional-looking results; however, they can be costly. Printing services such as FedEx (Fedex.com, 2013) or others will charge according to the size of the poster. Poster sizes may be regulated by the organization that is hosting a conference. This might be related to how much space there is for presentation. For example, printing charges for a 24" x 36" poster may cost more than $100 (depending on the printing options chosen and shipping and handling costs, with additional fees charged if it is requested to be a "rush"). This information may be found at FedEx's Web site (http://www.fedex.com/us/office/marketing/signsbanners/posters/packages.html).

General Information About Proposals

Most professional proposals are submitted online and are completed as "blind reviews," in which the reviewers do not know who has submitted the proposal. In the case of the AOTA, an online system such as the *OASIS—the Online Abstract Submission and Invitation System* is used in which the proposer submits his or her ideas for the paper, including an abstract and learning objectives. Several months later, the proposer receives an email response that will indicate whether the paper has been accepted or not. At that time, the proposer is made aware of the final score that is assigned by the reviewers (AOTA, 2013).

TIPS FOR SUCCESSFUL PRESENTATION SUBMISSIONS

Proposals should reflect the author's interest and enthusiasm for the subject. They should be thoughtfully written, as well as concise and clear. Learning objectives should be written that complete the phrase: "By the end of this presentation, the participant will be able to..." and should end with an action verb such as "explain" or "describe."

Topics that are too broad most likely will lessen the chance of acceptance. Researchers should be sure to do adequate research on the topic in advance so they are aware of the types of topics that are timely and have not been presented before. Rating and acceptance of submissions are usually done by experienced scholars and professionals in the field, so the author should be sure to design a proposal that has originality and the potential to explore a topic that has the potential to advance the profession.

For some proposals, the reviewers might be looking for a "theme." If this is the case, that will be outlined in the call for papers. If a theme is part of the criteria for acceptance for a particular conference, be sure that your topic is clearly aligned with the theme and that your explanation illustrates that linkage.

Above all, be sure that your proposal is well written, clear, and free of any grammatical or spelling errors. Proofread, proofread, and proofread again! It is also helpful to have someone else (a colleague within the field) proofread for you. *You* may know what you mean by a particular section of your proposal, but it might not be as clear as you think. Be willing to take constructive criticism and put your ego aside if you ask the opinion of others; just make sure you ask persons whose opinion you can trust.

SUBMITTING A CONFERENCE PROPOSAL

The method in which you submit a conference proposal will vary according to the method used by the reviewing body. Some are submitted via email, and others are submitted via online systems, such as the aforementioned OASIS system. In any event, be sure to follow the requirements of the proposal and make sure your credentials (and those of any co-presenters) are properly written. If the proposal is to be sent via email in an attachment, be sure to send it as a Word document because this format can be accessed by the majority of computers. Use of double spacing and a clear font (usually Times New Roman) is the preferred style. The document should be saved as a Portable Document Format (pdf) file because these files cannot be edited and are accessible by most computer operating systems.

If an electronic system is used, be aware of the character space limits, especially in the box that is usually included for the abstract. Be sure to make the best use of your limited characters in your writing so your proposal topic is clear to the reviewers. With these type of systems, you may be able to go in and out of the system at various times while you craft your proposal. You will most be issued a log in and password that you will need to access and edit your entry, so be sure to keep track of this information. The password and log in will most likely be auto generated by the system, so they may not be characters that are easy to remember. Either write them down or send them to yourself in an email so you can access your information more easily for later retrieval.

Presenting the Conference Paper

Congratulations if your paper is accepted! Now you are on to the next steps, which are even more daunting than the proposal. Koegel (2007) discusses the fact of being organized from the first notification of your acceptance. He uses the acronym of: OPEN UP as representing "...the six characteristics shared by exceptional presenters."

1. O: Be organized. Koegel believes that the message should be delivered in a structured flow, one that the audience can easily follow.

2. P: Be passionate. Exceptional presenters "exude enthusiasm and conviction." Convey a positive energy not just about the topic but also about the fact that you appreciate your audience.

3. E: Be engaging. Build rapport with the audience quickly and engage them immediately. An introduction or short personal anecdote informs your audience who you are, how you are qualified, and why they should listen to you!

4. N: Be natural. Exceptional presenters convey a conversational feel as they deliver their presentations. They also appear comfortable with their audience, and this comfort level in turn makes the audience more confident.

5. U: Understand your audience. Taking a poll of the audience (by a show of hands to various questions) can help you understand your audience. For example, in occupational therapy, it would be helpful to know how many participants in the audience are occupational therapists and how many are occupational therapy assistants.

6. P: Practice. Practice not only improves your delivery of a presentation, but it can also greatly lessen the "stage fright" that many are faced with just before stepping up to the podium. Some presenters memorize the opening and closing remarks so they maintain eye contact with the audience during these two crucial points of the presentation. In addition, if you are doing your presentation in a hotel or other type of conference room, it is important to visit the room the night before your presentation (if possible) so you can visualize how you will use the room. The day of the presentation, always arrive 1 hour early. Many professional conferences have "speaker's lounges" or other types of resources available if there are issues with any computer or audiovisual equipment. Arriving 1 hour early gives you the opportunity to make sure you are ready as your audience starts to arrive.

It is important to begin your presentation on time. It is not fair to force those in the audience who have arrived on time to wait for you to begin because some attendees come in late.

Last, if one is not provided for you by the persons who are sponsoring the conference, have an evaluation form ready for participants to complete after your presentation as they leave the room. Feedback can be a valuable tool for you the next time you do a presentation. Evaluations should contain comments on the content, delivery, currency of the topic, and general logistics (e.g., was the room temperature comfortable?).

SOME COMMENTS ABOUT THE USE OF POWERPOINT

PowerPoint can be a very useful tool when you are giving a presentation, but it should be considered just that—a tool! PowerPoint is an aid to a presentation; it should never *be* the presentation. The exterior content (what you say to the audience) should be different than the interior content of your slides. The notes function at the bottom of the slides (which are seen by the presenter and not by the audience) can be helpful in ensuring that you just do not read off the slides. Even the best PowerPoint presentation cannot take the place of your voice and eye contact with your audience!

As with any audiovisual tool, PowerPoint requires planning in order to be effective. Items to consider are your audience, the subject, and the type of presentation you are doing. For example, if you are doing a panel presentation, the group might decide to use the same slide design for better consistency and a better final product for the audience. Quality PowerPoint presentations are suitable for your audience, the subject, and the type of presentation. Strong opening slides should be crafted to engage the audience immediately at the beginning of the presentation. The opening slide should have the name of the presentation, the author, the date, and the name of the conference or event. The second slide should consist of an outline that serves as the table of contents, and this same slide may be used at the end of the presentation for review. Learning objectives of the presentation are generally the third and fourth slides. Logos are appropriate to use in footers and help to emphasize the speaker's professional affiliation.

As the presenter designs the content slides, there must be awareness that they are appropriate for the subject and the audience. For example, if you are presenting the findings of a research study that has slides with bar graphs and data tables, animated slides with figures flying in would be distracting. They might even be annoying to some in the audience and certainly would not add anything to your presentation. In this case, clear slides without any animation or long transitions would be most appropriate. If, on the other hand, you are doing a public relations piece that explains what occupational therapy is to a community group, then that would be the appropriate place for some fun graphics and animation.

Robinson (2003) made an excellent statement about the use of a laser pointer for reinforcement, which he expressed is most useful when you are illustrating figures and images but not as effective for text. He discussed several points worth thinking about in terms of the use of a laser pointer: (1) be aware of the length of time you leave the pointer on the slide (not too long; just use it for emphasis), (2) be aware of movement while you have the pointer in your hand so that you do not "fire" at the audience, and (3) be aware of keeping your hand steady when you hold the pointer. For the last point, Robinson suggested to hold the laser pointer at the edge of the lectern as you point with it which will help to steady your hand, and the laser will not move all around.

SPECIFICS REGARDING SLIDE DESIGN IN POWERPOINT: FONTS AND BACKGROUNDS

Fonts used for presentations should be clear and the size large enough that the audience can read. Use of "san serif" fonts is almost always the most appropriate. OWL defines a sans serif (or nonserif) font as one that has no "feet" (although both the OWL and others cannot claim the exact derivation of this term). This information can be found at the OWL's Web site at http://owl.english.purdue.edu/owl/resource/705/02. In essence, it means that the font style is more of a plain block style that does not have any additional "flair." The best examples of sans serif fonts are Calibri and Arial; this is why they are used most often in published works.

Most title slides are best written in a font size of 44, and subtitles are most suitable in a range from 28 to 34. It is distracting to the audience if different font styles are used. Lettering in bold or in italics is generally the preferred way to emphasize points. Bullets, if used, should be consistent. Do not mix alphabetical bullets with numerical bullets; use one or the other. Generally, numbers can be confusing unless you are trying to demonstrate a hierarchical relationship within a list. For example, if the slide is meant to show the prevalence of different types of diseases within a population, it would be appropriate to label the diagnosis that occurs the most with the value 1 and then list the remaining diagnoses with the appropriate sequential numbers.

In terms of the slide's background design, use of contrast allows for greater visibility. The suggestion is to use a light-colored lettering on a dark background or dark lettering on a light background. Keep in mind that to some in the audience, a white screen may cause glare. Colors often appear lighter when projected, and pastel colors may even appear to be white, depending on the projector. Always look at your slide design with a critical eye and imagine how you would react to it if you were in the audience. For example, use of red lettering on a

dark blue background can give the optical illusion of the words "dancing" on the page, and this cannot only be an annoyance to the audience but can also detract from the message on the slide. Finally, consistency in the design of the entire presentation creates a more professional appearance. The bottom line is that you want the audience to focus on your presentation, not on your background effects.

One common mistake made in PowerPoint slides is when presenters put too much text on one slide. An excess in text on a slide makes it difficult to read, especially if the presentation is being given in a large room that only has one screen. The goal of a PowerPoint presentation is to have the slides as a reference; the design should allow the audience to attend to what the presenter is saying; not to struggle to see what is up on the screen. Source citations should be included on the slide with the cited information, so be sure to leave room for the entire appropriate citation.

At the conclusion of your presentation, it is helpful to have a slide that says "thank you" or "Questions and Answers." This is a professional way of closing your presentation and letting your audience know that you are finished. Have you ever attended a presentation and the speaker stands there at the end and says something like, "Well, that's it!"? Don't you find that to be an awkward way to end a presentation? It almost makes it seem as though the end of the presentation was not planned at all. It does not leave the audience with a good impression. Conducting a question and answer period followed by a thank you to the audience is the most professional way to complete a presentation.

Be sure to be aware of what you are proficient at with the use of PowerPoint and keep the tips listed in this chapter in mind as you prepare your slides. Koegel (2007) reminds speakers to minimize eye contact with *objects* in the room (i.e., the screen) and maximize eye contact with the *people* in order to ensure an effective presentation. Always face forward to your audience; never turn your back while you glance at your slides for reference. To secure the audience's attention, leave time between slides and maintain eye contact with your audience. By following these tips and by practicing and knowing what is on your slides, you can deliver an effective PowerPoint presentation that will hold the attention of the audience from your first word to the final question!

Summary

This chapter has provided an overview of the definitions and importance of scholarly writing to the growth of the field of occupational therapy and to those who are fortunate enough to practice in this profession! The competence needed for the completion of scholarly writing was explored with an emphasis on the types of

Evidence-Based Research Chart

Topic	Evidence
Occupational therapy scholarship	AOTA, 2009, 2012
Scholarly writing	AOTA, 2009; Rocco & Hatcher, 2011
APA format for source citation	APA, 2010; Lipson, 2006
Plagiarism	Beins, 2012; Harris, 2005; Sutherland-Smith, 2008
Professional presentation	Koegel, 2007

scholarship available to occupational therapy practitioners. Discussion of the AOTA's *Centennial Vision* further illustrated why scholarly writing and the ultimate presentation of the work at conferences will advance the profession of occupational therapy for future generations of practitioners. Occupational therapy practitioners are charged with the responsibility of attaining the goals that were delineated by the leaders in the profession on the occasion of the 100th year of the profession. Occupational therapy scholarly writers must strive to be recognized as individuals who base their writings in sound, evidence-based science and who are competent in assisting the advancement of the profession into the next centennial.

Student Self-Assessment

1. What does "scholarship" consist of in the field of occupational therapy?

2. Identify the components that must be included in order to complete an article that will be submitted for a peer-reviewed journal.

3. How did this chapter help you to understand the definition of plagiarism? Can you explain how the appropriate use of citations lessens the chance of unintended plagiarism?

4. You have been given an assignment to do a 15-minute presentation on osteoarthritis. The professor requires that you include evidence-based data and that you create a PowerPoint presentation that will be given in class. What steps would take to plan this project? How would you design your PowerPoint slides?

Acknowledgments

I would like to thank Karen Jacobs, EdD, OTR/L, CPE, FAOTA, and Nancy MacRae, MS, OTR/L, FAOTA, for their guidance and support in the writing of this chapter.

Electronic Resources

- American Occupational Therapy Association: http://www.aota.org
- American Psychological Association: http://apastyle.org
- The Purdue Online Writing Lab: http://owl.english.purdue.edu
- Merriam-Webster Online Dictionary and Thesaurus: http://www.merriam-webster.com

References

Aitchison, C., & Lee, A. (2006). Research writing: Problems and pedagogies. *Teaching in Higher Education, 11,* 265-278.

American Occupational Therapy Association. (2007). AOTA's centennial vision and executive summary. *American Journal of Occupational Therapy, 61,* 613-614.

American Occupational Therapy Association. (2009). Scholarship in occupational therapy. *American Journal of Occupational Therapy, 63,* 790-796.

American Occupational Therapy Association. (2012). Guidelines for contributors to AJOT. *American Journal of Occupational Therapy, 6*(Suppl.), S104-S107.

American Occupational Therapy Association. (2013). Retrieved January 15, 2013, from http://www.aota.org

American Psychological Association. (2010). *Publication manual of the American Psychological Association.* Washington, DC: Author.

Arbesman, M., Leiberman, D., & Bondoc, S. (2012). Evidence exchange: Writing a critically appraised paper. *OT Practice, December 17,* 8.

Baehr, C., & Schaller, B. (2010). *Writing for the internet: A guide to real communication in virtual space.* Santa Barbara, CA: Greenwood Press

Barker, D. (2004). The scholarship of engagement: A taxonomy of five emerging practices. *Journal of Higher Education Outreach and Engagement, 9,* 123-127. Beins (2012).

Beins, B. C., (2012) *APA style simplified.* Hoboken: John Wiley & Sons. Retrieved from http://mercycollege.eblib.com/patron/FullRecord/aspx?p=822040

Belcher, W. L. (2009). *Writing your journal article in 12 weeks: A guide to academic publishing success.* Thousand Oaks, CA: Sage Publications.

Boyer, E. L. (1990). *Scholarship reconsidered: Priorities of the professoriate.* San Francisco, CA: Jossey-Bass.

Boyer, E. L. (1996). The scholarship of engagement. *Journal of Public Service and Outreach, 1,* 11-20.

Braveman, B. (2006). *Leading & managing occupational therapy services: An evidence-based approach.* Philadelphia, PA: F.A. Davis Company.

Braveman, B. H., Helfrich, C. A., & Fisher, G. S. (2001). Developing and maintaining community partnerships within "A scholarship of practice." *Occupational Therapy in Health Care, 15,* 109-125.

Dallimore, E. J., Hertenstein, J. H., & Platt, M. B. (2008). Using discussion pedagogy to enhance oral and written communication skills. *College Teaching, 56,* 163-172.

Dee, T. S., & Jacob, B. A. (2010). *Rational ignorance in education: A field experiment in student plagiarism,* National Bureau of Economic Research, working paper 15672. Retrieved from http://www.nber.org/papers/w15672

Fallahi, C. R., Wood, R. M., Austad, C. S., & Fallahi, H. (2006). A program for improving undergraduate psychology students' basic writing skills. *Teaching of Psychology, 33*(3), 171-175.

FedEx. (2013). Retrieved January 28, 2013, from http://www.fedex.com/us.

Harris (2005). *Using sources effectively: Strengthening your writing and avoiding plagiarism (2nd ed.).* Glendale, CA: Pyrczak Pub.

Koegel, T. J. (2007). *The exceptional presenter: A proven formula to open up and own the room.* Austin, TX: Greenleaf Book Group Press.

Lavelle, E., & Bushrow, K. (2007). Writing approaches of graduate students. *Educational Psychology, 27,* 807-822.

Lipson, C. (2006). *Cite right: A quick guide to citation styles—MLA, APA, Chicago, the sciences, professions, and more.* Chicago, IL: University of Chicago Press.

Merriam-Webster Online Dictionary. (2013). Retrieved February 1, 2013, from http://www.merriam-webster.com.

Purdue University. (2012). *Purdue online writing lab: OWL.* Retrieved from http://owl.english.purdue.edu.

Robinson, J. P. (2003, February 2012). *Presentation 101 for graduate students: A guide to giving a quality presentation.* Message posted to http://www.cyto.purdue.edu/education.

Rocco, T. S., & Hatcher, T. (2011). *The handbook of scholarly writing and publishing.* San Francisco, CA: Jossey-Bass.

Rocco, T. S., & Hatcher, T. (2011). *The handbook of scholarly writing and publishing (1st ed.)* Hoboken, NJ: Wiley.

Smith, D. L., & Gutman, S. A. (2011). Health literacy in occupational therapy practice and research. *American Journal of Occupational Therapy, 65*(4), 367-369.

Sutherland-Smith, W. (2008). *Plagiarism, the internet and student learning.* New York: Routledge.

Thesaurus.com. (2013). Retrieved January 24, 2013, from http://thesaurus.com.

Turn It In. (2013). Retrieved January 28, 2013, 2013, from http://turnitin.com.

University of Chicago Press. (2010). *The Chicago manual of style (16th ed.).* Chicago, IL: University of Chicago Press.

IX

PROFESSIONAL ETHICS, VALUES, AND RESPONSIBILITIES

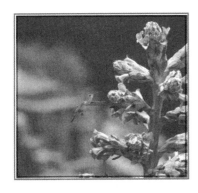

48

ETHICS AND ITS APPLICATION TO OCCUPATIONAL THERAPY PRACTICE

Gail M. Bloom, OTD, MA, OTR/L

ACOTE STANDARDS EXPLORED IN THIS CHAPTER
B.9.1, B.9.2

KEY VOCABULARY

- **Code of Ethics:** A collection of formal explicit statements forming a moral guide for an identified group outlining right and valued behavior, principles, and values.
- **Ethics:** A set of value-based principles to assist the individual in making moral decisions. Ethics examines how an individual *should* think and behave toward others.
- **Morality:** The accepted standards of right or wrong that direct the conduct of a person or a group.
- **Principles:** Basic rules of conduct.
- **Values:** Ethical principles that set a standard of quality or a worthwhile ideal.

Introduction

Occupational therapy is firmly rooted in ethical concepts and principles and has a long tradition of caring about morality-based social values. The earliest practitioners were concerned with concepts such as *autonomy* and *independence* and issues such as *meaningful* and *productive*. Occupational therapy professional values are fundamentally linked to *quality of life* (QOL) issues. Central to the practice of occupational therapy is a commitment to these ethical QOL issues. The promotion of maximum independence by enhancing functional ability and adapting the environment is basic to promoting QOL. The profession has always emphasized self-sufficiency through occupation that is meaningful to the individual.

Philosophers place an emphasis on concepts such as fairness, equality, goodness, justice, consequence, and obligation. These moral concepts provide a traditional foundation to create a practical, function-based approach

Jacobs, K., MacRae, N., & Sladyk, K. (Eds.).
*Occupational Therapy Essentials for
Clinical Competence, Second Edition* (pp. 629-645).
© 2014 SLACK Incorporated.

to ethics. This chapter begins by establishing a foundation of understanding through an examination of some basic ethical concepts. The chapter looks at societal groups and organizations for the structural hallmarks or characteristic building blocks necessary for the implementation of ethical principles. This chapter shows how everyday practice provides opportunity for the direct application of ethics.

Ethics and Its Application to Occupational Therapy Practice

In the rapidly changing health care environment, occupational therapy practitioners are confronted with complex ethical issues. As professionals, occupational therapy practitioners must take responsibility for understanding applicable policies, federal and state laws, and association principles. Occupational therapy practitioners must maintain high standards of *professional competence,* including an understanding of ethics. The moral aspects of practice require professionalism. Professional competencies include knowing how to obtain informed consent, knowing what to do if a client refuses intervention, and knowing how to communicate confidential material. Development of professional skills assists occupational therapy practitioners to make ethical decisions for moral behavior.

Occupational therapy and the study of ethics share common ground because both are concerned with *individual choice.* Both the ethical decision-making process and the clinical problem-solving approach of occupational therapy can rely on a process for function-based analysis. *Ethical reasoning* is a part of clinical decision making.

Critical thinking requires carefully weighing alternatives. Deliberate analysis is a part of solving problems. An implicit or explicit judgment guides decisions about which problems are worthy of attention. Ethical decision making is, of necessity, woven among the threads of clinical decision making. Ethical decision making is a mandatory component of clinical problem solving. Both involve the identification of the principles specific to the particular case situation, contemplation, negotiation, and reaching a resolution. The conceptual understanding of ethics is critical to decoding the complexity of specific situations. Occupational therapy practitioners should take all case-specific factors into consideration before making reasoned decisions. Daily clinical issues provide opportunity for the direct application of ethics in everyday practice. *Ethical action* is the product of ethical decision making.

An understanding of ethics can assist in sorting out complicated health and social issues.

The same ingredients can be useful for ethical problem solving in all areas of practice, including the clinical, corporate, and academic settings. Perhaps the secret recipe is seeking a balance of theoretical knowledge and practical application well seasoned with humanistic empathy and caring. An understanding of ethics helps occupational therapy practitioners know how to cope with QOL issues and quality of care problems.

A Foundation of Understanding

Essentially, ethics is a set of value-based principles to assist the individual in making moral decisions. *Ethics* examines how an individual should think and behave toward others. *Morality* is the accepted standard of right or wrong that directs the conduct of a person or group. Morality is learned early. Personal concepts of right and wrong are gathered from a variety of sources. The social environment is filled with influences that affect moral choice, including family, school, religion, and the media. A choice, or conversely, avoidance of a particular choice made as a mature adult could be influenced by moral rules learned as a child at home or in kindergarten (Fulghum, 1988): share, work cooperatively, do not cheat, treat others with respect. We learn morality by example from role models and by analogies shared through narratives (Cowley, 2005).

A basic rule of conduct is known as an ethical principle. An ethical *principle* that sets a standard of quality or a worthwhile ideal is a *value.* Most people consider certain values such as caring, honesty, and respect to be morally worthy. Tradition and custom have assigned worth to certain actions. Social norms set the expectation for certain behaviors and avoidance of other behaviors. Some social norms have been codified into law.

The practical application of knowledge is as fundamental to the study of ethics as it is to the practice of occupational therapy. There is an obligation to examine one's own personal values and belief system with recognition and insight of oneself as a moral agent. The honorable occupational therapy practitioner must have self-awareness. The process of becoming self-aware allows for an organization of one's belief system. The organization of ethical principles into an orderly system of beliefs assists the individual in making ethical decisions for determining rightness, morality, and praiseworthy behavior from wrongness, immorality, and blameworthy behavior. As an occupational therapy practitioner there is a social and legal *obligation* to consider the consequences of one's actions. A moral individual must focus on the questioning that results in making a decision to act or to not take action. Moral occupational therapy practitioners must focus on the case-specific human factors toward a process of clinical reasoning resulting in ethical decisions. An ethical decision is based on a thoughtful *judgment*, resulting in the production of action or the inhibition of action. Judgment is the act of deciding after considering alternatives. Ethics involves right and wrong conduct as determined by a reasoned thought process.

Theories of Fundamental Characteristics

Some philosophical schools of thought promote the idea that belief systems are based on basic rules. The *deontological theory of reasoning* relies on an acceptance of *universal law* or accepted truths. Proponents of these belief systems suggest that fundamental *objective principles* of morality exist. When making a decision, the fundamental principles of morality are examined for guidance to determine the best plan of action. An action is judged either "good" or "bad" because of the intrinsic nature of the action to be good or bad. There is an objective understanding of what is accepted as "good" or "bad." There is an obligation for action or inaction simply because some deeds are praiseworthy or blameworthy. Action is either right or wrong. One is obligated to a course of action that promotes goodness. There is an explicit call to duty. Awareness of moral standards is necessary in order to choose in accordance with inherent moral guides. The correct course of action can be determined by applying the appropriate obligatory rule to the situation. Rules based on universal law set *standards*. Universal imperatives include "natural order" and the Golden Rule. According to these sets of ethical rules, goodness or worth does not change with the circumstances of a specific situation.

For an example of this type of process, consider the concept of "fairness." To be "fair," all decisions must be based on a rule to treat all persons in an equitable, impartial way independent of any particular circumstances those persons might be facing. Therefore, fairness does not change with the circumstances of a specific situation. A standard of "justice" has a *duty* to be fair and equitable or it is "unjust" by definition.

Theories of Comparative Characteristics

Some philosophical schools of thought do not promote the idea that belief systems should be based on inherent and unchangeable basic rules. This type of *teleological theory* of reasoning does not rely on an acceptance of universal law or accepted truths. Proponents of these belief systems do not suggest that fundamental principles of morality exist. The teleological theory of reasoning

demands a *comparative* evaluation of the particular unique circumstances of a specific situation. These thinkers do not believe any rule can be valid for every possible application. Theories of teleological ethics apply a methodical process of reasoning to assess the *subjective nature* of "goodness" and "badness." One must define what is meant by "good." One must decide which action will result in the most good. Additionally, "bad" must be defined. Thought must be given to determine which action will result in the most harm. An *obligation* or duty to weigh the benefits and costs of any potential action must be considered with each event.

Consequentialism is based on the idea that the right or wrong action is determined by the result of that act. Actions have consequences, and consequences are compared to evaluate relative merit. *Moral worth* is determined with an evaluation of the *consequences* of an action. Careful weighing of all of the benefits and all the costs of an action is required before choosing an action judged most likely to maximize good relative to harm. An action is worthwhile if the resulting consequences are valued with more good consequences than bad consequences. The consequences of the action determine if its *outcome* is primarily good or bad. The outcome must be specified with a measurement of good as a defined goal. The outcome goals (or ends) are evaluated by rating the end product. Quite literally, "the ends justify the means." Ethical dilemma occurs with the acknowledgment that undesirable choices may lead to less than ideal alternatives or a need to choose between the lesser of unappealing options. A justification for action or inaction is derived from a review of options. Choosing one option will produce more benefit than selecting other options, and some options are more or less likely to produce more harm or less harm. A prediction must be made to determine *relative benefit* (or *utility*).

Utilitarianism is one type of teleological thought system. Utilitarian thinking compares benefits and costs with an emphasis on *utility*. Utility is something that provides a useful purpose. Decision making using utilitarian reasoning opts for the choice that promotes *the greatest good for the greatest number*. Utilitarianism emphasizes achieving the greatest benefit for the largest amount of individuals. A utilitarian considers the available resources and develops an objective standard for consequences. A utilitarian approach is reflected in a reliance on a standardized measurement. Contemplate the ethical guidance inherent in a QOL index, productivity report, and cost–benefit forecast. A form of utilitarianism examines the process rather than the final goal, or the "means towards the end" is evaluated. This type of thoughtful assessment relies on a comparison of situational variables. Analysis follows a separation of the whole into elemental parts because it is thought to be important to judge the "goodness" and "badness" of each of the components. This is an almost mathematical

Table 48-1.		
ETHICAL DECISION MAKING: **A SAMPLE OF A QUANTITATIVE PROCESS FOR ANALYSIS**		
Problem	**Pro**	**Con**
To splint or not to splint?	Avoid contractures Maintain skin integrity	Amount of fabrication time Several clients will not get therapy Cost of material On/off assistance needed Cleaning assistance needed
Result		
Do not make the splint.	Two pros or good idea components	Five cons or bad idea components

approach. Either a quantitative or a qualitative value is assigned to each situational variable. The variables are compared to resolve the ethical dilemma.

Ethical judgment is required when one thinks about factors such as the allocation of scarce resources. Occupational therapy practitioners rely on an implicit or explicit moral rule for guidance when determining who will get services. An ethical dilemma is present when an occupational therapy practitioner decides how to ration time because time constraints exist, and time is often a scarce resource in an occupational therapy clinic. For an example, an occupational therapy practitioner is worried about the amount of time required to fabricate a splint for one client because without sufficient time in the workday, several other clients will not be seen that day. Resolution of an ethical dilemma is based on the assumption that moral value can be determined with the categorization of the arguments for and against an action. A moral decision can be made by creating a list and then counting the pros and cons. Alternatively, a moral decision can be made with a numeric value placed on each variable for a total score. Let us first solve the problem using a quantitative utilitarian analysis. Table 48-1 uses a *quantitative process* for ethical decision making to resolve this issue. The action (splinting) is assessed to have two good components (pro) and five bad components (con) in our listing of situational characteristics specific to this dilemma. There are more arguments against the action. The larger amount of five situational variables on the con side of the equation necessitates a resolution against the action. The splint will not be made tomorrow.

Now we will solve the problem using a *qualitative utilitarian analysis*. We will see that using a qualitative analysis rather than a strictly quantitative analysis can lead to a very different result. Table 48-2 uses a qualitative process for ethical decision making to resolve this issue. The same situational characteristics specific to this dilemma are listed with a 10-point maximum quality rating scale for each factor. A quality rating is used to indicate relative benefit. The comparative numeric weight of the end

result will indicate whether an action should be pursued. The action (splinting) is assessed to have a total value of 19 favorable (pro) quality value points and a total of 13 against (con) quality value points in this situation. The larger amount of 19 points on the pro side of the equation necessitates a resolution in favor of the action. There is an obligation to perform the action in consideration because it will produce more value or benefit. The splint will be made tomorrow.

Theories of Relative Standards

Ethical relativism is another philosophical school of thought. An underlying question asks if any rule can be valid for all people all the time. Ethical relativism is formed around the assumption that rules to guide behavior *should* change relative to time and place. The values of the society in which people live are recognized as important for establishing norms and community traditions. Moral principles are expected to change over the course of time. Morality is viewed as not static but changing according to the accepted standards of a specific society at a specific point in time. Actions regarded as praiseworthy or blameworthy will be (and should be) different within various cultures, religions, and other communities. There is an acceptance that certain practices are valued as praiseworthy in some communities but that the same type of action would be condemned as blameworthy in other communities. Values differ because judgment of praiseworthy and blameworthy actions is a function of the social order.

Certain actions were socially acceptable in their time but judged immoral from our perspective looking back at the circumstances of history. Historical perspective can stimulate dialogue on the appropriateness of actions. Was child labor a rational socioeconomic product of its time? Were the massive legislative and institutional changes

	ETHICAL DECISION MAKING: A SAMPLE OF A QUALITATIVE PROCESS FOR ANALYSIS				
Problem	Pro	Quality Value		Con	Quality Value
To splint or not to splint?	Avoid Contractures Maintain skin integrity	10 9		Amount of fabrication time Several clients will not get therapy Cost of material On/off assistance needed Cleaning assistance needed	4 5 2 1 1
Total points		19			13
Result	Make the splint.				

Table 48-2.

leading to closing of hospitals and the deinstitutionalization and community integration efforts of persons with mental illness during the 1970s and 1980s justified? Well-intentioned people can disagree as to what is right or wrong. There are societal and cultural differences when judging the moral acceptability of life-sustaining measures, euthanasia, abortion, and numerous other topics of controversy. This type of reasoning can lead to incendiary debates. Ethical relativism does not provide universal rules for easy determination of good behavior.

Making a Distinction Between Ethical and Legal

It is important to note that there are distinct differences between the law and ethics; these terms are not interchangeable. The law and ethics are not one and the same. Legal considerations and ethical concerns are not necessarily the same. Of course, there are times when legal and ethical share the same compatible basis. There are instances when illegal and unethical are consistent. Unequal pay based on gender discrimination is both against the law and unethical. There are examples of legal actions that do not seem ethical. There are historical examples of legislation with unintended ramifications resulting in major unexpected ethical problems. Choices can be legally acceptable but not ethically appropriate. As an example, widespread commercial advertising promoting cheaply made toys to children is legal but not necessarily ethical in motivation. Conversely, illegal activity can be morally defensible. The story of Robin Hood robbing the rich to give to the poor is a classic example of an illegal action that can be defended as ethically acceptable.

Federal, state, and municipal governments have the power to pass legislation and implement policy through regulations. The forces of government have jurisdiction within their own borders. Each jurisdiction monitors for compliance and develops methods of enforcement.

Laws tend to differ from state to state. Age of maturity for minors and other laws intended to safeguard the rights of persons needing special protection vary across state borders. State licensure laws protecting the public by regulating the practice of health care providers, including occupational therapy practitioners, are somewhat different from state to state. It is important to know the state licensure laws in the location of your practice. Obligation exists for a professional to know the laws, regulations, and ethical principles in the community and the place of employment. Each type of work environment can have a set of guidelines specific to place, time, and person. Universities are required by federal law to develop and implement procedures for research, and they have faculty policies.

Legal concerns and ethical issues often overlap in the delivery of health care. Courts have decided that society has an obligation to protect life, and courts have ordered life-saving medical intervention for young persons with parents who refuse intervention. On occasion, the rights of the individual conflict with the rights of society. Both medical law and medical ethics (bioethics) are in dynamic change. New legislation and the latest court decisions interpreting existing legislation create a need for up-to-date understanding of law. Federal and state judicial systems consider and then rule on court cases creating revised analysis of constitutional rights and other laws. Courts analyze specific questions and make an official ruling based on the particular situation presented in the case. Precedent is set with interpretation of influential cases and subsequent generalization to similar situations. Past dilemmas offer guidance for handling current dilemmas.

Quality of Life

The idea of QOL is a multidimensional and complex variable that has different meaning for each individual. Good QOL is determined by the personal values of the individual. Subjective ideas for what makes a good QOL tend to change over time based on life experiences.

The concept of *health-related quality of life* (HRQOL) regards the factors that determine the presence or absence of health to be observable and measurable. HRQOL measures the impact of health on QOL. HRQOL measurement tools assess perceptions of wellness through ratings of physical health and mental health. HRQOL population studies can be used to provide insights into broad community needs as well as special populations in clinical settings. Diagnosis of disease, the intervention process, and the side effects of the intervention can disrupt coping strategies and occupational balance. When independence is limited or task accomplishment becomes compromised, occupational roles may be altered. HRQOL measurements assess perceptions of health status and activity performance. The presence of disability may result in limitations in functional independence and decreased opportunities for life satisfaction. QOL may be diminished from the perspective of the individual. Alternatively, enhanced perceptions of control over adverse situations may enhance positive adjustment and improve QOL. Changes in health status can encourage a personal self-assessment with exploration of standards measuring QOL and sometimes causing a reprioritizing of values. An understanding of meaningful engagement in occupation can help assess QOL beyond generalizations based on the presence of disability or cultural or gender implications. Relative independence in functional activities of daily living is not an adequate measure of HRQOL factors. QOL is more than an ability to perform self-care activities. Occupational therapy practitioners must assess beyond a fragmentation of component parts to adequately measure HRQOL.

Social policy often cannot keep pace with scientific discoveries. Advances in medical technology influence change in medical ethics. Improvements in medical technology now let us do the unimaginable. Life-sustaining techniques enable medical teams to prolong life in emergency departments, intensive care units, neonatal centers, and long-term care facilities. This creates an ethical dilemma highlighting QOL issues when the anticipated HRQOL and functional status are poor. The individual, family members, and health care professionals must sort through complex issues as they make important bioethical decisions for themselves or their loved ones.

Health Care Resource Allocation and Distribution

Community is a source of support representing fundamental access to basic resources. Conversely, community can be a source of barriers limiting access to essential material goods. Community suggests a context surrounding the individual with influence on available choices. Community standards create customs, beliefs, attitudes, expected behaviors, and normative social routines. Public policy establishes social infrastructure. Essential commodities such as housing, food, water, and education are considered basic rights in modern society. The quality and methods of distribution of fundamental commodities vary widely. *Health care disparities* exist because health care access and service allotment are not always defined as a *basic right*. Society does not grant equal access to health care services or equality to service delivery. Populations in remote rural locations have limited access to health care because of geographic location. Parts of the population have limited access to health care because of income status or financial limitations. Ethical health care issues focus on questions of *entitlement* (who can get service), *access* (which types of services are covered), and *allotment* (how many services). Access to health care, entitlement, and allotment are determined by public policy. *Equitable distribution* refers to the moral concept of *justice*. If we say that benefits should be distributed in fair proportions, then we must decide how "fair" is determined. Similar to other economic-based commodities, some say health care should be a basic right, but others disagree and say that health care is not a right. Many wonder if health care can be allocated or rationed effectively or efficiently. Whether health care can be rationed fairly is a question dependent on ethical judgment.

The overburdened health care system struggles with limited resources and rising expenses. In many places, "business as usual" means doing more with less. The perception of danger or crisis has been known to legitimize organizational behavior the larger society would judge as unethical. There have been instances of price controls having resulted in "padding" allowable expenses by ordering authorized but unnecessary procedures. An organization might be tempted to compromise or abandon values when threatening external forces influence decisions to conduct business outside of accepted standards. Temptation can lure some to increase profits while decreasing quality of service. As an example, some facilities unable to recruit skilled professionals because of staffing shortages have been known to hire untrained workers to fill the gaps for skilled therapeutic services.

Conflict between loyalty to recipients of services and loyalty to employer can result in an ethical "dilemma of the double agent" (Bruckner, 1987). Ethical unease can occur because health care providers have dual goals that could be in conflict: to provide quality services and to generate high profits. Serious ethical dilemmas arise when the role of clinical advocate is compromised against the role of income generator. Pressures for cost containment can influence a replacement of a decision for clinical service delivery with a decision based on financial or allocation factors. Dilemmas are created when practitioners feel that clinical excellence or social responsibility is in opposition to economic reality.

Quality care is the primary goal for occupational therapy practitioners and other care providers. Quality care can be defined as the best possible intervention resulting in the best outcome for the individual recipient of care. Who defines *quality?* The recipient of care, the provider of care, and the party who pays for the care determine quality.

Ethical issues include concern for modifications of service access, program costs, and reimbursement. Additional focus is placed on determination of approved services and eligibility for services. At least in part, medical decisions are based on somebody's value judgment. Course of action is planned after weighing the competing interests in terms of the benefits and costs to all stakeholders, including the client, facility, insurers, advocacy groups, lawyers, legislators, and society as a whole.

Managers of health care are expected to allocate resources, structure cost-effective practices, encourage efficiency, and increase productivity while simultaneously limiting costs. Incremental changes bring models of health care reform offering lessons for what to do and what not to do because lessons will be taught as innovative ideas are tried. Successes will be replicated, and deficiencies will need corrections as society continues to plan for a fair and affordable system of health care delivery. How do decisions about health care cost, program access, and service quality get made, and who should make them? Who is covered? What is covered? Who pays for it? How much is paid? Funding initiatives fluctuate depending on external macroenvironmental conditions and shifting environmental priorities. Innovations in biotechnology (e.g., new medications, experimental testing), civil emergencies because of the threat of terrorism or epidemic (e.g., tuberculosis, polio, influenza, measles), demographic changes, and weather-related disasters (e.g., hurricanes, floods) have had an impact on the amount of dollars available for public health programs as well as the types of health services funded.

Ultimately, decisions are always made. The moral agents expected to provide the structure for health care benefits and services are governments, businesses, and philanthropic organizations. Organizations in the business of health care service delivery are expected to provide quality services in an equitable way. As a society, we expect a health care business to conduct operations in a manner that creates some good, has social responsibility, and does not harm the greater community. We expect that an ethical society will strive to create a fair system because of a social obligation to maximize justice and equitable consequences. There is a belief that there will be an attempt to form a balance of more good over less harm. Generally accepted social principles form the philosophical foundation for medical ethics. The values that guide behavior in society at large are the basic standards used to make decisions in medical ethics. If fairness is an esteemed value in society as a whole, then fairness will also be an important factor for the resolution of medical ethical dilemmas. If compassion is an important social value, then empathy and caring will guide medical ethical decision making.

Direct Application in Everyday Practice

From corporations to street gangs, an expected obligation of *group membership* is an adoption of group values. All groups of all types assume member acceptance of group values. Group membership implies compliance with fundamental principles of the group. Behavioral norms are established through either formal or informal systems. The degree of formal structure does not determine the amount of internalization of values or the extent of compliance to rules. Regulations and laws are examples of formal methods of sharing group values with strong incentives for compliance. Custom and tradition are relatively informal methods of sharing group values, yet they have compelling authoritative commands for observance of principles. A sense of belonging to a group will foster adoption of group norms as personal values. Consequences for noncompliance include a wide variety of sanctions and penalties for infractions handed down in the form of restrictions, fines, or prison time. Compliance based merely on rule recognition rather than an internalized system of values has a focus on the threat of detection and punishment. Drivers who do not obey posted speed limits on interstate highways but slow down in the presence of a marked police vehicle demonstrate this observable truth.

Private entities such as professional associations or corporations create standards of conduct. It is not unusual for an organization policy to go beyond the minimum requirements set by legal standards. We can assume that just like individuals, organizations may rely on more than one type of value-based principle. Customs, principles, and regulations blend to define ethical behavior unique to an organization.

Attitudes and traditions are a part of organizational culture. The creation of an ethical work environment sets the tone for an organization. Constructing an ethical climate is most effective when the people who implement the policies and procedures cooperatively participate in their formation because a realistic, yet rigorous, set of ethical standards is more likely to be adhered to if there is a "buy-in" from those who must live under its authority. A proactive management can support ethical behavior by adopting a policy to lead by example. If management clearly supports ethical behavior, employees will be more likely to view an unethical action as unacceptable.

Either an implicit agreement or an explicit contract is established between an employer organization and its employees. Employees can expect a safe workplace environment, fair work conditions, and an equitable salary with benefits. There is a reasonable expectation of job satisfaction. It is incumbent upon employees to use performance skills and execute a fair amount of work in return.

Codes and Standards for Occupational Therapy

A *code of ethics* is a collection of formal explicit statements forming a moral guide for an identified group outlining right and valued behavior, principles, and values. Any formal statement can serve as a code of ethics if it provides group members with an outline of what is right and valued and defines underlying beliefs. A code of ethics creates recognition of the behaviors deemed good or bad within a group context. A code of ethics is a collection of value-based rules forming an impartial guide for making decisions by an identified group.

A code of ethics can be a stand-alone document or a component of an organization's policies and procedures manual. In many cases, a code of ethics is integrated into the organization's mission statement. Typically, an organization creates secondary documents such as an enforcement code to assist in interpretation and implementation of the code of ethics. These supplementary documents are generally safeguards built into the system to encourage compliance. Mechanisms for sanctions and penalties to deal with ethical misconduct in violation of principles specified in the code of ethics are provided in ancillary papers. Auxiliary supportive documents are commonly used to address specific issues as a need becomes evident.

The professional associations for occupational therapy practitioners have clearly identified the value-based principles important to the profession. The World Federation of Occupational Therapists (WFOT), National Board for Certification in Occupational Therapy (NBCOT), and American Occupational Therapy Association (AOTA) have a shared sense of which values are important and what constitutes good practice. In service of a mission with responsibility to protect the public interest, our professional organizations specify criteria for the appropriate conduct of all occupational therapy practitioners and define our responsibilities toward the recipients of occupational therapy services. Official documents for the use of members and nonmembers are available on each of our professional association's Web sites.

The WFOT Code of Ethics (see Appendix I) presents a general guide for "appropriate conduct . . . in any professional circumstance" (WFOT 2005). Categories highlighted are personal attributes, responsibility toward the recipient of occupational therapy services, collaboration, continued professional development, and promotion of the profession (WFOT, 2005).

The NBCOT Candidate/Certificant Code of Conduct (revised 2013) and the Procedures for The Enforcement of The NBCOT Candidate/Certificant Code of Conduct (revised 2013) "define and clarify" professional responsibilities in order to protect the public. The NBCOT requires certified occupational therapy practitioners and students compliance towards the seeking of "high standards for personal and professional conduct" (NBCOT, 2013). Violations can result in certification ineligibility for a specified time or sanctions such as monitoring or supervision. The NBCOT has the authority to impose penalties from a formal reprimand kept on record up to indefinite revocation of certification.

The AOTA has developed and adopted a series of documents to provide guidance for the occupational therapy practitioner. These documents of the AOTA represent a comprehensive ethics guide for all occupational therapy personnel (occupational therapists, occupational therapy assistants, and students). A set of principles for professional conduct is given in the Occupational Therapy Code of Ethics and Ethics Standards (2010b). The Standards of Practice for Occupational Therapy (AOTA, 2010c) provides practice guidelines for the delivery of occupational therapy services, defining minimum practice standards and giving the occupational therapy practitioner guidance for application of values and principles. Enforcement Procedures for the Occupational Therapy Code of Ethics and Ethics Standards (AOTA, 2010b) establishes a complaint process and sanctions as well as outlines the AOTA's ability to penalize AOTA members who violate the ethics standards. The AOTA's Societal Statement on Health Disparities is written in support of "advocacy to increase access to health services for persons in need"; this official document of the AOTA is an example of an auxiliary supportive document. Core Values and Attitudes of Occupational Therapy Practice (AOTA, 1993) is a supplemental document occupational therapy practitioners could use as an ethical guide. This document was integrated within the main content of the Occupational Therapy Code of Ethics and Ethics Standards (2010b).

The Occupational Therapy Code of Ethics and Ethics Standards (2010b) highlights the longstanding commitment of the profession to seven core values as first emphasized in Core Values and Attitudes of Occupational Therapy Practice (AOTA, 1993). Ethical values and morality-based attitudes form the core foundation for the practice of occupational therapy. These seven concepts are altruism, equality, freedom, justice, dignity, truth, and prudence.

1. Altruism is concerned with creating benefit for others.

2. Equality is the basis for impartial fairness.

3. Freedom is reflected in self-determination and the right to choose.

4. Justice is being objective and unbiased.

5. Dignity places emphasis on the unique characteristics of each person as valuable and worthy of respect.

6. Truth is a requirement for honesty and accuracy.

7. Prudence is the basis for cautious good sense.

The Occupational Therapy Code of Ethics and Ethics Standards (2010b) and the related official documents of the AOTA are intended to assist occupational therapy personnel with moral dilemmas and conflicts. A combination of deontological beliefs and teleological application principles are offered as guidance to sort through conflicting priorities in any type of work setting. With the Occupational Therapy Code of Ethics and Ethics Standards (2010b), there is a recognition that members of the profession will be called upon to make decisions regarding "situation-specific" ethical issues. The Occupational Therapy Code of Ethics and Ethics Standards (2010b) defines a set of principles: beneficence, nonmaleficence, autonomy, confidentiality, social justice, procedural justice, veracity, and fidelity.

- Principle 1 is based on the concept of *beneficence*. Maximize positive and good benefits. Perform with compassionate goodwill. Occupational therapy personnel are expected to provide services in a fair manner without discrimination.

- Principle 2 is based on the concept of *nonmaleficence*. Minimize or avoid causing harm. Occupational therapy personnel are called on to use good judgment and to refrain from taking part in actions that result in exploitation.

- Principle 3 is based on the double obligations of *autonomy* and *confidentiality*.

  ◊ The first is *autonomy*, free will or self-determination with respect for individuality. There is an obligation to collaborate and to follow the standards of informed consent.

  ◊ The second is *confidentiality*, the protection of privacy, information, and communication. This requires the establishment of a trusting relationship and guarding information shared in confidence. Discussions must be protected, taking care that conversations will not be overheard. Records are not to be disclosed except under conditions of authorized access in compliance with regulations. Computer security measures must be observed.

- Principle 4 requires *social justice* or *distributive justice*. Occupational therapy practitioners must advocate for fair distribution of resources.

- Principle 5 mandates *procedural justice,* a compliance with laws, regulations, and institutional rules.

- Principle 6 is *veracity*. There is an obligation for being truthful. Accurate and honest communication is a requirement.

- Principle 7 identifies a need for *fidelity*. An obligation exists for integrity and fairness in professional interactions.

Informed Consent

Principle 3 of the Occupational Therapy Code of Ethics and Ethics Standards (2010b) speaks to a concern with obtaining informed consent from recipients of services and participants in research. Although facility procedures may focus on signing an informed consent form, the key to true informed consent is the *process* of educating with appropriate, relevant, and truthful information so a *reasonable* person can make a decision regarding the *risk* (harm) and *options for success* (benefits). Informed consent is a process that acknowledges the service recipient's right to be directly involved in health care decisions. The informed consent process protects against unwanted intervention and allows for choice, including refusal to participate. Respect for the individual is fundamental to the concepts of self-determination and autonomy. The concept of informed consent is based on the principle of autonomy. Closely linked to beneficence, the process of informed consent relies on recognition of *self-determination*. A minimum of three components is widely recognized as necessary for informed consent:

1. Disclosure: Sufficient knowledge for making decisions

2. Competency: Sufficient capability to understand information

3. Voluntary: Sufficient freedom to choose

The occupational therapy practitioner must include the recipient of services as a full participant in the informed consent process. The practitioner must try to understand the situation from the perspective of the recipient of services. An active listening approach can allow the clinician to hear the preferences of the participant while avoiding a compromise to the values of the clinician or, more importantly, the client. Autonomy can be preserved with an appreciation of individual needs. A commitment for respect and honesty should be maintained. Collaboration is a requirement. A dynamic plan for communication should be standard procedure. Information must be shared in a manner that will facilitate communication. There is an obligation on the occupational therapy practitioner to ensure understanding and maximum comprehension. Allow for the asking of questions and answer with honesty.

The feelings, hopes, and fears of the individual must be considered within an environment that fosters open communication. Avoid prejudicing the selection process. Do not use coercive influence and avoid creating a sense of intimidation. Be aware of the unequal power between a caregiving professional and the recipient of care. The paternalistic sentiment of the health care professional's "knowing what is best" for the client is no longer meaningful in today's health care environment.

The practitioner has an obligation to clearly describe the preferred clinical alternative and the other options. The purpose of the recommended intervention must be presented. Available intervention alternatives must be offered. The probability of benefits and risks must be explained for all available options. An exhaustive list of every possible risk no matter how slight the probability is not required nor is it encouraged. Enough information must be given to allow a choice. The client has a right to either accept or refuse the recommended intervention. A refusal of intervention should be honored, but refusal does not necessarily mean the end of discussions because an exploration of the reason for refusal and consideration of alternatives is not only acceptable but also required.

The ability to give informed consent involves determination of competency by legal or common law standards. Capacity for reason and deliberation is required. There must be an ability to understand the treatment alternatives and appreciate the risks or benefits. It can be useful to look at *decisional capacity* instead of reliance on legal standards of *competence*. Strict adherence to legal standards can have the disadvantage of moving the responsibility for informed consent away from the recipient of service because of an impaired ability to communicate, degenerating or wavering mental status, or the person is a minor below the age of consent. Decisional capacity is based on the determination that the individual is capable of making a decision at a given time. How are intervention decisions made if the person does not have decisional capacity or is determined legally not competent? The question that should be asked in this type of case is, "What would the person do if able to decide independently?" Decisions should be made in the context of the individual's past values and preferences. Decisions should be consistent with earlier life choices. Conversations with family, friends, and staff at residential centers can lead to insights about preferences. Some states recognize a *health care proxy,* a family member or friend designated by the individual to make medical intervention decisions if the recipient of services is unable to make clinical care decisions and if the preferred option remains unknown. The designated health care proxy has the authority of making decisions on behalf of the individual. Decisions can be made according to the *best interests* determination when client wishes or attitudes are not known. Often the situation circumstances were not discussed with the surrogate decision maker or the person's wishes were not made clear. In some cases, the courts will assign a legal guardian to weigh all of the facts and determine what is in the client's best interest. *Substituted judgment* is a form of decision making asking, "If the client could tell us, what would the client's choice be in this situation?" The best intervention option is determined by deciding, "What would this person do in this specific situation?" It is putting yourself in the client's shoes and contemplating, "What if?" Again, the details of the specific situation must be considered. The situation-specific details necessitate the weighing of risks and benefits resulting in an examination of QOL issues. Decisions should not be based on age or presence of disability or generalized stereotypes.

Adherence to client autonomy respects the rights of the individual even if the individual chooses to abdicate decision-making control to another person. Each person and each family will have a unique experience based on family roles, education, immigration, assimilation, and personal patterns (Candib, 2002; Gold, 2004; Ho, 2006). Emphasis should be placed on expressed client values and expectations (Leino-Kilpi et al., 2003). It is important to avoid stereotypes and generalizations based on ethnicity. A respectful humanitarian position accommodates multicultural needs by meeting "traditional fundamental standards of ethics while respecting cultural and societal norms" (Crigger, Holcomb, & Weiss, 2001, p. 465).

The health care provider and the client might not speak the same language, creating linguistic challenges to obtaining informed consent. Terminology to describe pathology is lacking by western standards in many cultures (Crigger et al., 2001), making interpretation difficult. Translators have been known to create bias because of dialect or cross-cultural miscommunication (Barnes, Davis, Moran, Portillo, & Koenig, 1998; Crigger et al., 2001) with culture-based differences in maintaining hope (Barnes et al., 1998; Kagawa-Singer, 1993). The presence of unfamiliar translators taking part in personal, emotion-laden conversations can cause additional barriers to communication (Barnes et al., 1998). Family involvement in decision making can necessitate an interdependent approach to obtaining informed consent. Allowing the client to express a clear preference for another (or others) to contribute to the process for making decisions should be accepted as being as valid as an individual's own decision (Barnes et al., 1998; Ho, 2006). Authoritarian forcing of individual decision making is another form of paternalism (Candib, 2002; Ho, 2006). Some cultures believe the rights of the bigger community or family override the rights of the individual. In a family, the cultural expectation may motivate a husband to routinely make decisions on behalf of his wife (Crigger et al., 2001). Decisions by a leader are expected as the norm, and the client will assume a passive role in decisions, leaving authority and control to the expertise of the health care practitioner (Barnes et al., 1998). Some cultures avoid an overt discussion of dying or life-threatening illness. This cultural norm would lead to medical decision making by a trusted family member rather than directly by the client. "Partial disclosure" or "ambiguity" is widely practiced as a way to share information in an indirect manner (Candib, 2002). Only recently, medical culture in western traditions adopted the view that disclosure of life-threatening diagnosis was a beneficent act. In 1961, the majority of United States doctors did not disclose the diagnosis of cancer directly to clients; however, by the mid to late 1970s, most doctors disclosed as a routine practice (Candib, 2002; Gold, 2004).

Criticism of the informed consent form became widespread as facilities attempted to adopt more user-friendly documents. Similar to other medical documents, the informed consent form is viewed as too technical, too complicated, and too lengthy for the typical reader. Studies show that the document is often skimmed or not read in detail (Huntington & Robinson, 2007; Varnhagen et al., 2005). It is hypothesized that in addition to low readability, informed consent documents are not read because of a perception of low risk (Huntington & Robinson, 2007; Varnhagen et al., 2005) because the institution or clinician is trusted. True informed consent is not obtained even with a signature on a document when the document is not fully read and understood. Health messages developed according to universal accessibility standards clarify unfamiliar medical terminology and make complex concepts more comprehensible. Improved readability can be created with simpler text, decreased jargon and technological language, choice of font, and format clarity. Technical jargon should be avoided. At a minimum, terminology should be clearly defined, and layman's terms should be used whenever possible. Lack of comprehension can occur because of a language barrier, literacy level, cognitive deficit, or situation-specific anxiety. The demands of the medical environment can increase stress, often causing a barrier to communication. Attempt to decrease anxiety. Creating an informed consent document that meets universal accessibility standards for improving literacy can honor legal requirements and address ethical concerns for process.

Informed consent guidelines can be developed specific to the specialized needs of researchers. Although there are aspects of clinical informed consent similar to research informed consent, there are differences and implications to consider. The dual roles of researcher and clinician can cause confusion, conflict of interest, and the potential for coercion (Crigger et al., 2001).

Informed consent for research goes beyond the requirements of obtaining a signature on a permission form. Participants in a research study must be provided with sufficient information to understand the benefits and risks associated with becoming a research subject. Research participants have a right to stop participation in the activity under study. Commonly accepted practice

understands informed consent to be a process throughout the research participant's experience.

Moral fundamentalism accepts informed consent principles as universal and applicable throughout the world in all research situations (Crigger et al., 2001). Therefore, the protocol for obtaining informed consent should not be modified for populations in different geographic areas. *Moral multiculturalism* is in contrast to moral fundamentalism. A multicultural ethic does not seek absolutes but rather accepts a more situational approach that varies among communities. Therefore, protocol for obtaining informed consent should be modified to meet the cultural needs to place and time of the studied population.

Choices! Choices! Decisions! Decisions!

An *ethical dilemma* exists in a situation in which an argument can be made for opposing decisions or conflicting choices. Sometimes there is more than one "right" solution to a problem. There are situations when there is no clear indication of the "right or wrong" course of action. Rules might be vague or not well established. Sometimes partial good can be found in incompatible trade-offs. At times, dubious pathways lead to "good" end results. Other times, none of the available alternatives appears to be an acceptable option likely to result in a good ending. Rarely are there clearly defined problems with definitive solutions.

The role of ethics in occupational therapy is to assist the practitioner in solving complex problems when there is no clear identification of right or wrong or there is a need to identify the best alternative out of choices. Medical ethics can be a hodgepodge of incompatible values and conflicting regulations. Ethical dilemmas in health care reflect the moral conflicts of the larger society. Proponents and opponents can logically and passionately argue contradictory viewpoints on life and death issues.

Clinical ethics committees have been established in a number of health care facilities, and a study showed that facility employees are most likely to look to clinical ethics committees for legalistic guidance on informed consent and record keeping (Kerridge, Pearson, & Rolfe, 1998). Often dilemmas in the "typical" experience of occupational therapy practitioners are complex, involving a need for consensus among several participants and lasting an extended time period with repetition of episodes (Barnitt, 1998).

Ethical decision making in the work setting can "get stuck" while everyone with a stake in the process waits for someone else on the team to make a decision. Fear of malpractice or other litigation can slow the process further. Occupational therapy personnel are faced with ethical dilemmas along with the other professionals on the workplace team. In some cases, occupational therapy practitioners may feel excluded from the decision-making process; however, practitioners are encouraged to accept or develop a position of responsibility. All occupational therapy personnel inclusive of occupational therapists, occupational therapy assistants, and students have a duty to take an active role in the ethical decision-making process.

Ethics obligates one to judge. Ironically, adopting avoidance maneuvers, advocating for a neutral position, or having no judgment about anything will become a judgmental decision. Saying "I don't want to judge" is making a judgment. A course of action or inaction will result. Consequences will occur even without an acknowledgment of moral beliefs.

Moral occupational therapy practitioners identify and analyze ethical problems. An appropriate response to ethical problems is an exploration of choices. No two cases are ever identical, and "one size fits all" solutions do not exist. Emphasis cannot be placed on learning the "right" concept or replicating the "correct" action. Responsible decisions depend on thoughtful consideration of competing rights, obligations, values, and interests. Occupational therapy practitioners should consider and weigh conflicting and competing agendas, priorities, choices, values, and opinions of relevant stakeholders. The same practical thinking used outside the workplace to do the "right thing," such as being loyal to a friend or treating a grandparent with respect, is useful in the work setting. Act with goodwill, show compassion, and treat others with integrity and respect, or in other words, beneficence. Altruism is another way to express the importance of sharing. Equality and justice are based on fairness and point to distribution of scarce resources. There is an obligation to community. Do not cause harm and do not hurt anyone. Know the rules and follow them. Judgment necessitates a clarification of values and ethical principles.

The Ethical Decision SOAP

Is there a fair and just way to sort through conflicting principles to decide on a course of action—or inaction? How should an occupational therapy practitioner determine the best option? Identify the principles specific to the particular case situation, contemplate, negotiate, and reach a resolution. The ethical decision SOAP format is adapted for the purpose of resolving ethical dilemmas. A process for making ethical decisions is derived from clinical practice with a time-honored reporting method: the SOAP progress note.

How to Write an Ethical Decision SOAP

- Step 1: Create an initial problem list.
  - List the central problems or the most significant problems. What is the conflict? List all involved persons.
- Step 2: Subjective: Identify the subjective case-specific issues.
  - Identify the ethical issues or problems raised by the case-specific situation. It is critical to understand the clinical and social facts of the particular situation. Are the thoughts and wishes of the participants clear? Recognize the presence of feelings (e.g., acceptance, fear, worry, anger, ambivalence, other emotions). Clarify your own opinion and biases.
- Step 3: Objective: Gather objective case-relevant data.
  - Search the literature to identify similar situations. Determine the consensus of experts on prior cases. Examine the interpretation of law through court decisions. Find relevant department or organization procedures. Know professional guidelines and standards of practice. Determine relevant code of ethics principles.
- Step 4: Assess: Assess the situation.
  - Contemplate the relevant ethical principles as they apply to the specific people of the particular situation. Articulate the solution alternatives and realistic options.
  - Postulate all of the consequences of each choice. Weigh the competing interests, needs, risks, and benefits of all involved participants. Determine if the options are reasonable. Evaluate if resources for implementation of the alternatives are available.
- Step 5: Plan: Articulate a plan of action.
  - Plan for a practical and realistic solution. Formulate an overall strategy and schedule.
- Step 6: Implement the plan.
- Step 7: Evaluate the need to modify the plan.

Summary

Many occupational therapy personnel borrow from an assortment of ethical theories to arrive at a balanced approach to a moral making of decisions in the workplace. An eclectic approach is often used to make daily work decisions. The development of an ethical style or "personal compass" is an ongoing process.

Perhaps the highest standard for ethical decision making is a reliance on the principle of beneficence. Virtuous practitioners strive to maximize possible benefits in a fair way. "Superior quality" is a value judgment with an expectation for excellence. Value-based concepts such as dignity and respect can provide a foundation for service delivery.

Everyday occupational therapy practice is based on ethical judgments. Integrate an awareness of ethics into everyday practice. Moral reasoning strategies enhance clinical outcomes. Faced with increasing demands and decreasing resources, occupational therapy practitioners must cope with issues of quality, quantity, access, and allocation. Contemplate the pertinent ethical questions and the implications. Initiate conversations about the relevant moral principles. Proficiency with ethical knowledge develops ability when coping with real-world concerns.

Student Self-Assessment

1. Personal reflection: Where did you get your sense of morality? Write a four- or five-page biographical narrative describing your values and principles, linking the evolution of your standards to your personal history of past experiences and events.

2. Personal credo: Write your own code of ethics. Create a moral credo defining your personal system of philosophical beliefs.

3. Professional credo: Adapt your personal code of ethics to craft a professional doctrine suitable for use in work environments.

4. Small Group Exercises
    ◊ Exercise 1: Working in teams, think of a situation that raises an ethical dilemma. Concisely describe the situation using an objective descriptive style.
    ◊ Exercise 2: Brainstorm as many ideas as possible. Generate a list of alternative solutions to resolve the ethical dilemma described in Exercise 1.
    ◊ Exercise 3: List the relevant principles and values in the ethical dilemma described in Exercise 1.
    ◊ Exercise 4: Present a role play reflecting the attitudes, opinions, and feelings of the participants involved in the ethical dilemma described in Exercise 1.

5. Document review
    ◊ Option 1: Visit a local health care facility or human services agency. Request a mission statement, code of ethics, or patient bill of rights. Obtain a copy of any document that demonstrates moral concepts. Identify the main ethical principles or standards in the document(s).
    ◊ Option 2: Search the websites of two types of facilities that might provide occupational therapy services. You can choose a local hospital and a major teaching hospital, or you could select any combination of hospital, rehabilitation facility, home health agency, nursing home, school, or other place of service delivery for occupational therapy. Locate a mission statement, code of ethics, or patient bill of rights for both facilities. Compare the documents. Do they refer to the same values and standards? Describe two ethics-based components that are the same and two components that are different.

6. Ethics Case Study Projects
    ◊ Answer the following ethics case study questions for each case:
        * What is the most significant ethical dilemma? Explain your answer.
        * Which principles in the *Occupational Therapy Code of Ethics* apply to the case? Explain your answer.
        * Write an ethical decision SOAP.
        * Discuss the implications of allocation and distribution of resources.
    ◊ Case Study 1: Larry
        * Leaving the cafeteria after a late afternoon snack, you are rushing toward the elevator to get to a utilization review meeting when Larry, a nurse, taps your shoulder and with a big, friendly grin says, "I'm so glad that I ran into you. Let's ride back up to the unit together because I want your opinion about Mr. Stone's getting discharged next week." As the doors close on the crowded elevator, Larry looks at you and continues speaking, "So, I want to know if Mr. Stone can dress independently yet."
    ◊ Case Study 2: Edie
        * You work in the outpatient unit of a busy rehabilitation hospital. Dropped off in the parking lot by her mom, Edie always arrives promptly for her occupational therapy visits. She is being seen for intervention of a fracture to her left elbow after a slip on the stairs at her piano teacher's home. Her intervention time seems to be shorter than the hour duration because throughout the sessions, she chats about the numerous activities and events typical to an active 17-year-old high school student. Shortly before the end of today's session,

Edie confides that she has a handgun bought from another student.

◇ Case Study 3: Maddy

* You are a member of a geriatric medical behavioral assessment team in a large suburban hospital. One of your clients is an 80-year-old woman recuperating from a fall. The cause of her fall remains unknown. During her stay, Maddy presents as frightened, depressed, and anxious. She has ripped out her IVs repeatedly. She thwarts attempts made by staff to keep her seated in a chair and refuses to stay in her hospital bed. The staff considers her "a fall risk." She has multiple chronic conditions, including diabetes and arthritis. She is legally blind secondary to diabetic retinopathy. Significant hearing loss in both ears is somewhat compensated for with bilateral hearing aids. Never married, Maddy lives alone in the house that has been the family home for three generations. Maddy dedicated her adult life to caring for her frail, confused, and incontinent mother in her last years until she passed away about 10 years ago. Health insurance will not cover long-term home care services. Her small pension combined with her Social Security check makes her slightly over income for subsidized programs. Family members (a younger brother and a niece who, coincidentally, is a nurse on another unit) share responsibility of occasional visits, grocery shopping, and helping with mail for bill payments. Both relatives describe Maddy as strong, independent, self-reliant, and proud of it. The brother would like to see Maddy return to independent living in her own home as soon as possible. The niece is worried about Maddy returning home and has asked the assessment team to help decide for long-term planning. A transfer to a long-term care facility such as an assisted living facility, nursing home, or custodial care residence is a possibility being considered. Everyone who enters Maddy's room is asked the same question, "When can I go home?" One staff member said, "Sure, she wants to go home, but this would be for her own good; she will learn to like it." The multidisciplinary team looks to you, the occupational therapist, to determine the level of independent functioning with activities of daily living and to assess safety in the home. Will this client be safe at home? The discharge meeting starts.

◇ Case Study 4: The Roommate

* You have not seen your old roommate since graduation. You are meeting for a casual lunch on the following Sunday. Your roommate's family owns several skilled nursing facilities in a metropolitan center. After graduation, your friend's father asked you to work in the main facility where the corporate office is housed. After a few months of work at Sunny Meadows, it became obvious that the amount of actual therapy visits did not match what was documented in the medical record. Residents were wheeled into the large therapy area and then returned to the unit dayroom. You were instructed by the rehabilitation services director to document "slow progress" in the medical record so the residents appeared to need more intervention than actually required because health care insurers generally require termination of services if measurable progress halts.

◇ Case Study 5: Michael and Maria

* You are nearing the end of the number of home health visits allowed by Michael's health insurance plan. Michael, a 45-year-old carpenter who experienced a traumatic brain injury, is making measurable therapeutic gains during your home visits. Michael's wife, Maria, often accompanies her husband during the occupational therapy sessions in their kitchen. Maria is very worried, saying, "I don't want Michael to go downhill and lose his ability to do things. You know he is trying very hard! Can't you keep visiting? You know he has goals. Hope is important!"

◇ Case Study 6: Fred

* Fred is a 92-year-old man on your caseload. You are providing occupational therapy intervention after a hip fracture secondary to metastatic lung cancer. Fred has no remaining family. He has outlived his wife of 61 years. A drunk driver in a motor vehicle accident killed his only daughter on Christmas Eve 7 years ago. He is obviously depressed. He tells you that he doesn't want occupational therapy or more surgery, radiation therapy, or chemotherapy: "I just want to be left alone." The home health team has learned that his condition is considered terminal.

◇ Case Study 7: Juan

* Juan is well liked by the teachers of the residential school for his quick sense of humor

EVIDENCE-BASED RESEARCH CHART

Topic	Evidence
Moral conflict and ethical dilemmas	Barnitt, 1998; Foye, Kirschner, Brady Wagner, Stocking, & Siegler, 2002; Kälvemark, Höglund, Hansson, Westerholm, & Arnetz, 2004; Kassberg & Skär, 2008; Kirschner, Stocking, Wagner, Foye, & Siegler, 2001; Mukherjee, Brashler, Savage, & Kirschner, 2009; Scheirton, Mu, Lohman, & Cochran, 2007
Principles and values	Cox, 2012; Dige, 2009
Autonomy and independence	Cardol, De Jong, & Ward, 2002; Russell, Fitzgerald, Williamson, Manor, & Whybrow, 2002; Tamaru, McColl, & Yamasaki, 2007
Utilitarianism	Levack, 2009
Ethical decision making and reasoning	Dieruf, 2004; Martinez, 2000; Opacich, 1997

and compassionate demeanor. His obvious empathy for younger kids is frequently shown by his friendly attitude on the school playground. He is an artistically talented 16 year old with strong academic skills. Juan lives at the school because of a shortage of appropriate foster care homes. His short attention span and periodic fits of rage were too much for his teacher in the traditional classroom environment. Juan's teacher noticed cigarette burn marks along the insides of his arms. When questioned, he revealed he sometimes thought about suicide. Recently, the outpatient mental health unit intervention team completed retesting and tentatively made the diagnosis of bipolar disorder. Intervention suggestions include medication, individual counseling, and stress management techniques. After 2 months of intervention, Juan is saying he wants to quit school and is refusing to take medication. He complains that medication side effects always make him feel tired and thirsty. He says the worst part is no longer feeling "the flow of creativity" and that his "artistic energy is gone." The residential staff members are concerned because Juan is beginning to become "a loner," isolating himself in his bedroom.

You work for the occupational therapy team of the school department in a large urban community. Knowing occupational therapy can provide a range of interventions that could improve functional abilities in the school environment, you know you have a lot to offer kids like Juan. Shortly before his transfer to the residential school, the homeroom teacher requested an "occupational therapy consult for handwriting improvement." Initial contact with Juan was made in his old classroom, where sitting in a corner chair slouched into his oversized black hooded sweatshirt, he avoided eye contact. His only comments were, "My handwriting is just fine like it is. I don't want your help."

An invitation to Juan's IEP meeting arrived in today's mail. You look at your calendar to discover you already agreed to participate in another IEP meeting scheduled at the same time for a student who attends a different school. Sighing, you decide to write a memo to be read into the official meeting minutes outlining your thoughts and recommendations.

Electronic Resources

- AOTA: Frequently Asked Questions About Ethics: http://www.aota.org/Practitioners/Ethics/FAQs.aspx

- Bioethics Resources on the Web from National Institutes of Health: http://bioethics.od.nih.gov

- National Board for Certification in Occupational Therapy, How to File a Complaint: http://www.nbcot.org/index.php?option=com_content&view=article&id=24&Itemid=61

- National Reference Center for Bioethics Literature under the auspices of the Bioethics Research Library at Georgetown University: http://bioethics.georgetown.edu

- *Occupational Therapy Code of Ethics and Ethics Standards* (2010b) and related documents available on the AOTA Web site's sections for Practitioners, Educators/Researchers, Students, and About Occupational Therapy: http://aota.org/Practitioners/Ethics/Docs.aspx

- Presidential Commission for the Study of Bioethical Issues: http://bioethics.gov

- Tips on informed consent from Office for Protection from Research Risks, Office for Human Research Protections, U.S. Department of Health & Human Services: http://www.hhs.gov/ohrp/policy/ictips.html
- Virtual Mentor, American Medical Association: http://virtualmentor.ama-assn.org

References

American Occupational Therapy Association. (1993). Core values and attitudes of occupational therapy practice. *American Journal of Occupational Therapy, 47*, 1085-1086.

American Occupational Therapy Association. (2010a). Enforcement procedures for the occupational therapy code of ethics and ethics standards. *American Journal of Occupational Therapy, 64*.

American Occupational Therapy Association. (2010b). Occupational therapy code of ethics and ethics standards (2010). *American Journal of Occupational Therapy, 64*(Suppl.), S17-S26.

American Occupational Therapy Association. (2010c). Standards of practice for occupational therapy. *American Journal of Occupational Therapy, 64*.

American Occupational Therapy Association's Societal Statement on Health Disparities. (2011). The reference manual of the official documents of the American Occupational Therapy Association, Inc. *American Journal of Occupational Therapy, 65*(6 Suppl.).

Barnes, D. M., Davis, A. J., Moran, T., Portillo, C. J., & Koenig, B. A. (1998). Informed consent in a multicultural cancer patient population: Implications for nursing practice. *Nursing Ethics, 5*(5), 412-423.

Barnitt R. (1998). Ethical dilemmas in occupational therapy and physical therapy: a survey of practitioners in the UK National Health Service. *Journal of Medical Ethics, 24*(3), 193-199.

Bruckner, J. (1987). Physical therapists as double agents. Ethical dilemmas of divided loyalties. *Physical Therapy 67*(3), 383-387.

Candib, L. M. (2002). Truth telling and advance planning at the end of life: Problems with autonomy in a multicultural world. *Families, Systems and Health, 20*(3), 213-228.

Cowley, C. (2005). The dangers of medical ethics. *Journal of Medical Ethics, 31*, 739-742.

Crigger, N. J., Holcomb, L., & Weiss, J. (2001). Fundamentalism, multiculturalism and problems of conducting research with populations in developing nations. *Nursing Ethics, 8*(5), 459-468.

Fulghum, R. (1988). *All I really need to know I learned in kindergarten: Uncommon thoughts on common things* (pp. 6-7). New York, NY: Villard Books.

Gold, M. (2004). Is honesty always the best policy? Ethical aspects of truth telling. *Internal Medicine Journal, 34*, 578-580.

Ho, A. (2006). Family and informed consent in multicultural setting. *American Journal of Bioethics, 6*(1), 26-28.

Huntington, I., & Robinson, W. (2007). The many ways of saying yes and no: Reflections on the research coordinator's role in recruiting research participants and obtaining informed consent. *IRB: Ethics and Human Research, 29*(3), 6-10.

Kagawa-Singer, M. (1993). Redefining health: Living with cancer. *Social Science and Medicine, 37*(3), 295-304.

Kerridge, I. H., Pearson, S., & Rolfe, I. E. (1998). Determining the function of a clinical ethics committee: Making ethics work. *Journal of Quality in Clinical Practice, 18*, 117-124.

Leino-Kilpi, H., Valimaki, M., Dassen, T., Gasull, M., Lemonidou, C., Scott, P. A., et al. (2003). Perceptions of autonomy, privacy, and informed consent in the care of elderly people in five European countries: Comparison and implications for the future. *Nursing Ethics, 10*(1), 58-66.

National Board for Certification in Occupational Therapy. (2013). NBCOT candidate/certificant code of conduct.

National Board for Certification in Occupational Therapy. (2013) *Procedures for the enforcement of the NBCOT candidate/certificant code of conduct*. Revision November 14, 2011.

Varnhagen, C. K., Gushta, M., Daniels, J., Peters, T. C., Parmar, N., Law, D., et al. (2005). How informed is online informed consent? *Ethics and Behavior, 15*(1), 37-48.

World Federation of Occupational Therapists. (2005). *Code of ethics*. Western Australia, Australia: Author.

SELECTED LIST OF EVIDENCE-BASED PRACTICE RESOURCES

Moral Conflict and Ethical Dilemmas

Barnitt, R. (1998). Ethical dilemmas in occupational therapy and physical therapy: A survey of practitioners in the UK National Health Service. *Journal of Medical Ethics, 24*(3), 193-199.

Foye, S. J., Kirschner, K. L., Brady Wagner, L. C., Stocking, C., & Siegler, M. (2002) Ethical issues in rehabilitation: A qualitative analysis of dilemmas identified by occupational therapists. *Top Stroke Rehabilitation, 9*(3), 89-101.

Kälvemark, S., Höglund, A. T., Hansson, M. G., Westerholm, P., & Arnetz, B. (2004). Living with conflicts: Ethical dilemmas and moral distress in the health care system. *Social Science and Medicine, 58*(6), 1075-1084.

Kassberg, A. C., & Skär, L. (2008). Experiences of ethical dilemmas in rehabilitation: Swedish occupational therapists' perspectives. *Scandinavian Journal of Occupational Therapy, 15*(4), 204-211.

Kirschner, K. L., Stocking, C., Wagner, L. B., Foye, S. J., & Siegler, M. (2001) Ethical issues identified by rehabilitation clinicians. *Archives of Physical Medicine and Rehabilitation, 82*(12 Suppl. 2), S2-S8.

Mukherjee, D., Brashler, R., Savage, T. A., & Kirschner, K. L. (2009). Moral distress in rehabilitation professionals: Results from a hospital ethics survey. *PM & R, 1*(5), 450-458.

Scheirton, L. S., Mu, K., Lohman, H., & Cochran, T. M. (2007). Error and patient safety: ethical analysis of cases in occupational and physical therapy practice. *Medicine, Health Care and Philosophy, 10*(3), 301-311.

PRINCIPLES AND VALUES

Cox, D. J. (2012). From interdisciplinary to integrated care of the child with autism: The essential role for a code of ethics. *Journal of Autism and Developmental Disorders, 42*(12), 2729-2738.

Dige, M. (2009). Occupational therapy, professional development, and ethics. *Scandinavian Journal of Occupational Therapy, 16*(2), 88-98.

Autonomy and Independence

Cardol, M., De Jong, B, A,, & Ward, C. D. (2002). On autonomy and participation in rehabilitation. *Disability and Rehabilitation, 24*(18), 970-974; discussion 975-1004.

Russell, C., Fitzgerald, M. H., Williamson, P., Manor, D., & Whybrow, S. (2002). Independence as a practice issue in occupational therapy: The safety clause. *American Journal of Occupational Therapy, 56*(4), 369-379.

Tamaru, A., McColl, M. A., & Yamasaki, S. (2007). Understanding "independence": Perspectives of occupational therapists. *Disability and Rehabilitation, 29*(13), 1021-1033.

Utilitarianism

Levack, W. M. (2009). Ethics in goal planning for rehabilitation: A utilitarian perspective. *Clinical Rehabilitation, 23*(4), 345-351.

Ethical Decision Making and Reasoning

Dieruf, K. (2004). Ethical decision-making by students in physical and occupational therapy. *Journal of Allied Health, 3*(1), 24-30.

Martinez, R. (2000). A model for boundary dilemmas: Ethical decision-making in the patient-professional relationship. *Ethical Human Sciences and Services, 2*(1), 43-61.

Opacich, K. J. (1997). Moral tensions and obligations of occupational therapy practitioners providing home care. *American Journal of Occupational Therapy, 51*(6), 430-435.

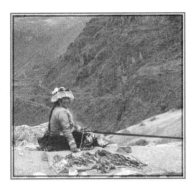

LOCAL TO GLOBAL RESOURCES FOR THE OCCUPATIONAL THERAPY PROFESSIONAL

Diane Sauter-Davis, MA, OTR/L

ACOTE STANDARDS EXPLORED IN THIS CHAPTER
B.6.6, B.9.2

KEY VOCABULARY

- **Attitude:** Your mindset or outlook.
- **Career:** A line of business or way of making a living.
- **Knowledge:** What one knows.

- **Profession:** An occupation requiring extensive education or specialized training.
- **Professional:** A person engaged in a profession.

Introduction

Have you ever really considered what it means to be "a professional"? How is a profession different from a career? A career is a line of business or a way of making a living. A career may or may not be a profession. Many people choose careers, but not all people choose professions.

The word *profession* is defined as "an occupation requiring extensive education or specialized training" (Encarta, 2009). This stems from the verb *to profess*—to declare public acknowledgement of something. To profess has been historically associated with religion and/or adherence to religious beliefs.

A professional is one who is engaged in a profession. Professionals engage in particular ways known and sanctioned by their profession. In occupational therapy, we

agree to specific ethics, language, and methods of engagement. Following these principles and employing professional behaviors is called *professionalization*.

If we look at these definitions, we begin to understand that being a professional is more than simply having knowledge and skill. A profession includes shared perspectives in knowledge, attitudes, and behaviors. Professionals demonstrate these shared beliefs, behaviors and standards.

- What is the value of professional knowledge, attitudes, and behaviors relative to being a professional?

- Knowledge is what you know, attitude is your mindset or outlook, and behavior is what you do or your actions. In order to be a "professional," these three things must be aligned and integrated. Employing one of these without the other limits an otherwise skillful practitioner.

Jacobs, K., MacRae, N., & Sladyk, K. (Eds.).
Occupational Therapy Essentials for Clinical Competence, Second Edition (pp. 647-662).

- How does this connect with the topic of professional associations? Why is participation in professional associations an important part of being a professional?

The following words are synonyms for *association*— organization, group, union, alliance, connection, and link (Encarta, 2009). The commonality of these terms leads us to believe that an association is a supportive network for a group of people with a similar declaration. Therefore, the knowledge, attitudes, and behaviors of professional members are shaped, in part, by the professional associations in which they participate. Belonging to an organization that believes in you and understands your mission is vital to your growth as a professional. Professional associations are groups that support, develop, and sustain your growth as a professional. They provide opportunities for networking, contributing, and promoting occupational therapy.

How Are Professions Shaped?

Professions are dynamic, interactive entities. They are open systems, much like humans are open systems. Associations affect and are affected by internal and external factors. The internal factors include member issues— member needs, member wants, member attitudes, and member behaviors, to name a few. External factors may include public perceptions, public policy, funding, and environmental demands.

More diversity within associations increases the opportunities for the members, and therefore the organization, to change and grow. These growth opportunities shape both the internal and external factors. Simply stated, if you want to affect the direction of your profession, an association is a place to begin!

Occupational Therapy Resources

In this chapter, you will become familiar with associations specific to occupational therapy, some general information about governing bodies and groups within the American Occupational Therapy Association (AOTA), and organizations related to occupational therapy that provide networking functions.

You will also learn the process of how a professional begins to participate in their profession. The following is a list of resources that will be discussed.

- Accreditation Council for Occupational Therapy Education (ACOTE)
- American Occupational Therapy Association (AOTA)
- The Fund to Promote Awareness of Occupational Therapy

- Affiliated State Association Presidents (ASAP) State Occupational Therapy Associations—all 50 states, Washington DC, and Puerto Rico have local associations
- American Occupational Therapy Political Action Committee (AOTAPAC)
- American Occupational Therapy Foundation (AOTF)
- World Federation of Occupational Therapists (WFOT)
- The Canadian Association of Occupational Therapists (CAOT)
- Australian Association of Occupational Therapists (OT Australia)
- Council for Occupational Therapists for the European Countries (COTEC)
- National Board for Certification in Occupational Therapy (NBCOT)
- Rehabilitation Engineering and Assistive Technology Society of North America (RESNA)
- American Society of Hand Therapists (ASHT)
- Human Factors and Ergonomics Society (HFES)

Accreditation Council for Occupational Therapy Education

Vision Statement

ACOTE is committed to the establishment, promotion, and evaluation of standards of excellence in occupational therapy education. To this end, ACOTE will lead in the development of effective collaborative partnerships with the communities of interest, both internal and external to the profession of occupational therapy, which are affected by its activities. (AOTA, 2008a)

Mission Statement

The mission of ACOTE is to foster the development and accreditation of quality occupational therapy education programs. By establishing rigorous standards for occupational therapy education, ACOTE supports the preparation of competent occupational therapy practitioners. (AOTA, 2008a)

ACOTE 2011 Standards for Accredited Educational Programs for the Occupational Therapist and the

Occupational Therapy Assistant determine that emerging occupational therapy practitioners must understand the value of professional associations. The standard addressed in this chapter is as follows:

> OT Standard B.9.2: Discuss and justify how the role of a professional is enhanced by knowledge of and involvement in international, national, state, and local occupational therapy associations and related professional associations and OTA Standard B.9.2: Explain and give examples of how the role of a professional is enhanced by knowledge of and involvement in international, national, state, and local occupational therapy associations and related professional Associations (ACOTE, 2012)

To completely appreciate the importance of this standard within the educational context, occupational therapy students must have a basic understanding of each organization and its relationship(s) to occupational therapy.

American Occupational Therapy Association

HISTORY OF THE AMERICAN OCCUPATIONAL THERAPY ASSOCIATION

AOTA is the nationally recognized professional association of more than 42,000 occupational therapists, occupational therapy assistants, and students of occupational therapy (AOTA, 2008b). The history of AOTA begins with the National Society for the Promotion of Occupational Therapy founded in 1917 and incorporated under the laws of the District of Columbia. The founders included a passionate group of advocates for occupation: William Rush Dunton, a psychiatrist who coined the term *occupation therapy* and served as the first president of the National Society for the Promotion of Occupational Therapy; Susan Tracy, an "occupational" nurse; George Barton, an architect by profession who contracted tuberculosis as an adult and became a firm believer in the value of occupation and occupational therapy; and Eleanor Clarke Slagle, an educator, social worker, and superintendent of occupational therapy at the Hull House (Padilla, 2005).

The *Essentials* were the skills deemed necessary for all occupational therapists in 1935. The term *essentials* was used by ACOTE through 1991 to recognize the criteria and guidelines established for all occupational therapy education (occupational therapist and occupational therapy assistant). ACOTE currently uses the term *standards* to connote the educational requirements for all entry-level occupational therapy practitioners.

AMERICAN OCCUPATIONAL THERAPY ASSOCIATION MISSION STATEMENT

> The American Occupational Therapy Association advances the quality, availability, use, and support of occupational therapy through standard-setting, advocacy, education, and research on behalf of its members and the public (AOTA, 2006).

AMERICAN OCCUPATIONAL THERAPY ASSOCIATION CENTENNIAL VISION

AOTA advances occupational therapy as the preeminent profession in promoting the health, productivity, and quality of life of individuals and society through the therapeutic application of occupation (Padilla, 2005). With extensive input from the membership over a 2-year period, the Centennial Vision statement adopted by the AOTA Board of Directors in January 2006 was approved by the Representative Assembly (RA) in April 2006.

"We envision that occupational therapy is a powerful, widely recognized, science-driven, and evidence-based profession with a globally connected and diverse workforce meeting society's occupational needs" (AOTA, 2006). This statement allows us to celebrate our past and to determine our future. In 2017, both AOTA and the profession will turn 100. How will you celebrate 100 years of occupational therapy? Where will occupational therapy be in the 21st century? What will you do to promote the occupational therapy profession of the future? Both the mission and the Centennial Vision help occupational therapy practitioners to understand the direction of their profession.

We can begin to see what the future holds for occupational therapy. What opportunities and threats face occupational therapy in the years ahead? What strengths do we have to position our profession for the future? What weaknesses must we acknowledge to grow, change, and respond effectively?

Figure 49-1 depicts the strategic efforts of AOTA from 2010 to 2013. Strategic plans are guiding statements set by organizations to assist them in achieving effective outcomes. This strategic plan describes the priorities that AOTA plans to use to assure that occupational therapy is well positioned for the future.

AMERICAN OCCUPATIONAL THERAPY ASSOCIATION GOVERNANCE STRUCTURE

AOTA as an Organization

AOTA is a nonprofit association that uses a system of paid and volunteer positions to systematically complete the work that needs to be done. AOTA utilizes a structure

At that time, the mission of the Association, as set forth in its Constitution, shall be to study and advance curative occupations for invalids and convalescents; to gather news of progress in occupational therapy and to use such knowledge to the common good; to encourage original research, to promote cooperation among occupational therapy societies, and with other agencies of rehabilitation.

About 3 years after its incorporation, the Association was urged by several leading physicians and authorities on hospital administration to establish a national register or directory of occupational therapists "for the protection of hospitals and institutions from unqualified persons posing as occupational therapists."

After careful consideration and on the advice of other national organizations in the field of medicine, the Association decided that the first step toward the establishment of a national register or directory was the establishment of minimum standards of training for occupational therapists.

In 1921, the name of the Association was changed to the American Occupational Therapy Association (AOTA). In 1923, accreditation of educational programs became a stated function of the AOTA, and basic educational standards were developed.

AOTA approached the Council on Medical Education of the American Medical Association (AMA) in 1933 to request cooperation in the development and improvement of educational programs for occupational therapists.

The Essentials of an Acceptable School of Occupational Therapy were adopted by the AMA House of Delegates in 1935. This action represented the first cooperative accreditation activity by the AMA. In 1958, AOTA assumed responsibility for approval of educational programs for the occupational therapy assistant. The standards on which accreditation was based were modeled after the Essentials established for baccalaureate programs.

In 1964, the AOTA/AMA collaborative relationship in accreditation was officially recognized by the National Commission on Accrediting (NCA). The NCA was a private agency serving as a coordinating agency for accrediting activities in higher education. Although it had no legal authority, it had great influence on educational accreditation through the listing of accrediting agencies it recommended to its members. The NCA continued its activities in a merger with the Federation of Regional Accrediting Commissions of Higher Education since January 1975. The new organization was the Council on Postsecondary Accreditation (COPA).

In 1990, AOTA petitioned the Committee on Allied Health Education and Accreditation (CAHEA) to include the accreditation of the occupational therapy assistant programs in the CAHEA system. Following approval of the change by the AMA Council on Medical Education, CAHEA petitioned both COPA and the U.S. Department of Education (USDE) for recognition as the accrediting body for occupational therapy assistant education.

In 1991, occupational therapy assistant programs, with approval status from the AOTA Accreditation Committee, became accredited by CAHEA/AMA in collaboration with the AOTA Accreditation Committee.

On January 1, 1994, the AOTA Accreditation Committee changed its name to the AOTA Accreditation Council for Occupational Therapy Education (ACOTE) and became operational as an accrediting agency independent of CAHEA/AMA.

During 1994, the ACOTE became listed by the USDE as a nationally recognized accrediting agency for professional programs in the field of occupational therapy. The ACOTE was also granted initial recognition by the Commission on Recognition of Postsecondary Accreditation (CORPA). CORPA was the nongovernmental recognition agency for accrediting bodies that was formed when the Council on Postsecondary Accreditation (COPA) dissolved in 1994.

On March 1, 1994, 197 previously accredited/approved and developing occupational therapy and occupational therapy assistant educational programs were transferred into the ACOTE accreditation system.

In a ballot election concluded October 31, 1994, the AOTA membership approved the proposed AOTA Bylaws Amendment that reflected the creation of AOTA's new accrediting body and establishment of the ACOTE as a standing committee of the AOTA Executive Board.

The Council on Higher Education Accreditation (CHEA) is presently the nongovernmental agency for accrediting bodies that replaced the Commission on Recognition of Postsecondary Accreditation (CORPA). In February, 1997, CHEA voted to accept CORPA's recognition status of ACOTE.

Reproduced with permission from American Occupational Therapy Association. (2009a). *History of AOTA accreditation.* Retrieved from www.aota.org/Educate/accredit/overview/38124.aspx

American Occupational Therapy Association Strategic Goals and Objectives 2010–2013

1. Building the profession's capacity to fulfill its potential and mission
   - Prepare occupational therapists and occupational therapy assistants for the 21st century.
   - Ensure a diverse workforce for multiple roles.
   - Increase the profession's research capacity and productivity.
   - Strengthen our capacity to influence and lead.
   - Enhance collaboration with international partners and state affiliates.
2. Demonstrating and articulating our value to individuals, organizations, and communities
   - Increase public understanding of the profession and its value in meeting diverse health and participation needs.
   - Support traditional occupational therapy roles and foster the development of emerging practice areas to help meet society's health, wellness, and quality of life needs.
   - Engage proactively with key external organizations and decision makers to assert occupational therapy leadership in essential areas of societal need.
3. Linking education, research, and practice
   - Promote stronger linkages and collaboration among the occupational therapy research, education, and practice communities.
   - Facilitate dissemination of occupational therapy knowledge to foster innovation in research, education, and practice.
   - Promote the dissemination and application of evidence-based knowledge.
4. Creating an inclusive community of members
   - Work to meet the needs of members across the diverse professional roles in practice, education, and research, and increase member satisfaction.
   - Expand outreach to occupational therapists, occupational therapy assistants, and students to grow membership.
   - Foster opportunities for active member participation, recognition, and leadership, and promote and develop volunteer leadership excellence.
5. Securing the financial resources to invest in the profession's ability to respond to societal needs
   - Actively monitor internal and environmental trends affecting operations.
   - Monitor current and prospective members' needs and expectations.
   - Exercise transparency and accountability in management practices.
   - Work to expand and diversify revenue streams.

Figure 49-1. AOTA Strategic Goals and Objectives 2010–2013. (Reprinted with permission from AOTA. Approved by the AOTA Board of Directors, 2012.)

that employs an executive director. This individual is a paid employee with experience running nonprofits and may or may not be an occupational therapy practitioner. An organizational chart helps to define the reporting mechanisms within an organization. The primary governance bodies of AOTA are outlined in Figure 49-2.

Governance Bodies

AOTA's governance system (Figure 49-3) consists of various and interdependent bodies. These include: Board of Directors, Organizational Advisors, Representative Assembly, Bodies of the Assembly, and the Associated Body of the Board.

The *Board of Directors* has the responsibility to govern the affairs of the Association in accordance with all duly vested statutory, corporate, and bylaws powers. There are voting members including four officers (President, Vice President, Secretary, and Treasurer), six Directors and the RA Speaker and four nonvoting members including the President-Elect, a Public Advisor, a Consumer Advisor and the AOTA Executive Director.

The purpose of the *Organizational Advisors* is to provide information to the Board regarding strategic planning and budgeting with respect to matters with the expertise of the specific Organizational Advisor. The advisors include Accreditation Council for Occupational Therapy Education (ACOTE) Chairperson, American Occupational Therapy Foundation (AOTF) President, American Occupational Therapy Association Political Action Committee (AOTPAC) Chairperson, Affiliated State Association Presidents (ASAP) Chairperson, Assembly of Student Delegates (ASD) Chairperson, and World Federation of Occupational Therapists (WFOT) Delegate.

The *Representative Assembly*, often referred to as the Assembly, is the legislative body of AOTA and is directly responsible for the policies affecting the direction of the profession.

The *Bodies of the Assembly* have the authority to establish bodies as necessary to carry out the purposes of the Representative Assembly. The Assembly establishes the

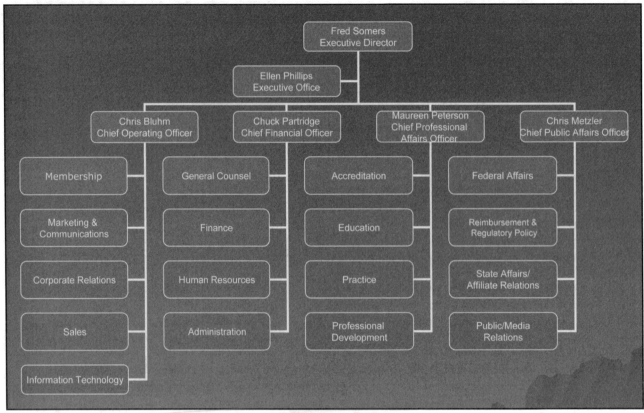

Figure 49-2. AOTA organizational chart. (Reprinted with permission from AOTA.)

membership criteria for all such bodies. The Association has the following entities:

- *Commission on Education (COE):* Promotes the quality of education for OTs and OTAs relative to educator, student, and consumer needs.

- *Commission on Practice (COP):* Promotes and guides best practice in and standards for occupational therapy relative to practitioner and consumer needs.

- *Ethics Commission (EC):* Serves the Association members and public through the identification, development, review, interpretation, and education of the AOTA Occupational Therapy Code of Ethics and Ethics Standards (2010) and to provide the process whereby the ethics of the Association are enforced.

- *Commission on Continuing Competence and Professional Development (CCCPD):* Promotes continuing competence and professional development in the profession in accordance with the Association's standards for continuing competence.

- *Agenda Committee:* Facilitates the business of the Assembly.

- *Bylaws, Policies, Procedures Committee (BPPC):* Reviews Association governance documents and

recommends changes to the appropriate body for their consideration.

- *Credentials Review and Accountability Committee (CRAC):* Ensures that Representatives and Alternate Representatives from each election area, including the OTAs and the ASD, meet the qualifications to be members of the Assembly.

- *Nominating Recognitions:* Prepares slates of eligible candidates for Association elections and solicits nominations and selects recipients for all Association recognitions and awards.

- *Special Interest Sections Council (SISC):* Coordinates and facilitates the activities of the Special Interest Sections (SISs) with the bodies of the Association.

- *Representative Assembly Coordinating Council (RACC):* Coordinates the activities and manages integrated projects of the COE, COP, EC, CCCPD, and SISC.

- *RA Leadership Team (RALT):* Plans, manages, and expedites the work of the Assembly.

- *Assembly of Student Delegates (ASD):* Provides an opportunity for student members to have input into decision making and actions of the Association, promotes well-being of students, and enhances students' knowledge and structure of the Association.

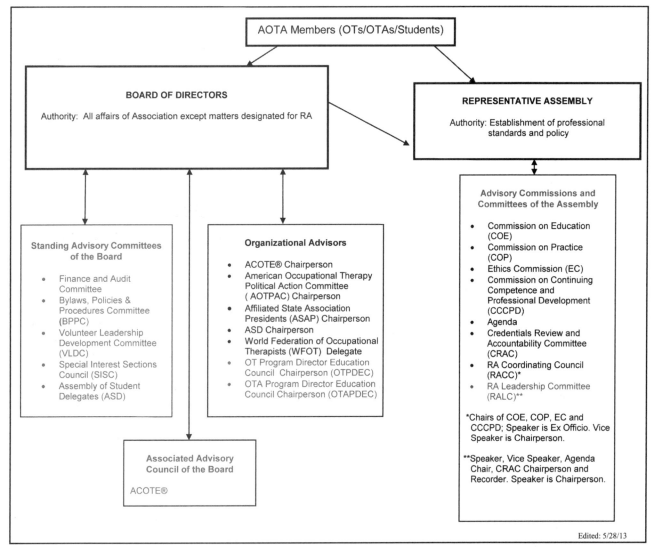

Figure 49-3. AOTA governance chart 2012–2013. (Reprinted with permission from AOTA.)

- *ACOTE* is the Associated Body of the Board whose purpose is to accredit occupational therapy educational programs and occupational therapy assistant educational programs. ACOTE establishes, approves, and administers educational standards to evaluate occupational therapy and occupational therapy assistant educational programs. ACOTE establishes its own policies and procedures (AOTA, 2012).

How Can You Get Involved?

How can you become a part of AOTA? What voice will you have in the future of your profession? You can become a member at any time. The fees are adjusted according to member categories and qualifications. Your membership cycle is unique to you. AOTA will invoice you at the same time each year. As a member, you receive the *American Journal of Occupational Therapy* (AJOT), *OT Practice*, and access to all SIS networks and subscriptions, as well as member-only Web site information. You can choose one printed *SIS Quarterly*. Students have two choices: Student Plus and Standard Student membership. As a Student Plus member, you receive full member benefits plus the Student Plus fieldwork list serve. You can be an active member of AOTA through the committee, surveys, or state leadership. It takes a diverse volunteer network to create a successful member association. You may have the skills needed to help your organization.

American Occupational Therapy Association Annual Conference and Exposition

AOTA holds its national conference and exposition each spring. The conference changes geographically each year to support all members' access. There are workshops, symposiums, and luncheons with experts. The exhibition hall is filled with an array of tools and resources for practitioners. There are opportunities to meet occupational therapy practitioners from around the nation and the world. Conference is a great opportunity to learn, network, and explore. You can find out more about occupational therapy, how to get involved, and about AOTA's conference on AOTA's Web site at www.aota.org.

WHY GET INVOLVED IN ANY PROFESSIONAL ORGANIZATION?

There are as many reasons to get involved in professional organizations as there are professions. The following are some of the reasons you will find to get involved:

- To direct health policy for occupational therapy
- To gain political power as a professional unit
- To stay informed and up to date
- To deliver best occupational therapy practice
- To secure occupational therapy as a profession for the future
- To contribute to your profession
- To advocate for your profession
- To share your skills with occupational therapy practitioners and non-occupational therapy practitioners alike

THE FUND TO PROMOTE AWARENESS OF OCCUPATIONAL THERAPY

The Fund to Promote Awareness of Occupational Therapy is an Independent 501C3 created by AOTA in 2002 with AOTA as the sole member. AOTA created the Fund as part of a long-term strategy to raise awareness of occupational therapy.

The Fund is committed to ongoing resource development to support targeted education, research, and professional development opportunities that will increase the public's understanding and utilization of occupational therapy services.

See updated personal testimonies about the value of being involved in a professional organization at the end of the chapter.

Their mission statement reads as follows: "The fund is committed to ongoing resource development to support targeted education, research, and professional development opportunities that will increase the public's understanding of occupational therapy. The Fund exists to achieve greater understanding, availability, and use of occupational therapy and to promote the profession's contributions to health, wellness, participation, productivity, and quality of life in society" (Fund to Promote Awareness of Occupational Therapy, n.d.).

The Fund's vision statement is as follows: "The Fund to Promote Awareness of Occupational Therapy facilitates society's understanding of and demand for occupational therapy and the profession's capacity to bring its virtues to more people in existing and future practice and policy environments" (Fund to Promote Awareness of Occupational Therapy, n.d.).

THE VALUE OF BELONGING TO ASSOCIATIONS—PERSONAL TESTIMONIES

Several case studies describing the value of belonging to Associations are included in the boxes.

Affiliated State Association Presidents

HISTORY

ASAP is a standing committee in the AOTA Bylaws. It is a body of the AOTA Board of Directors. ASAP began in 2001 with the Standing Committee called Chapter State Association Presidents (CSAP). CSAP and AOTA entered into an affiliation agreement. An affiliate is a professional organization of occupational therapists, occupational therapy assistants, and students that has been recognized by the national association. Affiliates represent members located within an individual state, commonwealth, the District of Columbia, or Puerto Rico (AOTA, 2009b). The name of the standing committee was changed to ASAP to reflect the affiliate status. A state becomes an affiliate of the AOTA through the process described in the *Affiliation Principles for AOTA and State Associations*. Continued recognition is dependent on compliance with the *Affiliation Principles* and termination can occur for the reasons and through the process described in the *Affiliation Principles* (AOTA, 2009b).

PURPOSE

The purpose of the affiliation is to foster communication and collaboration between AOTA and state associations (AOTA, 2009b).

MISSION

The mission of ASAP is to be the voice and resource that supports the practice of occupational therapy at the state level by representing state affiliate members to AOTA.

Communicating and networking with state affiliates as well as AOTA Training and mentoring state affiliate leadership Advising AOTA Board of Directors and RA. (AOTA, n.d.)

Over 49 Years in OT

My experience of over 49 years in occupational therapy practice began with studying at the Philadelphia School of Occupational Therapy, newly affiliated with the University of Pennsylvania. Two remarkable professors, Helen Willard and Clare Spackman, introduced me to the profession and the responsibilities of local, state, national, and international involvement. This is what I did, beginning with their firm philosophical base of what occupational therapy was and could provide to society.

My high school and undergraduate liberal arts education led me to interest in health, social issues, psychology, and cultural differences. In my clinical practice following postgraduate education and credentialing, I had the opportunity to meet many occupational therapists from other countries working in the United States. Association with them at State Association meetings informed me of programs in their countries and differences in practice perspectives and techniques. All of my classmates joined AOTA and learned more about different practices on the east and west coasts and internationally. I also learned from my participation on the Council on Practice and International Committee.

Following my independent extended travel in Europe, I received a fellowship to work in France, assisted by the AOTA and the World Rehabilitation Fund. This experience continued my association with AOTA, the French Occupational Therapy Association, and the World Federation of Occupational Therapists (WFOT). On return to the United States, I was able to continue all organization and association levels, which led to representing the Maine Occupational Therapy Association at the AOTA Representative Assembly, 2nd Alternate and 1st Alternate of the AOTA to the WFOT, to Chair the WFOT International Committee and to serve eventually as 1st Vice President of the WFOT.

My attention to the colleagues I met at all of these levels enabled me to have the opportunity to teach at two universities, to write for a major textbook, and to give presentations in this country and abroad. A further extension of these levels of occupational therapy experience was my representation of the WFOT to the Pan American Region of the World Health Organization.

My work interactively in this and other countries and my clinical practice has been enhanced by the initial strength of the philosophical base of occupational therapy in school. Working up the levels of organizations was a continual challenge and enlightenment of the possibilities of occupational therapy services to the variety of people and problems we have the privilege to meet. My life has been enriched by my involvement and practice of occupational therapy. I could not have made a better choice.

E. Anne Spencer, BA, OTR/L, MA, FAOTA

38 Years in OT

I entered the profession of Occupational Therapy in 1975 in a rural part of central Maine as a solo practitioner. Shortly into my career, I knew intuitively that I needed to connect with the OTs practicing in the area, but how to find them? Around this time, the Maine Occupational Therapy Association (MeOTA) was forming and that became the avenue for me to find other practitioners. Those first Maine state meetings drew fewer than 30 therapists but we were a hearty bunch—those relationships grew strong and steadfast over many years. We took on many key roles in developing our state association—we served as state officers, created our bylaws, grew our membership, collected dues, started a newsletter, sponsored continuing education opportunities, represented Maine to the AOTA, and worked with AOTA to develop our Maine OT Licensure. Seems like we did it all!

My first "official" duty in our State Association was to represent Maine to the AOTA Representative Assembly. This experience really clarified the critical connection between the "grass roots" state practitioners with the national organization. From this position, I shifted my commitment and served the State Association as the Legislative Committee Chair. I later served as the Continuing Education Chair and the State Association President.

Over these many years, the Maine OT Association has enabled me to network and collaborate with many colleagues across the state from all areas of OT practice. These professional relationships, based on mutual support and respect, have formed the cornerstone of my continuing competence as an OT practitioner. Now, 38 years later, I participate at the State Association Annual Conferences and serve on the State OT Licensure Board.

Kathy Adams, OTR/L, ATP

State Associations

Mission

The missions of all state occupational therapy associations are different, but all associations are designed to support members. The action statement of many State associations, similar to AOTA's mission, is to promote, foster, support, and advance occupational therapy within that particular state. State associations do not credential, license, certify, or enforce polices. The following is an example of a state mission: "The Maine Occupational Therapy Association [MeOTA] is committed to promoting the profession of Occupational Therapy and supporting all Occupational Therapy practitioners in the State of Maine" (MeOTA, 2006).

8 Years in OT

I graduated from Kennebec Valley Community College in 2004 and was excited to learn more about how my profession supported its practitioners and communities. Consequently, I became a member of MeOTA as a student, and I continued to be part of my state association long after graduation. As a new OT practitioner, I found myself employed in a large hospital, the new therapist among a very large group of clinicians. I soon discovered that this was the perfect environment for a young practitioner; I had 40+ seasoned therapists whom I could question, learn from, and call upon for help when I felt stuck. Clinically, this was a gift. Professionally, I at times felt adrift. All throughout college, I was strongly tied to our student OT group, and thoroughly enjoyed this connection to the "big picture" of occupational therapy practice. My intimate journey within the Maine OT community began. It was in school that I learned how valuable memberships and volunteering could be on a national level with AOTA, on a state level with the Maine Occupational Therapy Association (MeOTA) and locally with my alma mater's OTA advisory board. Along the way, I had champions who encouraged and helped me reach outside my comfort zone to become engaged in volunteering within my profession.

AOTA has supported me with tools, legislative support, and a framework to safely practice. However, it is the last of these two affiliations that allowed me to grow both personally and professionally with ever-increasing leadership roles. Entry into leadership originated with little steps during my first year in college as I joined my college's OTA advisory board as a student. Several years later I became its chair, which offered insight and involvement for its future OTA practitioners. Finally, teaching at the college as adjunct faculty brought it all full circle; it helped me become a better practitioner in practice.

When I first joined MeOTA, I served as a member of its conference committee. Eventually, I served on its executive board as the OTA representative. This position allowed me the opportunity to offer learning opportunities to all OT practitioners and representing the OT community with legislative insights and involvement with licensure feedback opportunities. OT practitioners have many opportunities to shape their own paths for involvement in occupational therapy; this has been mine.

Rebecca Cirillo, COTA/L, CAPS

5 Years in OT

I got involved in my state organization soon after graduation by serving as a regional representative for MeOTA. I felt that feeling of being adrift slowly fade away. I now felt tied to my profession in a way that connected the dots on a state and national level. I saw that the clinical successes I experienced needed to be communicated on a larger scale to our legislators to ensure reimbursement and future support for occupational therapy practice. I found that many of my fellow practitioners were struggling with the same issues, and together we could network and creatively solve these challenges. I found that my voice as an OT practitioner was much more powerful when combined with many others from across the state. I learned things about how legislative action really happens, and what membership in professional associations really does to advance and support my everyday practice as a clinician.

When the opportunity to serve as president of our state association came forward, I accepted that challenge, knowing that the skills I might acquire by serving and giving back in this way would only strengthen me as a clinician. While there are certainly challenging days, the lessons I have learned and professional relationships that have formed far outweigh the difficult days and frustrating moments. These opportunities through my state association continue to sharpen my professional skills, and also open doors to more opportunities for growth as an OT professional.

Carrie Beal, MS, OTR/L

Organizational Structure

Organizational structures of many state associations are similar to the organizational structure of AOTA. Some states hire Executive Directors or managers to fulfill leadership duties, but many rely on volunteer leadership elected by membership.

How Can You Get Involved in Your State Association?

Each state association is different, but all state associations have opportunities for involvement. State associations for occupational therapy provide a professional network for members. They serve the interests of members, represent the profession to the public, and promote access to occupational therapy.

State associations are volunteer organizations run by members, for members. Each membership year is unique to each state. It is important to find out the membership cycle for your state's association.

You can seek out information about how to contact your state association president or RA delegate on the AOTA Web site. You can also ask any occupational therapy program within your state how you can access your state's association Web site. There are many opportunities at the state level. Most positions within state associations are volunteer positions and all welcome participation from members. If you desire, you can belong to several state associations concurrently.

American Occupational Therapy Political Action Committee

WHAT IS A POLITICAL ACTION COMMITTEE?

A political action committee (PAC) is the legally sanctioned vehicle through which organizations, such as AOTA, can engage in otherwise prohibited political action and work to influence the outcome of Federal elections. The concept of PACs is described more thoroughly in Chapter 55, so we will include a brief description of AOTPAC: "AOTA hires its own lobbyist to represent occupational therapy issues on Capitol Hill. These people are knowledgeable about the legislative process and OT" (Stephens, 2006).

AOTPAC is a voluntary, nonprofit, unincorporated committee of members of AOTA. AOTPAC was authorized by the RA in 1976 and has been operational since the spring of 1978. The purpose of AOTPAC is to further the legislative aims of AOTA by influencing or attempting to influence the selection, nomination, election, or appointment of any individual to any Federal public office, and of any occupational therapist, registered, certified occupational therapy assistant, or occupational therapy student member of AOTA seeking election to public office at any level. The committee is not affiliated with any political party (AOTA, 2007a).

American Occupational Therapy Foundation

The American Occupational Therapy Foundation (AOTF) is a charitable, nonprofit organization created in 1965 to advance the science of occupational therapy and increase public understanding of its value. AOTF

gratefully acknowledges the support provided by AOTA in helping the profession build its capacity to engage in research that guides practice.

AOTA and AOTF have jointly funded occupational therapy research and secured competitive grant funding for research endeavors. AOTF offers over 70 scholarships each year through memorial endowments and partnerships with state associations. AOTF publishes *OTJR: Occupation, Participation and Health Journal* and maintains the content and maintenance of *OT SEARCH* through the Wilma L. West Library, which resides in the Foundation (AOTF, n.d.).

The profession of occupational therapy has networks of member organizations nationally and internationally designed to support and enhance the practice and profession of occupational therapy. These associations are vital to the future of occupational therapy. You can become a part of this integrated community at any time and participate at your comfort level. In turn, these associations will support you in your professional growth.

International Occupational Therapy Organizations

WORLD FEDERATION OF OCCUPATIONAL THERAPISTS

The World Federation of Occupational Therapists (WFOT) is the official international organization for the promotion of occupational therapy. It maintains the ethics of the profession and advances the practice and standards of occupational therapy internationally. It also promotes internationally recognized standards for the education of occupational therapists. WFOT supports and promotes occupational therapy around the world. Currently, there are 57 member countries, including the United States, one of the founding countries (AOTA, 2007b).

You can contribute to the global development and growth of the profession by joining as an individual member of WFOT through your AOTA membership. You will receive the WFOT professional journal (*The Bulletin*) twice a year and have an opportunity to engage in international projects. You can join WFOT by paying additional dues that are required with your AOTA membership. You can access the WFOT Web site at www.wfot.org.

THE CANADIAN ASSOCIATION OF OCCUPATIONAL THERAPISTS

CAOT provides services, products, events, and networking opportunities to help occupational therapists achieve excellence in their professional practice. In addition, CAOT provides national leadership to actively develop and promote the client-centered profession of occupational therapy in Canada and internationally.

The mission of CAOT is to advance excellence in occupational therapy. Their vision is that all people in Canada will value and have access to occupational therapy, and their values include integrity, accountability, respect, and equity (CAOT, n.d.). You can access CAOT at www.caot.ca.

The Australian Association

The vision of Occupational Therapy Australia is to "support our members by providing high-quality, relevant, equitable services focused on their needs." Their mission is to provide member benefits through access to local professional support and resources and through opportunities to contribute to, and shape, professional excellence (OTAUS, n.d.). For more information about OT Australia, go to www.otaus.com.au.

European Associations

The Council for Occupational Therapists for the European Countries (COTEC) is made up of delegates from European national associations of occupational therapists. It aims to develop, harmonize, and improve standards of professional practice and education, as well as to advance the theory of occupational therapy throughout Europe.

COTEC was initially established as a representative Committee of Occupational Therapists for the European Communities. It was founded in 1986 to coordinate the views of the national associations of occupational therapists of the then-Member States of the European Communities. In May 2001, the Committee passed a motion to change the name to Council for Occupational Therapists for the European Countries in view of the inclusion of countries that are not members of the European Union, but being part of Europe share the same aims.

COTEC represents 29 European Occupational Therapy Associations and more than 120,000 Occupational Therapists.

The national associations of a number of other European countries have observer status. All of these associations send delegates to the council meetings. The Council meets in plenary session twice a year to plan and coordinate the ongoing work. These meetings are held in different European countries and are arranged by each host association. You can access COTEC at www.cotec-europe.org.

Resource Organizations

National Board for Certification of Occupational Therapy

The National Board for Certification of Occupational Therapy (NBCOT) is not an association, but it is an important resource for all occupational therapy practitioners. NBCOT is a not-for-profit credentialing agency that provides certification for the occupational therapy profession. NBCOT serves the public interest by developing, administering, and continually reviewing a certification process that reflects current standards of competent practice in occupational therapy. NBCOT works with state regulatory authorities, providing information on credentials, disciplinary actions, and regulatory and certification renewal issues. NBCOT administers, develops, and continually reviews the certification process that reflects the current ACOTE standards.

The mission of NBCOT is to serve the public interest through the certification of occupational therapy practitioners (NBCOT, 2013).

The vision of NBCOT is to be internationally recognized, by all relevant stakeholders, as the premier organization for certifying occupational therapy practitioners and for promoting quality in the provision of occupational therapy services to consumers through the initial and ongoing certification of occupational therapy practitioners (NBCOT, 2013).

The following information includes some, but not all, of the other organizations/associations that might have occupational therapy practitioners as members. There are many associated organizations that support specific areas of interest and expertise.

Rehabilitation Engineering and Assistive Technology Society of North America

The Rehabilitation Engineering and Assistive Technology Society of North America (RESNA) is an example of an association that supports the needs of people with disabilities. Occupational therapy practitioners with an interest in assistive technology might join RESNA for education and support. RESNA is an interdisciplinary association of people with a common interest in technology and disability. RESNA's goal is to maximize the health and well-being of people with disabilities through technology. They do this through scientific, literary, professional, and educational activities. (RESNA, 2013).

AMERICAN SOCIETY OF HAND THERAPISTS

The American Society of Hand Therapists (ASHT) is a professional organization comprising licensed occupational and physical therapists who specialize in the treatment and rehabilitation of the upper extremity (ASHT, n.d.). Hand therapists are occupational or physical therapists who "through advanced study and experience specialize in treating individuals with conditions affecting the hands and upper extremities. A hand specialist may also have advanced certification as a Certified Hand Therapist (CHT)" (ASHT, n.d.).

HUMAN FACTORS AND ERGONOMICS SOCIETY

The mission of the HFES is to promote the discovery and exchange of knowledge concerning the characteristics of human beings that are applicable to the design of systems and devices of all kinds. The HFES considers how people function effectively in their activities and advocates the systematic use of this knowledge to achieve compatibility in the design of interactive systems of people, machines, and environments to ensure their effectiveness, safety, and ease of performance.

Summary

Becoming a professional does not just happen when you receive your diploma or your occupational therapy credential; you become a professional over time. Through collaboration, professional alliances, and engagement in your profession you will gain the knowledge and skill competence that makes you a 21st-century practitioner. The attitudes and behaviors of skillful practitioners shape the occupational therapy profession and are shaped, in part, by the professional associations in which they participate. Belonging to organizations that share your understanding of occupation, your philosophy of self-determination, and your beliefs of health and wellness is vital to your growth as a professional. Your professional associations are member focused, created to support you in your professional quest to be the best.

Student Self-Assessment

Reflection is a continuous process that creates connections and increases engagement. Reflection helps to create the context of experience. Taking the steps to get involved in your profession occurs best with commitment to reflection and competence. Reflective thinking is part of reflective action. It is the bridge between ideas and fact. It helps to integrate your knowledge, attitudes, and behaviors. Together, these are the characteristics of a critical thinking professional.

YOUR READINESS SELF-ASSESSMENT

Table 49-1 is based on reflective thinking. It is the first part of getting involved. It can help you to determine what your role can be in the occupational therapy profession and which level of belonging you may be ready for.

Table 49-2 will help you to determine how to get involved. This is your general action plan. Steps to become involved include the following: Decide to get involved. Determine how much time you can devote to any organization. Will you be a member, active member, leader, etc?

Table 49-1.			
READINESS SELF-ASSESSMENT			
	Knowledge min/mod/max	**Attitude yes/no**	**Behavior yes/no**
1. Are you excited about occupational therapy?			
2. Are you interested in networking?			
3. Are you looking for continuing education opportunities?			
4. Do you have the need for continuing education?			
5. Are you interested in professional development?			
6. Do you like to keep abreast of new information in the field?			
7. Are you looking to connect with other occupational therapy practitioners who have similar ideas about occupational therapy?			
8. Do you want to find out more about particular practice issues?			
9. Are you interested in developing leadership skills?			
10. Do you like small, grassroots organizations?			
11. Are you comfortable promoting occupational therapy?			
12. Would you like to have a mentor?			
13. Would you like to be a mentor?			
14. Do you know the difference between licensure, NBCOT and AOTA, and a state association?			
15. Do you understand how to pursue AOTA(Plus), NBCOT credentials, and licensure (CEUs)?			
16. Are you interested in how public policy affects you as an occupational therapy practitioner?			
17. Are you able to budget the needed funds? a) Can you afford up to $100/year for membership? b) Can you afford more than $100/year for membership?			
18. Do you have multiple competing financial interests?			
19. Are you interested in state, national, international issues (in this order)?			
20. Are you interested in national, state, international issues (in this order)?			
21. Are you interested in international issues and issues focusing on related occupational therapy issues?			
22. Are you planning to search for an occupational therapy job?			
23. Do you think membership makes a difference to your future employers?			
24. Do you think being involved makes a difference?			

- Yes to all: You are ready to engage in any and all association membership activities.
- No to all: You may not be ready to engage in your profession as a member. Review your decision to become a professional.
- Developing your Personal Involvement Plan may help you to determine a direction.
- Yes to 1–9; 11; 14; 17b; 18; 20–24: You are ready for AOTA or State membership.
- Yes to 1–13; 14; 17a; 19; 21–24: You may be better off starting at the state level. Build your connections and your financial resources.

Table 49-2.
PERSONAL INVOLVEMENT PLAN

Areas of Interest
Areas to Explore/Develop
Your Professional Goals
Method/Activity/Resources to Achieve Goal
Target Date
Date Completed Outcome
Adapted from 2006 ACOTE Standards (Form F)

- Determine the cost/benefit of belonging.
- How will you finance your decision?
- What will you gain from your membership?
- Contact organization by Web site, mail, email, or phone.
- Contact an occupational therapy friend, peer, and/or colleague and ask about the benefits of belonging.
- Fill out an application and pay your membership fee. Note your date of membership cycle on your calendar.
- Complete your Personal Involvement Plan. Set goals to explore your new role as a member and your new professional organization.
- Participate as you feel comfortable. Take advantage of the member opportunities. Join committees, contribute your expertise, and mentor a new peer.
- Provide feedback when asked.
- Be solution oriented, not problem focused.
- Enjoy being part of something bigger than yourself.
  - Design your own Personal Involvement Plan. Use the grid on page 664 to help you to determine a path to professional membership.
  - Discuss your readiness assessment with a peer. Develop a dialogue about your plan and your future success as an occupational therapy professional.
  - A. Discuss and justify how the role of a professional is enhanced by knowledge of and involvement in international, national, state, and local occupational therapy associations and related professional associations.
  - B. Now explain and give examples of how the role of a professional is enhanced by knowledge of and involvement in international, national, state, and local occupational therapy associations and related professional associations.

References

Accreditation Council on Occupational Therapy Education. (2012). *ACOTE standards and interpretive guidelines (August 2012).* American Occupational Therapy Association. Retrieved from http://www.aota.org/~/media/Corporate/Files/EducationCareers/Accredit/Policies/ACOTE%20Manual%202013.ashx.

American Occupational Therapy Association. (2006). *AOTA fact sheet: Continuing competence in the occupational therapy profession.* Retrieved from http://www.aota.org/-/media/Corporate/Files/Practice/OTAs/ContComp/CC%20Requirments%20Full%20Final%202012.ashx

American Occupational Therapy Association. (2007a). *American Occupational Therapy Political Action Committee.* Retrieved from http://www.aota.org/Practitioners/Advocacy/AOTPAC/About/36386.aspx

American Occupational Therapy Association. (2007b). *Frequently asked questions about WFOT.* Retrieved from http://www.aota.org/Practitioners/Resources/Intl/WFOT/40549.aspx

American Occupational Therapy Association. (2008a). *ACOTE guidelines and policy statements.* Retrieved from http://www.aota.org/Educate/Accredit/Policies/Policies.aspx

American Occupational Therapy Association. (2008b). *AOTPAC fact sheet.* Retrieved from http://www.aota.org/Practitioners/Advocacy/AOTPAC/About/36338.aspx

American Occupational Therapy Association. (2009a). *History of AOTA accreditation.* Retrieved from www.aota.org/Educate/accredit/overview/38124.aspx

American Occupational Therapy Association. (2009b). *Articles of incorporation: The official bylaws of the American Occupational Therapy Association, Inc.* Retrieved from http://www.aota.org/About/Core/Bylaws.aspx

American Occupational Therapy Association. (2012a). *About AOTA.* Retrieved from http://www.aota.org/About.aspx

American Occupational Therapy Association. (2012b). *Articles of incorporation: The official bylaws of the American Occupational Therapy Association, Inc.* (2012). Retrieved from http://www.aota.org/Governance/Bylaws.aspx?FT=.pdf

American Occupational Therapy Association. (n.d.). *Affiliated State Association Presidents (ASAP) and ASAP Steering Committee.* Retrieved from http://www.aota.org/Governance/Leadership/Leadership/ASAP.aspx

American Occupational Therapy Foundation. (n.d.). *About AOTF.* Retrieved from http://www.aotf.org/aboutaotf.aspx

American Society of Hand Therapists. (n.d.). *Consumer education.* Retrieved from http://www.asht.org/education/consumer.cfm

Canadian Association of Occupational Therapists. (n.d.). *About CAOT.* Retrieved from http://www.caot.ca/default.asp?pageid=2

Encarta. (2009). *"Profession."* Retrieved from http://encarta.msn.com/dictionary_1861736704/profession.html

Fund to Promote Awareness of Occupational Therapy. (n.d.). *About the Fund to Promote Awareness of Occupational Therapy.* Retrieved from www.promoteot.org/AF_AboutTheFund.html

Human Factors and Ergonomics Society. (n.d.). *About HFES.* Retrieved from http://www.hfes.org/web/AboutHFES/about.html

Maine Occupational Therapy Association. (2006). *MeOTA Member handbook.* Cumberland, ME: Author.

National Board for Certification in Occupational Therapy, Inc. *NBCOT®. About us.* Retrieved from http://www.nbcot.org/index.php?option=com_content&view=article&id=40&Itemid=

OT Australia. (n.d.). *Vision and purpose.* Retrieved from http://www.otaus.com.au/about/about-the-association

Padilla, R. (2005). *A professional legacy* (2nd ed.). Bethesda, MD: AOTA Press.

Rehabilitation Engineering and Assistive Technology Society of North America. (2009). *RESNA.* Retrieved from http://www.resna.org/aboutUs/aboutResna/

Stephens, L. (2006). What would the world be without political action? *OT Practice, 11*(10), 6. Retrieved from http://www.aota.org/pubs /otp/1997-2007/columns /capitalbriefing/2006/cb-061206.aspx

Suggested Readings

Braveman, B. (2006). *Leading and managing occupational therapy services.* Philadelphia, PA: F.A. Davis Company.

Hubbard, S. (2005). Professional organizations: Who should join? *American Journal of Occupational Therapy, 59*(1), 113–116.

Solomon, A., & Jacobs, K. (2003). *Management skills for the occupational therapy assistant.* Thorofare, NJ: SLACK Incorporated.

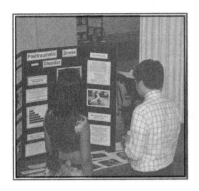

50

PROMOTING OCCUPATIONAL THERAPY TO OTHERS AND THE PUBLIC

Jan Rowe, DrOT, OTR/L, FAOTA

ACOTE STANDARDS EXPLORED IN THIS CHAPTER
B.9.3

KEY VOCABULARY

- **Advertisement:** Something that is shown or presented to the public to help sell a product or to make an announcement; a person or thing that shows how good or effective something is; the act or process of advertising (Merriam-Webster, n.d.).

- **Persuade:** The act of causing people to do or believe something; a particular type of belief or way of thinking (Merriam-Webster, n.d.).
- **Promote:** To help (something) happen, develop, or increase (Merriam-Webster, n.d.).

Introduction

In this chapter, we will discuss the importance of promoting our profession to survive the changes in health care and to be recognized in community participation. As students and occupational therapy practitioners, we need to be comfortable with our roles within the profession. In our profession, we also need to be able to define occupational therapy, regardless of our niche. Occupational therapy is "fine motor skills," "activities of daily living," "handwriting," and "community transportation," but it is also so much more! Occupation is core to our profession. Not using the word occupation in our definition of the profession is a big mistake. The

framework defines occupation as "goal-directed pursuits that typically extend over time, have meaning to the performance, and involve multiple tasks" (American Occupational Therapy Association [AOTA], 2008, p. 672). Students and practitioners alike have the power to educate the public about occupational therapy. Students learn to define occupational therapy for class assignments, during student occupational therapy association activities, in their fieldwork participation, and through state and national events.

Practitioners have daily opportunities to define and promote occupation to clients, stakeholders, organizations, and community members. Just how do we define occupation? Many think of occupational therapy very

Jacobs, K., MacRae, N., & Sladyk, K. (Eds.).
*Occupational Therapy Essentials for
Clinical Competence, Second Edition* (pp. 663-667).
© 2014 SLACK Incorporated.

narrowly. Jamnadas, Burns, and Paul (2001) reported that students from physician assistants and nursing professions had perceived knowledge about occupational therapy, but their awareness of the scope of the profession was very narrow. In fact, most of their knowledge regarded activities of daily living (ADL). These results imply that more information about our profession is needed with other professional programs as well as the general public. Additionally, in 1999, Barnhart interviewed different clinicians as part of her attempt to provide strategies for promotion of the profession. She found that therapists felt that the general public had a lack of awareness about occupational therapy, but certainly the specifics of what we do as occupational therapists are unknown to most (Barnhart, p. 26).

This chapter will explore promotion of our profession through the art of persuasion, advertisement, and assessing the profession's image. Two case studies will be used to explore how occupational therapy practitioners and students can promote the profession within society, in the business world, and to communities to answer the age-old question, "What is occupational therapy?"

Finally, this chapter will include a review of the literature to provide the reader with information on what has been done to promote our profession both within and external to our field. We will look at literature from occupational therapy as well as other health professions such as nursing and physical therapy. While some literature does exist on promotion of the profession, the majority of what was found was anecdotal or "tips for promotion." Image is also important to the survival of a profession. As occupational therapy practitioners, we have all had the question, "What is occupational therapy?" posed to us. Promotion of a person, product, or service relies on an image. What is our occupational therapy image? If a consistent, representative, and catchy image is lacking, consumers, colleagues, and communities will have difficulty remembering who we are and will therefore have difficulty establishing loyalty to our profession (Scarborough & Zimmerer, 2003).

Promotion

In order to effectively promote something, you need to have knowledge or awareness of the item or service, understand what it can do for you, and then believe in it (Barnhart, 1999). Promotion involves savvy persuasion of individuals or groups. Promotion also involves a level of advertisement. Persuasion and advertisement are done in many ways, depending on the personality and skills of the promoter (Scarborough & Zimmerer, 2003).

All occupational therapy practitioners know the value of "selling their goods." Our caseloads, number of community contracts, student recruitments for educational programs, and even number of clients in private practices depend on our skills of "selling." Personal, one-to-one selling does have a significant impact (Jacobs, 1998).

Consider the skills of school children selling candy in their neighborhood to promote and fundraise for a school band. Not all will be promotion savvy, but they believe in the band, and their belief is what drives them. As they make sale after sale, they learn that if you make others believe in your product, they will support it.

Persuasion

Acts of persuasion are as variable as the persuader. From the skills of a 6 year old to the skills of an educated, experienced occupational therapy practitioner, persuasion is powerful if effectively employed. Persuasion involves promotion and can include "publicity, personal selling, and advertising" (Scarborough & Zimmerer, 2003, p. 317). Timing is also included in the art of persuasion. As an effective persuader, you have to know when to pitch the idea, when to push or sell hard, and then when to quit. Leave the other party with just enough information (and contact numbers) and the feeling that this has all been under his or her control. Of course, there is also the strategy of the school child: "Believe it and they will buy." Do not stop talking until they buy the candy, agree to see an occupational therapy practitioner, or choose your educational program over others!

Is one-to-one selling of ideas, images, or services effective? Are we able to persuade our clients, customers, or communities that they need occupational therapy services? Consider the "partnership" that takes place during client-centered practice. In this relationship, there is mutual respect for both parties and an agreement to work together to achieve agreed-on goals. In this partnership, there is "buy-in" by the client and therapist in order to meet established goals. This is an example of one-to-one selling (Law & Mills, 1998). We also sell one to one when we provide our clients with the evidence that supports our practice. In this one-to-one selling, the client may have an empowered and positive experience with occupational therapy and become a loyal fan. In our education of communities and organizations, occupational therapy is further promoted. Group selling is possibly more powerful and effective than one-to-one selling. Overall, it seems that persuasion is not enough. Advertising our services has become more popular over the past several years. This has been achieved in the national awareness campaign with advertisements about occupational therapy appearing in *People Weekly, Family Circle, Better Homes and Gardens*, and *USA Today* (Jacobs, 1998, p. 620).

Advertisement

Advertising can have a significant impact for an individual, company, or profession. Advertisements have an agreed-on message by a paid sponsor (Jacobs, 1998, 2011;

Scarborough & Zimmerer, 2003). Advertisement includes "calling public attention to something, especially by emphasizing desirable qualities so as to arouse a desire to buy or patronize" (Merriam-Webster, 2006).

The AOTA has launched many advertisement campaigns over the decades. In the early years of our profession, members of AOTA and the founders published in journals like *The Modern Hospital* and *Maryland Psychiatric Quarterly* (Jacobs, 2011). In addition, there have been books written about being an occupational therapist such as *A Story of Occupational Therapy* by Betty Blake, and public service announcements by famous people (Jacobs, 2011).

You may be aware of the national advertisement campaign launched by AOTA in 1997. In the first phase of the campaign, paid messages appeared in a variety of well-known and common household magazines targeted to women between the ages of 35 and 55. In preparation for the sponsored ads, the marketing agency conducted interviews with occupational therapy practitioners to find out the answer to what their practice involved. The outcome was the byline "skills for the job of living" (Jacobs, 1998; Whiting, 1999). This was in effect a redirection of the question, "What is occupation?" The slogan "Occupational therapy: Skills for the job of living" has provided us mileage as a profession, but do more people actually understand the term *occupation*?

The answer is a resounding yes. According to Whiting (1999), there was a 44% increase in requests for information about occupational therapy from 1998 to 1999. In addition, "more than 16 million people, most of them members of our target audience, saw the ads" (p. 5). In the second phase of the ad campaign, the target audience included managed care organizations, long-term care facilities, and consumers (again, women between the ages of 35 and 55). The results again were very positive. The advertisements "reached over 2.6 million key decision makers in managed care and long-term care" (Whiting, 1999, p. 12). Hundreds of our practice guidelines were requested by people seeing the advertisements, and almost 1.5 million people saw the Internet ads. The advertising agency working for AOTA remarked that "this campaign has been a huge success!" (Whiting, p. 12).

In 2008, AOTA launched a new promotional campaign, which replaced the previous tag line with "Living Life to Its Fullest." Four years ago, the Nursing Association partnered with Johnson & Johnson (New Brunswick, NJ)—a well-known, family-oriented company. Partnering with a "household name" such as Johnson & Johnson has been a "win-win" situation for both parties. The nursing profession has had significant promotion as a result of the Johnson & Johnson advertisement campaign. Nursing has seen an increase in applicants to the professional educational programs, over 8 million dollars has been raised for nursing scholarships, and the first-ever "men in nursing scholarship" has been developed. Finally, there has been increased visibility for the profession overall (Johnson & Johnson, 2006). AOTA's partnership with L.L. Bean (Freeport, ME) to promote National School Backpack Awareness is one such example of partnership in occupational therapy.

The American Physical Therapy Association (APTA) has a national advertisement campaign as well. They are hoping to recruit physical therapist practitioners to promote their own practice or their company with "expertly crafted TV and radio commercials and corresponding print ad tailor-made for the Baby Boomers and Beyond audience whose lives are hindered by chronic aches and pains" (APTA, n.d.). Physical therapists can obtain copies of these commercials from the APTA with all components of the ad campaign, which can be personalized with therapists' contact information.

Our Image

When you think of our profession, what image comes to mind? It is one thing to define our profession in words; it is another to define our profession in images. Maybe the AOTA's logo is our profession's image. Or is our image based on the stories we read and pictures we see during AOTA's occupational therapy month each year? Perhaps our image is that of the annual backpack awareness campaign—Luminie, the lightening bug!

Many occupational therapy practitioners and students often have difficulty stating succinctly what we do in occupational therapy. We must explain to our clients and community what we do, the evidence behind why we do it, and the level of education needed to enter the profession. In the nursing discipline, Lusk (2000) found that nurses from the 1930s to 1950s were seen by the public as subordinate to physicians and hospital administrators. Overall, the nurses of the 1940s were seen as performing more complex activities when compared to the nurses of the 1930s and 1950s. The important message in this article is that nurses of that era were not seen as professional. In the profession of occupational therapy, we want the public to view us as professionals. Image, pride for the profession, and ensuring that people know what occupational therapy is are key.

The old adage "a picture is worth a thousand words" might be useful here. In an *OT Practice* issue, the Oklahoma State Association President, Suzanne Bowman, shows off her "OT Cruiser" (Collins, 2002, p. 11). Promoting occupational therapy visually is powerful. Not only does this type of promotion get people talking, but it also can and will convey pride in our profession. Wearing occupational therapy shirts and using pens, note pads, and drink holders with the occupational therapy logo are powerful ways to convey an image of the pride for our profession. Providing clients, consumers, students, and community stakeholders with visual images and "freebies" is a step in the right direction. To equate the profession with an image is memorable and can lead to building a loyal fan base.

General Promotion

When promoting anything or anyone, the same three principles apply: publicity, personal selling, and advertising (Scarborough & Zimmerer, 2003). We are all capable of doing any or all of these three things. Consider writing an article for *OT Practice* or a letter to the editor for your local newspaper. Sponsor an in-service or seminar for a local agency to promote occupational therapy or go to your child's school and talk to the classmates about occupational therapy. Speaking and "selling" to individuals is another approach. Becoming involved in the OT Global Day of Service (OTGDS) is an excellent way to promote the profession while learning what occupational therapists around the world are doing.

Personal selling for occupational therapy enlists the client-centered approach, but in general, personal selling is that one-to-one relationship between salesperson and consumer or customer. Developing the relationship is often what gives one company the "edge" over another. Having good interpersonal skills is a must when engaging in personal selling. Let the other person talk while you listen, be enthusiastic, pay attention to all details, and measure your success by the client's satisfaction. These are good strategies for effective practitioners as well, but in the end, we might have to resort to advertising our wares.

Advertising can encompass various media types, including magazines, newspapers, direct mail, radio, television, and now the Internet. We have previously discussed occupational therapy's past approach to advertising. These attempts will need to continue in assorted ways to ensure that we reach our target populations. The target populations will change over time depending on the message we are sending and, therefore, our media type will have to vary in order to reach our intended audience. Identify your audience and select the most appropriate media to reach them, then go for it!

Summary

This chapter, along with Chapter 35, provides an overview of promotional strategies that will assist in the marketing of occupational therapy to a broad and complex global community.

Student Self-Assessment

1. In 15 seconds or less, describe or define occupational therapy. How did you do? Did you get the words occupation, daily living skills, health promotion, and activities of daily living in there? If you were going to do this activity again, what would you change about your definition?

2. Occupational therapy is a diverse and wide-reaching profession. We often define the profession based on what our role is within the discipline. In order to promote the field of occupational therapy, you need to give your listeners a full range of what the profession is and what it can do for them. As another assignment, jot down the first 10 things that come to mind when you think about what an occupational therapist can do for a client, student, resident, community, or organization. What commonalities did you find in your lists? How often do you think about occupational therapy serving communities?

EVIDENCE-BASED RESEARCH CHART

Promotion Program	Activities	Evidence
Recruitment strategy; prospective occupational therapy students	Careers pack	Craik & Ross, 2003
National perspective about occupational therapy	Publication/presentation	Dickinson, 2003; Jacobs, 1998
Promotional ideas	"Mediaspeak"; National Awareness Campaign; Occupational therapy cruiser; Mass media to promote nursing	Collins, 2002; Walls, 1999; Whitehead, 2000; Whiting, 1999
Awareness/knowledge of occupational therapy; nursing	Marketing; survey	Barnhart, 1999; Jamnadas et al., 2001; Lusk, 2000
	Eleanor Clarke Slagle lecture	Jacobs, 2011

References

American Occupational Therapy Association. (2008). Occupational therapy practice framework: Domain and process, second edition. *American Journal of Occupational Therapy, 62,* 625-683.

American Physical Therapy Association. (n.d.). *Tools & resources.* Retrieved from http://www.apta.org/AM/Template.cfm?Section=Tools_and_Resources1&Template=/TaggedPage/TaggedPageDisplay.cfm&TPLID=322&ContentID=40239

Barnhart, P. D. (1999). Secrets of success: OTs share their strategies. *OT Practice, 4*(3), 26-30.

Collins, L. (2002). Easy ways to promote occupational therapy. *OT Practice, 8,* 11-14.

Craik, C., & Ross, F. (2003). Promotion of occupational therapy as career: A survey of occupational therapy managers. *British Journal of Occupational Therapy, 66*(2), 78-81.

Dickinson, R. (2003). Occupational therapy: A hidden treasure. *Canadian Journal of Occupational Therapy, 70*(3), 133-135.

Jacobs, K. (1998). Innovation to action: Marketing occupational therapy. *OT Practice, 52*(8), 618-620.

Jacobs, K. (2011). Eleanor Clarke Slagle lecture. PromOTing occupational therapy: Words, images and actions. *American Journal of Occupational Therapy, 66*(6), 652-671.

Jamnadas, B., Burns, J., & Paul, S. (2001). Understanding occupational therapy: Nursing and physician assistant students' knowledge about occupational therapy. *Occupational Therapy in Health Care, 14*(1), 13-27.

Johnson & Johnson. (2006). *The campaign for nursing's future: A progress report.* Retrieved from http://www.discovernursing.com/progressreport.pdf

Law, M., & Mills, J. (1998). Client-centered occupational therapy. In M. Law (Ed.), *Client-centered occupational therapy.* Thorofare, NJ: SLACK Incorporated.

Lusk, B. (2000). Pretty and powerless: Nurses in advertisements, 1930-1950. *Research in Nursing and Health, 23*(3), 229-236.

Merriam-Webster. (2006). *On-line dictionary* (10th ed.). Retrieved from http://www.merriam-webster.com

Scarborough, N. M., & Zimmerer, T. W. (2003). *Effective small business management: An entrepreneurial approach* (7th ed.). Upper Saddle River, NJ: Prentice Hall.

Walls, B. S. (1999). Sound bite: OT practitioners learn "mediaspeak." *OT Practice, 4*(7), 7, 20.

Whitehead, D. (2000). Using mass media within health-promoting practice: A nursing perspective. *Journal of Advanced Nursing, 32*(4), 807-816.

Whiting, F. (1999). PromOTing OT: Year two of the national awareness campaign. *OT Practice, 4*(6), 5, 12.

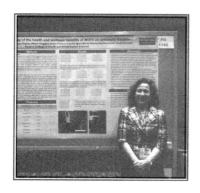

51

PROFESSIONAL DEVELOPMENT

Carol Reinson, PhD, OTR/L

ACOTE STANDARDS EXPLORED IN THIS CHAPTER
B.9.4

KEY VOCABULARY

- **Mentorship:** Defined by AOTA as a relationship between two people in which one person (the mentor) is dedicated to the personal and professional growth of the other (the mentee). The relationship is often mutually beneficial and collaborative, both parties participating willingly and knowingly in the development of the mentee.

- **Professional development:** The life-long process of assessing individual learning needs and interests, creating a professional development plan, and documenting professional development activities. These activities enhance one's knowledge of a specialty area, critical and ethical reasoning, and interpersonal and performance skills.

- **Professional identity:** Students develop a professional identity as an occupational therapy practitioner, aligning their professional judgments and decisions with the American Occupational Therapy Association (AOTA) Standards of Practice and the Occupational Therapy Code of Ethics.

- **Professional portfolio:** An autonomous, self-directed learning technique that unifies professional development and personal growth over a period of time. A collection of evidence-based activities that documents the successful completion of specific goals.

(continued)

Jacobs, K., MacRae, N., & Sladyk, K. (Eds.).
Occupational Therapy Essentials for
Clinical Competence, Second Edition (pp. 669-678).

Introduction

This chapter reviews the importance of professional development for students studying occupational therapy in institutions of higher learning. Educators can attest that learning to become or think like an occupational therapy practitioner is as much about learning how to use the clinical knowledge base and related practice skills as it is in appreciating the intellectual traits or virtues that support life-long learning. Intellectual traits or virtues promote meaningful reflection and include intellectual integrity, intellectual humility, confidence in reason, intellectual perseverance, fair-mindedness, intellectual courage, intellectual empathy, and intellectual autonomy (Paul & Elder, 2007). These characteristics are considered to be important components of higher-level critical thinking and are necessary to develop advanced clinical reasoning skills. The ability to integrate content knowledge, clinical experience, and evidence-based research with reflection is essential in meeting the diverse needs of clients. The need for lifelong learning and ongoing professional development has never been greater than it is today. It is important that students and practitioners alike be proactive and self-directed in creating professional development opportunities for themselves.

The aspiring occupational therapy student demonstrates significant personal and professional growth during a sustained period of preprofessional education. Students are involved in numerous formal and informal learning experiences that facilitate the socialization process into the profession (Collins, Harrison, Mason, & Lowden, 2011). Students need to be cognizant and actively engaged in this process to develop their own sense of professional identity and sense of self. A variety of strategies have been identified that promote professional identity, support ongoing professional development, and contribute to the profession of occupational therapy (Sladyk, 2010). These strategies include the following:

- Membership in international, national, state, and local occupational therapy associations
- Portfolio reviews
- Self-assessment and individual goal setting
- Mentoring
- Reflection
- Formal and informal professional development
- Networking and social media

Membership in Occupational Therapy Associations

Membership in international, national, state, and local occupational therapy associations should be the number one priority of all students, clinicians, educators, and researchers working in the field of occupational therapy. In particular, membership in the American Occupational Therapy Association (AOTA) is critical given the rapid changes in society, especially the newly revised American health care system. The most important feature of AOTA membership is the strong and effective legislative advocacy completed on behalf of its members and the clients that benefit from our services. AOTA is the official voice of occupational therapy, dedicated to promoting and defending the field now and in the future. AOTA assists with national public awareness initiatives such as the "Living Life to Its Fullest" campaign to educate the public, health care administrators, and policymakers about the range, scope, and value of occupational therapy services. They also advocate with state licensure boards to protect the field from being co-opted by other professional groups.

AOTA is the premiere storage house for all things related to occupational therapy. The organization supports high-quality and cost-effective continuing education opportunities needed for mandatory licensure for occupational therapists at all stages in their career. AOTA offers a multitude of tools and resources for practice, education, and research. Membership includes access to the *American Journal of Occupational Therapy (AJOT)*, the trade magazine *OT Practice,* 11 *Special Interest Sections Quarterly,* and the American Occupational Therapy Foundation's (AOTF) Wilma West Library. Membership carries a discount on books and self-study programs purchased through the AOTA marketplace (a great bargain for students building their own professional library).

The organization has a wealth of professional development tools to assist members with choosing professional development activities such as advanced board and specialty certification. Also, exclusive member discounts on insurance rates and other purchase offers are obtainable through AOTA as well. See www.aota.org for further information about AOTA, including their annual conference.

Portfolio Reviews

A professional portfolio is an autonomous, self-directed learning technique that unifies professional development and personal growth over a period of time. It is an active document that is reviewed and updated on an ongoing basis. A portfolio is both a "process" and an "end product," and as such requires honest self-appraisal and extensive reflection. The goal of reflection is to formulate future professional goals in a coherent and mindful manner. The portfolio may be in the form of an electronic document or a hardcopy review. Students are asked to provide concrete evidence that they meet a set of established criteria or desired outcomes. These outcomes can focus on a specific course or can be in the form of departmental objectives at the end of a student's program (Funk, 2007). For instance, an occupational therapy department may delineate the program goals for its students.

Students begin the process of reviewing both their formal educational experiences (previous course assignments) and informal personal experiences (volunteer work) in order to demonstrate clear and convincing evidence (artifacts) that they have achieved this goal or are working toward mastery. Possible artifacts might include a written "letter of necessity" to an insurance company, a podcast to announce occupational therapy month, and/or a needs assessment for an emerging community program. Students may discover upon reflection that they now fully understand the need for practitioners to be fluent in many forms of communication to increasingly diverse audiences. Students or practitioners decide that, in order to keep current in the field, they would like more information about telehealth practices or assistive technology and set a short-term goal to attend a formal workshop on the topic in the near future.

AOTA engages in a formal system of peer-reviewed portfolios to recognize those practitioners who meet the criteria for advanced Board and Specialty Certification. The criteria focus on the current knowledge of specialty area, critical and ethical reasoning, and interpersonal and performance skills. An occupational therapist can be awarded advanced Board Certification for Gerontology, Mental Health, Pediatrics, and Physical Rehabilitation. Occupational therapists and occupational therapy assistants (OT and OTA) can be awarded specialty certification in Driving and Community Mobility; Environmental Modification; Feeding, Eating, and Swallowing; Low Vision; and School Systems. It should be noted that the AOTA Official Documents have several documents detailing the skill set necessary to work in specialized areas of practice in occupational therapy such as the neonatal intensive care unit (NICU), adult vestibular treatment, and for the role of OT educator (AOTA, 2013). AOTA also has a Professional Development Tool (PDT) as a membership benefit so that occupational therapists can assess their own individual learning needs and interests, create a professional development plan, and document ongoing professional development activities. The ability to engage in portfolio review is an important strategy for students and practitioners to use in directing their career choices and establishing a professional identity. See Figure 51-1 for a detailed grading rubric for structuring professional portfolio feedback and Chapter 52 for more information on competence and professional development.

> **Sample Goal**
>
> Proficiency in oral and written communication for diverse audiences such as the public, consumers, other health care and educational practitioners, third-party payers, health care regulators, case managers, policy analysts and/or legislators, and for multiple purposes such as publication, service provision and justification, advocacy, grant writing, needs assessment and program proposal, public education, and research.

Self-Assessment and Individual Goal Setting

Donald Schon (1988) delivered a keynote address to the AOTA conference that introduced the concepts of "reflection in action" and "reflection on action" as the daily work of occupational therapy practitioners. At the time, he certainly (directly or indirectly) had an influence on the changing definitions of preservice training and continuing education, the critical role of ongoing self-assessment, and the future role of the "practitioner-researcher" in the field of occupational therapy. Currently, it is widely accepted that one's ability for self-assessment and reflection forms the basis of higher-level critical thinking and clinical reasoning skills.

The process of self-assessment should be fully grounded in the formative years of occupational therapy education. In fact, it is never too early to ask students to

Name: _____		
Criteria	**Score**	**Comments**
Artifacts and Evidence of Professional Standards • Does the selection of artifacts provide clear and convincing evidence that the student has achieved a true measure of professional competency with all departmental goals for occupational therapy? • Do individual artifacts meet expectations for quality and excellence? • Is there a diversity of artifacts throughout the presentation (i.e. use of summary sheets for long text documents; a wide-variety of multimedia; self-explanatory to reviewer, etc.)	(20)	
Reflections • Do the reflections clearly link the artifacts to the departmental goals? • Do the reflections demonstrate that the student has fully understood the relevance and meaning of each departmental goal? • Do the reflections demonstrate that the student has engaged in a process of self-analysis and self-discovery? • Do the reflections suggest that the student has mastered and fully integrated the core competencies expected of an entry-level occupational therapist? • Do the reflections include any future professional growth goals? • Do the reflections provide valuable insight into the student's unique characteristics and potential contributions to the field of OT?	(20)	
Artistic and Technological Impact • Do the layout and text elements provide a suitable canvas for the presentation of an e-portfolio? Are there unifying common threads? • Does the use of multimedia enhancements (photographs, graphics, sound, and/or video clips) enhance or distract from the content? • Have all audio and visual files been appropriately edited to ensure high technological quality? • Does the student demonstrate an appreciation for the aesthetics of color, imagery, and arrangement? • Does the tone and tempo of the presentation invite and captivate the audience? • Does the student demonstrate a unique sense of creativity and self-expression?	(20)	
Class Presentation and Personal Investment • Do you believe this presentation provides an accurate description of the student's abilities and competencies? • Does this student demonstrate an adequate comfort level with self-directed learning activities and educational risk-taking? • Were you able to determine the value of this assignment to the student? • Please rate: Creativity, innovation, special effects, charm • Does this student deserve extra credit for technological know-how? • Does this e-portfolio give you ideas about your own presentation? • Does the student demonstrate having successfully completed the first phase of the e-portfolio capstone project? • How does this e-portfolio compare to the other presentations? • Is this e-portfolio reflective of the student's "best" work? • Was the e-portoflio "user-friendly" and compatible with personal computers generally?	(20)	
Written, Oral, and Nonverbal Communication • Use of standard English for spelling, punctuation, and grammar? • Rate content, clarity, and organization of ideas. • Presentation skills: proper voice projection, clear pronunciation, etc. • Were proper APA guidelines for documentation followed? • Annoying mannerisms of speech and/or distracting body language? • Were the (13) department goals clearly delineated? • Were there unanswered questions or areas of concern not addressed?	(20)	
Outstanding Highlights: Suggestions for Improvement:	Final Grade: _____	

Figure 51-1. E-Portfolio grading rubric.

self-assess and reflect on professional behaviors while in the classroom and/or in the clinic. These professional behaviors are considered "hygiene" behaviors because they should be fully integrated in how students represent themselves and the field of occupational therapy on a daily basis. Professional behaviors may include (Kasar & Clark, 2000) the following:

- Dependability
- Professional presentation
- Initiative
- Empathy
- Cooperation
- Organization
- Clinical reasoning
- Supervisory process
- Verbal communication
- Written communication

Nagayda, Schindehette, and Richardson (2005) suggest that students begin learning self-assessment and individual goal setting by taking a "professional inventory" that lists the admirable traits of other professionals they respect. They can then decide to emulate one or more of these admirable traits by recognizing what changes they need to make in their own behaviors and set measureable short-term and long-term goals for themselves. Another strategy for gaining insight about oneself is to list the qualities that future employers are looking for in new graduates. The ability to engage in perspective taking of another viewpoint helps individuals to honestly appraise their own strengths and weaknesses. Portfolio review has also been shown to help students form a narrative professional identity and adds to the formation of a personal brand statement (Graves & Epstein, 2011). The development of one's professional identity can be realized through planned professional development activities and organized goal setting.

The field of occupational therapy has increasingly been concerned with how to assess one's ability "to think on your feet" and make ongoing changes to the treatment plan based on a client's individual needs. The AOTA Occupational Therapy Practice Framework (AOTA, 2008) provides a conceptual structure and assists in grading activities (up or down) to make them easier or more challenging for the client. A practitioner has to be consciously aware of discreet client responses during evaluation and treatment and use effective clinical reasoning skills to make ongoing changes. Teaching preprofessional students to gain self-awareness (about their own thinking) during a therapy session can be a challenge. The use of videotaping the interaction for later review with a mentor has been used with success. Another strategy is to implement fidelity measures that can be used

as a self-assessment tool during an occupational therapy intervention. See Figure 51-2 for a sample of play facilitation skills that can be used to assist the student or practitioner when trying to elicit a broad range of behaviors from a pediatric client (Linder, 2008).

Mentoring

A key ingredient for effective portfolio review and self-assessment techniques is personal and/or professional feedback from a trusted source. This relationship is called *mentorship* and it is generally conducted between an individual mentor and mentee. The relationship can be a formal, structured exchange or informal, such as helpful advice and support from family members or close friends. All mentoring relationships have an interpersonal focus and should be based on reciprocal respect, trust, and kindness. The mentor's feedback on professional issues should encourage higher-level critical thinking, problem solving, and resourcefulness in the mentee. Mentors that function as a coach need to provide ongoing encouragement, honesty, and redirection as necessary. The ability to be accessible and available to mentees on an as-needed basis is an important mentor responsibility.

The role of formal mentorship in professional development and career satisfaction in health care is well documented (Melnyk, 2007). Milner and Bossers (2005) identified expert knowledge, clinical experience, and guidance skills as desirable characteristics in a mentor. The mentor role often takes the form of helping students identify with the professional environment, navigate challenging situations, build self-confidence, and facilitate creative and independent thinking. Kuhaneck (2010) demonstrates qualitative evidence that mentors can facilitate increased professional involvement in the field, serve as matchmakers, open doors of opportunity, and teach mentees how to "pay it forward." Robertson and Savio (2003) point out that we are all on a professional development continuum and that no one person has the entire breadth and scope of knowledge and skills that exists in the field of occupational therapy. In reality, there is no singular pathway for ongoing professional development. Everyone can find personal and professional benefits by having a trusted mentor. A working contract that delineates the roles and responsibilities of mentors–mentees during research and scholarly activities is often desirable.

The model of mentorship and leadership in the area of sensory integration was the life's work of Dr. A. Jean Ayres and serves as a fine example of the importance of the mentoring process. She collaborated with 66 faculty researchers in her lifetime. Her legacy as an independent theorist, researcher, and innovator of a new practice model has had a significant and lasting effect on the field of occupational therapy (Burtner, Crowe, & Lopez, 2009;

Facilitation Strategies Checklist

Directions: Evaluate Your Skill Level in Being a Play Facilitator
[Needs Improvement] = 1   [Good] = 2   [Excellent] = 3

1. Environment promotes play through appropriate selection of toys (variety; number; level)? _____
2. Follows child's lead in selecting play materials that are interesting and meaningful? _____
3. Imitates the child when appropriate? _____
4. Reads child's cues and responds appropriately? _____
5. Adapts mode of communication to the necessary level of sensory input? _____
6. Waits for the child to play before initiating new activities or modeling behaviors? _____
7. Observes child's optimal behaviors and builds on strengths? _____
8. Uses aspects of play that are motivating to the child to regulate attention? _____
9. Responds to child's initiations? _____
10. Uses parallel play? _____
11. Emphasizes turn-taking? _____
12. Models slightly higher level of behaviors for the child? _____
13. Encourages exploration and creative use of objects? _____
14. Uses the following language strategies:
    • Mirroring (reflecting nonverbal expression)? _____
    • Parallel talk (talking about child's actions)? _____
    • Self-talk (commenting on own actions)? _____
    • Imitation (repeating child's vocalizations)? _____
    • Elaboration (adding new information to what child said)? _____
    • Corroborating (saying correctly what child has said in error)? _____
    • Expanding (building on child's words)? _____
    • Modeling (conversing without using the child's words)? _____
15. Modifies play to match child's capabilities? _____
16. Responds to child's affect? _____
17. Appears to enjoy the play interactions? _____

Figure 51-2. Transdisciplinary play-based assessment (TPBA). (Reprinted with permission from Toni Linder.)

Kuhaneck, 2010). See Figure 51-3 for a sample contract between a research mentor and mentee.

Reflection

The ability to have conscious awareness or knowledge of our own thinking process is termed *metacognition*. Paul and Elder (2007) describe several intellectual traits or virtues that provide incentives to think differently about what we know and understand about ourselves and the world (Table 51-1).

An individual must use field maturity and intellectual humility to judge one's own knowledge base, skill set, and personal attitudes. Individuals need to identify their own strengths, weaknesses, and professional aspirations in order to formulate short-term and long-term professional development goals.

Reflective inquiry should occur both in the midst of a treatment session (reflection in action) and after the treatment session (reflection on action) in order to achieve higher-level clinical reasoning skills and grow

professionally (Boyt Schell, 2008). It takes persistent, honest self-reflection to realize the true value of portfolio review, self-assessment and goal-setting, and mentoring relationships.

Wood (2011) introduced and applied the concept of *wayfinding* to the field of occupational therapy. She defines wayfinding as a dynamic process for finding one's path throughout one's career and in ways that strengthen the profession. She lists five strategies for helping occupational therapists navigate the ever-changing landscapes in our professional lives.

1. Lean into disorienting dilemmas and persevere.
2. Learn from those who illuminate the necessity of occupation.
3. Feed your intellectual curiosity about the field.
4. Find your empowering community.
5. Build robust communities through compelling occupational visions

Research Mentor Roles and Responsibilities

- Be available to meet with students on a regular basis. Guide student through transitions.
- Provide a learning environment that fosters respect, trust, and kindness. Display optimistic perspective.
- Respond to questions and written drafts within a reasonable timeframe (minimum 2 weeks for major pieces).
- Tailor level and type of assistance to match individual needs and interests.
- Function as a coach and provide ongoing encouragement, honesty, and redirection as necessary.
- Assist student with creating a reasonable timeline for research activities. Break down process in steps.
- Recommend and identify possible resources for the literature review.
- Provide referrals to content specialists, consultants, and learning support as appropriate.
- Provide assistance with designing the project, such as refining the research question, determining appropriate methodology, choosing variables and outcome measurement procedures.
- Check project for relevancy to the field of occupational therapy (the So-What Question).
- Critique written drafts with careful attention. Suggest strategies to improve organization, clarity, and style.
- Assist with interpretation and application of evidence/results to field of occupational therapy.
- Encourage critical thinking, problem solving, resourcefulness, and flexibility in student.
- Provide constructive criticism that is helpful to move student through the various stages of the research process.
- Encourage student to disseminate research findings in an appropriate forum.
- Monitor academic integrity, model ethical reasoning, and support design review board/institutional review board (DRB/IRB) decisions.
- Be willing to consult with occupational therapy colleagues, consultants, and/or content specialists on research-based issues.

Student Mentee Roles and Responsibilities

- Stay in contact with mentor on a regular basis!
- Respect mentor's time commitment and attend all meetings and classes fully prepared.
- Be honest with mentor regarding strengths, weaknesses, opportunities, and threats (SWOT).
- Fulfill responsibilities in an appropriate timeframe and meet established deadlines.
- Engage in self-directed learning and be *proactive* with requests for learning support.
- Articulate your personal and professional needs to mentor in a timely manner.
- Work on solving challenges during the project with guidance from mentor.
- Be fully committed to a 2-year project from initial stages through final dissemination activities.
- Choose an appropriate research topic that is both reasonable and meaningful. Be realistic!
- Conduct a systematic literature review and consult with content specialists for guidance as needed.
- Initiate ideas for choosing research question, purpose, and methodology and discuss these ideas with mentor.
- Respect contributions of others and carefully consider co-authorship of final product.
- Be aware of DRB/IRB guidelines, graduation requirements for BS/MS, and graduate school policies and procedures.
- Perform all phases of research process with academic integrity, ethical decision making, and self-reflection.
- Be prepared to work on phased writing assignments that may involve multiple revisions.
- Assume primary responsibility for the written manuscript including literature review, statement of problem, research question, methodology, results, and discussion.
- Understand and be willing to accept the financial costs of your proposed research project.
- Seek out external learning support for written communication needs (i.e., punctuation/grammar) and information literacy requirements.
- Engage in data collection procedures and quantitative and/or qualitative analyses with academic integrity.
- Disseminate findings in an appropriate forum.
- Trust the educational process and be willing to go with the flow. Remain flexible and fluid with thinking.
- Try not to personalize written or verbal feedback.
- Sets realistic expectations for self and others.
- Attempt to maintain positive attitude, sense of humor, and grow from past mistakes.

Figure 51-3. Research Mentor-Mentee Sample Contract.

Table 51-1.

INTELLECTUAL TRAITS IN METACOGNITION

Trait	Working Definition
Intellectual humility	Having the conscious awareness about the limits of one's knowledge.
Intellectual courage	Having a conscious need to face and fairly address ideas and beliefs.
Intellectual empathy	Having the conscious need to consider the perspectives of others vs. egocentrism.
Intellectual autonomy	Having rational control of one's beliefs, values, and inferences. Deciding on your own.
Intellectual integrity	Having intellectual standards and the need to be true to your own values and beliefs.
Intellectual perseverance	Having the need to struggle with confusion to achieve a deeper understanding.
Confidence in reason	Confidence in the process of rational thinking. Believing people can think for themselves.
Fair-mindedness	Having the awareness to entertain all viewpoints during rational problem solving.

Adapted from Paul, R., & Elder, L. (2007). *The miniature guide to critical thinking: Concepts and tools.* Dillon Beach, CA: Foundation for Critical Thinking Press, 1-24.

Formal and Informal Professional Development

FORMAL EDUCATION

The most highly recognized form of post-secondary education is to attend a public or private college or university and earn a credit-bearing college degree. AOTA's Accreditation Council for Occupational Therapy Education (ACOTE) currently accredits approximately 311 occupational therapy and occupational therapy assistant educational programs in the United States. This accrediting body is recognized by the United States Department of Education (USDE) and the Council for Higher Education Accreditation (CHEA). "In America, accreditation at the post-secondary levels performs a number of important functions, including the encouragement of efforts toward maximum educational effectiveness. The accrediting process requires institutions and programs to examine their goals, activities, and achievements; to consider the expert criticism and suggestions of a visiting team; and to determine internal procedures for action on recommendations from the accrediting agency" (www.aota.org). There are many types of post-secondary degrees available for prospective occupational therapy students. There are 2-year associate degrees for the occupational therapy assistant, 5-year master level entry degrees, post-professional master degrees for students having a bachelor degree in another field, and doctoral degrees. Currently, there are only five accredited entry-level occupational therapy doctoral programs in the country. The accreditation requirements of academic programs ensure that students are receiving a quality education in occupational therapy through careful monitoring from an external organization.

The National Board for Certification in Occupational Therapy (NBCOT) is the credentialing agency for occupational therapy. The NBCOT credentialing process is in place to protect the public by documenting entry-level competency, professional conduct, and ongoing professional development. All students must provide proof that they have graduated from an accredited occupational therapy or occupational therapy assistant college program before they can sit for the national exam in occupational therapy. The successful completion of the NBCOT examination is required for state licensure for practicing as an occupational therapist.

NBCOT requires ongoing Professional Development Units (PDUs) to keep an individual's occupational therapy certification current. Activities such as professional workshops, seminars, lectures, online courses, and/or conferences count towards continuing professional development. Interested occupational therapists should check ahead of attendance to make sure that the educational activity is AOTA approved for PDUs. AOTA offers an online Professional Development Tool (PDT) for members to document their history of continuing education. Both the Website at AOTA and NBCOT offer resources for individuals engaging in self-assessment, portfolio review, and reflection opportunities necessary for planning continuing education short-term and long-term goals. The standards for continuing competence in the field of occupational therapy include the following:

- Knowledge
- Critical reasoning
- Interpersonal abilities
- Performance skills
- Ethical reasoning

DOCTORAL DEGREES

The decision to obtain a doctoral degree is a major turning point in one's life. It takes commitment and resolve to persevere for several years on this long-term goal. Someone seriously considering a career in academia after working for a few years as a practitioner might entertain earning a research doctorate such as a PhD, EdD, or ScD at a Research I Institution. Some higher education institutions will only accept terminal research doctorates for rank and tenure decisions. These degrees can be in occupational therapy or related fields. The OTD (occupational therapy doctorate) can be used for career advancement in academia as well. It offers practitioners advanced study opportunities in specialty practice areas. The most important thing to remember is to do your homework regarding which degrees and programs best match your career goals and personal needs. The doctoral network in AOTA meets at the annual conference. This group can offer support and advice to those individuals thinking of earning a doctorate.

INFORMAL PROFESSIONAL DEVELOPMENT OPPORTUNITIES

Sladyk (2010) listed the following informal professional development opportunities:

- *AJOT*, SIS newsletters, *OT Practice* magazine
- AOTA annual conference
- Recently published books
- Online computer conference and online practice support with learning communities
- Participating in peer review
- Participating in research projects
- Self-study programs
- State occupational therapy associations and conferences
- Student conclave (NBCOT)
- Supervising Level I or II students
- Trade magazines in occupational therapy
- Volunteering to present a topic
- Work performance review
- Workplace in-services and journal clubs
- Workshops or seminars
- Writing for publication

There are forms available at AOTA and NBCOT to document these activities.

Networking and Social Media

The Internet (World Wide Web) offers many excellent opportunities for individuals to initiate or join a virtual online learning community. The digital world is especially valuable for therapists who practice as an independent entity or in rural, unpopulated regions. The learning communities can center on special practice issues or interests. Networking online facilitates professional development and international learning as well. The ability to network with others can open many doors for students and practitioners. A blog (short for Web log) can have a key role in professional development in a globalized community (Bodell, Hook, Penman, & Wade, 2009). All interaction should be professional even when using social media such as Facebook, LinkedIn, or Twitter. Nothing you put on the Web is confidential or private, and it is very difficult to remove once posted. Prospective employers can easily check you out on the Internet thus maintaining a professional image on the Web at all times is of utmost importance.

Summary

There is no singular pathway for ongoing professional development in the field of occupational therapy. There are numerous formal and informal professional development opportunities available for students and occupational therapy practitioners, including membership and involvement in international, national, state, and local occupational therapy associations; portfolio reviews; self-assessment and goal-setting; mentorship; reflection; and networking and social media. It is recommended that students actively seek out opportunities for ongoing personal and professional growth. Professional development requires a commitment to life-long learning and a passion for the field of occupational therapy.

References

American Occupational Therapy Association. (2008). Occupational therapy practice framework: Domain and process (2nd ed.). *American Journal of Occupational Therapy, 62*(6), 625-683.

American Occupational Therapy Association. (2003). *Professional development tool.* Bethesda, MD: Author.

American Occupational Therapy Association. (2013a). *Board and specialty certification.* Retrieved from http://aota.org/Practitioners/ProfDev/Certifcation

American Occupational Therapy Association. (2013b). *Member benefits and services.* Retrieved from http://aota.org/Benefits

Bodell, S., Hook, A., Penman, M., & Wade, W. (2009). Creating a learning community in today's world: How blogging can facilitate continuing professional development and international learning. *British Journal of Occupational Therapy, 72*(6), 279-281.

Boyt Schell, B. A. (2008). Becoming expert: The importance of reflection. *OT Practice, 13*(14), 20-21.

Burtner, P. A., Crowe, T. K., & Lopez, A. (2009). A model of mentorship in occupational therapy: The leadership of A. Jean Ayres. *Occupational Therapy in Health Care, 23*(3), 226-243.

Collins, M., Harrison, D., Mason, R., & Lowden, A. (2011). Innovation and creativity: Exploring human occupation and professional development in student education. *British Journal of Occupational Therapy, 74*(6), 304-308.

Funk, K. P. (2007). Student experiences of learning portfolios in occupational therapy education. *Occupational Therapy in Health Care, 21*(1/2), 175-184.

Graves, N., & Epstein, M. (2011). Eportfolio: A tool for constructing a narrative identity. *Business Communication Quarterly, 74*(3), 342-346.

Kasar, J., & Clark, N. (2000). Developing professional behaviors (ed). Baltimore, MD: SLACK Incorporated.

Kuhaneck, H. M. (2010). The importance of mentoring for the professional involvement of therapists specializing in Ayres Sensory Integration. *Sensory Integration Special Interest Section Quarterly, 33* (2)1-4.

Linder, T. (2008). *Transdisciplinary Play-based Assessment (2nd ed).* Baltimore, MD: Paul H. Brooks.

Melnyk, B. M. (2007). The latest evidence on the outcomes of mentoring. *Worldviews on Evidence-Based Nursing, 3,* 170-173.

Milner, T., & Bossers, A. (2005). Evaluation of the mentor-mentee relationship in an occupational therapy mentorship programme. *Occupational Therapy International, 11*(2), 96-111.

Milner, T., & Bossers, A. (2008). Evaluation of an occupational therapy mentorship program. *Canadian Journal of Occupational Therapy, 72*(4), 205-211.

Nagayda, J., Schindehette, S., & Richardson, J. (2005). *The professional portfolio in occupational therapy: Career development and continuing competence.* Thorofare, NJ: SLACK Incorporated.

Paul, R., & Elder, L. (2007). *The miniature guide to critical thinking: Concepts and tools.* Dillon Beach, CA: Foundation for Critical Thinking Press, 1-24.

Robertson, S. C., & Savio, M. C. (2003). Mentoring as professional development. *OT Practice, 8*(21), 12-16.

Schon, D. (1988). *Reflection in and on the practice of occupational therapy: A research perspective.* Paper presented at the Annual Conference of the American Occupational Therapy Association, Phoenix, AZ.

Sladyk, K. (2010). Professional development, In K. Sladyk, K. Jacobs, & N. MacRae (Eds.), *Occupational therapy essentials for clinical competence* (pp. 469-474). Thorofare, NJ: SLACK Incorporated.

Wood, W. (2011). Navigating the shifting sands of occupational therapy: Lessons from wise wayfinders. *New Zealand Journal of Occupational Therapy, 58*(1), 14-20.

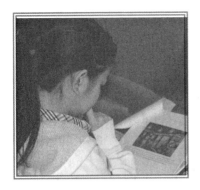

52

COMPETENCE AND PROFESSIONAL DEVELOPMENT

LEARNING FOR COMPLEXITY

Penelope A. Moyers, EdD, OT/L, BCMH, FAOTA

ACOTE STANDARDS EXPLORED IN THIS CHAPTER

B.9.6

KEY VOCABULARY

- **Competencies:** Explicit statements that define specific areas of expertise and are related to effective or superior performance in a job (Spencer & Spencer, 1993).
- **Continuing competence:** Refers to an individual's ongoing or life-long capacity to perform responsibilities as a part of one's professional role performance.
- **Continuing competency:** Focuses on an individual's actual performance in a particular situation according to standard as a part of one's current professional role performance.

- **Interprofessional collaborative practice:** "When multiple health workers from different professional backgrounds work together with patients, families, carers [sic], and communities to deliver the highest quality of care" (World Health Organization, 2010, p. 7).
- **Interprofessionality:** The process by which professionals reflect on and develop ways of practicing that provides an integrated and cohesive answer to the needs of the client/family/population" (Interprofessional Education Collaborative Expert Panel, 2011, p. 8).
- **Portfolios:** Archival of one's self-assessment processes, learning plans, evidence of engagement in selected learning methods, reflection on the learning process, and outcomes of the application of learning to practice.

(continued)

Jacobs, K., MacRae, N., & Sladyk, K. (Eds.).
Occupational Therapy Essentials for
Clinical Competence, Second Edition (pp. 679-691).
© 2014 SLACK Incorporated.

- **Professional development:** A process in which one plans and achieves excellence or establishes expertise in seeking a change in responsibilities, or when assuming more complex professional roles.

- **Self-assessment:** Provides the means to assess performance, abilities, and skills; to analyze demands and resources of the work environment; to interpret information about clients' outcomes; to reassess current learning goals; and to develop goals and plans for professional growth and continuing competence and competency.

"In Today's complex world, we must educate not merely for competence, but for capability (the ability to adapt to change, generate new knowledge, and continuously improve performance)."

—*Sarah W. Fraser and Trisha Greenhalgh*

Rapid redesign of health care delivery is being driven by the need to improve the experience of care in health care, social, and educational systems; improve the health of individuals and their families and populations; and reduce the per capita cost of health care and social services. These factors are often referred to as the "triple aim" in the reorganization of health care and social services. It is becoming quite clear that improvement in health care has to include a seamless integration with social services and community living. Additionally, in terms of the education of new health care professionals and current professionals, there is growing awareness of the importance of achieving team-based practice competencies as an essential public good in accomplishing this triple aim. Value-based health care and social services balance efficiency and effectiveness in terms of its cost and quality, which involves professionals working collaboratively with each other and their patients/clients within interdependent care systems. Consequently, the stakes for being competent as occupational therapists and occupational therapy assistants continue to rise not only with the focus on evidence-based practice (Moyers & Hinojosa, 2003), but also on interprofessional collaborative practice (Josiah Macy Jr. Foundation, 2013). According to the World Health Organization (2010), interprofessional collaborative practice occurs "when multiple health workers from different professional backgrounds work together with patients, families, carers [sic], and communities to deliver the highest quality of care" (p. 7).

While quality of care requires occupational therapy practitioners to prevent harm by ensuring that clients are not seriously injured during implementation of services due to practitioner neglect or malpractice or due to poor risk management, harm has a broader meaning. In addition, harm results when our clients receive ineffective intervention or intervention that is not as effective as an alternative method in improving occupational performance and participation in daily life. Occupational therapy practitioners who are ineffective in collaborative practice with key team members also create harm when they contribute to unnecessary team conflict, avoid addressing team conflict, do not examine effectiveness of their team performance, and are not reliable and dependable in carrying out team-assigned responsibilities. Harm also results from occupational therapy population- or organization-based services that are poorly designed, implemented, and evaluated. Services that are not interdependent with a range of systems and that do not incorporate input to constantly improve the quality of the client experience contribute to harm as well. The harm that occurs relates to the cost benefit of services in terms of the expenditures made for poor outcomes. Additionally, the client, organization, or population may have to assume other costs associated with intervention continuing over a longer duration than expected, with the additional burden for caregiving resulting from reduced performance in activities of daily living (ADL), with the loss of the worker role to support daily living, and with the possible reduction in the economic viability of the community if a large population or organization is negatively affected by ineffective programming. Policy for reimbursement of medically based services is beginning to incorporate the concept of paying for performance or the outcome achieved after intervention is delivered within a collaborative-based practice model (Sautter et al., 2007).

Because of the increasing pressure for accountability related to health care and social service outcomes, employers, third-party payers, community agencies, business, and industry all expect practitioners to remain competent and knowledgeable of the new developments in the field of occupational therapy, collaborative practice, and in related contextual areas involving local, state, national, and global communities. It is not acceptable to believe that an occupational therapist or occupational therapy assistant enters practice thoroughly trained, possessing all the knowledge needed throughout one's career. The career path taken should be punctuated with learning and knowledge management strategies to enhance professional development and continuing competence and competency in occupational therapy and in collaborative practice.

In this chapter, *Occupational Therapy Practice Framework: Domain and Process* (OTPF) (herein out referred to as the framework) will be used to understand the occupation of education (AOTA, 2008), particularly as learning is important for continuing competence and competency and professional development in occupational therapy and collaborative practice. These terms then are differentiated to highlight the three distinct purposes of the different types of learning. A model that proposes how change occurs and how assessment links collaborative practice performance, career growth, and learning is described. Based on a gap between actual and desired collaborative practice performance or gap between desired career development and actual career trajectory, a learning plan is developed that includes feasible strategies thought best to narrow these gaps and most likely to produce a measurable change in client daily life participation outcomes and in achievement of the practitioner's career goals. For collaborative practice, a team learning and development plan is necessary. The roles of administrators, team members and leaders, organizations, professional organizations, universities, continuing education providers, credentialing bodies, and government in fostering this model are described.

Education as an Occupation

"Lifelong learning means that education converges with (and is influenced by) work, family, and personal development."

—*Sarah W. Fraser and Trisha Greenhalgh*

Education in the framework (AOTA, 2008) addresses the "activities needed for learning and participating in the environment" (p. 632). One can be a learner beyond the formal education years when exploring learning needs and interests and participating in "classes, programs, and activities that provide instruction/training in identified areas of interest" (AOTA, p. 632). This chapter is concerned with the education related to the occupation of work after one has completed entry-level formal education as an occupational therapist or occupational therapy assistant. This life-long education throughout

one's career requires the practitioner to possess the necessary underlying body functions (movement-related, mental, and sensory) as well as performance skills (motor and praxis, sensory-perceptual, emotional regulation, cognitive, and communication and social). The occupational therapy practitioner has to have the ability to adapt new knowledge and skills, including advanced interprofessional competencies, to one's professional roles in order to be a successful learner and practice collaborator.

Learning as a part of the educational process is influenced by social, cultural, physical, virtual, temporal and personal contexts. For instance, the social expectations from the public and the profession are for the practitioner to be competent and up to date in the skills associated with providing a high-quality service, including collaboration with colleagues, clients, and team members. The organization in which one works may have a culture in which learning is left up to the individual practitioner rather than one that values learning as an aspect of organizational performance and collaborative practice. Depending on the learning preferences of the learner, the physical environment could be inadvertently designed where learning is inhibited instead of being facilitated. Often, virtual synchronous or asynchronous environments, whether in the form of online learning platforms, list serves and discussion groups, online courses, blogs, Web-based conferencing technology, and Web sites, are where learning occurs in order to accommodate geographical distance and a variety of schedule differences among learners. Thus, virtual contexts allow learners to individually address the temporal contextual needs of their daily life and biorhythms so that learning can occur at the most opportune time. The personal contextual factors of age, educational level, and socioeconomic status can influence learning in terms of the design of the education (e.g., education with expectations for large amounts of memorization may be difficult for older learners, or learners with young children may have less time to engage in educational offerings occurring over a long duration or requiring travel and overnight stays away from the family). Costs associated with the educational offering may deter participation as well (e.g., participating in some offerings may be cost prohibitive for practitioners with little employer support, lower salaries, and family financial pressures). Team-based learning is influenced by not only the confluence of personal contextual factors of the team members, but also by their access to technologically supported learning that bridges the time pressures when bringing team members together around a learning event. In addition, there is the added complication of what the team considers to be the focus of learning as individuals on the team will have competing interests, needs, and vision about how to improve client-centered care.

Competence, Competency, and Professional Development

The word *continuing* is typically combined with both competence and competency to denote a life-long learning process. Often, the terms *competence* and *competency* are used interchangeably, when in fact there is an important difference between these two concepts. Competence "refers to an individual's capacity to perform" professional responsibilities, whereas competency "focuses on an individual's actual performance in a particular situation" (McConnell, 2001, p. 14). Professional development is a process in which one plans and achieves excellence, establishes expertise, seeks a change in responsibilities, or assumes more complex professional roles (Moyers & Hinojosa, 2003). Continuing competence and competency are requirements for one's current professional responsibilities in a given role in contrast to professional development, which involves what one aspires to achieve regardless of one's present position or role. Professional development may not focus on what one needs to learn in order to perform better, but rather may address what one is interested in learning in order to advance one's career.

Continuing competence is designed to build capacity to perform one's responsibilities in the future for a given role. Occupational therapy practice and health care in general advances rapidly so that a practitioner who does not engage in continuing competence activities will become markedly out of date in a short amount of time. For example, if a new documentation system is going to be implemented, training would be needed to properly prepare for the change. Because neither the systems in which we work nor the external environment will ever be constant (Fraser & Greenhalgh, 2001), educating for capacity is very important.

Continuing competency, in contrast, ensures that the practitioner performs according to standard given that a distinctive set of variables dynamically interact, resulting in each client situation being unique. It is well known that practitioner performance is highly context dependent, such that the practitioner may have better outcomes in one situation compared to another similar situation (Handfield-Jones et al., 2002). With continuing competency, there is also an assumption that all practitioner skills and abilities fade with lack of practice, feedback, or team and administrative/system support.

Another factor important in understanding both continuing competence and competency is that there is not a linear relationship between learning and improved practice performance and changed capacity. Instead, there may be periods of time when there is either no improvement or even a slight decrease in performance. These periods of little change then may be followed by sudden jumps in practice performance (Handfield-Jones et al., 2002). Because most of practice is based on cognitively complex tasks, learning typically requires cognitive reorganization that may involve abandonment of previously held ideas and principles. Therefore the impact of learning on practice appears to occur in sudden leaps rather than through continuous and gradual change. Consequently, while practice performance improves in some areas, it may simultaneously deteriorate in others. When practicing in teams, learning among team members takes longer to integrate into a smooth practice change that significantly impacts client care. Team learning typically involves complex system change to support the changed work of the team.

Self-Assessment Model

The learning of currently practicing occupational therapists and occupational therapy assistants is different from learning obtained as students within their professional programs: the focus in the latter was on learning generalist practice and a core set of competencies, allowing few opportunities to learn any particular interest area in depth. Level 2 fieldwork and the first year or two on the job has been the time for specialized learning; more recently, the entry-level doctorate allows some time for delving into these interest areas. The first several years in a position in which intensive job training occurs, however, is complicated by the need to not only develop specialization but to focus learning efforts to enhance expected performance. The requirement is to simultaneously keep up with advances in these specialty areas as well as advances in quality improvement and team-based care. As a result, practitioners are expected to engage in and employers must facilitate a systematic approach to learning that considers learning styles, client populations, career stage, and influence of previous learning, while at the same time understanding the barriers and supports for application of new learning within practice, particularly within a climate of collaborative practice and quality improvement. Learning plans maximize the practitioner's educational efforts to enhance therapy and collaborative practice outcomes and to advance one's career (Wilkinson et al., 2002). Learning is thus a process to be managed, one that necessitates a dynamic approach to target the learning needs that arise from daily practice and from one's goals for career development.

In order to link practice performance with learning, the occupational therapist and occupational therapy assistant have to engage in a self-assessment process that increasingly involves their collaborative practice colleagues (Figure 52-1). "Self-assessment provides the means by which therapists and assistants develop goals and plans for professional growth, reassess current goals, assess performance, analyze demands and resources of

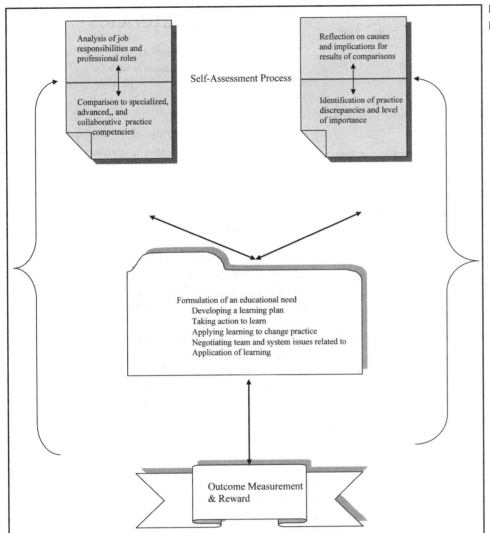

Figure 52-1. Linking practice performance and learning.

the work environment, and interpret information about the consumers' outcomes" (Moyers & Hinojosa, 2003, p. 484). Self-assessment for the development of a learning plan should primarily be formative in nature as summative assessments are mainly used for employee evaluation, certification programs, or licensure. Self-assessment answers the question, "What can I do to improve competence and competency in my job or role on a collaborative practice team?" Self-assessment can also answer the question of what is needed to advance one's career (Smith & Tillema, 2001). Self-assessment not only locates discrepancies in current practice compared to an ideal, but also validates what is going well. In terms of professional development, self-assessment ascertains strengths and how to further develop those strengths in preparation for career advancement.

Job Responsibilities and Client Outcomes

Self-assessment begins with an analysis of one's job responsibilities and roles, typically answering such questions as the following:

- What are my main responsibilities and roles?

- Within those roles, what are my most significant job tasks?

- What kinds of expertise are required to produce successful client outcomes?

- What are the criteria for successful performance?

Then, the self-assessment incorporates information from one's own work performance and would include answering such questions as the following:

- How do self outcomes data and team outcomes data inform my learning needs and that of my collaborative practice colleagues?
- Is improvement in my performance and the team's performance indicated?
- Are there systems problems and team collaboration issues that I can help modify?
- What can I do to improve efficiency and effectiveness of occupational therapy services and their interdependent integration within collaborative practice environments?

Self-assessment for professional development is slightly different and includes such questions as:

- What are my goals for my career?
- What roles will I need to develop?
- What kinds of tasks might be included in these roles?
- What skills and types of reasoning are involved in these tasks?
- What is my current skill level and reasoning ability in comparison to what might be required for these new tasks?
- What are the criteria for successful performance?

Generally, the practitioner learns to compare his or her current practice performance with some ideal or desired result. To be helpful, self-assessment for the practitioner requires the gathering of valid and reliable information about one's appropriateness and adequacy in working with clients in terms of helping them achieve occupational performance and participation goals within a collaborative practice environment. Self-assessments may include knowledge tests, skills checkouts, performance observations, case studies, self-reflection, peer ratings from team members, records audits, outcomes data, or consumer feedback (Ward, Gruppen, & Regehr, 2002). Self-assessment for professional development typically requires feedback from a mentor or from someone who is in a similar role in comparison to the one in which one hopes to assume.

The question is, how does one determine what is the desirable practice performance or desired level of professional skill development? This requires research into the existence of practice guidelines or standards, recommended competencies, protocols, professional benchmarks, expert recommendations, efficacy and effectiveness studies, and meta-analyses or systematic evidence reviews, as well as expectations of employers, team members, clients, third-party payers, and the public.

Competencies

Competencies are another type of standard guiding self-assessment. Competencies are explicit statements that define specific areas of expertise or competency (Decker, 1999), of which there are four types (Decker & Strader, 1997):

1. Generic across all jobs in an organization
2. Related to management, supervision, or leadership roles
3. Threshold or minimum requirements of a job
4. Specific to a job

A sample statement to illustrate how competencies are written is as follows: "Ability to select and use the most appropriate assessment instrument given the client's age, health and disability status, values, goals, and preferences for specific occupational performance outcomes." This is a threshold statement that could be written to be more specific to a specialized area of occupational therapy practice by referring to an age range or other demographics, diagnoses, type of occupational performance, or method of intervention.

The Interprofessional Education Collaborative Expert Panel (2011) has developed core competencies for interprofessional collaborative practice that all team practices should use to guide their competency and continuing competence. Within the report of the expert panel, the concept of interprofessionality was defined as "the process by which professionals reflect on and develop ways of practicing that provides an integrated and cohesive answer to the needs of the client/family/population" (p. 8). Because interprofessional practice has unique values, codes of conduct, and ways of working, competencies are categorized in a slightly different framework than that described by Decker. According to Barr (1998), professionals on a team have "common" or overlapping competencies, which are those expected of all health professionals. Each team member may overlap the competencies of other professionals on the team in varying ways depending on the professions involved and their scopes of practice, and on the expertise these professionals have developed within their various scopes. Overlapping competencies can be the source of interprofessional tensions, such as in the debate about overlapping competencies between occupational and physical therapists and speech and language pathologists. Overlap should not be seen automatically as negative; it is, in fact, an important strategy to extend the reach of a health profession whose practitioners are inaccessible for various reasons, or when reinforcement of interventions must occur throughout multiple client sessions.

Table 52-1.

CORE COMPETENCIES FOR
INTERPROFESSIONAL COLLABORATIVE PRACTICE

Interprofessional Competency Domain	Competency Statement
Values of Ethics of Interprofessional Practice	"Work with individuals of other professions to maintain a climate of mutual respect and shared values" (p. 19).
Roles and Responsibilities	"Use the knowledge of one's own role and those of other professions to appropriately assess and address the health care needs of the patients and populations served" (p. 21).
Interprofessional Communication	"Communicate with patients, families, communities, and other health professionals in a responsive and responsible manner that supports a team approach to the maintenance of health and the treatment of disease" (p. 23).
Teams and Teamwork	"Apply relationship-building values and the principles of team dynamics to perform effectively in different team roles to plan and deliver patient-/population-centered care that is safe, timely, efficient, effective, and equitable" (p. 25).

In addition, team members have "complementary" competencies that enhance the qualities of other professions in providing care. For instance, rehabilitation professionals work well together to achieve the outcomes for clients after a stroke, where gait, cognition, swallowing, and communication are addressed in ways that assist the occupational therapy practitioner's focus on occupational performance. Important for all team members are "collaborative" competencies, where each profession needs to work: (a) within a profession and among professions, (b) with patients and clients and their families, (c) with nonprofessionals and volunteers, and (d) within and between organizations and communities. These interprofessional competencies have been organized within domains with associated competency statements (Interprofessional Education Collaborative Expert Panel, 2011). Table 52-1 lists these competencies and their accompanying statements.

Discrepancies

Practice discrepancies uncovered through self-assessment do not always necessitate a change in practice, but careful analysis is needed to determine whether modification is needed. The practitioner reflects on why the difference exists as perhaps there are team, system, population, or other key circumstances that explain why one's results are dissimilar to the benchmarks. The size of the gap between what exists and what should occur in practice or in professional development contributes to motivation for change in that a small discrepancy may be overlooked as unimportant and a large discrepancy

may appear impossible to resolve (Handfield-Jones et al., 2002). Ultimately an educational need is identified that prompts development and implementation of a learning plan. The desired change has to be divisible into small, manageable learning steps.

Learning then has to be applied to practice to bring about a change with thought given to how to measure the impact of the learning application on client satisfaction and outcomes. Application to practice requires removal of team and system barriers and creation of system supports in which administration plays a key role. For instance, if the occupational therapist has learned how to administer a reliable and valid occupational performance assessment tool that has evidence for its effectiveness in developing occupation-based intervention, but there are not funds available to purchase the instrument, space to administer the evaluation, or time allowed to complete the evaluation, nor an intervention philosophy among team members that supports occupation-based practice, then the practitioner will be unable to apply this new learning. Similarly, learning will be difficult to apply to professional development if the new opportunities or roles are not available in one's employment or within one's professional roles.

Motivation for Learning

Motivation for learning is complicated and is dependent on one's understanding of the ethical nature inherent in the learning process. The competence of the occupational therapist and the occupational therapy assistant provides the moral justification for implementing occupational therapy processes and services (Moyers, 2005). Principle 1 of the American Occupational Therapy Association (AOTA) *Occupational Therapy Code of Ethics and Ethics Standards* (2010a) indicates the practitioner's responsibility for maintaining high standards of competence. In many states, mandatory continuing education is an aspect of licensure renewal. Similarly, the National Board for Certification in Occupational Therapy (NBCOT) has requirements for achievement of Professional Development Units (PDUs) in the renewal process for the practitioner to use the initials OTR or COTA, whichever is appropriate. The Joint Commission for Healthcare Organizations (JCHO), which accredits hospitals and other health care organizations, has standards that require all employees to update and demonstrate competence to carry out the job tasks assigned.

Motivation to engage in self-assessment and ongoing learning activities, in addition to external requirements of employers, credentialing and accrediting bodies, has an intrinsic component in that it is partially related to the virtues of being a "good" occupational therapist or occupational therapy assistant. The practitioner must display the integrity to self-assess as honestly as possible as a part of one's altruistic responsibility for providing optimal client services (Moyers, 2005). Prudence as a virtue facilitates the disciplined pursuit of competence in which there is a sincere effort to learn what will most likely contribute to excellent client outcomes and high levels of service satisfaction (Moyers, 2005). The practitioner must also have certain underlying abilities to support learning, such as the "requisite intellectual skill and cognitive complexity to understand and synthesize" information, the emotional ability to take risks in applying learning, and the relational abilities to inform clients and team members and to work within systems to implement learning application (p. 28). Obviously, learning application that leads to successful practice change in enhancing service outcomes has the potential for creating an iterative self-assessment process as the result of motivation derived from the quality improvement and collaborative practice process itself.

Development and Implementation of the Learning Plan

Given the complexity of the roles occupational therapists and occupational therapy assistants assume, the questions guiding the development and implementation of the learning plan, whether for continuing competency and competence or professional development, are listed in Table 52-2.

The job competencies thought most likely to lead to high-quality client outcomes are addressed in the

learning plan. These selected competencies are analyzed through the help of AOTA's *Standards for Continuing Competence* (2010b), which includes how knowledge, critical reasoning, interpersonal and performance skills, and ethical practice contribute to successful enactment of each competency. For instance, refer to the sample competency described earlier: to select and use the best assessment given the client's age, health and disability status, and goals for occupational performance. This competency requires *knowledge* of assessments available to measure the specific occupational performance. *Critical reasoning* involves the ability to select according to best evidence the assessment most likely to accurately and reliably assess the occupational performance of interest given the client's characteristics, values, and needs. The *performance skill* underlying this competency is the ability to administer the assessment according to standardization. Collaboratively selecting the assessment and explaining the evaluation process to promote client and team decision making is the requisite *interpersonal ability*. Weighing pragmatic issues of the evaluation process against client needs includes ethical *practice* ability.

Also, in order to develop an effective learning plan, one needs to be aware of the best methods for learning performance and interpersonal skills, gaining knowledge, and developing critical reasoning and ethical practice. For instance, reading may be appropriate for gaining knowledge, but does not compare to role-playing and simulation strategies that may be more effective in enhancing interpersonal abilities, particularly when improving team interactions and communication. Learning plans typically include learning goals, target dates for completion of the learning activities, specific learning activities, resources needed to implement the plan, how one plans to apply the learning to practice, and how one will determine the effectiveness of learning. Learning goals are derived from the learning needs identified in the self-assessment, related to the job competencies and AOTA's *Standards for Continuing Competence* (2010b), and lead to learning applied to practice.

In general, learning for competent performance against standards, for developing capacity, and for professional development must address the intricacy of today's practice environment, regardless of one's roles within that environment. Because occupational therapists and occupational therapy assistants assume roles in which problem solving occurs in complex environments, the cognitive processes are similar to creative thinking (Fraser & Greenhalgh, 2001). Therefore, learning approaches should be designed to facilitate the creative thinking involved in the ability to "appraise the situation as a whole, prioritize issues, and then integrate and make sense of many different sources of data to arrive at a solution" (p. 801). These creative learning approaches are nonlinear in nature or are designed to help learners capture a situation in its "holistic complexity" (p. 801).

Table 52-2. LEARNING QUESTIONS AND LEARNING PURPOSES			
Questions	**Continuing Competence**	**Continuing Competency**	**Professional Development**
Trigger for learning	Does trend information or forecasts indicate that a change in my typical and collaborative practice will be required in the future for my current role?	Is there a gap between my practice and collaborative practice outcomes and what is standard or what is ideal?	In order to assume another position, to be promoted, or to undertake professional leadership, what do I need to learn given my current skills and abilities?
Timing	When should learning occur given the likelihood that the prediction about future practice is feasible in my practice context?	When should learning occur given the importance of the standard to outcomes and to safety?	When should learning occur given my career goals and opportunities?
Content	What specific content for learning that might be applied in my collaborative practice context is suggested by the trend data or forecasts?	What specific evidence-based learning and collaborative practice content would most likely improve safety or outcomes in my practice?	What specific learning content would best prepare me for my future roles?
Learning methods and strategies	How should the learning be organized and delivered given the application feasibility issues and the collaborative practice context?	How should the learning be organized and delivered to ensure application to practice according to standard such that there most likely will be improvements in collaborative practice outcomes or safety?	How should the learning be organized and delivered to assist me in developing potentially applicable skills and abilities needed for assumption of other roles and responsibilities?
Location of learning	How important is learning in context of my practice and in collaboration with my team given that feasibility of application may or may not yet be determined?	How can I implement learning in the context of my practice so that I am able to apply the new learning to collaborative practice more effectively and efficiently?	How can I locate opportunities to apply learning so that skills and abilities will not erode before I reach my career goals?
Educational providers and role of employer	Who is producing the most up-to-date information on this trend and is conducting the latest research applicable to my collaborative practice?	How can I work with my employer and team to create learning opportunities within the context of my collaborative practice?	Is my employer supportive of my career goals and should I consider locating a mentor outside of work to help me get started?
Application	What aspect of the learning could be applied to collaborative practice in the near future? And, do I need more education and training before application?	What aspect of the learning must be applied to collaborative practice in order to better meet standards for safety and for outcomes?	What aspect of the learning could be implemented if I take advantage of upcoming career opportunities?
Context, environment, or system	What aspects of the collaborative practice context support or inhibit the feasibility of learning application in the near future?	What barriers in the collaborative practice context require removal and what supports should be put in place in order to assist me in meeting standards and achieving outcomes?	What barriers and supports in my professional context exist that would impact application of learning if I seek specific career opportunities?
Modifying context	What are the best strategies to enhance feasibility of learning being applied to collaborative practice in the near future?	What strategies would be effective in modifying the collaborative practice context to support immediate application of learning so that standards are met and outcomes are improved?	What do I need to do to make sure that I can take advantage of opportunities to apply new skills and abilities in order to meet my career goals?
Evaluation of the impact of learning	How will I know if my learning has made a difference in collaborative practice given questions of feasibility of application? Should I target evaluation primarily to change in knowledge?	How and when should the impact of learning on client outcomes be measured, or how will I know my learning has been effective in meeting collaborative practice standards?	What formative and summative skill and ability evaluations should I implement to give me feedback about my progress toward my career goals?

Nonlinear learning methods typically involve storytelling, case histories, reflection, and problem-based learning strategies. There is an emphasis on self-directed learning, in which the learner is supported in developing his or her own learning goals, receiving feedback, reflecting, and consolidating one's ideas. These self-directed learning goals avoid rigid and prescriptive content in that the subject matter may vary depending on the needs of the learner.

There also should be efforts to capture the benefits of informal and unplanned learning. Some examples of these informal learning methods include experiential learning (i.e., job shadowing or apprenticeships); networking opportunities; reflection exercises; list serves and discussion groups for professional interest groups; "teachback" opportunities, in which newly skilled practitioners teach others their shared understanding; and feedback on the application of the learning (Fraser & Greenhalgh, 2001, p. 802).

Self-directed learning, however, in collaborative practice requires modification to include team self-directed learning, in which the learning of the team as a whole takes precedence over individual learning needs. In addition, team-based learning is more likely to use work-based learning methods, in which adult learning approaches, small group work, and critical and active learning are central to the learning process (Cameron, Rutherford & Mountain, 2012). The strategies for team learning that occur within the work context include similar self-directed learning and informal methods described previously, but always includes clinical supervision, action learning through project work, and individual and team coaching/mentorship.

Portfolios

Portfolios archive the self-assessment process described in the model, including the reflection on the self-assessment to determine learning needs related to job-related competencies or to professional development aspirations (Tillema, 2001). The learning plan devised to address the learning needs is also housed in the portfolio, along with evidence of engagement in the various learning activities, such as specialty certifications or professional recognition and documentation of continuing education, coursework, publications, or presentations. Each of the learning activities is carefully appraised to ensure that the activity contributes to achievement of the learning competencies. The self-appraisal process answers the question: What evidence would best indicate my potential for possessing the competencies needed for practice?

The most complete portfolios are reflective in nature, as there is an examination of why one chose a particular learning activity and how participation in that activity affected one's practice relative to the specific competency.

Reflection connects learning application to practice with client outcomes. For instance, if the competency is about administering specialized assessments, then why was writing a case study chosen; how did constructing the case study contribute to knowing how and when to administer particular assessments; and how did the client evaluation experience change as the result of applying the learning to practice? Portfolios used to document one's continuing competence or competency or professional development processes are thus quite different in complexity and should not be considered the same as a scrapbook of personal and professional achievements, an archive of all one has ever done in one's life or career, or a collection of random continuing education certificates and program handouts. Portfolios can demonstrate the potential for continuing competence and competency, especially if requiring evidence of the following (Miller, 1990):

- Knowing
- Knowing how (knows the procedures or steps)
- Showing how (can do the procedures or steps)
- Actual doing (actually does the procedures in practice)

Even though portfolios have usefulness in determining potential for continuing competence and competency, safeguards to ensure the quality of the portfolio must be in place because the self-assessment (determining the learning need) and self-appraisal (selecting the best evidence of achieving the competency) skills of a health care professional may be limited under certain conditions. Health care professionals benefit from training in these self-evaluation processes, require experience over time, and need feedback from others who view their performance in order to become more skilled in self-assessment and in self-appraisal (Kruger & Dunning, 1999). Feedback is needed because high achievers tend to underestimate their abilities and low achievers tend to overestimate their abilities. However, persons who are incompetent may not only reach erroneous conclusions about their level of ability (overestimate), but they may also lack the metacognitive ability to realize their incompetence. Inherent within self-assessment and self-appraisal is the ability to accurately reflect on one's own practice to determine where further learning would be beneficial.

Roles of Stakeholders

A variety of stakeholders are interested in continuing competence and competency and professional development. The stakeholders in the professional community include occupational therapists and occupational therapy assistants, AOTA, state occupational therapy associations, state licensing boards, and NBCOT. Stakeholders

EVIDENCE-BASED RESEARCH CHART

Topic	Evidence
Self-assessment	Finlay & McLaren, 2009; Meretoja & Leino-Kilpi, 2003; Wilkinson, 2013; Wilkinson et al., 2002
Portfolios	Miller & Tuekam, 2011; Mills, 2009; Sowter, Cortis, & Clarke, 2011
Learning methods	Happell & Martin, 2004; Khomeiran, Yekta, Kiger, & Ahmadi, 2006; Landers, McWhorter, Krum, & Glovinsky, 2005; McQueen, Miller, Nivison, & Husband, 2006; Vachon & LeBlanc, 2013; Welch & Dawson, 2006; Williams, 2010
System barrier and facilitators	Price, Miller, Rahm, Brace, & Larson, 2010; Rappolt, Pearce, McEwen, & Polatajko, 2005; Sparrow, Ashford, & Heel, 2005

in the community at large include clients, the public, state and federal governments, third-party payers, accrediting bodies, other professional organizations, employers, team members, and educators. Some of these stakeholders, such as occupational therapists and occupational therapy assistants, are interested in continuing competence and competency as equally as they are concerned with professional development. Others are primarily interested in continuing competence and competency, with a secondary focus on professional development. Because of their missions to protect the public, state licensing boards and voluntary credentialing programs like NBCOT have a primary focus on continuing competence and competency. Professional development is encouraged as it intersects with ensuring that the public receives services from competent occupational therapists and occupational therapy assistants.

Providers of continuing education, such as state and national organizations and universities, need to help learners understand the competencies to be addressed in the offering, as well as incorporate learning activities that are more likely to lead to gains in knowledge, skills, or reasoning abilities. The providers should also help the learner devise a transfer of training plan, or how the practitioner hopes to apply the learning to collaborative practice contexts. Suggestions on how to measure the impact of the learning application should be made as well. The learning program should also incorporate time for periodic reflection about what one is learning and how that learning might improve practice.

Employers have a large role in the learning of their employees in terms of facilitating the self-assessment process, the use of portfolios, and the self-appraisal of learning activities. Careful consideration of the resources needed for learning should occur and should be reflected in the budgeting process in terms of ensuring that the employee has time for learning and the money needed to implement the learning plan. Employers are also in the best position to remove barriers to and to create supportive environments for the application of learning. This typically involves changes in the system and in the collaborative practice context so that new approaches and interventions can be tried and measured. Employers can also help employees obtain and interpret client outcomes data both in terms of identifying learning needs and assessing the success of learning application. Reward and incentive systems are also an important way that employers can facilitate the continuing competence and competency and professional development of their staff. Finally, employers are crucial in determining the competency of their employees as they can use observational methods to compare actual performance to standards.

Summary

Portfolios are an important aspect of continuing competence and competency and professional development. Portfolios document the self-assessment process when it becomes clear that a learning need is evident following a systematic investigative process. The learning need then leads to careful selection of learning activities thought more likely to produce an improvement in one or more competencies necessary for not only excellent, but collaborative, practice. Achieving these competencies through a focus on obtaining knowledge, skills, and reasoning abilities should result in a significant impact on client outcomes. Portfolios designed in this manner are powerful tools in facilitating formative assessment and effective learning; however, the challenge is ensuring that sufficient rigor is maintained throughout the portfolio self-assessment and self-appraisal processes. Portfolios are, more importantly, a way for ensuring that all occupational therapists and occupational therapy assistants undertake an active role in identifying and meeting their own learning needs as an aspect of continuous quality improvement within collaborative practice contexts typical of interdependent health care and social systems. Widespread, rigorous use of portfolios stands to greatly impact the profession in its ability to provide society with quality occupational therapy services.

Student Self-Assessment

1. Spend time reflecting on your career goals five years after you graduate. Identify generally what you would need to learn to achieve this career goal, the resources you would need, and how you would obtain these resources.

2. Suggest some ways that you could incorporate non-linear learning, self-directed learning, and team-based learning to augment what you are learning in a particular class.

3. Reflect on an unplanned learning event in which you experienced a change in your ability to analyze a client situation. Share this reflection in small groups.

4. If you worked with a practitioner who claimed never having time to read anything about occupational therapy, explain how this would be an ethical dilemma and how you would address this situation as a colleague.

References

American Occupational Therapy Association. (2008). *Occupational therapy practice framework: Domain and process* (2nd ed.). Bethesda, MD: AOTA Press.

American Occupational Therapy Association. (2010a). Occupational Therapy Code of Ethics and Ethics Standards (2010). *American Journal of Occupational Therapy, 64*(6), S17-S26. doi:10.5014/ajot.2010.64S17

American Occupational Therapy Association. (2010b). Standards: Standards for Continuing Competence, AOTA Standards for Continuing Competence. *American Journal of Occupational Therapy, 64*(6), S103-S105. doi: 10.5014/ajot.2010.64S103

Barr, H. (1998). Competent to collaborate: Towards a competency-based model for interprofessional education. *Journal of Interprofessional Care, 12*(2), 181-187.

Cameron, S., Rutherford, I., & Mountain, K. (2012). Debating the use of work-based learning and interprofessional education in promoting collaborative practice in primary care: A discussion paper. *Quality in Primary Care, 20*, 211-17.

Decker, P. J. (1999). The hidden competencies of health care: Why self-esteem, accountability, and professionalism may affect hospital customer satisfaction scores. *Hospital Topics, 77*(1), 14.

Decker, P. J., & Strader M. K. (1997). Beyond JCAHO: Using competency models to improve health care organizations, Part 1. *Hospital Topics. 75*(1), 23.

Finlay, K., & McLaren, S. (2009). Does appraisal enhance learning, improve practice and encourage continuing professional development? A survey of general practitioners' experiences of appraisal. *Quality in Primary Care, 17*, 387-395.

Fraser, S. W., & Greenhalgh, T. (2001). Complexity science. Coping with complexity: Education for capability. *British Medical Journal, 323*(6), 799-803.

Handfield-Jones, R. S., Mann, K. V., Challis, M. E., Hobma, S. O., Klass, D. F., McManus, I. C., . . . Wikinson, T. F. (2002). Linking assessment to learning: A new route to quality assurance in medical practice. *Medical Education, 36*, 949-958.

Happell, B., & Martin, T. (2004). Exploring the impact of the implementation of a nursing clinical development unit program: What outcomes are evident? *International Journal of Mental Health Nursing, 13*, 177-184.

Interprofessional Education Collaborative Expert Panel. (2011). *Core competencies for interprofessional collaborative practice: Report of an expert panel.* Washington, DC: Interprofessional Education Collaborative.

Josiah Macy Jr. Foundation. (2013). *Transforming patient care: Aligning interprofessional education with clinical practice redesign.* Retrieved from http://macyfoundation.org/publications/publication/aligning-interprofessional-education

Khomeiran, R. T., Yekta, Z. P., Kiger, A. M., & Ahmadi, F. (2006). Professional competence: Factors described by nurses as influencing their development. *International Nursing Review, 53*, 66-72.

Kruger, J., & Dunning, D. (1999). Unskilled and unaware of it: How difficulties in recognizing one's own incompetence lead to inflated self-assessments. *Journal of Personality and Social Psychology, 77*(6), 1121-1134.

Landers, M. R., McWhorter, J. W., Krum, L. L., & Glovinsky, D. (2005). Mandatory continuing education in physical therapy: Survey of physical therapists in states with and states without a mandate. *Physical Therapy, 85*, 861-871.

McConnell, E. A. (2001). Competence vs. competency. *Nursing Management, 32*(5),14.

McQueen, J., Miller, C., Nivison, C., & Husband, V. (2006). An investigation into the use of a journal club or evidence-based practice. *International Journal of Therapy and Rehabilitation, 13*, 311-317.

Meretoja, R., Leino-Kilpi, H. (2003). Comparison of competence assessments made by nurse managers and practicing nurses. *Journal of Nursing Management, 11*, 404-409.

Miller, G. E. (1990). The assessment of clinical skills/competence/performance. *Academic Medicine, 65*(Suppl.), S63-S67.

Miller, P., & Tuekam, R. (2011). The feasibility and acceptability of using a portfolio to assess professional competence. *Physiotherapy Canada, 63*(1), 78-85.

Mills, J. (2009). Professional portfolios and Australian registered nurses' requirements for licensure: Developing an essential tool. *Nursing & Health Sciences, 11*(2), 206-210.

Moyers, P. A. (2005). The ethics of competence. In R. B. Purtilo, G. M. Jensen, & C. B. Royeen (Eds.), *Educating for moral action: A sourcebook in health and rehabilitation ethics* (pp. 21-30). Philadelphia, PA: F.A. Davis Company.

Moyers, P. A., & Hinojosa, J. (2003). Continuing competency. In G. McCormack, E. Jaffe, & M. Goodman-Lavey (Eds.), *The occupational therapy manager* (4th ed., pp. 489). Bethesda, MD: AOTA Press.

Price, D. W., Miller, E. K., Rahm, A. K., Brace, N. E., & Larson, R. S. Assessment of barriers to changing practice as CME outcomes. *Journal of Continuing Education in the Health Professions, 30*(4), 237-245. doi: 10.1002/chp.20088

Rappolt, S., Pearce, K., McEwen, S., & Polatajko, H. J. (2005). Exploring organizational characteristics associated with practice changes following a mentored online educational module. *Journal of Continuing Education in the Health Professions, 25,* 116-124.

Sautter, K. M., Bokhour, B. C., White, B., Young, G. J., Burgess, J. F., Berlowitz, D., & Wheeler, J. R. C. (2007). The early experience of a hospital-based pay-for-performance program. *Journal of Healthcare Management, 52*(2), 95-107.

Smith, K., & Tillema, H. H. (2001). Long-term influences of portfolios on professional development. *Scandinavian Journal of Educational Research, 45*(2), 183-203.

Sowter, J., Cortis, J., & Clarke, D. (2011). The development of evidence based guidelines for clinical practice portfolios. *Nurse Education Today, 31*(8), 872-876.

Sparrow, J., Ashford, R., & Heel, D. (2005). A methodology to identify workplace features that can facilitate or impede reflective practice: A National Health Service UK study. *Reflective Practice, 6,* 189-197.

Spencer, L. M., & Spencer, S. M. (1993). *Competence at work.* New York, NY: John Wiley and Sons.

Tillema, H. H. (2001). Portfolios as developmental assessment tools. *International Journal of Training and Development, 5*(2), 1360-1376.

Vachon, B., & LeBlanc, J. (2011). Effectiveness of past and current critical incident analysis on reflective learning and practice change. *Medical Education, 45,* 894-904. doi: 10.1111/j.1365-2923.2011.04042.x

Ward, M., Gruppen, L., & Regehr, G. (2002). Measuring self-assessment: Current state of the art. *Advances in Health Sciences Education: Theory and Practice, 7,* 63-80.

Welch, A., & Dawson, P. (2006). Closing the gap: Collaborative learning as a strategy to embed evidence within occupational therapy practice. *Journal of Evaluation in Clinical Practice, 12,* 227-238.

Wilkinson, C. (2013). Competency assessment tools for registered nurses: An integrative review. *Journal of Continuing Education in Nursing, 44,* 31-37. doi: 10.3928/00220124-20121101-53

Wilkinson, T. J., Challins, M., Hobma, S. O., Newble, D. I., Parboosingh, J. T., Sibbald, R. G. & Wakeford, R. (2002). The use of portfolios for assessment of the competence and performance of doctors in practice. *Medical Education, 36*(10), 918-924,

Williams, C. (2010). Understanding the essential elements of work-based learning and its relevance to everyday clinical practice. *Journal of Nursing Management, 18,* 624-632. doi: 10.1111/j.1365-2834.2010.01141.x

World Health Organization. (2010). *Framework for action on interprofessional education and collaborative practice.* Retrieved from http://whqlibdoc.who.int/hq/2010/WHO_HRH_HPN_10.3_eng.pdf

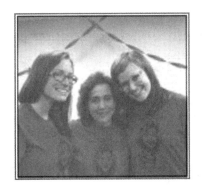

53

ROLES OF OCCUPATIONAL THERAPISTS

Thomas Fisher, PhD, OTR, CCM, FAOTA

ACOTE STANDARDS EXPLORED IN THIS CHAPTER
B.9.7–B.9.9

KEY VOCABULARY

- **Consultant:** Provider of services to an organization, individual, or group; not responsible for the outcome of the intervention.
- **Contractor:** Individual not employed by an agency but given a contract for specific services.
- **Educator:** Faculty member in an academic setting.

- **Entrepreneur:** One who is partially or completely self-employed.
- **Practitioner:** One who is engaged in providing direct, indirect, and/or consultative services.
- **Researcher:** Scientist contributing to a body of knowledge.
- **Roles:** Set of behaviors expected by a group.

Understanding the roles of occupational therapists is important for occupational therapy students, practitioners, educators, and researchers. The occupational therapy practitioner role(s) have evolved over the century and extend beyond reducing the effects of illness, injury, and disease on an individual to the promotion of health and wellness, enabling individuals and groups to increase control over and improve their health and well-being (Wilcock, 2003, 2006).

According to the Accreditation Council for Occupational Therapy Education (ACOTE, 2011), in order to be a competent contemporary occupational therapist in the 21st century, one needs to be able to do the following:

- Discuss and justify the varied roles of the occupational therapist as a practitioner, educator, researcher, consultant, and entrepreneur (Standard B.9.7).

- Explain and justify the importance of supervisory roles, responsibilities, and collaborative professional relationships between the occupational therapist and the occupational therapy assistant (Standard B.9.8).

- Describe and discuss professional responsibilities and issues when providing service on a contractual basis (Standard B.9.9).

Jacobs, K., MacRae, N., & Sladyk, K. (Eds.).
*Occupational Therapy Essentials for
Clinical Competence, Second Edition* (pp. 693-704).
© 2014 SLACK Incorporated.

Introduction

Christiansen and Baum (1997) define roles as "a set of behaviors that have some socially agreed upon function and for which there is an accepted code of norms" (p. 603). Through the years, occupational therapists' roles have expanded. Some occupational therapists are administrators of hospitals, deans in universities, risk managers, and/or case managers (Fisher, 1996).

The profession's official publication, *Occupational Therapy Practice Framework: Domain and Process* (AOTA, 2008), defines *roles* as "a set of behaviors expected by society, shaped by culture, and may be further conceptualized and defined by the client" (p. 643). Regardless of which point in the profession's history one is exploring, a primary focus of the occupational therapist has remained consistent: identifying strengths and barriers for individuals and/or groups as they function in their daily life roles. An occupational therapist assesses an individual's performance within a given role and designs intervention plans that address the skills needed for those specific roles in order for the individual to resume those roles that existed before the injury, illness, or disease. Through these interventions, an individual acquires or redevelops the skills necessary for role performance. The skills translate into habits of behavior. Within each role, individuals develop a repertoire of skills and habits necessary for successful performance. An individual performs many different roles during a lifetime.

An occupational therapist may assume several roles during a professional career. Each role is unique and has specific performance expectations. As occupational therapists, understanding and appreciating these roles and performance expectations are fundamental to being an occupational therapist in the 21st century. As a profession, we believe that roles not only shape what we do and how we look at the world but also allow us to know who we are.

Because of the many roles that shape our lives, we believe that roles provide us with an awareness of social identity and related obligations, as well as a framework for appreciating relevant situations and constructing appropriate behaviors. Roles support us in identifying our unique value and contribution to society (Kramer, Hinojosa, & Royeen, 2003). As occupational therapists, we address roles with the clients we serve. It is an essential component of the occupational therapy process.

In 2010, Scott encouraged occupational therapists to consider the desired roles that consumers of occupational therapy need or want to resume. She found that persons who have had liver transplants and are given the opportunity to share both what roles they value the most and when these roles are integrated into their intervention plan by the occupational therapist, there are better outcomes. She concluded that role participation is a part of social functioning. If the transplant client never moves beyond the patient role, his or her recovery is compromised.

Shannon (1985) addressed the broadening roles of occupational therapists in the continuity of care in a special edition of Occupational Therapy in Health Care. He expanded on an earlier discussion about occupational therapy beyond hospital-based occupational therapy practice. He reminded therapists to understand the political, economic, and cultural environment in which they practice regardless of their role. He suggested that they appreciate their holistic perspective and broad knowledge base, and he emphasized the unique opportunities that community practice brings.

Oakley, Kielhofner, Barris, and Reichler (1986) felt so strongly about this notion of roles that they developed a validated instrument: the Roles Checklist. This instrument was developed out of a need for occupational therapy to have a reliable and valid assessment focusing on several roles in which one engages. It provides the occupational therapist data about individuals' perception of themselves and their participation in roles throughout their life and the degree to which each role is valued. This instrument is used by occupational therapists in a variety of settings, primarily with adults. It addresses four dimensions of roles: "perceived incumbency (an individual's belief that he or she occupies a role), occupational role career (progression of roles throughout one's life), role balance (the ability to maintain sufficient important life roles without conflict or overload of role demand), and role value (degree that an individual attaches to a particular role)" (p. 159).

Henry and Coster (1997) investigated competency beliefs and occupational role behaviors among adolescents. They used the Model of Human Occupation as their theoretical underpinning and concluded that a person's occupational role behavior, be it adaptive or maladaptive, depends on the adolescents' academic ability, social competence, and physical competence.

Kao and Kellegrew (2000) discussed a similar notion of self-concept and academic achievement with adolescents and their role development. They found that young people who have successful experiences in their role as students have a better self-concept and outlook on life.

Braveman (Braveman & Page, 2012) concluded that roles help one to achieve identity and are associated with "who we are" (p. 40). He suggested that roles are critical for human development. Roles are how individuals see themselves, whether it is worker, student, son, granddaughter, and so on. When discussing or describing them, one will often share the responsibilities and obligations that are associated with the particular role. There are no other disciplines in the health and human services industry that explicitly address this component of humans. This is why it is so important for occupational therapy practitioners to address it in their interventions with clients and families.

In addition, an occupational therapist has the potential and opportunity to supervise and collaborate with occupational therapy assistants, thus expanding into the role of supervisor. This chapter's focus identifies specific roles and then addresses the role of supervisor and collaborator with occupational therapy assistants. At the end of this chapter, the responsibilities of the occupational therapist when service provision is on a contractual basis in the current service delivery systems will be addressed.

Roles

Each occupational therapist's employment setting, method of service delivery, competence, and professional development plan are interdependent and completely individualized. Frequently, an occupational therapist's position with an employer may include more than one role. For example, as an occupational therapy educator, the individual may also function as a researcher, service provider, and consultant. Another example would be an occupational therapist on an inpatient rehabilitation unit who could be functioning as a supervisor to the other occupational therapists, occupational therapy assistants, and students and/or as the team coordinator for the unit (e.g., stroke, spinal cord, brain injury) in addition to providing direct occupational therapy services. Therefore, the Roles Checklist is an occupational therapy assessment being used by practitioners and researchers with a variety of populations, individuals, and groups.

Dickerson (2008) summarized the instrument's properties, utility, and outcomes. The administration of the tool, which takes most clients 15 minutes to complete, yields a great wealth of information for the practitioner before developing the intervention plan. In each role, the occupational therapist has performance areas, as well as essential and marginal job functions. The essential functions are the major purposes of a position, whereas marginal functions are necessary to support the essential or major functions. The performance areas specify common activities and expectations associated with the role. As a competent contemporary occupational therapist, it is imperative that the individual perform the roles within the ethical code and standards of the profession (American Occupational Therapy Association [AOTA] Code of Ethics and Ethics Standards, 2010).

Regardless of the employment arrangement, therapists employed by the organization, independent contractor to the organization, or consultant to the organization, the professional responsibility of the occupational therapist to perform the role and provide services in an ethical and professional manner cannot be overemphasized.

Because of the profession's belief about roles and the variety of roles that occupational therapists assume during a career, the professional organization has addressed this officially. The AOTA has official documents (ACOTE, 2011) that support occupational therapists in understanding and appreciating the various roles and describe the supervision of occupational therapists and occupational therapy assistants. The following roles will be examined: practitioner, fieldwork educator, educator, researcher consultant, and entrepreneur.

Practitioner

In the United States, the term *occupational therapy practitioner* refers to both occupational therapists and occupational therapy assistants. For the purpose of this chapter, the discussion will be limited to the occupational therapist, given the text is addressing the educational standards for entry-level occupational therapists. Typically, occupational therapists progress along a continuum in clinical practice. They move from entry level to intermediate and then into advanced level based on experience, education, and practice skills. The essential function of the practitioner is to provide occupational therapy services that include assessments, interventions, program planning and implementation, discharge planning, and transition planning (AOTA, 2000). Services may be provided in direct, indirect, and/or consultative approaches. Within the role of practitioner, the occupational therapist may serve an administrative role or a patient/client educator role in addition to providing direct services.

In some settings, occupational therapy practitioners (therapists and assistants) provide services in groups. In fact, in mental health settings, acute rehabilitation settings, and many community settings (e.g., adult day programs, outpatient facilities, developmental disabilities centers), this is how occupational therapy services are delivered (Scaffa, 2001).

Occasionally, the practitioner may also function in the role of supervisor and/or fieldwork educator. In addition, there is an emerging role of care coordination or case manager which occupational therapists are well prepared to assume (Baldwin & Fisher, 2005; Fisher, 1996; Skinner & Kizziar, 2012).

Fieldwork Educator

With the additional role of fieldwork educator comes additional responsibilities for the therapist. The fieldwork educator needs not only to understand, value, and evaluate the provision of skilled services but also to understand the components of graduate professional education. This individual assists the student integration of classroom knowledge and application to practice. Performing both roles uses a variety of skills and requires additional knowledge. It is important to note that in occupational therapy, an occupational therapist is not permitted to supervise a level II fieldwork student until the therapist has practiced full-time for 1 year (ACOTE, 2011, Standard C.1.14). However, the therapist can begin taking level I students soon after graduation. In addition to these two roles, the occupational therapist might also provide an educational offering in the community to families of persons with disabilities, support groups, other health professionals, and so forth. This assists in explaining the continuum of providing occupational therapy education services to individuals and groups.

All of these functions and roles establish the contemporary role of practitioner in occupational therapy. Due to the shortage of educators, universities are presented with situations where fieldwork educators just meet the minimum standards to take students. Serving in these additional capacities is making the role of practitioner for occupational therapists increasingly challenging. Many organizations have productivity standards (e.g., long-term care facilities, home health) for their therapists. They must be able to charge for a minimum 6 to 7 hours of service a day. To have that level of client contact is challenging in today's fast-paced health care, social, and educational systems for most therapists. Those therapists who accept an additional role as fieldwork educator demonstrate a true commitment to the future of the profession. This underscores the professionalism of these practitioners.

Educator

At some point in one's career as an occupational therapist, an individual might consider a role as faculty member in an academic setting. This is different from being a fieldwork educator. Occasionally, the individual might be considered adjunct faculty by some universities. The profession, through the policymaking body of the organization (Representative Assembly), established a set of standards that articulate the competencies for individuals assuming the role as faculty member in a professional entry-level occupational therapist academic setting or a technical entry-level occupational therapy assistant program as faculty member. These were reaffirmed in the official document *A Descriptive Review of Occupational Therapy Education* (AOTA, 2007). This is a guide to occupational therapy education that was intended for the occupational therapy community to better understand occupational therapy education (doctorates, post doctorates, residencies, master's, and associate degrees).

Additionally, there are role documents for the program directors and academic fieldwork coordinators. These official documents articulate those competencies long suggested by scholars in the field of occupational therapy (Clark, 1987; Fidler, 1981; Jantzen, 1974; Mosey, 1998). They too believed that occupational therapists practicing in professional education have critical demands placed on them and that their performance influences practice, education, and research.

In fact, Bondoc (2005) suggested that professional accountability begins in the formative and formal educational years of the occupational therapist, thus making it critical that, as a profession, we recognize that graduate professional education needs to have those individuals who understand evidence-based education and practice. He articulated that education is a connection that binds the profession, and evidence-based education enhances that link. Because of this, it is no surprise that there was and still is a belief that therapists functioning in the role of occupational therapy educator should be held to certain standards. These standards are important to recognize and understand. Therefore, they are explicitly discussed in this chapter. The development of these standards and subsequent approval were not controversial. It was an expectation from the field. In the future, it would be useful to have similar competencies identified for other roles assumed by occupational therapists (e.g., consultant, researcher).

There are similar competencies for the role of the academic fieldwork coordinator. Like the faculty competencies, these competencies describe the values, knowledge, skills, and responsibilities needed for this role of academic fieldwork coordinator. The competencies for the faculty members and academic fieldwork coordinator in a professional-level occupational therapy program assist universities and colleges in determining and evaluating those routine functions of a faculty member in a professional entry-level program.

Competencies based on the *AOTA's Standards for Continuing Competence* (AOTA, 2000) describe those skills, responsibilities, obligations, and expertise/content knowledge in an area of occupational therapy service that the educator should possess. The standards are clear. The competencies to meet those standards are general statements that need not always be applied with each situation. Competencies may need to be modified. The AOTA cautions universities to consider these guidelines. The standards are knowledge, critical and ethical reasoning, interpersonal skills, and performance skills. Table 53-1 presents these standards.

In terms of the standard for *knowledge* and serving in the academic role, this standard goes on to declare that a faculty member must do the following:

- "Demonstrate the knowledge of how to facilitate student development toward leadership roles

- Develop a plan to continue competency in the breadth and depth of knowledge in the profession to incorporate student learning

- Facilitate effective learning processes that can be used to enhance the learning opportunities for students

Standard	Description	Example
Table 53-1.		
STANDARDS FOR CONTINUING COMPETENCE		
Knowledge	"Occupational therapy practitioners shall demonstrate understanding and comprehension of the information required for the multiple roles they assume" (p. 649).	• Regardless of setting, occupational therapists address the roles that clients assume during their everyday life.
Critical reasoning	"Occupational therapy practitioners shall employ reasoning processes to make sound judgments and decisions within the context of their roles" (p. 649).	• When presented with a client who is critically ill and has had multiple roles, the occupational therapist establishes a rapport with the client, and the client's support system determines an appropriate and safe intervention plan.
Ethical reasoning	"Occupational therapy practitioners shall identify, analyze, and clarify ethical issues of dilemmas in order to make responsible decisions within the changing context of their roles" (p. 650).	• Billing for services in a manner directed by the employer instead of that decision being made by the occupational therapist
Interpersonal skills	"Occupational therapy practitioners shall develop and maintain their professional relationships with others within the context of their roles" (p. 649).	• During team meetings (regardless of settings), the occupational therapist presents client-centered, occupation-based, theory-driven, and evidence-based assessments and interventions.
Performance skills	"Occupational therapy practitioners shall demonstrate the expertise, attitudes, proficiencies, and ability to competently fulfill their roles" (p. 649).	• During one's career, a professional development plan is established and revisited routinely.

Adapted from Accreditation Council for Occupational Therapy Education. (2006). *The reference manual of the official documents of the AOTA* (11th ed.). Bethesda, MD: AOTA Press.

• Develop a plan to continue proficiency in teaching through investigation, formal education, continuing education and self-investigation" (ACOTE, 2006, p. 649)

The standard of *critical reasoning* declares the faculty member must do the following:

• "Facilitate professional development in teaching through continuing education, research, or self-investigation

• Demonstrate the ability to effectively judge new materials, literature, and educational materials that enhance the lifelong learning of future occupational therapy practitioners

• Demonstrate the ability to critically integrate practice, theory, literature, and research for evidence-based practice

• Demonstrate the ability to critically evaluate curriculum and participate in curriculum development" (ACOTE, 2006, p. 649)

The *ethical reasoning* standard includes acting as a "role model of an occupational therapy advocate and change agent with professional and ethical behavior" (ACOTE, 2006, p. 650).

The *interpersonal skills* standard requires that the faculty member in an academic setting must do the following:

• "Project a positive image of the program both internally (within the college or university) and externally (within the community)

• Demonstrate a competent and positive attitude that will result in the mentoring of students in the beginning skills of scholarship, research, and/or service

• Effectively mentor and advise students and student groups

• Create a positive presence of occupational therapy in the university/college and community through service, scholarship, and/or educational experiences

• Effectively mentor other faculty members in their development of teaching, scholarship/research, and/or service

• Demonstrate positive interactions with diverse faculty, students, and others" (ACOTE, 2006, p. 649)

Finally, the standard for *performance skills* states that the faculty member must do the following:

• "Demonstrate the expertise to contribute to the growing body of knowledge in occupational therapy

- Demonstrate the ability to contribute to the profession, academic community, and/or society through service

- Demonstrate the ability to competently prepare ethical and competent practitioners for both traditional and emerging practice settings" (ACOTE, 2006, p. 649)

Similarly, the academic fieldwork coordinator has specific competencies articulated in the document *Role Competencies for an Academic Fieldwork Coordinator* (AOTA, 2000).

The competencies identified for each standard for the academic fieldwork coordinator that could be modified or may not apply to all situations are different from those for the faculty, even though the standards are the same. This was intentional by the Commission on Education of the AOTA. The roles and thus the responsibilities and competencies are different. In 2003, the Representative Assembly of the AOTA approved this document. This document was reviewed, and descriptions were integrated into another document in 2007 (AOTA, 2007). Within the *knowledge standard*, competencies recognized for the occupational therapist in the role of academic fieldwork coordinator that must be met are as follows:

- "Demonstrate the expertise to be able to facilitate the development of future leaders in occupational therapy through student development in supervised quality fieldwork settings

- Develop a plan to continue competency in the breadth and depth of knowledge in the profession to incorporate into student learning

- Develop a plan to promote effective learning processes for students in the program and associated fieldwork education sites

- Demonstrate competence to develop and maintain accurate and current knowledge of reimbursement issues, federal regulations concerning student services, legal issues concerning fieldwork experiences, and pertinent federal/state regulations such as the Americans With Disabilities Act (ADA)

- Demonstrate the competence to develop and maintain accurate and current knowledge in contractual agreements between colleges/universities and fieldwork sites

- Demonstrate the competence to develop and maintain proficiency in fieldwork coordination skills through investigation, formal education, continuing education, or self study" (AOTA, 2007, p. 653).

The *critical reasoning standard* has the following competencies:

- "Facilitate professional development in teaching/ fieldwork coordination through continuing education, research, or self-investigation

- Demonstrate the ability to effectively judge new materials, literature, and educational materials relating to fieldwork that enhance the lifelong learning for future occupational therapists

- Demonstrate the ability to critically integrate practice, theory, literature, and educational materials relating to fieldwork education sites

- Demonstrate the ability to critically evaluate the curriculum, particularly in terms of fieldwork education, for participation in curriculum development

- Demonstrate the ability to evaluate the interpersonal dynamics between occupational therapy practitioners and students to resolve issues and determine action plans" (AOTA, 2007, p. 653).

The *ethical reasoning standard* expects conformance to the following competencies:

- "Act as a role model as an occupational therapy advocate and change agent with professional and ethical behavior

- Clarify and analyze fieldwork issues within an ethical framework for positive resolution

- Identify and represent the educational and fieldwork settings accurately to ensure that legal contracts are appropriately documented" (AOTA, 2007, p. 654).

As with the *faculty standards and competencies*, there are performance skills and interpersonal skills standards. The performance skills competencies are as follows:

- "Demonstrate the ability to plan fieldwork experiences that will prepare ethical and competent practitioners for both traditional and emerging practice settings

- Demonstrate the expertise to develop fieldwork course objectives, course materials, and educational experiences that promote optimal learning for students

- Demonstrate the expertise to evaluate students' learning outcomes for fieldwork to meet the objectives of the program and the organization

- Demonstrate the ability to develop and implement a plan that effectively evaluates fieldwork educators and fieldwork sites to meet the objectives of the program and the organization

• Demonstrate the expertise to prepare, develop, and/or coordinate the legal contracts and associated issues for fieldwork establishment and maintenance

• Demonstrate the ability to design and implement a logical and justified system of fieldwork assignment for students and fieldwork educators

• Demonstrate the ability to plan and implement a plan that develops and maintains accurate documentation of student performance, collaboration with fieldwork settings and supervisors, and/or other documentation required for fieldwork experiences" (AOTA, 2007, p. 654).

Finally, the *standard related to interpersonal skills* requests that the academic fieldwork coordinator meet the following competencies:

• "Projects a positive image of the program both internally (within the college or university) and externally (within the community)

• Demonstrates a competent and positive attitude that will result in the development and mentoring of fieldwork educators

• Effectively mentors and advises students in relation to fieldwork education issues

• Effectively mediates interpersonal issues between students and fieldwork educators

• Demonstrates positive interactions with diverse faculty, fieldwork educators, and practitioners

• Demonstrates positive interactions with appropriate administrators and attorneys to facilitate contract negotiations" (AOTA, 2007, p. 653).

These role competency documents are the most defined competencies for any role an occupational therapist may assume. The AOTA established the Commission for Continuing Competency and Professional Development to develop and maintain specialty and board certifications in specific areas of practice. Certifications emerging through the work of the Commission are discussed elsewhere in this book.

For the AOTA to have engaged in this level of discussion and then adoption by the Representative Assembly are evidence supporting the notion that occupational therapists who want a professional career as a faculty member in an academic setting need to be committed to demonstrating the competencies presented earlier. The profession has articulated its beliefs about professional occupational therapy education and the competencies that should be demonstrated by occupational therapists in the role of faculty or academic fieldwork educator. Some individuals in the academic setting may pursue a career in the role of researcher. This role is one that all entry-level occupational therapists should understand and value.

Researcher

Another role that occupational therapists perform is that of researcher. Kielhofner (2006) suggested that occupational therapists who become researchers do this because they "find the process of discovery exhilarating and because they see how it enhances occupational therapy practice" (p. xiii). This specific role had less emphasis in earlier educational standards but then became recognized and required in the *Accreditation Council for Occupational Therapy Education 1998 Standards*. The current standards (ACOTE, 2011) affirm this educational need for research as the profession is now post-baccalaureate entry education (master's or clinical doctorate) for the professional occupational therapist. Because of research standards for entry level, the expectation for evidence-based practice, and the advancement of the profession, the role of researcher has gained focus by the profession. This particular role should continue to attract those individuals with the formal preparation, interest, and commitment to inquiry. Successful demonstration of the effectiveness and efficacy of occupational therapy interventions will continue during the 21st century.

Like other health professionals, occupational therapy acknowledged the need for research/evidence-based practice and scholarly activity. Because of this appreciation and understanding of the importance of research, the profession agreed that entry-level therapists needed to enter the profession with a graduate professional degree. Educational standards obligated academic programs to recruit and retain faculty with knowledge and skills who could teach this content and role-model the behavior of researcher. As the profession's number of faculty with doctorates increase, the number of faculty assuming the role of researcher/career scientist will also increase.

The major functions for the role of researcher at entry level are to collect, read, interpret, and apply scholarly information as it relates to occupational therapy. In addition to these functions, entry-level research skills include assuming responsibility for ethical concerns related to research and complying with the various institutional research boards and committees (AOTA, 2011).

As an individual progresses through the research career continuum, it is feasible for a therapist to acquire a research degree and assume the role exclusively as a researcher, scholar, or scientist. As a scholar, one possesses advanced knowledge and engages in the conceptualization of a research project, develops the proposal independently, and refines the study as needed. Research scholars in occupational therapy advance the profession of occupational therapy through their discovery, knowledge, and evidence. The Academy of Research, through the American Occupational Therapy Foundation, recognizes and inducts individuals who have made substantial contributions to occupational therapy through research.

Consultant

The role of consultant has been assumed by occupational therapy practitioners for some time. Many times, this is the role that the practitioner or researcher is asked to assume given the nature of the relationship. Organizations or individuals may wish to engage the occupational therapist as a consultant because the service requested is specific or the need for ongoing direct services is not necessary. Therefore, this role was addressed in the *Occupational Therapy Practice Framework* (AOTA, 2008) describing the consultation process for either the person, organization, or population.

The *Framework* describes consulting as "a type of intervention in which occupational therapy practitioners use their knowledge and expertise to collaborate with the client. The collaborative process involves identifying the problem, creating possible solutions, trying solutions, and altering them as necessary for effectiveness" (AOTA, 2011, p. 214).

Entrepreneur

Another role with which the entry-level occupational therapist should be familiar is that of entrepreneur. Entrepreneurs are either partially or fully self-employed individuals. They include those in private practice, independent contractors, and consultants. Because of the broad scope of services that these individuals may be providing, the structure of their organization may be sole proprietorship, partnership, corporation, group practice, or joint venture (AOTA, 2000, 2011). Independent contractors, consultants, and private practice owners are held to the same standard for demonstrating competencies as employees of an organization. This arrangement for demonstrating competence becomes a responsibility for both the contract employee and the employer contracting for the services. Regardless of what the employer or potential employer informs the occupational therapist, it is that individual's responsibility to perform in an ethical and professional manner.

In the role of entrepreneur, key performance areas for the entry-level occupational therapist have been identified. We will now discuss some of the advantages and disadvantages of each:

1. Sole proprietorship

- *Advantages:* Easiest and least expensive to organize; can be established, bought, sold, or terminated quickly; and size and structure can change and others (family) can be involved according to the proprietor's wishes

- *Disadvantages:* Both personal and business assets are at risk; mixing personal and business finances can make it more difficult to measure success; and conflicts or disagreements within the family can stagnate the business and delay needed decision making.

2. Partnerships

- *Advantages:* Relatively easy to establish; partners may combine resources; greater capacity for obtaining credit by partners as opposed to trying to do it solo

- *Disadvantages:* Personal assets of all partners are put at risk; business is disrupted upon the death or withdrawal of either partner.

3. Limited liability corporation (LLC)

- *Advantages:* Owners are provided a flexible form of business organization that provides liability protection comparable to the protection provided by incorporation; can be established at a moderate cost in a short time; all members, one or more members, or a non-member individual may manage an LLC.

- *Disadvantage:* Corporations are monitored by federal, state, and local agencies and so may require more paperwork to comply with regulations and incorporation may have higher taxes.

4. S corporations

- *Advantages:* Liability of stockholders is limited to their investment in the corporation; personal assets are protected; additional funds can be raised through the sale of stock.

- *Disadvantages:* Personal guarantees from officers/stockholders may be required; conflict can arise if a group of stockholders decide to join together to make change if the corporation has limited credit.

5. C corporations

- *Advantages:* Fractional ownership interests are easily accommodated in the initial offering of stock; purchase, sale, and gifting of stock make it possible for changes in ownership without disrupting the business and requires separation of finances and records to reduce inequity.

- *Disadvantages:* Conflict with a group of stockholders could stagnate decision making; paid benefits to stockholders may become costly and effect the business; personal guarantees from corporate officers may be required.

Braveman (2006) supported the role of entrepreneur when he shared the types of common businesses that occupational therapy practitioners can consider. He suggested that to assume the role of an entrepreneur, one needs to understand the various common types of businesses.

Collaboration With Occupational Therapy Assistants

In the 1950s, because of the demand for occupational therapy services and the time required to prepare professional occupational therapists, the profession created occupational therapy assistants in the United States (Crampton, 1958). Early on, the occupational therapy assistant education was designed for those individuals who were high school graduates or equivalent and employed as an occupational therapy aide. Many of the earlier occupational therapy assistant graduates were prepared to work in mental health occupational therapy. The training went from strictly technical to additional didactic instruction. Supervised clinical work (as it was called in earlier times) was mandatory. Throughout the history of occupational therapy assistant education, occupational therapists have been careful to include the assistant in the discussion, but recognizing that the professional occupational therapist had the formal educational preparation to understand the essence of occupation and its influence on humans (Hirama, 1986). Because of the appreciation of what the occupational therapy assistant brings to practice, the profession has routinely been a voice within the occupational therapy profession through representation within AOTA.

Occupational therapy assistants have more inclusion in the profession than other assistants have in their professions (i.e., medicine, physical therapy, nursing). For example, physical therapist assistants who are members of their professional organization are only allowed affiliate membership and have voice about policy through a separate body (American Physical Therapy Association [APTA], 2007). That separate body of physical therapist assistants has two persons in the House of Delegates representing the issues of the assistants. Occupational therapy assistants in the AOTA may run for any office of the association, with the exception of chairperson of the Commission on Education. That individual must be an occupational therapist with a doctoral degree. This is the criteria established by the Nominating Committee of the AOTA and approved by the Representative Assembly. In *Guidelines for Supervision, Roles, and Responsibilities During the Delivery of Occupational Therapy Services* (AOTA, 2009), it is stated that "the occupational therapy assistant delivers occupational therapy services under the supervision of and in partnership with the occupational therapist" (p. 173).

Collaborating with occupational therapy assistants has been and will continue to be a cost-effective method for delivering occupational therapy services. New models of services have emerged over the past decade. The use of occupational therapy assistants by occupational therapists has changed over time. However, regardless of the service model, the AOTA purports collaboration between occupational therapists and occupational therapy assistants as fundamental and necessary. In fact, ACOTE Standard B9.8 has required and continues to explicitly require professional entry-level academic programs for the occupational therapist to show evidence of how the programs are preparing students to collaborate with occupational therapy assistants (ACOTE, 2006, 2011; AOTA, 2000).

Throughout the decades, occupational therapists and occupational therapy assistants providing services together has been important to the profession and society (Hirama, 1986). Understanding and valuing this relationship is necessary for every occupational therapist and occupational therapy assistant. Because of this relationship, the need for the occupational therapist to possess supervision skills cannot be overemphasized. As discussed earlier, understanding the importance of the supervisory role and performing the functions of that role competently allow for a successful delivery of occupational therapy services. Being capable of meeting this understanding is an expectation and standard for accrediting an educational program (ACOTE, 2011). To accomplish this important expectation, it becomes necessary for professional entry-level programs to provide examples of the collaborative relationships during the didactic portion of the academic preparation, to have occupational therapy assistants on the faculty or used as guest lecturers, and to facilitate the exposure of student occupational therapists to occupational therapy assistants while doing both level I and II fieldwork. Over the past decade, many more occupational therapy practitioners have been contracting with organizations, such as school systems, to provide occupational therapy services.

Contractual Occupational Therapy Services

Understanding the responsibilities of a professional when providing occupational therapy services on a contract basis is paramount in the current environment. Green (2004) reported that the vacancy rate for occupational therapists in the past decade is more than 11%. As a result, organizations are willing to contract for services instead of hiring in-house staff. Because of the current environment—more demand than supply—some occupational therapists are transitioning from an employee of the organization to an independent contractor. When making this transition, there are several issues that the professional needs to understand. First, and most importantly, the independent contractor needs to adhere to the profession's code of ethics and standards of practice. Demonstrating a commitment to providing and continually improving occupational therapy services is a must. In this role as contractor, one needs to understand that not only does contracting allow autonomy, but it also requires the individual to be self-directed and goal oriented. Promoting the provision of the best possible quality of interventions for clients served is a primary goal of all occupational therapists; doing so also avoids litigation. In addition, lifelong learning, providing evidence-based interventions, and keeping current with the literature and technology are essential values for the contemporary occupational therapist.

As stated previously, occupational therapists who act as independent contractors or in some other way engage in a contractual arrangement to provide occupational therapy services are held to the same standards as permanent employees of an organization. This is such a fundamental practice parameter that the Joint Commission requires employers to manage contract services and its employees just as they manage their direct employees (Braveman, 2006). It is a shared responsibility between the occupational therapist and the agency with whom they contract. Establishing competency-based plans for all therapists, including contract therapists, helps identify the training that is needed and what should be assessed on a routine basis. For example, as an independent contractor to a free-standing rehabilitation hospital providing supplemental occupational therapy services, the contractor should be assessed on knowledge and skills related to the Functional Independence Measure (FIM), dysphagia, orthotic design and fabrication, and documentation. Because these are skills and knowledge that full-time, in-house staff need, so too should contract employees possess these capabilities.

A complete familiarity with and commitment to upholding the profession's code of ethics and standards of practice cannot be overemphasized. Obeying the code and standards of practice is an expectation. Ignorance is no excuse. Therefore, the contractual professional needs to engage in self-monitoring perhaps even to a greater extent than those employed by an organization. Currently, entry-level professional occupational therapy education is at the level of post-baccalaureate degree (either at the master's or doctorate level). However, because of the changing landscape in health care and societal needs, there are conversations about moving exclusively to the doctorate level. Simultaneously, there are a growing number and demand for individuals with doctoral degrees in occupational therapy. Those who have the Doctor of Occupational Therapy (OTD) credential have either achieved this level through their entry-level program or at the post-professional level. Individuals with this credential can advance their careers in leadership roles in education, practice, and translational or action research (Coppard, Berthelette, Gaffney, Muir, & Reitz, 2009; Leighty, 2011). There are discussions to mandate the entry level to the doctorate, but evidence for this change continues to be gathered. Some programs are already offering the doctorate at the entry level, whereas others are transitioning their master's programs to a doctorate. It is an institution's (university or college) choice. As this trend continues, roles and responsibilities will emerge and change.

Summary

Understanding the importance of roles assumed by occupational therapists is as important as valuing them from a client perspective. In this chapter, the varying roles of practitioner, researcher, educator, consultant, and entrepreneur were discussed. In addition, the importance of the collaborative relationship with occupational therapy assistants and appreciating the responsibilities associated with providing services on a contractual basis were presented. This chapter provided only an overview of issues related to one's role as an occupational therapist. It is the responsibility of occupational therapists to further explore and investigate their roles as they move through their careers. Table 53-2 provides definitions of roles and references to the role.

Student Self-Assessment

1. As you consider your career trajectory, what roles do you see yourself assuming?

2. During your professional education, including all your fieldwork experiences, what roles did you observe occupational therapists assuming? What are the knowledge and skills necessary to be successful in those roles?

3. Identify some roles you can see occupational therapists assuming that were not considered in this chapter.

Table 53-2.

VARIOUS ROLES OF THE OCCUPATIONAL THERAPIST

Topic	Definition	Reference
Educator	The role of educator is a practice area that some occupational therapists assume in their careers that can either be a core, full-time, or part-time position.	AOTA, 2007
Fieldwork educator	The person who supervises and educates entry level students during Level I or Level II Fieldwork.	Jacobs & McCormack, 2011
Researcher	One who finds discovering the science behind occupational therapy assessments, interventions, and outcomes important and wishes to contribute to the profession by building the science.	Kielhofner, 2006
Practitioner	An individual initially certified to practice as an OT or OTA, or licensed or regulated by a state, district, commonwealth, or territory of the United States to practice as an OT or OTA and who has not had that certification, license or registration revoked due to disciplinary action.	ACOTE, 2011
Entrepreneur	Either partially or fully self-employed individuals, including those in private practice, independent contractors, and consultants.	Braveman, 2006
Consultant	A practitioner, educator, or researcher who is asked to provide a specific service/intervention. The individual is not employed by the organization. As a consultant, one is not responsible for the outcome of the recommendation(s) made.	Braveman, 2006

References

Accreditation Council for Occupational Therapy Education. (2011). *Standards and interpretive guide for an accredited educational program for the occupational therapist.* Retrieved from www.aota.org

Accreditation Council for Occupational Therapy Education. (2006). The reference manual of the official documents of the AOTA (11th ed.). Bethesda, MD: AOTA Press.

American Occupational Therapy Association. (2000). Occupational therapy roles and career exploration and development: A companion guide to the Occupational Therapy Role Documents. In *The Reference Manual of the Official Documents of the American Occupational Therapy Association* (8th ed.). Bethesda, MD: AOTA Press.

American Occupational Therapy Association. (2004a). Role competencies for a professional-level occupational therapist faculty member in an academic setting. *American Journal of Occupational Therapy, 58*(6), 649-650.

American Occupational Therapy Association. (2004b). Role competencies for an academic fieldwork coordinator. *American Journal of Occupational Therapy, 58*(6), 653-654.

American Occupational Therapy Association. (2007). A descriptive review of occupational therapy education. *American Journal of Occupational Therapy, 61*(6), 672-677.

American Occupational Therapy Association. (2008). Occupational therapy practice framework: Domain and process (2nd ed.). *American Journal of Occupational Therapy, 62*(6), 625-688.

American Occupational Therapy Association. (2009). Guidelines for supervision, roles, and responsibilities during the delivery of occupational therapy services. *American Journal of Occupational Therapy, 63*(6), 797-803.

American Occupational Therapy Association Code of Ethics and Ethics Standards. (2010). *American Journal of Occupational Therapy, 64*(6), Online Supplement.

American Occupational Therapy Association. (2011b). *The reference manual of the official documents of the American Occupational Therapy Association.* Bethesda, MD: AOTA Press.

American Physical Therapy Association. (2007). *American Physical Therapy Association Web site.* Available at http://www.apta.org

Baldwin, T., & Fisher, T. F. (2005). Case management: Entry-level practice for occupational therapists. *Case Manager, 16*(4), 47-52.

Black, M. M. (1976). The occupational career. *American Journal of Occupational Therapy, 30*(4), 225-228.

Bondoc, S. (2005). Occupational therapy and evidence-based education. *Education Special Interest Section Quarterly, 15*(4), 1-4.

Braveman, B. (2006). *Leading & managing occupational therapy services: An evidence-based approach.* Philadelphia, PA: F.A. Davis Company.

Braveman, B., & Page, J. (2012). *Work: Promoting participation & productivity through occupational therapy.* Philadelphia, PA: F.A. Davis Company.

Bruce, M. A. G., & Borg, B. (2002). *Psychosocial frames of reference core for occupation-based practice* (3rd ed.). Thorofare, NJ: SLACK Incorporated.

Christiansen, C., & Baum, M. C. (1997). Glossary. In C. Christiansen & C. Baum (Eds.), *Occupational therapy: Enabling function and well-being* (2nd ed., pp. 591-606). Thorofare, NJ: SLACK Incorporated.

Clark, B. (1987). *The academic life: Small worlds, different worlds.* Princeton, NJ: Carnegie Foundation for the Advancement of Teaching.

Coppard, B., Berthelette, M., Gaffney, D., Muir, S., & Reitz, S. M. (2009). Why continue two points of entry education for occupational therapists? *OT Practice, 14*(4), 10-14.

Coster, W. (1998). Occupation-centered assessment of children. *American Journal of Occupational Therapy, 52*(5), 337-344.

Crampton, M. W. (1958). The recognition of occupational therapy assistants. *American Journal of Occupational Therapy, 12*, 269-275.

Dickerson, A. E. (2008). The role checklist. In B. J. Hemphill-Pearson (Ed.), *Assessments in occupational therapy mental health: An integrative approach* (2nd ed.). Thorofare, NJ: SLACK Incorporated.

Fidler, G. S. (1981). From crafts to competence. *American Journal of Occupational Therapy, 35*, 567-573.

Fisher, T. F. (1996). Roles and functions of a case manager. *American Journal of Occupational Therapy, 50*, 452-454.

Green, N. (2004). Demand and recruitment. *OT Practice, 9*(5),48.

Hirama, H. (1986). The COTA: A chronological review. In S. E. Ryan (Ed.), *The certified occupational therapist: Roles and responsibilities*. Thorofare, NJ: SLACK Incorporated.

Jacobs, K., & McCormack, G. (Eds.). (2011a). *The occupational therapy manager* (5th ed.). Bethesda, MD: AOTA Press.

Jantzen, A. C. (1974). Academic occupational therapy: A career specialty, 1973 Eleanor Clarke Slagle lecture. *American Journal of Occupational Therapy Association, 28*, 73-81.

Joint Commission on Accreditation of Healthcare Organizations. (2004). *Human resource standards applicability to contracted and volunteer personnel*. Retrieved from http://www.jointcommission.org/mobile/standards_information/jcfaqdetails.aspx?StandardsFAQId=344&StandardsFAQChapterId=66

Kao, C. C., & Kellegrew, D. H. (2000). Self concept, achievement and occupation in gifted Taiwanese adolescents. *Occupational Therapy International, 7*(2), 121-133.

Kielhofner, G. (2006). *Research in occupational therapy: Methods of inquiry for enhancing practice*. Philadelphia, PA: F.A. Davis Company.

Kramer, P., Hinojosa, J., & Royeen, C. B. (2003). *Perspectives in human occupation: Participation in life*. Philadelphia, PA: Lippincott Williams & Wilkins.

Leighty, J. (2011). The doctorate is in. *Today in OT, 4*(4), 10-12.

Mosey, A.C. (1998). The competent scholar. *American Journal of Occupational Therapy, 52*, 760-764.

Oakley, F., Kielhofner, G., Barris, R., & Reichler, R. (1986). The role checklist: Development and empirical assessment of reliability. *Occupational Therapy Journal of Research, 6*(3), 155-170.

Scaffa, M. (2001). *Occupational therapy in community-based practice settings*. Philadelphia, PA: F.A. Davis Company.

Scott, P. J. (2010). Participation in valued roles post-liver transplant. *British Journal of Occupational Therapy, 73*(11), 517-523.

Shannon, P. D. (1985). From another perspective: An overview of the issue. In F. S. Cromwell (Ed.), *The roles of occupational therapists in continuity of care*. New York, NY: Haworth Press.

Skinner, N., & Kizziar, B. K. (2012). The evolving role of care coordination in an acute care environment: Confirming the appropriate utilization of necessary services—separating tasks from process. *Case Management Society of America Today, 2*, 18-20.

Wilcock, A. A. (2003). Population interventions focused on health for all. In *Willard and Spackman's occupational therapy* (10th ed.). Hagerstown, MD: Lippincott Williams & Wilkins.

Wilcock, A. A. (2006). *An occupational perspective of health* (2nd ed.). Thorofare, NJ: SLACK Incorporated.

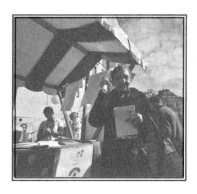

ETHICAL CONFLICT RESOLUTION

Susan C. Burwash, PhD, MSc(OT), OTR/L, OT(C)
and John W. Vellacott, EdD, MEd, BA

ACOTE STANDARDS EXPLORED IN THIS CHAPTER
B.9.10, B.9.11

KEY VOCABULARY

- **Bullying:** Unwanted, repetitive, aggressive behavior that may involve physical, verbal, relational, and/or electronic means of exerting power over another individual.
- **Conflict resolution:** Consciously used communication and problem-solving strategies for addressing conflict.
- **Ethical conflicts:** Disagreements between parties about the ethical resolution to a problem.

- **Ethical dilemmas:** Situations in which there are several alternatives, all of which are ethically somewhat problematic.
- **Moral distress:** Distress occurring when an individual knows what she or he should do but is not able to do it.
- **Moral residue:** Persisting feelings that arise over time from repeated experiences of moral distress.

Introduction

Occupational therapists and occupational therapy assistants work with people who typically seek our services because they or their loved ones are ill, may be suffering, and are unable to do what they need or want to do in their daily lives. Our role as occupational therapy practitioners is to help individuals with whom we work to regain hope for the future, to maintain, restore, or gain the skills they need, to modify how they do their occupations, and/or to make environmental modifications—all in the service of moving forward in their lives. Occupational therapy is, at its heart, an inherently moral undertaking. Thus, it should not be surprising that occupational therapy practitioners frequently encounter situations that call on them to recognize and resolve moral and ethical conflicts within practice.

Jacobs, K., MacRae, N., & Sladyk, K. (Eds.).
Occupational Therapy Essentials for
Clinical Competence, Second Edition (pp. 705-716).
© 2014 SLACK Incorporated.

Occupational therapy practitioners are guided by their personal morals as well as professional values and the expression of values that are contained in codes of ethics from national organizations (American Occupational Therapy Association [AOTA], 2010; see discussion in Chapter 48) and state licensing boards. However, no code of ethics is both broad and deep enough to provide specific guidance in every situation in which we encounter ethical conflicts and dilemmas. Furthermore, we work with clients, families, and other health care providers who may hold differing opinions about what is right or wrong and how individuals, groups, and communities should be. This work occurs within a variety of systems that are governed by laws, policies, and procedures that direct individuals working within them.

It is not surprising, then, that practitioners encounter ethical quandaries on a very regular basis. Respondents to a study done by Kyler (1998), which included occupational therapists, assistants, and students, reported frequent (21% daily, 31% weekly) instances where they had experienced ethical concerns. Slater and Brandt (2009) found high numbers of practitioners who had distress related to ethical issues, including reimbursement constraints, conflict with organizational policies, questionable decisions made by others, and conflicts about discharge decisions, among others. Kinsella, Park, Appiagyei, Chang, and Chow (2008) studied Canadian occupational therapy students' experiences of ethical tensions during fieldwork and found systemic constraints, conflicting values, observing questionable behavior, and failure to speak up as the most common themes reported in students' stories.

In this chapter, we will discuss ethical conflicts and ethical dilemmas—what they are, strategies for acting on these concerns (including the pros and cons of action), and general guidelines for reasoning through these challenging situations. We will also briefly explore the special case of bullying, given that this is something that occupational therapy practitioners' clients, or occupational therapy professionals themselves, may have experienced and be responding to. Resources for further learning will also be provided.

The Accreditation Council on Occupational Therapy Education (ACOTE, 2012) standard asks us to be able to competently identify, reason through, and take action (informal or formal) when we have either personal or organizational ethical issues. Although the primary focus of this chapter is on personal ethical conflicts and how they can be resolved, we acknowledge that ethical conflicts often arise from differences between individual practitioners and the organizations in which they work, and suggest that resolution of ethical issues rests on the shoulders of organizations as well as on practitioners.

Ethical Conflicts and Dilemmas

As described in Chapter 48, occupational therapy practice is guided by the principles of altruism, equality, freedom, justice, dignity, truth, and prudence. As noted, these principles guide us in everyday decisions about confidentiality, informed consent, and, more broadly, about the quality of life concerns that are central to occupational therapy practice. No matter how much we attend to following the code of ethics, we will face personal ethical conflicts and dilemmas that will sometimes cause distress.

ETHICAL CONFLICTS

Ethical conflicts arise when what we believe is the best resolution to a problem is either not in accordance with what another person involved in the situation believes and/or when our personal ethical standards collide with values we have committed ourselves to uphold as occupational therapy practitioners. For example, we might not agree with an individual's decision to refuse activities of daily living (ADL) skills training following a stroke because she or he expects that her or his family will provide significant support on a daily basis—an assumption that is part of the individual's cultural norms. Our professional values related to the importance of independence, our own valuing of independence, and the priorities of the health care systems in which we work may make it challenging for us to accept that a client might want to be dependent in ADL, or, more accurately perhaps, interdependent. Still, it would be possible, having talked with both the client and their caregiver(s), to use the code of ethics to explore this conflict and uphold the principles of freedom of choice. In so doing, the practitioner may decide to support this individual's decision and turn attention away from independence to working with the client and caregiver(s) to support them in completing ADL interdependently.

A frequently cited conflict from respondents in both Kyler (1998) and Slater and Brandt's (2009) studies was conflict arising from other health care professionals making or recommending discharge plans with which the occupational therapy practitioner disagreed. If the occupational therapy practitioner has strong doubts about the readiness of the client, family, or other caregivers for safe discharge to home, conflict could arise. Again, the code of ethics would provide guidance and direct the practitioner toward taking a stand, using altruism and prudence as guiding principles. Another example of an ethical conflict could occur when a practitioner is asked by his or her employer to use billing codes that do not accurately reflect services provided. In all of these examples, there is a choice that appears to clearly be more closely aligned with occupational therapy values and, in the last case, with legal requirements. Thus, the challenge to the practitioner is mostly in determining *how*, or *if*, action can be taken to address the conflict.

ETHICAL DILEMMAS

Ethical dilemmas, in comparison to ethical conflicts, are considerably more complex. They are defined as what happens when occupational therapy practitioners find themselves in situations where a decision must be made between two or more alternatives, *all* of which have considerable drawbacks (Epstein & Delgado, 2010). For instance, to go back to the example of discharge planning, a dilemma might be having to choose between recommending one of two discharge options, neither of which the client has chosen or is likely to provide the level of ongoing support that you know this client will need to continue to improve. Both options are available now within the client's home community and have a reputation for providing reasonably competent staff. Another example would be the dilemma faced by an occupational therapy practitioner when neither of three adaptive technology options for which funding is available are nearly as good as a more expensive option that is not covered by the client's insurance. A third common example could be balancing the competing demands of seeing more clients during a day but for less time each, or spending more time with certain clients and not seeing other clients that day. Ethical dilemmas can be large or small, but what marks them is the sense that there is no clear answer in the view of the person experiencing the dilemma. The challenge becomes if the practitioner can make a choice and on what grounds to pick one of several nonoptimal options.

Possible Responses to Ethical Tensions

Just as we have choices in how to address conflicts and dilemmas we encounter in our day-to-day lives outside work, we must also make informed choices within our workplaces about our available options. Most occupational therapy practitioners have had some experience with, or training in, assertive communication to address interpersonal conflicts. Many practitioners even teach social skills, including assertiveness, self-advocacy, and conflict resolution to clients. Our professional standards speak to the importance of occupational therapy practitioners acting as advocates for clients. Even so, the studies cited previously about ethical tensions suggest that occupational therapy practitioners sometimes struggle with taking ethical action. Students, in particular, are faced with tough decisions about whether to (1) ignore ethical issues that arise, (2) avoid discussing them with any of the involved parties and perhaps even their

supervising therapist, or (3) take the risk of addressing these issues and potentially jeopardizing successful completion of fieldwork. This ethical predicament has been observed not only in occupational therapy students but also in medical students (Caldicott & Faber-Langendoen, 2005; Lorris, Carpenter, & Miller, 2009), dietetics students (Tighe & Mainwaring, 2012), and nursing students (Callister, Luthy, Thompson, & Memmott, 2009), among others.

Each of these possible responses has some benefits and costs. Ignoring issues that arise or avoiding discussion of them may feel, particularly to students, like the safest choice. Finding a way to speak out may seem dangerous and requires careful consideration. Suggestions for how to address conflict are presented later in this chapter.

What Are the Costs of Not Addressing Conflict?

Although it may seem risky to speak up when you encounter ethical dilemmas or conflicts, there are also risks involved in ignoring or avoiding ethical concerns, or as Kinsella et al. (2008) call them, *ethical tensions*. Possible negative influences may affect not only clients and families but also colleagues, organizations, the community, and the occupational therapy profession. Jameton (1984) talks about *moral distress* as occurring when an individual knows what she should do but is not able to do it. Clinicians or students who see someone discharged who they clearly believe is not able to safely manage in the environment to which they are going, or who are unable to provide the number of therapy sessions that they believe will solidify gains made in a neuro-rehabilitation program, or who see a client being treated disrespectfully and do not intervene, might all suffer moral distress. Jameton (1984) and others (Webster & Bayliss, 2000) have labeled these long-term feelings as *moral residue*.

Much of the research on moral distress, and the long-term feelings arising from it, has focused on the nursing profession. This research has been briefly summarized by Kirk (2011). Epstein and Hamric (2009) note that nurses experiencing moral distress/moral residue may become morally numbed in the face of new ethical challenges. They often respond by withdrawing and feeling isolated from their colleagues, who they perceive to be better managing these tensions. They may choose more or less productive ways of registering their dissent. They may suffer from *compassion fatigue* or *burnout*. Compassion fatigue and burnout are associated with a variety of physical and behavioral symptoms that compromise clinician/caregiver health and well-being (Compassion Fatigue Solutions, 2013). Slater and Brandt's (2009) survey of occupational therapists who reported moral distress found that some had left jobs, were exploring other positions, or had even considered leaving the profession. More than half reported persistent feelings of guilt, anxiety, and depression as a result of these ethical tensions.

It is clear that unresolved ethical tensions will affect the clients with whom these clinicians are working. It can also affect health care organizations as a whole. Organizations and professional associations are recognizing this, although research on moral distress/residue's impact at the institutional level is somewhat sparse—after all, what organization wants to admit that situations leading to moral distress occur within their organization? Still, there have been institutional responses as organizations have recognized the levels of distress that are occurring. These will briefly be discussed later. However, our primary focus is at the individual practitioner level. Practitioners can often not completely address these concerns on their own. Kinsella et al. (2008) note "a need for greater attention to the ways in which macro-level policies can shape micro-level practices, and thus raise issues for occupational therapists" (pp. 180-181).

Individual and Organizational Strategies to Address Ethical Conflict

How can individuals and institutions, as well as professional associations and educational programs, help to reduce ethical tensions and address them when they arise? In this section, we review some general principles for conflict resolution and some specific strategies that have been developed for dealing with ethical conflict resolution. Some of the general guidelines for conflict resolution come from the work of those interested in improving assertiveness skills and/or nonviolent conflict resolution. Many occupational therapy practitioners may have learned some of these skills prior to entering their professional education or during their coursework. Taylor's (2008) *Intentional Relationship* text also offers some concrete strategies for occupational therapy practitioners when dealing with therapist–client conflicts. These strategies could be usefully reviewed when considering how to address ethical conflicts with other individuals in the practice setting. Although we review some of these approaches here, in our experience, students and clinicians report that knowing these skills alone is not always sufficient.

Assertive Communication

People communicate with one another through many different means—verbally, nonverbally, in writing, or in images. In therapy settings, the issue of communication arises in interactions between the practitioner and the client/family, other clinicians, administrators, billing authorities, and so forth. When conflict occurs during the communication process, the use of assertive communication skills can be a critical element in effectively managing the situation. Slater and Brandt (2009) note the crucial contribution that effective communication has in preventing and resolving conflicts. This aspect of the chapter will describe what assertive communication is and some specific approaches that occupational therapy practitioners can use in both their own practice and in assisting clients/families.

What Is Assertive Communication?

Hasan (2008) defines assertiveness as a mid-way point between passivity and aggression. He defines assertive communication as "the direct expression of an individual's ideas while respecting the rights of others in an atmosphere of trust" (p. 2). Similarly, Kubany, Richard, Bauer, and Muraoka (1992) consider assertiveness as the "expression of feelings, preferences or opinions in ways that respect the rights and opinions of others" (p. 337). Pipas (2010) likewise describes assertive communication as "the ability to represent to the world what you really are, to express what you feel, when you feel it necessary. It is the ability to express your feelings and your rights, respecting the feelings and rights of others" (p. 649). She notes that individuals who have mastered assertive communication skills are usually able to manage or reduce interpersonal conflicts in their lives. How does one communicate assertively? There are a number of possible techniques and approaches.

Preparing to Communicate Assertively

Before trying to communicate assertively, it is important to lay the groundwork for ensuring that the communication effort is successful. Barnette (2009) suggests the following steps:

1. *Assess the situation:* Before engaging in assertive communication, attempt to determine the possible consequences. Although assertive communication usually will result in a positive response, some people might react negatively to it. If that occurs, are you prepared to accept and address this response?

2. *Set the stage:* Remember that other individuals may be accustomed to interacting in a certain way. Being presented with a more assertive approach to communicating may be disconcerting or upsetting to them. Advising other people upfront and prefacing the conversation or communication with an acknowledgement that you may be communicating differently than you have in the past may be beneficial.

Assertive Communication Techniques

There are many different skills and techniques that can be applied to communicate assertively and effectively. Tillman (2007) breaks these down into three sets, which she summarizes as follows:

1. *Nonverbal:* These include such things as:

   - Eye contact (maintaining direct eye contact about 50% of the time)
   - Voice tone (well modulated)
   - Posture (straight and relaxed)
   - Facial expressions (reflecting your emotional state—smiling if happy, serious if angry, etc.)
   - Use of gestures (nodding or shaking head, avoiding aggressive gestures such as hands on hips, fists, etc.)
   - Nonverbal listening (attending to the person while he or she is speaking, leaning in slightly to show you are listening, etc.).

2. *Verbal:* The use of communication approaches such as:

   - Restatement (restating to the other person what you have heard)
   - Reflection (indicating what you saw, believe the other person said, and how you interpret it)
   - Clarification (asking the speaker to explain a point that he or she is trying to make)

3. *Interactive:* Assertive communication is a two-way street, with both parties responding and interpreting each other's verbal and nonverbal cues. To assist in this process, the individual can apply strategies such as:

   - Soft assertion (making statements that do not require anything of the listener, such as compliments and visual images)
   - Basic assertions (simple statements of what the speaker wants or does not want to happen)
   - Empathic assertions (attempts to communicate how he or she thinks the other person may be thinking or feeling)
   - Escalating assertions (a statement with a consequence attached to it)
   - Confrontive assertions (a statement made when an agreement has been violated)

Often, individuals engaging in assertive communications encounter resistance from the other party, who may not be responsive to the techniques described earlier. Barnette (2009) suggested some additional strategies for addressing challenges to assertive communication:

- *Broken record:* Keep repeating your point, using a low-level, pleasant voice. Do not get pulled into arguing or trying to explain yourself. This allows you to ignore manipulation, baiting, and irrelevant logic.

- *Fogging:* This is a way to deflect negative, manipulative criticism. You agree with some of the facts but retain the right to choose your behavior.

- *Content to process shift:* This means that you stop talking about the problem and bring up, instead, how the other person is behaving RIGHT NOW. Use it when someone is not listening or is trying to use humor or a distraction to avoid the issue.

- *Defusing:* Let someone cool down before discussing an issue.

- *Assertive inquiry/stop action:* This is similar to the content to process shift. "Let's hold it for a minute, something isn't working, what just happened? How did we get into this argument?" This approach helps to identify the real issue when the argument is actually about something bigger than the immediate topic. (p. 4)

Assertive communication involves the effective application of both verbal and nonverbal strategies to ensure that the individual is able to express his or her feelings, preferences, or opinions in a manner that is effective but that also respects the rights and opinions of others (Kubany et al., 1992). Assertive communicators are confident, direct, and honest but also willing to acknowledge the viewpoints of others (Kolb & Griffith, 2009). Effective and assertive communication can go a long way toward addressing and resolving conflict, whether it is about day-to-day differences or ethical issues.

Anticipating and Addressing Conflict Through the Use of the Intentional Relationship Model

Taylor (2008) discusses some of the anticipated conflicts that clinicians may experience and strategies for dealing with these conflicts. Anticipating what she calls the "inevitable interpersonal events of therapy" (p. 117) and having the skills to understand the client, understand oneself, and being able to shift modes (i.e., from educating mode to empathizing mode) can prevent or reduce clinician–client conflicts. She also briefly addresses other instances of conflict and provides advice on how to resolve these conflicts, as well as provides learning activities designed to further develop these skills. She links the modes to the ethical principles outlined by AOTA and describes how using these modes can help the practitioner meet these ethical standards.

A Process for Addressing Ethical Tensions and Moral Distress

The American Association of Critical-Care Nurses (AACN, 2008) outlines a helpful process for those experiencing and addressing ethical conflict. This "4A's" model asks that we do the following:

1. *Ask:* Reflect on whether we are experiencing moral distress as the result of ethical conflicts or dilemmas.

2. *Affirm:* Validate our experience with trusted others, decide that we are willing to take care of ourselves, and review our professional obligations.

3. *Assess:* Determine the personal and environmental factors contributing to distress, the severity of distress, our willingness to take action, and pros/cons of taking action.

4. *Act:* Prepare, act, and maintain the change you have initiated.

These steps are described in more detail and additional tools provided in the AACN publication *The 4A's to Rise Above Moral Distress* (available at no charge) on the AACN Web site (see the Electronic Resources section for the URL).

Other Suggestions for Dealing With Ethical Conflicts

Epstein and Delgado (2010) summarize some strategies for addressing moral distress in a variety of work settings. Being willing to speak up, being intentional, being accountable, ensuring that you have support from colleagues, focusing on the system and not just on individuals, and participating in or designing interdisciplinary ethics workshops are all strategies that they suggest may help. The institution with which they are affiliated has instituted a Moral Distress Consult Service specifically to address these concerns. Most large institutions will have a medical ethicist on staff; such individuals can also be very helpful when individual action seems overwhelming or has not been successful. Ethicist Hilde Nelson (1995) suggests the importance of addressing issues as part of what she calls a "chosen community"; she believes that it is in these communities of peers that individuals can further develop moral agency.

Student clinicians who encounter ethical conflicts and dilemmas should, ideally, address these first with their supervising therapist and also with their educational institutions' fieldwork coordinator. It is important to have support as you work through what is happening and what your next step should be. Document what you are experiencing. Reflect on your options and the pluses and minuses of each. Consider whether the 4A process mentioned previously might help you in your decision making. Many educational programs offer some form of fieldwork "debriefing" sessions following fieldwork. Use these as an opportunity to share your experiences and get support and advice from faculty and student colleagues. Brown and Gillespie (1997) used "theatre of the oppressed" techniques to assist occupational therapy students in practicing moral courage in response to ethical tensions. In this approach, the individual who has experienced ethical tensions describes the incident to peers, who help her or him act out the incident. During subsequent repetitions of the scene, observers may take the part of the protagonist to show alternative ways of dealing with the situation differently.

The Special Case of Bullying and Conflict Resolution

Conflict takes many forms, and resolving conflicts in a professional and ethical manner is a critical skill for all helping professionals. However, some types of conflict present more challenging issues than others. One such example is the behavior known as bullying. Bullying, in all its manifestations, has been the topic of much attention within the media, academia, and society at large in recent years. Bullying is increasingly being recognized as a problematic and destructive phenomenon that is present in many aspects of society, including education, academia, the online world, the workplace, and within institutional settings. Bullying is the most common form of violence in our society (Blazer, 2005) and is a phenomenon that is experienced across the age spectrum. Bullying in childhood and adolescence (especially bullying in school settings and online), bullying in adulthood (particularly in workplace settings), and bullying among and to the aged (especially within institutional care settings) are common. Occupational therapy practitioners, in their varied roles, can be called upon as key interveners in addressing bullying behaviors and its impacts across a wide range of settings.

Bullying: Definitions

Although the underlying causes or origins of bullying behavior are not fully understood (Strandmark & Hallberg, 2007), there are many different definitions of what constitutes bullying, depending on the population and setting. In children and adolescents, the U.S. Department of Health and Human Services (2013) defines bullying as "unwanted, aggressive behavior" among school-age children that involves a real or perceived power imbalance. The behavior is repeated, or has the potential to be repeated, over time. Bullying includes actions such as making threats, spreading rumors, attacking someone physically or verbally, and excluding someone from a group on purpose. The National Association of School Psychologists (2012) defines bullying as "unwanted, repetitive, and aggressive behavior marked by an imbalance of power. It can take on multiple forms, including physical (e.g., hitting), verbal (e.g., name calling or making threats), relational (e.g., spreading rumors), and electronic (e.g., texting, social networking)" (p. 1).

Most research in adult bullying has focused on the workplace. Bullying in the workplace is usually more covert than overt, and the construct normally excludes direct physical violence (Bulutlar & Oz, 2009). Rayner and Keashly (2004) identify a range of behaviors as signifying bullying, including social isolation, undermining of professional status, tampering with tools or equipment that people need to do their jobs, intimidation, micromanagement of one's work duties, and personal attacks on credibility. Georgakopoulos, Wilkin, and Kent (2011), building on Leymann and Gustafsson's (1996) constructs, identify workplace bullying as a form of psychological violence that is continuously and persistently repeated and is done with malice.

Bullying among and upon the aged is a relatively new area of research and to date has focused primarily on older adults within institutional care facilities (Mapes, 2011). Bullying within this context often involves passive-aggressive behaviors such as gossiping and whispering but is occasionally compounded by direct physical contact and violence, something atypical among younger adults (Bonifas, in Mapes, 2011).

Other definitions of bullying focus less on the age of bully or victim, and more on societal or racial characteristics. Fox and Stallworth (2004) include racial and ethnic bullying under the construct, arguing that racism is often expressed overtly through bullying behaviors. Other researchers focus on the differences in power between perpetrator and victim as the key dynamic (Carbo, 2012; Strandmark & Hallberg, 2007). For example, Jenkins (2011) differentiates between bullying and normal conflict by noting the power imbalance between the perpetrator and victim, as the victim is placed in an increasingly inferior position to the bully. Jenkins (2011) also notes the role of intent, where the perpetrator deliberately intends to inflict harm of some form on the victim. This behavior can be predatory in nature, with the bully deliberately targeting individuals who he or she knows to be vulnerable.

Bullying: Prevalence

As noted earlier, bullying is prevalent across age groups. The Centers for Disease Control and Prevention (2012), citing a 2011 nationally representative sample of youth in grades 9 through 12, found that 20.1% reported being bullied on school property in the 12 months preceding

the survey, and 16.2% reported being bullied electronically (email, chat room, Web site, texting) in the 12 months preceding the survey. The National Association of School Psychologists (2012), while acknowledging that there is a lack of consensus in the research literature on the prevalence of bullying due to challenges faced with differing methodologies, nonetheless estimates that approximately 70% to 80% of school-age children have been involved in bullying, either as perpetrator, victim, or bystander.

In adults, the U.S. Workplace Bullying Survey (Workplace Bullying Institute, 2007) estimates that up to 37% of workers in the United States have experienced some form of workplace bullying—that is, up to 54 million working Americans. The costs to organizations and the economy at large are estimated in the billions of dollars per year (Gardner & Johnson, 2001; Sypher, 2004) through increased absenteeism, turnover, decreased staff commitment, job satisfaction, and productivity (Bulutlar & Oz, 2009; Hague, Skogstad, & Einarsen, 2007). But it is the personal costs to individual workers that are the most alarming. Negative and, in some cases, severe impacts to an individual's physical and psychological health can occur, including anxiety, depression, burnout, frustration, eating disorders, heart disease, and stomach ailments (Keashly & Neuman, 2004). Workplace bullying is a silent epidemic causing untold harm to millions of people.

The prevalence of bullying among seniors is difficult to estimate given the diversity of the population and settings. Researchers estimates that up to 20% of seniors residing in institutional settings have experienced some form of peer-to-peer bullying (Mapes, 2011; Searson, 2012). Perfett (2013) notes that in institutional environments such as retirement homes or other senior settings, bullying tends to occur more readily because resources are being shared. She also argues that elderly bullies often are reflecting lifelong personality traits, although dementia and other age-related cognitive impairments could also result in behaviors that mimic bullying even though they may not be done with intent.

ETHICAL CONSIDERATIONS IN BULLYING

Rhodes, Pullen, Vickers, Clegg, and Pitsis (2010) note that "bullying is not a simple phenomenon, and nor is it necessarily easy to detect, identify, and categorize" (p. 96). Because the term *bullying* encompasses such a wide range of behaviors and environments, the ethical considerations for occupational therapy practitioners are many and varied. Although each situation is unique, there are a number of common ethical considerations that can be clustered, which are discussed next.

Individual

Victims of bullying often seek, or are referred to, assistance from professionals who are perceived as having some ability to intervene or otherwise assist the individual. In these cases, the potential intervener is faced with a number of ethical considerations. Some are associated with the professional role of the intervener, such as professional ethical guidelines, professional skill levels, scope of practice, and so forth. Other ethical considerations are more specific to the situation at hand.

- Can the intervention be effective?
- Does the intervener have the authority (official or inferred) to be effective?
- Could the intervention make things worse?

Functioning as an intervener in bullying situations is not without risks, and the phrase from the Hippocratic Oath, "First, do no harm," should be a driving ethical consideration for any potential intervention.

Organizational

A considerable amount of research undertaken in the area of bullying has focused on the ethical issues of the organizations in which the bullying takes place. This is particularly true when looking at bullying within the workplace or within senior care facilities. Bullying activities are often seen in the context of poor management (Ontario Safety Association for Community and Healthcare, 2010). Rhodes et al. (2010) argue that another common response is to place responsibility solely on the perpetrator, the so-called bad apple syndrome, which minimizes the organization's ethical responsibility. Other researchers contend that the high-performance expectations and high-pressure environments within today's educational and work environments can predispose some individuals to bullying behaviors (Yamada, 2008).

Regardless of causal factors within the organization, there is concurrence across the literature that organizations have a moral, ethical, and legal responsibility to ensure the prevention of bullying, and to have policies and mechanisms in place to address specific instances should they occur (Bulultar & Oz, 2009; Carbo, 2012; Chartered Institute of Personnel and Development, 2004; Fox & Stallworth, 2004; Ontario Safety Association for Community and Healthcare, 2010; Rhodes et al., 2010; Yamada, 2008).

ETHICAL INTERVENTIONS TO ADDRESS BULLYING

Interventions to address bullying can be divided into two different categories: (1) preventative, which attempts to establish organizational and environmental constraints that reduce the probability that bullying will occur, and (2) responsive, which attempts to address current or ongoing cases of bullying and ameliorate, to the degree possible, the negative impacts to the victim.

Preventive

Much of the research on bullying focuses on the role of the organization in creating a safe environment wherein bullying behaviors are not only discouraged but also one where they are effectively prevented. Naturally, the differing environments in which the occupational therapy practitioner works and the victim resides will determine the type and scope of preventative interventions possible.

Bennett (2009), citing Harris, Petrie, and Willoughby (2002), identifies a number of elements necessary for effective prevention of bullying in schools: (1) a warm, positive environment with involved adults; (2) policies setting firm limits on unacceptable behavior; (3) a commitment by administration and staff to consistent application of nonhostile, nonphysical sanctions on offenders; and (4) active engagement by authoritative (but not authoritarian) adults (p. 14). Cecil and Molnar-Main (2011), in their review of the literature, identify a number of elements to an effective anti-bullying approach within schools, including (1) a whole systems approach that engages school, community, and family environments; (2) specific activities and measures tailored for the particular setting; (3) the adequate monitoring of program implementation, including multiple sources of data; (4) effective and ongoing school staff training; (5) educating parents and engaging them in bullying prevention efforts; (6) clearly delineated disciplinary methods; and (7) sufficient program duration (p. 2).

For adults, particularly within workplace settings, much of the research on prevention of bullying has focused on the role of the employing organization. Bulultar and Oz (2009) argue that the most effective way of preventing workplace bullying is through the establishment of an "ethical climate," encompassing a caring organizational climate combined with a principle-led approach to ethical decision making within the organization. Together, these will produce an organizational environment in which bullying is actively discouraged. Yamada (2008) proposes a two-pronged approach for organizations seeking to prevent workplace bullying. One prong emphasizes a values-based approach to leadership by the organization's managers, which emphasizes honesty and mutual respect at all levels, promotes a level of trust that reduces feelings of helplessness by victims, and supports the belief that organizational leaders can be approached for help. The other prong focuses on educational and policy responses, with information being provided to staff to assist in the recognition of workplace bullying among peers and superiors, combined with clearly identified policies, procedures, and sanctions to address cases of workplace bullying.

Fox and Stallworth (2004) identify four ethical considerations that organizations must address to prevent workplace bullying: (1) recognizing that workplace bullying exists and that there are environmental factors within the organization that can prevent or encourage bullying behaviors, (2) establishing internal policies and procedures that impose serious and prompt sanctions on workplace bullies, (3) developing effective conflict management and dispute resolution mechanisms to deal with complaints of workplace bullying, and (4) supporting anti-bullying efforts at the legislative and community levels.

Preventative measures for bullying to and among older adults is a relatively new area of study and closely linked to research on elder abuse and neglect. Fallon (2006), in her review of the literature and international best practices, identifies preventative interventions at both the systemic and organizational level:

1. Guidelines on the development and implementation of multi-agency policies and procedures to protect vulnerable adults from abuse

2. Specific adult protection legislation

3. Drawing on community resources to provide a coordinated response; advocacy programs premised on a philosophy that the least restrictive and intrusive interventions should be used

Citing Keys (2003), Fallon refers to three major themes emerging from the literature: (1) a multidisciplinary approach, (2) a commitment to preventative measures in addition to direct responses to individual cases, and (3) local/community-level responses.

Responsive

Ethical responses or interventions to addressing specific cases of bullying are varied both in terms of approaches and effectiveness. These will hinge in large part on the specifics of the school, workplace, or institution and the individuals involved.

In school situations, a vast range of resources are available both online and in the educational and occupational therapy literature to assist practitioners in developing effective responses to specific cases of bullying by and among children. Of particular note is the work done by Terry Olivas-De La O, a COTA/L (Figure 54-1) in California who has made anti-bullying initiatives one of the primary goals of her work. Some of what she does is described on her Web site (http://familysuccessbydesign.org/dontfighthugtight/). Her work includes organizing a yearly Young Woman's Summit, which seeks to provide young women with leadership skills to address bullying within their schools and communities.

Some other relevant discussions of possible ways in which occupational therapy practitioners can address bullying can be found at these sites:

- AOTA on bullying prevention: http://www.aota.org/en/Practice/Children-Youth/Emerging-Niche/Bullying.aspx

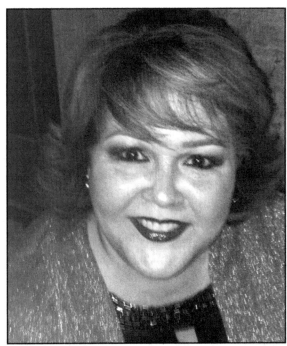

Figure 54-1. Terry Olivas-De La O, COTA/L, ROH, founder and CEO, Family Success by Design.

- Virtual Chat on occupational therapy and bullying prevention: http://www.talkshoe.com/talkshoe/web/audioPop.jsp?episodeId=380320&cmd=apop

- Facebook page for occupational therapists against bullying: https://www.facebook.com/lowdownonbullying

In terms of workplace bullying, Jenkins (2011) notes that mediation (either external or internal) can at times be an effective tool, particularly if supported by legislative or policy authority that helps balance the power discrepancy between parties. Official processes, such as legal proceedings or (in the case of unionized environments) collective agreement grievance procedures are sometimes effective in addressing bullying behaviors or at least intimidating bullies from continuing (Fox & Stallworth, 2004). Training the victim on skills in effective conflict management and bullyproofing are sometimes effective in challenging or managing the bullying behaviors (Ontario Safety Association for Community and Healthcare, 2010), although Strandmark and Hallberg (2007) caution that the power imbalance in many work environments can result in such strategies backfiring by provoking the bully to assert dominance. Lastly, and unfortunately, in situations where neither organizational nor external supports or interveners are available, and personal conflict management and bullyproofing strategies prove ineffective, the victim may need to evaluate the possibility of personally leaving the abusive environment. Workplace bullying is highly complex and involves a host of factors, including personality types, organizational structure, leadership and management styles, cultural values, race, gender, and power. Navigating this minefield and helping the victim (or yourself) is neither easy nor always successful. However, in today's increasingly competitive and globalized work environment, workplace bullying is a phenomenon that will not be going away any time soon.

Effective responses for the cases of bullying among older adults are again determined in large part by the environment in which the behavior is taking place, such as institutional, community, or independent living settings. Perfett (2013) suggests that providing education and training to seniors who are experiencing bullying behaviors on how to manage bullies may be effective. These strategies include the following :

- Determining if the setting has a set of rules or policies in place to address bullying, what they encompass, and how they are enforced

- Discussing the issue with supervisors, staff, or other professionals such as senior advocates or ombudsmen, clergy, social workers, or a family member

- Developing support networks

- Being understanding of the bully, particularly if dementia or other forms of cognitive impairment are evident

- Ignoring or walking away from the bullying

Bullying by staff, family members, or other individuals who are in a position of power over the senior is more complex and may require interventions based on organization policies, legal standards or codes, or even criminal investigations. Occupational therapy practitioners engaged in these types of interventions should reference the ethical guidelines of their professional association and the policies and procedures in place within their own organizational settings.

Bullying is highly complex and involves a host of factors, including personality types, organizational structure, leadership and management styles, cultural values, race, gender, and power. Navigating this minefield and helping the victim (or yourself) is neither easy nor always successful. However, bullying is an issue that will continue to present itself to occupational therapy practitioners in a variety of settings. Being able to ethically address and assist your clients is a key skill in effectively dealing with this destructive behavior.

Summary

In this chapter, we have examined conflict—particularly ethical conflict. We have discussed how conflict impacts individuals and organizations, and possible responses to conflict. The use of a variety of skills, including assertive communication, and strategies for ethical conflict resolution were reviewed. The special case of bullying and how individual clinicians as well as the organizations they work for, or in, can address bullying was also discussed. It is the authors' hope that students and clinicians will explore these ideas and find them useful when they encounter ethical conflicts in their practice.

Electronic Resources

- AACN handbook on addressing moral distress: http://www.aacn.org/WD/Practice/Docs/4As_to_Rise_Above_Moral_Distress.pdf

- Conflict resolution skills: http://www.helpguide.org/mental/eq8_conflict_resolution.htm

- Nonviolent communication: http://www.cnvc.org/

- Dealing with workplace bullying: http://occupational-therapy.advanceweb.com/student-and-new-grad-center/student-top-story/dealing-with-workplace-bullies.aspx

Student Self-Assessment

1. Describe the differences between ethical conflicts and ethical dilemmas.

2. Given your context, review local, state, or national regulations regarding bullying.

3. How comfortable are you with resolving conflict? Think of a situation in which you have experienced ethical distress. Describe what happened, what you did, and what you would hope to do differently next time. If possible, share this with a trusted colleague. Ask the colleague to suggest other possible resolutions.

4. How would you describe your approaches to assertively communicating, and how would you deal with someone who is actively resistant to your interpersonal communication styles?

References

American Association of Critical-Care Nurses. (2008). *The 4A's to rise above moral distress*. Retrieved from http://www.aacn.org/WD/Practice/Docs/4As_to_Rise_Above_Moral_Distress.pdf

Accreditation Council on Occupational Therapy Education. (2012). *ACOTE standards and interpretive guidelines (August 2012)*. American Occupational Therapy Association. Retrieved from http://www.aota.org/Education/Careers/Accreditation/StandardsReview.aspx

American Occupational Therapy Association. (2010). *Occupational therapy code of ethics and ethics standards.* Retrieved from http://www.aota.org/en/Practice/Ethics.aspx

Barnette, V. (2009). Assertive communication. Retrieved from http://www.uiowa.edu/ucs/asertcom.shtml

Bennett, C. (2009). *Literature review of bullying at schools.* Winnipeg, Manitoba, Canada: University of Manitoba.

Blazer, C. (2005). *Literature review on bullying.* Miami, FL: Miami-Dade County Public Schools.

Brown, K. H., & Gillespie, D. (1997). "We become brave by doing brave acts": Teaching moral courage through the theatre of the oppressed. *Literature and Medicine, 16,* 108-120.

Bulutlar, F., & Oz, E. U. (2009). The effects of ethical climates on bullying behavior in the workplace. *Journal of Business Ethics, 86,* 273-298.

Caldicott, C., & Faber-Langendoen, K. (2005). Deception, discrimination and fear of reprisal: Lessons in ethics from third-year medical students. *Academic Medicine, 80,* 866-873.

Callister, L., Luthy, K., Thompson, P., & Memmott, R. (2009). Ethical reasoning in baccalaureate nursing students. *Nursing Ethics, 16,* 499-510.

Carbo, J. (2012). *Exploring solutions in workplace bullying.* Retrieved from http://www.aabri.com/OC2012Manuscripts/OC12037.pdf

Cecil, H., & Molnar-Main, S. (2011). *Olweus bullying prevention program in high schools: A review of the literature. Center for Schools and Communities Research Brief No. 5.* Retrieved from http://www.Center-School.org

Centers for Disease Control and Prevention. (2012). *Youth violence: Facts at a glance.* Retrieved from http://www.cdc.gov/violenceprevention/pdf/yv-datasheet-a.pdf

Chartered Institute of Personnel and Development. (2004). *Managing conflict at work: A guide for line managers.* Retrieved from http://www.cardiff.ac.uk/humrs/staffinfo/organisationaldevelopment/leadership/dashboard/Managing%20Conflict%20at%20Work%20-%20a%20guide%20for%20line%20managers.pdf

Compassion Fatigue Solutions. (2013). *Running on empty: Compassion fatigue in professionals.* Retrieved August 30, 2013, from http://compassionfatigue.ca/article-to-recommend/

Epstein, E., & Delgado, S. (2010). Understanding and addressing moral distress. *Online Journal of Issues in Nursing, 15,* 1.

Epstein, E., & Hamric, A. (2009). Moral distress, moral residue and the crescendo effect. *Journal of Clinical Ethics, 20,* 330-342.

Fallon, P. (2006). Elder abuse and/or neglect: literature review. Centre for Social Research and Evaluation: Te Pakapū Rangahau Arotaki Hapori, Ministry of Social Development, Wellington, New Zealand.

Fox, S., & Stallworth, L. E. (2004). Employee perceptions of internal conflict management programs and ADR processes in preventing and resolving incidents of workplace bullying: Ethical challenges for decision makers in organizations. *Employee Rights and Employment Policy Journal of Chicago-Kent College of Law, 8,* 375-405.

Gardner, S., & Johnson, P. R. (2001). The leaner meaner workplace: Strategies for handling bullies at work. *Employee Relations Today, 28*(2), 23-36.

Georgakopoulos, A., Wilkin, L., & Kent, B. (2011). Workplace bullying: A complex problem in contemporary organizations. *International Journal of Business and Social Science, 2*(3), 1-20.

Hague, L. J., Skogstad, A., & Einarsen, S. (2007). Relationships between stressful work environments and bullying: Results of a large representative study. *Work and Stress, 21*(3), 220-242.

Harris, S., Petrie, G., & Willoughby, W. (2002). Bullying among 9th graders: An exploratory study. *NASSP Bulletin, 86*(630), 3-14.

Hasan, S. (2008). Instructional design and assessment: A tool to teach communication skills to pharmacy students. *American Journal of Pharmaceutical Education, 72*(3), 1-9.

Jameton, A. (1984). *Nursing practice: The ethical issues.* Englewood Cliffs, NJ: Prentice Hall.

Jenkins, M. (2011). Practice note: Is mediation suitable for complaints of workplace bullying? *Conflict Resolution Quarterly, 29*(1), 25-38.

Keashly, L., & Neuman, J. H. (2004). Bullying in the workplace: Its impact and management. *Employment Policy, 83*(3), 335-373.

Keys, F. (2003). *Responding to elder abuse and neglect: Assessment and referral procedures.* Wellington, New Zealand: Office for Senior Citizens.

Kinsella, E. A., Park, A., Appiagyei, J., Chang, E., & Chow, D. (2008). Through the eyes of students: Ethical tensions in occupational therapy practice. *Canadian Journal of Occupational Therapy, 75,* 176-183.

Kirk, S. (2011). *Moral distress: A literature review. Arizona Bioethics Network.* Retrieved from http://abnbp.tapslhi.org/wp-content/uploads/2011/05/Moral-Distress.pdf

Kolb, S. M., & Griffith, A. C. S. (2009). I'll repeat myself again: Empowering students through assertive communication skills. *Teaching Exceptional Children, 41*(3), 32-36.

Kubany, E. S., Richard, D. C., Bauer, G. S., & Muraoka, M. Y. (1992). Impact of assertive and accusatory communication of distress and anger: A verbal component analysis. *Aggressive Behavior, 18,* 337-347.

Kyler, P. (1998). Putting everyday ethics into practice. *OT Practice, 3,* 36-40.

Leymann, H., & Gustafsson, A. (1996). Mobbing at work and the development of post-traumatic stress disorders. *European Journal of Work and Organizational Psychology, 5,* 251-276.

Lorris, K. D., Carpenter, R. O., & Miller, B. M. (2009). Moral distress in the third year of medical school: A descriptive review of student case reflections. *American Journal of Surgery, 197,* 107-112.

Mapes, D. (2011). *Mean old girls: Seniors who bully.* Retrieved from http://www.nbcnews.com/id/41353544/ns/health-aging/%20-%20.UQ8_--jZq_4#.UvJboPldXQg

Mathieu, F. (2009). *Signs and symptoms of compassion fatigue and vicarious trauma.* Compassion Fatigue Solutions. Retrieved August 30, 2013, from http://compassionfatigue.ca/signs-and-symptoms-of-compassion-fatigue-and-vicarious-trauma/

National Association of School Psychologists. (2012). *A framework for school-wide bullying prevention and safety.* Retrieved from http://www.nasponline.org/resources/bullying/Bullying_Brief_12.pdf

Nelson, H. (1995). Resistance and insubordination. *Hypatia, 10,* 23-40.

Ontario Safety Association for Community and Healthcare. (2010). *Bullying in the workplace: A handbook for the workplace.* Toronto, Ontario, Canada: HealthForce Ontario.

Perfett, M. (2013). *Senior bullying: Cliques, harassment, ostracism prevalent among elders.* Retrieved from http://www.thebesttimes.org/aaa/elder_abuse/0811_senior_bullying.shtml

Pipas, M. D. (2010). Assertive communication skills. *Anales Universitatis Apulensis Series Oeconomica, 12*(2), 649-656.

Rayner, C., & Keashly, L. (2004). Bullying at work: A perspective from Britain and North America. In S. Fox & P. E. Spector (Eds.), *Counterproductive work behavior: Investigations of actors and targets* (pp. 271-296). Washington, DC: American Psychological Association.

Rhodes, C., Pullen, A., Vickers, M. H., Clegg, S. R., & Pitsis, A. (2010). Violence and workplace bullying: What are an organization's moral responsibilities? *Administrative Theory and Praxis, 32*(1), 96-115.

Searson, L. (2012). *Senior bullying.* Retrieved from http://www.retirement-living.com/senior-bullying/

Slater, D., & Brandt, L. (2009). Combating moral distress. *OT Practice, 14,* 13-16.

Strandmark, M., & Hallberg, L. R. M. (2007). The origin of workplace bullying: Experiences from the perspective of bully victims in the public service sector. *Journal of Nursing Management, 15,* 332-341.

Sypher, B. D. (2004). Reclaiming civil discourse in the workplace. *Southern Communications Journal, 69*(3), 257-270.

Taylor, R. (2008). *The intentional relationship: Occupational therapy and use of self.* Philadelphia, PA: F.A. Davis Company.

Tighe B., & Mainwaring J. (2012). The bioethical experiences of student dietitians on their final clinical placement. *Journal of Human Nutrition and Dietetics, 26*(2), 198-203. doi: 10.1111/jhn.12007

Tillman, L. D. (2007). *Effective communication: Speaking up assertively.* Retrieved from http://www.speakupforyourself.com/Powerpoint/BasicAssertiveCommunication.pps

U.S. Department of Health and Human Services. (2013). *Bullying definition.* Retrieved from http://www.stopbullying.gov/what-is-bullying/definition/index.html

Webster, G. C., & Baylis, F. (2000). Moral residue. In S. B. Rubin & L. Zoloth (Eds.), *Margin of error: The ethics of mistakes in the practice of medicine* (p. 208). Hagerstown, MD: University Publishing Group.

Workplace Bullying Institute. (2007). U.S. Workplace Bullying Survey.

Yamada, D. C. (2008). Workplace bullying and ethical leadership. *Journal of Values-Based Leadership, 1*(2), 49. Retrieved from http://papers.ssrn.com/sol3/papers.cfm?abstract_id=1301554

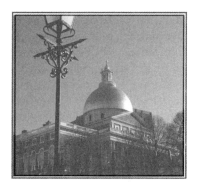

55

ADVOCACY IN OCCUPATIONAL THERAPY

Amy Jo Lamb, OTD, OTR/L, FAOTA

ACOTE STANDARDS EXPLORED IN THIS CHAPTER
B.2.3, B.6.4, B.9.13

KEY VOCABULARY

- **Advocacy:** To speak up for or plead the case of another.
- **Coalition:** Individuals or groups joining forces together for a common cause.
- **Grassroots advocacy:** A group effort of like-minded individuals working together to achieve a desired outcome.
- **Policy:** Principle or rule to guide decisions and achieve outcomes.

Introduction

Occupational therapy is an integral part of today's dynamic health care system. However, as a profession we are consistently challenged to keep our place in the system. We are consistently advocating for appropriate reimbursement in a health care market that is full of competition and low on resources. We diligently work to demonstrate the value and skill occupational therapy brings to the treatment of clients. In this current era of health care reform, it is vital that we communicate the message that occupational therapy is an investment worth making. We must make the occupational therapy voice heard for our clients, for our profession, and in the larger context of health care reforms. Occupational therapy enables meaningful participation that allows people to "live life to the fullest." As occupational therapy professionals, we must be aware of the changes currently affecting our practice and the system at large, and keep a laser-like focus for our advocacy efforts.

Advocacy Defined

Advocacy means to speak up, or to plead the case of another (Webster-Merriam, 2011). For a practitioner, this may mean speaking up for a client who could benefit from continued services or for an occupational therapy department to be included in a new program within your organization. For a professional association, such as the American Occupational Therapy Association (AOTA), this means championing a cause on behalf of the people it serves, and asking people to help in carrying out the

Jacobs, K., MacRae, N., & Sladyk, K. (Eds.).
Occupational Therapy Essentials for
Clinical Competence, Second Edition (pp. 717-723).
© 2014 SLACK Incorporated.

organization's mission. Examples of advocacy include voicing positions about the rights or benefits to which someone is entitled or taking action to ensure that institutions work appropriately.

Why is advocacy important to the occupational therapy profession? Advocacy is about getting listened to, being at the table when decisions are made, and being heard by people who make decisions (Daly, 2011). It is essential for the voices of occupational therapy practitioners to be heard at tables where decisions are being made regarding clients and populations who can benefit from our services. Policymakers, employers, consumers, advocacy groups, health care and education professionals, and the insurance industry will better understand the value of occupational therapy through the advocacy efforts of the profession.

History of Advocacy in Occupational Therapy

EARLY EFFORTS

The pioneers of occupational therapy believed in the profession and were staunch advocates for it. They fought for the survival of occupational therapy because they believed in the benefits of the services. They wanted to create a base for future generations of occupational therapy professionals to build on. Quiroga (1995, p. 15) states that "in the early 1900's the founders defined the profession's boundaries, developed theories of practice, increased the number of practitioners, strategized to convince the American public and the medical world the value of occupational therapy, built many institutions in which to train practitioners and treat patients, and established standards for training and practice." These efforts of our profession's pioneers are examples of their role in advocating for occupational therapy.

Several individuals were extremely active in the advancement and expansion of the occupational therapy profession. Eleanor Clark Slagle, for example, was active in advocacy with medical professionals to help bring to light the importance of occupational therapy intervention in mental health care as well as tuberculosis prevention and care. These efforts helped occupational therapy move into the medical arena of health care. Quiroga (1995, p. 46) reports that "Slagle made it her business to contact people in other cities who were beginning to see, as she did, that her work had the potential to become its own profession." Contacting people and promoting the benefits of occupational therapy was a demonstration of her involvement in advocacy for the profession and its potential clients.

William Rush Dunton, Jr., a psychiatrist who has come to be known as the "father of occupational therapy," was also instrumental in the advancement of the profession. Quiroga (1995) reported that Dunton participated in nationwide struggles to raise the status of psychiatry in American medicine. He viewed making occupational therapy a profession as an important step in that direction, for he believed that the new profession combined a scientific approach with humanitarian values. Together, Dunton and Slagle were active in the establishment of our first national association, the National Society for the Promotion of Occupational Therapy (NSPOT). This association today is known as the American Occupational Therapy Association (AOTA). Establishing the first national association was a direct result of advocacy efforts and a first step for occupational therapy toward becoming a distinct profession.

Susan Tracy was another advocate of the profession. Tracy is credited for shaping the identity of the new profession by training newcomers to the field, widening the settings in which occupational therapy was practiced, and exposing a variety of clients to the services we provide. In addition, she also helped carve a place for the profession in early 20th-century America (Quiroga, 1995). Susan Tracy was an advocate for the profession through her attempts to train future therapists with a broader domain of practice.

In her 1967 Eleanor Clark Slagle lecture, Wilma West encouraged occupational therapy leaders and professionals to direct advocacy efforts to meet the needs of society. West cited two major purposes of a profession: "to meet external obligations to society" and "to meet the internal loyalties to members on the other" (1967, p. 184). "Responsibility for awareness and interpretation of those changes which affect any part of our profession, and responsibility for whatever group action is appropriate to facilitate or hasten adjustment to change." She went on to state that "both as individuals and as a professional group we should be assuming a far more frequent and contributing part in the planning of health services. It will be mandatory that we do so if we are to have a part in shaping our own development" (West, 1967, p. 187). These words continue to provide direction for the profession today.

Occupational therapy was a valuable profession in the past, we are a valuable profession today, and we have every opportunity to continue to be a valuable part of the health care system in the future. To succeed in this ever-changing environment, occupational therapy professionals will need to be advocates within the larger conversation of reform. Some of the changes we see today are different than those faced by our founders, while some are similar. Nonetheless, it is our time to take charge to fight for the same roots of the profession that our founders fought for so many years ago.

Instrumental Legislation

Occupational therapy is included in numerous pieces of legislation that have been instrumental in opening doors and opportunity for occupational therapy; our inclusion is a direct result of advocacy by association leaders and grassroots advocates. These laws have been very influential in the services provided by occupational therapy as well as the rights our clients are entitled to.

The Individuals with Disabilities Education Act (IDEA, 1990) was a landmark piece of legislation that made a place for occupational therapy in the schools and assisted in the reimbursement for such services. Occupational therapy is a related service under Part B of IDEA and provides services to children with special education needs.

The American With Disabilities Act (ADA) was another landmark piece of legislation shifting the way in which society views persons with disabilities. ADA played a vital role in changing social attitudes about health, disease, and disability since its inception. This legislation has impacted the occupational therapy profession and provided standards to increase accessibility for persons with disability.

The Medicare system was established as an amendment to the Social Security Act of 1965. This landmark legislation provided health insurance to persons who were 65 and older and those under 65 with specific diagnoses. Later, advocacy efforts of the AOTA were successful in including occupational therapy as a reimbursable service under both Medicare Part A and Part B.

The Patient Protection and Affordable Care Act (PPACA) was passed in 2010. This law is intended to expand health care coverage to about 31 million uninsured Americans through a combination of cost controls, subsidies, and mandates. The PPACA also includes ideas to change the current health care system to improve coordination and patient outcomes as well as to achieve savings. The PPACA delineates essential health benefits, outlining parameters of what insurance plans participating in the exchanges are required to meet and cover. At a minimum, the ten essential health benefits include ambulatory patient services, emergency services, hospitalization, maternity and newborn care, mental health and substance use disorder, prescription drugs, rehabilitative and habilitative services and devices, laboratory services, preventive and wellness services and chronic disease management, and pediatric services including oral and vision (PPACA, 2010). While implementation of the PPACA is currently underway, occupational therapy finds advocacy opportunities in three of these essential health benefit categories: rehabilitative and habilitative services and devices, preventive and wellness services and chronic disease management, and mental health and substance use disorder.

These are examples of federal laws that have made improvements in the access to services provided by occupational therapy practitioners. Without the advocacy efforts of our professional association and occupational therapy professionals, these pieces of legislation may have advanced without the inclusion of occupational therapy.

A Changing Society

It is essential for us to examine the societal context in which we live, work, and play to understand what advocacy is needed to promote occupational therapy. The United States health care system is undergoing reforms emphasizing systems that support increased efficiency in the health care system, increased quality of services provided, and decreased costs. There is a growing emphasis on creating a culture of personal responsibility for one's health and attempts to shift the system to focus on prevention and wellness. There is a shift toward primary care in an effort to reduce costs and increase system efficiency. We face continuing challenges to our reimbursement structure and system as it currently exists. This context of the U.S. health care system is essential for us to understand in our advocacy efforts. It is imperative that as we grow as a profession we set our path within the external societal issues we face. Occupational therapy practitioners will be required to go beyond performing direct services and step forward to articulate a clear message outlining the value and distinctiveness of occupational therapy.

The AOTA has provided a vision statement for where occupational therapy will be in its centennial year of 2017. It states, "We envision that occupational therapy is a powerful, widely recognized, science-driven, and evidence-based profession with a globally connected and diverse workforce meeting society's occupational needs" (AOTA, 2006). The Centennial Vision provides occupational therapy professionals with a laser-like focus for their advocacy efforts moving forward.

Importance of Grassroots Advocacy

Grassroots advocacy is a group effort of like-minded individuals working together to achieve a desired outcome. Grassroots advocacy may occur as part of our daily practice, within our professional organizations, and at the health systems level. As occupational therapy professionals, our grassroots advocacy efforts are enhanced when we share a clear and consistent message with our target audience.

Therapy Level

Earlier, we defined advocacy as the act of speaking up for or pleading the case of another. This definition clearly fits the grassroots advocacy efforts of occupational therapy practitioners in their daily practice. This may occur in clinical, education, community-based or research settings depending on where you put your occupational therapy knowledge and skills to work on a daily basis.

In our practice, we often engage in advocacy on behalf of the clients we serve as well as assisting them in developing their own advocacy voice. When we ensure that clients have access to the services for which they are eligible, we are advocating. When we make the client's requests known to other members of the health care team, we are promoting coordinated care through our advocacy efforts. When we take complex information and provide the necessary client education to increase the client's understanding and ability to apply the information, we are being advocates. When we take the time to explain the role of occupational therapy in our setting to our clients, we are serving as advocates. Opportunities for advocacy are endless in our daily practice, regardless of what setting that may be.

Professional Level

Advocacy at the professional level provides a necessary and important link to our daily practice and our recognition at the health systems level. This type of advocacy occurs in a variety of settings as well. Professional advocacy may occur in clinical practice when we educate potential referral sources about the role of occupational therapy in our setting. Engaging in program development to provide occupational therapy services to a specific population or group to enhance quality of life is professional advocacy. Educating insurance companies on the role of occupational therapy in certain areas can lead to decreased denials and increased payments for service, a direct result from professional advocacy efforts. Participating in coalitions in which we use our occupational therapy knowledge to promote services for individuals and populations that meet societal needs is another example of high-value professional advocacy.

Health Systems Level

The health systems level is where public policy is introduced, debated, and passed; it can influence the practice of occupational therapy and the individuals/populations that we serve. It is not always a logical process, as it is more often than not influenced by politics. This should not discourage occupational therapy professionals. Instead, this should motivate us to share our message. We, the members of the profession, are the experts in occupational therapy. Policymakers do not know or understand the profession. It is our responsibility to share the occupational therapy message with these influential individuals to ensure that laws are supportive of occupational therapy practice. There are several important points to remember regarding this health systems level of advocacy: policy impacts every area of occupational therapy practice, professional associations are essential in our advancement, and occupational therapy is a wise investment in the U.S. health services system.

Policy impacts every area of occupational therapy practice, regardless of age or setting. The Individuals with Disabilities Act supports our practice in school-based settings. The American with Disabilities Act supports our work in accessibility design, and home and work modifications to support independence in daily life. Inclusion under Medicare laws supports occupational therapy practice in numerous settings with older adults and created a path for inclusion with other third-party reimbursement systems. The Patient Protection and Affordable Care Act recognized the value of occupational therapy in the essential benefits package with the inclusion of rehabilitation and habilitation, as well as our roles in wellness and prevention and working with persons with mental health and substance use disorders. Recognizing the link between policy and practice is essential for every occupational therapy professional in today's context. Articulating the value of occupational therapy through grassroots advocacy efforts is the responsibility of every practitioner, educator, and researcher.

Professional associations are essential in our advancement as a profession. Having a strong national professional organization is a fundamental key to advocacy success. Without the advocacy efforts of our national association, occupational therapy may not have been included in the policies we have already discussed in this chapter. Without these policies in place, our practice would be limited. A healthy state association is equally important to the profession of occupational therapy as our national association. All politics are local. Federal law often filters down to states for implementation. It is then that our state occupational therapy associations step forward and make the occupational therapy voice heard, protecting our practice and promoting our profession. Therefore, a simple first step to being an occupational therapy advocate is to be a member of both your national and state occupational therapy associations. In doing so, you provide the associations with the necessary resources they need to protect and advance the practice of occupational therapy and the clients that we serve each day.

Occupational therapy is a part of the solution to the challenges of the United States health services system and a wise investment for policymakers. In 2010, the President of the United States signed into law the PPACA, which sets forth a plan to restructure the United States health services system. A foundational concept of the PPACA is often referred to as the triple aim of health care reform (Berwick, Nolan, & Whittington, 2008) to control costs, improve quality, and increase efficiency. With occupational therapy professionals engaging in advocacy efforts, we can strategically position ourselves with the triple aim. Occupational therapy provides the necessary services to individuals and populations to allow them to live, work, and play at their highest level of independence, which is valuable in controlling costs. Occupational therapy improves quality of care by utilizing evidence-based assessments and interventions to increase a person's functional status and enhance quality of life. Occupational therapy can increase the efficiency of the system by using our distinct skill set as we examine clients across the contexts in which they live, work, and play to appropriately evaluate risks, make recommendations, and engage in intervention to decrease potential unnecessary utilization of the system.

The engagement in grassroots advocacy is a professional obligation for all occupational therapy professionals. Toto (2012) offered practical advice for practitioners emphasizing the importance of recognizing our individual strengths and seeking advocacy opportunities for our talents; whether within an organization, a state, or at the national level, we all have a role to take. When we all participate in the process, share a consistent message, and provide the highest quality of care possible in our daily practice, our impact will be significant.

Effective Advocacy Tips

It all begins with an idea. Whether it is an idea for a new program to be developed or a policy to be introduced, it all begins at this basic point. After an idea has been generated and the science supporting it has been identified, the idea needs to become a reality. That is where advocacy comes in. Effective advocates are passionate. As occupational therapy professionals, we must be passionate about our message and the work that we do. This passion can serve as a driver for moving occupational therapy forward.

CLEARLY COMMUNICATE YOUR MESSAGE

Prepare before meetings and plan ahead what you would like to say. AOTA has helpful one-page fact sheets and talking points on many of the key legislative issues for occupational therapy; using and distributing such resources ensures that a consistent message is communicated from the profession. Create a talking-point guide for a laser-like focus on the essential points you want the decision maker to understand. Share only these essential points and avoid getting lost in some of the interesting, but nonessential, information. Do not get discouraged if you need to deliver the message more than once to decision makers. Often a message will need to be heard multiple times in alternative ways prior to action taking place. Be patient, prepared, and focused. View every

---

Practical Examples of Advocacy

- Becoming a member of the national and state associations
- Helping the state legislative committee advocate
- Participating in political action committees
- Providing testimony to issues relevant to areas of practice
- Writing letters to state and federal representatives about health issues
- Drafting fact sheets about the profession's role in health care
- Inviting legislators to visit your facility to provide a first-hand experience

Advocacy Dos

- Establish an ongoing relationship and reputation for reliability.
- Treat the person as a friend/intelligent person.
- Be specific and know your facts.
- Provide a brief, clearly written summary of position.
- Request specific action.
- Be sure to express thanks for opportunity to advocate.

Advocacy Don'ts

- Don't try to talk with people when they are obviously in a hurry.
- Don't be argumentative or abrasive.
- Don't overload them with written material.
- Don't assume that they are familiar with your issues.
- Don't bluff if you don't know the answer to a question.
- Don't talk about too many issues at once.
- Don't be late
- Don't threaten a legislator with votes.

---

meeting as an opportunity to strengthen relationships, deepen understanding, and broaden support.

STORIES HAVE IMPACT

Telling stories is a powerful way to deliver a message. The use of stories is very valuable in advocacy efforts. We become engrossed in stories. We can take a complex concept and break it down in a way that decision makers can relate to through stories. A story can paint a vivid picture and message that will be remembered long after we leave

EVIDENCE-BASED RESEARCH CHART

Issue	Evidence
Foundation of advocacy	AOTA, 2006; Quiroga, 1995; West, 1968
Effective advocacy	AOTA, 2012; Daly, 2011; Field, Gauld, & Laurence, 2012; Toto, 2012
Future Directions for Advocacy	Berwick, Nolan, & Whittington, 2008; Bisognano & Kenney, 2012; Weissert & Weissert, 2012

the meeting. Identify a powerful story from practice with links to the area that you are focusing your advocacy on and practice sharing that story with a colleague. Finally, when in a meeting with a decision maker, clearly and confidently share this story as a way to personalize the message that you are delivering, showcasing your occupational therapy expertise.

NETWORK

Networking and advocacy go hand in hand. Advocates are constantly looking to expand their network and meet new people. Develop a network with key decision makers and their staff before you need to approach them for support on an issue. Send them a congratulatory note when they win an election or take a leadership position. Attend meetings and events that they are a part of and stop to talk with them at the end. The goal of networking and building this relationship is not only for you to advance an issue but also so that they know you are a valuable resource for advice on issues in your area of expertise.

SPEAK WITH CONFIDENCE

Remember that you are the expert in occupational therapy. You have the message they need to hear—they have a problem and you have a solution. Have confidence in the message you are sharing. Using language that is accessible to people outside of our profession is important in crafting our message to avoid misunderstandings. Using inclusive language is also important so that decision makers recognize that you intend to work with them to achieve a common goal. Finally, do not forget to ask what outcome decision makers want from the meeting. Perhaps you want their support on a particular piece of legislation or a program you are proposing; to receive you must first ask. If you do not ask the answer will always be no. Let the decision maker clearly know what it is that you advocate and propose possible solutions.

Summary

Advocacy has been foundational to occupational therapy since our inception, positioning us for success in the U.S. health care and educational systems. Advocacy is also about empowerment. Our profession is empowered by the recognition of policymakers who understand the value occupational therapy brings to the greater systems at hand. Our professionals are empowered by the contributions that they have made to improve the system and ensure access for the clients we serve. Our clients are empowered through participation in occupational therapy. Decisions being made today will drive the practice of tomorrow; the time is now for occupational therapy professionals to make their voices heard and be a part of the process.

Electronic Resources

- American Occupational Therapy Association: www.aota.org
- The Showalter Group: www.showaltergroup.com
- AOTA's Guide to Promotion and Advocacy: http://www.aota.org/~/media/Corporate/Files/Publications/OTP/OTP/2012-Issues/OTP%20Vol%2017%20Issue%2019.ashx

References

Advocacy. (2011) In *Merriam-Webster Online Dictionary*. Retrieved from http://www.m-w.com/dictionary/advocacy

American Occupational Therapy Association. (2006). *The road to the centennial vision*. Retrieved from http://www.aota.org/News/Centennial.aspx

American Occupational Therapy Association. (2012). *AOTA's guide to promotion and advocacy*. Retrieved from http://www.aota.org/pubs/otp/2012-issues/otp-102912.aspx?ft=.pdf

Americans with Disabilities Act (ADA). (1990). Pub. L. No. 101-336, 104 Stat 328.

Berwick, D. M., Nolan, T. W., & Whittington, J. (2008). The triple aim: Care, health, and cost. *Health Affairs, 27*, 759-769. PubMed http://dx.doi.org/10.1377/hlthaff.27.3.759

Bisognano, M., & Kenney, C. (2012). *Pursuing the triple aim.* San Francisco, CA: Jossey-Bass.

Daly, J. (2011). *Advocacy: Championing ideas and influencing others.* New Haven, CT: Yale University Press.

Field, P., Gauld, R., & Laurence, M. (2012). Evidence-informed health policy: The crucial role of advocacy. *International Journal of Clinical Practice, 66*(4), 337-341.

Individuals with Disabilities Education Act. Pub. L. 101-476, 20 U.S.C., Chapter 33. (1990).

Merriam-Webster. (2011). Advocacy. Retrieved from http://www.m-w.com/dictionary/advocacy

Patient Protection and Affordable Care Act, Pub. L. 111–148, § 3502, 124 Stat. 119, 124 (2010).

Quiroga, V. (1995). *Occupational therapy: The first 30 years—1900 to 1930.* Bethesda, MD: AOTA Press.

Toto, P. (2012). Be an occupational therapy superhero. *OT Practice, 17*(7), 9-12.

Weissert, W. G., & Weissert, C. S. (2012). *Governing health: The politics of health policy.* Baltimore, MD: John Hopkins University Press.

West, W. M. (1968). Professional responsibility in times of change. *American Journal of Occupational Therapy, 22*(1), 175-189.

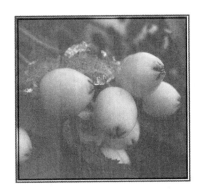

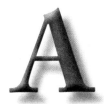

2011 ACCREDITATION COUNCIL FOR OCCUPATIONAL THERAPY EDUCATION STANDARDS AND INTERPRETIVE GUIDE

Reproduced with permission from the American Occupational Therapy Association.

Jacobs, K., MacRae, N., & Sladyk, K. (Eds.).
Occupational Therapy Essentials for Clinical Competence, Second Edition (pp. 725-768).
© 2014 SLACK Incorporated.

2011 Accreditation Council for Occupational Therapy Education (ACOTE®) Standards and Interpretive Guide
(effective July 31, 2013)
January 2012 Interpretive Guide Version

STANDARD NUMBER	ACCREDITATION STANDARDS FOR A DOCTORAL-DEGREE-LEVEL EDUCATIONAL PROGRAM FOR THE OCCUPATIONAL THERAPIST	ACCREDITATION STANDARDS FOR A MASTER'S-DEGREE-LEVEL EDUCATIONAL PROGRAM FOR THE OCCUPATIONAL THERAPIST	ACCREDITATION STANDARDS FOR AN ASSOCIATE-DEGREE-LEVEL EDUCATIONAL PROGRAM FOR THE OCCUPATIONAL THERAPY ASSISTANT
PREAMBLE	The rapidly changing and dynamic nature of contemporary health and human services delivery systems provides challenging opportunities for the occupational therapist to use knowledge and skills in a practice area as a direct care provider, consultant, educator, manager, leader, researcher, and advocate for the profession and the consumer.	The rapidly changing and dynamic nature of contemporary health and human services delivery systems requires the occupational therapist to possess basic skills as a direct care provider, consultant, educator, manager, researcher, and advocate for the profession and the consumer.	The rapidly changing and dynamic nature of contemporary health and human services delivery systems requires the occupational therapy assistant to possess basic skills as a direct care provider, educator, and advocate for the profession and the consumer.
	A graduate from an ACOTE-accredited doctoral-degree-level occupational therapy program must	A graduate from an ACOTE-accredited master's-degree-level occupational therapy program must	A graduate from an ACOTE-accredited associate-degree-level occupational therapy assistant program must
	• Have acquired, as a foundation for professional study, a breadth and depth of knowledge in the liberal arts and sciences and an understanding of issues related to diversity.	• Have acquired, as a foundation for professional study, a breadth and depth of knowledge in the liberal arts and sciences and an understanding of issues related to diversity.	• Have acquired an educational foundation in the liberal arts and sciences, including a focus on issues related to diversity.
	• Be educated as a generalist with a broad exposure to the delivery models and systems used in settings where occupational therapy is currently practiced and where it is emerging as a service.	• Be educated as a generalist with a broad exposure to the delivery models and systems used in settings where occupational therapy is currently practiced and where it is emerging as a service.	• Be educated as a generalist with a broad exposure to the delivery models and systems used in settings where occupational therapy is currently practiced and where it is emerging as a service.
	• Have achieved entry-level competence through a combination of academic and fieldwork education.	• Have achieved entry-level competence through a combination of academic and fieldwork education.	• Have achieved entry-level competence through a combination of academic and fieldwork education.
	• Be prepared to articulate and apply occupational therapy theory and evidence-based evaluations and interventions to achieve expected outcomes as related to occupation.	• Be prepared to articulate and apply occupational therapy principles and intervention tools to achieve expected outcomes as related to occupation.	• Be prepared to articulate and apply occupational therapy principles and intervention tools to achieve expected outcomes as related to occupation.
	• Be prepared to articulate and apply therapeutic use of occupations with individuals or groups for the purpose of participation in roles and situations in home, school, workplace, community, and other settings.	• Be prepared to articulate and apply therapeutic use of occupations with individuals or groups for the purpose of participation in roles and situations in home, school, workplace, community, and other settings.	• Be prepared to articulate and apply therapeutic use of occupations with individuals or groups for the purpose of participation in roles and situations in home, school, workplace, community, and other settings.
	• Be able to plan and apply occupational therapy interventions to address the physical, cognitive, psychosocial, sensory, and other aspects of performance in a variety of contexts and	• Be able to plan and apply occupational therapy interventions to address the physical, cognitive, psychosocial, sensory, and other aspects of performance in a variety of contexts and environments to support engagement in everyday	• Be able to apply occupational therapy interventions to address the physical, cognitive, psychosocial, sensory, and other aspects of performance in a variety of contexts and environments to support engagement in everyday

STANDARD NUMBER	ACCREDITATION STANDARDS FOR A DOCTORAL-DEGREE-LEVEL EDUCATIONAL PROGRAM FOR THE OCCUPATIONAL THERAPIST	ACCREDITATION STANDARDS FOR A MASTER'S-DEGREE-LEVEL EDUCATIONAL PROGRAM FOR THE OCCUPATIONAL THERAPIST	ACCREDITATION STANDARDS FOR AN ASSOCIATE-DEGREE-LEVEL EDUCATIONAL PROGRAM FOR THE OCCUPATIONAL THERAPY ASSISTANT
	environments to support engagement in everyday life activities that affect health, well-being, and quality of life.	life activities that affect health, well-being, and quality of life.	life activities that affect health, well-being, and quality of life.
	• Be prepared to be a lifelong learner and keep current with evidence-based professional practice.	• Be prepared to be a lifelong learner and keep current with evidence-based professional practice.	• Be prepared to be a lifelong learner and keep current with the best practice.
	• Uphold the ethical standards, values, and attitudes of the occupational therapy profession.	• Uphold the ethical standards, values, and attitudes of the occupational therapy profession.	• Uphold the ethical standards, values, and attitudes of the occupational therapy profession.
	• Understand the distinct roles and responsibilities of the occupational therapist and occupational therapy assistant in the supervisory process.	• Understand the distinct roles and responsibilities of the occupational therapist and occupational therapy assistant in the supervisory process.	• Understand the distinct roles and responsibilities of the occupational therapist and occupational therapy assistant in the supervisory process.
	• Be prepared to effectively communicate and work interprofessionally with those who provide care for individuals and/or populations in order to clarify each member's responsibility in executing components of an intervention plan.	• Be prepared to effectively communicate and work interprofessionally with those who provide care for individuals and/or populations in order to clarify each member's responsibility in executing components of an intervention plan.	• Be prepared to effectively communicate and work interprofessionally with those who provide care for individuals and/or populations in order to clarify each member's responsibility in executing components of an intervention plan.
	• Be prepared to advocate as a professional for the occupational therapy services offered and for the recipients of those services.	• Be prepared to advocate as a professional for the occupational therapy services offered and for the recipients of those services.	• Be prepared to advocate as a professional for the occupational therapy services offered and for the recipients of those services.
	• Be prepared to be an effective consumer of the latest research and knowledge bases that support practice and contribute to the growth and dissemination of research and knowledge.	• Be prepared to be an effective consumer of the latest research and knowledge bases that support practice and contribute to the growth and dissemination of research and knowledge.	
	• Demonstrate in-depth knowledge of delivery models, policies, and systems related to the area of practice in settings where occupational therapy is currently practiced and where it is emerging as a service.		
	• Demonstrate thorough knowledge of evidence-based practice.		
	• Demonstrate active involvement in professional development, leadership, and advocacy.		
	• Relate theory to practice and demonstrate synthesis of advanced knowledge in a practice area through completion of a culminating project.		

STANDARD NUMBER	ACCREDITATION STANDARDS FOR A DOCTORAL-DEGREE-LEVEL EDUCATIONAL PROGRAM FOR THE OCCUPATIONAL THERAPIST	ACCREDITATION STANDARDS FOR A MASTER'S-DEGREE-LEVEL EDUCATIONAL PROGRAM FOR THE OCCUPATIONAL THERAPIST	ACCREDITATION STANDARDS FOR AN ASSOCIATE-DEGREE-LEVEL EDUCATIONAL PROGRAM FOR THE OCCUPATIONAL THERAPY ASSISTANT
	• Develop in-depth experience in one or more of the following areas through completion of a doctoral experiential component: clinical practice skills, research skills, administration, leadership, program and policy development, advocacy, education, and theory development.		
FOR ALL STANDARDS LISTED BELOW, IF ONE COMPONENT OF THE STANDARD IS NONCOMPLIANT, THE ENTIRE STANDARD WILL BE CITED. THE PROGRAM MUST DEMONSTRATE COMPLIANCE WITH ALL COMPONENTS OF THE STANDARD IN ORDER FOR THE AREA OF NONCOMPLIANCE TO BE REMOVED.			

SECTION A: GENERAL REQUIREMENTS

A.1.0.   SPONSORSHIP AND ACCREDITATION

STANDARD NUMBER	DOCTORAL-DEGREE-LEVEL (OCCUPATIONAL THERAPIST)	MASTER'S-DEGREE-LEVEL (OCCUPATIONAL THERAPIST)	ASSOCIATE-DEGREE-LEVEL (OCCUPATIONAL THERAPY ASSISTANT)
A.1.1.	The sponsoring institution(s) and affiliates, if any, must be accredited by the recognized regional accrediting authority. For programs in countries other than the United States, ACOTE will determine an alternative and equivalent external review process.	The sponsoring institution(s) and affiliates, if any, must be accredited by the recognized regional accrediting authority. For programs in countries other than the United States, ACOTE will determine an alternative and equivalent external review process.	The sponsoring institution(s) and affiliates, if any, must be accredited by a recognized regional or national accrediting authority.
A.1.2.	Sponsoring institution(s) must be authorized under applicable law or other acceptable authority to provide a program of postsecondary education and have appropriate doctoral degree–granting authority.	Sponsoring institution(s) must be authorized under applicable law or other acceptable authority to provide a program of postsecondary education and have appropriate degree–granting authority.	Sponsoring institution(s) must be authorized under applicable law or other acceptable authority to provide a program of postsecondary education and have appropriate degree-granting authority, or the institution must be a program offered within the military services.
A.1.3.	Accredited occupational therapy educational programs may be established only in senior colleges, universities, or medical schools.	Accredited occupational therapy educational programs may be established only in senior colleges, universities, or medical schools.	Accredited occupational therapy assistant educational programs may be established only in community, technical, junior, and senior colleges; universities; medical schools; vocational schools or institutions; or military services.
A.1.4.	The sponsoring institution(s) must assume primary responsibility for appointment of faculty, admission of students, and curriculum planning at all locations where the program is offered. This would include course content, satisfactory completion of the educational program, and granting of the degree. The sponsoring institution(s) must also be responsible for the coordination of classroom teaching and supervised fieldwork practice and for providing assurance that the practice activities assigned to students in a fieldwork setting are appropriate to the program.	The sponsoring institution(s) must assume primary responsibility for appointment of faculty, admission of students, and curriculum planning at all locations where the program is offered. This would include course content, satisfactory completion of the educational program, and granting of the degree. The sponsoring institution(s) must also be responsible for the coordination of classroom teaching and supervised fieldwork practice and for providing assurance that the practice activities assigned to students in a fieldwork setting are appropriate to the program.	The sponsoring institution(s) must assume primary responsibility for appointment of faculty, admission of students, and curriculum planning at all locations where the program is offered. This would include course content, satisfactory completion of the educational program, and granting of the degree. The sponsoring institution(s) must also be responsible for the coordination of classroom teaching and supervised fieldwork practice and for providing assurance that the practice activities assigned to students in a fieldwork setting are appropriate to the program.
	THE DEGREES MOST COMMONLY CONFERRED ARE THE OCCUPATIONAL THERAPY DOCTORATE (OTD) AND DOCTOR OF OCCUPATIONAL THERAPY (DrOT).	*THE DEGREES MOST COMMONLY CONFERRED ARE THE MASTER OF OCCUPATIONAL THERAPY (MOT), MASTER OF SCIENCE IN OCCUPATIONAL THERAPY (MSOT), AND MASTER OF SCIENCE (MS). PROGRAMS OFFERING COMBINED BACCALAUREATE/MASTER'S (BS/MS OR BS/MOT) DEGREES ARE STRONGLY*	*THE DEGREES MOST COMMONLY CONFERRED ARE THE ASSOCIATE OF APPLIED SCIENCE (AAS) AND ASSOCIATE OF SCIENCE (AS).*

STANDARD NUMBER	ACCREDITATION STANDARDS FOR A DOCTORAL-DEGREE-LEVEL EDUCATIONAL PROGRAM FOR THE OCCUPATIONAL THERAPIST	ACCREDITATION STANDARDS FOR A MASTER'S-DEGREE-LEVEL EDUCATIONAL PROGRAM FOR THE OCCUPATIONAL THERAPIST	ACCREDITATION STANDARDS FOR AN ASSOCIATE-DEGREE-LEVEL EDUCATIONAL PROGRAM FOR THE OCCUPATIONAL THERAPY ASSISTANT
A.1.5.	The program must • Inform ACOTE of the transfer of program sponsorship or change of the institution's name within 30 days of the transfer or change. • Inform ACOTE within 30 days of the date of notification of any adverse accreditation action taken to change the sponsoring institution's accreditation status to probation or withdrawal of accreditation. • Notify and receive ACOTE approval for any significant program changes prior to the admission of students into the new/changed program. • Inform ACOTE within 30 days of the resignation of the program director or appointment of a new or interim program director. • Pay accreditation fees within 90 days of the invoice date. • Submit a Report of Self-Study and other required reports (e.g., Interim Report, Plan of Correction, Progress Report) within the period of time designated by ACOTE. All reports must be complete and contain all requested information. • Agree to a site visit date before the end of the period for which accreditation was previously awarded. • Demonstrate honesty and integrity in all interactions with ACOTE.	*ENCOURAGED TO AVOID USING "BACCALAUREATE IN OCCUPATIONAL THERAPY" AS THE BACCALAUREATE PORTION OF THE DEGREE NAME TO AVOID CONFUSING THE PUBLIC. DEGREE NAMES FOR THE BACCALAUREATE PORTION OF THE PROGRAM MOST COMMONLY USED ARE "BACCALAUREATE IN HEALTH SCIENCES," "BACCALAUREATE IN ALLIED HEALTH," "BACCALAUREATE IN OCCUPATIONAL SCIENCE," AND "BACCALAUREATE IN HEALTH STUDIES."* The program must • Inform ACOTE of the transfer of program sponsorship or change of the institution's name within 30 days of the transfer or change. • Inform ACOTE within 30 days of the date of notification of any adverse accreditation action taken to change the sponsoring institution's accreditation status to probation or withdrawal of accreditation. • Notify and receive ACOTE approval for any significant program changes prior to the admission of students into the new/changed program. • Inform ACOTE within 30 days of the resignation of the program director or appointment of a new or interim program director. • Pay accreditation fees within 90 days of the invoice date. • Submit a Report of Self-Study and other required reports (e.g., Interim Report, Plan of Correction, Progress Report) within the period of time designated by ACOTE. All reports must be complete and contain all requested information. • Agree to a site visit date before the end of the period for which accreditation was previously awarded. • Demonstrate honesty and integrity in all interactions with ACOTE.	The program must • Inform ACOTE of the transfer of program sponsorship or change of the institution's name within 30 days of the transfer or change. • Inform ACOTE within 30 days of the date of notification of any adverse accreditation action taken to change the sponsoring institution's accreditation status to probation or withdrawal of accreditation. • Notify and receive ACOTE approval for any significant program changes prior to the admission of students into the new/changed program. • Inform ACOTE within 30 days of the resignation of the program director or appointment of a new or interim program director. • Pay accreditation fees within 90 days of the invoice date. • Submit a Report of Self-Study and other required reports (e.g., Interim Report, Plan of Correction, Progress Report) within the period of time designated by ACOTE. All reports must be complete and contain all requested information. • Agree to a site visit date before the end of the period for which accreditation was previously awarded. • Demonstrate honesty and integrity in all interactions with ACOTE.
	THE INSTITUTION AND THE ACCREDITED PROGRAM WILL BE ADVISED THAT THE PROGRAM IS ON ADMINISTRATIVE PROBATIONARY ACCREDITATION WHEN THE PROGRAM DOES NOT COMPLY WITH ONE OR MORE OF THE ABOVE ADMINISTRATIVE REQUIREMENTS FOR MAINTAINING ACCREDITATION. THE POLICIES AND PROCEDURES FOR ADMINISTRATIVE PROBATIONARY ACCREDITATION ARE DETAILED IN ACOTE POLICY IV.C., "CLASSIFICATION OF ACCREDITATION CATEGORIES." *THE PROGRAM IS ALSO RESPONSIBLE FOR COMPLYING WITH THE CURRENT REQUIREMENTS OF ALL ACOTE POLICIES, INCLUDING THE REQUIREMENT FOR THE PROGRAM TO SUBMIT A LETTER OF INTENT TO SEEK ACCREDITATION FOR AN ADDITIONAL LOCATION AT LEAST 12 MONTHS PRIOR TO THE PLANNED ADMISSION OF STUDENTS INTO THAT ADDITIONAL LOCATION.*		

STANDARD NUMBER	ACCREDITATION STANDARDS FOR A DOCTORAL-DEGREE-LEVEL EDUCATIONAL PROGRAM FOR THE OCCUPATIONAL THERAPIST	ACCREDITATION STANDARDS FOR A MASTER'S-DEGREE-LEVEL EDUCATIONAL PROGRAM FOR THE OCCUPATIONAL THERAPIST	ACCREDITATION STANDARDS FOR AN ASSOCIATE-DEGREE-LEVEL EDUCATIONAL PROGRAM FOR THE OCCUPATIONAL THERAPY ASSISTANT
A.2.0.	**ACADEMIC RESOURCES**		
A.2.1.	The program must identify an individual as the program director who is assigned to the occupational therapy educational program on a full-time basis. The director may be assigned other institutional duties that do not interfere with the management and administration of the program. The institution must document that the program director has sufficient release time to ensure that the needs of the program are being met.	The program must identify an individual as the program director who is assigned to the occupational therapy educational program on a full-time basis. The director may be assigned other institutional duties that do not interfere with the management and administration of the program. The institution must document that the program director has sufficient release time to ensure that the needs of the program are being met.	The program must identify an individual as the program director who is assigned to the occupational therapy educational program on a full-time basis. The director may be assigned other institutional duties that do not interfere with the management and administration of the program. The institution must document that the program director has sufficient release time to ensure that the needs of the program are being met.
	THE STANDARD DOES NOT ALLOW THE APPOINTMENT OF CO-DIRECTORS.		
A.2.2.	The program director must be an initially certified occupational therapist who is licensed or otherwise regulated according to regulations in the state(s) or jurisdiction(s) in which the program is located. The program director must hold a doctoral degree awarded by an institution that is accredited by a regional accrediting body recognized by the U.S. Department of Education (USDE). The doctoral degree is not limited to a doctorate in occupational therapy. *A DOCTORAL DEGREE THAT WAS AWARDED PRIOR TO JULY 1, 2013, FROM AN INSTITUTION THAT WAS NOT REGIONALLY ACCREDITED IS CONSIDERED ACCEPTABLE TO MEET THIS STANDARD.* *FOR DEGREES FROM INSTITUTIONS IN COUNTRIES OTHER THAN THE UNITED STATES, ACOTE WILL DETERMINE AN ALTERNATIVE AND EQUIVALENT EXTERNAL REVIEW PROCESS.*	The program director must be an initially certified occupational therapist who is licensed or otherwise regulated according to regulations in the state(s) or jurisdiction(s) in which the program is located. The program director must hold a doctoral degree awarded by an institution that is accredited by a regional accrediting body recognized by the U.S. Department of Education (USDE). The doctoral degree is not limited to a doctorate in occupational therapy. *A DOCTORAL DEGREE THAT WAS AWARDED PRIOR TO JULY 1, 2013, FROM AN INSTITUTION THAT WAS NOT REGIONALLY ACCREDITED IS CONSIDERED ACCEPTABLE TO MEET THIS STANDARD.* *FOR DEGREES FROM INSTITUTIONS IN COUNTRIES OTHER THAN THE UNITED STATES, ACOTE WILL DETERMINE AN ALTERNATIVE AND EQUIVALENT EXTERNAL REVIEW PROCESS.*	The program director must be an initially certified occupational therapist or occupational therapy assistant who is licensed or otherwise regulated according to regulations in the state(s) or jurisdiction(s) in which the program is located. The program director must hold a minimum of a master's degree awarded by an institution that is accredited by a regional or national accrediting body recognized by the U.S. Department of Education (USDE). The master's degree is not limited to a master's degree in occupational therapy. *A MASTER'S DEGREE THAT WAS AWARDED PRIOR TO JULY 1, 2013, FROM AN INSTITUTION THAT WAS NOT REGIONALLY OR NATIONALLY ACCREDITED IS CONSIDERED ACCEPTABLE TO MEET THIS STANDARD.* *FOR DEGREES FROM INSTITUTIONS IN COUNTRIES OTHER THAN THE UNITED STATES, ACOTE WILL DETERMINE AN ALTERNATIVE AND EQUIVALENT EXTERNAL REVIEW PROCESS.*
A.2.3.	The program director must have a minimum of 8 years of documented experience in the field of occupational therapy. This experience must include • Clinical practice as an occupational therapist; • Administrative experience including, but not limited to, program planning and implementation, personnel management, evaluation, and budgeting; • Scholarship (e.g., scholarship of application, scholarship of teaching and learning); and • At least 3 years of experience in a full-time academic appointment with teaching responsibilities at the postbaccalaureate level.	The program director must have a minimum of 8 years of documented experience in the field of occupational therapy. This experience must include • Clinical practice as an occupational therapist; • Administrative experience including, but not limited to, program planning and implementation, personnel management, evaluation, and budgeting; • Scholarship (e.g., scholarship of application, scholarship of teaching and learning); and • At least 3 years of experience in a full-time academic appointment with teaching responsibilities at the postsecondary level.	The program director must have a minimum of 5 years of documented experience in the field of occupational therapy. This experience must include • Clinical practice as an occupational therapist or occupational therapy assistant; • Administrative experience including, but not limited to, program planning and implementation, personnel management, evaluation, and budgeting; • Understanding of and experience with occupational therapy assistants; and • At least 1 year of experience in a full-time academic appointment with teaching responsibilities at the postsecondary level.

STANDARD NUMBER	ACCREDITATION STANDARDS FOR A DOCTORAL-DEGREE-LEVEL EDUCATIONAL PROGRAM FOR THE OCCUPATIONAL THERAPIST	ACCREDITATION STANDARDS FOR A MASTER'S-DEGREE-LEVEL EDUCATIONAL PROGRAM FOR THE OCCUPATIONAL THERAPIST	ACCREDITATION STANDARDS FOR AN ASSOCIATE-DEGREE-LEVEL EDUCATIONAL PROGRAM FOR THE OCCUPATIONAL THERAPY ASSISTANT
A.2.4.	The program director must be responsible for the management and administration of the program, including planning, evaluation, budgeting, selection of faculty and staff, maintenance of accreditation, and commitment to strategies for professional development.	The program director must be responsible for the management and administration of the program, including planning, evaluation, budgeting, selection of faculty and staff, maintenance of accreditation, and commitment to strategies for professional development.	The program director must be responsible for the management and administration of the program, including planning, evaluation, budgeting, selection of faculty and staff, maintenance of accreditation, and commitment to strategies for professional development.
A.2.5.	*(No related Standard)*	*(No related Standard)*	In addition to the program director, the program must have at least one full-time equivalent (FTE) faculty position at each accredited location where the program is offered. This position may be shared by up to three individuals who teach as adjunct faculty. These individuals must have one or more additional responsibilities related to student advisement, supervision, committee work, program planning, evaluation, recruitment, and marketing activities.
A.2.6.	The program director and faculty must possess the academic and experiential qualifications and backgrounds (identified in documented descriptions of roles and responsibilities) that are necessary to meet program objectives and the mission of the institution.	The program director and faculty must possess the academic and experiential qualifications and backgrounds (identified in documented descriptions of roles and responsibilities) that are necessary to meet program objectives and the mission of the institution.	The program director and faculty must possess the academic and experiential qualifications and backgrounds (identified in documented descriptions of roles and responsibilities) that are necessary to meet program objectives and the mission of the institution.
A.2.7.	The program must identify an individual for the role of academic fieldwork coordinator who is specifically responsible for the program's compliance with the fieldwork requirements of Standards Section C.1.0 and is assigned to the occupational therapy educational program as a full-time faculty member as defined by ACOTE. The academic fieldwork coordinator may be assigned other institutional duties that do not interfere with the management and administration of the fieldwork program. The institution must document that the academic fieldwork coordinator has sufficient release time to ensure that the needs of the fieldwork program are being met. This individual must be a licensed or otherwise regulated occupational therapist. Coordinators must hold a doctoral degree awarded by an institution that is accredited by a USDE-recognized regional accrediting body.	The program must identify an individual for the role of academic fieldwork coordinator who is specifically responsible for the program's compliance with the fieldwork requirements of Standards Section C.1.0 and is assigned to the occupational therapy educational program as a full-time faculty member as defined by ACOTE. The academic fieldwork coordinator may be assigned other institutional duties that do not interfere with the management and administration of the fieldwork program. The institution must document that the academic fieldwork coordinator has sufficient release time to ensure that the needs of the fieldwork program are being met. This individual must be a licensed or otherwise regulated occupational therapist. Coordinators must hold a minimum of a master's degree awarded by an institution that is accredited by a USDE-recognized regional accrediting body.	The program must identify an individual for the role of academic fieldwork coordinator who is specifically responsible for the program's compliance with the fieldwork requirements of Standards Section C.1.0 and is assigned to the occupational therapy assistant educational program as a full-time faculty member as defined by ACOTE. The academic fieldwork coordinator may be assigned other institutional duties that do not interfere with the management and administration of the fieldwork program. The institution must document that the academic fieldwork coordinator has sufficient release time to ensure that the needs of the fieldwork program are being met. This individual must be a licensed or otherwise regulated occupational therapist or occupational therapy assistant. Coordinators must hold a minimum of a baccalaureate degree awarded by an institution that is accredited by a USDE-recognized regional or national accrediting body.

STANDARD NUMBER	ACCREDITATION STANDARDS FOR A DOCTORAL-DEGREE-LEVEL EDUCATIONAL PROGRAM FOR THE OCCUPATIONAL THERAPIST	ACCREDITATION STANDARDS FOR A MASTER'S-DEGREE-LEVEL EDUCATIONAL PROGRAM FOR THE OCCUPATIONAL THERAPIST	ACCREDITATION STANDARDS FOR AN ASSOCIATE-DEGREE-LEVEL EDUCATIONAL PROGRAM FOR THE OCCUPATIONAL THERAPY ASSISTANT
	A DOCTORAL DEGREE THAT WAS AWARDED PRIOR TO JULY 1, 2013, FROM AN INSTITUTION THAT WAS NOT REGIONALLY ACCREDITED IS CONSIDERED ACCEPTABLE TO MEET THIS STANDARD. *FOR DEGREES FROM INSTITUTIONS IN COUNTRIES OTHER THAN THE UNITED STATES, ACOTE WILL DETERMINE AN ALTERNATIVE AND EQUIVALENT EXTERNAL REVIEW PROCESS.*	*A MASTER'S DEGREE THAT WAS AWARDED PRIOR TO JULY 1, 2013, FROM AN INSTITUTION THAT WAS NOT REGIONALLY ACCREDITED IS CONSIDERED ACCEPTABLE TO MEET THIS STANDARD.* *FOR DEGREES FROM INSTITUTIONS IN COUNTRIES OTHER THAN THE UNITED STATES, ACOTE WILL DETERMINE AN ALTERNATIVE AND EQUIVALENT EXTERNAL REVIEW PROCESS.*	*A BACCALAUREATE DEGREE THAT WAS AWARDED PRIOR TO JULY 1, 2013, FROM AN INSTITUTION THAT WAS NOT REGIONALLY OR NATIONALLY ACCREDITED IS CONSIDERED ACCEPTABLE TO MEET THIS STANDARD.* *FOR DEGREES FROM INSTITUTIONS IN COUNTRIES OTHER THAN THE UNITED STATES, ACOTE WILL DETERMINE AN ALTERNATIVE AND EQUIVALENT EXTERNAL REVIEW PROCESS.*
A.2.8.	Core faculty who are occupational therapists or occupational therapy assistants must be currently licensed or otherwise regulated according to regulations in the state or jurisdiction in which the program is located. Faculty in residence and teaching at additional locations must be currently licensed or otherwise regulated according to regulations in the state or jurisdiction in which the additional location is located.	Core faculty who are occupational therapists or occupational therapy assistants must be currently licensed or otherwise regulated according to regulations in the state or jurisdiction in which the program is located. Faculty in residence and teaching at additional locations must be currently licensed or otherwise regulated according to regulations in the state or jurisdiction in which the additional location is located.	Core faculty who are occupational therapists or occupational therapy assistants must be currently licensed or otherwise regulated according to regulations in the state or jurisdiction in which the program is located. Faculty in residence and teaching at additional locations must be currently licensed or otherwise regulated according to regulations in the state or jurisdiction in which the additional location is located.
A.2.9.	*(No related Standard)*	*(No related Standard)*	In programs where the program director is an occupational therapy assistant, an occupational therapist must be included on faculty and contribute to the functioning of the program through a variety of mechanisms including, but not limited to, teaching, advising, and committee work. In a program where there are only occupational therapists on faculty who have never practiced as an occupational therapy assistant, the program must demonstrate that an individual who is an occupational therapy assistant or an occupational therapist who has previously practiced as an occupational therapy assistant is involved in the program as an adjunct faculty or teaching assistant.
A.2.10.	All full-time faculty teaching in the program must hold a doctoral degree awarded by an institution that is accredited by a USDE-recognized regional accrediting body. The doctoral degree is not limited to a doctorate in occupational therapy.	The majority of full-time faculty who are occupational therapists or occupational therapy assistants must hold a doctoral degree. All full-time faculty must hold a minimum of a master's degree. All degrees must be awarded by an institution that is accredited by a USDE-recognized regional accrediting body. The degrees are not limited to occupational therapy. For an even number of full-time faculty, at least half must hold doctorates. The program director is counted as a faculty member.	All occupational therapy assistant faculty who are full-time must hold a minimum of a baccalaureate degree awarded by an institution that is accredited by a USDE-recognized regional or national accrediting body.

STANDARD NUMBER	ACCREDITATION STANDARDS FOR A DOCTORAL-DEGREE-LEVEL EDUCATIONAL PROGRAM FOR THE OCCUPATIONAL THERAPIST	ACCREDITATION STANDARDS FOR A MASTER'S-DEGREE-LEVEL EDUCATIONAL PROGRAM FOR THE OCCUPATIONAL THERAPIST	ACCREDITATION STANDARDS FOR AN ASSOCIATE-DEGREE-LEVEL EDUCATIONAL PROGRAM FOR THE OCCUPATIONAL THERAPY ASSISTANT
	A DOCTORAL DEGREE THAT WAS AWARDED PRIOR TO JULY 1, 2013, FROM AN INSTITUTION THAT WAS NOT REGIONALLY ACCREDITED IS CONSIDERED ACCEPTABLE TO MEET THIS STANDARD. *FOR DEGREES FROM INSTITUTIONS IN COUNTRIES OTHER THAN THE UNITED STATES, ACOTE WILL DETERMINE AN ALTERNATIVE AND EQUIVALENT EXTERNAL REVIEW PROCESS.*	*A DOCTORAL OR MASTER'S DEGREE THAT WAS AWARDED PRIOR TO JULY 1, 2013, FROM AN INSTITUTION THAT WAS NOT REGIONALLY ACCREDITED IS CONSIDERED ACCEPTABLE TO MEET THIS STANDARD.* *FOR DEGREES FROM INSTITUTIONS IN COUNTRIES OTHER THAN THE UNITED STATES, ACOTE WILL DETERMINE AN ALTERNATIVE AND EQUIVALENT EXTERNAL REVIEW PROCESS.*	*A BACCALAUREATE DEGREE THAT WAS AWARDED PRIOR TO JULY 1, 2013, FROM AN INSTITUTION THAT WAS NOT REGIONALLY OR NATIONALLY ACCREDITED IS CONSIDERED ACCEPTABLE TO MEET THIS STANDARD.* *FOR DEGREES FROM INSTITUTIONS IN COUNTRIES OTHER THAN THE UNITED STATES, ACOTE WILL DETERMINE AN ALTERNATIVE AND EQUIVALENT EXTERNAL REVIEW PROCESS.*
A.2.11.	The faculty must have documented expertise in their area(s) of teaching responsibility and knowledge of the content delivery method (e.g., distance learning).	The faculty must have documented expertise in their area(s) of teaching responsibility and knowledge of the content delivery method (e.g., distance learning).	The faculty must have documented expertise in their area(s) of teaching responsibility and knowledge of the content delivery method (e.g., distance learning).
		EVIDENCE OF EXPERTISE IN TEACHING ASSIGNMENTS MIGHT INCLUDE DOCUMENTATION OF RECENT CONTINUING EDUCATION, RELEVANT EXPERIENCE, FACULTY DEVELOPMENT PLAN REFLECTING ACQUISITION OF NEW CONTENT, INCORPORATION OF FEEDBACK FROM COURSE EVALUATIONS, AND OTHER SOURCES.	
A.2.12.	For programs with additional accredited location(s), the program must identify a faculty member who is an occupational therapist as site coordinator at each location who is responsible for ensuring uniform implementation of the program and ongoing communication with the program director.	For programs with additional accredited location(s), the program must identify a faculty member who is an occupational therapist as site coordinator at each location who is responsible for ensuring uniform implementation of the program and ongoing communication with the program director.	For programs with additional accredited location(s), the program must identify a faculty member who is an occupational therapist or occupational therapy assistant as site coordinator at each location who is responsible for ensuring uniform implementation of the program and ongoing communication with the program director.
A.2.13.	The occupational therapy faculty at each accredited location where the program is offered must be sufficient in number and must possess the expertise necessary to ensure appropriate curriculum design, content delivery, and program evaluation. The faculty must include individuals competent to ensure delivery of the broad scope of occupational therapy practice. Multiple adjuncts, part-time faculty, or full-time faculty may be configured to meet this goal. Each accredited additional location must have at least one full-time equivalent (FTE) faculty member.	The occupational therapy faculty at each accredited location where the program is offered must be sufficient in number and must possess the expertise necessary to ensure appropriate curriculum design, content delivery, and program evaluation. The faculty must include individuals competent to ensure delivery of the broad scope of occupational therapy practice. Multiple adjuncts, part-time faculty, or full-time faculty may be configured to meet this goal. Each accredited additional location must have at least one full-time equivalent (FTE) faculty member.	The occupational therapy assistant faculty at each accredited location where the program is offered must be sufficient in number and must possess the expertise necessary to ensure appropriate curriculum design, content delivery, and program evaluation. The faculty must include individuals competent to ensure delivery of the broad scope of occupational therapy practice. Multiple adjuncts, part-time faculty, or full-time faculty may be configured to meet this goal. Each accredited additional location must have at least one full-time equivalent (FTE) faculty member.
A.2.14.	Faculty responsibilities must be consistent with and supportive of the mission of the institution.	Faculty responsibilities must be consistent with and supportive of the mission of the institution.	Faculty responsibilities must be consistent with and supportive of the mission of the institution.
A.2.15.	The faculty–student ratio must permit the achievement of the purpose and stated objectives for laboratory and lecture courses, be compatible with accepted practices of the institution for similar programs, and ensure student and consumer safety.	The faculty–student ratio must permit the achievement of the purpose and stated objectives for laboratory and lecture courses, be compatible with accepted practices of the institution for similar programs, and ensure student and consumer safety.	The faculty–student ratio must permit the achievement of the purpose and stated objectives for laboratory and lecture courses, be compatible with accepted practices of the institution for similar programs, and ensure student and consumer safety.
A.2.16.	Clerical and support staff must be provided to the program, consistent with institutional practice, to meet	Clerical and support staff must be provided to the program, consistent with institutional practice, to meet	Clerical and support staff must be provided to the program, consistent with institutional practice, to meet

STANDARD NUMBER	ACCREDITATION STANDARDS FOR A DOCTORAL-DEGREE-LEVEL EDUCATIONAL PROGRAM FOR THE OCCUPATIONAL THERAPIST	ACCREDITATION STANDARDS FOR A MASTER'S-DEGREE-LEVEL EDUCATIONAL PROGRAM FOR THE OCCUPATIONAL THERAPIST	ACCREDITATION STANDARDS FOR AN ASSOCIATE-DEGREE-LEVEL EDUCATIONAL PROGRAM FOR THE OCCUPATIONAL THERAPY ASSISTANT
	programmatic and administrative requirements, including support for any portion of the program offered by distance education.	programmatic and administrative requirements, including support for any portion of the program offered by distance education.	programmatic and administrative requirements, including support for any portion of the program offered by distance education.
A.2.17.	The program must be allocated a budget of regular institutional funds, not including grants, gifts, and other restricted sources, sufficient to implement and maintain the objectives of the program and to fulfill the program's obligation to matriculated and entering students.	The program must be allocated a budget of regular institutional funds, not including grants, gifts, and other restricted sources, sufficient to implement and maintain the objectives of the program and to fulfill the program's obligation to matriculated and entering students.	The program must be allocated a budget of regular institutional funds, not including grants, gifts, and other restricted sources, sufficient to implement and maintain the objectives of the program and to fulfill the program's obligation to matriculated and entering students.
A.2.18.	Classrooms and laboratories must be provided that are consistent with the program's educational objectives, teaching methods, number of students, and safety and health standards of the institution, and they must allow for efficient operation of the program.	Classrooms and laboratories must be provided that are consistent with the program's educational objectives, teaching methods, number of students, and safety and health standards of the institution, and they must allow for efficient operation of the program.	Classrooms and laboratories must be provided that are consistent with the program's educational objectives, teaching methods, number of students, and safety and health standards of the institution, and they must allow for efficient operation of the program.
A.2.19.	If the program offers distance education, it must include • A process through which the program establishes that the student who registers in a distance education course or program is the same student who participates in and completes the program and receives academic credit, • Technology and resources that are adequate to support a distance-learning environment, and • A process to ensure that faculty are adequately trained and skilled to use distance education methodologies.	If the program offers distance education, it must include • A process through which the program establishes that the student who registers in a distance education course or program is the same student who participates in and completes the program and receives academic credit, • Technology and resources that are adequate to support a distance-learning environment, and • A process to ensure that faculty are adequately trained and skilled to use distance education methodologies.	If the program offers distance education, it must include • A process through which the program establishes that the student who registers in a distance education course or program is the same student who participates in and completes the program and receives academic credit, • Technology and resources that are adequate to support a distance-learning environment, and • A process to ensure that faculty are adequately trained and skilled to use distance education methodologies.
A.2.20.	Laboratory space provided by the institution must be assigned to the occupational therapy program on a priority basis. If laboratory space for occupational therapy lab classes is provided by another institution or agency, there must be a written and signed agreement to ensure assignment of space for program use.	Laboratory space provided by the institution must be assigned to the occupational therapy program on a priority basis. If laboratory space for occupational therapy lab classes is provided by another institution or agency, there must be a written and signed agreement to ensure assignment of space for program use.	Laboratory space provided by the institution must be assigned to the occupational therapy assistant program on a priority basis. If laboratory space for occupational therapy assistant lab classes is provided by another institution or agency, there must be a written and signed agreement to ensure assignment of space for program use.
A.2.21.	Adequate space must be provided to store and secure equipment and supplies.	Adequate space must be provided to store and secure equipment and supplies.	Adequate space must be provided to store and secure equipment and supplies.
A.2.22.	The program director and faculty must have office space consistent with institutional practice.	The program director and faculty must have office space consistent with institutional practice.	The program director and faculty must have office space consistent with institutional practice.
A.2.23.	Adequate space must be provided for the private advising of students.	Adequate space must be provided for the private advising of students.	Adequate space must be provided for the private advising of students.
A.2.24.	Appropriate and sufficient equipment and supplies must be provided by the institution for student use and for the didactic, supervised fieldwork, and	Appropriate and sufficient equipment and supplies must be provided by the institution for student use and for the didactic and supervised fieldwork	Appropriate and sufficient equipment and supplies must be provided by the institution for student use and for the didactic and supervised fieldwork

STANDARD NUMBER	ACCREDITATION STANDARDS FOR A DOCTORAL-DEGREE-LEVEL EDUCATIONAL PROGRAM FOR THE OCCUPATIONAL THERAPIST	ACCREDITATION STANDARDS FOR A MASTER'S-DEGREE-LEVEL EDUCATIONAL PROGRAM FOR THE OCCUPATIONAL THERAPIST	ACCREDITATION STANDARDS FOR AN ASSOCIATE-DEGREE-LEVEL EDUCATIONAL PROGRAM FOR THE OCCUPATIONAL THERAPY ASSISTANT
	experiential components of the curriculum.	components of the curriculum.	components of the curriculum.
A.2.25.	Students must be given access to and have the opportunity to use the evaluative and treatment methodologies that reflect both current practice and practice in the geographic area served by the program.	Students must be given access to and have the opportunity to use the evaluative and treatment methodologies that reflect both current practice and practice in the geographic area served by the program.	Students must be given access to and have the opportunity to use the evaluative and treatment methodologies that reflect both current practice and practice in the geographic area served by the program.
A.2.26.	Students must have ready access to a supply of current and relevant books, journals, periodicals, computers, software, and other reference materials needed for the practice areas and to meet the requirements of the curriculum. This may include, but is not limited to, libraries, online services, interlibrary loan, and resource centers.	Students must have ready access to a supply of current and relevant books, journals, periodicals, computers, software, and other reference materials needed to meet the requirements of the curriculum. This may include, but is not limited to, libraries, online services, interlibrary loan, and resource centers.	Students must have ready access to a supply of current and relevant books, journals, periodicals, computers, software, and other reference materials needed to meet the requirements of the curriculum. This may include, but is not limited to, libraries, online services, interlibrary loan, and resource centers.
A.2.27.	Instructional aids and technology must be available in sufficient quantity and quality to be consistent with the program objectives and teaching methods.	Instructional aids and technology must be available in sufficient quantity and quality to be consistent with the program objectives and teaching methods.	Instructional aids and technology must be available in sufficient quantity and quality to be consistent with the program objectives and teaching methods.
A.3.0.	**STUDENTS**		
A.3.1.	Admission of students to the occupational therapy program must be made in accordance with the practices of the institution. There must be stated admission criteria that are clearly defined and published and reflective of the demands of the program.	Admission of students to the occupational therapy program must be made in accordance with the practices of the institution. There must be stated admission criteria that are clearly defined and published and reflective of the demands of the program.	Admission of students to the occupational therapy assistant program must be made in accordance with the practices of the institution. There must be stated admission criteria that are clearly defined and published and reflective of the demands of the program.
A.3.2.	Institutions must require that program applicants hold a baccalaureate degree or higher prior to admission to the program.	(No related Standard)	(No related Standard)
A.3.3.	Policies pertaining to standards for admission, advanced placement, transfer of credit, credit for experiential learning (if applicable), and prerequisite educational or work experience requirements must be readily accessible to prospective students and the public.	Policies pertaining to standards for admission, advanced placement, transfer of credit, credit for experiential learning (if applicable), and prerequisite educational or work experience requirements must be readily accessible to prospective students and the public.	Policies pertaining to standards for admission, advanced placement, transfer of credit, credit for experiential learning (if applicable), and prerequisite educational or work experience requirements must be readily accessible to prospective students and the public.
A.3.4.	Programs must document implementation of a mechanism to ensure that students receiving credit for previous courses and/or work experience have met the content requirements of the appropriate doctoral Standards.	Programs must document implementation of a mechanism to ensure that students receiving credit for previous courses and/or work experience have met the content requirements of the appropriate master's Standards.	Programs must document implementation of a mechanism to ensure that students receiving credit for previous courses and/or work experience have met the content requirements of the appropriate occupational therapy assistant Standards.
A.3.5.	Criteria for successful completion of each segment of the educational program and for graduation must be given in advance to each student.	Criteria for successful completion of each segment of the educational program and for graduation must be given in advance to each student.	Criteria for successful completion of each segment of the educational program and for graduation must be given in advance to each student.

STANDARD NUMBER	ACCREDITATION STANDARDS FOR A DOCTORAL-DEGREE-LEVEL EDUCATIONAL PROGRAM FOR THE OCCUPATIONAL THERAPIST	ACCREDITATION STANDARDS FOR A MASTER'S-DEGREE-LEVEL EDUCATIONAL PROGRAM FOR THE OCCUPATIONAL THERAPIST	ACCREDITATION STANDARDS FOR AN ASSOCIATE-DEGREE-LEVEL EDUCATIONAL PROGRAM FOR THE OCCUPATIONAL THERAPY ASSISTANT
A.3.6.	Evaluation content and methods must be consistent with the curriculum design; objectives; and competencies of the didactic, fieldwork, and experiential components of the program.	Evaluation content and methods must be consistent with the curriculum design, objectives, and competencies of the didactic and fieldwork components of the program.	Evaluation content and methods must be consistent with the curriculum design, objectives, and competencies of the didactic and fieldwork components of the program.
A.3.7.	Evaluation must be conducted on a regular basis to provide students and program officials with timely indications of the students' progress and academic standing.	Evaluation must be conducted on a regular basis to provide students and program officials with timely indications of the students' progress and academic standing.	Evaluation must be conducted on a regular basis to provide students and program officials with timely indications of the students' progress and academic standing.
A.3.8.	Students must be informed of and have access to the student support services that are provided to other students in the institution.	Students must be informed of and have access to the student support services that are provided to other students in the institution.	Students must be informed of and have access to the student support services that are provided to other students in the institution.
A.3.9.	Advising related to professional coursework, fieldwork education, and the experiential component of the program must be the responsibility of the occupational therapy faculty.	Advising related to professional coursework and fieldwork education must be the responsibility of the occupational therapy faculty.	Advising related to coursework in the occupational therapy assistant program and fieldwork education must be the responsibility of the occupational therapy assistant faculty.
A.4.0.	OPERATIONAL POLICIES		
A.4.1.	All program publications and advertising—including, but not limited to, academic calendars, announcements, catalogs, handbooks, and Web sites—must accurately reflect the program offered.	All program publications and advertising—including, but not limited to, academic calendars, announcements, catalogs, handbooks, and Web sites—must accurately reflect the program offered.	All program publications and advertising—including, but not limited to, academic calendars, announcements, catalogs, handbooks, and Web sites—must accurately reflect the program offered.
A.4.2.	Accurate and current information regarding student and program outcomes must be readily available to the public on the program's Web page. At a minimum, the following data must be reported for the previous 3 years: • Total number of program graduates • Graduation rates. The program must provide the direct link to the National Board for Certification in Occupational Therapy (NBCOT) program data results on the program's home page.	Accurate and current information regarding student and program outcomes must be readily available to the public on the program's Web page. At a minimum, the following data must be reported for the previous 3 years: • Total number of program graduates • Graduation rates. The program must provide the direct link to the National Board for Certification in Occupational Therapy (NBCOT) program data results on the program's home page.	Accurate and current information regarding student and program outcomes must be readily available to the public on the program's Web page. At a minimum, the following data must be reported for the previous 3 years: • Total number of program graduates, • Graduation rates. The program must provide the direct link to the National Board for Certification in Occupational Therapy (NBCOT) program data results on the program's home page.
A.4.3.	The program's accreditation status and the name, address, and telephone number of ACOTE must be published in all of the following materials used by the institution: catalog, Web site, and program-related brochures or flyers available to prospective students. A link to www.acoteonline.org must be provided on the program's home page.	The program's accreditation status and the name, address, and telephone number of ACOTE must be published in all of the following materials used by the institution: catalog, Web site, and program-related brochures or flyers available to prospective students. A link to www.acoteonline.org must be provided on the program's home page.	The program's accreditation status and the name, address, and telephone number of ACOTE must be published in all of the following materials used by the institution: catalog, Web site, and program-related brochures or flyers available to prospective students. A link to www.acoteonline.org must be provided on the program's home page.

SAMPLE WORDING: "THE OCCUPATIONAL THERAPY/OCCUPATIONAL THERAPY ASSISTANT PROGRAM IS ACCREDITED BY THE ACCREDITATION COUNCIL FOR OCCUPATIONAL THERAPY EDUCATION (ACOTE) OF THE AMERICAN OCCUPATIONAL THERAPY ASSOCIATION (AOTA), LOCATED AT 4720 MONTGOMERY LANE, PO BOX 31220, BETHESDA, MD 20824-1220. ACOTE'S TELEPHONE NUMBER, C/O AOTA, IS (301) 652-AOTA."

STANDARD NUMBER	ACCREDITATION STANDARDS FOR A DOCTORAL-DEGREE-LEVEL EDUCATIONAL PROGRAM FOR THE OCCUPATIONAL THERAPIST	ACCREDITATION STANDARDS FOR A MASTER'S-DEGREE-LEVEL EDUCATIONAL PROGRAM FOR THE OCCUPATIONAL THERAPIST	ACCREDITATION STANDARDS FOR AN ASSOCIATE-DEGREE-LEVEL EDUCATIONAL PROGRAM FOR THE OCCUPATIONAL THERAPY ASSISTANT
A.4.4.	All practices within the institution related to faculty, staff, applicants, and students must be nondiscriminatory.	All practices within the institution related to faculty, staff, applicants, and students must be nondiscriminatory.	All practices within the institution related to faculty, staff, applicants, and students must be nondiscriminatory.
A.4.5.	Graduation requirements, tuition, and fees must be accurately stated, published, and made known to all applicants. When published fees are subject to change, a statement to that effect must be included.	Graduation requirements, tuition, and fees must be accurately stated, published, and made known to all applicants. When published fees are subject to change, a statement to that effect must be included.	Graduation requirements, tuition, and fees must be accurately stated, published, and made known to all applicants. When published fees are subject to change, a statement to that effect must be included.
A.4.6.	The program or sponsoring institution must have a defined and published policy and procedure for processing student and faculty grievances.	The program or sponsoring institution must have a defined and published policy and procedure for processing student and faculty grievances.	The program or sponsoring institution must have a defined and published policy and procedure for processing student and faculty grievances.
A.4.7.	Policies and procedures for handling complaints against the program must be published and made known. The program must maintain a record of student complaints that includes the nature and disposition of each complaint.	Policies and procedures for handling complaints against the program must be published and made known. The program must maintain a record of student complaints that includes the nature and disposition of each complaint.	Policies and procedures for handling complaints against the program must be published and made known. The program must maintain a record of student complaints that includes the nature and disposition of each complaint.
A.4.8.	Policies and processes for student withdrawal and for refunds of tuition and fees must be published and made known to all applicants.	Policies and processes for student withdrawal and for refunds of tuition and fees must be published and made known to all applicants.	Policies and processes for student withdrawal and for refunds of tuition and fees must be published and made known to all applicants.
A.4.9.	Policies and procedures for student probation, suspension, and dismissal must be published and made known.	Policies and procedures for student probation, suspension, and dismissal must be published and made known.	Policies and procedures for student probation, suspension, and dismissal must be published and made known.
A.4.10.	Policies and procedures for human-subject research protocol must be published and made known.	Policies and procedures for human-subject research protocol must be published and made known.	Policies and procedures for human-subject research protocol must be published and made known (if applicable to the program).
A.4.11.	Programs must make available to students written policies and procedures regarding appropriate use of equipment and supplies and for all educational activities that have implications for the health and safety of clients, students, and faculty (including infection control and evacuation procedures).	Programs must make available to students written policies and procedures regarding appropriate use of equipment and supplies and for all educational activities that have implications for the health and safety of clients, students, and faculty (including infection control and evacuation procedures).	Programs must make available to students written policies and procedures regarding appropriate use of equipment and supplies and for all educational activities that have implications for the health and safety of clients, students, and faculty (including infection control and evacuation procedures).
A.4.12.	A program admitting students on the basis of ability to benefit (defined by the USDE as admitting students who do not have either a high school diploma or its equivalent) must publicize its objectives, assessment measures, and means of evaluating the student's ability to benefit.	A program admitting students on the basis of ability to benefit (defined by the USDE as admitting students who do not have either a high school diploma or its equivalent) must publicize its objectives, assessment measures, and means of evaluating the student's ability to benefit.	A program admitting students on the basis of ability to benefit (defined by the USDE as admitting students who do not have either a high school diploma or its equivalent) must publicize its objectives, assessment measures, and means of evaluating the student's ability to benefit.
A.4.13.	Documentation of all progression, retention, graduation, certification, and credentialing requirements must be published and made known to applicants. A statement on the program's Web site about the potential impact of a felony conviction on a	Documentation of all progression, retention, graduation, certification, and credentialing requirements must be published and made known to applicants. A statement on the program's Web site about the potential impact of a felony conviction on a	Documentation of all progression, retention, graduation, certification, and credentialing requirements must be published and made known to applicants. A statement on the program's Web site about the potential impact of a felony conviction on a

STANDARD NUMBER	ACCREDITATION STANDARDS FOR A DOCTORAL-DEGREE-LEVEL EDUCATIONAL PROGRAM FOR THE OCCUPATIONAL THERAPIST	ACCREDITATION STANDARDS FOR A MASTER'S-DEGREE-LEVEL EDUCATIONAL PROGRAM FOR THE OCCUPATIONAL THERAPIST	ACCREDITATION STANDARDS FOR AN ASSOCIATE-DEGREE-LEVEL EDUCATIONAL PROGRAM FOR THE OCCUPATIONAL THERAPY ASSISTANT
	graduate's eligibility for certification and credentialing must be provided. SAMPLE WORDING: "GRADUATES OF THE PROGRAM WILL BE ELIGIBLE TO SIT FOR THE NATIONAL CERTIFICATION EXAMINATION FOR THE OCCUPATIONAL THERAPIST, ADMINISTERED BY THE NATIONAL BOARD FOR CERTIFICATION IN OCCUPATIONAL THERAPY (NBCOT). AFTER SUCCESSFUL COMPLETION OF THIS EXAM, THE GRADUATE WILL BE AN OCCUPATIONAL THERAPIST, REGISTERED (OTR). IN ADDITION, MOST STATES REQUIRE LICENSURE TO PRACTICE; HOWEVER, STATE LICENSES ARE USUALLY BASED ON THE RESULTS OF THE NBCOT CERTIFICATION EXAMINATION. A FELONY CONVICTION MAY AFFECT A GRADUATE'S ABILITY TO SIT FOR THE NBCOT CERTIFICATION EXAMINATION OR ATTAIN STATE LICENSURE."	graduate's eligibility for certification and credentialing must be provided. SAMPLE WORDING: "GRADUATES OF THE PROGRAM WILL BE ELIGIBLE TO SIT FOR THE NATIONAL CERTIFICATION EXAMINATION FOR THE OCCUPATIONAL THERAPIST, ADMINISTERED BY THE NATIONAL BOARD FOR CERTIFICATION IN OCCUPATIONAL THERAPY (NBCOT). AFTER SUCCESSFUL COMPLETION OF THIS EXAM, THE GRADUATE WILL BE AN OCCUPATIONAL THERAPIST, REGISTERED (OTR). IN ADDITION, MOST STATES REQUIRE LICENSURE TO PRACTICE; HOWEVER, STATE LICENSES ARE USUALLY BASED ON THE RESULTS OF THE NBCOT CERTIFICATION EXAMINATION. A FELONY CONVICTION MAY AFFECT A GRADUATE'S ABILITY TO SIT FOR THE NBCOT CERTIFICATION EXAMINATION OR ATTAIN STATE LICENSURE."	graduate's eligibility for certification and credentialing must be provided. SAMPLE WORDING: "GRADUATES OF THE PROGRAM WILL BE ELIGIBLE TO SIT FOR THE NATIONAL CERTIFICATION EXAMINATION FOR THE OCCUPATIONAL THERAPY ASSISTANT, ADMINISTERED BY THE NATIONAL BOARD FOR CERTIFICATION IN OCCUPATIONAL THERAPY (NBCOT). AFTER SUCCESSFUL COMPLETION OF THIS EXAM, THE GRADUATE WILL BE A CERTIFIED OCCUPATIONAL THERAPY ASSISTANT (COTA). IN ADDITION, MOST STATES REQUIRE LICENSURE TO PRACTICE; HOWEVER, STATE LICENSES ARE USUALLY BASED ON THE RESULTS OF THE NBCOT CERTIFICATION EXAMINATION. A FELONY CONVICTION MAY AFFECT A GRADUATE'S ABILITY TO SIT FOR THE NBCOT CERTIFICATION EXAMINATION OR ATTAIN STATE LICENSURE."
A.4.14.	The program must have a documented and published policy to ensure that students complete all graduation, fieldwork, and experiential component requirements in a timely manner. This policy must include a statement that all Level II fieldwork and the experiential component of the program must be completed within a time frame established by the program. SAMPLE WORDING: "STUDENTS MUST COMPLETE ALL LEVEL II FIELDWORK AND THE EXPERIENTIAL COMPONENT OF THE PROGRAM WITHIN [XX] MONTHS FOLLOWING COMPLETION OF THE DIDACTIC PORTION OF THE PROGRAM."	The program must have a documented and published policy to ensure that students complete all graduation and fieldwork requirements in a timely manner. This policy must include a statement that all Level II fieldwork must be completed within a time frame established by the program. SAMPLE WORDING: "STUDENTS MUST COMPLETE ALL LEVEL II FIELDWORK WITHIN [XX] MONTHS FOLLOWING COMPLETION OF THE DIDACTIC PORTION OF THE PROGRAM."	The program must have a documented and published policy to ensure that students complete all graduation and fieldwork requirements in a timely manner. This policy must include a statement that all Level II fieldwork must be completed within a time frame established by the program. SAMPLE WORDING: "STUDENTS MUST COMPLETE ALL LEVEL II FIELDWORK WITHIN [XX] MONTHS FOLLOWING COMPLETION OF THE DIDACTIC PORTION OF THE PROGRAM."
A.4.15.	Records regarding student admission, enrollment, fieldwork, and achievement must be maintained and kept in a secure setting. Grades and credits for courses must be recorded on students' transcripts and permanently maintained by the sponsoring institution.	Records regarding student admission, enrollment, fieldwork, and achievement must be maintained and kept in a secure setting. Grades and credits for courses must be recorded on students' transcripts and permanently maintained by the sponsoring institution.	Records regarding student admission, enrollment, fieldwork, and achievement must be maintained and kept in a secure setting. Grades and credits for courses must be recorded on students' transcripts and permanently maintained by the sponsoring institution.

A.5.0.   STRATEGIC PLAN AND PROGRAM ASSESSMENT

For programs that are offered at more than one location, the program's strategic plan, evaluation plan, and results of ongoing evaluation must address each program location as a component of the overall plan.

STANDARD NUMBER	DOCTORAL	MASTER'S	ASSOCIATE
A.5.1.	The program must document a current strategic plan that articulates the program's future vision and guides the program development (e.g., faculty recruitment and professional growth, scholarship, changes in the curriculum design, priorities in academic resources,	The program must document a current strategic plan that articulates the program's future vision and guides the program development (e.g., faculty recruitment and professional growth, scholarship, changes in the curriculum design, priorities in academic resources,	The program must document a current strategic plan that articulates the program's future vision and guides the program development (e.g., faculty recruitment and professional growth, scholarship, changes in the curriculum design, priorities in academic resources,

STANDARD NUMBER	ACCREDITATION STANDARDS FOR A DOCTORAL-DEGREE-LEVEL EDUCATIONAL PROGRAM FOR THE OCCUPATIONAL THERAPIST	ACCREDITATION STANDARDS FOR A MASTER'S-DEGREE-LEVEL EDUCATIONAL PROGRAM FOR THE OCCUPATIONAL THERAPIST	ACCREDITATION STANDARDS FOR AN ASSOCIATE-DEGREE-LEVEL EDUCATIONAL PROGRAM FOR THE OCCUPATIONAL THERAPY ASSISTANT
	procurement of fieldwork and experiential component sites). A program strategic plan must be for a minimum of a 3-year period and include, but need not be limited to, • Evidence that the plan is based on program evaluation and an analysis of external and internal environments. • Long-term goals that address the vision and mission of both the institution and the program, as well as specific needs of the program. • Specific measurable action steps with expected timelines by which the program will reach its long-term goals. • Person(s) responsible for action steps. • Evidence of periodic updating of action steps and long-term goals as they are met or as circumstances change.	procurement of fieldwork sites). A program strategic plan must be for a minimum of a 3-year period and include, but need not be limited to, • Evidence that the plan is based on program evaluation and an analysis of external and internal environments. • Long-term goals that address the vision and mission of both the institution and the program, as well as specific needs of the program. • Specific measurable action steps with expected timelines by which the program will reach its long-term goals. • Person(s) responsible for action steps. • Evidence of periodic updating of action steps and long-term goals as they are met or as circumstances change.	procurement of fieldwork sites). A program strategic plan must be for a minimum of a 3-year period and include, but need not be limited to, • Evidence that the plan is based on program evaluation and an analysis of external and internal environments. • Long-term goals that address the vision and mission of both the institution and the program, as well as specific needs of the program. • Specific measurable action steps with expected timelines by which the program will reach its long-term goals. • Person(s) responsible for action steps. • Evidence of periodic updating of action steps and long-term goals as they are met or as circumstances change.
A.5.2.	The program director and each faculty member who teaches two or more courses must have a current written professional growth and development plan. Each plan must contain the signature of the faculty member and supervisor. At a minimum, the plan must include, but need not be limited to, • Goals to enhance the faculty member's ability to fulfill designated responsibilities (e.g., goals related to currency in areas of teaching responsibility, teaching effectiveness, research, scholarly activity). • Specific measurable action steps with expected timelines by which the faculty member will achieve the goals. • Evidence of annual updates of action steps and goals as they are met or as circumstances change. • Identification of the ways in which the faculty member's professional development plan will contribute to attaining the program's strategic goals.	The program director and each faculty member who teaches two or more courses must have a current written professional growth and development plan. Each plan must contain the signature of the faculty member and supervisor. At a minimum, the plan must include, but need not be limited to, • Goals to enhance the faculty member's ability to fulfill designated responsibilities (e.g., goals related to currency in areas of teaching responsibility, teaching effectiveness, research, scholarly activity). • Specific measurable action steps with expected timelines by which the faculty member will achieve the goals. • Evidence of annual updates of action steps and goals as they are met or as circumstances change. • Identification of the ways in which the faculty member's professional development plan will contribute to attaining the program's strategic goals.	The program director and each faculty member who teaches two or more courses must have a current written professional growth and development plan. Each plan must contain the signature of the faculty member and supervisor. At a minimum, the plan must include, but need not be limited to, • Goals to enhance the faculty member's ability to fulfill designated responsibilities (e.g., goals related to currency in areas of teaching responsibility, teaching effectiveness, research, scholarly activity). • Specific measurable action steps with expected timelines by which the faculty member will achieve the goals. • Evidence of annual updates of action steps and goals as they are met or as circumstances change. • Identification of the ways in which the faculty member's professional development plan will contribute to attaining the program's strategic goals.
	THE PLAN SHOULD REFLECT THE INDIVIDUAL FACULTY MEMBER'S DESIGNATED RESPONSIBILITIES (E.G., EVERY PLAN DOES NOT NEED TO INCLUDE SCHOLARLY ACTIVITY IF THIS IS NOT PART OF THE FACULTY MEMBER'S RESPONSIBILITIES. SIMILARLY, IF THE FACULTY MEMBER'S PRIMARY ROLE IS RESEARCH, HE OR SHE MAY NOT NEED A GOAL RELATED TO TEACHING EFFECTIVENESS).		
A.5.3.	Programs must routinely secure and document sufficient qualitative and quantitative information to allow for meaningful analysis about the extent to	Programs must routinely secure and document sufficient qualitative and quantitative information to allow for meaningful analysis about the extent to	Programs must routinely secure and document sufficient qualitative and quantitative information to allow for meaningful analysis about the extent to

STANDARD NUMBER	ACCREDITATION STANDARDS FOR A DOCTORAL-DEGREE-LEVEL EDUCATIONAL PROGRAM FOR THE OCCUPATIONAL THERAPIST	ACCREDITATION STANDARDS FOR A MASTER'S-DEGREE-LEVEL EDUCATIONAL PROGRAM FOR THE OCCUPATIONAL THERAPIST	ACCREDITATION STANDARDS FOR AN ASSOCIATE-DEGREE-LEVEL EDUCATIONAL PROGRAM FOR THE OCCUPATIONAL THERAPY ASSISTANT
	which the program is meeting its stated goals and objectives. This must include, but need not be limited to, • Faculty effectiveness in their assigned teaching responsibilities. • Students' progression through the program. • Student retention rates. • Fieldwork and experiential component performance evaluation. • Student evaluation of fieldwork and the experiential component experience. • Student satisfaction with the program. • Graduates' performance on the NBCOT certification exam. • Graduates' job placement and performance as determined by employer satisfaction. • Graduates' scholarly activity (e.g., presentations, publications, grants obtained, state and national leadership positions, awards).	which the program is meeting its stated goals and objectives. This must include, but need not be limited to, • Faculty effectiveness in their assigned teaching responsibilities. • Students' progression through the program. • Student retention rates. • Fieldwork performance evaluation. • Student evaluation of fieldwork experience. • Student satisfaction with the program. • Graduates' performance on the NBCOT certification exam. • Graduates' job placement and performance as determined by employer satisfaction.	which the program is meeting its stated goals and objectives. This must include, but need not be limited to, • Faculty effectiveness in their assigned teaching responsibilities. • Students' progression through the program. • Student retention rates. • Fieldwork performance evaluation. • Student evaluation of fieldwork experience. • Student satisfaction with the program. • Graduates' performance on the NBCOT certification exam. • Graduates' job placement and performance as determined by employer satisfaction.
A.5.4.	Programs must routinely and systematically analyze data to determine the extent to which the program is meeting its stated goals and objectives. An annual report summarizing analysis of data and planned action responses must be maintained.	Programs must routinely and systematically analyze data to determine the extent to which the program is meeting its stated goals and objectives. An annual report summarizing analysis of data and planned action responses must be maintained.	Programs must routinely and systematically analyze data to determine the extent to which the program is meeting its stated goals and objectives. An annual report summarizing analysis of data and planned action responses must be maintained.
	THE INTENT OF STANDARD A.5.4 IS THAT PROGRAMS PREPARE AN ANNUAL REPORT THAT SUMMARIZES AN ANALYSIS OF DATA COLLECTED ABOUT THE EXTENT TO WHICH THE PROGRAM IS MEETING ITS STATED GOALS AND OBJECTIVES AS REQUIRED BY STANDARD A.5.3 (E.G., FACULTY EFFECTIVENESS IN THEIR ASSIGNED TEACHING RESPONSIBILITIES; STUDENTS' PROGRESSION THROUGH THE PROGRAM, STUDENT RETENTION RATES, FIELDWORK PERFORMANCE EVALUATION, STUDENT EVALUATION OF FIELDWORK EXPERIENCE, STUDENT SATISFACTION WITH THE PROGRAM, GRADUATES' PERFORMANCE ON THE NBCOT CERTIFICATION EXAM, GRADUATES' JOB PLACEMENT, AND PERFORMANCE AS DETERMINED BY EMPLOYER SATISFACTION).		
A.5.5.	The results of ongoing evaluation must be appropriately reflected in the program's strategic plan, curriculum, and other dimensions of the program.	The results of ongoing evaluation must be appropriately reflected in the program's strategic plan, curriculum, and other dimensions of the program.	The results of ongoing evaluation must be appropriately reflected in the program's strategic plan, curriculum, and other dimensions of the program.
A.5.6.	The average pass rate over the 3 most recent calendar years for graduates attempting the national certification exam within 12 months of graduation from the program must be 80% or higher (regardless of the number of attempts). If a program has less than 25 test takers in the 3 most recent calendar years, the program may include test takers from additional years until it reaches 25 or until the 5 most recent calendar years are included in the total.	The average pass rate over the 3 most recent calendar years for graduates attempting the national certification exam within 12 months of graduation from the program must be 80% or higher (regardless of the number of attempts). If a program has less than 25 test takers in the 3 most recent calendar years, the program may include test takers from additional years until it reaches 25 or until the 5 most recent calendar years are included in the total.	The average pass rate over the 3 most recent calendar years for graduates attempting the national certification exam within 12 months of graduation from the program must be 80% or higher (regardless of the number of attempts). If a program has less than 25 test takers in the 3 most recent calendar years, the program may include test takers from additional years until it reaches 25 or until the 5 most recent calendar years are included in the total.
	PROGRAMS THAT DID NOT HAVE CANDIDATES WHO SAT FOR THE EXAM IN EACH OF THE 3 MOST RECENT CALENDAR YEARS MUST MEET THE REQUIRED 80% PASS RATE EACH YEAR UNTIL DATA FOR 3 CALENDAR YEARS ARE AVAILABLE.		*PROGRAMS THAT DID NOT HAVE CANDIDATES WHO SAT FOR THE EXAM IN EACH OF THE 3 MOST RECENT CALENDAR YEARS MUST MEET THE REQUIRED 80% PASS*

STANDARD NUMBER	ACCREDITATION STANDARDS FOR A DOCTORAL-DEGREE-LEVEL EDUCATIONAL PROGRAM FOR THE OCCUPATIONAL THERAPIST	ACCREDITATION STANDARDS FOR A MASTER'S-DEGREE-LEVEL EDUCATIONAL PROGRAM FOR THE OCCUPATIONAL THERAPIST	ACCREDITATION STANDARDS FOR AN ASSOCIATE-DEGREE-LEVEL EDUCATIONAL PROGRAM FOR THE OCCUPATIONAL THERAPY ASSISTANT
A.6.0.	**CURRICULUM FRAMEWORK**		
	The curriculum framework is a description of the program that includes the program's mission, philosophy, and curriculum design.		
A.6.1.	The curriculum must ensure preparation to practice as a generalist with a broad exposure to current practice settings (e.g., school, hospital, community, long-term care) and emerging practice areas (as defined by the program). The curriculum must prepare students to work with a variety of populations including, but not limited to, children, adolescents, adults, and elderly persons in areas of physical and mental health.	The curriculum must include preparation for practice as a generalist with a broad exposure to current practice settings (e.g., school, hospital, community, long-term care) and emerging practice areas (as defined by the program). The curriculum must prepare students to work with a variety of populations including, but not limited to, children, adolescents, adults, and elderly persons in areas of physical and mental health.	The curriculum must include preparation for practice as a generalist with a broad exposure to current practice settings (e.g., school, hospital, community, long-term care) and emerging practice areas (as defined by the program). The curriculum must prepare students to work with a variety of populations including, but not limited to, children, adolescents, adults, and elderly persons in areas of physical and mental health.
A.6.2.	The curriculum must include course objectives and learning activities demonstrating preparation beyond a generalist level in, but not limited to, practice skills, research skills, administration, professional development, leadership, advocacy, and theory.	*(No related Standard)*	*(No related Standard)*
A.6.3.	The occupational therapy doctoral degree must be awarded after a period of study such that the total time to the degree, including both preprofessional and professional preparation, equals at least 6 FTE academic years. The program must document a system and rationale for ensuring that the length of study of the program is appropriate to the expected learning and competence of the graduate.	The program must document a system and rationale for ensuring that the length of study of the program is appropriate to the expected learning and competence of the graduate.	The program must document a system and rationale for ensuring that the length of study of the program is appropriate to the expected learning and competence of the graduate.
A.6.4.	The curriculum must include application of advanced knowledge to practice through a combination of experiential activities and a culminating project.	*(No related Standard)*	*(No related Standard)*
A.6.5.	The statement of philosophy of the occupational therapy program must reflect the current published philosophy of the profession and must include a statement of the program's fundamental beliefs about human beings and how they learn.	The statement of philosophy of the occupational therapy program must reflect the current published philosophy of the profession and must include a statement of the program's fundamental beliefs about human beings and how they learn.	The statement of philosophy of the occupational therapy assistant program must reflect the current published philosophy of the profession and must include a statement of the program's fundamental beliefs about human beings and how they learn.
A.6.6.	The statement of the mission of the occupational therapy program must be consistent with and supportive of the mission of the sponsoring institution. The program's mission statement should explain the unique nature of the program and how it helps fulfill or advance the mission of the sponsoring institution, including religious missions.	The statement of the mission of the occupational therapy program must be consistent with and supportive of the mission of the sponsoring institution. The program's mission statement should explain the unique nature of the program and how it helps fulfill or advance the mission of the sponsoring institution, including religious missions.	The statement of the mission of the occupational therapy assistant program must be consistent with and supportive of the mission of the sponsoring institution. The program's mission statement should explain the unique nature of the program and how it helps fulfill or advance the mission of the sponsoring institution, including religious missions.
A.6.7.	The curriculum design must reflect the mission and philosophy of both the occupational therapy program and the institution and must provide the basis for	The curriculum design must reflect the mission and philosophy of both the occupational therapy program and the institution and must provide the	The curriculum design must reflect the mission and philosophy of both the occupational therapy assistant program and the institution and must provide the

STANDARD NUMBER	ACCREDITATION STANDARDS FOR A DOCTORAL-DEGREE-LEVEL EDUCATIONAL PROGRAM FOR THE OCCUPATIONAL THERAPIST	ACCREDITATION STANDARDS FOR A MASTER'S-DEGREE-LEVEL EDUCATIONAL PROGRAM FOR THE OCCUPATIONAL THERAPIST	ACCREDITATION STANDARDS FOR AN ASSOCIATE-DEGREE-LEVEL EDUCATIONAL PROGRAM FOR THE OCCUPATIONAL THERAPY ASSISTANT
	program planning, implementation, and evaluation. The design must identify curricular threads and educational goals and describe the selection of the content, scope, and sequencing of coursework.	program planning, implementation, and evaluation. The design must identify curricular threads and educational goals and describe the selection of the content, scope, and sequencing of coursework.	basis for program planning, implementation, and evaluation. The design must identify curricular threads and educational goals and describe the selection of the content, scope, and sequencing of coursework.
A.6.8.	The program must have clearly documented assessment measures by which students are regularly evaluated on their acquisition of knowledge, skills, attitudes, and competencies required for graduation.	The program must have clearly documented assessment measures by which students are regularly evaluated on their acquisition of knowledge, skills, attitudes, and competencies required for graduation.	The program must have clearly documented assessment measures by which students are regularly evaluated on their acquisition of knowledge, skills, attitudes, and competencies required for graduation.
A.6.9.	The program must have written syllabi for each course that include course objectives and learning activities that, in total, reflect all course content required by the Standards. Instructional methods (e.g., presentations, demonstrations, discussion) and materials used to accomplish course objectives must be documented. Programs must also demonstrate the consistency between course syllabi and the curriculum design.	The program must have written syllabi for each course that include course objectives and learning activities that, in total, reflect all course content required by the Standards. Instructional methods (e.g., presentations, demonstrations, discussion) and materials used to accomplish course objectives must be documented. Programs must also demonstrate the consistency between course syllabi and the curriculum design.	The program must have written syllabi for each course that include course objectives and learning activities that, in total, reflect all course content required by the Standards. Instructional methods (e.g., presentations, demonstrations, discussion) and materials used to accomplish course objectives must be documented. Programs must also demonstrate the consistency between course syllabi and the curriculum design.

SECTION B: CONTENT REQUIREMENTS
The content requirements are written as expected student outcomes. Faculty are responsible for developing learning activities and evaluation methods to document that students meet these outcomes.

STANDARD NUMBER	DOCTORAL	MASTER'S	ASSOCIATE
B.1.0.	FOUNDATIONAL CONTENT REQUIREMENTS Program content must be based on a broad foundation in the liberal arts and sciences. A strong foundation in the biological, physical, social, and behavioral sciences supports an understanding of occupation across the lifespan. If the content of the Standard is met through prerequisite coursework, the application of foundational content in sciences must also be evident in professional coursework. The student will be able to	FOUNDATIONAL CONTENT REQUIREMENTS Program content must be based on a broad foundation in the liberal arts and sciences. A strong foundation in the biological, physical, social, and behavioral sciences supports an understanding of occupation across the lifespan. If the content of the Standard is met through prerequisite coursework, the application of foundational content in sciences must also be evident in professional coursework. The student will be able to	FOUNDATIONAL CONTENT REQUIREMENTS Program content must be based on a broad foundation in the liberal arts and sciences. A strong foundation in the biological, physical, social, and behavioral sciences supports an understanding of occupation across the lifespan. If the content of the Standard is met through prerequisite coursework, the application of foundational content in sciences must also be evident in professional coursework. The student will be able to
B.1.1.	Demonstrate knowledge and understanding of the structure and function of the human body to include the biological and physical sciences. Course content must include, but is not limited to, biology, anatomy, physiology, neuroscience, and kinesiology or biomechanics.	Demonstrate knowledge and understanding of the structure and function of the human body to include the biological and physical sciences. Course content must include, but is not limited to, biology, anatomy, physiology, neuroscience, and kinesiology or biomechanics.	Demonstrate knowledge and understanding of the structure and function of the human body to include the biological and physical sciences. Course content must include, but is not limited to, anatomy, physiology, and biomechanics.
B.1.2.	Demonstrate knowledge and understanding of human development throughout the lifespan (infants, children, adolescents, adults, and older adults). Course content must include, but is not limited to,	Demonstrate knowledge and understanding of human development throughout the lifespan (infants, children, adolescents, adults, and older adults). Course content must include, but is not limited to,	Demonstrate knowledge and understanding of human development throughout the lifespan (infants, children, adolescents, adults, and older adults). Course content must include, but is not limited to,

STANDARD NUMBER	ACCREDITATION STANDARDS FOR A DOCTORAL-DEGREE-LEVEL EDUCATIONAL PROGRAM FOR THE OCCUPATIONAL THERAPIST	ACCREDITATION STANDARDS FOR A MASTER'S-DEGREE-LEVEL EDUCATIONAL PROGRAM FOR THE OCCUPATIONAL THERAPIST	ACCREDITATION STANDARDS FOR AN ASSOCIATE-DEGREE-LEVEL EDUCATIONAL PROGRAM FOR THE OCCUPATIONAL THERAPY ASSISTANT
	developmental psychology.	developmental psychology.	developmental psychology.
B.1.3.	Demonstrate knowledge and understanding of the concepts of human behavior to include the behavioral sciences, social sciences, and occupational science. Course content must include, but is not limited to, introductory psychology, abnormal psychology, and introductory sociology or introductory anthropology.	Demonstrate knowledge and understanding of the concepts of human behavior to include the behavioral sciences, social sciences, and occupational science. Course content must include, but is not limited to, introductory psychology, abnormal psychology, and introductory sociology or introductory anthropology.	Demonstrate knowledge and understanding of the concepts of human behavior to include the behavioral and social sciences (e.g., principles of psychology, sociology, abnormal psychology) and occupational science.
B.1.4.	Apply knowledge of the role of sociocultural, socioeconomic, and diversity factors and lifestyle choices in contemporary society to meet the needs of individuals and communities. Course content must include, but is not limited to, introductory psychology, abnormal psychology, and introductory sociology or introductory anthropology.	Demonstrate knowledge and appreciation of the role of sociocultural, socioeconomic, and diversity factors and lifestyle choices in contemporary society. Course content must include, but is not limited to, introductory psychology, abnormal psychology, and introductory sociology or introductory anthropology.	Demonstrate knowledge and appreciation of the role of sociocultural, socioeconomic, and diversity factors and lifestyle choices in contemporary society (e.g., principles of psychology, sociology, and abnormal psychology).
B.1.5.	Demonstrate an understanding of the ethical and practical considerations that affect the health and wellness needs of those who are experiencing or are at risk for social injustice, occupational deprivation, and disparity in the receipt of services.	Demonstrate an understanding of the ethical and practical considerations that affect the health and wellness needs of those who are experiencing or are at risk for social injustice, occupational deprivation, and disparity in the receipt of services.	Articulate the ethical and practical considerations that affect the health and wellness needs of those who are experiencing or are at risk for social injustice, occupational deprivation, and disparity in the receipt of services.
B.1.6.	Demonstrate knowledge of global social issues and prevailing health and welfare needs of populations with or at risk for disabilities and chronic health conditions.	Demonstrate knowledge of global social issues and prevailing health and welfare needs of populations with or at risk for disabilities and chronic health conditions.	Demonstrate knowledge of global social issues and prevailing health and welfare needs of populations with or at risk for disabilities and chronic health conditions.
B.1.7.	Apply quantitative statistics and qualitative analysis to interpret tests, measurements, and other data for the purpose of establishing and/or delivering evidence-based practice.	Demonstrate the ability to use statistics to interpret tests and measurements for the purpose of delivering evidence-based practice.	Articulate the importance of using statistics, tests, and measurements for the purpose of delivering evidence-based practice.
B.1.8.	Demonstrate an understanding of the use of technology to support performance, participation, health and well-being. This technology may include, but is not limited to, electronic documentation systems, distance communication, virtual environments, and telehealth technology.	Demonstrate an understanding of the use of technology to support performance, participation, health and well-being. This technology may include, but is not limited to, electronic documentation systems, distance communication, virtual environments, and telehealth technology.,	Demonstrate an understanding of the use of technology to support performance, participation, health and well-being. This technology may include, but is not limited to, electronic documentation systems, distance communication, virtual environments, and telehealth technology.
B.2.0. BASIC TENETS OF OCCUPATIONAL THERAPY Coursework must facilitate development of the performance criteria listed below. **The student will be able to**			
B.2.1.	Explain the history and philosophical base of the profession of occupational therapy and its importance in meeting society's current and future occupational needs.	Articulate an understanding of the importance of the history and philosophical base of the profession of occupational therapy.	Articulate an understanding of the importance of the history and philosophical base of the profession of occupational therapy.
B.2.2.	Explain the meaning and dynamics of occupation and activity, including the interaction of areas of	Explain the meaning and dynamics of occupation and activity, including the interaction of areas of	Describe the meaning and dynamics of occupation and activity, including the interaction of areas of

STANDARD NUMBER	ACCREDITATION STANDARDS FOR A DOCTORAL-DEGREE-LEVEL EDUCATIONAL PROGRAM FOR THE OCCUPATIONAL THERAPIST	ACCREDITATION STANDARDS FOR A MASTER'S-DEGREE-LEVEL EDUCATIONAL PROGRAM FOR THE OCCUPATIONAL THERAPIST	ACCREDITATION STANDARDS FOR AN ASSOCIATE-DEGREE-LEVEL EDUCATIONAL PROGRAM FOR THE OCCUPATIONAL THERAPY ASSISTANT
	occupation, performance skills, performance patterns, activity demands, context(s) and environments, and client factors.	occupation, performance skills, performance patterns, activity demands, context(s) and environments, and client factors.	occupation, performance skills, performance patterns, activity demands, context(s) and environments, and client factors.
B.2.3.	Articulate to consumers, potential employers, colleagues, third-party payers, regulatory boards, policymakers, other audiences, and the general public both the unique nature of occupation as viewed by the profession of occupational therapy and the value of occupation to support performance, participation, health, and well-being.	Articulate to consumers, potential employers, colleagues, third-party payers, regulatory boards, policymakers, other audiences, and the general public both the unique nature of occupation as viewed by the profession of occupational therapy and the value of occupation to support performance, participation, health, and well-being.	Articulate to consumers, potential employers, colleagues, third-party payers, regulatory boards, policymakers, other audiences, and the general public both the unique nature of occupation as viewed by the profession of occupational therapy and the value of occupation support performance, participation, health, and well-being.
B.2.4.	Articulate the importance of balancing areas of occupation with the achievement of health and wellness for the clients.	Articulate the importance of balancing areas of occupation with the achievement of health and wellness for the clients.	Articulate the importance of balancing areas of occupation with the achievement of health and wellness for the clients.
B.2.5.	Explain the role of occupation in the promotion of health and the prevention of disease and disability for the individual, family, and society.	Explain the role of occupation in the promotion of health and the prevention of disease and disability for the individual, family, and society.	Explain the role of occupation in the promotion of health and the prevention of disease and disability for the individual, family, and society.
B.2.6.	Analyze the effects of heritable diseases, genetic conditions, disability, trauma, and injury to the physical and mental health and occupational performance of the individual.	Analyze the effects of heritable diseases, genetic conditions, disability, trauma, and injury to the physical and mental health and occupational performance of the individual.	Understand the effects of heritable diseases, genetic conditions, disability, trauma, and injury to the physical and mental health and occupational performance of the individual.
B.2.7.	Demonstrate task analysis in areas of occupation, performance skills, performance patterns, activity demands, context(s) and environments, and client factors to formulate an intervention plan.	Demonstrate task analysis in areas of occupation, performance skills, performance patterns, activity demands, context(s) and environments, and client factors to formulate an intervention plan.	Demonstrate task analysis in areas of occupation, performance skills, performance patterns, activity demands, context(s) and environments, and client factors to implement the intervention plan.
B.2.8.	Use sound judgment in regard to safety of self and others and adhere to safety regulations throughout the occupational therapy process as appropriate to the setting and scope of practice.	Use sound judgment in regard to safety of self and others and adhere to safety regulations throughout the occupational therapy process as appropriate to the setting and scope of practice.	Use sound judgment in regard to safety of self and others and adhere to safety regulations throughout the occupational therapy process as appropriate to the setting and scope of practice.
B.2.9.	Express support for the quality of life, well-being, and occupation of the individual, group, or population to promote physical and mental health and prevention of injury and disease considering the context (e.g., cultural, personal, temporal, virtual) and environment.	Express support for the quality of life, well-being, and occupation of the individual, group, or population to promote physical and mental health and prevention of injury and disease considering the context (e.g., cultural, personal, temporal, virtual) and environment.	Express support for the quality of life, well-being, and occupation of the individual, group, or population to promote physical and mental health and prevention of injury and disease considering the context (e.g., cultural, personal, temporal, virtual) and environment.
B.2.10.	Use clinical reasoning to explain the rationale for and use of compensatory strategies when desired life tasks cannot be performed.	Use clinical reasoning to explain the rationale for and use of compensatory strategies when desired life tasks cannot be performed.	Explain the need for and use of compensatory strategies when desired life tasks cannot be performed.
B.2.11.	Analyze, synthesize, evaluate, and apply models of occupational performance.	Analyze, synthesize, and apply models of occupational performance.	Identify interventions consistent with models of occupational performance.

STANDARD NUMBER	ACCREDITATION STANDARDS FOR A DOCTORAL-DEGREE-LEVEL EDUCATIONAL PROGRAM FOR THE OCCUPATIONAL THERAPIST	ACCREDITATION STANDARDS FOR A MASTER'S-DEGREE-LEVEL EDUCATIONAL PROGRAM FOR THE OCCUPATIONAL THERAPIST	ACCREDITATION STANDARDS FOR AN ASSOCIATE-DEGREE-LEVEL EDUCATIONAL PROGRAM FOR THE OCCUPATIONAL THERAPY ASSISTANT
B.3.0.	**OCCUPATIONAL THERAPY THEORETICAL PERSPECTIVES** The program must facilitate the development of the performance criteria listed below. The student will be able to		
B.3.1.	Evaluate and apply theories that underlie the practice of occupational therapy.	Apply theories that underlie the practice of occupational therapy.	Describe basic features of the theories that underlie the practice of occupational therapy.
B.3.2.	Compare, contrast, and integrate a variety of models of practice and frames of reference that are used in occupational therapy.	Compare and contrast models of practice and frames of reference that are used in occupational therapy.	Describe basic features of models of practice and frames of reference that are used in occupational therapy.
B.3.3.	Use theories, models of practice, and frames of reference to guide and inform evaluation and intervention.	Use theories, models of practice, and frames of reference to guide and inform evaluation and intervention.	Discuss how occupational therapy history and occupational therapy theory, and the sociopolitical climate influence practice.
B.3.4.	Analyze and discuss how occupational therapy history, occupational therapy theory, and the sociopolitical climate influence and are influenced by practice.	Analyze and discuss how occupational therapy history, occupational therapy theory, and the sociopolitical climate influence practice.	*(No related Standard)*
B.3.5.	Apply theoretical constructs to evaluation and intervention with various types of clients in a variety of practice contexts and environments, including population-based approaches, to analyze and effect meaningful occupation outcomes.	Apply theoretical constructs to evaluation and intervention with various types of clients l a variety of practice contexts and environments to analyze and effect meaningful occupation outcomes.	*(No related Standard)*
B.3.6.	Articulate the process of theory development in occupational therapy and its desired impact and influence on society.	Discuss the process of theory development and its importance to occupational therapy.	*(No related Standard)*
B.4.0.	**SCREENING, EVALUATION, AND REFERRAL** The process of screening, evaluation, referral, and diagnosis as related to occupational performance and participation must be culturally relevant and based on theoretical perspectives, models of practice, frames of reference, and available evidence. In addition, this process must consider the continuum of need from individuals to populations The program must facilitate development of the performance criteria listed below. The student will be able to	**SCREENING, EVALUATION, AND REFERRAL** The process of screening, evaluation, and referral as related to occupational performance and participation must be culturally relevant and based on theoretical perspectives, models of practice, frames of reference, and available evidence. In addition, this process must consider the continuum of need from individuals to populations The program must facilitate development of the performance criteria listed below. The student will be able to	**SCREENING AND EVALUATION** The process of screening and evaluation and participation must be conducted under the supervision of and in cooperation with the occupational therapist and must be culturally relevant and based on theoretical perspectives, models of practice, frames of reference, and available evidence. The program must facilitate development of the performance criteria listed below. The student will be able to
B.4.1.	Use standardized and nonstandardized screening and assessment tools to determine the need for occupational therapy intervention. These tools include, but are not limited to, specified screening tools; assessments; skilled observations; occupational histories; consultations with other professionals; and interviews with the client, family, significant others, and community.	Use standardized and nonstandardized screening and assessment tools to determine the need for occupational therapy intervention. These tools include, but are not limited to, specified screening tools; assessments; skilled observations; occupational histories; consultations with other professionals; and interviews with the client, family, significant others, and community.	Gather and share data for the purpose of screening and evaluation using methods including, but not limited to, specified screening tools; assessments; skilled observations; occupational histories; consultations with other professionals; and interviews with the client, family, and significant others.

STANDARD NUMBER	ACCREDITATION STANDARDS FOR A DOCTORAL-DEGREE-LEVEL EDUCATIONAL PROGRAM FOR THE OCCUPATIONAL THERAPIST	ACCREDITATION STANDARDS FOR A MASTER'S-DEGREE-LEVEL EDUCATIONAL PROGRAM FOR THE OCCUPATIONAL THERAPIST	ACCREDITATION STANDARDS FOR AN ASSOCIATE-DEGREE-LEVEL EDUCATIONAL PROGRAM FOR THE OCCUPATIONAL THERAPY ASSISTANT
B.4.2.	Select appropriate assessment tools on the basis of client needs, contextual factors, and psychometric properties of tests. These must be culturally relevant, based on available evidence, and incorporate use of occupation in the assessment process.	Select appropriate assessment tools on the basis of client needs, contextual factors, and psychometric properties of tests. These must be culturally relevant, based on available evidence, and incorporate use of occupation in the assessment process.	Administer selected assessments using appropriate procedures and protocols (including standardized formats) and use occupation for the purpose of assessment.
B.4.3.	Use appropriate procedures and protocols (including standardized formats) when administering assessments.	Use appropriate procedures and protocols (including standardized formats) when administering assessments.	*(No related Standard)*
B.4.4.	Evaluate client(s)' occupational performance in activities of daily living (ADLs), instrumental activities of daily living (IADLs), education, work, play, rest, sleep, leisure, and social participation. Evaluation of occupational performance using standardized and nonstandardized assessment tools includes • The occupational profile, including participation in activities that are meaningful and necessary for the client to carry out roles in home, work, and community environments. • Client factors, including values, beliefs, spirituality, body functions (e.g., neuromuscular, sensory and pain, visual, perceptual, cognitive, mental) and body structures (e.g., cardiovascular, digestive, nervous, genitourinary, integumentary systems). • Performance patterns (e.g., habits, routines, rituals, roles). • Context (e.g., cultural, personal, temporal, virtual) and environment (e.g., physical, social). • Performance skills, including motor and praxis skills, sensory–perceptual skills, emotional regulation skills, cognitive skills, and communication and social skills.	Evaluate client(s)' occupational performance in activities of daily living (ADLs), instrumental activities of daily living (IADLs), education, work, play, rest, sleep, leisure, and social participation. Evaluation of occupational performance using standardized and nonstandardized assessment tools includes • The occupational profile, including participation in activities that are meaningful and necessary for the client to carry out roles in home, work, and community environments. • Client factors, including values, beliefs, spirituality, body functions (e.g., neuromuscular, sensory and pain, visual, perceptual, cognitive, mental) and body structures (e.g., cardiovascular, digestive, nervous, genitourinary, integumentary systems). • Performance patterns (e.g., habits, routines, rituals, roles). • Context (e.g., cultural, personal, temporal, virtual) and environment (e.g., physical, social). • Performance skills, including motor and praxis skills, sensory–perceptual skills, emotional regulation skills, cognitive skills, and communication and social skills.	Gather and share data for the purpose of evaluating client(s)' occupational performance in activities of daily living (ADLs), instrumental activities of daily living (IADLs), education, work, play, rest, sleep, leisure, and social participation. Evaluation of occupational performance includes • The occupational profile, including participation in activities that are meaningful and necessary for the client to carry out roles in home, work, and community environments. • Client factors, including values, beliefs, spirituality, body functions (e.g., neuromuscular, sensory and pain, visual, perceptual, cognitive, mental) and body structures (e.g., cardiovascular, digestive, nervous, genitourinary, integumentary systems). • Performance patterns (e.g., habits, routines, rituals, roles). • Context (e.g., cultural, personal, temporal, virtual) and environment (e.g., physical, social). • Performance skills, including motor and praxis skills, sensory–perceptual skills, emotional regulation skills, cognitive skills, and communication and social skills.
B.4.5.	Compare and contrast the role of the occupational therapist and occupational therapy assistant in the screening and evaluation process along with the importance of and rationale for supervision and collaborative work between the occupational therapist and occupational therapy assistant in that process.	Compare and contrast the role of the occupational therapist and occupational therapy assistant in the screening and evaluation process along with the importance of and rationale for supervision and collaborative work between the occupational therapist and occupational therapy assistant in that process.	Articulate the role of the occupational therapy assistant and occupational therapist in the screening and evaluation process along with the importance of and rationale for supervision and collaborative work between the occupational therapy assistant and occupational therapist in that process.
B.4.6.	Interpret criterion-referenced and norm-referenced standardized test scores on the basis of an understanding of sampling, normative data, standard and criterion scores, reliability, and validity.	Interpret criterion-referenced and norm-referenced standardized test scores on the basis of an understanding of sampling, normative data, standard and criterion scores, reliability, and validity.	*(No related Standard)*

STANDARD NUMBER	ACCREDITATION STANDARDS FOR A DOCTORAL-DEGREE-LEVEL EDUCATIONAL PROGRAM FOR THE OCCUPATIONAL THERAPIST	ACCREDITATION STANDARDS FOR A MASTER'S-DEGREE-LEVEL EDUCATIONAL PROGRAM FOR THE OCCUPATIONAL THERAPIST	ACCREDITATION STANDARDS FOR AN ASSOCIATE-DEGREE-LEVEL EDUCATIONAL PROGRAM FOR THE OCCUPATIONAL THERAPY ASSISTANT
B.4.7.	Consider factors that might bias assessment results, such as culture, disability status, and situational variables related to the individual and context.	Consider factors that might bias assessment results, such as culture, disability status, and situational variables related to the individual and context.	(No related Standard)
B.4.8.	Interpret the evaluation data in relation to accepted terminology of the profession, relevant theoretical frameworks, and interdisciplinary knowledge.	Interpret the evaluation data in relation to accepted terminology of the profession and relevant theoretical frameworks.	(No related Standard)
B.4.9.	Evaluate appropriateness and discuss mechanisms for referring clients for additional evaluation to specialists who are internal and external to the profession.	Evaluate appropriateness and discuss mechanisms for referring clients for additional evaluation to specialists who are internal and external to the profession.	Identify when to recommend to the occupational therapist the need for referring clients for additional evaluation.
B.4.10.	Document occupational therapy services to ensure accountability of service provision and to meet standards for reimbursement of services, adhering to the requirements of applicable facility, local, state, federal, and reimbursement agencies. Documentation must effectively communicate the need and rationale for occupational therapy services.	Document occupational therapy services to ensure accountability of service provision and to meet standards for reimbursement of services, adhering to the requirements of applicable facility, local, state, federal, and reimbursement agencies. Documentation must effectively communicate the need and rationale for occupational therapy services.	Document occupational therapy services to ensure accountability of service provision and to meet standards for reimbursement of services, adhering to the requirements of applicable facility, local, state, federal, and reimbursement agencies. Documentation must effectively communicate the need and rationale for occupational therapy services.
B.4.11.	Articulate screening and evaluation processes for all practice areas. Use evidence-based reasoning to analyze, synthesize, evaluate, and diagnose problems related to occupational performance and participation.	(No related Standard)	(No related Standard)
B.5.0.	INTERVENTION PLAN: FORMULATION AND IMPLEMENTATION The process of formulation and implementation of the therapeutic intervention plan to facilitate occupational performance and participation must be culturally relevant; reflective of current and emerging occupational therapy practice; based on available evidence; and based on theoretical perspectives, models of practice, and frames of reference. In addition, this process must consider the continuum of need from individual- to population-based interventions. The program must facilitate development of the performance criteria listed below. The student will be able to	INTERVENTION PLAN: FORMULATION AND IMPLEMENTATION The process of formulation and implementation of the therapeutic intervention plan to facilitate occupational performance and participation must be culturally relevant; reflective of current occupational therapy practice; based on available evidence; and based on theoretical perspectives, models of practice, and frames of reference. The program must facilitate development of the performance criteria listed below. The student will be able to	INTERVENTION AND IMPLEMENTATION The process of intervention to facilitate occupational performance and participation must be done under the supervision of and in cooperation with the occupational therapist and must be culturally relevant, reflective of current occupational therapy practice, and based on available evidence. The program must facilitate development of the performance criteria listed below. The student will be able to
B.5.1.	Use evaluation findings based on appropriate theoretical approaches, models of practice, frames of reference, and interdisciplinary knowledge. Develop occupation-based intervention plans and strategies (including goals and methods to achieve them) on the basis of the stated needs of the client as well as data	Use evaluation findings based on appropriate theoretical approaches, models of practice, and frames of reference to develop occupation-based intervention plans and strategies (including goals and methods to achieve them) on the basis of the stated needs of the client as well as data gathered during the evaluation process in collaboration with the client	Assist with the development of occupation-based intervention plans and strategies (including goals and methods to achieve them) on the basis of the stated needs of the client as well as data gathered during the evaluation process in collaboration with the client and others. Intervention plans and strategies must be culturally relevant, reflective of current occupational

STANDARD NUMBER	ACCREDITATION STANDARDS FOR A DOCTORAL-DEGREE-LEVEL EDUCATIONAL PROGRAM FOR THE OCCUPATIONAL THERAPIST	ACCREDITATION STANDARDS FOR A MASTER'S-DEGREE-LEVEL EDUCATIONAL PROGRAM FOR THE OCCUPATIONAL THERAPIST	ACCREDITATION STANDARDS FOR AN ASSOCIATE-DEGREE-LEVEL EDUCATIONAL PROGRAM FOR THE OCCUPATIONAL THERAPY ASSISTANT
	gathered during the evaluation process in collaboration with the client and others. Intervention plans and strategies must be culturally relevant, reflective of current occupational therapy practice, and based on available evidence. Interventions address the following components: • The occupational profile, including participation in activities that are meaningful and necessary for the client to carry out roles in home, work, and community environments. • Client factors, including values, beliefs, spirituality, body functions (e.g., neuromuscular, sensory and pain, visual, perceptual, cognitive, mental) and body structures (e.g., cardiovascular, digestive, nervous, genitourinary, integumentary systems). • Performance patterns (e.g., habits, routines, rituals, roles). • Context (e.g., cultural, personal, temporal, virtual) and environment (e.g., physical, social). • Performance skills, including motor and praxis skills, sensory–perceptual skills, emotional regulation skills, cognitive skills, and communication and social skills.	and others. Intervention plans and strategies must be culturally relevant, reflective of current occupational therapy practice, and based on available evidence. Interventions address the following components: • The occupational profile, including participation in activities that are meaningful and necessary for the client to carry out roles in home, work, and community environments. • Client factors, including values, beliefs, spirituality, body functions (e.g., neuromuscular, sensory and pain, visual, perceptual, cognitive, mental) and body structures (e.g., cardiovascular, digestive, nervous, genitourinary, integumentary systems). • Performance patterns (e.g., habits, routines, rituals, roles). • Context (e.g., cultural, personal, temporal, virtual) and environment (e.g., physical, social). • Performance skills, including motor and praxis skills, sensory–perceptual skills, emotional regulation skills, cognitive skills, and communication and social skills.	therapy practice, and based on available evidence. Interventions address the following components: • The occupational profile, including participation in activities that are meaningful and necessary for the client to carry out roles in home, work, and community environments. • Client factors, including values, beliefs, spirituality, body functions (e.g., neuromuscular, sensory and pain, visual, perceptual, cognitive, mental) and body structures (e.g., cardiovascular, digestive, nervous, genitourinary, integumentary systems). • Performance patterns (e.g., habits, routines, rituals, roles). • Context (e.g., cultural, personal, temporal, virtual) and environment (e.g., physical, social). • Performance skills, including motor and praxis skills, sensory–perceptual skills, emotional regulation skills, cognitive skills, and communication and social skills.
B.5.2.	Select and provide direct occupational therapy interventions and procedures to enhance safety, health and wellness, and performance in ADLs, IADLs, education, work, play, rest, sleep, leisure, and social participation.	Select and provide direct occupational therapy interventions and procedures to enhance safety, health and wellness, and performance in ADLs, IADLs, education, work, play, rest, sleep, leisure, and social participation.	Select and provide direct occupational therapy interventions and procedures to enhance safety, health and wellness, and performance in ADLs, IADLs, education, work, play, rest, sleep, leisure, and social participation.
B.5.3.	Provide therapeutic use of occupation, exercises, and activities (e.g., occupation-based intervention, purposeful activity, preparatory methods).	Provide therapeutic use of occupation, exercises, and activities (e.g., occupation-based intervention, purposeful activity, preparatory methods).	Provide therapeutic use of occupation, exercises, and activities (e.g., occupation-based intervention, purposeful activity, preparatory methods).
B.5.4.	Design and implement group interventions based on principles of group development and group dynamics across the lifespan.	Design and implement group interventions based on principles of group development and group dynamics across the lifespan.	Implement group interventions based on principles of group development and group dynamics across the lifespan.
B.5.5.	Provide training in self-care, self-management, health management and maintenance, home management, and community and work integration.	Provide training in self-care, self-management, health management and maintenance, home management, and community and work integration.	Provide training in self-care, self-management, health management and maintenance, home management, and community and work integration.
B.5.6.	Provide development, remediation, and compensation for physical, mental, cognitive, perceptual, neuromuscular, behavioral skills, and sensory functions (e.g., vision, tactile, auditory, gustatory, olfactory, pain, temperature, pressure,	Provide development, remediation, and compensation for physical, mental, cognitive, perceptual, neuromuscular, behavioral skills, and sensory functions (e.g., vision, tactile, auditory, gustatory, olfactory, pain, temperature, pressure,	Provide development, remediation, and compensation for physical, mental, cognitive, perceptual, neuromuscular, behavioral skills, and sensory functions (e.g., vision, tactile, auditory, gustatory, olfactory, pain, temperature, pressure,

STANDARD NUMBER	ACCREDITATION STANDARDS FOR A DOCTORAL-DEGREE-LEVEL EDUCATIONAL PROGRAM FOR THE OCCUPATIONAL THERAPIST	ACCREDITATION STANDARDS FOR A MASTER'S-DEGREE-LEVEL EDUCATIONAL PROGRAM FOR THE OCCUPATIONAL THERAPIST	ACCREDITATION STANDARDS FOR AN ASSOCIATE-DEGREE-LEVEL EDUCATIONAL PROGRAM FOR THE OCCUPATIONAL THERAPY ASSISTANT
	vestibular, proprioception).	vestibular, proprioception).	vestibular, proprioception).
B.5.7.	Demonstrate therapeutic use of self, including one's personality, insights, perceptions, and judgments, as part of the therapeutic process in both individual and group interaction.	Demonstrate therapeutic use of self, including one's personality, insights, perceptions, and judgments, as part of the therapeutic process in both individual and group interaction.	Demonstrate therapeutic use of self, including one's personality, insights, perceptions, and judgments, as part of the therapeutic process in both individual and group interaction.
B.5.8.	Develop and implement intervention strategies to remediate and/or compensate for cognitive deficits that affect occupational performance.	Develop and implement intervention strategies to remediate and/or compensate for cognitive deficits that affect occupational performance.	Implement intervention strategies to remediate and/or compensate for cognitive deficits that affect occupational performance.
B.5.9.	Evaluate and adapt processes or environments (e.g., home, work, school, community) applying ergonomic principles and principles of environmental modification.	Evaluate and adapt processes or environments (e.g., home, work, school, community) applying ergonomic principles and principles of environmental modification.	Adapt environments (e.g., home, work, school, community) and processes, including the application of ergonomic principles.
B.5.10.	Articulate principles and be able to design, fabricate, apply, fit, and train in assistive technologies and devices (e.g., electronic aids to daily living, seating and positioning systems) used to enhance occupational performance and foster participation and well-being.	Articulate principles of and be able to design, fabricate, apply, fit, and train in assistive technologies and devices (e.g., electronic aids to daily living, seating and positioning systems) used to enhance occupational performance and foster participation and well-being.	Articulate principles of and demonstrate strategies with assistive technologies and devices (e.g., electronic aids to daily living, seating and positioning systems) used to enhance occupational performance and foster participation and well-being.
B.5.11.	Provide design, fabrication, application, fitting, and training in orthotic devices used to enhance occupational performance and participation. Train in the use of prosthetic devices, based on scientific principles of kinesiology, biomechanics, and physics.	Provide design, fabrication, application, fitting, and training in orthotic devices used to enhance occupational performance and participation. Train in the use of prosthetic devices, based on scientific principles of kinesiology, biomechanics, and physics.	Provide fabrication, application, fitting, and training in orthotic devices used to enhance occupational performance and participation, and training in the use of prosthetic devices.
B.5.12.	Provide recommendations and training in techniques to enhance functional mobility, including physical transfers, wheelchair management, and mobility devices.	Provide recommendations and training in techniques to enhance functional mobility, including physical transfers, wheelchair management, and mobility devices.	Provide training in techniques to enhance functional mobility, including physical transfers, wheelchair management, and mobility devices.
B.5.13.	Provide recommendations and training in techniques to enhance community mobility, including public transportation, community access, and issues related to driver rehabilitation.	Provide recommendations and training in techniques to enhance community mobility, including public transportation, community access, and issues related to driver rehabilitation.	Provide training in techniques to enhance community mobility, including public transportation, community access, and issues related to driver rehabilitation.
B.5.14.	Provide management of feeding, eating, and swallowing to enable performance (including the process of bringing food or fluids from the plate or cup to the mouth, the ability to keep and manipulate food or fluid in the mouth, and swallowing assessment and management) and train others in precautions and techniques while considering client and contextual factors.	Provide management of feeding, eating, and swallowing to enable performance (including the process of bringing food or fluids from the plate or cup to the mouth, the ability to keep and manipulate food or fluid in the mouth, and swallowing assessment and management) and train others in precautions and techniques while considering client and contextual factors.	Enable feeding and eating performance (including the process of bringing food or fluids from the plate or cup to the mouth, the ability to keep and manipulate food or fluid in the mouth, and the initiation of swallowing) and train others in precautions and techniques while considering client and contextual factors.

STANDARD NUMBER	ACCREDITATION STANDARDS FOR A DOCTORAL-DEGREE-LEVEL EDUCATIONAL PROGRAM FOR THE OCCUPATIONAL THERAPIST	ACCREDITATION STANDARDS FOR A MASTER'S-DEGREE-LEVEL EDUCATIONAL PROGRAM FOR THE OCCUPATIONAL THERAPIST	ACCREDITATION STANDARDS FOR AN ASSOCIATE-DEGREE-LEVEL EDUCATIONAL PROGRAM FOR THE OCCUPATIONAL THERAPY ASSISTANT
B.5.15.	Demonstrate safe and effective application of superficial thermal and mechanical modalities as a preparatory measure to manage pain and improve occupational performance, including foundational knowledge, underlying principles, indications, contraindications, and precautions.	Demonstrate safe and effective application of superficial thermal and mechanical modalities as a preparatory measure to manage pain and improve occupational performance, including foundational knowledge, underlying principles, indications, contraindications, and precautions.	Recognize the use of superficial thermal and mechanical modalities as a preparatory measure to improve occupational performance. On the basis of the intervention plan, demonstrate safe and effective administration of superficial thermal and mechanical modalities to achieve established goals while adhering to contraindications and precautions.
	SKILLS, KNOWLEDGE, AND COMPETENCIES FOR ENTRY-LEVEL PRACTICE ARE DERIVED FROM AOTA PRACTICE DOCUMENTS AND NBCOT PRACTICE ANALYSIS STUDIES. SUPERFICIAL THERMAL MODALITIES INCLUDE, BUT ARE NOT LIMITED TO, HYDROTHERAPY/WHIRLPOOL, CRYOTHERAPY (COLD PACKS, ICE), FLUIDOTHERAPY™, HOT PACKS, PARAFFIN, WATER, AND INFRARED. MECHANICAL MODALITIES INCLUDE, BUT ARE NOT LIMITED TO, VASOPNEUMATIC DEVICES AND CONTINUOUS PASSIVE MOTION *THE WORD "DEMONSTRATE" DOES NOT REQUIRE THAT A STUDENT ACTUALLY PERFORM THE TASK TO VERIFY KNOWLEDGE AND UNDERSTANDING. THE PROGRAM MAY SELECT THE TYPES OF LEARNING ACTIVITIES AND ASSESSMENTS THAT WILL INDICATE COMPLIANCE WITH THE STANDARD.* *FOR INSTITUTIONS IN STATES WHERE REGULATIONS RESTRICT THE USE OF PHYSICAL AGENT MODALITIES, IT IS RECOMMENDED THAT STUDENTS BE EXPOSED TO THE MODALITIES OFFERED IN PRACTICE TO ALLOW STUDENTS KNOWLEDGE AND EXPERIENCE WITH THE MODALITIES IN PREPARATION FOR THE NBCOT EXAMINATION AND FOR PRACTICE OUTSIDE OF THE STATE IN WHICH THE EDUCATIONAL INSTITUTION RESIDES.*		
B.5.16.	Explain the use of deep thermal and electrotherapeutic modalities as a preparatory measure to improve occupational performance, including indications, contraindications, and precautions.	Explain the use of deep thermal and electrotherapeutic modalities as a preparatory measure to improve occupational performance, including indications, contraindications, and precautions.	*(No related Standard)*
	SKILLS, KNOWLEDGE, AND COMPETENCIES FOR ENTRY-LEVEL PRACTICE ARE DERIVED FROM AOTA PRACTICE DOCUMENTS AND NBCOT PRACTICE ANALYSIS STUDIES. DEEP THERMAL MODALITIES INCLUDE, BUT ARE NOT LIMITED TO, THERAPEUTIC ULTRASOUND AND PHONOPHORESIS. ELECTROTHERAPEUTIC MODALITIES INCLUDE, BUT ARE NOT LIMITED TO, BIOFEEDBACK, NEUROMUSCULAR ELECTRICAL STIMULATION, FUNCTIONAL ELECTRICAL STIMULATION, TRANSCUTANEOUS ELECTRICAL NERVE STIMULATION, ELECTRICAL STIMULATION FOR TISSUE REPAIR, HIGH-VOLTAGE GALVANIC STIMULATION, AND IONTOPHORESIS.		
B.5.17.	Develop and promote the use of appropriate home and community programming to support performance in the client's natural environment and participation in all contexts relevant to the client.	Develop and promote the use of appropriate home and community programming to support performance in the client's natural environment and participation in all contexts relevant to the client.	Promote the use of appropriate home and community programming to support performance in the client's natural environment and participation in all contexts relevant to the client.
B.5.18.	Demonstrate an understanding of health literacy and the ability to educate and train the client, caregiver, family and significant others, and communities to facilitate skills in areas of occupation as well as prevention, health maintenance, health promotion, and safety.	Demonstrate an understanding of health literacy and the ability to educate and train the client, caregiver, family and significant others, and communities to facilitate skills in areas of occupation as well as prevention, health maintenance, health promotion, and safety.	Demonstrate an understanding of health literacy and the ability to educate and train the client, caregiver, and family and significant others to facilitate skills in areas of occupation as well as prevention, health maintenance, health promotion, and safety.
B.5.19.	Apply the principles of the teaching–learning process using educational methods to design experiences to address the needs of the client, family, significant others, communities, colleagues, other health providers, and the public.	Apply the principles of the teaching–learning process using educational methods to design experiences to address the needs of the client, family, significant others, colleagues, other health providers, and the public.	Use the teaching–learning process with the client, family, significant others, colleagues, other health providers, and the public. Collaborate with the occupational therapist and learner to identify appropriate educational methods.

STANDARD NUMBER	ACCREDITATION STANDARDS FOR A DOCTORAL-DEGREE-LEVEL EDUCATIONAL PROGRAM FOR THE OCCUPATIONAL THERAPIST	ACCREDITATION STANDARDS FOR A MASTER'S-DEGREE-LEVEL EDUCATIONAL PROGRAM FOR THE OCCUPATIONAL THERAPIST	ACCREDITATION STANDARDS FOR AN ASSOCIATE-DEGREE-LEVEL EDUCATIONAL PROGRAM FOR THE OCCUPATIONAL THERAPY ASSISTANT
B.5.20.	Effectively interact through written, oral, and nonverbal communication with the client, family, significant others, communities, colleagues, other health providers, and the public in a professionally acceptable manner.	Effectively interact through written, oral, and nonverbal communication with the client, family, significant others, colleagues, other health providers, and the public in a professionally acceptable manner.	Effectively interact through written, oral, and nonverbal communication with the client, family, significant others, colleagues, other health providers, and the public in a professionally acceptable manner.
B.5.21.	Effectively communicate, coordinate, and work interprofessionally with those who provide services for individuals, organizations, and/or populations in order to clarify each member's responsibility in executing components of an intervention plan.	Effectively communicate and work interprofessionally with those who provide services to individuals, organizations, and/or populations in order to clarify each member's responsibility in executing an intervention plan.	Effectively communicate and work interprofessionally with those who provide services to individuals and groups in order to clarify each member's responsibility in executing an intervention plan.
B.5.22.	Refer to specialists (both internal and external to the profession) for consultation and intervention.	Refer to specialists (both internal and external to the profession) for consultation and intervention.	Recognize and communicate the need to refer to specialists (both internal and external to the profession) for consultation and intervention.
B.5.23.	Grade and adapt the environment, tools, materials, occupations, and interventions to reflect the changing needs of the client, the sociocultural context, and technological advances.	Grade and adapt the environment, tools, materials, occupations, and interventions to reflect the changing needs of the client, the sociocultural context, and technological advances.	Grade and adapt the environment, tools, materials, occupations, and interventions to reflect the changing needs of the client and the sociocultural context.
B.5.24.	Select and teach compensatory strategies, such as use of technology and adaptations to the environment, that support performance, participation, and well-being.	Select and teach compensatory strategies, such as use of technology and adaptations to the environment, that support performance, participation, and well-being.	Teach compensatory strategies, such as use of technology and adaptations to the environment, that support performance, participation, and well-being.
B.5.25.	Identify and demonstrate techniques in skills of supervision and collaboration with occupational therapy assistants and other professionals on therapeutic interventions.	Identify and demonstrate techniques in skills of supervision and collaboration with occupational therapy assistants and other professionals on therapeutic interventions.	Demonstrate skills of collaboration with occupational therapists and other professionals on therapeutic interventions.
B.5.26.	Demonstrate use of the consultative process with groups, programs, organizations, or communities.	Understand when and how to use the consultative process with groups, programs, organizations, or communities.	Understand when and how to use the consultative process with specific consumers or consumer groups as directed by an occupational therapist.
B.5.27.	Demonstrate care coordination, case management, and transition services in traditional and emerging practice environments.	Describe the role of the occupational therapist in care coordination, case management, and transition services in traditional and emerging practice environments.	Describe the role of the occupational therapy assistant in care coordination, case management, and transition services in traditional and emerging practice environments.
B.5.28.	Monitor and reassess, in collaboration with the client, caregiver, family, and significant others, the effect of occupational therapy intervention and the need for continued or modified intervention.	Monitor and reassess, in collaboration with the client, caregiver, family, and significant others, the effect of occupational therapy intervention and the need for continued or modified intervention.	Monitor and reassess, in collaboration with the client, caregiver, family, and significant others, the effect of occupational therapy intervention and the need for continued or modified intervention, and communicate the identified needs to the occupational therapist.

STANDARD NUMBER	ACCREDITATION STANDARDS FOR A DOCTORAL-DEGREE-LEVEL EDUCATIONAL PROGRAM FOR THE OCCUPATIONAL THERAPIST	ACCREDITATION STANDARDS FOR A MASTER'S-DEGREE-LEVEL EDUCATIONAL PROGRAM FOR THE OCCUPATIONAL THERAPIST	ACCREDITATION STANDARDS FOR AN ASSOCIATE-DEGREE-LEVEL EDUCATIONAL PROGRAM FOR THE OCCUPATIONAL THERAPY ASSISTANT
B.5.29.	Plan for discharge, in collaboration with the client, by reviewing the needs of the client, caregiver, family, and significant others; available resources; and discharge environment. This process includes, but is not limited to, identification of client's current status within the continuum of care; identification of community, human, and fiscal resources; recommendations for environmental adaptations; and home programming to facilitate the client's progression along the continuum toward outcome goals.	Plan for discharge, in collaboration with the client, by reviewing the needs of the client, caregiver, family, and significant others; available resources; and discharge environment. This process includes, but is not limited to, identification of client's current status within the continuum of care; identification of community, human, and fiscal resources; recommendations for environmental adaptations; and home programming to facilitate the client's progression along the continuum toward outcome goals.	Facilitate discharge planning by reviewing the needs of the client, caregiver, family, and significant others; available resources; and discharge environment, and identify those needs to the occupational therapist, client, and others involved in discharge planning. This process includes, but is not limited to, identification of community, human, and fiscal resources; recommendations for environmental adaptations; and home programming.
B.5.30.	Organize, collect, and analyze data in a systematic manner for evaluation of practice outcomes. Report evaluation results and modify practice as needed to improve client outcomes.	Organize, collect, and analyze data in a systematic manner for evaluation of practice outcomes. Report evaluation results and modify practice as needed to improve client outcomes.	Under the direction of an administrator, manager, or occupational therapist, collect, organize, and report on data for evaluation of client outcomes.
B.5.31.	Terminate occupational therapy services when stated outcomes have been achieved or it has been determined that they cannot be achieved. This process includes developing a summary of occupational therapy outcomes, appropriate recommendations, and referrals and discussion of postdischarge needs with the client and with appropriate others.	Terminate occupational therapy services when stated outcomes have been achieved or it has been determined that they cannot be achieved. This process includes developing a summary of occupational therapy outcomes, appropriate recommendations, and referrals and discussion of post-discharge needs with the client and with appropriate others.	Recommend to the occupational therapist the need for termination of occupational therapy services when stated outcomes have been achieved or it has been determined that they cannot be achieved. Assist with developing a summary of occupational therapy outcomes, recommendations, and referrals.
B.5.32.	Document occupational therapy services to ensure accountability of service provision and to meet standards for reimbursement of services. Documentation must effectively communicate the need and rationale for occupational therapy services and must be appropriate to the context in which the service is delivered.	Document occupational therapy services to ensure accountability of service provision and to meet standards for reimbursement of services. Documentation must effectively communicate the need and rationale for occupational therapy services and must be appropriate to the context in which the service is delivered.	Document occupational therapy services to ensure accountability of service provision and to meet standards for reimbursement of services. Documentation must effectively communicate the need and rationale for occupational therapy services and must be appropriate to the context in which the service is delivered.
B.5.33.	Provide population-based occupational therapy intervention that addresses occupational needs as identified by a community.	*(No related Standard)*	*(No related Standard)*

B.6.0.   CONTEXT OF SERVICE DELIVERY
Context of service delivery includes the knowledge and understanding of the various contexts, such as professional, social, cultural, political, economic, and ecological, in which occupational therapy services are provided. The program must facilitate development of the performance criteria listed below. The student will be able to

STANDARD NUMBER	ACCREDITATION STANDARDS FOR A DOCTORAL-DEGREE-LEVEL EDUCATIONAL PROGRAM FOR THE OCCUPATIONAL THERAPIST	ACCREDITATION STANDARDS FOR A MASTER'S-DEGREE-LEVEL EDUCATIONAL PROGRAM FOR THE OCCUPATIONAL THERAPIST	ACCREDITATION STANDARDS FOR AN ASSOCIATE-DEGREE-LEVEL EDUCATIONAL PROGRAM FOR THE OCCUPATIONAL THERAPY ASSISTANT
B.6.1.	Evaluate and address the various contexts of health care, education, community, political, and social systems as they relate to the practice of occupational therapy.	Evaluate and address the various contexts of health care, education, community, political, and social systems as they relate to the practice of occupational therapy.	Describe the contexts of health care, education, community, and social systems as they relate to the practice of occupational therapy.
B.6.2.	Analyze the current policy issues and the social, economic, political, geographic, and demographic	Analyze the current policy issues and the social, economic, political, geographic, and demographic	Identify the potential impact of current policy issues and the social, economic, political, geographic, or

STANDARD NUMBER	ACCREDITATION STANDARDS FOR A DOCTORAL-DEGREE-LEVEL EDUCATIONAL PROGRAM FOR THE OCCUPATIONAL THERAPIST	ACCREDITATION STANDARDS FOR A MASTER'S-DEGREE-LEVEL EDUCATIONAL PROGRAM FOR THE OCCUPATIONAL THERAPIST	ACCREDITATION STANDARDS FOR AN ASSOCIATE-DEGREE-LEVEL EDUCATIONAL PROGRAM FOR THE OCCUPATIONAL THERAPY ASSISTANT
	factors that influence the various contexts for practice of occupational therapy.	factors that influence the various contexts for practice of occupational therapy.	demographic factors on the practice of occupational therapy.
B.6.3.	Integrate current social, economic, political, geographic, and demographic factors to promote policy development and the provision of occupational therapy services.	Integrate current social, economic, political, geographic, and demographic factors to promote policy development and the provision of occupational therapy services.	(No related Standard)
B.6.4.	Advocate for changes in service delivery policies, effect changes in the system, and identify opportunities to address societal needs.	Articulate the role and responsibility of the practitioner to advocate for changes in service delivery policies, to effect changes in the system, and to identify opportunities in emerging practice areas.	Identify the role and responsibility of the practitioner to advocate for changes in service delivery policies, to effect changes in the system, and to recognize opportunities in emerging practice areas.
B.6.5.	Analyze the trends in models of service delivery, including, but not limited to, medical, educational, community, and social models, and their potential effect on the practice of occupational therapy.	Analyze the trends in models of service delivery, including, but not limited to, medical, educational, community, and social models, and their potential effect on the practice of occupational therapy.	(No related Standard)
B.6.6.	Integrate national and international resources in education, research, practice, and policy development.	Utilize national and international resources in making assessment or intervention choices and appreciate the influence of international occupational therapy contributions to education, research, and practice.	(No related Standard)
B.7.0.	LEADERSHIP AND MANAGEMENT Leadership and management skills include principles and applications of leadership and management theory. The program must facilitate development of the performance criteria listed below. The student will be able to	MANAGEMENT OF OCCUPATIONAL THERAPY SERVICES Management of occupational therapy services includes the application of principles of management and systems in the provision of occupational therapy services to individuals and organizations. The program must facilitate development of the performance criteria listed below. The student will be able to	ASSISTANCE WITH MANAGEMENT OF OCCUPATIONAL THERAPY SERVICES Assistance with management of occupational therapy services includes the application of principles of management and systems in the provision of occupational therapy services to individuals and organizations. The program must facilitate development of the performance criteria listed below. The student will be able to
B.7.1.	Identify and evaluate the impact of contextual factors on the management and delivery of occupational therapy services for individuals and populations.	Describe and discuss the impact of contextual factors on the management and delivery of occupational therapy services.	Identify the impact of contextual factors on the management and delivery of occupational therapy services.
B.7.2.	Identify and evaluate the systems and structures that create federal and state legislation and regulations and their implications and effects on practice and policy.	Describe the systems and structures that create federal and state legislation and regulations and their implications and effects on practice.	Identify the systems and structures that create federal and state legislation and regulations and their implications and effects on practice.
B.7.3.	Demonstrate knowledge of applicable national requirements for credentialing and requirements for licensure, certification, or registration under state laws.	Demonstrate knowledge of applicable national requirements for credentialing and requirements for licensure, certification, or registration under state laws.	Demonstrate knowledge of applicable national requirements for credentialing and requirements for licensure, certification, or registration under state laws.
B.7.4.	Demonstrate knowledge of various reimbursement systems (e.g., federal, state, third party, private payer), appeals mechanisms, and documentation requirements that affect society and the practice of	Demonstrate knowledge of various reimbursement systems (e.g., federal, state, third party, private payer), appeals mechanisms, and documentation requirements that affect the practice of occupational	Demonstrate knowledge of various reimbursement systems (e.g., federal, state, third party, private payer) and documentation requirements that affect

STANDARD NUMBER	ACCREDITATION STANDARDS FOR A DOCTORAL-DEGREE-LEVEL EDUCATIONAL PROGRAM FOR THE OCCUPATIONAL THERAPIST	ACCREDITATION STANDARDS FOR A MASTER'S-DEGREE-LEVEL EDUCATIONAL PROGRAM FOR THE OCCUPATIONAL THERAPIST	ACCREDITATION STANDARDS FOR AN ASSOCIATE-DEGREE-LEVEL EDUCATIONAL PROGRAM FOR THE OCCUPATIONAL THERAPY ASSISTANT
	occupational therapy.	therapy.	the practice of occupational therapy.
B.7.5.	Demonstrate leadership skills in the ability to plan, develop, organize, and market the delivery of services to include the determination of programmatic needs and service delivery options and formulation and management of staffing for effective service provision.	Demonstrate the ability to plan, develop, organize, and market the delivery of services to include the determination of programmatic needs and service delivery options and formulation and management of staffing for effective service provision.	Demonstrate the ability to participate in the development, marketing, and management of service delivery options.
B.7.6.	Demonstrate leadership skills in the ability to design ongoing processes for quality improvement (e.g., outcome studies analysis) and develop program changes as needed to ensure quality of services and to direct administrative changes.	Demonstrate the ability to design ongoing processes for quality improvement (e.g., outcome studies analysis) and develop program changes as needed to ensure quality of services and to direct administrative changes.	Participate in the documentation of ongoing processes for quality improvement and implement program changes as needed to ensure quality of services.
B.7.7.	Develop strategies for effective, competency-based legal and ethical supervision of occupational therapy and non–occupational therapy personnel.	Develop strategies for effective, competency-based legal and ethical supervision of occupational therapy and non–occupational therapy personnel.	Identify strategies for effective, competency-based legal and ethical supervision of nonprofessional personnel.
B.7.8.	Describe the ongoing professional responsibility for providing fieldwork education and the criteria for becoming a fieldwork educator.	Describe the ongoing professional responsibility for providing fieldwork education and the criteria for becoming a fieldwork educator.	Describe the ongoing professional responsibility for providing fieldwork education and the criteria for becoming a fieldwork educator.
B.7.9.	Demonstrate knowledge of and the ability to write program development plans for provision of occupational therapy services to individuals and populations.	(No related Standard)	(No related Standard)
B.7.10.	Identify and adapt existing models or develop new service provision models to respond to policy, regulatory agencies, and reimbursement and compliance standards.	(No related Standard)	(No related Standard)
B.7.11.	Identify and develop strategies to enable occupational therapy to respond to society's changing needs.	(No related Standard)	(No related Standard)
B.7.12.	Identify and implement strategies to promote staff development that are based on evaluation of the personal and professional abilities and competencies of supervised staff as they relate to job responsibilities.	(No related Standard)	(No related Standard)

B.8.0.   SCHOLARSHIP
Promotion of scholarly endeavors will serve to describe and interpret the scope of the profession, establish new knowledge, and interpret and apply this knowledge to practice. The program must facilitate development of the performance criteria listed below. The student will be able to

STANDARD NUMBER	DOCTORAL	MASTER'S	ASSOCIATE
B.8.1.	Articulate the importance of how scholarly activities contribute to the development of a body of knowledge relevant to the profession of occupational therapy.	Articulate the importance of how scholarly activities contribute to the development of a body of knowledge relevant to the profession of occupational therapy.	Articulate the importance of how scholarly activities and literature contribute to the development of the profession.

STANDARD NUMBER	ACCREDITATION STANDARDS FOR A DOCTORAL-DEGREE-LEVEL EDUCATIONAL PROGRAM FOR THE OCCUPATIONAL THERAPIST	ACCREDITATION STANDARDS FOR A MASTER'S-DEGREE-LEVEL EDUCATIONAL PROGRAM FOR THE OCCUPATIONAL THERAPIST	ACCREDITATION STANDARDS FOR AN ASSOCIATE-DEGREE-LEVEL EDUCATIONAL PROGRAM FOR THE OCCUPATIONAL THERAPY ASSISTANT
B.8.2.	Effectively locate, understand, critique, and evaluate information, including the quality of evidence.	Effectively locate, understand, critique, and evaluate information, including the quality of evidence.	Effectively locate and understand information, including the quality of the source of information.
B.8.3.	Use scholarly literature to make evidence-based decisions.	Use scholarly literature to make evidence-based decisions.	Use professional literature to make evidence-based practice decisions in collaboration with the occupational therapist.
B.8.4.	Select, apply, and interpret basic descriptive, correlational, and inferential quantitative statistics and code, analyze, and synthesize qualitative data.	Understand and use basic descriptive, correlational, and inferential quantitative statistics and code, analyze, and synthesize qualitative data.	*(No related Standard)*
B.8.5.	Understand and critique the validity of research studies, including their design (both quantitative and qualitative) and methodology.	Understand and critique the validity of research studies, including their design (both quantitative and qualitative) and methodology.	*(No related Standard)*
B.8.6.	Design a scholarly proposal that includes the research question, relevant literature, sample, design, measurement, and data analysis.	Demonstrate the skills necessary to design a scholarly proposal that includes the research question, relevant literature, sample, design, measurement, and data analysis.	*(No related Standard)*
B.8.7.	Implement a scholarly study that evaluates professional practice, service delivery, and/or professional issues (e.g., Scholarship of Integration, Scholarship of Application, Scholarship of Teaching and Learning).	Participate in scholarly activities that evaluate professional practice, service delivery, and/or professional issues (e.g., Scholarship of Integration, Scholarship of Application, Scholarship of Teaching and Learning). *THE INTENT OF STANDARD B.8.7 IS TO EMPHASIZE THE "DOING" PART OF THE RESEARCH PROCESS THAT CAN SUPPORT BEGINNING RESEARCH SKILLS IN A PRACTICE SETTING. SYSTEMATIC REVIEWS THAT REQUIRE ANALYSIS AND SYNTHESIS OF DATA MEET THE REQUIREMENT FOR THIS STANDARD. NARRATIVE REVIEWS DO NOT MEET THIS STANDARD.* *A CULMINATING PROJECT RELATED TO RESEARCH IS NOT REQUIRED FOR THE MASTER'S LEVEL. IF IT IS CONSISTENT WITH THE PROGRAM'S CURRICULUM DESIGN AND GOALS, THE PROGRAM MAY CHOOSE TO REQUIRE A CULMINATING RESEARCH LEARNING ACTIVITY (E.G., SYSTEMATIC REVIEW OF LITERATURE, FACULTY-LED RESEARCH ACTIVITY, STUDENT RESEARCH PROJECT).*	Identify how scholarly activities can be used to evaluate professional practice, service delivery, and/or professional issues (e.g., Scholarship of Integration, Scholarship of Application, Scholarship of Teaching and Learning).
B.8.8.	Write scholarly reports appropriate for presentation or for publication in a peer-reviewed journal. Examples of scholarly reports would include position papers, white papers, and persuasive discussion papers.	Demonstrate skills necessary to write a scholarly report in a format for presentation or publication.	Demonstrate the skills to read and understand a scholarly report.
B.8.9.	Demonstrate an understanding of the process of locating and securing grants and how grants can serve as a fiscal resource for scholarly activities.	Demonstrate an understanding of the process of locating and securing grants and how grants can serve as a fiscal resource for scholarly activities.	*(No related Standard)*

STANDARD NUMBER	ACCREDITATION STANDARDS FOR A DOCTORAL-DEGREE-LEVEL EDUCATIONAL PROGRAM FOR THE OCCUPATIONAL THERAPIST	ACCREDITATION STANDARDS FOR A MASTER'S-DEGREE-LEVEL EDUCATIONAL PROGRAM FOR THE OCCUPATIONAL THERAPIST	ACCREDITATION STANDARDS FOR AN ASSOCIATE-DEGREE-LEVEL EDUCATIONAL PROGRAM FOR THE OCCUPATIONAL THERAPY ASSISTANT
B.8.10.	Complete a culminating project that relates theory to practice and demonstrates synthesis of advanced knowledge in a practice area.	(No related Standard)	(No related Standard)

B.9.0. PROFESSIONAL ETHICS, VALUES, AND RESPONSIBILITIES

Professional ethics, values, and responsibilities include an understanding and appreciation of ethics and values of the profession of occupational therapy. The program must facilitate development of the performance criteria listed below. The student will be able to

STANDARD NUMBER	ACCREDITATION STANDARDS FOR A DOCTORAL-DEGREE-LEVEL EDUCATIONAL PROGRAM FOR THE OCCUPATIONAL THERAPIST	ACCREDITATION STANDARDS FOR A MASTER'S-DEGREE-LEVEL EDUCATIONAL PROGRAM FOR THE OCCUPATIONAL THERAPIST	ACCREDITATION STANDARDS FOR AN ASSOCIATE-DEGREE-LEVEL EDUCATIONAL PROGRAM FOR THE OCCUPATIONAL THERAPY ASSISTANT
B.9.1.	Demonstrate knowledge and understanding of the American Occupational Therapy Association (AOTA) *Occupational Therapy Code of Ethics and Ethics Standards* and AOTA *Standards of Practice* and use them as a guide for ethical decision making in professional interactions, client interventions, and employment settings.	Demonstrate knowledge and understanding of the American Occupational Therapy Association (AOTA) *Occupational Therapy Code of Ethics and Ethics Standards* and AOTA *Standards of Practice* and use them as a guide for ethical decision making in professional interactions, client interventions, and employment settings.	Demonstrate knowledge and understanding of the American Occupational Therapy Association (AOTA) *Occupational Therapy Code of Ethics and Ethics Standards* and AOTA *Standards of Practice* and use them as a guide for ethical decision making in professional interactions, client interventions, and employment settings.
B.9.2.	Discuss and justify how the role of a professional is enhanced by knowledge of and involvement in international, national, state, and local occupational therapy associations and related professional associations.	Discuss and justify how the role of a professional is enhanced by knowledge of and involvement in international, national, state, and local occupational therapy associations and related professional associations.	Explain and give examples of how the role of a professional is enhanced by knowledge of and involvement in international, national, state, and local occupational therapy associations and related professional associations.
B.9.3.	Promote occupational therapy by educating other professionals, service providers, consumers, third-party payers, regulatory bodies, and the public.	Promote occupational therapy by educating other professionals, service providers, consumers, third-party payers, regulatory bodies, and the public.	Promote occupational therapy by educating other professionals, service providers, consumers, third-party payers, regulatory bodies, and the public.
B.9.4.	Identify and develop strategies for ongoing professional development to ensure that practice is consistent with current and accepted standards.	Discuss strategies for ongoing professional development to ensure that practice is consistent with current and accepted standards.	Discuss strategies for ongoing professional development to ensure that practice is consistent with current and accepted standards.
B.9.5.	Discuss professional responsibilities related to liability issues under current models of service provision.	Discuss professional responsibilities related to liability issues under current models of service provision.	Identify professional responsibilities related to liability issues under current models of service provision.
B.9.6.	Discuss and evaluate personal and professional abilities and competencies as they relate to job responsibilities.	Discuss and evaluate personal and professional abilities and competencies as they relate to job responsibilities.	Identify personal and professional abilities and competencies as they relate to job responsibilities.
B.9.7.	Discuss and justify the varied roles of the occupational therapist as a practitioner, educator, researcher, policy developer, program developer, advocate, administrator, consultant, and entrepreneur.	Discuss and justify the varied roles of the occupational therapist as a practitioner, educator, researcher, consultant, and entrepreneur.	Identify and appreciate the varied roles of the occupational therapy assistant as a practitioner, educator, and research assistant.
B.9.8.	Explain and justify the importance of supervisory roles, responsibilities, and collaborative professional relationships between the occupational therapist and the occupational therapy assistant.	Explain and justify the importance of supervisory roles, responsibilities, and collaborative professional relationships between the occupational therapist and the occupational therapy assistant.	Identify and explain the need for supervisory roles, responsibilities, and collaborative professional relationships between the occupational therapist and the occupational therapy assistant.

STANDARD NUMBER	ACCREDITATION STANDARDS FOR A DOCTORAL-DEGREE-LEVEL EDUCATIONAL PROGRAM FOR THE OCCUPATIONAL THERAPIST	ACCREDITATION STANDARDS FOR A MASTER'S-DEGREE-LEVEL EDUCATIONAL PROGRAM FOR THE OCCUPATIONAL THERAPIST	ACCREDITATION STANDARDS FOR AN ASSOCIATE-DEGREE-LEVEL EDUCATIONAL PROGRAM FOR THE OCCUPATIONAL THERAPY ASSISTANT
B.9.9.	Describe and discuss professional responsibilities and issues when providing service on a contractual basis.	Describe and discuss professional responsibilities and issues when providing service on a contractual basis.	Identify professional responsibilities and issues when providing service on a contractual basis.
B.9.10.	Demonstrate strategies for analyzing issues and making decisions to resolve personal and organizational ethical conflicts.	Demonstrate strategies for analyzing issues and making decisions to resolve personal and organizational ethical conflicts.	Identify strategies for analyzing issues and making decisions to resolve personal and organizational ethical conflicts.
B.9.11.	Demonstrate a variety of informal and formal strategies for resolving ethics disputes in varying practice areas.	Explain the variety of informal and formal systems for resolving ethics disputes that have jurisdiction over occupational therapy practice.	Identify the variety of informal and formal systems for resolving ethics disputes that have jurisdiction over occupational therapy practice.
B.9.12.	Describe and implement strategies to assist the consumer in gaining access to occupational therapy and other health and social services.	Describe and discuss strategies to assist the consumer in gaining access to occupational therapy services.	Identify strategies to assist the consumer in gaining access to occupational therapy services.
B.9.13.	Demonstrate advocacy by participating in and exploring leadership positions in organizations or agencies promoting the profession (e.g., AOTA, state occupational therapy associations, World Federation of Occupational Therapists, advocacy organizations), consumer access and services, and the welfare of the community.	Demonstrate professional advocacy by participating in organizations or agencies promoting the profession (e.g., AOTA, state occupational therapy associations, advocacy organizations).	Demonstrate professional advocacy by participating in organizations or agencies promoting the profession (e.g., AOTA, state occupational therapy associations, advocacy organizations).

SECTION C: FIELDWORK EDUCATION AND DOCTORAL EXPERIENTIAL COMPONENT

C.1.0: FIELDWORK EDUCATION

Fieldwork education is a crucial part of professional preparation and is best integrated as a component of the curriculum design. Fieldwork experiences should be implemented and evaluated for their effectiveness by the educational institution. The experience should provide the student with the opportunity to carry out professional responsibilities under supervision of a qualified occupational therapy practitioner serving as a role model. The academic fieldwork coordinator is responsible for the program's compliance with fieldwork education requirements. The academic fieldwork coordinator will

STANDARD NUMBER	DOCTORAL-DEGREE-LEVEL	MASTER'S-DEGREE-LEVEL	ASSOCIATE-DEGREE-LEVEL
C.1.1.	Ensure that the fieldwork program reflects the sequence and scope of content in the curriculum design in collaboration with faculty so that fieldwork experiences strengthen the ties between didactic and fieldwork education.	Ensure that the fieldwork program reflects the sequence and scope of content in the curriculum design in collaboration with faculty so that fieldwork experiences strengthen the ties between didactic and fieldwork education.	Ensure that the fieldwork program reflects the sequence and scope of content in the curriculum design in collaboration with faculty so that fieldwork experiences strengthen the ties between didactic and fieldwork education.
C.1.2.	Document the criteria and process for selecting fieldwork sites, to include maintaining memoranda of understanding, complying with all site requirements, maintaining site objectives and site data, and communicating this information to students.	Document the criteria and process for selecting fieldwork sites, to include maintaining memoranda of understanding, complying with all site requirements, maintaining site objectives and site data, and communicating this information to students.	Document the criteria and process for selecting fieldwork sites, to include maintaining memoranda of understanding, complying with all site requirements, maintaining site objectives and site data, and communicating this information to students.
C.1.3.	Demonstrate that academic and fieldwork educators collaborate in establishing fieldwork objectives and communicate with the student and fieldwork educator about progress and performance during fieldwork.	Demonstrate that academic and fieldwork educators collaborate in establishing fieldwork objectives and communicate with the student and fieldwork educator about progress and performance during fieldwork.	Demonstrate that academic and fieldwork educators collaborate in establishing fieldwork objectives and communicate with the student and fieldwork educator about progress and performance during fieldwork.

STANDARD NUMBER	ACCREDITATION STANDARDS FOR A DOCTORAL-DEGREE-LEVEL EDUCATIONAL PROGRAM FOR THE OCCUPATIONAL THERAPIST	ACCREDITATION STANDARDS FOR A MASTER'S-DEGREE-LEVEL EDUCATIONAL PROGRAM FOR THE OCCUPATIONAL THERAPIST	ACCREDITATION STANDARDS FOR AN ASSOCIATE-DEGREE-LEVEL EDUCATIONAL PROGRAM FOR THE OCCUPATIONAL THERAPY ASSISTANT
C.1.4.	Ensure that the ratio of fieldwork educators to students enables proper supervision and the ability to provide frequent assessment of student progress in achieving stated fieldwork objectives.	Ensure that the ratio of fieldwork educators to students enables proper supervision and the ability to provide frequent assessment of student progress in achieving stated fieldwork objectives.	Ensure that the ratio of fieldwork educators to students enables proper supervision and the ability to provide frequent assessment of student progress in achieving stated fieldwork objectives.
C.1.5.	Ensure that fieldwork agreements are sufficient in scope and number to allow completion of graduation requirements in a timely manner in accordance with the policy adopted by the program as required by Standard A.4.14.	Ensure that fieldwork agreements are sufficient in scope and number to allow completion of graduation requirements in a timely manner in accordance with the policy adopted by the program as required by Standard A.4.14.	Ensure that fieldwork agreements are sufficient in scope and number to allow completion of graduation requirements in a timely manner in accordance with the policy adopted by the program as required by Standard A.4.14.
C.1.6.	The program must have evidence of valid memoranda of understanding in effect and signed by both parties at the time the student is completing the Level I or Level II fieldwork experience. (Electronic memoranda of understanding and signatures are acceptable.) Responsibilities of the sponsoring institution(s) and each fieldwork site must be clearly documented in the memorandum of understanding.	The program must have evidence of valid memoranda of understanding in effect and signed by both parties at the time the student is completing the Level I or Level II fieldwork experience. (Electronic memoranda of understanding and signatures are acceptable.) Responsibilities of the sponsoring institution(s) and each fieldwork site must be clearly documented in the memorandum of understanding.	The program must have evidence of valid memoranda of understanding in effect and signed by both parties at the time the student is completing the Level I or Level II fieldwork experience. (Electronic memoranda of understanding and signatures are acceptable.) Responsibilities of the sponsoring institution(s) and each fieldwork site must be clearly documented in the memorandum of understanding.
	IF A FIELD TRIP, OBSERVATION, OR SERVICE LEARNING ACTIVITY IS USED TO COUNT TOWARD PART OF LEVEL I FIELDWORK, THEN A MEMORANDUM OF UNDERSTANDING IS REQUIRED. IF A FIELD TRIP, OBSERVATION, OR SERVICE LEARNING ACTIVITY IS NOT USED TO COUNT TOWARD PART OF LEVEL I FIELDWORK, THEN NO MEMORANDUM OF UNDERSTANDING IS REQUIRED. *WHEN A MEMORANDUM OF UNDERSTANDING IS ESTABLISHED WITH A MULTISITE SERVICE PROVIDER (E.G., CONTRACT AGENCY, CORPORATE ENTITY), THE ACOTE STANDARDS DO NOT REQUIRE A SEPARATE MEMORANDUM OF UNDERSTANDING WITH EACH PRACTICE SITE.*	*IF A FIELD TRIP, OBSERVATION, OR SERVICE LEARNING ACTIVITY IS USED TO COUNT TOWARD PART OF LEVEL I FIELDWORK, THEN A MEMORANDUM OF UNDERSTANDING IS REQUIRED. IF A FIELD TRIP, OBSERVATION, OR SERVICE LEARNING ACTIVITY IS NOT USED TO COUNT TOWARD PART OF LEVEL I FIELDWORK, THEN NO MEMORANDUM OF UNDERSTANDING IS REQUIRED.* *WHEN A MEMORANDUM OF UNDERSTANDING IS ESTABLISHED WITH A MULTISITE SERVICE PROVIDER (E.G., CONTRACT AGENCY, CORPORATE ENTITY), THE ACOTE STANDARDS DO NOT REQUIRE A SEPARATE MEMORANDUM OF UNDERSTANDING WITH EACH PRACTICE SITE.*	
C.1.7.	Ensure that at least one fieldwork experience (either Level I or Level II) has as its focus psychological and social factors that influence engagement in occupation.	Ensure that at least one fieldwork experience (either Level I or Level II) has as its focus psychological and social factors that influence engagement in occupation.	Ensure that at least one fieldwork experience (either Level I or Level II) has as its focus psychological and social factors that influence engagement in occupation.
The goal of Level I fieldwork is to introduce students to the fieldwork experience, to apply knowledge to practice, and to develop understanding of the needs of clients. The program will			
C.1.8.	Ensure that Level I fieldwork is integral to the program's curriculum design and include experiences designed to enrich didactic coursework through directed observation and participation in selected aspects of the occupational therapy process.	Ensure that Level I fieldwork is integral to the program's curriculum design and include experiences designed to enrich didactic coursework through directed observation and participation in selected aspects of the occupational therapy process.	Ensure that Level I fieldwork is integral to the program's curriculum design and include experiences designed to enrich didactic coursework through directed observation and participation in selected aspects of the occupational therapy process.
C.1.9.	Ensure that qualified personnel supervise Level I fieldwork. Examples may include, but are not limited to, currently licensed or otherwise regulated occupational therapists and occupational therapy assistants, psychologists, physician assistants, teachers, social workers, nurses, and physical therapists.	Ensure that qualified personnel supervise Level I fieldwork. Examples may include, but are not limited to, currently licensed or otherwise regulated occupational therapists and occupational therapy assistants, psychologists, physician assistants, teachers, social workers, nurses, and physical therapists.	Ensure that qualified personnel supervise Level I fieldwork. Examples may include, but are not limited to, currently licensed or otherwise regulated occupational therapists and occupational therapy assistants, psychologists, physician assistants, teachers, social workers, nurses, and physical therapists.

STANDARD NUMBER	ACCREDITATION STANDARDS FOR A DOCTORAL-DEGREE-LEVEL EDUCATIONAL PROGRAM FOR THE OCCUPATIONAL THERAPIST	ACCREDITATION STANDARDS FOR A MASTER'S-DEGREE-LEVEL EDUCATIONAL PROGRAM FOR THE OCCUPATIONAL THERAPIST	ACCREDITATION STANDARDS FOR AN ASSOCIATE-DEGREE-LEVEL EDUCATIONAL PROGRAM FOR THE OCCUPATIONAL THERAPY ASSISTANT
C.1.10.	Document all Level I fieldwork experiences that are provided to students, including mechanisms for formal evaluation of student performance. Ensure that Level I fieldwork is not substituted for any part of Level II fieldwork.	Document all Level I fieldwork experiences that are provided to students, including mechanisms for formal evaluation of student performance. Ensure that Level I fieldwork is not substituted for any part of Level II fieldwork.	Document all Level I fieldwork experiences that are provided to students, including mechanisms for formal evaluation of student performance. Ensure that Level I fieldwork is not substituted for any part of Level II fieldwork.
	The goal of Level II fieldwork is to develop competent, entry-level, generalist occupational therapists. Level II fieldwork must be integral to the program's curriculum design and must include an in-depth experience in delivering occupational therapy services to clients, focusing on the application of purposeful and meaningful occupation and management of occupational therapy services. It is recommended that the student be exposed to a variety of clients across the lifespan and to a variety of settings. The program will		**The goal of Level II fieldwork is to develop competent, entry-level, generalist occupational therapy assistants. Level II fieldwork must be integral to the program's curriculum design and must include an in-depth experience in delivering occupational therapy services to clients, focusing on the application of purposeful and meaningful occupation. It is recommended that the student be exposed to a variety of clients across the lifespan and to a variety of settings. The program will**
C.1.11.	Ensure that the fieldwork experience is designed to promote clinical reasoning and reflective practice, to transmit the values and beliefs that enable ethical practice, and to develop professionalism and competence in career responsibilities.	Ensure that the fieldwork experience is designed to promote clinical reasoning and reflective practice, to transmit the values and beliefs that enable ethical practice, and to develop professionalism and competence in career responsibilities.	Ensure that the fieldwork experience is designed to promote clinical reasoning appropriate to the occupational therapy assistant role, to transmit the values and beliefs that enable ethical practice, and to develop professionalism and competence in career responsibilities.
C.1.12.	Provide Level II fieldwork in traditional and/or emerging settings, consistent with the curriculum design. In all settings, psychosocial factors influencing engagement in occupation must be understood and integrated for the development of client-centered, meaningful, occupation-based outcomes. The student can complete Level II fieldwork in a minimum of one setting if it is reflective of more than one practice area, or in a maximum of four different settings.	Provide Level II fieldwork in traditional and/or emerging settings, consistent with the curriculum design. In all settings, psychosocial factors influencing engagement in occupation must be understood and integrated for the development of client-centered, meaningful, occupation-based outcomes. The student can complete Level II fieldwork in a minimum of one setting if it is reflective of more than one practice area, or in a maximum of four different settings.	Provide Level II fieldwork in traditional and/or emerging settings, consistent with the curriculum design. In all settings, psychosocial factors influencing engagement in occupation must be understood and integrated for the development of client-centered, meaningful, occupation-based outcomes. The student can complete Level II fieldwork in a minimum of one setting if it is reflective of more than one practice area, or in a maximum of three different settings.
C.1.13.	Require a minimum of 24 weeks' full-time Level II fieldwork. This may be completed on a part-time basis, as defined by the fieldwork placement in accordance with the fieldwork placement's usual and customary personnel policies, as long as it is at least 50% of an FTE at that site.	Require a minimum of 24 weeks' full-time Level II fieldwork. This may be completed on a part-time basis, as defined by the fieldwork placement in accordance with the fieldwork placement's usual and customary personnel policies, as long as it is at least 50% of an FTE at that site.	Require a minimum of 16 weeks' full-time Level II fieldwork. This may be completed on a part-time basis, as defined by the fieldwork placement in accordance with the fieldwork placement's usual and customary personnel policies, as long as it is at least 50% of an FTE at that site.

STANDARD NUMBER	ACCREDITATION STANDARDS FOR A DOCTORAL-DEGREE-LEVEL EDUCATIONAL PROGRAM FOR THE OCCUPATIONAL THERAPIST	ACCREDITATION STANDARDS FOR A MASTER'S-DEGREE-LEVEL EDUCATIONAL PROGRAM FOR THE OCCUPATIONAL THERAPIST	ACCREDITATION STANDARDS FOR AN ASSOCIATE-DEGREE-LEVEL EDUCATIONAL PROGRAM FOR THE OCCUPATIONAL THERAPY ASSISTANT
C.1.14.	Ensure that the student is supervised by a currently licensed or otherwise regulated occupational therapist who has a minimum of 1 year full-time (or its equivalent) of practice experience subsequent to initial certification and who is adequately prepared to serve as a fieldwork educator. The supervising therapist may be engaged by the fieldwork site or by the educational program.	Ensure that the student is supervised by a currently licensed or otherwise regulated occupational therapist who has a minimum of 1 year full-time (or its equivalent) of practice experience subsequent to initial certification and who is adequately prepared to serve as a fieldwork educator. The supervising therapist may be engaged by the fieldwork site or by the educational program.	Ensure that the student is supervised by a currently licensed or otherwise regulated occupational therapist or occupational therapy assistant (under the supervision of an occupational therapist) who has a minimum of 1 year full-time (or its equivalent) of practice experience subsequent to initial certification and who is adequately prepared to serve as a fieldwork educator. The supervising therapist may be engaged by the fieldwork site or by the educational program.
C.1.15.	Document a mechanism for evaluating the effectiveness of supervision (e.g., student evaluation of fieldwork) and for providing resources for enhancing supervision (e.g., materials on supervisory skills, continuing education opportunities, articles on theory and practice).	Document a mechanism for evaluating the effectiveness of supervision (e.g., student evaluation of fieldwork) and for providing resources for enhancing supervision (e.g., materials on supervisory skills, continuing education opportunities, articles on theory and practice).	Document a mechanism for evaluating the effectiveness of supervision (e.g., student evaluation of fieldwork) and for providing resources for enhancing supervision (e.g., materials on supervisory skills, continuing education opportunities, articles on theory and practice).
C.1.16.	Ensure that supervision provides protection of consumers and opportunities for appropriate role modeling of occupational therapy practice. Initially, supervision should be direct and then decrease to less direct supervision as appropriate for the setting, the severity of the client's condition, and the ability of the student.	Ensure that supervision provides protection of consumers and opportunities for appropriate role modeling of occupational therapy practice. Initially, supervision should be direct and then decrease to less direct supervision as appropriate for the setting, the severity of the client's condition, and the ability of the student.	Ensure that supervision provides protection of consumers and opportunities for appropriate role modeling of occupational therapy practice. Initially, supervision should be direct and then decrease to less direct supervision as appropriate for the setting, the severity of the client's condition, and the ability of the student.
C.1.17.	Ensure that supervision provided in a setting where no occupational therapy services exist includes a documented plan for provision of occupational therapy services and supervision by a currently licensed otherwise regulated occupational therapist with at least 3 years' full-time or its equivalent of professional experience. Supervision must include a minimum of 8 hours of direct supervision each week of the fieldwork experience. An occupational therapy supervisor must be available, via a variety of contact measures, to the student during all working hours. An on-site supervisor designee of another profession must be assigned while the occupational therapy supervisor is off site.	Ensure that supervision provided in a setting where no occupational therapy services exist includes a documented plan for provision of occupational therapy services and supervision by a currently licensed or otherwise regulated occupational therapist with at least 3 years' full-time or its equivalent of professional experience. Supervision must include a minimum of 8 hours of direct supervision each week of the fieldwork experience. An occupational therapy supervisor must be available, via a variety of contact measures, to the student during all working hours. An on-site supervisor designee of another profession must be assigned while the occupational therapy supervisor is off site.	Ensure that supervision provided in a setting where no occupational therapy services exist includes a documented plan for provision of occupational therapy assistant services and supervision by a currently licensed or otherwise regulated occupational therapist or occupational therapy assistant (under the direction of an occupational therapist) with at least 3 years' full-time or its equivalent of professional experience. Supervision must include a minimum of 8 hours of direct supervision each week of the fieldwork experience. An occupational therapy supervisor must be available, via a variety of contact measures, to the student during all working hours. An on-site supervisor designee of another profession must be assigned while the occupational therapy supervisor is off site.

STANDARD NUMBER	ACCREDITATION STANDARDS FOR A DOCTORAL-DEGREE-LEVEL EDUCATIONAL PROGRAM FOR THE OCCUPATIONAL THERAPIST	ACCREDITATION STANDARDS FOR A MASTER'S-DEGREE-LEVEL EDUCATIONAL PROGRAM FOR THE OCCUPATIONAL THERAPIST	ACCREDITATION STANDARDS FOR AN ASSOCIATE-DEGREE-LEVEL EDUCATIONAL PROGRAM FOR THE OCCUPATIONAL THERAPY ASSISTANT
C.1.18.	Document mechanisms for requiring formal evaluation of student performance on Level II fieldwork (e.g., the AOTA *Fieldwork Performance Evaluation for the Occupational Therapy Student* or equivalent).	Document mechanisms for requiring formal evaluation of student performance on Level II fieldwork (e.g., the AOTA *Fieldwork Performance Evaluation for the Occupational Therapy Student* or equivalent).	Document mechanisms for requiring formal evaluation of student performance on Level II fieldwork (e.g., the AOTA *Fieldwork Performance Evaluation for the Occupational Therapy Assistant Student* or equivalent).
C.1.19.	Ensure that students attending Level II fieldwork outside the United States are supervised by an occupational therapist who graduated from a program approved by the World Federation of Occupational Therapists and has 1 year of experience in practice.	Ensure that students attending Level II fieldwork outside the United States are supervised by an occupational therapist who graduated from a program approved by the World Federation of Occupational Therapists and has 1 year of experience in practice.	Ensure that students attending Level II fieldwork outside the United States are supervised by an occupational therapist who graduated from a program approved by the World Federation of Occupational Therapists and has 1 year of experience in practice.
	C.2.0. DOCTORAL EXPERIENTIAL COMPONENT **The goal of the doctoral experiential component is to develop occupational therapists with advanced skills (those that are beyond a generalist level). The doctoral experiential component shall be an integral part of the program's curriculum design and shall include an in-depth experience in one or more of the following: clinical practice skills, research skills, administration, leadership, program and policy development, advocacy, education, or theory development.** **The student must successfully complete all coursework and Level II fieldwork and pass a competency requirement prior to the commencement of the doctoral experiential component. The specific content and format of the competency requirement is determined by the program. Examples include a written comprehensive exam, oral exam, NBCOT certification exam readiness tool, and the NBCOT practice exams.**		
C.2.1.	Ensure that the doctoral experiential component is designed and administered by faculty and provided in setting(s) consistent with the program's curriculum design, including individualized specific objectives and plans for supervision.	*(No related Standard)*	*(No related Standard)*
C.2.2.	Ensure that there is a memorandum of understanding that, at a minimum, includes individualized specific objectives, plans for supervision or mentoring, and responsibilities of all parties.	*(No related Standard)*	*(No related Standard)*
C.2.3.	Require that the length of this doctoral experiential component be a minimum of 16 weeks (640 hours). This may be completed on a part-time basis and must be consistent with the individualized specific objectives and culminating project. No more than 20% of the 640 hours can be completed outside of	*(No related Standard)*	*(No related Standard)*

STANDARD NUMBER	ACCREDITATION STANDARDS FOR A DOCTORAL-DEGREE-LEVEL EDUCATIONAL PROGRAM FOR THE OCCUPATIONAL THERAPIST	ACCREDITATION STANDARDS FOR A MASTER'S-DEGREE-LEVEL EDUCATIONAL PROGRAM FOR THE OCCUPATIONAL THERAPIST	ACCREDITATION STANDARDS FOR AN ASSOCIATE-DEGREE-LEVEL EDUCATIONAL PROGRAM FOR THE OCCUPATIONAL THERAPY ASSISTANT
	the mentored practice setting(s). Prior fieldwork or work experience may not be substituted for this experiential component.		
C.2.4.	Ensure that the student is mentored by an individual with expertise consistent with the student's area of focus. The mentor does not have to be an occupational therapist.	(No related Standard)	(No related Standard)
	MENTORING IS DEFINED AS A RELATIONSHIP BETWEEN TWO PEOPLE IN WHICH ONE PERSON (THE MENTOR) IS DEDICATED TO THE PERSONAL AND PROFESSIONAL GROWTH OF THE OTHER (THE MENTEE). A MENTOR HAS MORE EXPERIENCE AND KNOWLEDGE THAN THE MENTEE. THE PROGRAM MUST HAVE A SYSTEM TO ENSURE THAT MENTOR HAS DEMONSTRATED EXPERTISE IN ONE OR MORE OF THE FOLLOWING AREAS IDENTIFIED AS THE STUDENT'S FOCUSED AREA OF STUDY: CLINICAL PRACTICE SKILLS, RESEARCH SKILLS, ADMINISTRATION, LEADERSHIP, PROGRAM AND POLICY DEVELOPMENT, ADVOCACY, EDUCATION, OR THEORY DEVELOPMENT.		
C.2.5.	Document a formal evaluation mechanism for objective assessment of the student's performance during and at the completion of the doctoral experiential component.	(No related Standard)	(No related Standard)

GLOSSARY

Accreditation Standards for a Doctoral-Degree-Level Educational Program for the Occupational Therapist,
Masters-Degree-Level Educational Program for the Occupational Therapist, and
Associate-Degree-Level Educational Program for the Occupational Therapy Assistant

Definitions given below are for the purposes of these documents.

ABILITY TO BENEFIT: A phrase that refers to a student who does not have a high school diploma or its recognized equivalent, but is eligible to receive funds under the Title IV Higher Education Act programs after taking an independently administered examination and achieving a score, specified by the Secretary of the U.S. Department of Education (USDE), indicating that the student has the ability to benefit from the education being offered.

ACADEMIC CALENDAR: The official institutional document that lists registration dates, semester/quarter stop and start dates, holidays, graduation dates, and other pertinent events. Generally, the academic year is divided into two major semesters, each approximately 14 to 16 weeks long. A smaller number of institutions have quarters rather than semesters. Quarters are approximately 10 weeks long; there are three major quarters and the summer session.

ACTIVITY: A term that describes a class of human actions that are goal directed (AOTA, 2008b).

ADVANCED: The stage of being beyond the elementary or introductory.

AFFILIATE: An entity that formally cooperates with a sponsoring institution in implementing the occupational therapy educational program.

AREAS OF OCCUPATION: Activities in which people engage: activities of daily living, instrumental activities of daily living, rest and sleep, education, work, play, leisure, and social participation.

ASSIST: To aid, help, or hold an auxiliary position.

BODY FUNCTIONS: The physiological functions of body systems (including psychological functions).

BODY STRUCTURES: Anatomical parts of the body such as organs, limbs, and their components.

CARE COORDINATION: The process that links clients with appropriate services and resources.

CASE MANAGEMENT: A system to ensure that individuals receive appropriate health care services.

CLIENT: The term used to name the entity that receives occupational therapy services. Clients may include (1) individuals and other persons relevant to the client's life including family, caregivers, teachers, employers, and others who may also help or be served indirectly; (2) organizations, such as businesses, industries, or agencies; and (3) populations within a community (AOTA, 2008b).

CLIENT-CENTERED SERVICE DELIVERY: An orientation that honors the desires and priorities of clients in designing and implementing interventions.

CLIENT FACTORS: Factors that reside within the client and that may affect performance in areas of occupation. Client factors include body functions and body structures.

CLINICAL REASONING: Complex multifaceted cognitive process used by practitioners to plan, direct, perform, and reflect on intervention.

COLLABORATE: To work together with a mutual sharing of thoughts and ideas.

COMPETENT: To have the requisite abilities/qualities and capacity to function in a professional environment.

CONSUMER: The direct and/or indirect recipient of educational and/or practitioner services offered.

CONTEXT/CONTEXTUAL FACTORS AND ENVIRONMENT:

CONTEXT: The variety of interrelated conditions within and surrounding the client that influence performance. Contexts include cultural, personal, temporal, and virtual aspects.

ENVIRONMENT: The external physical and social environment that surrounds the client and in which the client's daily life occupations occur.

CONTEXT OF SERVICE DELIVERY: The knowledge and understanding of the various contexts in which occupational therapy services are provided.

CRITERION-REFERENCED: Tests that compare the performance of an individual to that of another group, known as the *norm group*.

CULMINATING PROJECT: A project that is completed by a doctoral student that demonstrates the student's ability to relate theory to practice and to synthesize advanced knowledge in a practice area.

CURRICULUM DESIGN: An overarching set of assumptions that explains how the curriculum is planned, implemented, and evaluated. Typically, a curriculum design includes educational goals and curriculum threads and provides a clear rationale for the selection of content, the determination of scope of content, and the sequence of the content. A curriculum design is expected to be consistent with the mission and philosophy of the sponsoring institution and the program.

CURRICULUM THREADS: Curriculum threads, or *themes*, are identified by the program as areas of study and development that follow a path through the curriculum and represent the unique qualities of the program, as demonstrated by the program's graduates. Curriculum threads are typically based on the profession's and program's vision, mission, and philosophy (e.g., occupational needs of society, critical thinking/professional reasoning, diversity/globalization . (AOTA, 2008a).

DIAGNOSIS: The process of analyzing the cause or nature of a condition, situation, or problem. Diagnosis as stated in Standard B.4.0. refers to the occupational therapist's ability to analyze a problem associated with occupational performance and participation.

DISTANCE EDUCATION: Education that uses one or more of the technologies listed below to deliver instruction to students who are separated from the instructor and to support regular and substantive interaction between the students and the instructor, either synchronously or asynchronously. The technologies may include

- The Internet;
- One-way and two-way transmissions through open broadcast, closed circuit, cable, microwave, broadband lines, fiber optics, satellite, or wireless communications devices;
- Audio conferencing; or
- Video cassettes, DVDs, and CD-ROMs, if the cassettes, DVDs, or CD-ROMs are used in a course.

DRIVER REHABILITATION: Specialized evaluation and training to develop mastery of specific skills and techniques to effectively drive a motor vehicle independently and in accordance with state department of motor vehicles regulations.

ENTRY-LEVEL OCCUPATIONAL THERAPIST: The outcome of the occupational therapy educational and certification process; an individual prepared to begin generalist practice as an occupational therapist with less than 1 year of experience.

ENTRY-LEVEL OCCUPATIONAL THERAPY ASSISTANT: The outcome of the occupational therapy educational and certification process; an individual prepared to begin generalist practice as an occupational therapy assistant with less than 1 year of experience.

FACULTY:

FACULTY, CORE: Persons who are resident faculty, including the program director, appointed to and employed primarily in the occupational therapy educational program.

FACULTY, FULL TIME: Core faculty members who hold an appointment that are full-time, as defined by the institution, and whose job responsibilities include teaching and/or contributing to the delivery of the designed curriculum regardless of the position title (e.g., full-time instructional staff and clinical instructors would be considered faculty).

FACULTY, PART TIME: Core faculty members who hold an appointment that is considered by that institution to constitute less than full-time service and whose job responsibilities include teaching and/or contributing to the delivery of the designed curriculum regardless of the position title.

FACULTY, ADJUNCT: Persons who are responsible for teaching at least 50% of a course and are part-time, nonsalaried, non-tenure-track faculty members who are paid for each class they teach.

FIELDWORK COORDINATOR: Faculty member who is responsible for the development, implementation, management, and evaluation of fieldwork education.

FRAME OF REFERENCE: A set of interrelated, internally consistent concepts, definitions, postulates, and principles that provide a systematic description of a practitioner's interaction with clients. A frame of reference is intended to link theory to practice.

FULL-TIME EQUIVALENT (FTE): An equivalent position for a full-time faculty member (as defined by the institution). A full-time equivalent can be made up of no more than 3 individuals.

GRADUATION RATE: The total number of students who graduated from a program within 150% of the published length of the program, divided by the number of students on the roster who started in the program.

HABITS: "Automatic behavior that is integrated into more complex patterns that enable people to function on a day-to-day basis" (Neidstadt & Crepeau, 1998).

HEALTH LITERACY: Degree to which individuals have the capacity to obtain, process, and understand basic health information and services needed to make appropriate health decisions (National Network of Libraries of Medicine, 2011).

INTERPROFESSIONAL COLLABORATIVE PRACTICE: "Multiple health workers from different professional backgrounds working together with patients, families, careers, and communities to deliver the highest quality of care"(World Health Organization, 2010).

MEMORANDUM OF UNDERSTANDING (MOU): A document outlining the terms and details of an agreement between parties, including each parties' requirements and responsibilities. A memorandum of understanding may be signed by any individual who is authorized by the institution to sign fieldwork memoranda of understanding on behalf of the institution.

MENTORING: A relationship between two people in which one person (the mentor) is dedicated to the personal and professional growth of the other (the mentee). A mentor has more experience and knowledge than the mentee.

MISSION: A statement that explains the unique nature of a program or institution and how it helps fulfill or advance the goals of the sponsoring institution, including religious missions.

MODALITIES: Application of a therapeutic agent, usually a physical agent modality.

DEEP THERMAL MODALITIES: Modalities such as therapeutic ultrasound and phonophoresis.

ELECTROTHERAPEUTIC MODALITIES: Modalities such as biofeedback, neuromuscular electrical stimulation, functional electrical stimulation, transcutaneous electrical nerve stimulation, electrical stimulations for tissue repair, high-voltage galvanic stimulation, and iontophoresis.

MECHANICAL MODALITIES: Modalities such as vasopneumatic devices and continuous passive motion.

SUPERFICIAL THERMAL MODALITIES: Modalities such as hydrotherapy, whirlpool, cryotherapy, fluidotherapy, hot packs, paraffin, water, and infrared.

MODEL OF PRACTICE: The set of theories and philosophies that defines the views, beliefs, assumptions, values, and domain of concern of a particular profession or discipline. Models of practice delimit the boundaries of a profession.

OCCUPATION: "Activities . . . of everyday life, named, organized and given value and meaning by individuals and a culture. Occupation is everything that people do to occupy themselves, including looking after themselves . . . enjoying life . . . and contributing to the social and economic fabric of their communities" (Law, Polatajko, Baptiste, & Townsend, 1997).

OCCUPATIONAL PROFILE: An analysis of a client's occupational history, routines, interests, values, and needs to engage in occupations and occupational roles.

OCCUPATIONAL THERAPY: The art and science of applying occupation as a means to effect positive, measurable change in the health status and functional outcomes of a client by a qualified occupational therapist and/or occupational therapy assistant (as appropriate).

OCCUPATIONAL THERAPY PRACTITIONER: An individual who is initially credentialed as an occupational therapist or an occupational therapy assistant.

PARTICIPATION: Active engagement in occupations.

PERFORMANCE PATTERNS: Patterns of behavior related to daily life activities that are habitual or routine. Performance patterns include habits, routines, rituals, and roles.

PERFORMANCE SKILLS: Features of what one does, not what one has, related to observable elements of action that have implicit functional purposes. Performance skills include motor and praxis, sensory/perceptual, emotional regulation, cognitive, and communication and social skills.

PHILOSOPHY: The underlying belief and value structure for a program that is consistent with the sponsoring institution and which permeates the curriculum and the teaching learning process.

POPULATION-BASED INTERVENTIONS: Interventions focused on promoting the overall health status of the community by preventing disease, injury, disability, and premature death. A population-based health intervention can include assessment of the community's needs, health promotion and public education, disease and disability prevention, monitoring of services, and media interventions. Most interventions are tailored to reach a subset of a population, although some may be targeted toward the population at large. Populations and subsets may be defined by geography, culture, race and ethnicity, socioeconomic status, age, or other characteristics. Many of these characteristics relate to the health of the described population (Keller, Schaffer, Lia-Hoagberg, & Strohschein, 2002).

PREPARATORY METHODS: Intervention techniques focused on client factors to help a client's function in specific activities.

PROGRAM DIRECTOR (associate-degree-level occupational therapy assistant): An initially certified occupational therapist or occupational therapy assistant who is licensed or credentialed according to regulations in the state or jurisdiction in which the program is located. The program director must hold a minimum of a master's degree.

PROGRAM DIRECTOR (master's-degree-level occupational therapist): An initially certified occupational therapist who is licensed or credentialed according to regulations in the state or jurisdiction in which the program is located. The program director must hold a doctoral degree.

PROGRAM DIRECTOR (doctoral-degree-level occupational therapist): An initially certified occupational therapist who is licensed or credentialed according to regulations in the state or jurisdiction in which the program is located. The program director must hold a doctoral degree.

PROGRAM EVALUATION: A continuing system for routinely and systematically analyzing data to determine the extent to which the program is meeting its stated goals and objectives.

PURPOSEFUL ACTIVITY: "An activity used in treatment that is goal directed and that the [client] sees as meaningful or purposeful" (Low, 2002).

RECOGNIZED REGIONAL OR NATIONAL ACCREDITING AUTHORITY: Regional and national accrediting agencies recognized by the USDE and/or the Council for Higher Education Accreditation (CHEA) to accredit postsecondary educational programs/institutions. The purpose of recognition is to ensure that the accrediting agencies are reliable authorities for evaluating quality education or training programs in the institutions they accredit.

Regional accrediting bodies recognized by USDE:

- Accrediting Commission for Community and Junior Colleges, Western Association of Schools and Colleges (ACCJC/WASC)
- Accrediting Commission for Senior Colleges and Universities, Western Association of Schools and Colleges (ACSCU/WASC)
- Commission on Colleges, Southern Association of Colleges and Schools (SACS)
- Commission on Institutions of Higher Education, New England Association of Schools and Colleges (CIHE/NEASC)
- Higher Learning Commission, North Central Association of Colleges and Schools (HLC)
- Middle States Commission on Higher Education, Middle States Association of Colleges and Schools (MSCHE)
- Northwest Commission on Colleges and Universities (NWCCU)

National accrediting bodies recognized by USDE:

- Accrediting Bureau of Health Education Schools (ABHES)
- Accrediting Commission of Career Schools and Colleges (ACCSC)
- Accrediting Council for Continuing Education and Training (ACCET)
- Accrediting Council for Independent Colleges and Schools (ACICS)
- Council on Occupational Education (COE)
- Distance Education and Training Council Accrediting Commission (DETC)

REFLECTIVE PRACTICE: Thoughtful consideration of one's experiences and knowledge when applying such knowledge to practice. Reflective practice includes being coached by professionals.

RELEASE TIME: Period when a person is freed from regular duties, especially teaching, to allow time for other tasks or activities.

RETENTION RATE: A measure of the rate at which students persist in their educational program, calculated as the percentage of students on the roster, after the add period, from the beginning of the previous academic year who are again enrolled in the beginning of the subsequent academic year.

SCHOLARSHIP: "A systematic investigation . . . designed to develop or to contribute to generalizable knowledge" (45 CFR § 46). Scholarship is made public, subject to review, and part of the discipline or professional knowledge base (Glassick, Huber, & Maeroff, 1997). It allows others to build on it and further advance the field (AOTA, 2009).

SCHOLARSHIP OF DISCOVERY: Engagement in activity that leads to the development of "knowledge for its own sake." The Scholarship of Discovery encompasses original research that contributes to expanding the knowledge base of a discipline (Boyer, 1990).

SCHOLARSHIP OF INTEGRATION: Investigations making creative connections both within and across disciplines to integrate, synthesize, interpret, and create new perspectives and theories (Boyer , 1990).

SCHOLARSHIP OF APPLICATION: Practitioners apply the knowledge generated by Scholarship of Discovery or Integration to address real problems at all levels of society (Boyer, 1990). In occupational therapy, an example would be the application of theoretical knowledge to practice interventions or to teaching in the classroom.

SCHOLARSHIP OF TEACHING AND LEARNING: ""Involves the systematic study of teaching and/or learning and the public sharing and review of such work through presentations, publications, and performances" (McKinney, 2007, p. 10).

SKILL: The ability to use one's knowledge effectively and readily in execution or performance.

SPONSORING INSTITUTION: The identified legal entity that assumes total responsibility for meeting the minimal standards for ACOTE accreditation.

STRATEGIC PLAN: A comprehensive plan that articulates the program's future vision and guides the program development (e.g., faculty recruitment and professional growth, changes in the curriculum design, priorities in academic resources, procurement of fieldwork sites). A program's strategic plan must include, but need not be limited to,

- Evidence that the plan is based on program evaluation and an analysis of both the institution and program, as well as specific needs of the program,
- Long-term goals that address the vision and mission of both the institution and program, as well as specific needs of the program,
- Specific measurable action steps with expected timelines by which the program will reach its long-term goals,
- Person(s) responsible for action steps, and
- Evidence of periodic updating of action steps and long-term goals as they are met or as circumstances change.

SUPERVISE: To direct and inspect the performance of workers or work.

SUPERVISION, DIRECT: Supervision that occurs in real time and offers both audio and visual capabilities to ensure opportunities for timely feedback.

SUPERVISOR: One who ensures that tasks assigned to others are performed correctly and efficiently.

THEORY: A set of interrelated concepts used to describe, explain, or predict phenomena.

TRANSFER OF CREDIT: A term used in higher education to award a student credit for courses earned in another institution prior to admission to the occupational therapy or occupational therapy assistant program.

References

American Occupational Therapy Association. (2008a). *Occupational therapy model curriculum.* Bethesda MD: Author. Retrieved from www.aota.org/Educate/EdRes/COE/Other-Education-Documents/OT-Model-Curriculum.aspx

American Occupational Therapy Association. (2008b). Occupational therapy practice framework: Domain and process (2nd ed.). *American Journal of Occupational Therapy, 62,* 625–683.

American Occupational Therapy Association. (2009). Scholarship in occupational therapy. *American Journal of Occupational Therapy, 63,* 790–796. http://dx.doi.org/10.5014/ajot.63.6.790

Boyer, E. L. (1990). *Scholarship reconsidered: Priorities of the professoriate.* San Francisco: Jossey-Bass.

Crepeau, E. B., Cohn, E., & Schell, B. (Eds.). (2008). *Willard and Spackman's occupational therapy* (11th ed.). Philadelphia: Lippincott Williams & Wilkins.

Glassick, C. E., Huber, M. T., & Maeroff, G. I. (1997). *Scholarship assessed: Evaluation of the professoriate.* San Francisco: Jossey-Bass.

Interprofessional Education Collaborative Expert Panel. (2011). *Core competencies for interprofessional collaborative practice: Report of an expert panel.* Washington, DC: Interprofessional Education Collaborative.

Keller, L., Schaffer, M., Lia-Hoagberg, B., & Strohschein S. (2002). Assessment, program planning and evaluation in population-based public health practice. *Journal of Public Health Management and Practice, 8*(5), 30–44.

Law, M., Polatajko, H., Baptiste, W., & Townsend, E. (1997). Core concepts of occupational therapy. In E. Townsend (Ed.), *Enabling occupation: An occupational therapy perspective* (pp. 29–56). Ottawa, ON: Canadian Association of Occupational Therapists.

Low, J. (2002). Historical and social foundations for practice. In C. A. Trombly & M. V. Radomski (Eds.), *Occupational therapy for physical dysfunction* (5th ed., pp. 17–30). Philadelphia: Lippincott Williams & Wilkins.

McKinney, K. (2007). *Enhancing learning through the scholarship of teaching and learning.* San Francisco: Jossey-Bass.

National Network of Libraries of Medicine. (2011). *Health literacy.* Retrieved February 3, 2012, from http://nnlm.gov/outreach/consumer/hlthlit.html

Schon, D. A. (1987). *Educating the reflective practitioner.* San Francisco: Jossey-Bass.

Public welfare: Protection of human subjects, 45 CFR § 46 (2005).

U.S. Department of Education (2011). *Funding Your Education: The Guide to Federal Student Aid, 2012-13.* Retrieved February 3, 2012, from http://studentaid.ed.gov/students/attachments/siteresources/12-13_Guide.pdf.

World Health Organization. (2010). *Framework for action on interprofessional education and collaborative practice.* Geneva: Author. Retrieved from http://whqlibdoc.who.int/hq/2010/WHO_HRH_HPN_10.3_eng.pdf.

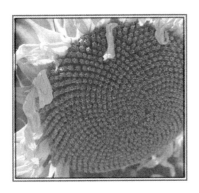

B

ASSESSMENT TOOL GRID

Jacobs, K., MacRae, N., & Sladyk, K. (Eds.).
*Occupational Therapy Essentials for
Clinical Competence, Second Edition* (pp. 769-786).
© 2014 SLACK Incorporated.

Assessment Tool Grid
Amy Peluso Burns
Printed with permission from the author.

Foundations for Functional Activity

Name of Assessment tool, Author, and Publication date	Standardized	Validity/ Reliability	Setting Used	Areas Assessed	Age Group
Balance/Posture/Mobility					
Berg Scale *Measures 14 balance items. Includes sitting and standing unsupported, sit-to-stand, transfers, picking up objects from floor, and turning.*	No	Valid and Reliable	Home or clinic setting	Transfers, sitting, standing, balance	Adult/elderly
Functional Reach Test *Simple way to measure standing balance. Measures the difference between arm's length and maximal forward reach.*	Yes	Valid and Reliable	Wall and tape measure needed	Reaching and balance	Adult/elderly
Modified Gait Abnormality Rating Scale (GARS) *Seven item assessment of gait, stepping and arm movements, staggering foot contact, hip ROM, shoulder extension, etc.*	No		Room to walk	Hip ROM, foot contact, staggering, arm/leg symmetry, guarding	Adult/elderly
Timed Get Up and Go (TGUG) *Measures the overall time to complete a series of functionally important tasks. Helps to identify clients with balance deficits.*	No	Valid and Reliable	Room to walk 10 feet; chair	Balance, posture, mobility	Adult/elderly
Tinetti *Measures a client's gait and balance.*	No	Inter-rater reliability	Room to walk 10 feet; chair	Balance and gait	Adult/elderly
Cognition					
Autobiographical Memory Interview (AMI) *Interview recalling events from the clients' past including school, wedding, children, etc.*	Yes	Valid and Reliable	Quiet environment with minimal distractions	Memory, retrograde amnesia	Adult/elderly
Bay Area Functional Performance Evaluation (BaFPE) *Assesses how a client might function in task-oriented settings and settings with social interaction. Uses sea shells, design blocks, and associated items.*	Yes	Valid and Reliable	Seated at table	Memory, organization, attention span	Adult/elderly
Behavioral Inattention Test *Assesses unilateral visual neglect. Includes card sorting, article reading, figure/shape copying, etc.*	Yes	Valid and Reliable	Quiet environment with minimal distractions	Unilateral visual neglect, picture recalling, line crossing, article reading, phone dialing	Adult/elderly

Brown ADD Scale *Assesses executive function impairments associated with ADD/ADHD and related problems.*	Yes	Valid and Reliable	Quiet environment with minimal distractions	Attention, listening skills	Age 3 to adult
Cognitive Assessment of Minnesota (CAM) *Assesses the cognitive abilities of adults with neurological impairments.*	Yes	Valid and Reliable	Quiet room	Attention, memory, visual neglect	Ages 18 to 70
Contextual Memory Test *Assesses awareness of memory capacity, strategy use, and recall in adults with memory dysfunction.*	Yes	Valid and Reliable	Quiet room with minimal distraction	Memory, awareness of memory capacity, recall of line drawings	Adult/elderly
Glasgow Coma Scale *Measures response of eyes, verbal response, and motor response in numerical levels.*	No	Reliable	In hospital	Alertness, awareness, verbal response, motor response	All ages
King-Devick Test of Oculomotor Speed and Accuracy (K-D) *Assesses residual oculomotor functions in a clinical setting, and its components can also be used for vision therapy training purposes as well.*	Yes	Valid and Reliable	Quiet environment with minimal distractions	eye tracking skills, general motor skills	Ages 6 to 14
Leiter International Performance Scale - Revised (Leiter-R) *A non-verbal test to assess cognitive functions in children and adolescents.*	Yes	Valid and Reliable	Individual setting, comfortable for the client	Intellectual ability, memory, attention	Ages 2 to 20 years, 11 months
Lowenstein Occupational Therapy Cognitive Assessment (LOTCA) (also LOTCA-Geriatric) *Assesses clients with neurological deficits and mental health issues. Tests orientation, visual/spatial perception, praxis, visuomotor. Includes cards, blocks, pegboard.*	Yes	Valid and Reliable	Quiet environment with minimal distractions	Orientation, perception, praxis, visuomotor, organization, thinking operations	Adult/elderly
Luria-Nebraska Neuropsychological Battery *Reading numbers, writing words, differentiate hard/soft touch, sounds. Provides a pattern analysis of strengths and weakness across areas of brain function.*	Yes	Valid and Reliable	Quiet environment with minimal distractions	Numbers, reading, writing, touching	All ages
Mini-Mental Status Evaluation (MMSE) *Used to assess cognitive function.*	Yes	Valid and Reliable	Seated at table	Brain injury, writing, reading, drawing	Ages 18+

Ranchos Los Amigos (Developed at the Rancho Los Amigos Hospital in California by the Head Injury Treatment Team) *Medical scale, assesses the level of recovery of a client with a brain injury and those recovering from a coma.*	No	Reliable	In hospital	Alertness, awareness	All ages
Rivermead Behavioral Memory Test (RBMT-II) *Assessment of gross memory impairments encountered by clients in their everyday lives. Identifies everyday memory problems and monitors change over time.*	Yes	Valid and Reliable	Quiet environment with minimal distractions	Memory: immediate and recall	Ages 16+
Severe Impairment Battery *Evaluates cognitive abilities at the lower end of the range (severely impaired dementia client). Allows for non-verbal and partially correct responses.*	Yes	Valid and Reliable	Quiet environment with minimal distractions	Memory, completing simple actions	Adult/elderly
Test of Everyday Attention *Measures selective attention, sustained attention, and attentional switching. Includes map search, telephone search, elevator counting, etc.*	Yes	Valid and Reliable	Quiet room; table and chairs	Everyday materials (map searching, phone skills, etc.)	Ages 18 to 80
Dexterity					
Jebsen-Taylor Hand Function Test *Assesses a broad range of hand functions used in daily activities. A seven-part test that uses common items such as paper clips, cans, pencils, etc.*	Yes	Reliable	Seated, requires adequate lighting	Writing, page turning, lifting small/large objects, simulated feeding	Ages 20 to 94
Manipulative Aptitude Test *Measures hand/arm/finger dexterity and speed through sorting and assembling.*	Yes	Valid and Reliable	Seated at a table or desk	Dexterity, manipulative aptitude, dominant hand	Ages 13+
Minnesota Rate of Manipulation *Assesses unilateral and bilateral manual dexterity along with eye-hand coordination. Provides information on standing tolerance, sustained neck flexion, weight bearing, and repetitive reach.*	Yes	Valid and Reliable	Table and chair	Manual dexterity, turning, displacing	Ages 13+
Nine Hole Peg *Client places nine dowels in nine holes while being timed.*	Yes	Valid and Reliable	Table and chair	Finger dexterity	Ages 20+
O'Connor Finger Dexterity Test *Requires hand placement of 3 pins per hole.*	Yes		Table and chair	Predictor of rapid manipulation	Ages 13+

O'Connor Tweezer Dexterity Test *Measures the speed with which a client can puck up pins with a tweezer, one at a time, and place the pin into a small hole.*	Yes		Table and chair	Finger dexterity, fine motor coordination, speed, eye-hand coordination	Ages 13+
Pennsylvania Bi-manual Worksample *Assesses finger dexterity of both hands, as well as gross movements of both arms.*	Yes	Reliable	Table and chair	Finger dexterity of both hands, gross movements of both arms, eye-hand coordination	Ages 16+
Purdue Pegboard *Assesses gross movement of hands/fingers/arms, as well as fingertip dexterity.*	Yes	Valid and Reliable	Table and chair	Gross movement of hands, fingers, and arms; fingertip dexterity	Ages 5+
Range of Motion *Measurement of the achievable distance between the flexed position and the extended position of a particular joint or muscle group.*	Yes	Valid, not 100% reliable	Comfortable for client, chair/mat	Biomechanical	All ages
Rosenbusch Test of Finger Dexterity *Measures the speed of inter-digital manipulation of each hand separately.*	Yes	Valid and Reliable	Table and chair	Manipulation of all parts of the hand	All ages
Strength Testing *The strength of each muscle group is measured on a scale of 0/5 to 5/5.*	Yes	Valid, not 100% reliable	Comfortable for client, chair/mat	Biomechanical	All ages

Motor/cognition/coping/self-help (Pediatric)

Battelle Developmental Inventory, Second Edition, (BDI-2) *Developmental assessment for early childhood. Screening, diagnosis, and evaluation of early development.*	Yes	Valid and Reliable	Familiar to child; little to no auditory and visual distractions	Personal-social, motor, adaptive, communication, cognitive (all with sub-domains too)	Birth to age 8
Bayley Scales of Infant Development (BIDS) *Measures the mental and motor development and tests the behavior of infants.*	Yes	Valid and Reliable	Quiet environment with minimal distractions	Performance in occupation, performance skills, context, activity demands	Ages 1 to 42 months
Behavioral-Characteristics Progression (BCP) *Curriculum-based assessment and planning tool for use by special education professionals serving children and adults who are functioning between the developmental ages of 1 to 14 years.*	No	Valid and Reliable	Comfortable for child	Self-help, fine motor, gross motor, academic, etc.	Ages 1 to 14
Bruininks-Oseretoky of Motor Proficiency *Comprehensive index of motor proficiency as well as separate measures of both gross and fine motor skills.*	Yes	Valid and Reliable	Gym	Motor	Ages 4.5 to 14.5

The Carolina Curriculum for Infants and Toddlers with Special Needs, Second Edition (CCITSN) *Designed for children who have mild to severe special needs and who function in the birth to 24-month developmental range.*	Yes	Valid and Reliable	Comfortable for child	Cognition, communication, social adaptation, fine motor, gross motor	Birth to age 2
The Carolina Curriculum for Preschoolers with Special Needs (CCPSN) *Designed for children who have mild to severe special needs and who function in the 2- to 5-year developmental range.*	Yes	Valid and Reliable	Comfortable for child	Cognition, communication, social adaptation, fine motor, gross motor	Ages 2 to 5
Coping-Inventory *Assesses the behavior patterns and skills used by children and adults to meet personal needs and adapt to the demands of their environment.*	No	Self-rated and observation	Variety of environments	Two forms of coping behavior, self and environment	Ages 3+
First Step (FirstSTEp) *Screening test for evaluating pre-schooler.*	Yes	Valid and Reliable	Public schools, public health situations, pediatrician's office	IDEA domains: cognition, communication, and motor	Ages 2 years, 9 months to 6 years, 2 months
Early Coping Inventory *Assesses the coping-related behavior of children.*	No	Observation form	Comfortable for child	Sensorimotor, reactive behavior, self-initiated behavior	Ages 4 to 36 months
Hawaii Early Learning Profile (HELP) *Test is helpful to see development of child throughout periods of time.*	Criterion referenced	Valid and Reliable	Comfortable for child	Cognition, language, gross motor, fine motor, social-emotional, self-help, regulatory, sensory organization	Birth to age 3 and preschool
Infant-Toddler and Family Instrument (ITFI) and Manual *Helps to evaluate the strengths and vulnerabilities of children and their families.*		Valid and Reliable	Family environment, comfortable	Gross and fine motor, social and emotional, language, coping and self-help	Ages 6 months to 3 years
Kent Inventory of Developmental Skills (KIDS) *Provides a clear picture of a child's development status and relative strengths and needs.*	Yes	Valid and Reliable	Familiar to child; home	Cognitive, motor, communication, self-help, social	Birth to 15 months, or up to age 6 when severe developmental disabilities are present
Mullen Scales of Early Learning *Provides a complete picture of cognitive and motor ability.*	Yes	Valid and Reliable	Clinic and school setting	Visual, linguistic, motor, distinguish between receptive and expressive processing	Birth to 68 months

Peabody Developmental Motor Scales, Second Edition, (PDMS-2) *Measures both gross and fine motor skills.*	Yes	Valid and Reliable	Quiet environment with minimal distractions	Motor (gross and fine)	Birth to age 7
Pediatric Evaluation of Disability Inventory (PEDI) *Assesses key functional capabilities and performance.*	Yes	Valid and Reliable	Natural environment for child	Self-care, mobility, social function	Ages 6 months to 7 years
PEERAMID-2 *Assesses a child's performance in five different areas of development.*	Yes	n/a	Quiet, comfortable	Fine motor/ graphomotor function, language function, gross motor function, memory function, and visual processing	School Grades 4 to 10
Pediatric Examination of Educational Readiness (PEER) *Assesses the preschooler's performance in six areas.*	Yes	n/a	Quiet, child comfortable, no parents	Orientation, gross motor, visual-fine motor, sequential, linguistic, and preacademic learning	Ages 4 to 6
Pediatric Extended Exam at Three (PEET) *Assesses a child's performance in five basic areas of development.*	Yes	n/a	Quiet, comfortable, low visual stim, supportive	Gross motor, language, visual-fine motor, memory, and intersensory integration	Age 3
Pediatric Early Elementary Exam (PEEX-2) *Assesses a child's performance in five different areas of development.*	Yes	n/a	quiet, comfortable, sit to left or right of child at table	Fine motor/ graphomotor function, language function, gross motor function, memory function, and visual processing function	Ages 6 to 9
Posture and Fine Motor Assessments (PFMAI) *Designed to identify motor delays in infants and to monitor progress in the first year of life.*	Yes	Valid and Reliable	Familiar, child only in diaper	Motor	Ages 2 to 12 months
Quick Neurological Screening Test - II, Revised Edition *Designed for use in screening for early identification of disabilities*	Norms suggest cutoff scores	Some Validity and Reliability	Table and chairs, room to walk	Hand skill, discrimination, eye tracking, sound patterns, movements	Ages 5+
Temperament and Atypical Behavior Scale (TABS) *Early Childhood Indicators of Developmental Dysfunction*	Norm referenced	Valid and Reliable	Parent may be able to complete independently, or with help from professional	Sensory regulation, attachment behaviors	Ages 11 to 71 months
Test of Gross Motor Development (TGMD-2) *Measures gross motor abilities that develop in early life*	Yes	Valid and Reliable	School (Open and large area)	Gross motor	Ages 3 to 10

Toddler Infant Motor Eval (TIME) *Evaluates children who have atypical motor development.*	Yes	Valid and Reliable	Quiet environment with minimal distractions	Motor	Birth to 42 months
Play					
Adolescent Role Assessment (ARA) *Gathers information on the adolescent's occupational role involvement over time and across domains.*	No	Scores lack internal consistency	Comfortable for client	Social integration, school, roles, play, family	Ages 13 to 20
Adolesant Leisure Interest Profile *Asks adolescent to report his or her interest and/or participation in a variety of age-appropriate leisure activities.*	No	Self-report, Valid and Reliable	Comfortable for child	Sports, outdoor, summer, winter, indoor, creative	Ages 12 to 21
Infant Preschool Play Assessment Scale (I-PAS) *Systematically observes children at play and in other routines or natural environments.*	Criterion referenced	Valid and Reliable	Comfortable for child	Social, sensorimotor, memory, gross motor, communication, motivation, problem solving	Birth to 5 years
Kid Play Profile *Asks child to report his or her interest and/or participation in a variety of age-appropriate leisure activities.*	No	Self-report, Valid and Reliable	Comfortable for child	Sports, outdoor, summer, winter, indoor, creative	Ages 6 to 9
Knox Preschool Play Scale (KPPS) *Preschoolers can be observed during free play, and a play age can be computed.*	Yes	Valid and Reliable	Comfortable for child, classroom setting	Space management, material management, imitation, participation	Preschoolers
Preteen Play Profile *Asks preteen to report his or her interest and/or participation in a variety of age-appropriate leisure activities.*	No	Self-report, Valid and Reliable	Comfortable for child	Sports, outdoor, summer, winter, indoor, creative	Ages 9 to 12
Takata Play History (TPH) *Probes past and actual play history that relate to sensory integration function.*	No	Valid and Reliable	Comfortable for child	Sensorimotor, symbolic, dramatic, games, recreational	All children
Test of Playfulness (ToP) *The information gathered provides a clue on inner drive and response to just right challenges, socialization, and play.*	No	Valid and Reliable	Indoors and outdoors	Intrinsic motivation, internal control, freedom to suspend reality	Ages 18 months+
Transdiciplinary Play-Based Assessment *Allows children to initiate and engage in play activities that are natural and enjoyable.*	Norm referenced	Valid and Reliable	Environment comfortable to child	Cognitive, social-emotional, communication, language, and sensorimotor	Infancy to age 6
Sensation/Edema					
Tactile Activity Kit *Versatile tool for sensory integration therapy.*	No	Not Valid, Not Reliable	Table-top	Tactile stimulation, discrimination, and desensitization	All ages

Volumeter *Fill container with water, measure the displaced water of both hands.*	No		Countertop or table; need access to water faucet	Edema, swelling of UE	All ages
Sensory					
DeGangi-Berk Test of Sensory Integration (TSI) *Measures overall sensory integration, as well as postural control, bilateral motor integration, and reflex integration.*	Yes	Valid and Reliable	Environment comfortable for child	Vestibular function; postural control, bilateral motor integration, reflex integration	Ages 3 to 5
Sensory Integration and Praxis Tests (SIPT) *Measures sensory processing deficits related to learning and behavior problems.*	Yes	Valid and Reliable	Environment comfortable for child	Visual, tactile, kinesthetic perception, motor performance	Ages 4 to 8
Sensory Processing Measure *Provides a complete picture of children's sensory processing difficulties at school and at home.*	Yes	Valid and Reliable	Home Form by caregiver in the home; School Forms by staff in multiple school environments	Sensory processing, praxis, social participation	Ages 5 to 12
Sensory Profile *Measures children's responses to sensory events in everyday life.*	Yes	Valid and Reliable	Environment comfortable for child	Modulation of sensory input across sensory systems, behavioral/emotional responses associated with sensory processing	Ages 3 to 10
Sensory Profile: Infant/Toddler *Examines patterns in children who are at risk or have specific disabilities.*	Yes	Valid and Reliable	Environment comfortable for child	Modulation of sensory input across sensory systems, behavioral/emotional responses associated with sensory processing	Birth to 36 months
Sensory Profile: Adolescent/Adult *Identifies sensory processing patterns and effects on functional performance.*	Based on normative information	Valid and Reliable	Environment comfortable for child	Modulation of sensory input across sensory systems, behavioral/emotional responses associated with sensory processing	Ages 11+
Sensory Profile School Companion *Assesses children's sensory processing information related to school performance.*	Yes	Valid and Reliable	Environment comfortable for child	Classroom behavior and performance	Ages 3 to 11

Test of Sensory Function in Infants (TSFI) *Objective assessment to determine whether, and to what extent, an infant has sensory processing deficits.*	Yes	Valid and Reliable	Individually administered, simple interaction with the infant, infant can be seated on parent's lap	Deep pressure, visual tactile integration, adaptive motor function, ocular motor control, reactivity to vestibular stimulation	Ages 4 to 18 months

Vision/Visual Perceptual

Benton Visual Form Discrimination *Assesses the ability to discriminate between complex visual configurations. Book of line drawings.*	No	Valid	Quiet environment with minimal distractions	Neglect, neuropsycho-logical	Adult/elderly
Developmental Test of Visual-Motor Integration (VMI) *Visuomotor skills are tested as the student copies a series of shapes in a test booklet.*	Yes	Valid and Reliable	Seated at desk/table, lighting, free of distraction	Visual perceptual	Ages 3+
Developmental Test of Visual Perception (DTVP-2) *Measures visual perception and motor integration skills.*	Yes	Valid and Reliable	Seated at desk/table, lighting, free of distraction	Pure visual perception (no motor response) and visual-motor integration	Ages 4 to 10
Hooper Visual Organization Test (VOT) *Ability to visually integrate information into whole perceptions through the use of line drawings arranged in puzzles.*	Yes	Valid and Reliable	Quiet environment with minimal distractions	Organization of visual stimuli	Ages 13+
McDowell Visual Screening Kit *Allows vision testing of very young or severely disabled children.*	Screening	Valid and Reliable	Comfortable for child	Distance visual acuity, near point acuity, ocular alignment, color perception, ocular function	Ages 2.5 to 5.5
Motor-Free Visual Perception Test (MVPT-3) *Assesses overall visual perceptual ability.*	Yes	Valid and Reliable	Seated at table Adequate light and free from distraction	Visual perceptual	Ages 4+
STROOP Color and Word Test *Reading aloud colored words. The words themselves are names of colors, but the actual color is different than the name.*	Yes	Valid and Reliable	Quiet environment with minimal distractions	Brain function and planning	Ages 15+
Test of Visual Motor Skills *Assesses a child's ability to transcribe geometric forms.*	Yes	Valid and Reliable	Seated at desk/table, individually or in groups	Eye-hand coordination skills	Ages 3 to 14
Test of Visual Motor Skills (UPPER) *Measures visual motor functioning using 16 geometric figures.*	Yes	Valid and Reliable	Seated at table Adequate light and free from distraction	Visual motor	Ages 12 to 40

Test of Visual-Perceptual Skills (non-motor) (TVPS-R) *Measures seven areas of visual-perception skills.*	Yes	Valid and Reliable	Seated at desk/table, lighting, free of distraction	Visual discrimination/ memory, visual spatial relationships, visual form-constancy, visual sequential memory, visual figure ground, visual closure	Ages 4 to 13
Warren's Brain Injury Visual Assessment Battery for Adults (biVABA) *Assessment of visual processing ability after a brain injury.*	Yes	Valid and Reliable	Comfortable for client	Visual perceptual processing, oculomotor function, how function is affected	Post CVA or head/brain injury

ADLs and IADL					
Name of Assessment tool, Author, and Publication date	**Standardized**	**Validity/ Reliability**	**Setting Used**	**Areas Assessed**	**Age**
Allen Cognitive Level Test (ACL) *Leather lacing test.*	Yes	Valid and Reliable	Environment with minimal distractions and good lighting	Problem solving, sequencing	Adults/elderly
Arnadottir Occupational Therapy Neurobehavioral Evaluation (A-one) *Determines the impact of neurobehavioral impairments on activities of daily living and mobility tasks using a five-point scale.*	Yes	Valid and Reliable	Clinic or home setting	ADLs, severity of neurobehavioral impairment, occupational performance	Adults/elderly
Assessment of Motor and Process Skills (AMPS) *Observational assessment, measures the quality of a person's ADLs. Rates the effort, efficiency, safety, and independence of ADL motor/process skills. *Training required.*	Yes	Valid and Reliable	Various conditions	IADLs, motor skills and processing skills	Adults/elderly
Assessment of Occupational Functioning (AOF) *Assesses the functional capacity of residents in long-term treatment settings who have physical and/or psychiatric problems.*	Yes	Valid and Reliable	Comfortable for the client	IADLs, MOHO, volition, habituation, performance	Ages 13+
Barthel Index *Assesses self-care functions in older adults.*	No	Predictive validity	Individual or group evaluation	Self-care	Adults/elderly
Canadian Occupational Performance Measure (COPM) *Individualized outcome measure designed to detect changes in self-perception of occupational performance over time.*	Yes, but not norm referenced	Valid and Reliable	Comfortable for client	Occupational performances and perception	All ages
Comprehensive Occupational Therapy Evaluation (COTE) *Developed in an acute psychiatric setting. Identifies 25 OT-related behaviors within three categories (general behavior, interpersonal behavior, and task behavior).*	Yes	Valid and Reliable	Quiet environment with minimal distractions	Behavior	All ages
Direct Assessment of Functional Abilities (DAFA) *Direct measurement of the instrumental activities of daily living. Used to determine functional deficits in clients with mild cognitive impairment.*	Yes	Valid and Reliable	Clinic setting, cafeteria, gift shop, and exam room	IADLs	Adults/elderly

Functional Independent Measure (FIM) *Scale (range from 1 to 7) that measures a client's ability to function with independence. Collected upon admission to rehabilitation unit, upon discharge, and after discharge.*	Yes	Valid and Reliable	Clinic or home setting	ADLs, self-care, communication, cognitive function	Adults/elderly
Independent Living Scales (ILS) *Offers assessment, daily living skills, self-advocacy training, and support with issues that challenge the independence of a client.*	Yes	Valid and Reliable	Table and chairs; can be bedside	IADL, memory, orientation, money management, health, safety, etc.	Ages 65+
Index of Activities of Daily Living (ADL) *Assesses functional status as a measurement of the client's ability to perform activities of daily living independently. *No longer in print, may still be seen in some clinics.*	Yes	Valid and Reliable	Inpatient observations	ADL, biological and psychological function	Ages 65+
Kitchen Task Assessment (KTA) *Measures organization, planning, and judgment skills through common kitchen tasks.*	Yes	Valid and Reliable	Kitchen/ cooking environment	IADL, initiation, organization, sequencing, judgment, safety	Adults/elderly
Klein-Bell Activities of Daily Living Scale *Assesses age-related changes in activities of daily living ability. *No longer in print, may still be seen in some clinics.*	Yes	Valid and Reliable	General rehabilitation setting	ADLs	Adults/elderly
Kohlman Evaluation of Living Skills (KELS) *Ability to function in 17 basic living skills. Assesses skills in five areas: self-care, safety and health, money management, transportation/ telephone, and work/leisure.*	Yes	Valid and Reliable	Table and chairs	Self-care, safety and health, money management, transportation, telephone, work, leisure	Adults/elderly
Level of Rehabilitation Scale (LORS-II) *Evaluates the success of inpatient rehabilitation programs.*	Yes	Valid and Reliable	Hospital rehabilitation units	ADLs	Adults/elderly
Milwaukee Evaluation of Daily Living Skills (MEDLS) *Information from clients and families; establishes baseline behaviors necessary to develop treatment plans and guide intervention in regard to daily living skills.*	No	Valid and Reliable	Home environment	ADLs, including communication, personal care, clothing care, etc.	Adult/elderly

Occupational Circumstances Assessment and Interview Rating Scale (OCAIRS) *A 40-minute interview that analyzes the extent and nature of a client's occupational adaptation and participation.*	No	Valid and Reliable	Comfortable for the client	MOHO, volitional, habituation, performance	Ages 13+
Occupational Performance History Interview (OPHI-II) *Interview that gathers the appreciation of a client's life history, the direction in which they want to take their life, as well as the impact of a disability on their life.*	Yes	Valid and Reliable	Comfortable for client	Occupational roles, daily routine, critical life events	Adolescents and adults
Pre-Feeding Skills Checklist *Manual for feeding assessment and intervention.*	No	Valid and Reliable	Quiet environment with minimal distractions	Feeding positions, types, quantity, sucking, movements	Ages 1 to 24 months
Performance Assessment of Self-care Skills (PASS) *Performance-based observation tool covering functional mobility, personal care, and IADLs. Measures short term functional change in elderly after hospitalization. *Requires 2-day training workshop.*	Criterion referenced	Valid and Reliable	Clinic and home version	IADLs	Adult/elderly
Role-Checklist *Assesses the values that clients place on their occupational roles.*	Yes	Valid and Reliable	Comfortable for client	MOHO, habituation subsystem	Ages 13+
Routine Task Inventory (RTI-II) *Measures the level of performance in activities of daily living through observation and questioning.*	No	Valid and Reliable	Clinic or home setting	ADLs, effect of cognitive impairment on task performance	Adult/elderly
Occupational Self Assessment *This is a self-assessment of perceptions of strengths and weaknesses relative to occupational functioning.*	Yes	Valid and Reliable	Comfortable for the client	MOHO, volitional, habituation, performance	Ages 16+
Environmental Evaluations					
Enabler *Norm-based environment assessment, developed to assess the accessibility of housing and its close surroundings.*	Yes	Valid and Reliable	Home environment and close surroundings	IADLs, neurological, musculoskeletal, psychological, movement, cognition, physical	All ages
Home Observation for Measurement of the Environment *Measures the quality and quantity of stimulation and support available to a child in the home environment.*	Yes	Valid and Reliable	Home environment	Interaction, environment	Ages 3 to 15

Education

Name of Assessment tool, Author, and Publication date	Standardized	Validity/ Reliability	Setting Used	Areas Assessed	Age
Occupational Therapy Psychosocial Assessment of Learning (OT PAL) *Designed to examine the environmental factors to determine the best "fit" between a child and his or her environment.*	No	Content validity	Classroom	Volition, habituation, and environmental fit within the classroom setting	Ages 6 to 12
School Function Assessment *Measures school-related functional skills.*	Yes	Valid and Reliable	School setting	Participation, task supports, activity performance, adaptations	School grades 1 to 6

Handwriting

Denver Handwriting Analysis (DHA)	No	Valid and Reliable	Classroom	Fine motor, visual motor, auditory	School grades 3 to 8
Erhardt Developmental Prehension Assessment (EDPA) *Designed for charting the prehensile development of a child.*	Yes	Valid and Reliable	Quiet environment with minimal distractions	Positional-reflexive, cognitively directed, pre-writing skills	Birth to 15 months
Evaluation Tool of Children's Handwriting (ETCH) *Evaluates six different areas of children's handwriting.*	Yes	Valid and Reliable	Quiet environment with minimal distractions	Alphabet production, numerical writing, near/far point copying, dictation, sentence composition	School grades 1 to 6
Minnesota Handwriting Assessment *Used to analyze handwriting skills.*	Yes	Valid and Reliable	Quiet environment with minimal distractions	Legibility, form, alignment, size, spacing	1st and 2nd grade
Observation of Handwriting Skills *Looks at the functional handwriting performance of the student in the classroom. Helps to identify areas that could impact handwriting or academic performance.*	No	Valid and Reliable	Quiet environment with minimal distractions	Gross and fine motor, visual motor, visual memory	Kindergarten and 1st grade-age

Work and Retirement

Name of Assessment tool, Author, and Publication date	Standardized	Validity/ Reliability	Setting Used	Areas Assessed	Age
Worker Environment Impact Scale (WEIS) *Assesses environmental characteristics that facilitate successful employment experiences. Goal is to maximize the "fit" of the worker and his or her skill to the job environment.*	No	Fair Validity and Reliability	Comfortable for the client	Space-related issues, fit of environment	Ages 16+
Worker Role Interview (WRI) *Identifies psychosocial and environmental factors that influence a client's ability to return to work.*	Yes	Valid and Reliable	Work, comfortable for client	Physical evaluation, essential job functions, psychosocial capacity to return to work	Ages 16+

Leisure (many ADL/IADL evaluations include leisure)

Name of Assessment tool, Author, and Publication date	Standardized	Validity/ Reliability	Setting Used	Areas Assessed	Age
Adolescent Leisure Interest Profile *Asks adolescent to report his or her interest and/or participation in a variety of age-appropriate leisure activities.*	No	Self-report, Valid and Reliable	Comfortable for the client	Sports, outdoor, summer, winter, indoor, creative	Ages 12 to 21
Adolescent Role Assessment (ARA) *Gathers information on the adolescent's occupational role involvement over time and across domains.*	No	Scores lack internal consistency	Comfortable for the client	Social integration, school, roles, play, family	Ages 13 to 20

Social Participation					
Name of Assessment tool, Author, and Publication date	Standardized	Validity/ Reliability	Setting Used	Areas Assessed	Age
Coping Inventory *Profiles coping styles, as well as behaviors, that facilitate or interfere with adaptive coping. Self-administered and profiled.*	No	Self-report and observation	Comfortable for the client	Sensorimotor, reactive behavior, self-initiated behavior, adaptive coping	Ages 15+
Life Satisfaction Index *Looking at five factors that make up total life satisfaction (pleasure, meaningfulness, feeling of success, self-image, happiness).*	Yes	Valid and Reliable	Comfortable for the client	Activity, developmental theory, internal satisfaction	Ages 50 to 90
Occupational Questionnaire (OQ) *Self-report assessment. Client documents the main activity in which he or she engages for each half-hour throughout the morning/day/evening and identifies each activity as work, ADL, recreation, or rest. Explores the meaning of leisure from the client's perspective.*	Yes	Valid and Reliable	Clinic or home setting	IADLs, volition, activity pattern, life satisfaction, interests, values, personal causation	Ages 13+
Social Profile *Assessment of activity participation, social interaction, and membership roles in a group.*	No	Valid and Reliable; Ongoing research	Activity focused	Individualized to client choices	Adolescents and adults
Volitional Questionnaire *Observational assessment, gathers information on a client's volition.*	Yes	Valid	Observations are context specific: leisure, work, ADL environments	MOHO, volition subsystem, work, leisure, intrinsic motivation, values, interests	Ages 16+

Wellness

Name of Assessment tool, Author, and Publication date	Standardized	Validity/ Reliability	Setting Used	Areas Assessed	Age
Engagement in Meaningful Activities Survey (EMAS) *Clients read statements about activities, put an 'X' in the box that best describes them (never to always).*	Yes, for research purposes only	Valid and Reliable	Comfortable for the client	Activities	Adult/elderly
Measure of Sub-Acute Rehabilitation Potential *Uses a five-point rating scale to assess health status, history, hope, help, health efforts.*	No		90-day type clinical setting	Health status, history, hope, help, health efforts	Adult/elderly
Stress Management Questionnaire (SMQ) *Identification of symptoms linked to stress and coping strategies that aid in the reduction of stress.*	Yes	Valid and Reliable	Comfortable for the client	Coping, stressors, behavioral theory	Adult/elderly

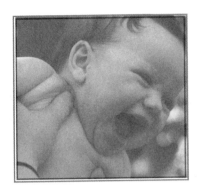

ASSESSMENTS IN PLAY AND LEISURE

Jacobs, K., MacRae, N., & Sladyk, K. (Eds.).
Occupational Therapy Essentials for
Clinical Competence, Second Edition (pp. 787-794).
© 2014 SLACK Incorporated.

Play Assessments

CHILD-INITIATED PRETEND PLAY ASSESSMENT

Ages	Children 3 to 7 years of age
Purpose	Measures the quality of spontaneous pretend play (Bundy, 2005)
Format/ Procedure	Observation of play in two 15-minute sessions. Assesses three items—elaborate play actions, substitutions, and imitated actions. Involves imaginative play with typical toys and symbolic, unstructured play. Author recommends that the administrator should be professionally trained to work with children (Bundy, 2005)
Psychometric Properties	Scoring manual is unpublished. Internal consistency = not reported. Interrater reliability (involves use of videotapes): elaborate play actions 0.96 or 0.98; substitutions 1.00 or 0.97; imitated actions 0.98 to 1.00; Test-retest reliability: elaborate play actions $r = 0.73$ to $r = 0.85$; substitutions $r = 0.56$ to $r = 0.57$. Distribution of the remaining items was not normal. Content validity has been established via expert review, and play items were tested for developmental sensitivity and gender neutrality; Construct validity = not reported (Bundy, 2005). Interrater reliability also established at kappa 0.7 (Swindells & Stagnitti, 2006)

CHILDREN'S PLAYFULNESS SCALE

Ages	Preschool- and toddler-aged children
Purpose	Measures the predisposition to be playful
Format/ Procedure	Twenty-three item instrument categorized into five areas of playfulness: physical spontaneity, social spontaneity, cognitive spontaneity, manifest joy, and sense of humor. Rater scored based on observations
Psychometric Properties	Interrater reliability ranged from 0.92 to 0.97; Test-retest reliability ranged from 0.84 to 0.88 at 1 month, 0.88 to 0.92 at 3 months, and 0.89 to 0.95 between the two intervals. Internal consistency for the scales ranged from 0.80 to 0.89 and 0.88 overall. Content validity based on playfulness research; Construct validity reported (Asher, 1996)

(REVISED) KNOX PRESCHOOL PLAY SCALE

Ages	Children 0 to 6 years of age
Purpose	Provides child's capacity for play and some information regarding play interests. Has been used for both diagnostic purposes and as an outcome measure for intervention (Bundy, 2005)
Format/ Procedure	Observation of play inside and outside in familiar settings and with familiar toys and peers. Four dimensions of play are observed: space management, material management, imitation, and participation. Administered in two 30-minute observations (Bundy, 2005; Sturgess, 1997)
Psychometric Properties	Not standardized as administration occurs in familiar environments. Internal consistency-not reported; Interrater reliability-coefficients ranged from $r = 0.88$ to $r = 0.996$; $P = 0.0001$; Test-retest reliability-coefficients range from $r = 0.91$ to $r = 0.965$; $P = 0.0001$; content validity has been established via an extensive review of the literature; Construct validity-not reported (Bundy, 2005; Rodger & Ziviani, 1999; Stagnitti, 2004)

PENN INTERACTIVE PEER PLAY SCALE

Ages	Preschool and kindergarten age in disadvantaged urban areas
Purpose	Developed to assess peer play interactions in disadvantaged urban children at risk for experiencing disconnection between school and home life (Fantuzzo & Hampton, 2000)
Format/ Procedure	Parallel versions of parent and teacher rating scales, with preschool and kindergarten versions. The parent versions assess play in the home and neighborhood, and the teacher version examines play in structured and unstructured school activities. Each version is composed of 32 items indicating the frequency the behavior is observed during free play within the preceding 2 months in three constructs: play interaction, play disruption, and play disconnection (Fantuzzo & Hampton)
Psychometric Properties	Each construct demonstrated a Cronbach alpha reliability of 0.90, 0.91, and 0.87. Inter-rater reliability of each construct was 0.84, 0.81, and 0.74. Content validity based on theoretical research. Congruence among test items was established (Fantuzzo & Hampton)

PLAY HISTORY

Ages	0 to 16 years
Purpose	Caregiver perspective of children's play; a tool for intervention planning
Format/ Procedure	Semi-structured interview administered to parents and/or caregivers; gather information on past play experiences and actual play; records play in five epochs—sensorimotor, symbolic, and simple constructive; dramatic; complex constructive; pre-game; and recreational. Each section is divided into four elements: materials, actions, people, and setting (Bundy, 2005; Sturgess, 1997; Taylor, Menarchek-Fetkovich, & Day, 2000)
Psychometric Properties	Test-retest reliability coefficient was 0.77 with section coefficients ranging from 0.41 to 0.78; Inter-rater reliability using videotaped interviews was 0.91 with section coefficients ranging from 0.58-0.85. Reliability was higher for typically developing children than children with disabilities (Behnke & Menarchek-Fetkovich, 1984); content validity based on theoretical research (Bundy; Taylor et al.)

PLAY IN EARLY CHILDHOOD EDUCATION SYSTEM

Ages	Early childhood
Purpose	To develop a standardized procedure for assessment and coding of play in preschoolers
Format/ Procedure	Still being developed
Psychometric Properties	Relatively new assessment that is still being developed and standardized. Research is limited. However, initial studies indicate reliability of the assessment. Content validity is reported by the authors secondary to development based on empirical research (Kelly-Vance & Ryalls, 2005)

SYMBOLIC PLAY TEST

Ages	Ages 1 to 3
Purpose	Developed to assess functional play skills typically demonstrated in children between 12 and 36 months (Power & Radcliffe, 2000)
Format/ Procedure	Children are observed in several modes of play, including tactile exploration, self-orientation, and doll orientation. Four sets of toys are presented in a specific manner. Administration takes approximately 15 to 20 minutes, and raw scores are obtained and converted to a developmental age (Power & Radcliffe). Assesses symbolic play to determine whether language development relates to difficulties with symbolism or concept formation (Sturgess, 1997)
Psychometric Properties	Split-half reliability coefficients were corrected by the Spearman-Brown formula and ranged from 0.52 to 0.92. Reliability coefficients at the 15- and 18-month age levels were low (0.57 and 0.52, respectively), borderline at the 12-, 21-, and 36-month levels (0.74-0.79), and acceptable at the 24- and 30-month levels (greater than 0.90). Test-retest reliability was 0.72 at 3 months. Floor and ceiling effects affect validity. Normative data was obtained on 137 children, with much of the testing occurring on the same children. This included seven age ranges with small sample sizes within each range (Power & Radcliffe)

TEST OF PLAYFULNESS

Ages	3 months to 15 years
Purpose	Captures the four playfulness components: intrinsic motivation, internal control, freedom from some constraints of reality, and framing (Bundy, 2005)
Format/ Procedure	29 observational items; each item is scored 0 to 3 reflecting extent, intensity, or skill. Administered during 15 to 20 minutes of free play in a familiar environment. Author urges administration in more than one environment (Bundy, 2005); The Test of Playfulness continues to be developed and researched (Stagnitti, 2004)
Psychometric Properties	Internal consistency—Cronbach's alpha was near 1.00; Interrater reliability—Rasch model goodness of fit; Test-retest reliability is being established and is not yet published; Content validity has been established via an extensive review of the literature; Construct validity—28/29 items demonstrate acceptable goodness of fit statistics using Rasch analysis (Bundy, 2005)

The Test of Playfulness (ToP) is not commercially available, but may be obtained by contacting the author, Anita Bundy, ScD, OTR, School of Occupation and Leisure Sciences, University of Sydney, PO Box 170, Lidcombe NSW, Australia, bookspublishing@slackinc.com (Bundy, 2005).

TRANSDISCIPLINARY PLAY-BASED ASSESSMENT 2ND EDITION

Ages	Children 0 to 6 years of age
Purpose	Captures the four playfulness components: intrinsic motivation, internal control, freedom from some constraints of reality, and framing (Bundy, 2005; Linder, 2000)
Format/ Procedure	29 observational items; each item is scored 0 to 3 reflecting extent, intensity, or skill. Administered during 15 to 20 minutes of free play in a familiar environment. Author urges administration in more than one environment (Bundy, 2005; Linder, 2000)
Psychometric Properties	Internal consistency—Cronbach's alpha was near 1.00; Interrater reliability—Rasch model goodness of fit; Test-retest reliability is being established and is not yet published; Content validity has been established via an extensive review of the literature; Construct validity—28/29 items demonstrate acceptable goodness of fit statistics using Rasch analysis (Bundy, 2005; Linder, 2000)

Leisure Assessments

ACTIVITY CARD SORT

Ages	Adults with and without cognitive impairment
Purpose	Originally designed to identify activity level for adults with Alzheimer's Disease; has been used with different populations. Includes Healthy Older Adult version, Institutional version, and Recovering version (Connolly, Law, & MacGuire, 2005)
Format/ Procedure	80 photo cards; caregiver or client sorts into categories. Categories vary depending upon version administered; Israeli version has been developed
Psychometric Properties	Test-retest reliability 0.897 (Baum & Edwards, 2001); internal consistency for Israeli version: high for IADL (0.82) and cultural activities (0.80) and moderate for low physical activities (0.66) and high physical activities (0.61) (Katz, Karpin, Lak, Furman, & Hartman-Maeir, 2003). Content and construct validity reported (Connolly et al., 2005)

CHILDREN'S ASSESSMENT OF PARTICIPATION AND ENJOYMENT

Ages	From ages 6 to 21; should be able to sort/categorize (Connolly et al., 2005)
Purpose	Identify participation in/enjoyment of daily activities
Format/ Procedure	55 item instrument; divided into five scales: recreational, active physical, social, skill-based, and self-improvement/educational. Can be categorized into formal and informal activities. Measures participation in five areas: diversity of activity, intensity/frequency, with whom activity occurs, where activity occurs, and enjoyment of activity. Includes two versions: self-administered and interviewer-assisted (Connolly et al.)
Psychometric Properties	Test-retest reliability ranges from 0.12 to 0.86. Internal consistency ranged from 0.32 to 0.62. Content, construct, and criterion validity are reported (Connolly et al.)

INTEREST CHECKLIST/ACTIVITY CHECKLIST

Ages	Adolescent to adult
Purpose	Identify an individual's level of interest in leisure activities
Format/ Procedure	Original Interest Checklist included 80 items in five categories: manual skills, physical sports, social recreation, ADL, and cultural/educational (Matsutsuyu, 1969). Revised and renamed Activity Checklist contains 60 items in four categories: sports and physical tasks, intellectual and musical tasks, social tasks, and fine manual tasks and homemaking (Katz, 1988). Both are self-report instruments with level of interest rating.
Psychometric Properties	Test retest reliability at three weeks ranged from 0.84 to 0.92 for each category and 0.92 overall (Asher, 1996); internal consistency has not been reported. Testing on content validity has revealed mixed results (Connolly et al., 2005).

LEISURE ACTIVITY PROFILE

Population	Diagnosis of alcoholism
Purpose	Time use measurement of individuals with alcoholism; identifies dysfunctional patterns of leisure activities related to alcohol use (Mann & Talty, 1990)
Format/ Procedure	38 item instrument; 19 related to alcohol consumption. Self-report or interviewer administration. Client reports time spent in activities, with whom activities occur, enjoyment, and alcohol consumption during activities
Psychometric Properties	Test retest reliability $r = 0.90$ to $r = 0.94$. Internal consistency not reported. Content and construct validity reported (Connolly et al., 2005)

LEISURE ASSESSMENT INVENTORY

Population	Adults with mental retardation
Purpose	Measures leisure behavior for adults with mental retardation
Format/ Procedure	Contains four indices based upon a conceptual definition of leisure: The Leisure Activity Participation Index reflects a person's leisure repertoire and involves 50 picture-cued activity cards; the Leisure Preference and Leisure Interest Indices represent 2 different aspects of choice making to assess the perceived degree of well-being, self-worth, and self-determination experienced during leisure; and the Leisure Constraints Index measures the degree in which internal and external constraints inhibit engagement in new leisure activities. Administered using a structured, three-part interview (Hawkins, Ardovino, & Hsieh, 1998)
Psychometric Properties	Reliability: Leisure Activity Participation ($r = 0.84$, $P < 0.01$), Leisure Preference ($r = 0.53$, $P < 0.01$), Leisure Interest ($r = 0.77$, $P < 0.01$), and Leisure Constraints ($r = 0.48$, $P < 0.01$); Content validity at $P < 0.01$ for each index

LEISURE ATTITUDE SCALE

Population	
Purpose	To examine leisure attitude
Format/ Procedure	36 item instrument; three subscales assessing various aspects of attitude, including cognitive, affective, and behavioral subscales; Elderly version modified from original and includes 26 items measuring desired leisure, perceived leisure, self definition through work or leisure, affinity for leisure, and society's role in leisure planning. Can be administered as an interview or questionnaire (Teaff, Ernst, & Ernst, 1982)
Psychometric Properties	Overall reliability 0.95; subscales reliability: Cognitive 0.89; Affective 0.90; Behavioral 0.91 (Siegenthaler & O'Dell, 2000)

LEISURE BOREDOM SCALE

Ages	Adolescents and young adults
Purpose	Assess perception of boredom relative to leisure opportunities
Format/ Procedure	16-item self-report instrument rating relative to boredom
Psychometric Properties	Test-retest reliability $r = 0.73$ with 95% confidence interval; Moderate Cohen's Kappa for seven items (0.41 to 0.52); fair for two items (0.32 to 0.38); Internal consistency reported at 0.85; 0.86, 0.88; Construct validity reported (Connolly et al., 2005).

LEISURE COMPETENCE MEASURE

Ages	Adults
Purpose	Evaluates changes in leisure functioning
Format/ Procedure	Service provider rating based on observation, interview, and review of records; eight subscales including Leisure Awareness, Leisure Attitude, Leisure Skills, Cultural/Social Behaviors, Interpersonal Skills, Community Integration Skills, Social Contact, and Community Participation. Takes approximately 1 hour to administer
Psychometric Properties	No test-retest reliability reported; Inter-rater reliability = 0.91 overall and 0.71-0.91 for subscales; Internal consistency—Cronbach's Alpha 0.92; Content validity reported (Connolly et al., 2005)

LEISURE DIAGNOSTIC BATTERY [1]

Ages	Individuals with adapted IQ of 80 and higher; mental age 12 and older; Rancho Los Amigos level of seven and higher; mild to no orientation disability (Connolly et al., 2005)
Purpose	Identify client's leisure capacity
Format/ Procedure	Comprised of four assessments: Leisure Attitude Measure (LAM), Leisure Interest Measure (LIM), Leisure Motivation Scale (LMS), and Leisure Satisfaction Measure (LSM). Leisure Attitude Measure assesses leisure attitude on cognitive, affective, and behavioral levels; Leisure Interest Measure assesses interest in eight areas: physical, outdoor, mechanical, artistic, service, social, cultural, and reading. Leisure Motivation Scale includes 48 item Full Scale and 32 item Short Scale measuring client motivation; Leisure Satisfaction Measure assesses six satisfaction subscales: psychological, educational, social, relaxation, physiological, and aesthetic. Self report instruments
Psychometric Properties	Test-retest not reported. Internal consistency: LAM: 0.89-0.94; LIM: 0.87 overall, poor internal reliability in artistic domain, acceptable in all others; LMS: Authors report strong internal reliability (Beard & Ragheb, 1983); LSM: overall reliability 0.93; Content validity reported for all four assessments; Construct validity reported for LAM and LSM; Criterion validity reported for LAM (Connolly et al., 2005)

LEISURE DIAGNOSTIC BATTERY [2]

Ages	One version for youth with disabilities; one for adults
Purpose	Assess perception of freedom and barriers to participation in leisure
Format/ Procedure	147 item Full Forms (A and C; youth and adults, respectively) related to control, competence, needs, playfulness, barriers, and knowledge. 25-item Short Form (B). Both forms are self-report instruments.
Psychometric Properties	Test retest (Form A) 0.72. Internal consistency 0.83 to 0.94 (Form A), 0.89 to 0.94 (Form B), and 0.90 to 0.96 (Form C). Content and construct validity reported for Form A (Connolly et al., 2005)

LEISURE SATISFACTION SCALE

Ages	Adults
Purpose	To examine leisure satisfaction and the extent in which individuals perceive their needs are being met through participation in leisure activities
Format/ Procedure	Self report measure; Original version: 51 item instrument; six subscales assessing satisfaction, including Psychological, Educational, Social, Relaxational, Physiological, and Aesthetic subscales; Short Form: 24 item instrument; same six subscales as original version
Psychometric Properties	Test-retest reliability not reported; One study reports reliability at 0.96 (Siegenthaler & O'Dell, 2000); Internal consistency ranged from 0.86 to 0.92 for subtest and overall 0.96 (original version) and 0.93 (short form). Content validity reported (Connolly et al., 2005)

PREFERENCES FOR ACTIVITIES OF CHILDREN	
Ages	From ages 6 to 21; should be able to sort/categorize (Connolly et al., 2005)
Purpose	Identify activity preferences
Format/ Procedure	55 item instrument; five activity scales: Recreational, Active Physical, Social, Skill-Based, and Self-Improvement/Educational in two domains: formal and informal activities. Can be self administered or inter-viewer-assisted (Connolly et al., 2005)
Psychometric Properties	Test-retest reliability not reported; Intenal consistency ranged from 0.67 to 0.84. Content validity reported; Construct validity related to participation outcome variables ($r < 0.01$); correlations with CAPE ranged from 0.22 to 0.61 (Connolly et al., 2005)

References

Asher, I. E. (1996). *Occupational therapy assessment tools: An annotated index* (2nd ed.). Bethesda, MD: AOTA Press.

Baum, C. M., & Edwards, D. (2001). *Activity card sort*. St. Louis, MO: Washington University at St. Louis.

Beard, J. G., & Ragheb, M. G. (1983). Measuring leisure motivation. *Journal of Leisure Research, 15*(3), 219-228.

Behnke, C. J., & Menarchek-Fetkovich, M. M. (1984). Examining the reliability and validity of the Play History. *American Journal of Occupational Therapy, 38*(2), 94-100.

Bundy, A. C. (2005). Measuring play performance. In M. Law, C. Baum, & W. Dunn (Eds.), *Measuring occupational performance: Supporting best practice in occupational therapy* (2nd ed., pp. 129-150). Thorofare, NJ: SLACK Incorporated.

Connolly, K., Law, M., & MacGuire, B. (2005). Measuring leisure performance. In M. Law, W. Dunn, & C. Baum (Eds.), *Measuring occupational performance: Supporting best practice in occupational therapy* (2nd ed., pp. 249-276). Thorofare, NJ: SLACK Incorporated.

Fantuzzo, J. W., & Hampton, V. R. (2000). Penn Interactive Peer Play Scale: A parent and teacher rating system for young children. In K. Gitlin-Weiner, S. Sandgrund, & C. Schaefer (Eds.), *Play diagnosis and assessment* (2nd ed., pp. 599-620). New York, NY: John Wiley & Sons.

Hawkins, B. A., Ardovino, P., & Hsieh, C. (1998). Validity and reliability of the Leisure Assessment Inventory. *Mental Retardation, 36*(4), 303-313.

Katz, N. (1988). Interest checklist: A factor analytical study. *Occupational Therapy in Mental Health, 8*(1), 45-55.

Katz, N., Karpin, H., Lak, A., Furman, T., & Hartman-Maeir, A. (2003). Participation in occupational performance: Reliability and validity of the Activity Card Sort. *Occupational Therapy Journal of Research, 23*(1), 10-17.

Kelly-Vance, L., & Ryalls, B. O. (2005). A systematic, reliable approach to play assessment in preschoolers. *School Psychology International, 26*(4), 398-412.

Linder, T. (2000). Transdisciplinary play-based assessment. In K. Gitlin-Weiner, S. Sandgrund, & C. Schaefer (Eds.), *Play diagnosis and assessment* (2nd ed., pp. 139-166). New York, NY: John Wiley & Sons.

Mann, W. C., & Talty, P. (1990). Leisure Activity Profile: Measuring use of leisure time by persons with alcoholism. *Occupational Therapy in Mental Health, 10*(4), 31-41.

Matsutsuyu, J. S. (1969). The Interest Checklist. *American Journal of Occupational Therapy, 23*, 323-328.

Power, T. J., & Radcliffe, J. (2000). Assessing the cognitive ability of infants and toddlers through play: The Symbolic Play Test. In K. Gitlin-Weiner, A. Sandgrund, & C. Schaefer (Eds.), *Play diagnosis and assessment* (2nd ed., pp. 58-79). New York, NY: John Wiley & Sons.

Rodger, S., & Ziviani, J. (1999). Play-based occupational therapy. *International Journal of Disability, Development, and Education, 46*(3), 337-365.

Siegenthaler, K. L., & O'Dell, I. (2000). Leisure attitude, leisure satisfaction, and perceived freedom in leisure within family dyads. *Leisure Sciences, 22*(4), 281-296.

Stagnitti, K. (2004). Understanding play: The implications for play assessment. *Australian Occupational Therapy Journal, 51*, 3-12.

Sturgess, J. L. (1997). Current trends in assessing children's play. *British Journal of Occupational Therapy, 60*(9), 410-414.

Swindells, D., & Stagnitti, K. (2006). Pretend play and parents' view of social competence: The construct validity of the Child-Initiated Pretend Play Assessment. *Australian Occupational Therapy Journal, 53*, 314-324.

Taylor, K. M., Menarchek-Fetkovich, M., & Day, C. (2000). The Play History interview. In K. Gitlin-Weiner, S. Sandgrund, & C. Schaefer (Eds.), *Play diagnosis and assessment* (2nd ed., pp. 114-138). New York, NY: John Wiley & Sons.

Teaff, J. D., Ernst, N. W., & Ernst, M. (1982). Elderly Leisure Attitude Scale. In D. J. Mangen & W. A. Peterson (Eds.), *Research instruments in social gerontology: Vol. 2. Social roles and social participation* (pp. 498-499; 535-537). Minneapolis, MN: University of Minnesota Press.

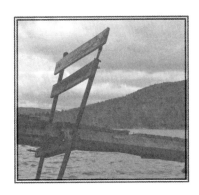

D

Intervention Plan Outline

Jacobs, K., MacRae, N., & Sladyk, K. (Eds.).
Occupational Therapy Essentials for
Clinical Competence, Second Edition (pp. 795-796).
© 2014 SLACK Incorporated.

Intervention Plan

Client's name:
Age:
Date of plan:
How long will sessions be? Where? When?:

Diagnosis:

Background information:

Precautions:

Strengths and weaknesses:

Goals and objectives:

Frame of reference:

- Principles of the frame of reference that will be used to design intervention:

- Rationale for using frame of reference:

- Evidence to support using frame of reference with this type of client:

Sample activity selection:

Progression of activities—how will they be graded and adapted?:

Equipment needs:

Safety concerns:

Describe the role of the occupational therapy practitioner according to the frame of reference:

Describe what is expected of the client:

Other:

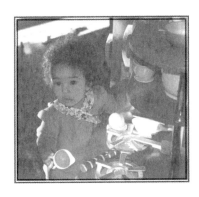

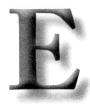

SAMPLE OF AN
INDIVIDUAL EDUCATION PLAN

Barbara J. Steva, MS, OTR/L

Jacobs, K., MacRae, N., & Sladyk, K. (Eds.).
Occupational Therapy Essentials for
Clinical Competence, Second Edition (pp. 797-803).
© 2014 SLACK Incorporated.

Maine Unified Special Education Regulations (MUSER) IX.3.G.

Maine
Department of
Education

INDIVIDUALIZED EDUCATION PROGRAM (IEP)

SAU/School/Grade or CDS Placement: Arundel, Kennebunk, Kennebunkport Regional School Unit 21 / Mildred L Day School / 01

Date IEP Sent to Parent: 5/23/2013

Date of Meeting:	05/02/2013
Effective Date of IEP:	5/6/2013 – 5/1/2014
Date of Annual IEP Review:	5/1/2014
Date of Re-evaluation:	4/28/2016
Date(s) of Amended IEP:	N/A
Case Manager:	▊▊▊▊

1. CHILD INFORMATION

Child's Name: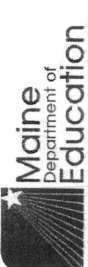

Date of Birth: 8/11/2005   Age: 7

School/Program: Mildred L Day School   Grade: 01

Parent Information:

State Agency Client: Yes ☐   No ☒

2. DISABILITY (MUSER) VII.2

☐ Autism
☐ Developmental Delay (ages 3-5)
☐ Hearing Impairment
☐ Other Health Impairment
☒ Specific Learning Disability

☐ Deaf-Blindness
☐ Developmental Delay (Kindergarten)
☐ Intellectual Disability
☐ Orthopedic Impairment
☐ Traumatic Brain Injury

☐ Deafness
☐ Emotional Disturbance
☐ Multiple Disabilities(list concomitant disabilities)
☐ Speech/Language Impairment
☐ Visual Impairment (Including Blindness)

Child's Name: ▉

3. CONSIDERATIONS

In developing each child's IEP, the IEP team must consider – MUSER.IX.3.C.

A. Concerns of parents for enhancing the education of their child. MUSER IX.3.C.(1)(b)

▉ is pleased with the results of the evaluation. She is happy that ▉ will be receiving services. She expressed that it is frustrating sometimes when she is unable to help him understand information. She said that he is very uncoordinated but is very active at home.

B. Results of the initial evaluation or most recent evaluation of the child. MUSER IX.3.C.(1)(c)

April 2013:

WISC-IV: Verbal Comprehension Composite Score 98, 45%; Perceptual Reasoning Composite Score 90, 25%; Working Memory Composite Score 83, 13%; Processing Speed Composite Score 70, 2%; Full Scale Composite Score 83, 13%.

WRMT: Readiness SS 83, 13%; Basic Skills 70, 2%; Reading Comprehension 81, 10%; Total Reading 70, 2%.

KeyMath3: Basic Concepts SS 97, 42%; Operations 90, 25%; Applications 88, 21%; Total Test Composite 89, 23%.

Peabody Picture Vocabulary Test-4: SS 140, 99.6%
Expressive Vocabulary Test-2: SS 112, 79%
CELF-4: Core Language Score SS 102, 55%; Receptive Language Index 117, 87%; Expressive Language Index 101, 53%; Language Content Index 121, 92%; Language Structure Index 106, 66%.

Beery Developmental Test of Visual Motor Integration-6: Visual Motor Integration SS 71, 3%; Visual Perception 104,61%; Motor Coordination Unable to Score. Bruininks-Oseretsky Test of Motor Proficiency-2: Fine Motor Precision 9; Fine Motor Integration 10; Manual Dexterity 14; Upper Limb Coordination 16; Fine Manual Control 37, 10%; Manual Coordination 50, 50%; Motor Free Visual Perception Test 95, 37%.

C. Strengths of the child. MUSER IX.3.C.(1)(a)

▉ has great communication skills with adults. Has strength in expressive and receptive language skills.

D. Needs of the child – academic, developmental, and functional. MUSER IX.3.C.(1)(d)

Academic: Due to his weaknesses in Processing Speed and Working Memory ▉ requires specially designed instruction in Reading and Writing to access the General Education Curriculum.

Developmental: ▉s poor muscle strength through his core muscles impacts his ability to maintain a stable base on which to build refined fine motor control needed to complete academic tasks at a level consistent with same age and grade level peers.

Functional: Due to his difficulty with forming peer relations and anxious behaviors ▉ will benefit from Social Work services to help access the general education curriculum.

Child's Name: ▓▓▓▓

Consideration of Special Factors: The IEP Team must - MUSER IX.3.C.(2)

E. In the case of a child whose behavior impedes the child's learning or that of others consider the use of positive behavioral interventions and supports and other strategies to address the behavior. MUSER IX.3.C.(2)(a)

Check if not needed [x]   **If needed, indicate where it is addressed in the IEP.**

F. In the case of a child with limited English proficiency, consider the language needs of the child as those needs relate to the child's IEP. MUSER IX.3.C.(2)(b)

Check if not needed [x]   **If needed, indicate where it is addressed in the IEP.**

G. In the case of a child who is blind or visually impaired, provide for instruction in Braille and the use of Braille unless the IEP Team determines, after an evaluation of the child's reading and writing skills, needs, and appropriate reading and writing media (including an evaluation of the child's future needs for instruction in Braille or the use of Braille), that instruction in Braille or the use of Braille is not appropriate for the child. MUSER IX.3.C.(2)(c)

Check if not needed [x]   **If needed, indicate where it is addressed in the IEP.**

H. Consider the communication needs of the child, and in the case of a child who is deaf or hard of hearing, consider the child's language and communication needs, opportunities for direct communication with peers and professional personnel in the child's language and communication mode, academic level, and full range of needs including opportunities for direct instruction in the child's language and communication mode. MUSER IX.3.C.(2)(d)

Check if not needed [ ]   **If needed, indicate where it is addressed in the IEP.**
FM System as needed in the regular education classroom only.

I. Consider whether the child needs assistive technology devices and services. MUSER IX.3.C.(2)(e)

Check if not needed [x]   **If needed, indicate where it is addressed in the IEP.**

Child's Name: ▆▆▆

4. PRESENT LEVELS OF ACADEMIC AND FUNCTIONAL PERFORMANCE   MUSER IX.3.A.(1)(a)(i)&(ii)

A statement of Present levels of academic achievement and functional performance.

Goal ID: 21622   Academic
Currently, ▆▆ independently uses a Powerplan to initiate the writing process 15% of the time as measured by Teacher Observations.

Goal ID: 21621   Academic
Currently, ▆▆ has a grade equivalent score of <1.0 on Oral Reading Fluency as measured by the WRMT-III.

Goal ID: 21620   Academic
Currently, ▆▆ has a Basic Reading Skills grade equivalent score of <1.0 as measured by WRMT-III.

Goal ID: 21702   OT
Currently, ▆▆ uses bilateral coordination and graded motions to cut 1/16" lines, containing at least two directional changes, with no more than 2 deviations from the line, 10% of trials.

Goal ID: 21700   OT
Currently, ▆▆ demonstrates the ability to plan, sequence, and carry out a motor task, requiring right and left side and upper and lower extremity coordination, 20% of the time.

Goal ID: 21699   OT
Currently, ▆▆ independently creates and constructs projects (including gathering needed materials and sequencing of steps), involving 4 or more steps from a model, 30% of the time.

Goal ID: 21689   OT
Currently, ▆▆ writes demonstrating spontaneous letter formation 83% of the time. The expectation for the end of first grade is 96%.
Currently, ▆▆ writes demonstrating appropriate placement on and within the writing lines 75% of the time. The expectation for the end of first grade is 88%.

Goal ID: 21618   PT
▆▆ runs around the gym 1 time without slowing down or stopping

Goal ID: 21617   PT
▆▆ will accesses 5 climbing items on the playground.

Goal ID: 21616   PT
▆▆ will sits upright on the floor and table top in a crossed legged pattern without leaning on arms for supports less than 30 seconds at a time.

Goal ID: 21615   PT
▆▆ squats to stand 4 times without the support of his hands

Goal ID: 21614   PT
▆▆ does not complete an exercise program.

Goal ID: 21639   Social/Emotional
Currently, ▆▆ is able to focus 50% of the time.

Goal ID: 21637   Social/Emotional
Based on staff reports ▆▆ interacts with peers appropriately 25% of the time.

How the child's disability affects the child's involvement and progress in the general education curriculum. For preschool children, as appropriate, how the disability affects the child's participation in appropriate activities.

▆▆ has weaknesses in Processing Speed and Working Memory. He needs specially designed instruction in reading, writing, Physical Therapy, and Occupational Therapy in order to access the general education curriculum. ▆▆ has difficulty interacting with peers and making peer relationships and this adversely effects his academic setting.

Child's Name: ▮▮▮

5. ANNUAL GOAL(S)

A statement of measurable annual goals, including academic and functional goals, designed to: meet the child's needs that result from the child's disability to enable the child to be involved in and make progress in the general education curriculum which must be for children 3-5 aligned with the Early Learning Guidelines and for children 5-20 aligned with the system of Maine's Learning Results; and meet each of the child's other educational needs that result from the child's disability. The IEP shall reflect the individual goals to successfully meet the content standards of the system of Maine's Learning Results in addition to any other diploma requirements applicable to all secondary children pursuant to 20-A MRSA §4722.
Include below a statement of how the child's progress toward meeting the annual goals will be measured. MUSER IX.3.A.(1)(b)&(c).

Measurable Annual Goal	* 1, 2, 3, 4 For Pre School only	How Goal will be Measured	** PROGRESS
Goal ID: 21702 OT - Given therapeutic activities ▮▮▮ will use bilateral coordination and graded motions to cut 1/16" lines, containing at least two directional changes, with no more than 2 deviations from the line, 60% of trials, by May 2014.	N/A	Clinical data collection, informal assessment, work samples and observation of functional daily performance.	6/20/2013 12/6/2013 3/21/2014
Goal ID: 21700 OT - Given therapeutic activities to improve planning and dissociation of body parts, ▮▮▮ will demonstrate the ability to plan, sequence, and carry out a motor task, requiring right and left side and upper and lower extremity coordination, 60% of the time, by May 2014.	N/A	clinical data collection, informal assessment, and observation of functional daily performance	6/20/2013 12/6/2013 3/21/2014
Goal ID: 21699 OT - Given visual and verbal cues as needed and a completed model, ▮▮▮ will independently create and construct projects (including gathering needed materials and sequencing of steps), involving 4 or more steps from a model, 60% of the time, by May 2014.	N/A	clinical data colledtion, informal assessment, work samples and observation of functional daily performance	6/20/2013 12/6/2013 3/21/2014
Goal ID: 21689 OT - Given direct intervention, ▮▮▮ will write a minimum of two sentences, demonstrating spontaneous letter formation and correct letter height, spacing and placement within the writing lines, 90% of the time, by May 2014.	N/A	clinical data collection, informal assessment, work samples, and observation of functional daily performance	6/20/2013 12/6/2013 3/21/2014

Child's Name: ▓▓▓

7. SPECIAL EDUCATION AND RELATED SERVICES MUSER IX.3.A.(1)(d) & IX.3.A.(1)(g)

Special Education Services	Position Responsible	Location	Frequency	Duration Beginning/Ending Date
Specially Designed Instruction Reading and Writing	Special Educator	Special ed.	5 times per Week for 1 hour and 30 minutes	5/6/2013 to 5/1/2014

Related Services	Position Responsible	Location	Frequency	Duration Beginning/Ending Date
Social Work Service	Social Worker	Special ed.	2 times per Week for 30 minutes	5/6/2013 to 5/1/2014
Occupational Therapy	Occupational Therapist	Special ed.	2 times per Week for 30 minutes	5/6/2013 to 5/1/2014
Physical Therapy Services	Physical Therapist	Special ed.	2 times per Week for 30 minutes	5/6/2013 to 5/1/2014

9. LEAST RESTRICTIVE ENVIRONMENT

What percentage of time is this child with non-disabled children?
68%

An explanation of the extent, if any, to which the child will not participate with non disabled children in the regular class and in extracurricular and other nonacademic activities: MUSER IX.3.A.(1)(e)

▓▓▓ will participate in all regular education activities/settings with the exception of 5x1.5 hours per week of Specially Designed Instruction in Reading and Writing, 2x 30 minutes per week of Social Work, 2x30 minutes per week of Occupational Therapy, and 2x30 minutes per week of Physical Therapy.

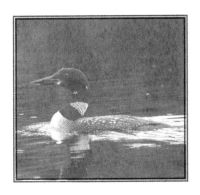

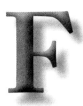

AMERICAN OCCUPATIONAL THERAPY
ASSOCIATION CODE OF ETHICS AND
ETHICS STANDARDS

*Reproduced with permission from the
American Occupational Therapy Association.*

Jacobs, K., MacRae, N., & Sladyk, K. (Eds.).
*Occupational Therapy Essentials for
Clinical Competence, Second Edition* (pp. 805-816).
© 2014 SLACK Incorporated.

Occupational Therapy Code of Ethics and Ethics Standards (2010)

PREAMBLE

The American Occupational Therapy Association (AOTA) *Occupational Therapy Code of Ethics and Ethics Standards (2010)* ("Code and Ethics Standards") is a public statement of principles used to promote and maintain high standards of conduct within the profession. Members of AOTA are committed to promoting inclusion, diversity, independence, and safety for all recipients in various stages of life, health, and illness and to empower all beneficiaries of occupational therapy. This commitment extends beyond service recipients to include professional colleagues, students, educators, businesses, and the community.

Fundamental to the mission of the occupational therapy profession is the therapeutic use of everyday life activities (occupations) with individuals or groups for the purpose of participation in roles and situations in home, school, workplace, community, and other settings. "Occupational therapy addresses the physical, cognitive, psychosocial, sensory, and other aspects of performance in a variety of contexts to support engagement in everyday life activities that affect health, well being, and quality of life" AOTA, 2004). Occupational therapy personnel have an ethical responsibility primarily to recipients of service and secondarily to society.

The *Occupational Therapy Code of Ethics and Ethics Standards (2010)* was tailored to address the most prevalent ethical concerns of the profession in education, research, and practice. The concerns of stakeholders including the public, consumers, students, colleagues, employers, research participants, researchers, educators, and practitioners were addressed in the creation of this document. A review of issues raised in ethics cases, member questions related to ethics, and content of other professional codes of ethics were utilized to ensure that the revised document is applicable to occupational therapists, occupational therapy assistants, and students in all roles.

The historical foundation of this Code and Ethics Standards is based on ethical reasoning surrounding practice and professional issues, as well as on empathic reflection regarding these interactions with others (see e.g., AOTA, 2005, 2006). This reflection resulted in the establishment of principles that guide ethical action, which goes beyond rote following of rules or application of principles. Rather, *ethical action* is a manifestation of moral character and mindful reflection. It is a commitment to benefit others, to virtuous practice of artistry and science, to genuinely good behaviors, and to noble acts of courage.

While much has changed over the course of the profession's history, more has remained the same. The profession of occupational therapy remains grounded in seven core concepts, as identified in the *Core Values and Attitudes of Occupational Therapy Practice* (AOTA, 1993): *altruism, equality, freedom, justice, dignity, truth,* and *prudence. Altruism* is the individual's ability to place the needs of others before their own. *Equality* refers to the desire to promote fairness in interactions with others. The concept of *freedom* and personal choice is paramount in a profession in which the desires of the client must guide our interventions. Occupational therapy practitioners, educators, and researchers relate in a fair and impartial manner to individuals with whom they interact and respect and adhere to the applicable laws and standards regarding their area of practice, be it direct care, education, or research *(justice).* Inherent in the practice of occupational therapy is the promotion and preservation of the individuality and *dignity* of the client, by assisting him or her to engage in occupations that are meaningful to him or her regardless of level of disability. In all situations, occupational therapists, occupational therapy assistants, and students must provide accurate information, both in oral and written form (*truth*). Occupational therapy personnel use their clinical and ethical reasoning skills, sound judgment, and reflection to make decisions to direct them in their area(s) of practice (*prudence*). These seven core values provide a foundation by which occupational therapy personnel guide their interactions with others, be they students, clients, colleagues, research participants, or communities. These values also define the ethical principles to which the profession is committed and which the public can expect.

The *Occupational Therapy Code of Ethics and Ethics Standards* (*2010*) is a guide to professional conduct when ethical issues arise. Ethical decision making is a process that includes awareness of how the outcome will impact occupational therapy clients in all spheres. Applications of Code and Ethics Standards Principles are considered situation-specific, and where a conflict exists, occupational therapy personnel will pursue responsible efforts for resolution. These Principles apply to occupational therapy personnel engaged in any professional role, including elected and volunteer leadership positions.

The specific purposes of the *Occupational Therapy Code of Ethics and Ethics Standards (2010)* are to

1. Identify and describe the principles supported by the occupational therapy profession.

2. Educate the general public and members regarding established principles to which occupational therapy personnel are accountable.

3. Socialize occupational therapy personnel to expected standards of conduct.

4. Assist occupational therapy personnel in recognition and resolution of ethical dilemmas.

The *Occupational Therapy Code of Ethics and Ethics Standards (2010)* define the set of principles that apply to occupational therapy personnel at all levels:

DEFINITIONS
*   **Recipient of service:** Individuals or groups receiving occupational therapy.
*   **Student:** A person who is enrolled in an accredited occupational therapy education program.
*   **Research participant:** A prospective participant or one who has agreed to participate in an approved research project.
*   **Employee:** A person who is hired by a business (facility or organization) to provide occupational therapy services.
*   **Colleague:** A person who provides services in the same or different business (facility or organization) to which a professional relationship exists or may exist.
*   **Public:** The community of people at large.

BENEFICENCE

Principle 1. Occupational therapy personnel shall demonstrate a concern for the well-being and safety of the recipients of their services.

Beneficence includes all forms of action intended to benefit other persons. The term *beneficence* connotes acts of mercy, kindness, and charity (Beauchamp & Childress, 2009). Forms of beneficence typically include altruism, love, and humanity. Beneficence requires taking action by helping others, in other words, by promoting good, by preventing harm, and by removing harm. Examples of beneficence include protecting and defending the rights of others, preventing harm from occurring to others, removing conditions that will cause harm to others, helping persons with disabilities, and rescuing persons in danger (Beauchamp & Childress, 2009).

Occupational therapy personnel shall

A. Respond to requests for occupational therapy services (e.g., a referral) in a timely manner as determined by law, regulation, or policy.

B. Provide appropriate evaluation and a plan of intervention for all recipients of occupational therapy services specific to their needs.

C. Reevaluate and reassess recipients of service in a timely manner to determine if goals are being achieved and whether intervention plans should be revised.

D. Avoid the inappropriate use of outdated or obsolete tests/assessments or data obtained from such tests in making intervention decisions or recommendations.

E. Provide occupational therapy services that are within each practitioner's level of competence and scope of practice (e.g., qualifications, experience, the law).

F. Use, to the extent possible, evaluation, planning, intervention techniques, and therapeutic equipment that are evidence-based and within the recognized scope of occupational therapy practice.

G. Take responsible steps (e.g., continuing education, research, supervision, training) and use careful judgment to ensure their own competence and weigh potential for client harm when generally recognized standards do not exist in emerging technology or areas of practice.

H. Terminate occupational therapy services in collaboration with the service recipient or responsible party when the needs and goals of the recipient have been met or when services no longer produce a measurable change or outcome.

I. Refer to other health care specialists solely on the basis of the needs of the client.

J. Provide occupational therapy education, continuing education, instruction, and training that are within the instructor's subject area of expertise and level of competence.

K. Provide students and employees with information about the Code and Ethics Standards, opportunities to discuss ethical conflicts, and procedures for reporting unresolved ethical conflicts.

L. Ensure that occupational therapy research is conducted in accordance with currently accepted ethical guidelines and standards for the protection of research participants and the dissemination of results.

M. Report to appropriate authorities any acts in practice, education, and research that appear unethical or illegal.

N. Take responsibility for promoting and practicing occupational therapy on the basis of current knowledge and research and for further developing the profession's body of knowledge.

NONMALEFICENCE

Principle 2. Occupational therapy personnel shall intentionally refrain from actions that cause harm.

Nonmaleficence imparts an obligation to refrain from harming others (Beauchamp & Childress, 2009). The principle of nonmaleficence is grounded in the practitioner's responsibility to refrain from causing harm, inflicting injury, or wronging others. While beneficence requires action to incur benefit, nonmaleficence requires non-action to avoid harm (Beauchamp & Childress, 2009). Nonmaleficence also includes an obligation to not impose risks of harm even if the potential risk is without malicious or harmful intent. This principle often is examined under the context of *due care*. If the standard of due care outweighs the benefit of treatment, then refraining from treatment provision would be ethically indicated (Beauchamp & Childress, 2009).

Occupational therapy personnel shall

A. Avoid inflicting harm or injury to recipients of occupational therapy services, students, research participants, or employees.

B. Make every effort to ensure continuity of services or options for transition to appropriate services to avoid abandoning the service recipient if the current provider is unavailable due to medical or other absence or loss of employment.

C. Avoid relationships that exploit the recipient of services, students, research participants, or employees physically, emotionally, psychologically, financially, socially, or in any other manner that conflicts or interferes with professional judgment and objectivity.

D. Avoid engaging in any sexual relationship or activity, whether consensual or nonconsensual, with any recipient of service, including family or significant other, student, research participant, or employee, while a relationship exists as an occupational therapy practitioner, educator, researcher, supervisor, or employer.

E. Recognize and take appropriate action to remedy personal problems and limitations that might cause harm to recipients of service, colleagues, students, research participants, or others.

F. Avoid any undue influences, such as alcohol or drugs, that may compromise the provision of occupational therapy services, education, or research.

G. Avoid situations in which a practitioner, educator, researcher, or employer is unable to maintain clear professional boundaries or objectivity to ensure the safety and well-being of recipients of service, students, research participants, and employees.

H. Maintain awareness of and adherence to the Code and Ethics Standards when participating in volunteer roles.

I. Avoid compromising client rights or well-being based on arbitrary administrative directives by exercising professional judgment and critical analysis.

J. Avoid exploiting any relationship established as an occupational therapist or occupational therapy assistant to further one's own physical, emotional, financial, political, or business interests at the expense of the best interests of recipients of services, students, research participants, employees, or colleagues.

K. Avoid participating in bartering for services because of the potential for exploitation and conflict of interest unless there are clearly no contraindications or bartering is a culturally appropriate custom.

L. Determine the proportion of risk to benefit for participants in research prior to implementing a study.

AUTONOMY AND CONFIDENTIALITY

Principle 3. Occupational therapy personnel shall respect the right of the individual to self-determination.

The principle of autonomy and confidentiality expresses the concept that practitioners have a duty to treat the client according to the client's desires, within the bounds of accepted standards of care and to protect the client's confidential information. Often *autonomy* is referred to as the *self-determination* principle. However, respect for autonomy goes beyond acknowledging an individual as a mere agent and also acknowledges a "person's right to hold views, to make choices, and to take actions based on personal values and beliefs" (Beauchamp & Childress, 2009, p. 103). Autonomy has become a prominent principle in health care ethics; the right to make a determination regarding care decisions that directly impact the life of the service recipient should reside with that individual. The principle of autonomy and confidentiality also applies to students in an educational program, to participants in research studies, and to the public who seek information about occupational therapy services.

Occupational therapy personnel shall

A. Establish a collaborative relationship with recipients of service including families, significant others, and caregivers in setting goals and priorities throughout the intervention process. This includes full disclosure of the benefits, risks, and potential outcomes of any intervention; the personnel who will be providing the intervention(s); and/or any reasonable alternatives to the proposed intervention.

B. Obtain consent before administering any occupational therapy service, including evaluation, and ensure that recipients of service (or their legal representatives) are kept informed of the progress in meeting goals specified in the plan of intervention/care. If the service recipient cannot give consent, the practitioner must be sure that consent has been obtained from the person who is legally responsible for that recipient.

C. Respect the recipient of service's right to refuse occupational therapy services temporarily or permanently without negative consequences.

D. Provide students with access to accurate information regarding educational requirements and academic policies and procedures relative to the occupational therapy program/educational institution.

E. Obtain informed consent from participants involved in research activities, and ensure that they understand the benefits, risks, and potential outcomes as a result of their participation as research subjects.

F. Respect research participant's right to withdraw from a research study without consequences.

G. Ensure that confidentiality and the right to privacy are respected and maintained regarding all information obtained about recipients of service, students, research participants, colleagues, or employees. The only exceptions are when a practitioner or staff member believes that an individual is in serious foreseeable or imminent harm. Laws and regulations may require disclosure to appropriate authorities without consent.

H. Maintain the confidentiality of all verbal, written, electronic, augmentative, and non-verbal communications, including compliance with HIPAA regulations.

I. Take appropriate steps to facilitate meaningful communication and comprehension in cases in which the recipient of service, student, or research participant has limited ability to communicate (e.g., aphasia or differences in language, literacy, culture).

J. Make every effort to facilitate open and collaborative dialogue with clients and/or responsible parties to facilitate comprehension of services and their potential risks/benefits.

SOCIAL JUSTICE

Principle 4. Occupational therapy personnel shall provide services in a fair and equitable manner.

Social justice, also called *distributive justice,* refers to the fair, equitable, and appropriate distribution of resources. The principle of social justice refers broadly to the distribution of all rights and responsibilities in society (Beauchamp & Childress, 2009). In general, the principle of social justice supports the concept of achieving justice in every aspect of society rather than merely the administration of law. The general idea is that individuals and groups should receive fair treatment and an impartial share of the benefits of society. Occupational therapy personnel have a vested interest in addressing unjust inequities that limit opportunities for participation in society (Braveman & Bass-Haugen, 2009). While opinions differ regarding the most ethical approach to addressing distribution of health care resources and reduction of health disparities, the issue of social justice continues to focus on limiting the impact of social inequality on health outcomes.

Occupational therapy personnel shall

A. Uphold the profession's altruistic responsibilities to help ensure the common good.

B. Take responsibility for educating the public and society about the value of occupational therapy services in promoting health and wellness and reducing the impact of disease and disability.

C. Make every effort to promote activities that benefit the health status of the community.

D. Advocate for just and fair treatment for all patients, clients, employees, and colleagues, and encourage employers and colleagues to abide by the highest standards of social justice and the ethical standards set forth by the occupational therapy profession.

E. Make efforts to advocate for recipients of occupational therapy services to obtain needed services through available means.

F. Provide services that reflect an understanding of how occupational therapy service delivery can be affected by factors such as economic status, age, ethnicity, race, geography, disability, marital status, sexual orientation, gender, gender identity, religion, culture, and political affiliation.

G. Consider offering *pro bono* ("for the good") or reduced-fee occupational therapy services for selected individuals when consistent with guidelines of the employer, third-party payer, and/or government agency.

PROCEDURAL JUSTICE

Principle 5. Occupational therapy personnel shall comply with institutional rules, local, state, federal, and international laws and AOTA documents applicable to the profession of occupational therapy.

Procedural justice is concerned with making and implementing decisions according to fair processes that ensure "fair treatment" (Maiese, 2004). Rules must be impartially followed and consistently applied to generate an unbiased decision. The principle of procedural justice is based on the concept that procedures and processes are organized in a fair manner and that policies, regulations, and laws are followed. While *the law* and *ethics* are not synonymous terms, occupational therapy personnel have an ethical responsibility to uphold current reimbursement regulations and state/territorial laws governing the profession. In addition, occupational therapy personnel are ethically bound to be aware of organizational policies and practice guidelines set forth by regulatory agencies established to protect recipients of service, research participants, and the public.

Occupational therapy personnel shall

A. Be familiar with and apply the Code and Ethics Standards to the work setting, and share them with employers, other employees, colleagues, students, and researchers.

B. Be familiar with and seek to understand and abide by institutional rules, and when those rules conflict with ethical practice, take steps to resolve the conflict.

C. Be familiar with revisions in those laws and AOTA policies that apply to the profession of occupational therapy and inform employers, employees, colleagues, students, and researchers of those changes.

D. Be familiar with established policies and procedures for handling concerns about the Code and Ethics Standards, including familiarity with national, state, local, district, and territorial procedures for handling ethics complaints as well as policies and procedures created by AOTA and certification, licensing, and regulatory agencies.

E. Hold appropriate national, state, or other requisite credentials for the occupational therapy services they provide.

F. Take responsibility for maintaining high standards and continuing competence in practice, education, and research by participating in professional development and educational activities to improve and update knowledge and skills.

G. Ensure that all duties assumed by or assigned to other occupational therapy personnel match credentials, qualifications, experience, and scope of practice.

H. Provide appropriate supervision to individuals for whom they have supervisory responsibility in accordance with AOTA official documents and local, state, and federal or national laws, rules, regulations, policies, procedures, standards, and guidelines.

I. Obtain all necessary approvals prior to initiating research activities.

J. Report all gifts and remuneration from individuals, agencies, or companies in accordance with employer policies as well as state and federal guidelines.

K. Use funds for intended purposes, and avoid misappropriation of funds.

L. Take reasonable steps to ensure that employers are aware of occupational therapy's ethical obligations as set forth in this Code and Ethics Standards and of the implications of those obligations for occupational therapy practice, education, and research.

M. Actively work with employers to prevent discrimination and unfair labor practices, and advocate for employees with disabilities to ensure the provision of reasonable accommodations.

N. Actively participate with employers in the formulation of policies and procedures to ensure legal, regulatory, and ethical compliance.

O. Collect fees legally. Fees shall be fair, reasonable, and commensurate with services delivered. Fee schedules must be available and equitable regardless of actual payer reimbursements/contracts.

P. Maintain the ethical principles and standards of the profession when participating in a business arrangement as owner, stockholder, partner, or employee, and refrain from working for or doing business with organizations that engage in illegal or unethical business practices (e.g., fraudulent billing, providing occupational therapy services beyond the scope of occupational therapy practice).

VERACITY

Principle 6. Occupational therapy personnel shall provide comprehensive, accurate, and objective information when representing the profession.

Veracity is based on the virtues of truthfulness, candor, and honesty. The principle of *veracity* in health care refers to comprehensive, accurate, and objective transmission of information and includes fostering the client's understanding of such information (Beauchamp & Childress, 2009). Veracity is based on respect owed to others. In communicating with others, occupational therapy personnel implicitly promise to speak truthfully and not deceive the listener. By entering into a relationship in care or research, the recipient of service or research participant enters into a contract that includes a right to truthful information (Beauchamp & Childress, 2009). In addition, transmission of information is incomplete without also ensuring that the recipient or participant understands the information provided. Concepts of veracity must be carefully balanced with other potentially competing ethical principles, cultural beliefs, and organizational policies. Veracity ultimately is valued as a means to establish trust and strengthen professional relationships. Therefore, adherence to the Principle also requires thoughtful analysis of how full disclosure of information may impact outcomes.

Occupational therapy personnel shall

A. Represent the credentials, qualifications, education, experience, training, roles, duties, competence, views, contributions, and findings accurately in all forms of communication about recipients of service, students, employees, research participants, and colleagues.

B. Refrain from using or participating in the use of any form of communication that contains false, fraudulent, deceptive, misleading, or unfair statements or claims.

C. Record and report in an accurate and timely manner, and in accordance with applicable regulations, all information related to professional activities.

D. Ensure that documentation for reimbursement purposes is done in accordance with applicable laws, guidelines, and regulations.

E. Accept responsibility for any action that reduces the public's trust in occupational therapy.

F. Ensure that all marketing and advertising are truthful, accurate, and carefully presented to avoid misleading recipients of service, students, research participants, or the public.

G. Describe the type and duration of occupational therapy services accurately in professional contracts, including the duties and responsibilities of all involved parties.

H. Be honest, fair, accurate, respectful, and timely in gathering and reporting fact-based information regarding employee job performance and student performance.

I. Give credit and recognition when using the work of others in written, oral, or electronic media.

J. Not plagiarize the work of others.

FIDELITY

Principle 7. Occupational therapy personnel shall treat colleagues and other professionals with respect, fairness, discretion, and integrity.

The principle of fidelity comes from the Latin root *fidelis* meaning loyal. *Fidelity* refers to being faithful, which includes obligations of loyalty and the keeping of promises and commitments (Veatch & Flack, 1997). In the health professions, fidelity refers to maintaining good-faith relationships between various service providers and recipients. While respecting fidelity requires occupational therapy personnel to meet the client's reasonable expectations (Purtillo, 2005), Principle 7 specifically addresses fidelity as it relates to maintaining collegial and organizational relationships. Professional relationships are greatly influenced by the complexity of the environment in which occupational therapy personnel work. Practitioners, educators, and researchers alike must consistently balance their duties to service recipients, students, research participants, and other professionals as well as to organizations that may influence decision-making and professional practice.

Occupational therapy personnel shall

A. Respect the traditions, practices, competencies, and responsibilities of their own and other professions, as well as those of the institutions and agencies that constitute the working environment.

B. Preserve, respect, and safeguard private information about employees, colleagues, and students unless otherwise mandated by national, state, or local laws or permission to disclose is given by the individual.

C. Take adequate measures to discourage, prevent, expose, and correct any breaches of the Code and Ethics Standards and report any breaches of the former to the appropriate authorities.

D. Attempt to resolve perceived institutional violations of the Code and Ethics Standards by utilizing internal resources first.

E. Avoid conflicts of interest or conflicts of commitment in employment, volunteer roles, or research.

F. Avoid using one's position (employee or volunteer) or knowledge gained from that position in such a manner that gives rise to real or perceived conflict of interest among the person, the employer, other Association members, and/or other organizations.
G. Use conflict resolution and/or alternative dispute resolution resources to resolve organizational and interpersonal conflicts.
H. Be diligent stewards of human, financial, and material resources of their employers, and refrain from exploiting these resources for personal gain.

References

American Occupational Therapy Association. (1993). Core values and attitudes of occupational therapy practice. *American Journal of Occupational Therapy*, *47*, 1085–1086.

American Occupational Therapy Association. (2005). Occupational therapy code of ethics (2005). *American Journal of Occupational Therapy, 59,* 639–642.

American Occupational Therapy Association. (2006). Guidelines to the occupational therapy code of ethics. *American Journal of Occupational Therapy, 60*, 652–658.

American Occupational Therapy Association. (2004). Policy 5.3.1: Definition of occupational therapy practice for State Regulation. *American Journal of Occupational Therapy, 58,* 694-695.

Beauchamp, T. L., & Childress, J. F. (2009). *Principles of biomedical ethics* (6th ed.). New York: Oxford University Press.

Braveman, B., & Bass-Haugen, J. D. (2009). Social justice and health disparities: An evolving discourse in occupational therapy research and intervention. *American Journal of Occupational Therapy, 63,* 7–12.

Maiese, M. (2004). *Procedural justice.* Retrieved July 29, 2009, from http://www.beyondintractability.org/essay/procedural_justice/

Purtillo, R. (2005). *Ethical dimensions in the health professions* (4th ed.). Philadelphia: Elsevier/Saunders.

Veatch, R. M., & Flack, H. E. (1997). *Case studies in allied health ethics.* Upper Saddle River, NJ: Prentice-Hall.

Authors

Ethics Commission (EC):

Kathlyn Reed, PhD, OTR, FAOTA, MLIS, Chairperson
Barbara Hemphill, DMin, OTR, FAOTA, FMOTA, Chair-Elect
Ann Moodey Ashe, MHS, OTR/L
Lea C. Brandt, OTD, MA, OTR/L
Joanne Estes, MS, OTR/L
Loretta Jean Foster, MS, COTA/L
Donna F. Homenko, RDH, PhD
Craig R. Jackson, JD, MSW
Deborah Yarett Slater, MS, OT/L, FAOTA, Staff Liaison

Adopted by the Representative Assembly 2010CApr17.

Note. This document replaces the following rescinded Ethics documents 2010CApril18: the Occupational *Therapy Code of Ethics (2005)* (*American Journal of Occupational Therapy, 59,* 639–642); the *Guidelines to the Occupational Therapy Code of Ethics* (*American Journal of Occupational Therapy, 60,* 652–658); and the *Core Values and Attitudes of Occupational Therapy Practice* (*American Journal of Occupational Therapy, 47,* 1085–1086).

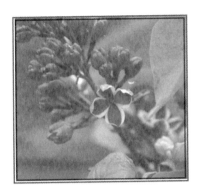

G

PROCEDURES FOR THE ENFORCEMENT OF THE NATIONAL BOARD FOR CERTIFICATION IN OCCUPATIONAL THERAPY CANDIDATE/CERTIFICANT CODE OF CONDUCT

Reproduced with permission from the
National Board for Certification in Occupational Therapy

Jacobs, K., MacRae, N., & Sladyk, K. (Eds.).
Occupational Therapy Essentials for
Clinical Competence, Second Edition (pp. 817-824).
© 2014 SLACK Incorporated.

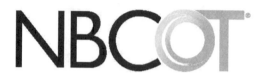

PROCEDURES FOR THE ENFORCEMENT OF THE NBCOT® CANDIDATE/CERTIFICANT CODE OF CONDUCT

SECTION A. Preamble

In exercising its responsibility for promoting and maintaining standards of professional conduct in the practice of occupational therapy and in order to protect the public from those practitioners whose behavior falls short of these standards, the National Board for Certification in Occupational Therapy, Inc. ("NBCOT®," formerly known as "AOTCB") has adopted a Candidate/Certificant Code of Conduct. The NBCOT has adopted these procedures for resolving issues arising under the Candidate/Certificant Code of Conduct with respect to persons who have been certified by the NBCOT or who have applied for such certification. These procedures are intended to enable the NBCOT, through its Qualifications and Compliance Review Committee ("QCRC"), comprised of both professional and public members, QCRC Chair, (or Co-Chair when Chair is unavailable) and Staff to act fairly in the performance of its responsibilities to the public as a certifying agency, and to ensure that the rights of candidates and certificants are protected.

SECTION B. Basis for Sanction

A violation of the Candidate/Certificant Code of Conduct provides basis for action and sanction under these Procedures.

SECTION C. Sanctions

1. Violations of the Candidate/Certificant Code of Conduct may result in one or more of the following sanctions:

    a. Ineligibility for certification, which means that an individual is barred from becoming certified by the NBCOT, either indefinitely or for a certain duration.

    b. Reprimand, which means a formal expression of disapproval, which shall be retained in the certificant's file, but shall not be publicly announced.

    c. Censure, which means a formal expression of disapproval which is publicly announced.

    d. Probation, which means continued certification is subject to fulfillment of specified conditions, e.g., monitoring, education, supervision, and/or counseling.

    e. Suspension, which means the loss of certification for a certain duration, after which the individual may be required to apply for reinstatement.

    f. Revocation, which means permanent loss of certification.

2.   All sanctions other than reprimand shall be announced publicly, in accordance with Section D.10. All sanctions other than reprimand shall be disclosed in response to inquiries in accordance with Section D.10.

SECTION D.   Procedures For The Enforcement of
The Candidate/Certificant Code of Conduct

1. Jurisdiction

The NBCOT has jurisdiction over all individuals who have been certified as an OCCUPATIONAL THERAPIST REGISTERED OTR (OTR®) henceforth OTR, or CERTIFIED OCCUPATIONAL THERAPY ASSISTANT COTA (COTA®) henceforth COTA, or who have applied for certification, or have applied for Occupational Therapist Eligibility Determination (OTED) to take the NBCOT Certification Examination for OTR. In addition, NBCOT has jurisdiction over all individuals who have applied for an Early Determination Review to determine eligibility to take the Certification Examination for OTR or COTA; Jurisdiction, in this case, is for the limited purpose of acting upon a request for an Early Determination.

2. Initiation of the Review Process

The NBCOT Staff ("Staff") shall initiate the process upon receipt by the NBCOT of information indicating that an individual subject to NBCOT's jurisdiction may have violated the Candidate/Certificant Code of Conduct. Receipt of such information shall be considered a complaint for the purposes of these procedures, regardless of the source.

3. Staff Investigation and Action

a. Staff shall review all complaints and investigate these complaints, as it deems appropriate.

b. Staff may review any evidence, which it deems appropriate and relevant.

    i.   If Staff determines that the evidence does not support the allegation(s), no file shall be opened and the complainant shall be notified of the Staff's decision.

    ii. If Staff determines that the evidence does support the allegation(s) and decides to investigate, the subject of the complaint shall be notified. This notification shall be in writing and shall include a description of the complaint. The subject of the complaint shall have thirty (30) days from the date notification is sent to respond in writing to the complaint. The Staff may extend this period up to an additional thirty (30) days upon request, provided sufficient justification for the extension is given.

    iii. In addition to providing a written response to the complaint and as part of the investigative process, the subject may request a telephone conference with an NBCOT representative. The purpose of this call is to give the subject an additional opportunity to verbally provide information about the case. The subject may also submit additional written information or documentation.

c. Upon the completion of its investigation, Staff shall either:

i. Dismiss the case due to insufficient evidence, the matter being insufficiently serious, or other reasons as may be warranted. The qualifications and compliance review shall be considered closed at the time such decision is made; or

ii. Present a proposed sanction to the QCRC Chair in the form of a disciplinary action agreement. At the discretion of the Chair additional members, both professional and public, may be asked to assist with the decision making process prior to taking the case to the full Committee.

4.   Voluntary Forfeiture

The subject of a complaint may voluntarily forfeit his or her certification. This forfeiture must be submitted in writing and can be made, at any time, while the complaint is either under active investigation or when disciplinary action has been taken by the NBCOT but the terms of the sanction remain incomplete.

Staff will advise the Qualifications and Compliance Review Committee (QCRC) Chair of any voluntary forfeiture.

If the subject requests reinstatement of certification, after voluntary forfeiture, the subject must meet all of the following requirements:

a. submit reinstatement of certification request in writing
b. satisfy current certification examination eligibility requirements (including academic and fieldwork requirements) and
c. re-take and pass the national certification examination

Further, any pending investigation will be resumed upon request to regain certification.

If the subject's certification is voluntarily forfeited, public notice may be given in accordance with Section D.10 of these procedures.

5.   Non-Response (Noncomplaint-Inactive)

If the subject does not respond to investigative inquiries, the subject's certification will be placed on Noncompliant-Inactive status in accordance with Section 9.

Staff will advise the QCRC Chair of this action.

If the subject requests reinstatement of certification, after being placed on Non Compliant-Inactive status, the subject must meet all of the following requirements:

    a. submit reinstatement of certification request in writing

    b. satisfy current certification renewal requirements, and

    c. cooperate with and provide written response and supporting documentation to the NBCOT investigative inquiry

6.   <u>QCRC Chair Review and Procedures for Disciplinary Action Agreement</u>

Staff shall prepare a case summary of its investigation along with the disciplinary action agreement for the QCRC Chair to consider. The report shall include the basis for Staff's findings, as well as any written responses, or other materials submitted in relation to the investigation of the complaint.

If Staff and the QCRC Chair are not able to reach agreement on the proposed sanction, the Chair will schedule a meeting of the QCRC to review and determine final conditions and terms of the disciplinary action agreement.

If the QCRC Chair and Staff are in agreement on the proposed sanction, Staff shall forward the disciplinary action agreement to the subject.

The subject may either:

a. Accept the disciplinary action agreement and thereby waive his/her right to a hearing. The disciplinary action agreement will be sent to the subject in writing. To accept the agreement, the subject must sign, date and return the agreement to NBCOT. Upon the subject's acceptance of the disciplinary action agreement, the qualifications and compliance process shall be considered closed. The public notification standards of Section D.10 are applicable if the settlement contains a sanction that warrants such announcement be made; or

b. Not accept the disciplinary action agreement and request a hearing before the QCRC. Request for a hearing must be submitted by the subject in writing.

    At the hearing:

      i. The subject of the complaint may be represented at the hearing by his/her legal counsel, or any other individual of his or her choosing.

      ii. The subject of the complaint shall be solely responsible for all of his/her own expenses related to the hearing. Hearings can be conducted via teleconference call or in person at the sole discretion of the QCRC. Should the subject cancel the hearing, he/she must notify the QCRC of the cancellation no less than fifteen (15) days prior to the hearing date. Should the subject cancel the hearing within fifteen (15) days of the hearing date or not appear at the scheduled hearing, all costs associated with the preparation of the hearing shall be paid by the subject (e.g. court reporting fees, teleconference fees, hearing manual preparation fees).

iii. The subject of the complaint shall provide the QCRC with any and all materials he/she may wish to include for the hearing no less than fifteen (15) days prior to the hearing date.

Following the hearing, Staff shall notify (in writing) the complainant and the subject of the complaint of the QCRC's decision within thirty (30) days of the decision. The decision shall take effect immediately unless otherwise provided by the QCRC.

c. If the subject fails to respond to the disciplinary action agreement, within thirty (30) days after the agreement has been sent to the subject, conditions and terms of the agreement take effect immediately.

7. Appeals Process

Within thirty (30) days after the notification of the QCRC's decision, any individual(s) sanctioned by the QCRC at the hearing may appeal the hearing decision to the NBCOT Directors. A notice of appeal, which must be in writing and signed by the subject, shall be sent by the subject to the NBCOT Chairperson in care of the President/Chief Executive Officer. The basis for the appeal shall be fully explained in this notice.

The Chairperson shall form an Appeals Panel within thirty (30) days after receipt of the notice of appeal. The Appeals Panel shall be comprised of three (3) NBCOT Directors and shall include at least one (1) OTR or one (1) COTA and one (1) public member. Members of the QCRC who participated in any aspect of the proceedings related to the complaint shall not serve on the Appeals Panel.

An appeal must relate to evidence, issues and procedures that are part of the record of the QCRC hearing and decision. The appeal may also address the substance of the disciplinary action. However, the Panel may in its discretion consider additional evidence.

Within fifteen (15) days after the notice of appeal is received by the Appeals Panel, the Panel shall provide the subject with an opportunity to schedule a hearing. The subject may be represented at the hearing by legal counsel or any other individual of his/her choosing. The subject shall be solely responsible for all of his/her own expenses related to the hearing.

Within fifteen (15) days after the appeals hearing or if the subject elects not to request a formal hearing, the Panel shall decide the appeal and notify the Chairperson of its decision.

The Appeals Panel may either:

a. Affirm the QCRC's disciplinary action agreement;

b. Deny the QCRC's disciplinary action agreement;

c. Refer the case back to the Staff for further investigation and resolution with full right of appeal; or

    d. Modify the QCRC's disciplinary action agreement, but not in a manner that would be more adverse to the subject.

The Chairperson shall promptly notify the subject of the Appeals Panel's decision. The decision of the Appeals Panel shall be final.

8.   Cooperation with NBCOT Enforcement Procedures

Failure to respond to any aspect of the Enforcement Procedures, will be considered a violation of the Candidate/Certificant Code of Conduct, Principle 2, and is sufficient grounds for the imposition of sanction by the NBCOT.

9.   Noncompliant-Inactive

Individuals who do not satisfy the NBCOT certification renewal requirements by their scheduled renewal date, or who are non-responsive to NBCOT investigative inquiries are "Noncompliant-Inactive" and CANNOT a) identify themselves to the public as an OCCUPATIONAL THERAPIST REGISTERED (OTR) or CERTIFIED OCCUPATIONAL THERAPY ASSISTANT (COTA) or b) use the OTR or COTA credential after their name.

10.   Announcement of Sanction

If an individual's certification status is voluntarily forfeited, suspended or revoked, or he/she is censured or placed on probation, occupational therapy state regulatory bodies shall be notified and an announcement included on its web site and in one or more publications of general circulation to persons engaged or otherwise interested in the profession of occupational therapy. The NBCOT may also disclose its final decision, including ineligibility for certification, to others as it deems appropriate, including, but not limited to, persons inquiring about the status of an individual's certification, employers, third party payers and the general public.

11.   Notification

All notifications referred to in these procedures shall be in writing and if the subject does not respond, shall be by confirmation of signature, return receipt mail, unless otherwise indicated. Subjects of complaints who live outside of the U.S. may be given additional time to respond to any notifications they are sent, as determined by the Staff in its discretion.

12.   Records and Reports

At the completion of this procedure, all records and reports shall be returned to the Staff. The complete files in the qualifications and compliance review proceedings shall be maintained.

13. Expedited Action

The NBCOT may expedite a matter by shortening any notice or response period provided for under these procedures if the responsible party determines in its sole discretion that shortening the period is appropriate in order to protect against the possibility of harm to recipients of occupational therapy services.

In matters where the severity of the allegations and evidence provided warrant such action in order to protect the public, the NBCOT may authorize immediate suspension/revocation of certification. The subject will be duly notified of the action and given fifteen (15) days to contest the suspension or revocation.

14. Standard Of Proof

The NBCOT shall take disciplinary action against an individual only where there is clear and convincing evidence of a violation of the Candidate/Certificant Code of Conduct.

15. Special Accommodations

The NBCOT recognizes the definition of disability as defined by the Americans with Disabilities Act (ADA) and acknowledges the provisions and protections of the Act. The NBCOT shall offer hearings related to qualifications and compliance review or the appeals process in a site and manner, which is architecturally accessible to persons with disabilities or offer alternative arrangements for such individuals.

An individual with a documented disability may request special accommodations for a hearing by providing reasonable advance notice to the NBCOT of his or her disability and of the modifications or aids needed at the hearing at his or her own expense.

16. Amendment to Procedures

These procedures may be amended at any time by the NBCOT Directors.

Revision: November 14 , 2011   © Copyright 2013 NBCOT, Inc.

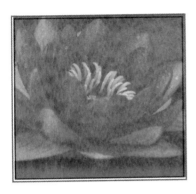

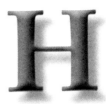

NATIONAL BOARD FOR CERTIFICATION IN OCCUPATIONAL THERAPY COMPLAINT FORM

Reproduced with permission from the
National Board for Certification in Occupational Therapy

Jacobs, K., MacRae, N., & Sladyk, K. (Eds.).
Occupational Therapy Essentials for
Clinical Competence, Second Edition (pp. 825-827).
© 2014 SLACK Incorporated.

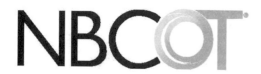

COMPLAINT FORM

1.   **Complaint is filed against:**

Name: _____ Telephone: _____

Address: _____ NBCOT Cert #: _____

2.   **Person filing complaint (complainant):**

Name: _____ Telephone: _____

Address: _____

3.   **Complainant's relationship with the person against whom the complaint is being filed (e.g., supervisor, co-worker, patient, etc.):**

4.   **Summary of complaint (in your own words – who, what, where, when, why, and how): [Use additional sheets if needed].**

5.   **Other persons with knowledge of the incident(s) giving rise to this complaint:**

Name: _____ Telephone: _____

Address: _____

Name: _____ Telephone: _____

Address: _____

(see reverse side)

6. Other agencies or organizations you have submitted this complaint to (i.e., state licensing boards, Medicare, AOTA, police or other authorities, etc.):

7. State in your own words how this incident(s) relates to the NBCOT's "Candidate/Certificant Code of Conduct" (use additional sheets if needed):

_____

_____

_____

_____

_____

_____

_____

_____

_____

_____

_____

_____   _____

Complainant Signature   **Date**

(Note: Complete separate form for each complaint or complainant)

Revision Date: 01/02/2013   © Copyright 2013, NBCOT, Inc.

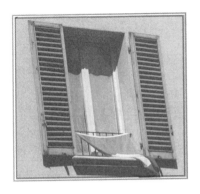

WORLD FEDERATION OF OCCUPATIONAL THERAPISTS CODE OF ETHICS

Reproduced with permission from the
World Federation of Occupational Therapists

Jacobs, K., MacRae, N., & Sladyk, K. (Eds.).
Occupational Therapy Essentials for
Clinical Competence, Second Edition (pp. 829-830).
© 2014 SLACK Incorporated.

WORLD FEDERATION of OCCUPATIONAL THERAPISTS (WFOT)

CODE OF ETHICS

This code describes the general categories of appropriate conduct for occupational therapists in any professional circumstance. It is understood that each member association will have a detailed code of ethics particular to its needs.

Personal Attributes

Occupational therapists demonstrate personal integrity, reliability, open-mindedness and loyalty in all aspects of their professional role.

Responsibility towards the Recipient of Occupational Therapy Services

Occupational therapists approach all persons receiving their services with respect and have regard for their individual situations. Occupational therapists shall not discriminate against these persons on the basis of race, colour, impairment, disability, national origin, age, gender, sexual preference, religion, political beliefs or status in society.

The values, preferences and ability to participate of persons receiving occupational therapy will be taken into account in providing services.

Confidentiality of the persons' personal information is guaranteed and any personal details are passed on only with that person's consent.

Professional Conduct in Collaborative Practice

Occupational therapists recognise the need for inter-professional collaboration and respect the unique contributions of other professions. Occupational therapists' contribution to inter-professional collaboration is based on occupational performance as it affects the health and well-being of people.

Developing Professional Knowledge

Occupational therapists participate in professional development through life-long learning and apply their acquired knowledge and skills in their professional work which is based on the best available evidence.

When participating in research occupational therapists respect the ethical implications involved.

Promotion and Development

Occupational therapists are committed to the improvement and development of the profession in general. They are also concerned with ethically promoting occupational therapy to the public, other professional organisations and government bodies at regional, national and international levels.

GLOSSARY

ABA design: A single case experimental design where (A) baseline data is measured, (B) intervention provided, and (C) measurement repeated.

AbleData: A federally sponsored Web site that organizes and tracks adaptive tools and provides an overview of a wide range of assistive devices across a wide spectrum of functions.

abstract: Summary of an article or paper containing the most important points of each subsection.

activities of daily living (ADL): An area of occupation; "Activities that are oriented toward taking care of one's own body (adapted from Rogers & Holm, 1994, pp. 181-202). ADL also is referred to as basic activities of daily living (BADL) and personal activities of daily living (PADL). These activities are fundamental to living in a social world; they enable basic survival and well-being' (Christiansen & Hammecker, 2001, p. 156)" (AOTA, 2008, p. 631).

activity/activities: The execution of a task or action by an individual (WHO, 2001); "a term that describes a class of human actions that are goal directed" (AOTA, 2008, p. 669).

activity demands: Requirements specific to the activity and independent of the person.

ADA Amendments Act (2008) (ADAAA): This federal act amended the Americans with Disabilities Act of 1990. The changes, which apply to both the ADA and the Rehabilitation Act, include an updated definition of the term "disability" which clarifies and broadens the words used in order to protect more people under the ADA and other Federal disability nondiscrimination laws. The definition of *major life activities* was expanded to include bodily functions, which allows many people with internal function disorders such as gastrointestinal disorders, cancer, sleep disorders, insulin-dependent diabetes, and heart disease to now be covered under the ADA. The act also required the Equal Employment Opportunity Commission (EEOC) to adopt the changes into their regulations in order to protect the rights of a greater number of employees.

adaptation (when used as an outcome): "The response approach the client makes encountering an occupational challenge. 'This change is implemented when the individual's customary response approaches are found inadequate for producing some degree of mastery over the challenge' (Schultz & Schkade, 1997, p. 474)" (AOTA, 2008, p. 630).

adapting: To make suitable to or fit for a specific use or situation (Dictionary.com); to change something (i.e., the demands of the activity) so that the client is successful.

advertisement: To make something known; to make publicly and generally known; to announce publicly especially by a printed notice or a broadcast; to call public attention to especially by emphasizing desirable qualities so as to arouse a desire to buy or patronize (Merriam-Webster, 2006).

advertising: "A specific communication task to be accomplished with a specific audience in mind in a specific target market during a specific period of time. The advertisement goals are based on achieving one of four aims: to inform, to persuade, to remind, or to reinforce" (Kotler, 2003, p. 312).

advocacy: To speak up for or plead the case of another.

affordable insurance exchange: A new transparent, competitive insurance marketplace where individuals and small businesses can purchase affordable and qualified health benefit plans.

American Psychological Association (APA) format: The standard format used in health science literature for in-text citation and reference information.

Americans with Disabilities Act (ADA): A Federal law that prevents discrimination against individuals with disabilities.

analysis of occupational performance: A multi-step process conducted by the occupational therapist. Based on a select model and/or frame(s) of reference, the occupational therapist analyzes the occupational profile in conjunction with other occupational therapists' assessments to formulate hypotheses about which factors encourage as well as disrupt the client's successful engagement in occupations and in daily life activities.

analysis of variance (ANOVA): A statistical procedure used to measure differences between measurements.

annotated bibliography: A citation and short summary.

autism: A complex developmental disability that typically appears during the first 3 years of life and affects a person's ability to communicate, read facial expressions, and interact with others. Autism is defined by a certain set of behaviors including repetitive actions, self-stimulation (rocking, hand flapping, spinning, etc.), avoidance of eye contact, and echoalia. Autism is a spectrum disorder that affects individuals differently and to varying degrees. Developmental disorder characterized by a severely reduced ability to communicate and emotionally relate to other people; self-absorption.

autistic spectrum disorders (ASDs): Common name for a variety of autistic disorders. Autism spectrum disorders are a group of developmental disabilities that can cause significant social, communication, and behavioral challenges. ASDs affect individuals differently and the spectrum includes those who are severely affected and experience great difficulty in communicating and building relationships, in addition to those with more mild forms such as Asperger's, who mainly have difficulty with obsessive interests and social situations.

applied research: Research directed toward the solution of specified practical problems in delineated areas, or to achieve practical goals (Kerlinger, 1979).

applied theory: The results of applied research, intended to address problems of practical interest.

areas of occupation: The variety of meaningful activities in which people engage, including the following categories: activities of daily living, instrumental activities of daily living, education, work, play, leisure, and social participation (AOTA, 2008).

arts and crafts movement: A transformation of the American lifestyle, created in response to workers and their working environments, to restore the relationship between nature and creativity.

aspiration: The entry of secretions, fluids, food, or any foreign substance below the vocal cords and into the lungs that may result in aspiration pneumonia and may be fatal (AOTA, 2007).

assessment: Specific tools, instruments, or procedures used to obtain data during the evaluative process.

assistive technology: Devices that augment or extend a user's ability to function in the task environment.

associative level participation: Consists of approaching others briefly in verbal or nonverbal interactions.

assumptions: Broad general statements that are taken for granted for the sake of argument.

attitude: Your mindset or outlook.

backward chaining: A technique that teaches the last part of a task first, thus ensuring success. Once the last part is learned, the next to last part is taught, until the entire task is learned.

basic cooperative level participation: Includes selecting longer activities or tasks of mutual interest and following the norms or rules of interaction in play or work.

basic research: Systematic study to test theory and to understand relations among phenomena without consideration of application of the results (Kerlinger, 1979).

bed mobility: Safely and effectively moving in bed for comfort, skin integrity, and function.

behavioral response: Ability to express oneself in a social situation using independently generated verbal and nonverbal cues.

benchmark: Quantifiable measures of the outcomes of a process used as comparisons to current targets for improvement (Braveman, 2006).

body functions and structures: Physiologic and psychological aspects of individual systems, including anatomic parts (WHO, 2001).

body mechanics: The utilization of appropriate muscles and positions to complete heavy work safely and efficiently (Brookside Associates, 2007).

bolus: Food or liquid in a mass form (AOTA, 2007).

bullying: Unwanted, repetitive, aggressive behavior that may involve physical, verbal, relational, and/or electronic means of exerting power over another individual.

care coordination: A process that facilitates the linkage of individuals and their families with appropriate services and resources in a coordinated effort to achieve good health.

career: A line of business or way of making a living.

caring: A set of feelings, attitudes, and actions that convey respect, hope, and care toward others.

case management: A collaborative process that assesses, plans, implements, coordinates, monitors, and evaluates the options and services required to meet the client's health and human services needs.

case mix groups (CMGs): A term that classifies client discharges into diagnostic categories.

certified occupational therapy assistant: Professional personnel who work under the supervision of an occupational therapist and deliver occupational therapy intervention in partnership with occupational therapists.

circadian process: The process within our body that uses environmental cues (light/dark cycle) to train the body to have the ability of knowing when to sleep even if there are no environmental cues present at a given time.

client: A specific person, family of an identified person, or a population who is the recipient of occupational therapy services; The term used to name the entity that receives occupational therapy services. Clients may include the following: (1) individuals and other persons relevant to the individual's life including family, caregivers, teachers, employers, and others who may also help or be served indirectly; (2) organizations such as business, industries, or agencies; and (3) populations within a community (AOTA, 2008; Moyers & Dale, 2007).

client-centered approach: "An orientation that honors the desires and priorities of clients in designing and implementing interventions (adapted from Dunn, 2000a, p. 4)" (AOTA, 2008, p. 670).

client-centered care: Therapeutic interventions where the person who is receiving services has a major role in the decision making regarding his or her care. The practitioner takes a collaborative rather than an authoritative role.

client-centered practice: A partnership between a client and therapist that serves to empower a client toward reaching goals of his or her own choosing; "an approach to therapy that supports a respectful partnership between therapists and clients" (Law, Baptiste, & Mills, 1995, p. 256). Client-centered practice includes the following concepts: (1) recognition of each client's unique perspective; (2) a shift in power toward the client having more say in defining and directing intervention; (3) a shift to an enablement intervention model; (4) an understanding of the importance of the influence on intervention of the client's culture, preferences, interests, roles, and environments; (5) an understanding of the importance of flexible and dynamic interventions that emphasize learning and problem solving; and (6) respect for the client's values regardless of whether these are shared by the therapist.

client factors: Body functions, body structures, spirituality, values, and beliefs required to complete an activity; those factors residing within the client that may affect performance in areas of occupation (AOTA, 2008).

clinical education: The full scope of application experiences that focus on the development of students' practice skills.

clinical instructor: On-site supervisor for practical experiences; assists all parties in recognizing that these individuals are part of the students' education, thus offering the title of instructor.

clinical pathway: A method used in health care settings as a way of organizing, evaluating, and limiting variations in expected client care secondary to diagnosis and other client-specific factors.

clinical reasoning: Complex cognitive process composed of various types of reasoning.

cluster sampling: When a researcher collects data from groups of participants.

coalition: Individuals or groups joining forces together for a common cause.

Code of Ethics: A collection of formal explicit statements forming a moral guide for an identified group outlining right and valued behavior, principles, and values.

cognitive behavioral therapy: A therapy approach that is used when a practitioner is aiming to change the way a client thinks about something; this is done using the assumption that the way in which we think about a situation controls how we feel and in turn controls our actions and the consequences to those actions.

co-occupations: Activities that involve the social interaction of two or more persons.

collaboration: Both parties have their perspectives and beliefs, but individual goals are put aside to do what is best for the situation and the organization, not what is best for the respective parties.

community mobility: Engaging in mobility resulting in successful participation in the community (AOTA, 2008).

compensation: Changing the way a person completes an activity so that they can be successful given their current situation.

competencies: Explicit statements defining specific areas of expertise; are related to effective or superior performance in a job (Spencer & Spencer, 1993).

compromise: Both parties work together and each side concedes a portion of their viewpoint in order to arrive at an agreement and to resolve the conflict.

concept: An idea or notion formed by mentally combining characteristics (Reed & Sanderson, 1999).

conceptual models in occupational therapy: Graphic or schematic representations of concepts and assumptions that explain why the profession works as it does (Reed & Sanderson, 1999).

concurrent validity: A form of criterion-related validity that shows differences between participants at the time of the measure.

conditional reasoning: Holistic approach to understanding the person, his or her illness, and intervention.

conflict resolution: The ability to identify conflict, to understand the various approaches, and to arrive at a resolution that is beneficial to all parties.

confounding variable: A factor other than the controlled variables that influences the study's results.

construct: Models of assembled relationships between or among two or more concepts (Depoy & Gitlin, 2005).

construct validity: The relationship of one construct to another, such as the relationship of the scores on two different but similar assessments.

consultation: The provision of advice or information; The exchange of ideas with an expert who is called on for professional advice (AOTA, 1994).

content analysis: Process of analyzing written words as data.

contexts: Environmental factors or social environments that influence a specific client's participation in occupations (AOTA, 2008); the circumstances in which an event occurs; a setting (Dictionary.com); "refers to a variety of interrelated conditions within and surrounding the client that influence performance. Contexts include cultural, personal, temporal, and virtual" (AOTA, 2008); the multitude of factors that can define the situation in which leadership takes place.

continuing competence: Refers to an individual's ongoing or lifelong capacity to perform responsibilities as a part of one's professional role performance.

continuing competency: Focuses on an individual's actual performance in a particular situation compared to a standard as a part of one's current professional role performance.

contractor: A person who provides services on a contractual basis.

control group: Participants in an experimental research design who receive no intervention.

convenient sample: Sample of participants that is easily available to the researcher.

correlational coefficient: A measurement of the direction and magnitude of a relationship of two variables.

counter-transference: When one person, usually the therapist, accepts the role the client has placed on him or her.

criterion referenced: The client's score can be compared to a set of specific skills or skill components of standard performance rather than a normative group.

cultural competence: A process of gaining self-awareness, knowledge and awareness of others, and the skills necessary to interact effectively and sensitively in communicating with diverse groups of people (Wells & Black, 2000).

culturally competent care: The process of interacting collaboratively and effectively with culturally diverse clients in order to provide culturally sensitive assessments and interventions.

culture: "Refers to learned behaviors, values, norms, and symbols that are passed from generation to generation within a society" (Loveland, 1999, p. 18).

DAP format: A format for documentation that includes description, assessment, and plan.

data: Any numerical result of research; always written in the plural form (i.e., "data are").

decubitus ulcers: Pressure sores due to excessive pressure on or shearing of the skin.

deep thermal agents: Those procedures or interventions that use a form of energy capable of raising tissue temperature to a depth of up to 5 cm.

deglutition: Consuming of solids or liquids in a normal sensorimotor process (Jenks & Smith, 2006, p. 610).

deinstitutionalization: The closing of mental hospitals and residential institutions, which resulted in mentally ill clients joining the community.

demographics: "Data related to the size and growth rate of populations in different cities, regions, and nations; age distribution and ethnic mix; educational levels; household patterns; and regional characteristics and movements" (Kotler, 2003, p. 100).

dependent variable: one or more clinical findings, behaviors, personal attributes, or internal experiences that are measured in research; the dependent variable might be hypothesized to change as the result of the independent variable or to differ between independent variable groupings.

disability: Medical and social construct related to the paradox of describing individual capacity (ability and impairment) and community capacity (attitudes and resources; Finkelstein, 1991).

discharge: The termination of therapy services.

discontinuation note: A note that summarizes the course of a client's intervention and includes recommendations for the future.

disease: "A disorder with a specific cause and recognizable signs and symptoms; any bodily abnormality or failure to function properly, except that resulting directly from physical injury" (Encyclopedia.com, 2008).

documentation: The legal and professional responsibility of recording occupational therapy service delivery and outcomes.

driver rehabilitation: A form of therapy that focuses on evaluation and intervention in the occupation of driving a vehicle.

durable medical equipment (DME): Medically necessary equipment that can be provided to a client to increase safety and independence in the home. Examples include hospital beds, wheelchairs, and walkers. Items such as grab bars, reachers, and long-handled sponges are not considered DME. All covered DME requires a physician prescription.

dysphagia: Difficulty with swallowing or the inability to swallow (Jenks & Smith, 2006).

eating: The ability to manipulate and swallow food and liquids (Jenks & Smith, 2006).

education: "Includes activities needed for learning and participating in the environment" (AOTA, 2008, p. 632).

educational activities: Tasks that facilitate learning (i.e., reading, writing, and math).

educator: A faculty member in an academic setting (AOTA, 2004a).

effect size: Magnitude of the effect; the strength and magnitude of a relationship between two variables.

effective communication: The artful interplay between listening and speaking with attention to both verbal and nonverbal communication, coupled with awareness and sensitivity to human diversity.

electrotherapeutic agent: Those procedures or interventions that are systematically applied to modify specific client factors that may be limiting occupational performance; use of electricity and the electromagnetic spectrum to facilitate tissue healing, improve muscle strength and endurance, decrease edema, modulate pain, decrease the inflammatory process, and modify the healing process and are used as an adjunctive method to occupation (Bracciano, 2007).

empathy: A process of reaching for true understanding of the experiences and feelings of another person.

employment interests and pursuits: Identifying and selecting work opportunities based on assets, limitations, likes, and dislikes relative to work (adapted from Mosey, 1996, p. 342).

employment seeking and acquisition: Identifying and recruiting for job opportunities; completing, submitting, and reviewing appropriate application materials; preparing for interviews; participating in interviews and following up afterward; discussing job benefits; and finalizing negotiations.

enteral tube feedings: Tubes that deliver nutrition directly to the gastrointestinal system (Morris & Klein, 2000).

entrepreneur: Partially or fully self-employed individuals. Includes those in private practice, independent contractors, and consultants (AOTA, 2000).

environment: The external physical and social environment that surrounds the client and in which the client's daily life occupations occur.

environmental factors: Contextual factors extrinsic to the individual such as the physical, social, and attitudinal environment in which people live and conduct their lives (WHO, 2001).

epistemology: The dynamics of knowing (Hooper, 2006); how we know what we know.

ergonomics: Study of the "fit" between human and environment.

error variance: The variance left over after all of the studied variance is accounted for.

ethical dilemmas: Situations in which there are several alternatives, all of which are ethically somewhat problematic.

ethical reasoning: Making sure one selects the morally justifiable decisions.

ethics: The study of right and wrong conduct as determined by reasonable thought processes.

evaluation: "The process of obtaining and interpreting data necessary for intervention. This includes planning for and documenting the evaluation process and results" (Brayman et al., 2005, p. 663).

evidence-based occupational therapy: Intervention "based on client information and a critical review of relevant research, expert consensus, and past experience" (CAOT, 1999).

exceptional educational need (EEN): Determination that a student exhibits a disability or handicapping condition that prevents educational progress.

executive skills: High-level cognitive skills that involve planning, problem solving, cognitive flexibility, judgment/insight, and self-monitoring.

experience sampling method: The use of an electronic device that randomly beeps throughout the day and requires the subject to record data regarding the quality of experience, associated challenges, and kind of activity in which he or she is engaged.

external validity: The degree to which the study's results can be generalized to another population.

F-test: A statistical measure used in ANOVA.

face validity: The degree to which experts in the area would agree that a measurement appears to measure what it says it does. Also called *content validity*.

feeding: Setting up, arranging, and bringing food or fluid from a plate or a cup to the mouth (AOTA, 2007).

fieldwork educator: This individual assists the student's integration of classroom knowledge and application to practice. Not permitted to supervise a Level II fieldwork student until they have practiced full-time for one year (ACOTE, 1999).

FIP format: A format of documentation that includes findings, interpretation, and plan.

flow experience: The way people describe their state of mind when consciousness is harmoniously ordered and they want to pursue whatever they are doing for its own sake.

formal educational participation: Including the categories of academic (e.g., math, reading, working on a degree), nonacademic (e.g., recess, lunchroom, hallway), extracurricular (e.g., sports, band, cheerleading, dance), and vocational (prevocational and vocational) participation.

frame of reference: System of compatible concepts from theory which guides a plan of action within a specific occupational therapy domain of concern (Mosey, 1986); a set of ideas, in terms of which other ideas are interpreted or assigned meaning (Dictionary.com); frames of reference provide intervention guidelines and help practitioners know what to do in practice; provide information on the nature of function/dysfunction, intervention strategies, principles guiding intervention, assessments, and expected outcomes; and define who would benefit from the intervention.

framing: The method through which a player offers cues about how he or she wishes to be treated during play (Bateson, 1972).

freedom to suspend reality: The child is able to defer the restrictions of realistic play and use his or her imagination to take on new roles and identities (Bundy, 1997; Rubin, Fein, Vandenberg, 1983); the ability to participate in make-believe activities or pretend play (Bundy, 1997).

frequency: Number of participants who have a specific score.

fun: "That which provides mirth and amusement; enjoyment; playfulness" (Parham & Fazio, 1997, p. 250).

function: The ability to perform meaningful activities and tasks that involve body structure, body functions, activities, and participation (WHO, 2001).

functional mobility: "Moving from one position to another during performance of everyday activities" (AOTA, 2008, p. 631).

funding agencies: Federal, state, local, or community organizations; corporations; foundations; and trusts offering monetary support to develop programs or run research projects.

gastroesophageal reflux disease (GERD): "Reflux of food, medication, liquids, and gastric juice from the stomach into the esophagus" (AOTA, 2007, p. 698).

gastroesophageal scintigraphy: Sometimes referred to as a *milk scan,* this medical test looks at stomach emptying as well as extent and severity of reflux (Morris & Klein, 2000).

gastrostomy tube (G-tube): Bypasses the mouth and is surgically inserted directly into the stomach.

goal: Outcome measure of progress.

grading: Changing aspects of an activity to make it easier or more difficult.

grants: Monies disbursed by a funding agency to another agency or person for the purpose of a specific program, research study, or products.

grassroots advocacy: A group effort of like-minded individuals working together to achieve a desired outcome.

health: "A complete state of physical, mental, and social well-being, and not just the absence of disease or infirmity" (WHO, 1947, p. 29).

Health Insurance Portability and Accountability Act of 1996 (HIPAA): Title I of HIPAA protects health insurance coverage for workers and their families when they change or lose their jobs. Title II of HIPAA, known as the Administrative Simplification (AS) provisions, requires the establishment of national standards for electronic health care transactions and national identifiers for providers, health insurance plans, and employers. The act gives the right to privacy to individuals from age 12 through 18. The provider must have a signed disclosure from the affected individual before giving out any information on provided health care to anyone, including parents. The administrative simplification provisions also address the security and privacy of health data.

health literacy: Ability to find, understand, and use information to make health-related decisions.

health promotion: Actions or activities that support the enhancement of health and well-being.

hi-tech: Devices, often electronic or electric, commonly more expensive and often customized according to the user's needs.

holistic approach: Perceiving interrelated components as one whole unit that cannot be subdivided into parts.

human factors engineering: *See* ergonomics.

humanism: A philosophical approach recognizing the basic goodness of being human and the uniqueness of each individual.

ideational apraxia: A complete loss of the ability to do a task due to a perceptual disorder.

ideomotor apraxia: Ability to carry out a task automatically but inability to simulate the task or do it on command due to a perceptual disorder.

impairments: Problems in body function or structure (WHO, 2001).

inclusion: The act of including and providing intervention to students with disabilities in the regular education classroom; Adapting the environment for persons with disabilities to be successful in occupations, roles, and activities with others.

independent t-test: T-test performed on independent groups of participants' scores to measure differences between the scores.

independent variable: A factor in research such as an intervention that can be manipulated by the investigator; also, a stable characteristic of individuals by which they can be grouped.

individual education plan (IEP): Written, legal document developed by the individual education team, incorporating the student's strengths and need areas as well as goals and objectives for intervention.

informal personal educational needs or interests exploration (beyond formal education): Identifying topics and methods for obtaining topic-related information or skills.

informal personal education participation: "Participating in classes, programs, and activities that provide instruction or training in identified areas of interest" (AOTA, 2008, p. 632).

instrumental activities of daily living (IADL): An area of occupation; "activities to support daily life within the home and community that often require more complex interactions than self-care used in ADL" (AOTA, 2008, p. 631).

interactive reasoning: Involves understanding the client as a holistic human being and looking at issues from the client's perspective.

interdependence: Reciprocal reliance on others.

interprofessional: A group of professions whose communication is collaborative, goals are shared between members, and are all responsible for team efforts (MacRae & Dyer, 2005).

interprofessional education: When two or more professions learn with, from, and about each other to improve collaboration and the quality of care (Center for the Advancement of Interprofessional Education, 2010 definition).

internal control: The player is in control of the materials, play interactions, and some aspect of the outcome (Bundy, 1997; Connor, Williamson, & Seipp, 1978); the extent to which the child is in control of his or her actions and, to some aspect, the outcome of the activity (Bundy, 1997).

internal validity: The degree to which the researcher's conclusions are accurate.

International Classification of Diseases (ICD-10): International framework for coding health conditions including diseases, disorders, and injuries.

International Classification of Functioning, Disability, and Health (ICF): International framework for coding components of health and functioning.

interprofessional collaborative practice: "When multiple health workers from different professional backgrounds work together with patients, families, carers [sic], and communities to deliver the highest quality of care" (World Health Organization, 2010, p. 7).

intervention plan: A collaborative listing of client-oriented actions meant to enhance occupational performance with specific targeted outcomes based on select models, frames of reference, and evidence.

intrinsic motivation: What drives a child to participate in an activity for pleasure rather than extrinsic reward (Bundy, 1993); the self-initiation or drive to action that is rewarded by the activity itself, rather than some external reward (Bundy, 1997).

jejunostomy tube: Placed directly into the jejunum (the central of the three divisions of the small intestine), bypassing the stomach.

job performance: Including work skills and patterns; time management; relationships with co-workers, managers, and customers; creation, production, and distribution of products and services; initiation, sustainment, and completion of work; and compliance with work norms and procedures.

judgment: The act of deciding after consideration of alternatives.

"just right" challenge: When the challenge of a task does not exceed the abilities of the client to meet the challenge.

kinesthesia: The sense of movement of one's body or part of one's body (e.g., joint or limb) in space.

knowledge: What one knows.

leadership: The ability to engage and influence others to facilitate and embrace meaningful change through careful consideration of individual and societal contexts in the embodiment of a shared vision.

least restrictive environment: An educational environment most like a regular education classroom; Developing a natural environment that enhances a person's occupational performance in as self-structured a format as possible.

legislative process: The path through which a bill becomes a law. Involves hearings in Congressional/Statehouse committees, votes by committee members and, if passed, voting on the floor of the legislative body.

leisure: "A nonobligatory activity that is intrinsically motivated and engaged in during discretionary time, that is, time not committed to obligatory occupations such as work, self-care or sleep" (Parham & Fazio, 1997, p.250).

leisure activities: "Nonobligatory, discretionary, and intrinsically rewarding activities" (AOTA, 2004b, p. 674).

level I fieldwork: Introductory practical experiences to expose students to a variety of practice settings.

level II fieldwork: Practical experiences created to develop competent, entry-level occupational therapists and occupational therapy assistants.

lobbyist: A person who attempts to influence the legislative process by providing information.

low-tech: Device that is easily fabricated or obtained.

maintenance: Ensuring continued competence through the use of external devices, templates, or skill retraining despite expectations of potential or eventual declines in occupational performance.

managed care: A variety of methods of financing and organizing the delivery of health care in which costs are contained by controlling the provision of services.

manager: An individual often responsible for task-specific functions within an organization.

marketing: "The process of planning and executing the conception, price, promotion, and distribution of ideas, goods, and services to create exchanges that satisfy individual and organizational objectives" (Bennett, 1995, p. 21).

mature level participation: Combines basic and supportive cooperative participation, and is focused on task completion and social interaction.

mean: Mathematical average of a set of scores.

meaningful occupation: A valued activity that contributes to identity, well-being, and quality of life.

measures of central tendency: Frequency, mean, mode, median.

measures of variability: Descriptive statistics of range, variance, and standard deviation.

median: Middle score of a range.

mentorship: Defined by AOTA as a relationship between two people in which one person (the mentor) is dedicated to the personal and professional growth of the other (the mentee). The relationship is often mutually beneficial and collaborative, both parties participating willingly and knowingly in the development of the mentee.

meta-analysis: Statistical analysis to integrate the results of several studies on one topic.

mode: The most common score in a range.

modeling: Demonstration of behavior.

models of practice: A set of ideas in terms of which other ideas are interpreted or assigned meaning; provides an overview of the occupational therapy philosophy and process. Models of practice help practitioners organize thinking.

monitoring: The act of observing a client's response to intervention.

moral distress: Distress occurring when an individual knows what she or he should do but is not able to do it.

moral residue: Persisting feelings that arise over time from repeated experiences of moral distress.

moral treatment: An approach to the treatment of what was called *madness* in the middle to late 19th century that was characterized by an "optimistic view of human nature, and influenced by enlightenment humanism and pietistic evangelicalism... [which at its] core was the belief that if treated like rational beings within a rational environment, the insane would regain their reason" (Lilleleht, 2002, p. 169).

moral treatment movement: A theory based on the respect and dignity for all humans and their need to participate in daily occupations.

morality: The accepted standards of right or wrong that direct the conduct of a person or a group.

moratorium: A temporary freeze on the implementation of a piece of legislation.

multiple regression analysis: A statistical measure that allows one variable to predict another.

narrative reasoning: Utilized to learn about the client's life story.

nasogastric tube: A feeding tube inserted through the oral pharyngeal area supplying liquid nutrition by passing the mouth.

natural environments: The context in which an individual lives.

naturalistic observation: Observation of behavior as it occurs naturally without the researcher interfering.

neuroscience-based treatment: Founded primarily on the idea that "the brain can be studied empirically" (Cohen & Reed, 1995, p. 562). In neuroscience, the brain is considered a dynamic system that includes virtually all of the underlying physiological and neurological processes that support human performance. An understanding of these processes supports the development of occupational therapy models of practice.

nonlinear dynamics: A framework for analyzing unpredictable, self-organizing systems concerning people and their context.

nonverbal communication: Communication through eye contact, tone of voice, facial expression, body language, and posture.

norm referenced: Client scores can be compared to a specific "normative" group utilized during test development.

NPO (nil per os): Latin for "nothing by mouth"; no food, liquid, or medication is to be given orally (Avery-Smith, 2002).

objective: Building blocks needed to achieve a larger goal.

occupation: Everyday activities and occupations that people find meaningful and purposeful (Moyers & Dale, 2007); "'goal-directed pursuits that typically extend over time have meaning to the performance, and involve multiple tasks" (Christiansen, Baum, & Bass-Haugen, 2005, p. 548); "daily activities that reflect cultural values, provide structure to living, and meaning to individuals; these activities meet human needs for self-care, enjoyment, and participation in society" (Crepeau, Cohn, & Schell, 2003, p. 1031); "activities that people engage in throughout their daily lives to fulfill their time and give life meaning. Occupations involve mental abilities and skills, and may or may not have an observable physical dimension" (Hinojosa & Kramer, 1997, p. 865); "[a]ctivities…of everyday life, named, organized, and given value and meaning by individuals and a culture. Occupation is everything people do to occupy themselves including looking after themselves…enjoying life…and contributing to the social and economic fabric of their communities" (Law, Polatajko, Baptiste, & Townsend, 1997, p. 32); "a dynamic relationship among an occupational form, a person with a unique developmental structure, subjective meanings and purpose, and the resulting occupational performance" (Nelson & Jepson Thomas, 2003, p. 90); "occupations are defined in the science as chunks of daily activity that can be named in the lexicon of the culture" (Zemke & Clark, 1996, p. vii)" (AOTA, 2008, p. 672).

occupation-based: Refers to providing intervention that includes the actual occupation (activities in which the client engages, in its actual context).

occupation-based activity: Activity meaningful to the person, which is conducted in the actual context.

occupation-based model: Proposed interaction of person, environment, and occupation that guide the organization of occupational therapy practice (Cole & Tufano, 2008).

occupational justice: "Justice related to opportunities and resources required for occupational participation sufficient to satisfy personal needs and full citizenship" (Christiansen & Townsend, 2004, p. 278); "to experience meaning and enrichment in one's occupations; to participate in a range of occupations for health and social inclusion; to make choices and share decision-making power in daily life; and to receive equal privileges for diverse participation in occupations (Townsend & Wilcock, 2004)" (AOTA, 2008, p. 630).

occupational performance: The ability to carry out activities of daily life including activities of daily living, education, work, play, leisure, and social participation (AOTA, 2008).

occupational performance model: A framework for understanding the individual's dynamic experience in daily occupations within the environment (Baum & Law, 1995).

occupational profile: An initial interview process that may be formal and/or informal. It is meant to reveal the client's personal history, daily living patterns, interests, values, and needs, while highlighting problems from the client's perspective concerning the performance of occupations and daily living activities. At its conclusion, the client is asked to prioritize his or her goals for occupational therapy intervention; "a summary of the client's occupational history, patterns of daily living, interests, values, and needs" (AOTA, 2008, p. 649).

occupational therapy: A health and wellness profession enabling people to participate in the everyday activities they want and need to do.

occupational therapy practitioners: Term used to encompass occupational therapists and occupational therapy assistants.

optimal experience: Alternate term for "flow experience."

organizations: Not limited to but includes agencies, businesses, corporations, industries, for-profits, nonprofits, or practices that receive occupational therapy services or consultations.

outlier: An extreme score that falls far from the mean score.

P **value:** The alpha score of the probability of a type I error.

paired t-test: T-test performed on paired groups of participants' scores to measure differences between the scores.

paradigm: A shared vision encompassing fundamental assumptions and beliefs which serves as the cultural core of the profession (Kielhofner, 2004).

parallel level participation: Play, activity, or work carried out side by side, without interaction, with others present.

parenteral tube feedings: Tubes that deliver nutrition via bypassing the gastrointestinal system to deliver nutrition into the bloodstream (Morris & Klein, 2000).

participation: Involvement in life situations and activities that include the capacity to execute and perform tasks (WHO, 2001).

partnerships in health: Collaborations with individuals and community members that have a central mission to enhance health and well-being.

Patient Protection and Affordable Care Act (2010) (PPACA; "ObamaCare"): This United States federal statute is aimed at decreasing the number of uninsured Americans and reducing the overall costs of health care. It includes mandates, subsidies, and tax credits to employers and individuals with the goal of increasing the coverage rate and streamlining the delivery of health care. Insurance companies are now required to cover all applicants and offer the same rates regardless of pre-existing conditions or gender. Sometimes referred to as *ObamaCare*, the act also includes telehealth provisions that create ways to promote evidence-based medicine and patient engagement, report on quality and cost measures, and coordinate care through the use of telehealth, remote patient monitoring, and other such enabling technologies. The PPACA directs the new Center for Medicare and Medicaid Innovation (CMI), to explore as a care model how to facilitate inpatient care at local hospitals through the use of electronic monitoring by specialists. The legislation also provides states with a "health home" option for chronic conditions that include the use of health information technology in providing health home services including the use of wireless patient technology to improve coordination and management of care and increased patient adherence to recommendations made by their provider.

Pearson correlation coefficient: The most common measure of relationships between two factors.

peer review: A process in which a panel of experts in the field is responsible for judging the merit of a proposal for a scholarly publication or presentation.

performance context: Environment in which occupational performance occurs, including the physical environment, available resources, sensory input, temporal and societal influences, or the presence or availability of caregivers.

performance in areas of occupation: Activities of daily living, instrumental activities of daily living, education, work, play, social participation, leisure, rest, and sleep (AOTA, 2008).

performance patterns: Habits, roles, and routines providing structure to day-to-day living. Performance patterns also include rituals that can be spiritual, cultural, or societal in nature and give meaning to the client (AOTA, 2008).

performance skills: Skills needed to participate in areas of occupation including motor, process, and communication/interaction skills (AOTA, 2008); "observable, concrete goal-directed actions clients use to engage in daily life occupations (Fisher, 2006). Performance skills are learned and developed over time and are situated in context. Multiple aspects such as the context in which the occupation is performed, the specific demands of the activity being attempted, and the client's body functions and structures affect the client's ability to acquire or demonstrate performance skills" (AOTA, 2008, p. 639).

personal factors: Contextual factors intrinsic to the individual such as attributes of age, gender, and social status (WHO, 2001).

persuade: To move by argument, entreaty, or expostulation to a belief, position, or course of action; to plead with (Merriam-Webster, 2006).

pH probe: Medical test used to help identify the amount and severity of gastroesophageal reflux (Morris & Klein, 2000).

philosophy: A fundamental belief (Meyer, 1977).

physical agent modalities: Procedures and interventions that are systematically applied to modify specific client factors that may be limiting occupational performance and use various forms of energy in order to modulate pain; modify tissue healing; increase tissue extensibility; modify skin and scar tissue; decrease edema, inflammation, or occupational performance secondary to musculoskeletal or integumentary conditions; and are used as an adjunctive method to occupation (Bracciano, 2008).

physical transfers: Teaching a client who uses a wheelchair to move from one surface to another.

pilot test: Trial run of a study to evaluate for problems in future experiments.

plagiarism: The use of information that was created by another individual as though it were original.

play: "Any spontaneous or organized activity that provides enjoyment, entertainment, amusement or diversion" (Parham & Fazio, 1997, p. 252).

play activities: "Spontaneous and organized activities that promote pleasure, amusement, and diversion" (AOTA, 2004b, p. 674).

playfulness: "A play temperament that is comprised of intrinsic motivation, internal control, freedom to suspend reality, and framing; A behavioral or personality trait characterized by flexibility, manifest joy, and spontaneity" (Parham & Fazio, 1997, p. 252).

policy: Principle or rule to guide decisions and achieve outcomes.

populations: Groups within communities that have a commonality such as, but not limited to, brain injury, diabetes, refugees, or prisoners of war that receive occupational therapy services.

positioning: Ensuring and/or placing an individual in an ergonomically correct posture, one that enables occupational performance.

post hoc tests: Statistical tests used to follow up significant findings.

postulate: A theoretical statement that suggests how two or more concepts are related (Mosey, 1986).

practice skills: Repetition of an ability to improve the consistency of performance; components of occupations.

practitioner: Provides occupational therapy services including assessments, interventions, program planning and implementation, discharge planning, and transition planning (AOTA, 2000).

pragmatic reasoning: Used to understand the practical issues that may have an impact on the situation with the person and the person's family.

pragmatism: A philosophical view that knowledge grows through change and adaptation and is best gained through practical application and experience (Breines, 1987).

preparatory activity: Repetitive techniques to get a client ready to perform (e.g., stretching, mental review).

pretest sensitization: Participants completing the pretest complicates the post-test results.

principles: Basic rules of conduct.

probability: Likelihood of finding the same results in repeated studies.

procedural reasoning: Focuses on client performance and diagnosis.

profession: An occupation requiring extensive education or specialized training.

professional: A person engaged in a profession.

professional development: Ongoing plan to ensure practice is current and based on best known practices; a process where one plans and achieves excellence or establishes expertise in seeking a change in responsibilities, or when assuming more complex professional roles.

professional identity: Students develop a professional identity as an occupational therapy practitioner, aligning their professional judgments and decisions with the American Occupational Therapy Association (AOTA) Standards of Practice and the Occupational Therapy Code of Ethics.

professional presentation: An oral report of research findings or other evidence-based practice information.

professional portfolio: A collection of evidence demonstrating that practice is current and based on best known practices; an archival of one's self-assessment processes, learning plans, evidence of engagement in selected learning methods, reflection on the learning process, and outcomes of the application of learning to practice.

promote: Further the progress of (something, especially a cause, venture, or aim); support or actively encourage.

promotion: Advance in station, rank, or honor; to advance (a student) from one grade to the next higher grade; to contribute to the growth or prosperity of, promote international understanding; to help bring (as in an enterprise) into being; to present (merchandise) for buyer acceptance through advertising, publicity, or discounting (Merriam-Webster, 2006).

proposal: The collective materials used to apply for a grant, including an application and supporting documents.

proprioception: The sense of one's body or parts of one's body (e.g., joint or limb) in space.

Prospective Payment System (PPS): Created by the Balanced Budget Act of 1997 as a method for controlling costs. Payment for skilled service is made on a daily rate, chosen based on certain admission criteria indicating an estimated level of need.

psychometrics: The study of psychological and behavioral measurement.

qualitative research: Exploratory gathering of in-depth, detailed descriptions of problems or conditions from the point of view of the group or individual experiencing them in order to discover themes and their interrelationships or linkages.

quality assessment: A measure of quality against standards.

quality improvement: Management philosophy and method for structuring problem solving.

quantitative research: Use of the scientific method to gather data that can be expressed numerically and analyzed statistically in order to describe population characteristics and/or determine the relationship between one or more independent and dependent variables.

range: Measure of variability between the highest and lowest scores.

real life: Individuals' description and interpretation of their life.

recreation: Adult play or activities whose purpose is to "regenerate energy to support the worker role" (Glantz & Richman, 2001, p. 249).

reductionistic approach: Perceiving many individual parts that make up the whole, which may be studied and dealt with separately or interchangeably.

referral: Making a professional judgment to have another occupational therapy specialist, discipline, or facility evaluate the client; the practice of directing an initial request for service or changing the degree and direction of service (Agnes, 1999).

reflection: A useful tool in analyzing thoughts and actions that assists practitioners to justify interventions and gives practitioners the ability to learn from experience.

reflective listening: A process of listening to both the verbal and emotional content of a speaker and verbalizing both the feelings and attitudes sensed behind the spoken words to the speaker (Davis, 2006).

rehabilitation movement: Began with a change in the way society viewed those with handicaps to individuals who could become independent and contributing members of the community.

related service: Services that may be required for a student to benefit from special education. Service providers include occupational therapy, physical therapy, social work, and school health services.

reliability: Accuracy and stability of a measure; The dependability and consistency of a measurement.

remediation: Helping clients regain skills and abilities.

researcher: An individual who "find[s] the process of discovery exhilarating because they see how it enhances occupational therapy practice" (Kielhofner, 2006).

resource utilization groups (RUG): Categories used in PPS that describe the amount of service clients will need.

retirement preparation and adjustment: Determining aptitudes, developing interests and skills, and selecting appropriate avocational pursuits.

rigor: Close adherence to experimental research methodology; in broader usage, embedding of sound principles and practices—agreed upon by the scientific community—into each step of the quantitative or qualitative research process in order to ensure trustworthiness of results.

safety: Practices that reduce the risk of adverse incidents.

sample: A selection from a population.

sampling error: The difference between the sample's scores and what the whole population would have scored.

scaffolding: Foundation of prerequisite skills.

scientific reasoning: Involves the logical thinking about the nature of the client's problems and the optimal course of action in treatment.

scholarship: Research activities designed to build the knowledge base of occupational therapy so as to further advance practice and teaching.

scholarly practice: Evidence-based practice; Using the knowledge base of the profession in occupational therapy practice and teaching.

scholarly reports: Documents that are written by reflective practitioners for the advancement of a profession.

screening: The process of gathering and reviewing data with the intent to determine if additional evaluative procedures are warranted.

seating systems: Selection and utilization of a comfortable, supportive wheelchair or chair seat that encourages symmetry, skin integrity, and occupational performance.

self-assessment: Provides the means to assess performance, abilities, and skills; to analyze demands and resources of the work environment; to interpret information about clients' outcomes; to reassess current learning goals; and to develop goals and plans for professional growth and continuing competence and competency.

simulation: Creating as realistic as possible situations to allow learners to practice and apply skills.

site: Facility offering clinical affiliations to students.

SOAP note format: Documentation format that includes four parts in documenting a client's intervention: subjective, objective, assessment, and plan.

social participation: A person's performance of meaningful roles and occupations within preferred social groups such as families, classrooms, work teams, organizations, and communities (Cole & Donohue, 2011); Consists of verbal and interpersonal activity interactions among people.

standard deviation: A measurement of variability; a description of how far from the mean a score is.

standard precautions: A form of infection control based on the assumption that all bodily substances may transmit infectious diseases.

statistical significance: The likelihood that the finding is not due to error.

suck, swallow, breathe synchrony: The smooth coordination of sucking, swallowing, and breathing into rhythmic patterns to allow for efficient and effective eating (Case-Smith & Humphry, 2005).

superficial thermal agent: Those procedures or interventions that are capable of raising or decreasing the temperature of superficial tissue to a therapeutic level.

supervisee: One who receives direction and undergoes evaluation by a qualified practitioner.

supervision: A reciprocal process involving the supervisor and supervisee aimed at the improvement of performance.

support: The provision of services that enable clients to achieve maximum occupational performance.

supportive cooperative level participation: Consists of interactions that express feelings and emotions designed to foster social cohesion in a group.

t-test: A statistical measure of the difference between two means.

tacit: Involves learning and skill, but not in a way that can be written down.

taxonomy: A system of classification.

technology: "The branch of knowledge that deals with the creation and use of technical means and their interrelation with life, society, and the environment, drawing upon such subjects as industrial arts, engineering, applied science, and pure science" (Flexner, 1987, p. 1950).

telehealth: The application of evaluative, consultative, preventative, and therapeutic services delivered through telecommunication and information technologies (AOTA, 2013).

test-retest reliability: Consistency of a score of repeated measures over time.

theoretical constructs: Visible and non-visible ideas and explanations that form into a concept.

theory: Describes, explains, and predicts behavior and/or the relationships between concepts or events.

therapeutic use of self: A practitioner's intuitive nature that derives from one's personality traits, self-awareness, and personal experiences; understanding of human behavior; and observations through the use of the five senses. The practitioner makes conscious use of this nature to engage and impact a therapeutic relationship and foster a meaningful experience for the client.

transference: When one person, usually the client, places a role on another, usually the therapist.

transition services: A results-oriented process that facilitates movement between settings and providers based on changing client needs. This term is most often used in the school setting but is an essential part of care coordination across the continuum.

TriAlliance of Health and Rehabilitation Professions: "The TriAlliance is the largest constituency of health and rehabilitation professionals representing the professions of occupational therapy, physical therapy, audiology and speech-language pathology. In 1988, informal meetings began among the Presidents and Executive Directors of the American Occupational Therapy Association (AOTA), the American Physical Therapy Association (APTA), and the American Speech-Language-Hearing Association (ASHA)" (APTA, 2000).

type I error: Finding that the independent variable had an effect when it did not.

type II error: Finding that the independent variable did not have an effect when it did.

universal design: Principles that seek to promote access to and use of structures and tools across the lifespan.

utilization review: A look-over of care/services that were provided in a particular case to ascertain necessity, efficiency, and effectiveness.

validity: Generalizability of a measure to the general population; the extent to which a measurement measures what it is intended to measure.

values: Principles that set a standard of quality or a worthwhile ideal.

variability: The degree to which scores differ from each other.

variance: An index or score of variability that explains the differences between factors.

videofluoroscopy: A primary imaging technique for detailed dynamic assessment of oral, pharyngeal, and upper esophageal phases of a swallow (Arvedson, Brodsky, & Christensen, 2002); also known as *modified barium swallow*.

volunteer exploration: Determining community causes, organizations, or opportunities for unpaid 'work' in relationship to personal skills, interests, location, and time available.

volunteer participation: Performing unpaid 'work' activities for the benefit of identified selected causes, organizations, or facilities" (AOTA, 2008, p. 632).

well-being: The state of being content, comfortable, and satisfied with one's self, relationships, and quality of life.

wellness: A dynamic way of life that involves actions, values, and attitudes that support or improve both health and quality of life (AOTA, 2001).

wellness programs: A program intended to improve and promote health and fitness that is typically offered through the workplace, although insurance plans can offer them directly to their enrollees. The program allows employers or plans to offer employees premium discounts, cash rewards, gym memberships, and other incentives to participate. The Affordable Care Act creates new incentives to promote employer wellness programs and encourage opportunities to support healthier workplaces

wheelchair management: Selection, utilization, and functional mobility of the wheelchair.

work: "Includes activities needed for engaging in remunerative employment or volunteer activities" (Mosey, 1996, p. 341):

References

Accreditation Council for Occupational Therapy Education. (1999). Standards for an accredited educational program for the occupational therapist. *American Journal of Occupational Therapy, 53,* 575-581.

Agnes, M. (Ed.). (1999). *Webster's new world college dictionary* (4th ed.). New York, NY: Macmillan.

American Occupational Therapy Association. (1994). Occupational Therapy Code of Ethics. *American Journal of Occupational Therapy, 48,* 1037-1038.

American Occupational Therapy Association. (2000). Occupational therapy roles and career exploration and development: A companion guide to the Occupational Therapy Role Documents. In the *reference manual of the official documents of the American Occupational Therapy Association* (8th ed.). Bethesda, MD: Author.

American Occupational Therapy Association. (2001). Position paper: Occupational therapy in the promotion of health and the prevention of disease and disability statement. *American Journal of Occupational Therapy, 55*(6), 656-660.

American Occupational Therapy Association. (2004a). Role competencies for a professional-level occupational therapist faculty member in an academic setting. *American Journal of Occupational Therapy, 58*(6), 649-650.

American Occupational Therapy Association. (2004b). Scope of practice. *American Journal of Occupational Therapy, 58*(6), 673-677.

American Occupational Therapy Association. (2007). Specialized knowledge and skills in eating and feeding for occupational therapy practice. *American Journal of Occupational Therapy, 61,* 686-700.

American Occupational Therapy Association. (2008). Occupational therapy practice framework: Domain and process (2nd ed.). *American Journal of Occupational Therapy, 62,* 625-683.

American Physical Therapy Association. (2000). TriAlliance to explore Medicare alternative payment methods. Retrieved from http://www.apta.org/AM/Template.cfm?Section = Home &TEMPLATE=/CM/ContentDisplay.cfm &CONTENTID =30620

Arvedsen, J. C., Brodsky, L., & Christensen, S. (2002). Instrumental evaluation of swallowing. In J. C. Arvedsen & L. Brodsky (Eds.), *Pediatric swallowing and feeding assessment and management* (2nd ed., pp. 341-388). Albany, NY: Singular Publishing Group.

Avery-Smith, W. (2002). Dysphagia. In C. A. Trombly & M. V. Radomski (Eds.), *Occupational therapy for physical dysfunction* (pp. 1091-1109). Philadelphia, PA: Lippincott Williams & Wilkins.

Bateson, G. (1972). Toward a theory of play and fantasy. In G. Bateson (Ed.), *Steps to an ecology of the mind* (pp. 14-20). New York, NY: Bantam.

Baum, C., & Law, M. (1995). Occupational performance: Occupational therapy's definition of function. *American Journal of Occupational Therapy, 49,* 1019.

Bennett, P. D. (Ed.). (1995). *Dictionary of marketing terms* (2nd ed.). Chicago, IL: American Marketing Association.

Bracciano, A. (2008). *Physical agent modalities: Theory and application for the occupational therapist.* Thorofare, NJ: SLACK Incorporated.

Braveman, B. (2006). *Leading & managing occupational therapy services: An evidence-based approach.* Philadelphia, PA: F.A. Davis Company.

Brayman, S. J., Roley, S. S., Clark, G. F., DeLany, J. V., Garza, E. R., Radomski, M. V., et al. (2005). Standards of practice for occupational therapy. *American Journal of Occupational Therapy, 59*(6), 663-665.

Brookside Associates Multi-Media Edition. (2007). Nursing Fundamentals I. Retrieved from http://www.brookside-press.org/Products/Nursing_Fundamentals_1/Index.htm

Breines, E. (1987). Pragmatism as a foundation for occupational therapy curricula. *American Journal of Occupational Therapy, 47*, 522-525.

Bundy, A. C. (1993). Assessment of play and leisure: Delineation of the problem. *American Journal of Occupational Therapy, 47*, 217-222.

Bundy, A. C. (1997). Play and playfulness: What to look for. In L. D. Parham & L. S. Fazio (Eds.), *Play in occupational therapy for children* (pp. 52-66). St. Louis, MO: Mosby.

Canadian Association of Occupational Therapists. (1999). Joint position statement on evidence-based occupational therapy. Retrieved from http://www.caot.ca/default.asp?ChangeID =166& pageID =156

Case-Smith, J., & Humphry, R. (2005). Feeding intervention. In J. Case-Smith (Ed.), Occupational therapy for children (5th ed., pp. 481-520). St. Louis, MO: Elsevier Mosby.

Center for the Advancement of Interprofessional Education. (2010). Interprofession education: A definition. Retrieved from www.caipe.org.uk/us/defining-ipe

Christiansen, C. H., & Townsend, E. A. (2004). *Introduction to occupation: The art and science of living.* Upper Saddle River, NJ: Prentice Hall.

Cohen, H., & Reed, K. L. (1995). The historical development of neuroscience in physical rehabilitation. *American Journal of Occupational Therapy, 50*(7), 561-568.

Cole, M., & Donohue, M. (2011). *Social participation and occupation: In schools, clinics, and communities.* Thorofare, NJ: SLACK Incorporated.

Cole, M., & Tufano, R. (2008). *Applied theories in occupational therapy.* Thorofare, NJ: SLACK Incorporated.

Connor, F. P., Williamson, G. G., & Siepp, J. M. (Eds.). (1978). *Program guide for infants and toddlers with neuromotor and other developmental disabilities.* New York, NY: Teachers College.

Davis, C. M. (2006). *Patient practitioner interaction: An experiential manual for developing the art of health care* (4th ed.). Thorofare, NJ: SLACK Incorporated.

Depoy, E., & Gitlin, L. (2005). *Introduction to research: Understanding and applying multiple strategies* (3rd ed.). New York, NY: Mosby.

Dictionary.com. Retrieved from http://dictionary.reference.com

Encyclopedia.com. (2008). Disease. In Oxford dictionary of nursing. Oxford University Press. Retrieved from http://www.encyclopedia.com/doc/1O62-disease.html

Finkelstein, V. (1991). Disability: An administrative challenge? In M. Oliver (Ed.), *Social work: Disabled people and disabling environments* (pp. 19-39). London, England: Jessica Kingsley.

Flexner, S. B. (Ed.). (1987). *The Random House dictionary of the English language, unabridged* (2nd ed.). New York, NY: Random House.

Glantz, C. H., & Richman, N. (2001). Leisure activities. In L. W. Pedretti & M. B. Early (Eds.), *Occupational therapy practice skills for physical dysfunction* (5th ed., pp. 249-256). St. Louis, MO: Mosby.

Hooper, B. (2006). Epistemological transformation in occupational therapy: Educational implications and challenges. *Occupational Therapy Journal of Research, 26*, 15-24.

Jenks, K. N., & Smith, G. (2006). Eating and swallowing. In H. M Pendleton & W. Schultz-Krohn (Eds.), *Pedretti's occupational therapy practice skills for physical dysfunction* (6th ed., pp. 609-645). St. Louis, MO: Mosby.

Kerlinger, F. (1979). *Behavioral research: A conceptual approach.* New York, NY: Holt, Rinehart, & Winston.

Kielhofner, G. (2004). *Conceptual foundations of occupational therapy* (3rd ed.). Philadelphia, PA: F.A. Davis Company.

Kielhofner, G. (2006). *Research in occupational therapy: Methods of inquiry for enhancing practice.* Philadelphia, PA: F.A. Davis Company.

Kotler, P. (2003). *A framework for marketing management* (2nd ed.). Upper Saddle River, NJ: Prentice Hall.

Law, M., Baptiste, S., & Mills, J. (1995). Client-centered practice: What does it mean and does it make a difference? *Canadian Journal of Occupational Therapy, 62*, 250-257.

Lilleleht, E. (2002). Progress and power: Exploring the disciplinary connections between moral treatment and psychiatric rehabilitation. *Philosophy, Psychiatry, & Psychology, 9*(2), 167-182.

Loveland, C. A. (1999). The concept of culture. In R. L. Leavitt (Ed.), *Cross-cultural rehabilitation: An international perspective* (pp. 15-24). London, England: Saunders.

MacRae, N., & Dyer, J. (2005). Collaborative teaching methods for health professionals. *Occupational therapy in health care, 19*(3), 93-103.

Merriam-Webster. (2006). On-line dictionary (10th ed.). Retrieved from http://www.merriam-webster.com

Meyer, A. (1977). The philosophy of occupational therapy. *American Journal of Occupational Therapy, 31*, 639-642. (Original work published in 1922).

Morris, S. E., & Klein, M. D. (2000). *Pre-feeding skills: A comprehensive resource for mealtime development* (2nd ed.). Austin, TX: Therapy Skills Builders.

Mosey, A. C. (1986). *Psychosocial components of occupational therapy.* New York, NY: Raven Press.

Moyers, P. A., & Dale, L. M. (2007). *The guide to occupational therapy practice.* Bethesda, MD: AOTA Press.

Parham, L. D., & Fazio, L. S. (1997). *Play in occupational therapy for children.* St. Louis, MO: Mosby.

Reed, K., & Sanderson, S. (1999). *Concepts of occupational therapy* (4th ed.). Baltimore, MD: Lippincott Williams & Wilkins.

Rubin, K. H., Fein, G. G., & Vandenberg, B. (1983). Play. In P. H. Mussen (Ed.), *Handbook of child psychology: Vol. 4. Socialization, personality, and social development* (4th ed., pp. 693-774). New York, NY: Wiley.

Spencer, L. M., & Spencer, S. M. (1993). *Competence at work.* New York, NY: John Wiley and Sons.

Wells, S. A., & Black, R. M. (2000). *Cultural competency for health professionals.* Bethesda, MD: AOTA Press.

World Health Organization. (1947). Constitution of the World Health Organization. *Chronicle for the World Health Organization, 1*(1),29-40.

World Health Organization. (2001). *ICF: International Classification of Functioning, Disability and Health.* Geneva, Switzerland: Author.

Financial Disclosures

Ali Kae Arsenault has no financial or proprietary interest in the materials presented herein.

Bethany Augustoni has not disclosed any relevant financial relationships.

Diane P. Bergey has no financial or proprietary interest in the materials presented herein.

Caryn Birstler Husman has no financial or proprietary interest in the materials presented herein.

Dr. Roxie M. Black has no financial or proprietary interest in the materials presented herein.

Dr. Gail M. Bloom has no financial or proprietary interest in the materials presented herein.

Dr. Jessica J. Bolduc has no financial or proprietary interest in the materials presented herein.

Dr. Alfred G. Bracciano is co-founder of PAMPCA, LLC, a company that provides continuing education for occupational therapists.

Dr. Susan C. Burwash has no financial or proprietary interest in the materials presented herein.

Lisa L. Clark has no financial or proprietary interest in the materials presented herein.

Marilyn B. Cole has no financial or proprietary interest in the materials presented herein.

Dr. Jeffrey L. Crabtree has no financial or proprietary interest in the materials presented herein.

William R. Croninger has no financial or proprietary interest in the materials presented herein.

Danielle J. Cropley has no financial or proprietary interest in the materials presented herein.

Betsy DeBrakeleer has not disclosed any relevant financial relationships.

Dr. Mary V. Donohue has not disclosed any relevant financial relationships.

Dr. Nancy Doyle has no financial or proprietary interest in the materials presented herein.

Julie Eldredge has not disclosed any relevant financial relationships.

Dr. Verna G. Eschenfelder has not disclosed any relevant financial relationships.

Dr. Thomas Fisher has no financial or proprietary interest in the materials presented herein.

Erica A. Flagg has not disclosed any relevant financial relationships.

Dr. Kathleen Flecky has no financial or proprietary interest in the materials presented herein.

Jan Froehlich has not disclosed any relevant financial relationships.

Dr. Heather Goertz has not disclosed any relevant financial relationships.

Michelle Goulet has no financial or proprietary interest in the materials presented herein.

Dr. Kristin B. Haas has no financial or proprietary interest in the materials presented herein.

Dory E. Holmes has no financial or proprietary interest in the materials presented herein.

Dr. Karen Jacobs has no financial or proprietary interest in the materials presented herein.

Bevin J. Journey has not disclosed any relevant financial relationships.

Tara Kaminski has no financial or proprietary interest in the materials presented herein.

Dr. Rosalie M. King has no financial or proprietary interest in the materials presented herein.

Dr. Lisa J. Knecht-Sabres has no financial or proprietary interest in the materials presented herein.

Dr. Amy Jo Lamb has no financial or proprietary interest in the materials presented herein.

John E. Lane, Jr. has no financial or proprietary interest in the materials presented herein.

Barbara Larson has no financial or proprietary interest in the materials presented herein.

Dr. Kathryn M. Loukas has no financial or proprietary interest in the materials presented herein.

Nancy MacRae has no financial or proprietary interest in the materials presented herein.

James Marc-Aurele has no financial or proprietary interest in the materials presented herein.

Dr. Scott McNeil has no financial or proprietary interest in the materials presented herein.

Dr. Penelope A. Moyers has no financial or proprietary interest in the materials presented herein.

Dr. Julie Ann Nastasi has no financial or proprietary interest in the materials presented herein.

Dr. Linda H. Niemeyer has no financial or proprietary interest in the materials presented herein.

Dr. Claudia E. Oakes has no financial or proprietary interest in the materials presented herein.

Dr. Jane O'Brien has no financial or proprietary interest in the materials presented herein.

Dr. Carol Reinson has no financial or proprietary interest in the materials presented herein.

Michael E. Roberts has no financial or proprietary interest in the materials presented herein.

Dr. Regula H. Robnett has no financial or proprietary interest in the materials presented herein.

Dr. Jan Rowe has no financial or proprietary interest in the materials presented herein.

Marie C. Roy has not disclosed any relevant financial relationships.

Diane Sauter-Davis has no financial or proprietary interest in the materials presented herein.

Julie Savoyski has no financial or proprietary interest in the materials presented herein.

Courtney S. Shufelt has no financial or proprietary interest in the materials presented herein.

Dr. Karen Sladyk has not disclosed any relevant financial relationships.

Dr. Wendy B. Stav has no financial or proprietary interest in the materials presented herein.

Barbara J. Steva has no financial or proprietary interest in the materials presented herein.

Dr. Christine Sullivan has no financial or proprietary interest in the materials presented herein.

Roseanna Tufano has not disclosed any relevant financial relationships.

Dr. Nicolaas van den Heever has no financial or proprietary interest in the materials presented herein.

Dr. Lori Vaughn has no financial or proprietary interest in the materials presented herein.

Dr. John W. Vellacott has not disclosed any relevant financial relationships.

Dr. Kristin Winston has not disclosed any relevant financial relationships.

Patricia A. Wisniewski has no financial or proprietary interest in the materials presented herein.

Briana Youland has no financial or proprietary interest in the materials presented herein.

INDEX